Springer
Specialist
Surgery
Series

Other titles in this grouping include:

Transplantation Surgery edited by Hakim & Danovitch, 2001
Upper Gastrointestinal Surgery edited by Fielding & Hallissey, 2004

Springer
London
Berlin
Heidelberg
New York
Hong Kong
Milan
Paris
Tokyo

Anne J. Moore and David W. Newell (Eds)

Neurosurgery

Principles and Practice

Series Editor: John Lumley

Springer

Anne J. Moore, MB BS, BSc, FRCS
South West Neurosurgery Centre
Derriford Hospital
Plymouth, UK

David W. Newell
Department of Neurological Surgery
University of Washington Medical Center
Harborview Medical Center
Seattle, WA, USA

British Library Cataloguing in Publication Data
Neurosurgery. – (Springer specialist surgery series)
1. Nervous system – Surgery
I. Moore, Anne J. II. Newell, David W.
617.4′8

Library of Congress Cataloging-in-Publication Data
Neurosurgery/Anne J. Moore and David W. Newell, eds.
p. ; cm. – (Springer specialist surgery series)
Includes bibliographical references.

1. Nervous system – Surgery. I. Moore, Anne J., 1958– II. Newell, David W. III. Series.
[DNLM: 1. Neurosurgery. 2. Neurosurgical Procedures. WL 368 N49511 2004]
RD593.N4172 2004
617.4′8–dc21 2003054444

ISBN 978-1-84996-881-2 Springer London Berlin Heidelberg

Springer is part of Springer Science+Business Media
springeronline.com

Softcover reprint of the hardcover 1st edition 2005

Typeset by Florence Production, Stoodleigh, Devon, England
Printed and bound at Kyodo Printing Co (S'pore) Pte Ltd
28/3830-543210 Printed on acid-free paper SPIN 10839760

Preface

This book provides coverage of a broad range of topics in the field of neurosurgery, for residents and registrars in training and for recent graduates of training programs. As neurosurgical training incorporates expertise from centers worldwide, there is a need to have input from specialists in neurosurgery from various countries. This text is a compilation by expert authors in the USA and the UK to provide information on the basic knowledge and clinical management required for optimal care of neurosurgical patients.

The text is an up-to-date synopsis of the field of neurosurgery from American and British perspectives, which covers the most common clinical conditions encountered by neurosurgeons. The chapters are organized under broad topics, including investigative studies, perioperative care, the role of newer techniques and the management of tumors, vascular and traumatic lesions. Additional topics are then covered, including pediatrics, spine and peripheral nerve lesions, as well as functional neurosurgery and infections. We anticipate that trainees will find this information useful for certification examinations and recent graduates of neurosurgical training programs can utilize this text as an update of the most important neurosurgical topics.

Anne J. Moore
Plymouth, UK

David W. Newell
Seattle, USA

Contents

I – Investigations

II – Perioperative Care

III – Techniques

IV – Tumors

V – Vascular

VI – Trauma

VII – Hydrocephalus

VIII – Pediatrics

IX – Spine

X – Peripheral and Cranial Nerves

XI – Functional Neurosurgery

XII – Infection

Contributors

Bizhan Aarabi MD, FRCS, FACSC
Department of Neurosurgery
R Adams Cowley Shock Trauma Center
University of Maryland School of Medicine
Baltimore, MD
USA

Ellsworth C Alvord Jr, MD
Department of Pathology
Neuropathology Laboratory
University of Washington School of Medicine
Harborview Medical Center
Seattle, WA
USA

Sepideh Amin-Hanjani MD
Harvard Medical School
Massachusetts General Hospital
Neurosurgery Service
Boston, MA
USA

Robert E Anderson BS
Mayo Medical School
Department of Neurological Surgery
Mayo Clinic
Rochester, MN
USA

Kristian Aquilina FRCS
Department of Neurosurgery
Beaumont Hospital
Dublin, Ireland

June Bendall RN
The Wolfson Medical Rehabilitation Centre
London, UK

Mitchell S Berger MD
Department of Neurological Surgery
University of California, San Francisco
School of Medicine
San Francisco, CA
USA

Gavin Wayne Britz MD
Department of Neurological Surgery
University of Washington
Harborview Medical Center
Seattle, WA
USA

Katherine Brosnan MBBS, FRCA
Pain Clinic
Atkinson Morley's Hospital
London
UK

Mark G Burnett MD
Department of Neurosurgery
Hospital of the University of Pennsylvania
Philadelphia, PA
USA

Christopher L Chandler BSc, MB BS, FRCS(SN)
Department of Neurosurgery
King's College Hospital
London
UK

Roger A Chisholm MA, MB, BChir, MRCP, FRCR
Salford Royal Hospitals NHS Trust
Salford
Greater Manchester
UK

Andrew G Clifton MA (Oxon), MRCP, FRCR
Neuroradiology
Atkinson Morley Wing
St. George's Hospital
London, UK

Anna DePold Hohler MD
Department of Neurology
Madigan Army Medical Center
Tacoma, WA
USA

Aaron S Dumont MD
Department of Neurological Surgery
University of Virginia Health Sciences Center
Charlottesville, VA
USA

Philip Edwards PhD
Department of Radiological Sciences
Medical School of Guy's, King's and
St Thomas' Hospitals
King's College London
London
UK

Howard M Eisenberg MD
Department of Neurosurgery
University of Maryland School of Medicine
Baltimore, MD
USA

Richard G Ellenbogen MD
Department of Neurological Surgery
University of Washington School of Medicine
Children's Hospital & Regional Medical
Center
Seattle, WA
USA

Fred J Epstein MD
Hyman-Newman Institute for Neurology and
Neurosurgery
Pediatric Neurosurgery
Beth Israel Medical Center, Singer Division
New York, NY
USA

James J Evans MD
Department of Neurosurgery
Thomas Jefferson University
Philadelphia, PA
USA

Jonathan A Friedman MD
Section of Neurosurgery
Dartmouth Hitchcock Medical Center
Lebanon, NH
USA

Russell Geyer MD
Department of Pediatrics
University of Washington School of Medicine
Children's Hospital & Regional Medical
Center
Seattle, WA
USA

Mladen Golubic MD, PhD
Brain Tumor Institute and
Department of Neurosurgery
The Cleveland Clinic Foundation
Cleveland, OH
USA

Robert Goodkin MD
Department of Neurological Surgery
University of Washington School of Medicine
Seattle, WA
USA

Gerald Grant MD
Department of Neurosurgery
University of Washington
Seattle, WA
USA

Joan P Grieve MBBS, FRCS (SN)
Victor Horsley Department of Neurosurgery
The National Hospital for Neurology and
Neurosurgery
London
UK

W S Lal Gunasekera MBBS, FRCS, PhD
Hurstwood Park Neurological Centre
Haywards Heath
West Sussex
UK

Stephen J Haines MD
Department of Neurological Surgery
Medical University of South Carolina
Charleston, SC
USA

David G Hardy BSc, MA, MB, ChB,
FRCS (Ed), FRCS
Addenbrookes NHS Trust
Cambridge, Cambridgeshire
UK

Griffith R Harsh IV, MD, MA, MBA
Stanford Medical School
Neurosurgical Oncology
Stanford Medical Center
Stanford University
Stanford, CA
USA

Tom Hollway BA, MBBS, FRCS
Pain Clinic
Atkinson Morley's Hospital
London
UK

David G Hughes MBBS, MRCP, FRCR
Department of Neuroradiology
Greater Manchester Neurosciences Centre
Hope Hospital
Salford
Greater Manchester
UK

George I Jallo MD
Pediatric Neurosurgery
Johns Hopkins University
Baltimore, MD
USA

John A Jane Jr, MD
Department of Neurological Surgery
University of Virginia Health Sciences Center
Charlottesville, VA
USA

John A Jane Sr, MD, PhD
David D Weaver Professor & Chairman
Department of Neurological Surgery
University of Virginia Health Sciences Center
Charlottesville, VA
USA

Francis R Johns DMD, MD
Department of Plastic Surgery
Aestique Medical Center
Greensburg, PA
USA

G Evren Keles MD
Department of Neurological Surgery
University of California, San Francisco
School of Medicine
San Francisco, CA
USA

Andras A Kemeny FRSC, MD
The National Centre for Stereotactic
Radiosurgery
Royal Hallamshire Hospital
Sheffield
South Yorkshire
UK

Richard S C Kerr BSc, MS, FRCS
Oxford Skull Base Unit
Radcliffe Infirmary
Oxford
Oxfordshire
UK

Vini G Khurana MD, PhD
Department of Neurological Surgery
Mayo Clinic
Rochester, MN
USA

Neil D Kitchen MD, FRCS (SN)
Victor Horsley Department of Neurosurgery
The National Hospital for Neurology and
Neurosurgery
London
UK

Michel Kliot MD
Department of Neurological Surgery
University of Washington
Seattle VA Puget Sound Health System
Seattle
USA

Karl F Kothbauer MD
Division of Neurosurgery
Department of Surgery
Kantonsspital Luzern
Lucerne
Switzerland

Maryke A Kraayenbrink MRCP, FRCA
Department of Anesthesia
St George's Hospital
London, UK

Charlie Kuntz MD
Department of Neurological Surgery
University of Cincinnati
Cincinnati, OH
USA

Sandeep Kunwar MD
Department of Neurological Surgery
University of California, San Francisco
School of Medicine
San Francisco, CA
USA

Arthur M Lam MD, FRCPC
Departments of Anesthesiology and
Neurological Surgery
Harborview Medical Center
University of Washington
Seattle, WA
USA

Joung H Lee MD
Brain Tumor Institute and
Department of Neurosurgery
The Cleveland Clinic Foundation
Cleveland, OH
USA

Peter D Le Roux MD, FACS
Department of Neurosurgery
The Hospital of the University of Pennsylvania
Philadelphia, PA
USA

Kant Y K Lin MD
Department of Plastic Surgery
University of Virginia Health Sciences Center
Charlottesville, VA
USA

David A Lundin MD
Department of Neurological Surgery
University of Washington Medical Center
Seattle, WA
USA

Paul J Marcotte MD, FACS, FRCS(C)
Department of Neurosurgery
The Hospital of the University of Pennsylvania
Philadelphia, PA
USA

Henry Marsh MA, MBBS, FRCS
Department of Neurosurgery
Atkinson Morley's Hospital
London, UK

Gregory R McAnulty BA, FRCA
Department of Anesthesia
St George's Hospital
London, UK

Todd McCall MD
Department of Neurosurgery
University of Washington
Seattle, WA
USA

Rajesh Mehta MD
Department of Neurosurgery
University of Maryland Medical System
Baltimore, MD
USA

Fredric B Meyer MD
Mayo Medical School
Department of Neurological Surgery
Mayo Clinic
Rochester, MN
USA

Christopher A Milford BA, FRCS
Oxford Skull Base Unit
Radcliffe Infirmary
Oxford, Oxfordshire
UK

Anne J Moore MBBS, BSc, FRCS
South West Neurosurgery Centre
Derriford Hospital
Plymouth
Devon
UK

David W Newell MD
Department of Neurological Surgery
Harborview Medical Center
Seattle, WA
USA

Richard K Osenbach MD
Assistant Professor of Neurosurgery
Duke University Medical Center
Durham, NC
USA

Charles E Polkey MD, FRCS
Department of Neurosurgery
King's College Hospital
London
UK

Michael P Powell MA, MBBS, FRCS
Victor Horsley Department of Neurosurgery
The National Hospital for Neurology and Neurosurgery
London
UK

Jonathan Punt MB, BS, FRCS, FRCPCH
Children's Brain Tumor Research Centre
Academic Department of Child Health
University of Nottingham
Nottingham
UK

Matthias W R Radatz MD
The National Centre for Stereotactic Radiosurgery
Royal Hallamshire Hospital
Sheffield, South Yorkshire
UK

Robert C Rostomily MD
University of Washington Medical Center
Department of Neurological Surgery
Seattle, WA
USA

Jeremy G Rowe
The National Centre for Stereotactic Radiosurgery
Royal Hallamshire Hospital
Sheffield, South Yorkshire
UK

Stephen M Russell MD
Department of Neurosurgery
New York University School of Medicine
New York, NY
USA

Ali Samii MD
University of Washington School of Medicine
Department of Neurology
Seattle Veterans Administration Medical Center
Seattle, WA
USA

Christopher I Shaffrey MD
Department of Neurological Surgery and Orthopedic Surgery
University of Washington Medical Center
Seattle, WA
USA

Cheng-Mei Shaw MD
Department of Pathology
Neuropathology Laboratory
University of Washington School of Medicine
Harborview Medical Center
Seattle, WA
USA

Daniel L Silbergeld MD
University of Washington Medical Center
Department of Neurological Surgery
Seattle, WA
USA

Alexander M Spence MD
University of Washington Medical Center
Department of Neurology
Seattle, WA
USA

Richard J Stacey MBBS
Department of Neurosurgery
Radcliffe Infirmary
Oxford, Oxfordshire
UK

Simon Stapleton MD, FRCS(SN)
Department of Neurosurgery
Atkinson Morley's Hospital
London
UK

Kevin L Stevenson MD
Pediatric Neurosurgery
Children's Healthcare of Atlanta
Atlanta, GA
USA

Anthony Strong MA, DM, FRCSEd
Department of Neurosurgery
Medical School of Guy's, King's and St Thomas' Hospitals
King's College London
London, UK

John Suh MD
Brain Tumor Institute and
Department of Radiation Oncology
The Cleveland Clinic Foundation
Cleveland, OH
USA

Derek A Taggard MD
Department of Neurosurgery
University of Iowa
Iowa City, IA
USA

Dominic N P Thompson MB, BS, BSc, FRCS(SN)
Department of Neurosurgery
Great Ormond Street Hospital for Children NHS Trust
London
UK

Vincent C Traynelis MD
Department of Neurosurgery
University of Iowa Hospital
Iowa City, IA
USA

Dennis A Velez MD
Department of Neurological Surgery
University of Washington School of Medicine
Seattle, WA
USA

Allen E Waziri MD
Neurological Surgery
Columbia University
New York, NY
USA

Peter C Whitfield BM, PhD,FRCS (SN)
South West Neurosurgical Unit
Derriford Hospital
Plymouth, Devon
UK

Tessa L Whitton BM, FRCA
Department of Anesthesiology
Harborview Medical Center
University of Washington
Seattle, WA
USA

Joseph R Zunt MD, MPH
Department of Neurology
Harborview Medical Center
University of Washington School of Medicine
Seattle, WA
USA

I
Investigations

1

Neurophysiology

Allen E. Waziri, Derek A. Taggard and
Vincent C. Traynelis

Summary

The goal of this chapter is to provide a brief description and critical review of the various intraoperative monitoring techniques available to the modern neurosurgeon.

Introduction

Since the mid-1960s, neurosurgeons have been increasingly dedicated to utilizing technology that allows for the monitoring of neurological integrity and assessment of progress towards operative goals while a procedure is under way. Most neurosurgical procedures bear the risk of permanent neurological injury and, in the worst cases, devastation. In an attempt to reduce such morbidity, numerous methods of intraoperative monitoring have been created to guide the neurosurgeon in altering operative activity in a way that will prevent or minimize neurological damage. Ideally, these monitoring techniques involve minimal additional risks to the patient. There are a number of methods that have been in use for several decades and are well described. In addition, experimental techniques are being developed to provide further insight into the neurophysiological changes associated with surgical manipulation of the nervous system.

The ideal intraoperative monitoring tool satisfies several technical criteria. First is the ability to detect neurological damage at an early and reversible stage. Second, any modifications of the operative technique to allow for monitoring must not interfere with the surgeon's ability to achieve the operative goal. Components of the monitoring system should be easy to use and provide consistent, reliable data. The information obtained should be resistant to variables of the operative environment, such as depth of anesthesia, choice of anesthetic agents, temperature, or electrical artifact. Last, the neurological function or region being monitored must be that which is placed at risk by the operative procedure. The goal of intraoperative monitoring is to provide the surgeon with information that will guide or improve the current procedure as well as subsequent procedures. All currently available techniques fulfill these ideals to variable degrees.

In addition to the theoretical goals of intraoperative monitoring, there are a number of practical issues that must be taken into consideration if such techniques are to be used efficiently and successfully. Appropriate technical and analytical assistance is required from individuals who are thoroughly familiar with the particular technique to be used. The positioning of the patient and the monitoring equipment must be optimized to allow for the gathering of useful data without disruption of the surgical field or approach. The equipment to be used should be in excellent working order and calibrated for the particular needs of each case. Finally, potential sources of interference that could mask or prohibit data acquisition, such as operating lights or other emitters of radiated electrical activity, should be minimized pre-operatively.

This chapter attempts to provide a brief description and discussion of intraoperative monitoring techniques that are currently used by neurosurgeons, some of which have been utilized with great success over the years, and others which remain in an experimental phase. Intraoperative imaging and image-guidance will be covered in Chapter 7.

Electroencephalography

Electroencephalography (EEG) monitors and records spontaneously generated electrical potentials originating from the various surface cortical regions of the brain. EEG was first utilized as an intraoperative monitoring technique in 1965. It has subsequently grown in popularity owing to readily available equipment, familiar and consistent technique, relative simplicity of pre-operative set-up, and well- characterized patterns of response to various states of neurological function.

Traditional EEG relies on the application of a standard grid of scalp electrodes that are positioned using the International 10–20 Scalp Electrode Placement System (Fig. 1.1). Data are typically gathered from both cerebral hemispheres. Appropriate personnel, including an individual trained in interpretation of the ongoing recordings, are required to apply the electrodes and maintain the system throughout the surgical procedure. Conventional EEG recording generates a great deal of data and requires continuous monitoring by a trained individual; therefore, there has been some interest in developing computer-based methods of real-time EEG analysis. Several methods of digitally processing EEG signals with subsequent computer analysis have been described, which utilize Fourier transforms to provide spectral power representations that are easier to interpret than the raw EEG data (known as compressed spectral array, or CSA). However, there has been concern over the failure of CSA to detect mild changes that could be detected with analog EEG monitoring, and the simplified data provided by CSA are more likely to be complicated by artifacts introduced by the operative environment. This may be alleviated by comparison of selected segments of raw data with the histograms generated by the computer.

The primary utility of intraoperative EEG is in monitoring for the presence of prolonged and

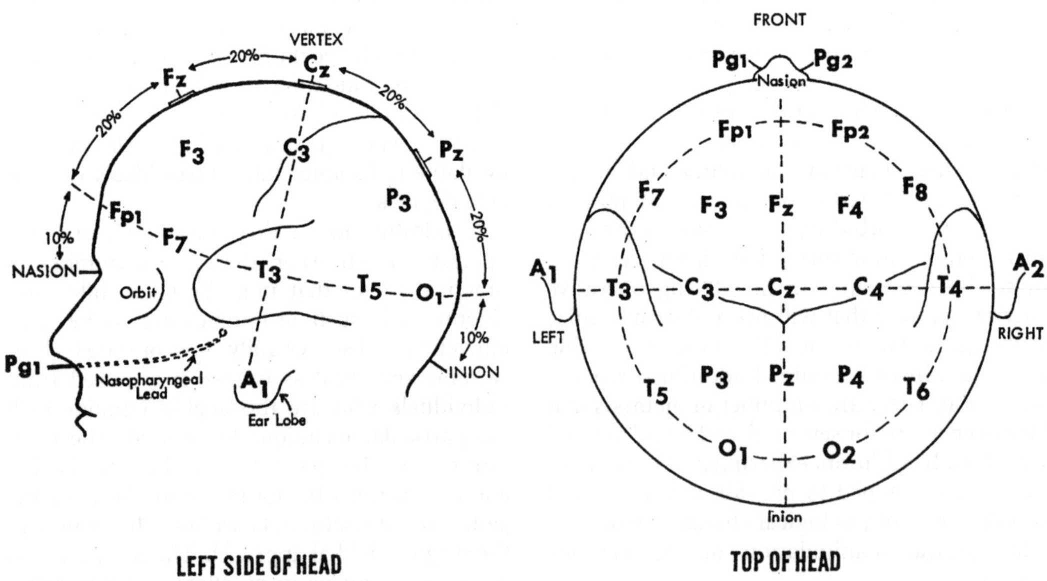

Fig. 1.1. The International 10–20 Scalp Electrode Placement System used to obtain electroencephalographic recordings, as viewed from the left side and top of the head.

significant ischemia of the brain related to various surgical manipulations. Numerous studies have demonstrated that synaptic transmission is abolished when cerebral blood flow (CBF) decreases below 15 ml/100 g/min, and the ability of the neuron to maintain its membrane potential fails when flow drops below 10 ml/100 g/min. At this level, permanent neurological damage may ensue within minutes if blood flow remains reduced. Unilateral hemispheric ischemia will abrogate EEG activity within about 20 seconds. However, permanent neuronal damage, which can be detected by potassium efflux, does not begin to occur until 5 minutes post ischemia. Surgical trials in humans have demonstrated that major EEG changes occur with drops in CBF below 10 ml/100 g/min, while more minor changes occur with flows of 10–18 ml/100 g/min. The EEG pattern generally remains stable at flows of 25 ml/100 g/min or greater. Zampella et al. demonstrated that only 5% of patients will have demonstrable EEG changes at flows of 20 ml/100 g/min, while 31% of patients showed these changes at flows of less than 13 ml/100 g/min [1]. The crucial role of EEG lies in identifying the "ischemic penumbra", which is the pathophysiological state of acute ischemia in which neurons are non-functional but still alive and salvageable by reperfusion. As EEG is capable of detecting this state of cerebral ischemia prior to the development of permanent damage, it can be an extremely valuable technique in monitoring procedures that may result in reduced blood flow. In general, EEG has been shown to be more sensitive and to show more rapid changes than the recording of somatosensory-evoked potentials for alerting the surgeon to potentially harmful manipulations, although the rate of false-positives is higher.

Importantly, EEG is particularly sensitive to anesthesia. Most anesthetic agents, including the halogenated gases, thiopental, midazolam, etomidate and propofol, cause similar EEG changes. At doses below the minimum alveolar concentration (MAC), widespread, frontally predominant, fast rhythms appear. Increasing doses are generally characterized by a disappearance of these alpha rhythms with concurrent appearance of a beta rhythm, followed by a progressive slowing towards theta and delta rhythms. Deep anesthesia is associated with a burst–suppression pattern, and at the deepest levels measurable potentials may disappear altogether. Although the effects of different anesthetics differ slightly at lower doses in terms of the particular patterns seen, slowing with burst–suppression is the common feature of all of these drugs. Anesthetic-induced EEG changes should be seen bilaterally and symmetrically over both cerebral cortices.

Intraoperative use of EEG during neurosurgery has primarily been used in the monitoring of ischemic changes associated with carotid endarterectomy (CEA). Recordings are typically obtained pre-operatively, at induction, intermittently during dissection, and continuously during cross-clamp occlusion of the internal carotid artery (ICA). Indications of significant ischemia may potentially mandate use of a shunt during the period of cross-clamping. Considering that the use of a shunt increases operative risk, related to either the potential for embolism or prolongation of operative time, the surgeon is required to balance these concerns with the benefits of shunting. A retrospective study by Salvian et al. compared a large cohort of patients who had undergone CEA either with routine shunting (n = 92) or with selective shunting using EEG changes as the indicator (n = 213). Of the selectively shunted group, only 16% had EEG changes that led to shunting. Post-operatively, 4 of the 92 patients who were routinely shunted had major stroke. In contrast, the selectively shunted group had only one case of post-operative stroke, suggesting that the use of EEG in determining the need for shunting may significantly reduce the risk of post-operative neurological deficit [2].

The two major EEG changes predictive of cerebral ischemia are: (1) slowing with decreased amplitude in the ischemic hemisphere, and (2) attenuation of the anesthetic-induced fast rhythms. EEG changes may be classified as major or moderate, with total or near-complete attenuation of 8–15 Hz activity and/or at least a doubling of delta activity of 1 Hz or less representing major changes. These alterations typically involve the ipsilateral hemisphere but can also be seen bilaterally or exclusively in the contralateral hemisphere. Moderate changes include amplitude attenuation of at least 50% or an increase in delta activity of 1 Hz or greater. When alterations of the recorded activity occur, whether major or moderate, they generally begin within minutes of cross-clamping the ICA. Nearly all of the major EEG changes that occur upon cross-clamping will reverse with placement of a shunt.

It has been suggested that EEG monitoring has a high false- positive rate in predicting stroke during CEA, thus unnecessarily subjecting many patients to the risks of shunt placement. However, the sum of the data on EEG monitoring in the setting of CEA indicates that it can identify the subset of patients at risk of clamp-induced ischemic insult. Redekop and Ferguson described a cohort of 293 patients who underwent routine CEA without shunting. Eight percent of these individuals demonstrated major EEG changes following clamping of the ICA; of this subset, 18% had immediate post-operative deficits, compared with only 1% of the individuals who did not have clamp-related EEG changes [3]. Another large retrospective analysis demonstrated similar success with the use of intraoperative EEG during CEA; stroke occurred in only 0.3% of patients who had been monitored with EEG during their procedure (and who had shunts placed upon the appearance of significant EEG changes), compared with a stroke incidence of 2.3% in the non-monitored group [4].

It has been pointed out that the predictive value of EEG monitoring, as measured by the actual number of strokes associated with major alterations of EEG patterns, is relatively low. There are a number of factors that are relevant to this issue. The threshold between tolerable ischemia and irreversible infarction does not clearly correlate with changes in the EEG patterns. Time is also a significant variable. A patient may well tolerate relative ischemia for the short time in which the ICA is cross-clamped during endarterectomy; however, if such ischemia were to persist for a greater length of time, permanent injury could result.

Obviously, the utility of standard methods of EEG, which require the placement of a grid of scalp electrodes, is limited by specific requirements of the operative approach, so these methods are of very little practical utility for a large proportion of intracranial cases. In addition, EEG monitoring loses efficacy in cases performed under deep hypothermic circulatory arrest (e.g. complex intracranial aneurysm); in fact, EEG activity ceases at brain temperatures of 19–26°C. Conversely, the disappearance of EEG activity has been used as a method to assess the adequacy of cooling in cases where deep hypothermic circulatory arrest is required. It has been proposed that a total of 3 minutes of electrocerebral silence (ECS) is an adequate endpoint for the assessment of therapeutic hypothermia.

Electrocorticography

Electrocorticography (ECoG) has been used as a tool to identify loci of epileptiform activity or to delineate regions of eloquent cortex. As with EEG, ECoG records electrical potentials that are generated by the changing oscillatory activity of cortical neuronal groups. Unlike EEG, however, ECoG uses depth electrodes or surface electrode "grids" that are placed in direct contact with the cortical tissue, allowing for much finer spatial resolution of cortical electrical activity. Synchronous neuronal activity must be within approximately 6 cm^2 of the cortical surface in order to be detectable by scalp electrodes, while ECoG is able to detect epileptiform discharges outside of this radius. As with standard EEG, the interpretation of intraoperative ECoG is complicated by the effects of anesthetic agents.

The traditional use of intraoperative ECoG has been dedicated to the identification and demarcation of the limits of resectable epileptogenic foci, primarily based on the detection of interictal epileptiform activity. There has been no agreement, however, on which interictal discharges are predictive of continued risk of epileptiform activity. A study evaluating the implications of residual epileptogenic discharges following tumor resection suggested that surgical irritation of the cortex could induce such activity; furthermore, such discharges were not predictive of post-operative clinical seizures [5]. In addition, ECoG may not be helpful in determining whether such discharges are independent of, or propagated from, another site. The most widely accepted use of ECoG in epilepsy surgery has been in cases of extratemporal partial seizures, where it has been used routinely to set the boundaries of tissue resection. The use of ECoG in temporal lobe procedures has been more dependent on individual institutional philosophy, as some centers employ standard resection strategies or depend on pre-operative delineation of the epileptogenic focus. The use of post-excisional ECoG is also variable, although the chances of seizure-free outcome are improved if there is no evidence of persistent epileptiform activity following resection. A comprehensive discussion about the use of ECoG in the management of primary epilepsy remains beyond the scope of this chapter.

Somatosensory Evoked Potentials

Neurosurgical monitoring of sensory evoked potentials (SEPs) relies on the recognition of characteristic alterations in the excitable properties of compromised neurons. These alterations generally occur before the onset of irreversible damage and can thus theoretically guide or alter the subsequent surgical technique. Evoked potential recordings, in contrast to those obtained via EEG, can only be generated via the use of external stimuli of various means. In general, SEPs used in intraoperative monitoring are generated by applying a peripheral stimulus to the particular sensory modality that carries its signal through the neurological region at risk, with recordings being taken at standardized points along the afferent pathway that allow for the assessment of both amplitude and latency of the signal. These stimuli can take the form of peripheral nerve shocks for somatosensory evoked potentials (SSEPs), trains of auditory clicks for brainstem auditory evoked potentials (BAEPs), or flashes of light for visual evoked potentials (VEPs). Waveforms of the SEPs are amplified and undesirable background noise may be filtered out. Prolongation of signal latency or decreased amplitude suggests diminished function at some point along the sensory pathway.

For the interpretation of SSEP data, adequate analysis of the waveforms requires averaging of at least 100 responses to provide reliable and clear waveform morphology. The rate of stimulation is usually 4–5 Hz, which minimizes acquisition time without inducing attenuation of the cortical response. Therefore, feedback can be provided to the surgeon about every 30–60 seconds. It is optimal to perform bilateral recordings, which allows the contralateral hemisphere to serve as an internal control. Components of the evoked response recording are labeled as either positive or negative, relative to a reference electrode, followed numerically by their modal peak latency in milliseconds. As an example, characteristic median nerve SSEP waves should include N13, P14, N20, P20 and P25 peaks (Fig. 1.2). The clival area generates the N13 deflection and reflects activation of the caudal medial lemniscus. Thalamocortical afferent activity is represented by the P14 wave, and N20 is associated with activation of cortical neurons in the primary somatosensory cortex. The latency difference between N13 and N20 is referred to as the "central conduction time" (CCT).

There are several variables that must be taken into consideration when using SSEP during neurosurgical procedures. Factors that can alter SSEP performance intraoperatively include anesthetic depth and type, patient temperature, blood pressure, limb positioning, and specific placement of stimulator and recording electrodes. In general, anesthetics cause an attenuation of the cortical components of the SSEP, such as N20, while the subcortical components remain resistant. Wave amplitudes are reduced and latencies are prolonged in a dose-related manner, particularly with the halogenated agents. Several exceptions include etomidate and ketamine, which can enhance the amplitude of the cortical components. Baseline recordings are crucial for evaluating changes that occur as a result of the operative procedure; individuals with carotid stenosis often demonstrate prolonged baseline CCTs and decreased amplitudes of various cortical responses.

SSEP monitoring has been used as an indicator of cerebral ischemia in much the same way as EEG. However, SSEP has several advantages over EEG as an intraoperative monitoring technique, which include greater relative resistance to general anesthesia, fewer electrode sites, and comparative ease of recording and interpretation. Generally, reductions in SSEP amplitudes are initiated by decreased cerebral oxidative mechanisms rather than by permanent neuronal damage. Decreases in CBF leading to SSEP changes parallel those causing noticeable EEG changes. Fisher et al. summarized a series of seven studies that analyzed outcomes of CEA as a function of SSEP changes. Of the total of 3,028 patients in all studies, 5.6% demonstrated a significant decline of SSEP as a direct result of surgical manipulation. Among these individuals,

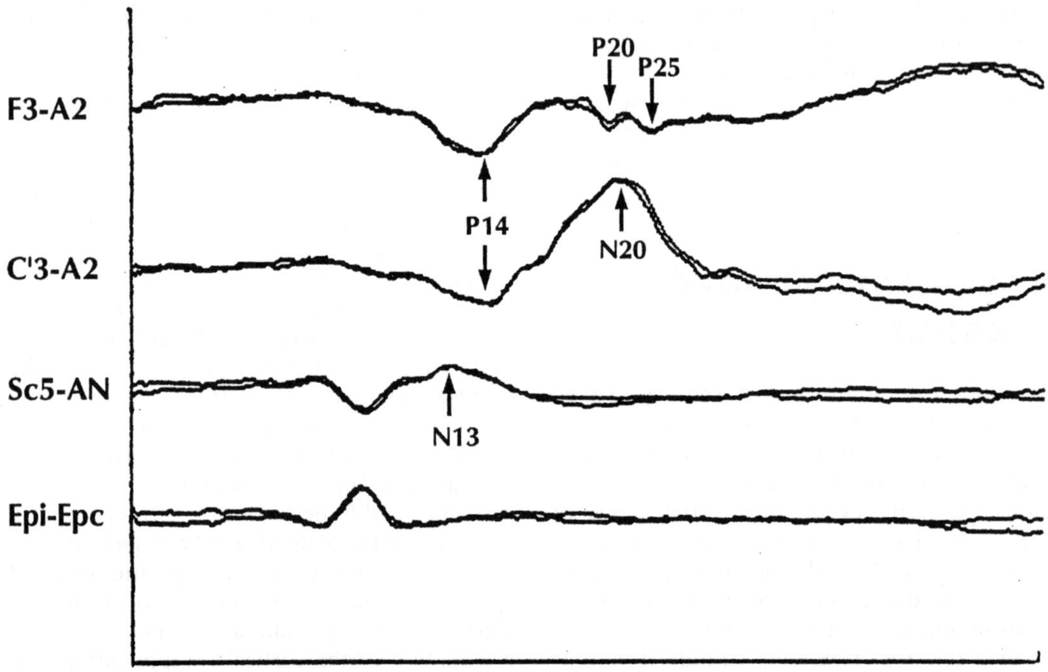

Fig. 1.2. Normal somatosensory evoked potentials detected after stimulation of the right median nerve. The central conduction time is calculated as the difference between the N13 and N20 peaks.

20% developed significant post-operative deficit. This number may have been larger had not a number of the patients with SSEP changes undergone shunting as a result of those changes [6]. Severe, irreversible SSEP changes appear to be a rare but ominous sign. This occurred in less than 1% of cases in a series of 994 CEAs; however, all awoke with neurological sequelae [7]. In contrast to EEG, no study has been performed with the intent to delineate the false-positive rate of SSEP monitoring – as it relates to stroke – if a shunt is not placed.

When cerebral ischemia occurs with the application of a clamp upon the ICA, characteristic changes occur in the N20, P25 and N30 components of the SSEP. A defined sequence of alterations, or stages, that occur with progressive ischemia has been described. Amplitude reduction combined with latency progression of N30 represents mild, or stage 1, ischemic change. Stage 2, or moderate, changes include the disappearance of N30 as well as amplitude reductions of N20 and P25 up to 50%. Severe, or stage 3, changes are defined by the loss of P25 with the concomitant progression of increasing latency and amplitude reduction of N20. Guerit describes a similar system, which recommends shunt placement whenever moderate-to-severe SSEP alterations occur within 7 minutes after cross-clamping, and he suggests that some cases of mild-to-moderate SSEP change may be due to drops in blood pressure rather than to the ischemic effects of cross-clamping [8].

Experience of others has supported the sensitivity of N20 and P25 to ischemic insults, and amplitude reductions have proven to be more predictive than latency increases. Most surgeons who rely on SSEPs place a shunt when the N20-P25 complex decreases by 50% or rapidly disappears with clamping of the ICA. These changes typically recover when flow is re-established through the shunt. Overall, the correlation of SSEP changes to clinical outcome is quite good. Neurological dysfunction is remarkably rare in the setting of SSEP with little or no change. In the series by Haupt and Horsch, only one of the 994 patients suffered a stroke in the face of normal SSEPs. As with EEG, clamp-induced changes in SSEPs occur in about 20–30% of monitored cases. It is important to note that temporary ischemia, whether due to intended or accidental vessel occlusion, does not immediately give rise to alterations in the relevant SSEP [7].

SSEP monitoring has also been shown to be useful during intracranial procedures that directly or indirectly contribute to ischemia, including aneurysm clipping or manipulation and retraction of various brain structures. Isolated vascular territories can be assessed through judicious selection of the stimulus location to be used for SSEP. Regions of cortex subserved by the ICA and MCA can be monitored by stimulation through the median nerve; in addition, the median nerve can be used to assess flow to the thalamic segment of the somatosensory pathway, an area provided for by the PCA. Posterior tibial nerve SSEP has been used for monitoring the territory of the ACA, although concurrent monitoring of the median nerve may be necessary for adequate detection of ischemia involving the dependent regions of the recurrent artery of Huebner. In assessing the posterior circulation, isolated monitoring of either SSEP or BAEP during vertebrobasilar aneurysm clipping may be of little use, as ischemia due to basilar perforator occlusion may not affect the auditory or somatosensory pathways traversing the brainstem; however, if used in combination, SSEP and BAEP monitoring may enhance the ability to detect brainstem ischemia.

Currently, prospective data comparing EEG and SSEP monitoring for reversible ischemia and patient outcomes do not exist. On a theoretical level, EEG monitors a larger area of the cerebral cortex and does not require time averaging of signals. However, Fava et al. have suggested that SSEP monitoring, in addition to EEG, enhances the overall predictive value of monitoring during CEA. Patients ($n = 151$) with EEG changes indicating significant ischemia were shunted only if severe SSEP changes occurred within the first few minutes after vessel occlusion. Fewer shunts were placed using this protocol than if EEG were used independently. No patient with significant EEG changes in conjunction with insignificant SSEP changes had a post-operative deficit. Patients who were shunted did well, with the exception of subjects whose ischemia was felt to be embolic and who awoke with new deficit [9]. Guerit suggests that SSEP may be superior to EEG in the determination of ECS in cases using deep hypothermic circulatory arrest, as the SSEP is much less sensitive to environmental electrical noise and is therefore better suited to identifying true ECS [8].

SSEP has also been used for functional localization in the cerebral cortex, most particularly in defining the central sulcus, via the use of phase reversal. SSEPs recorded simultaneously from the precentral and postcentral gyri exhibit typical responses of reversed polarity (Fig. 1.3). The evoked potential from the precentral gyrus is a biphasic positive-negative waveform, compared with the mirror image of the postcentral gyrus, which is negative-positive. The typically recorded response in the postcentral gyrus following median nerve stimulation is a negative deflection with a latency period of 20 ms (N20) followed by a positive deflection at 30 ms (P30). Precentral recordings reveal somewhat lower amplitude deflections that mirror the sensory strip recordings (characteristically, a P22 component followed by an N33 deflection). The precise etiology of these potentials and phase reversal is not fully understood. Brodman's area 3b, located on the primary sensory cortex along

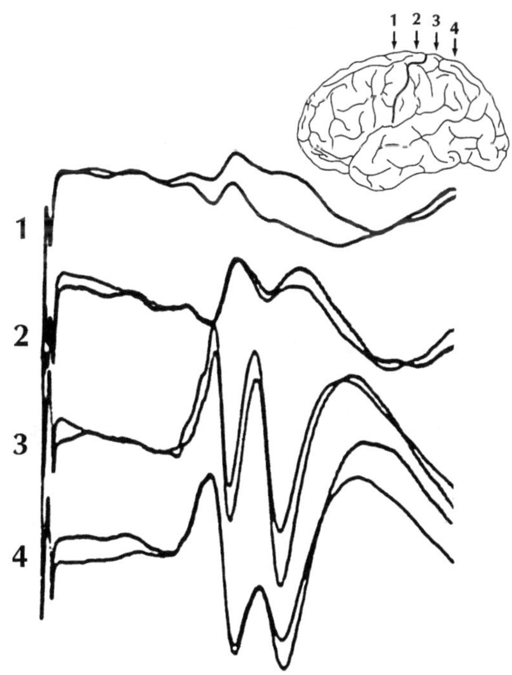

Fig. 1.3. Phase reversal across the central sulcus in response to contralateral median nerve stimulation. The reversal in polarity is evident when comparing leads 2 and 3, positions that bridge the central sulcus (darkened for emphasis).

the posterior wall of the central sulcus, receives sensory impulses from the thalamus. This region at least partially contributes to the generation of the N20 wave. Neurons within the precentral gyrus are thought to be responsible for generating the P22 deflection, as ablation of the postcentral gyrus does not eliminate this component of the SSEP. The P22 wave probably results from direct projections from the thalamus to the motor strip, but may be influenced by association fibers from area 3b.

SSEPs may also be recorded at the spinal level to monitor for insult to neurological tissues during spinal surgery, assuming that the location of peripheral stimulation is optimized to assess the level of cord at risk during a particular procedure (Fig. 1.4). SSEP monitoring is commonly used during a number of spinal procedures, including correction of scoliosis, resection of spinal AVM or tumor, therapeutic embolization of spinal AVMs, correction of spinal instability, and therapy for syringomyelia. Changes in spinal SSEP after the placement of hardware can suggest a need for changes in positioning of the hardware. Electrodes may be placed in the subarachnoid or epidural space, on the interspinous ligament, or attached to a spinous process. With the exception of subarachnoid leads, these leads may be placed percutaneously or at the site of surgical exposure. Recording evoked potentials at the spinal level has some advantages over cortically recorded SSEPs. Spinal evoked potentials have larger amplitudes, and repetition rates may be increased (which can reduce acquisition time). In addition, SSEPs recorded from the spinal cord are more resistant to the effects of anesthetic agents than are cortically detected SSEPs.

While median nerve stimulation has been commonly used for monitoring SSEP during cervical spine procedures, caudal portions of the cervical cord may not receive appropriate coverage with this modality. The ulnar nerve may offer more complete representation of lower cervical levels. For procedures placing the thoracic or lumbar cord at risk, SSEPs generated through the posterior tibial or common peroneal nerves can be used. Recordings taken simultaneously from both the upper and lower limb may allow for an internal control in certain procedures; specifically, evoked potentials that are lost from both the upper and lower extremity during a procedure which places the thoracic cord at risk suggest a technical error in stimu-

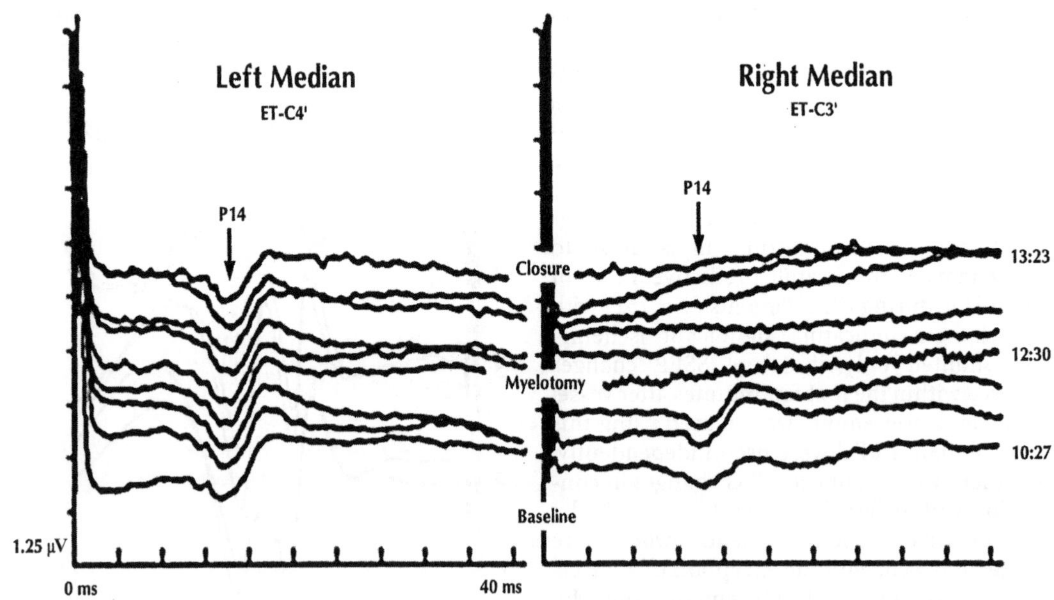

Fig. 1.4. Left and right median nerve somatosensory evoked potentials in a patient who underwent laminectomy and exposure of an intradural, intramedullary tumor of the cervical spine. The right P14 waveform is initially diminished at baseline and then is permanently lost during the midline myelotomy. Left-sided tracings are unaffected. The patient awoke with a permanent right hemi-proprioceptive loss.

lation or recording. However, if only lower extremity responses were lost in this case, the surgeon would be more suspicious of injury to the thoracic cord.

A large (n = 51,263), multicenter retrospective survey examining the role of SSEP monitoring in scoliosis surgery suggested a 50% reduction in the rate of neurological defects related to the procedure in patients who had intraoperative SSEP monitoring. The rate of false-negatives was remarkably low in this survey (0.06%), and the authors concluded that spinal SSEP was effective for detecting more than 90% of intraoperative neurological deficits [10]. Others have suggested that SSEPs may be useful in the assessment of compromising mechanical factors or decreases in relative blood flow to the spinal cord. A small study (n = 13) performed on patients with syringomyelia, treated with syringo-subarachnoid shunting, demonstrated a rapid improvement in spinal SSEPs following decompression of the syrinx. This improvement correlated with increased local blood flow to these regions, and the patients had postoperative improvement in their symptoms [11].

However, larger trials have not demonstrated similar consistency. Falsely positive SSEP changes are relatively common [10]. In a review of 182 cervical spine procedures, complete loss of evoked potential recordings occurred in 33 subjects and was associated with post-operative deficit in only 50% of these cases [12]. Partial loss of response was even less predictive, providing an overall specificity of only 27%. Further, false-negative recordings have been described. A large retrospective survey of nearly 190 spine surgeons who routinely used intraoperative SSEP monitoring found that nearly 30% of combined post-operative deficits seen in their patients occurred in the absence of observed spinal SSEP changes [13]. Confoundingly, recordings may show improvement during a case without correlation to post-operative neurological improvement. Positive changes to SSEP waveforms may reassure the surgeon intraoperatively, while several studies have demonstrated that improvement of SSEP amplitude or latency appears to be of little post-operative clinical significance.

It has been suggested that the use of SSEP monitoring in spinal surgery may be augmented with the concurrent use of another monitoring technique (such as motor evoked potentials). However, at this time there is no consensus as to the efficacy of isolated intraoperative spinal SSEP monitoring.

Monitoring techniques for surgery of the lumbosacral spine have also been reported. In an attempt to reduce the limited morbidity associated with lumbosacral diskectomy or pedicle screw fixation of the lumbosacral spine, some surgeons monitor nerve root function in the lower extremity during the procedure. Again, no clear efficacy has been demonstrated by controlled study.

Spinal Stimulation

Electrical stimulation of the spinal cord, both directly and indirectly, has been well described over the last decade as an additional method for monitoring the integrity of the descending tracts during surgical manipulation of the spine. The evoked motor responses, termed "neurogenic motor evoked potentials" (NMEPs), can be followed by recording from the sciatic nerve at the popliteal fossa bilaterally or by monitoring for myogenic responses in the lower limbs. The electrodes used to evoke NMEPs can be placed in several locations rostral to the region to be manipulated, including the epidural space, the spinous processes, or in a position that allows for percutaneous stimulation. Direct stimulation through pedicle screws has also been attempted as a means of assessing impingement upon, or damage to, nerve roots owing to misalignment of the hardware.

A recent study evaluated the efficacy of each of these electrode positions in 50 patients undergoing posterior thoracic or thoracolumbar procedures with instrumentation. The findings demonstrated excellent results for each method; however, epidural placement of the stimulating electrodes was found to be most reliable in terms of the acquisition of initial NMEPs and in maintaining those NMEPs throughout the procedure [14]. The use of electrodes placed on the spinous processes or in the epidural space often requires enlargement of the surgical field and placement of the electrodes within the surgical field, which can result in some inconvenience.

A comparison of NMEP and SSEP was performed by Pereon et al. in a consecutive series of 112 patients undergoing surgical correction of spinal deformity, in which both NMEPs and SSEPs were generated and monitored. In three of the cases, surgical manipulation resulted in sudden loss of both NMEPs and SSEPs. In these cases, the electrodes used for elicitation of NMEP were moved along the spinal cord until the precise level of involvement was appreciated, with subsequent laminectomy and decompression at that level. Two of the three patients exhibiting evoked potential loss were asymptomatic following the procedure, while a third was left paraplegic. However, in two additional operations, isolated changes in NMEP were seen without a concomitant change in SSEP. In both of these cases, the surgical procedure was altered accordingly and potential neurological damage was avoided. In addition, the data from NMEP monitoring, requiring no time averaging, were acquired more quickly than data from SSEP, allowing for more timely interventions in the face of pending injury [15].

Monitoring of sacral root innervation to the anal and urethral sphincters can be performed with either evoked potential monitoring or by manometric recordings. In cases of tethered cord or tumor resection, a comprehensive strategy for monitoring has been proposed, which provides coverage from L2 to S4 [16]. This system uses a combination of SSEP monitoring from tibial nerve and nerve root stimulation with electromyographic (EMG) recordings of muscle from the sphincters and relevant leg musculature. The proposed benefit is an ability to differentiate functional neural tissue from non-functional or fibrous tissue. Despite the successful application of these various monitoring techniques, there has been no controlled study documenting improved neurological outcomes in these cases, and the circumstances in which lumbosacral spinal cord monitoring is efficacious have not been well defined.

Motor Evoked Potentials

Identification of the primary motor cortex and the specifics of the motor homunculus can be accomplished via the use of cortical electrical or magnetic stimulation, using concomitant EMG recording to assess a response to the evoked potential in the periphery. Electrical stimulation is performed with single surface electrodes or electrode grids that are placed in direct contact with the cortex. Transcranial electrical stimulation is remarkably painful, due to current flow across the scalp. Therefore, non-anesthetized recordings are not feasible. Furthermore, transcranial electrical stimulation is contraindicated in patients with a history of seizure or an EEG suggestive of seizure tendency. Magnetically induced motor evoked potentials (MEPs) are generated by passing a changing current through a coil held perpendicular to the cortical surface, which induces a magnetic force perpendicular to the electrical field. Transcranial magnetic stimulation (TMS) of the cortex is painless, may be obtained both pre- and intraoperatively, and does not require averaging for analytical purposes. However, this method is cumbersome, expensive and non-specific with regard to the cortex it stimulates.

MEPs are exquisitely sensitive to the effects of anesthetics. It has been conclusively demonstrated that isoflurane will abolish MEPs generated by either electrical or magnetic stimulation of the cortex. Barbiturates, propofol and benzodiazepines exert a strong depressive effect on MEPs; etomidate causes a milder depression that eventually returns to baseline. Anesthetics that have been shown to have little or no effect on MEP are halothane, fentanyl and ketamine. MEPs generated by stimulation of the spinal cord avoid the cortical effects of these anesthetics and will remain intact. Cortical MEPs may be difficult to generate in young children, in whom the motor cortex is relatively inexcitable.

Enhanced patient outcome has not been clearly documented with the use of MEPs in controlled trials. A retrospective study reviewed the resections of 130 intramedullary tumors performed with the assistance of MEP recordings. The results suggested that gross total resection of these tumors was more likely when MEP monitoring was used; however, no clear reduction in morbidity or improvement in patient outcome related to monitoring was demonstrated [17].

In addition to assessing cortical elements of the motor system, MEP may prove to be a valuable technique in the assessment of intraoperative risk to the motor pathways of the brainstem and spinal cord. Considering that sensory impulses travel in the posterior tracts of the spinal cord and the lateral aspects of the brainstem, isolated monitoring of SSEP is incomplete for assessing the integrity of all spinal pathways.

The use of simultaneous MEP and SSEP monitoring has been suggested for this purpose and has been studied to a limited extent. Nagle et al. reviewed a series of 116 cases involving surgical manipulation of the spinal cord or column in which simultaneous intraoperative SSEP and MEP monitoring was utilized. Significant intraoperative changes in both SSEP and MEP patterns occurred in eight of these patients. An additional patient had isolated MEP changes. All patients with intraoperative changes awoke with post-operative deficit. Therefore, the authors support simultaneous use of both MEP and SSEP monitoring to achieve parallel, independent monitoring of spinal function [18]. Additional data from another series of patients undergoing surgical correction of spinal deformity suggested that relevant intraoperative changes are acquired in a more timely fashion with MEP than with SSEP [15].

Cortical Mapping Techniques

Functional areas other than the primary motor cortex can be localized with electrically or magnetically driven cortical mapping techniques. Preservation of language function is a primary concern when performing dominant temporal lobe resections. Investigations that have mapped cortical regions subserving functional speech have demonstrated considerable variability in the specific location of these areas along the superior and medial temporal gyri. Resections of the dominant temporal lobe using standardized strategies have the potential to significantly damage the patient's ability to speak or, alternatively, underestimate the potential limits of resection, depending on the exact location of language areas.

The most reliable and widely used technique for identifying cortical language areas involves direct electrical stimulation of cortex that is putatively involved in functional speech. Numerous studies have shown that electrical stimulation of speech-related cortex will interfere with language tasks, generally resulting in anomia or a complete abrogation of speech. Electrical-stimulation language mapping is typically carried out in awake patients. When circumstances dictate that a resection be carried out under general anesthesia, an initial craniotomy can be performed to place indwelling surface electrode grids over the brain regions to be mapped. Following recovery from this initial procedure, detailed language-mapping protocols are carried out via the externalized electrical leads. After language mapping has been completed, with all functionally important cortical sites identified, the patient is returned to the operating room for electrode removal and an appropriately guided resection under general anesthesia.

Safe and effective language mapping is accomplished via direct electrical stimulation of the cortex at strengths that are below the after-discharge (AD) threshold. ADs are abnormal cortical discharges that are evoked by focal electrical stimulation and which persist beyond the period of stimulation. Electrocorticographic recording electrodes must be positioned immediately adjacent to the site of electrical stimulation in order to detect ADs. Stimulation strengths with the potential to evoke ADs are also capable of evoking local seizure activity. This can render stimulation mapping uninterpretable or, at worst, precipitate a generalized seizure. Typically, electrical stimuli are delivered via a hand-held probe and consist of pulse trains of charge-balanced square waves (0.2 ms duration, 50 Hz). The patient is instructed to carry out a variety of language tasks (e.g. object identification, word repetition, counting, execution of verbal commands) as disruptive electrical stimuli are delivered to various cortical surface sites. Sites that are associated with changes in speech and comprehension are identified and can be spared during the subsequent surgical resection.

Microelectrode Recording/Stimulation

Neurosurgical treatment options for the various movement disorders have been under investigation for a number of decades. Parkinson's disease has perhaps received the greatest amount of attention, partly owing to unsatisfactory long-term outcomes with current medical therapies, improved understanding of the pathophysiological connections relevant to Parkinson's disease, and advances in monitoring techniques relevant to these procedures. These cases generally involve either ablation or deep-brain stimulation of the motor thalamus, the globus pallidus or the subthalamic nucleus via stereotactic electrode placement; more recently, stem cell transplantation has emerged as a potential treatment option. Precise advancement and the final position of electrodes used for ablation or stimulation are of paramount importance in reducing post-operative morbidity as well as ensuring the best chance for therapeutic success. The primary method used over the last decade for this purpose is electrophysiological monitoring of the brain structures that are traversed by the microelectrode during the procedure.

The microelectrode mapping technique relies on the development of a "physiological map" based on the known spontaneous firing rate and pattern of particular neuronal groups and the predictable pattern changes that are related to various stimuli. The internal capsule and optic tract can be identified through the recording of firing changes related to sensory stimuli such as limb movement or flashes of light, respectively. As the recording/stimulating electrode is advanced, the physiological map that is developed can be correlated to a standardized stereotactic atlas or thin-slice high-resolution MRI images from the particular patient. Once this map is developed, lesion or stimulation electrode placement can occur with maximum precision.

The proven utility of microelectrode recording for increasing accuracy and decreasing morbidity in ablation or deep-brain stimulator placement is somewhat unclear. Although the vast majority of surgeons performing these procedures utilize microelectrode guidance, a critical review of the relevant literature compiled by Hariz and Fodstad questioned this practice. They noted that rates of severe complications and mortality appeared to be higher when microelectrodes were used, rather than MRI-based guidance, for either ablative or stimulatory purposes, while concomitant gains in accuracy and efficacy of the procedure were not seen. Their final conclusion focused on the need for a prospective, randomized trial comparing micro- and macroelectrodes in movement disorder surgery [19].

Brainstem Auditory Evoked Potentials

The recording of cortical potentials related to auditory stimuli has proven to be difficult. In many patients, the primary auditory cortex is located deep within the Sylvian fissure. This location generates potentials whose dipole is perpendicular to the cortical surface, thereby rendering them undetectable by surface or scalp electrodes. However, detection and analysis of BAEPs have been developed for a number of neurosurgical procedures involving areas that are traversed by the ascending auditory signal, including both extra-axial (nerve) and intra-axial (brainstem) tissues. These procedures include resection of vestibular schwannomas, microvascular decompression of cranial nerves, retrolabyrinthine vestibular neurectomy, clipping of basilar artery aneurysms, treatment of posterior fossa AVMs, and resection of tumors residing in the cerebellopontine angle (CPA) or brainstem.

BAEPs are generated via the presentation of trains of clicks to one or both ears, resulting in an afferent signal that can be detected by scalp electrodes as it passes through the vestibulocochlear nerve, lower brainstem and midbrain. As with SSEP, changes in waveform amplitude or prolongation of signal latency are suggestive of impending or actual damage to the pathway, and persistent loss of the BAEP is more indicative of permanent damage than transient loss. Pre-operative assessment must be performed to obtain the baseline performance of the ascending auditory pathway for each individual prior to surgical manipulation. In most cases, hundreds or even thousands of responses to rapid (10–30 Hz) stimuli are averaged to obtain high quality waveforms. There are five major peaks, numbered I–V, which are particularly relevant in the analysis of BAEPs (Fig. 1.5). These waves are thought to be generated from the proximal eighth cranial nerve (I), the entry zone into the brainstem (II), the cochlear nuclear complex (III), the superior olive (IV), and the contralateral lemniscus or nucleus (V). These associations become important in the operating room, as brainstem ischemia may prolong the latency of peak V but leave peaks I and III essentially unaffected. Although it is possible to record directly from an exposed eighth nerve, the

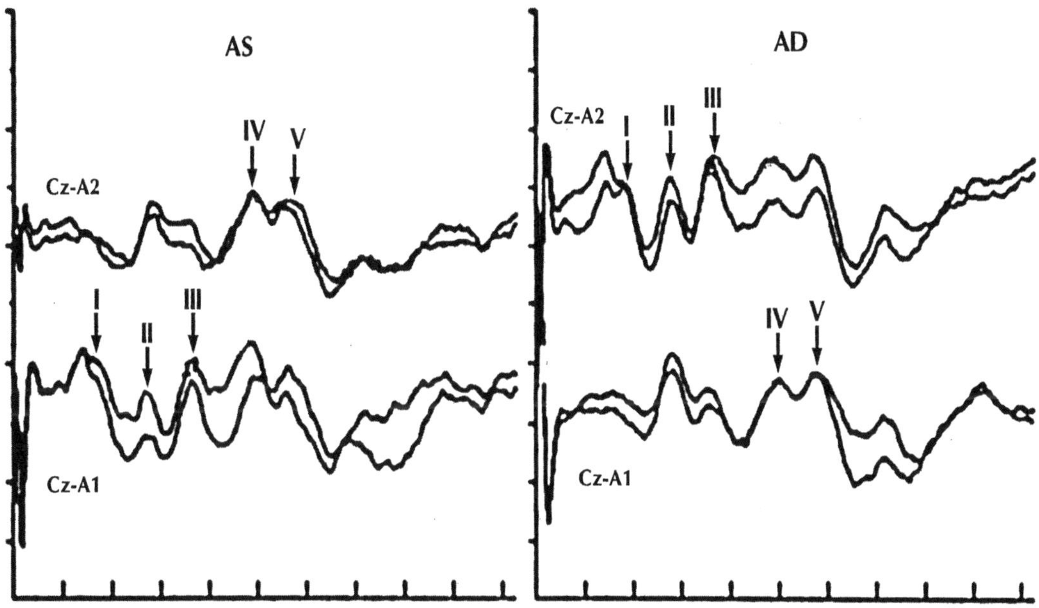

Fig. 1.5. Normal brainstem auditory evoked potentials with labeling of peaks I–V. During CPA surgery, peak V commonly exhibits a gradual prolongation of latency and reduction of amplitude that is not predictive of hearing loss (AS = left ear, AD = right ear).

potentials detected in this fashion are difficult to record and fail to provide insight into the functional status of ascending pathways in the brainstem.

The most frequent indication for the use of BAEP monitoring has been in the resection of vestibular schwannomas. There are a number of steps in the surgical procedure that are known to place auditory function at risk, including opening of the dura, cerebellar retraction, coagulation of tumor vessels, and removal of tumor present in the auditory canal, particularly from the most lateral portion. A series presented by Fischer et al. demonstrated that hearing was preserved in an average of 45% of patients who underwent resection of a vestibular schwannoma with concomitant recording of BAEP; this number was variable depending on the particular grade of the tumor [20]. Similar findings were described by Fahlbusch et al. in a series of 61 patients who underwent resection of large vestibular schwannomas via a lateral suboccipital approach with pre-operative and intraoperative BAEP monitoring. In this cohort, hearing was preserved in approximately 43% of patients in the early post-operative phase; however, a number of patients had subsequent decreases in hearing, resulting in a decrease in the final number of hearing-intact individuals to 27% [21]. BAEP monitoring has also been used in cases focusing on microvascular decompression of the facial or trigeminal nerves. Both retrospective and prospective studies have suggested that post-operative hearing loss can be reduced in these cases with the use of BAEP monitoring before and during the procedure.

Changes in BAEP that have been referred to as significant indicators of post-operative hearing loss are: decreases in waveform amplitude of 50%, prolongation of waveform latency of 10% or greater, and dramatic alterations in waveform morphology. Obviously, disappearance of the waveform is most concerning and is most likely to correlate with subsequent loss of hearing. Upon exposure of the CPA, wave V may exhibit prolonged latency and amplitude reduction that gradually continues until the potential is lost. When wave V is lost, no prediction of post-operative hearing can be made. If the potential is unchanged throughout surgery, the patient's post-operative auditory function will be stable. Loss of wave I occurs more acutely over minutes and is always associated with loss of wave V; return of this potential will occur within 15 minutes or will not return at all. If it fails to reappear within this time, hearing will inevitably be lost. Hearing will be preserved if both waves remain unaffected.

Cranial Nerve Monitoring

The most extensive experience with brainstem and cranial nerve monitoring has come from procedures involving the CPA. Various sensory and motor functions of the cranial nerves can be monitored in an attempt to preserve function or to assist intraoperative decision making. As previously, sensory nerves are typically monitored with evoked potentials and motor nerves with EMG recordings. The theoretical rationale for monitoring spontaneous EMG activity relies on the property that thermal, mechanical or metabolic irritation of the intracranial portion of a cranial motor nerve will lead to a predictable and measurable activity in the innervated muscle.

Logistically, intraoperative EMG monitoring of muscles innervated by the various cranial nerves is relatively simple. Needle insertion into the appropriate muscle is preferable to surface electrode placement for increasing the sensitivity and specificity of the system. Intramuscular electrodes increase the sensitivity of detection for spontaneous EMG activity, while surface electrodes are more appropriate for the assessment of compound muscle action potentials (CMAPs). Most systems amplify and convert the muscle action potential to audible signals that are immediately available to the surgical team. A variety of probes are available for the purposes of stimulation. Both constant current and constant voltage stimulation paradigms exist, and both have been used effectively and safely. Monopolar and bipolar stimulating electrodes are available, with the latter providing more focal stimulation. Finally, appropriate communication with the anesthesiologist is crucial, as EMG potentials will be abrogated by significant neuromuscular blockade.

The efficacy of facial nerve monitoring in reducing post-operative facial palsy during CPA tumor surgery is well established. Monitoring during vestibular schwannoma resection is particularly crucial, as up to 78% of these cases involve an impairment of the facial nerve. Facial nerve activity is usually recorded from the ipsilateral frontalis, orbicularis oculi, orbicularis oris, and/or mentalis muscles. EMG responses have been classified as either spontaneous or evoked. Spontaneous activity is common with the onset of monitoring, generally characterized by low-amplitude, low-density unit potentials presenting as steady trains or small repetitive bursts. Evoked responses, which are more common, are further subdivided into three patterns. "Pulse patterns" result from purposeful stimulation of the facial nerve with the stimulating probe and have a frequency identical to that generated by the stimulator. A second response, the "burst pattern", results from mechanical, chemical or thermal stimuli. Such alterations of nerve firing occur soon after the inciting event, with the observed pattern consisting of short (<1 s) bursts of synchronous motor activity. The final type of activity, known as the train pattern, presents as groups of asynchronous discharges with durations of several minutes. These potentials may have a latency of seconds to minutes after the aggravating event occurs. Traction on the nerve is usually the causative event, but chemical or thermal irritation may also be responsible. Activity may also be seen if cold irrigation fluid is used. The train pattern is most concerning as an indicator of potential or current damage to the nerve; the effect is typically delayed and outlasts the stimulus that incited it.

Post-operative function of the facial nerve can be predicted based on stimulation studies performed prior to wound closure. Inability to produce facial motion with high current stimulation is predictive of post-operative paralysis. When stimulation of more than 3.0 mA in a constant voltage setting is required to produce facial movement, post-operative palsy of the seventh cranial nerve is expected. However, potential for recovery exists if the nerve is intact. Good movement induced by 0.05–0.2 mA at the brainstem has been correlated with normal or minimal paresis of the facial nerve. Using a constant current setting, elevation of stimulus threshold to 0.2 or 0.3 V following the procedure is usually associated with good post-operative function of the nerve. However, threshold potentials greater than 0.3 V may be indicative of post-operative loss of function.

Antidromic stimulation of the facial nerve is also possible via the use of a hand-held electrode placed in the surgical field, with nerve stimulation at the stylomastoid foramen. This technique is advantageous in cases where neuromuscular blockade is required; however, continuous monitoring of nerve function is obviously extremely difficult, and a certain amount of inconvenience is added due to the need to introduce a hand-held device into the surgical field.

EMG monitoring of the facial nerve has also been an important part of procedures performed to relieve hemifacial spasm. Abnormal muscle response to stimulation of the appropriate branch of the facial nerve, which is typically seen in this patient population, disappears when the nerve is released from the offending vessel. This finding has been associated with good post-operative outcomes, while perseverance of an abnormal response parallels residual post-operative spasm.

Intraoperative monitoring of the other cranial nerves is also possible. Needle electrodes can be placed into any of the extraocular muscles, thereby monitoring cranial nerves III, IV and VI. The masseter or temporalis serve as recording sites for the motor division of the trigeminal nerve. Electrodes placed into the soft palate or posterior pharyngeal musculature can be used to monitor the function of cranial nerve IX. However, great care must be taken when stimulating these motor fibers, as some of them innervate the carotid body and stimulation may result in bradycardia or hypotension. Similarly, vagal monitoring, using electrodes placed endoscopically into the vocal cords or cricothyroid muscle, may also result in marked bradycardia, arrythmias or alterations of blood pressure. The absence of vagal activity, as recorded in laryngeal muscles, can be used to determine whether posterior pharyngeal recordings are attributable to cranial nerve IX rather than to nerve X. EMG recordings from either the trapezeus or sternocleidomastoid muscles will indicate activity of cranial nerve XI; however, stimulus intensity should be kept low to minimize the possibility of forceful jerking of the head with resulting trauma at the pin sites. Electrodes placed in the tongue allow for recording of evoked potentials from hypoglossal stimulation.

Visual Evoked Potentials

There has been interest in developing a reliable method of measuring and interpreting visual evoked potentials (VEPs) for use during procedures that could compromise elements of the visual pathway from the retina to the occipital cortex. Optic stimuli have been traditionally delivered through LED-emitting goggles or fitted contact lenses. There have been very few studies assessing the role of VEP monitoring in neurosurgical procedures, perhaps due to the enormous variation in observed waveform characteristics in conjunction with persistently unreliable recordings. Preliminary results have been mixed, but the overriding consensus suggests that the use of VEP monitoring is not justified as a technique owing to this extensive variability. It has been demonstrated that alterations in VEP have very poor sensitivity and specificity for the prediction of post-operative visual changes. Therefore, this technique remains primarily in the experimental arena.

Measurement of Cerebral Blood Flow

Two major methods have been devised for the purpose of primary quantification of CBF. As opposed to EEG or SSEP monitoring, which give a secondary glimpse of CBF by detecting physiological changes that occur owing to decreases in flow, direct measurement of flow would hypothetically provide more rapid and relevant intraoperative feedback. The first of these methods relies on measuring the clearance of an injectable tracer from brain tissue. The tracer that has been used for this purpose, due to its relative insolubility in water and rapid diffusion across the blood–brain barrier, is 133Xe. Typically, clearance is detected with a hand-held sensor placed over the region of interest following injection of the tracer into the ICA. A clearance curve is generated and the area under the curve is used for calculating CBF. The use of 133Xe for CBF measurement during CEA has been well described. Sundt has reported the greatest experience with regional CBF (rCBF) measurements during CEA [22]. It is primarily his analysis of nearly 2,200 monitored patients that supports shunt placement for flows of less than 18–20 ml/100 g/min. Others have questioned the efficacy of measuring rCBF during CEA. Zampella et al. performed EEG monitoring and rCBF measurements during 431 consecutive

CEAs without shunting [1]. No correlation was found between rCBF measurements and neurological morbidity or overall complication rate.

A second method of measuring CBF relies on near-infrared spectroscopy to assess cerebral oxygenation status. Also known as "cerebral oximetry", this technique measures changes in the levels of oxygenated, deoxygenated and total hemoglobin as well as oxidized cytochrome in the local cerebral blood supply. The advantage of using the near-infrared spectrum is that this wavelength of light passes easily through the extracranial tissues, allowing for non-invasive monitoring. However, variations in anatomy or extra- to intracranial collateral blood supply can make interpretation of the results somewhat difficult. The sensor patch is placed over the forehead on the ipsilateral side and continuous measurements of regional cerebral oxygen saturation (rSO_2) are obtained. Several studies have assessed the utility of cerebral oximetry as a monitoring technique during CEA; results have been mixed and it is clear that significant improvements need to be made to this technique before it can be used with any consistency for intraoperative monitoring.

Intraoperative Ultrasound

B-mode ultrasound began to be used by neurosurgeons soon after it became available in the early 1980s. It quickly proved its value for localizing lesions, delineating normal and pathological anatomy, guiding instrumentation, and identifying residual tumor following resection. It can be particularly useful for localizing intramedullary spinal cord pathology. More recently, stereotactic intraoperative ultrasound has been employed as an adjunct during surgical procedures using image guidance. As intraoperative "shift" can instill significant error into these systems, real-time ultrasound imaging can be compared with the pre-operative scans used for image guidance, and appropriate corrections can be made.

Transcranial Doppler (TCD) ultrasound has been used for the intraoperative assessment of flow velocities and detection of embolic events during CEA by insonation of the terminal ICA, MCA or ACA through a temporal window. A large study ($n = 1058$) of patients undergoing CEA with intraoperative TCD monitoring concluded that microemboli detected during dissection/wound closure, decreases of MCA velocities equal to or greater than 90%, and increases of pulsatility index of 100% or more were significantly associated with post-operative stroke [23].

Microvascular Doppler has several intraoperative uses, including evaluation of flow in the carotid artery following CEA, documentation of graft patency in cases of EC–IC bypass, and assessment of flow in an aneurysm and adjacent vessels before and after clip application.

Intraoperative Angiography

Intraoperative angiography is used during a wide range of neurovascular procedures including aneurysm clipping, AVM resection, and EC–IC bypass. The imaging procedure itself is identical to non-operative angiography; however, patient positioning and preparation and the use of radiolucent stabilizing equipment are crucial for the successful use of this technique in the operating room. The potential complications are similar to those seen during non-operative cerebral angiography, namely groin hematoma, femoral artery thrombosis, stroke and vasospasm.

The utility of intraoperative angiography has been documented by several studies. In a series of 115 patients undergoing various neurovascular procedures with angiography, the operative procedure was altered in 19 of these cases owing to concerns raised by the intraoperative angiogram, while only 2 of the 115 patients had a post-operative complication that could potentially have been related to angiography [24].

Peripheral Nerve Monitoring

Peripheral nerve monitoring relies primarily on EMG recordings, nerve conduction velocity (NCV), nerve action potentials (NAPs) and SSEPs, all of which are performed in the same fashion as during routine non-operative evaluation of nerve function. These techniques can be used to assess the pre-operative function of the nerve, as related to pathological changes, in addition to allowing for the monitoring of functional status of the nerve during surgical manipulation. Sources of insult to the nerve, capable of instigating changes detectable with these techniques, include compression, laceration, stretching or ischemia.

EMG recordings are particularly helpful in establishing the location, severity and extent of a peripheral nerve problem. The recording electrode is placed into the belly of the muscle innervated by the peripheral nerve that is pathologically involved or placed at risk by surgical manipulation. During the procedure, nerve integrity can be monitored by proximal application of an electrical stimulus with assessment of the resulting muscle activity through EMG recordings. This technique can also be used to demonstrate the identity of a nerve by the pattern of muscle responses seen after stimulation.

NCVs can be used to specifically localize a region of pathological change in a peripheral nerve. Measurement of NCVs requires the placement of stimulating and recording electrodes along the length of the nerve of interest. Relevant pathology can be localized by measuring the conduction time (and therefore velocity) and amplitude of an action potential passing through a particular segment of the nerve. A decrease in velocity suggests a problem with myelination (seen in entrapment syndromes) whilst a diminished amplitude is indicative of axonal loss. Sensory and motor fibers cannot be delineated by this method. Direct stimulation of a lesion may be extremely helpful in differentiating between pathological nervous tissue (e.g. neuroma) and normal nervous tissue and for guiding the appropriate limits of surgical resection.

Typically, bipolar stimulation is used for optimal focusing of the stimulus current. Hooked electrodes can be used, which allow for the nerve to be lifted free of surrounding tissue in a gentle fashion, thereby minimizing stimulus artifact due to volume conduction. Adequate stimulation can be accomplished using a setting of 50 V (constant current) or 10 mA (constant voltage) for a duration of 0.05 ms. Greater current may be necessary in cases where the nerve is fibrotic or has decreased myelination. In general, the recording electrode must be placed at a minimum of 5 cm from the stimulation electrode; if the distance is smaller, any relevant NAP may be obscured by shock artifact. NAPs will not be affected by general anesthetics or neuromuscular blockade. However, local ischemia, as caused by application of a tourniquet, may result in obliteration of the NAP. Circulation should be restored for a minimum of 20 minutes before reliable NAPs can be recorded.

In a review of 25 years of experience, including more than 2,000 patients, Kline and Happel found that recording intraoperative NAPs was essential to surgical decision making and successful outcome. When a NAP could be successfully recorded across a lesion in continuity, 93% of patients had good recovery of function following neurolysis. If the NAP failed to cross the region of pathology, the dysfunctional tissue could be resected and repaired with satisfactory results in nearly two-thirds of cases [25].

Conclusions

To assure the greatest possible success of any of the aforementioned intraoperative monitoring techniques, a number of factors need to be considered on a case-by-case basis. Cooperation and communication between the surgeon, anesthesiologist and physiologist or technician responsible for collection and interpretation of the monitoring data are paramount for accurate intraoperative information. The operative team must be dedicated to the proper set-up and use of the monitoring equipment, although the preparation may take a few extra moments, in order to maximize data acquisition and avoid the unlikely possibility of harm related to the monitoring process itself. Similarly, the monitoring team should maintain an unobtrusive presence in the operating room and provide no unnecessary distraction or delay to the procedure. Appropriate selection of a particular technique for a given case is crucial and the surgeon must be willing to change his operative technique if the appropriate warning signs become apparent. Finally, it is important to note that no form of intraoperative monitoring guarantees a good post-operative result, even in the absence of the relevant warning signs.

Key Points

- *Various techniques for intraoperative neurophysiological monitoring are available to neurosurgeons for use during procedures that involve both the central and peripheral nervous system.*
- *Some of these techniques have a proven utility and play an integral role during a number of neurosurgical cases. Other techniques are used as a matter of personal preference or remain in the experimental realm.*
- *Several of these methods, particularly EEG and SSEP monitoring, are effective at demonstrating neurophysiological changes attributable to ischemia, and therefore are of use in procedures that place the CBF at risk.*
- *Techniques such as SSEP, MEP, BAEP, EMG and NCV recording allow for monitoring of afferent or efferent activity through regions of the nervous system placed at risk by neurosurgical manipulation.*
- *Monitoring/mapping of cortical functions can be performed using techniques such as phase reversal, microelectrode recording or cortical stimulation (either electrical or magnetic).*

References

1. Zampella E, Morawetz RB, McDowell HA, Zeiger HE, Varner PD, McKay RD et al. The importance of cerebral ischemia during carotid endarterectomy. Neurosurgery 1991;29:727–30.
2. Salvian AJ, Taylor DC, Hsiang YN et al. Selective shunting with EEG monitoring is safer than routine shunting for carotid endarterectomy. Cardiovasc Surg 1997;5: 481–5.
3. Redekop G, Ferguson G. Correlation of contralateral stenosis and intraoperative electroencephalogram change with risk of stroke during carotid endarterectomy. Neurosurgery 1992;30:191–4.
4. Plestis KA, Loubser P, Mizrahi EM, Kantis G, Jiang ZD, Howell JF. Continuous electroencephalographic monitoring and selective shunting reduces neurologic morbidity rates in carotid endarterectomy. J Vasc Surg 1997; 25:620–8.
5. Schwartz TH, Bazil CW, Forgione M, Bruce JN, Goodman RR. Do reactive post-resection "injury" spikes exist? Epilepsia 2000;41:1463–8.
6. Fisher RS, Raudzens P, Nunemacher M. Efficacy of intraoperative neurophysiological monitoring. J Clin Neurophysiol 1995;12:97–109.
7. Haupt WF, Horsch S. Evoked potential monitoring in carotid surgery: a review of 994 cases. Neurology 1992; 42:835–8.
8. Guerit JM. Neuromonitoring in the operating room: why, when, and how to monitor? Electroencephalogr Clin Neurophysiol 1998;106:1–21.
9. Fava E, Bortolani E, Ducati A, Schieppati M. Role of SEP in identifying patients requiring temporary shunt during carotid endarterectomy. Electroencephalogr Clin Neurophysiol 1992;84:426–32.
10. Nuwer MR, Dawson EG, Carlson LG, Kanim LE, Sherman JE. Somatosensory evoked potential spinal cord monitoring reduces neurologic deficits after scoliosis surgery: results of a large multicenter survey. Electroencephalogr Clin Neurophysiol 1995;96:6–11.
11. Milhorat TH, Kotzen RM, Capocelli AL Jr, Bolognese P, Bendo AA, Cottrell JE. Intraoperative improvement of somatosensory evoked potentials and local spinal cord blood flow in patients with syringomyelia. J Neurosurg Anesthesiol 1996;8:208–15.
12. May DM, Jones SJ, Crockard HA. Somatosensory evoked potential monitoring in cervical surgery: identification of pre- and intraoperative risk factors associated with neurological deterioration. J Neurosurg 1996; 85:566–73.
13. Dawson EG, Sherman JE, Kanim LE, Nuwer MR. Spinal cord monitoring. Results of the Scoliosis Research Society and the European Spinal Deformity Society survey. Spine 1991;16:S361–4.
14. Wilson-Holden TJ, Padberg AM, Parkinson JD, Bridwell KH, Lenke LG, Bassett GS. A prospective comparison of neurogenic mixed evoked potential stimulation methods: utility of epidural elicitation during posterior spinal surgery. Spine 2000;25:2364–71.
15. Pereon Y, Bernard JM, Fayet G, Delecrin J, Passuti N, Guiheneuc P. Usefulness of neurogenic motor evoked potentials for spinal cord monitoring: findings in 112 consecutive patients undergoing surgery for spinal deformity. Electroencephalogr Clin Neurophysiol 1998; 108:17–23.
16. Kothbauer K, Schmid UD, Seiler RW, Eisner W. Intraoperative motor and sensory monitoring of the cauda equina. Neurosurgery 1994;34:702–7.
17. Kothbauer K, Deletis V, Epstein FJ. Intraoperative spinal cord monitoring for intramedullary surgery: an essential adjunct. Pediatr Neurosurg 1997;26:247–54.
18. Nagle KJ, Emerson RG, Adams DC et al. Intraoperative monitoring of motor evoked potentials: a review of 116 cases. Neurology 1996;47:999–1004.
19. Hariz MI, Fodstad H. Do microelectrode techniques increase accuracy or decrease risks in pallidotomy and deep brain stimulation? A critical review of the literature. Stereotact Funct Neurosurg 1999;72:157–69.
20. Fischer G, Fischer C, Remond J. Hearing preservation in acoustic neurinoma surgery. J Neurosurg 1992;76: 910–17.
21. Fahlbusch R, Neu M, Strauss C. Preservation of hearing in large acoustic neurinomas following removal via suboccipito-lateral approach. Acta Neurochir (Wien) 1998; 140:771–7.
22. Sundt TM. The ischemic tolerance of neural tissue and the need for monitoring and selective shunting during carotid endarterectomy. Stroke 1983;14:93–8.
23. Ackerstaff RG, Moons KG, van de Vlasakker CJ et al. Association of intraoperative transcranial doppler monitoring variables with stroke from carotid endarterectomy. Stroke 2000;31:1817–23.

24. Barrow DL, Boyer KL, Joseph GJ. Intraoperative angiography in the management of neurovascular disorders. Neurosurgery 1992;30:153–9.

25. Kline DG, Happel LT. A quarter century's experience with intraoperative nerve action potential recording. Can J Neurol Sci 1993;20:3–10.

2

Neuroradiology and Ultrasound

David G. Hughes

With a contribution on Ultrasound by

Roger Chisholm

Summary

Neuroradiology utilises a wide range of imaging modalities in the diagnosis and treatment of CNS pathologies. MRI is the investigation of choice for most neuroradiological imaging. CT remains the foremost modality in the emergency situation, and is superior to MRI in the visualisation of calcification, bone detail and acute hemorrhage. Angiography should be considered for all patients without a clear cause of hemorrhage and who are surgical candidates. Digital subtraction angiography is currently the gold standard in the investigation of subarachnoid hemorrhage, but in the future MRA and CTA will replace it. Technological advances are moving towards less invasive imaging modalities, supported by functional and physiological data. Ultrasound is the primary investigation in a neonate with an enlarging head and will reliably diagnose ventriculomegaly. It is accurate in the assessment of internal carotid artery stenosis for potential carotid endarterectomy patients.

Introduction

Neuroradiology has evolved as a subspecialty of radiology by the application of different radiological techniques to the investigation of clinical problems related to the central nervous system (CNS) and spine. Initially limited to radiographs, a number of techniques became available that required skill in performance and interpretation, demanding the establishment of "neuroradiology". We now have a core of imaging modalities that allow ever more accurate diagnosis, and increasingly treatment, of CNS pathologies. These modalities include radiographs, computed tomography (CT), magnetic resonance imaging (MRI), angiography, ultrasound, nuclear medicine, myelography and interventional neuroradiology. These present a complex permutation of possible investigation of given clinical conditions that may be further influenced by local availability and expertise.

This chapter will review these imaging modalities and discuss the basic principles, indications, weaknesses and complications illustrated by clinical examples. A comprehensive imaging review of neurological disease is not possible in the length of this chapter and the reader is referred to recent neuroradiological textbooks for further reading [1, 2].

Radiographs

Radiographs, once the only investigation available, are nearly redundant in modern neuroradiology. The use of skull radiographs has been greatly reduced even in trauma, and are now used in the UK as part of a triage exercise in minor head injury cases to decide on the safe discharge of a patient.

A person who has sustained a mild head injury, has no skull fracture, is Glasgow Coma Scale 15 and has adequate support at home can be discharged with a head injury advice chart. Even in this situation there is a case for CT scanning, the limiting factors being radiation dosage (ten times that of skull radiographs) and extensive workload to the CT scanner. There may be a role for skull radiographs in mild trauma to exclude a depressed skull fracture that is suspected from the mechanism of injury. The skull radiograph is still requested in myeloma and renal bone disease "screens".

Radiographs of the spine can be more helpful. They still form the basis of trauma cervical spine imaging "clearing the spine", although there are advocates of CT in this role if the patient is already undergoing CT of another part of the body.

A vast number of radiographs are still used in the assessment of neck and back pain. The yield of significant abnormalities is generally very low; in low back pain it is more productive if the use of radiographs is limited to the young patient (under 20 years) for the detection of spondylolisthesis (Fig. 2.1) and to older patients (over 55 years) where metastasis is more likely. Degenerative disease seen on a radiograph correlates poorly with clinical signs and symptoms. Where surgical management of degenerative disease is considered, then there is a case for MRI only [3].

Computed Tomography

The first patient to be scanned using CT was at Atkinson Morley's Hospital in London in 1972. The technology invented by Sir Godfrey Hounsfield [4] (an engineer at the Central Research Laboratories, EMI, England) was the single most important development in neuroradiology.

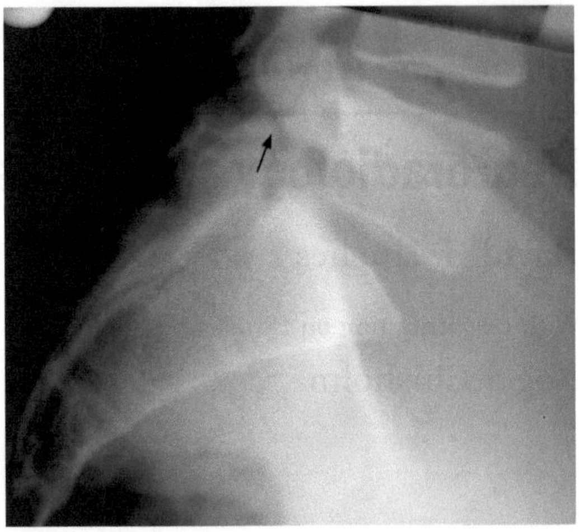

Fig. 2.1. Lateral radiograph of the lumbosacral junction. Defect in the pars interarticularis of L5 is clearly shown (arrow).

There have been great improvements since the early machines, with excellent resolution and very fast scanning times, making it possible to scan a head in a few seconds. Although MRI is superior in the investigation of most neurological and spinal diseases, CT scanners are both readily available in virtually all hospitals and very cost effective, so they are widely used as the workhorse of neuroimaging. CT remains the foremost imaging modality in the emergency situation. This applies particularly to trauma, where intracranial hematoma can be rapidly assessed in the unstable patient and where, in the case of polytrauma, other areas such as the cervical spine or abdomen can be scanned. CT is superior to MRI in the visualization of calcification, bone detail and acute hemorrhage.

The CT appearances of hematoma are well recognized in the acute phase, being of higher attenuation than the adjacent brain. In hyperacute hematoma, areas of low density may be seen consistent with active bleeding before a clot has formed. The appearance of the hematoma changes to become the same density as brain and eventually lower (Table 2.1). This typical evolution of hematoma can be altered by clotting disorder, anticoagulation, low haemocrit and anemia, when the acute hematoma can be isodense with brain in 50% of cases [5].

The presence of fluid–fluid levels within an extra-axial hematoma often represents acute hemorrhage with a chronic bleed. Fluid levels within a parenchymal hematoma are not only

Table 2.1. CT appearances of hematoma (relative to brain)

Phase	Time	Attenuation
Hyperacute	Minutes to hours	Hyperdense with hypodense areas
Acute	Hours to 1 week	Hyperdense
Subacute	1–6 weeks	Isodense
Chronic	>6 weeks	Hypodense

seen in hemorrhagic tumors but also in any of the many causes of cerebral hemorrhage.

Low-density extra-axial collections are not necessarily hematomas. Empyemas are low density with mass effect and, when subdural, may expand the interhemispheric fissure (Fig. 2.2). Often the patient is more clinically unwell than would be suggested by the size of the collection. Intravenous contrast typically causes enhancement of a surrounding membrane, which may aid diagnosis. Contrast medium is used routinely in CT scanning, particularly if there is a possibility of infection, tumor or vascular lesion. Unnecessary use should be avoided, e.g. in acute trauma or hydrocephalus, as there is a risk of serious reaction in 1 in 2,500 injections [6].

When subarachnoid hemorrhage (SAH) mixes with CSF, the attenuation of the hematoma is reduced, becoming the same as brain. Therefore smaller SAHs will be subtle with apparent effacement of sulci and cisterns – an appearance that should not be mistaken for brain swelling. CT will detect 95% of SAHs within 24 hours of the ictus. A reliable indirect sign is the presence of mild hydrocephalus. After 1 week, CT is much less reliable as the density of the hematoma is significantly reduced.

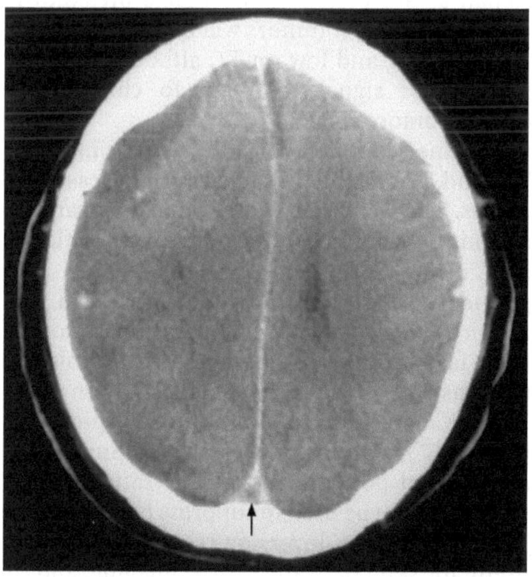

Fig. 2.2. CT scan post i.v. contrast. Low-density subdural collection with mass effect. Note fluid in the interhemispheric fissure, which suggests a subdural empyema. This is complicated by a sagittal sinus thrombosis (arrow points to the delta sign).

Current CT scanners use multislice techniques of acquisition, allowing greater coverage in shorter times. This reduces any movement artifact and facilitates CT angiography as a significant length of vessel can be scanned while the bolus of contrast medium passes through. Reformation of the scans can be performed in several ways, such as multi-planar reconstructions, maximum intensity projections, volume-rendered images or even "fly through" endoluminal views. CT angiography (CTA) has been used to demonstrate carotid artery disease, intracranial vascular anatomy, including arteriovenous malformations (AVMs), and aneurysms [7] and is now frequently used as a first investigation of SAH. The three-dimensional images obtained can be used to decide between an endovascular or open neurosurgical operation on an aneurysm. It is useful in the emergency situation when a large hematoma has been demonstrated and when there is a suspicion of an underlying vascular lesion. CTA in this situation may demonstrate an underlying aneurysm, enabling the patient to proceed rapidly to evacuation of the clot and clipping of the aneurysm without the delay of organizing a formal angiogram.

CTA requires the administration of iodinated contrast media and also for the patient to lie very still during the scan time of approximately 30 seconds.

A large aneurysm may be apparent on the initial CT scan as blood within the aneurysm is less dense than the surrounding hematoma (Fig. 2.3).

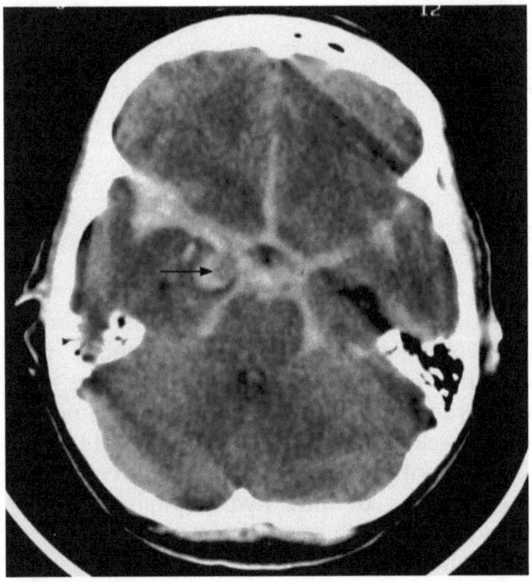

Fig. 2.3. CT scan demonstrating extensive subarachnoid hematoma with the lower density aneurysm lumen visible (arrow).

The ability of CT to detect subtle calcification and show excellent bone detail highlights its use as an adjunct to MRI. Detection of calcification within a tumor may aid the differential diagnosis. Subtle calcification may not be apparent on an MR scan but is obvious on a CT scan, which may lead to the diagnosis of tuberous sclerosis in the investigation of epilepsy. Skull base detail is very well shown on a CT scan and is complementary to MRI in fully defining complex lesions of this region. This ability to define bone detail is also very useful in spinal imaging, particularly in trauma, to define and classify fractures. Reconstruction of data into sagittal and coronal planes is easily achieved and adds essential information on alignment and extent of abnormality.

Magnetic Resonance Imaging

The principles of nuclear magnetic resonance were first described in the 1930s by C.J. Gorter and used extensively as spectroscopy to study physical and chemical properties of matter. It was not until the late 1970s that images of human anatomy were produced and the technique became known as "magnetic resonance imaging". Extensive development has enabled MRI to become the investigation of choice for most neuroradiological imaging.

The quantum mechanics and mathematics that attempt to explain MRI are beyond this author and are not required for image interpretation. An understanding of the simplified principles and the various sequences produced is necessary [2, 8].

From a practical view of image interpretation, we need to know what is white, black or gray on a particular MR sequence. These are summarized in Table 2.2. Fat, very proteinaceous tissues, certain degradation products of hemorrhage, and gadolinium influence free protons to produce high signal on T1 weighting. Gray and white matter will be intermediate signal, but white will be slightly higher signal because of its increased fat content. Brain edema and most pathologies will be intermediate signal, i.e. grey, and CSF will be black.

On T2 weighting, CSF is high signal and gray matter is higher signal than white matter. Air and cortical bone are very low signal owing to the small amount of free protons in these. Arterial blood flow and certain venous flow will present no signal (flow void) on standard spin-echo sequences. Most pathologies will be high signal, as are certain hemorrhagic breakdown products. So most tumors will be high signal on T2 weighting and low on T1, although atypical patterns of signal can help to characterize certain tumors (Fig. 2.4).

Routine scanning with MRI usually involves T1- and T2-weighted sequences in at least two planes. The weighting can be gained by various scanning techniques, including conventional spin echo (CSE), fast spin echo (FSE) and gradient echo (GE). Acquisitions can be acquired in two- or three-dimensional modes. Very fast scanning is possible with techniques such as echo-planar imaging (EPI) or half-Fourier acquisition single-shot turbo spin-echo ("HASTE"), although they may be limited by artifact and poor signal-to-noise ratio. Special sequences can be used to suppress fat, such as in "STIR" (short tau inversion recovery), which is useful for skull base and orbital imaging, and to suppress CSF, as in "FLAIR" (fluid-attenuated inversion recovery), which increases the conspicuity of lesions at brain–CSF interfaces. More recently, specialized applications of MR scan-

Table 2.2. Signal intensity on MRI

Substance	On T1 weighting	On T2 weighting
Water	Black	White
Fat	White	Gray/white
White matter	Gray	Gray/black
Gray matter	Gray/black	Gray/white
Bone		
Cortex	Black	Black
Marrow	White	Gray/white
Calcification	Gray/white	Black
Intervertebral disk	Gray	White
Air	Black	Black
Hematoma	See Table 2.3	
Most pathology	Gray/black	White

Signal intensity (SI) dictates appearance on a gray scale. High signal is white; low signal is black. Substance is often compared to the SI of gray matter.

ning include: functional (f)MRI [9], MR spectroscopy (MRS) [10], MR-guided therapy (MRT) [11], and perfusion and diffusion MRI [12].

Use of Contrast Media

Gadolinium, a rare earth metal, is used frequently in MRI. The paramagnetic properties of gadolinium affect free protons and hence shorten T1-weighted signal. It is not the gadolinium that is being visualized but its effect on free protons. Where there are increased concentrations of gadolinium, this will result in high signal, i.e. enhancement, on T1 weighting. It highlights areas of blood–brain barrier breakdown, areas of inflammation and increased vascularity. Marked enhancement is visible normally in the pituitary, the choroid plexus, the nasal mucosa and turbinates, and in slow-flowing blood in vessels. Contrast enhancement is used frequently to improve detection and definition of tumors, infection, meningeal disease, vascular disease and the "post-operative spine". Gadolinium is an extremely safe substance and has been used in millions of cases worldwide with side-effects that are less common and less severe than with the iodinated contrast media used in CT.

MRI of Intracranial Hemorrhage

The appearances of hemorrhage on MRI demonstrate the possible permutations of signal

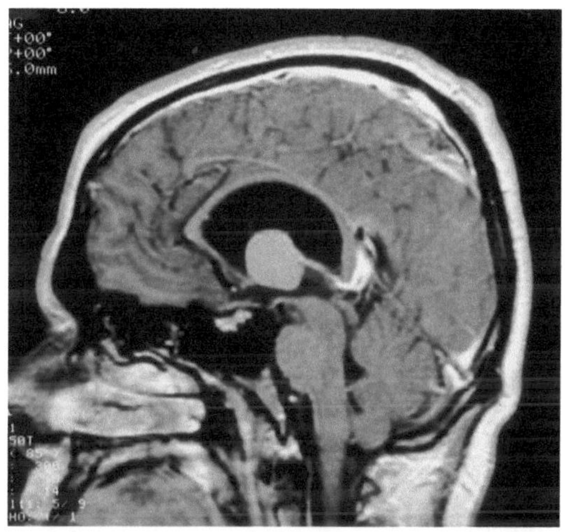

a

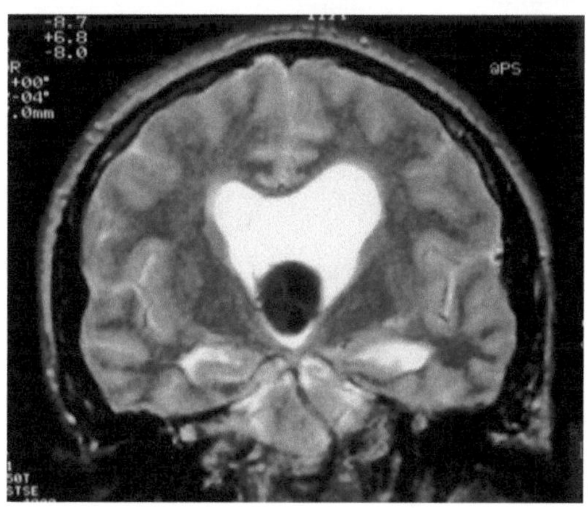

b

Fig. 2.4 a–b MRI scan for severe intermittent headaches. **a** Sagittal T1 with a high-signal mass in the region of the foramen of Monro. **b** Coronal FSE T2, with a low-signal mass. The position and signal changes are characteristic of a colloid cyst.

pattern, making its more detailed explanation worthwhile as a model for understanding the principles of MR signal characteristics (Table 2.3). These are affected by many factors both intrinsic to the hemorrhage and related to MR scanning. Operator-dependent factors include strength of magnet, pulse sequence (e.g. SE, GE, EPI, etc.) and parameters set, such as the repetition time (TR) and the echo time (TE). Intrinsic factors are multifactorial but the hemoglobin oxidation state and red cell morphology are the most important.

Parenchymal Hematomas

Hyperacute Stage

Within minutes of the hemorrhage, intact red cells will contain oxyhemogloblin and there will be protein-rich serum and platelets. The appearances are non-specific and virtually indistinguishable from any brain lesion that causes increased water content of the brain, i.e. white on T2 and gray/black on T1.

Acute Stage

Within the first few hours, deoxyhemoglobin is formed, which is paramagnetic. This particularly affects the T2 relaxation, resulting in marked reduction in signal (black) on T2 weighting, but has little effect on T1. The low signal is accentuated on GE sequences because of the susceptibility effect.

Subacute Stage

After several days, methemoglobin forms, which is initially intracellular and gives rise to high signal on T1 weighting but remains low on T2. As the cells hemolyze, extracellular methemoglobin accumulates in the hematoma, which is very high signal on both T1- and T2-weighted images. Throughout these stages there will be an admixture of products present. In large hematomas, the center will be hypoxic, delaying hemoglobin desaturation. High signal occurs from the outside of the hematoma and progresses inwards with time (Fig. 2.5a, b).

Chronic Stage

Edema and mass effect will disappear and the end-stage products of ferritin and hemosiderin form, which are very low on T2 weighting, particularly GE T2. Macrophages laden with these iron storage products will remain for years in the wall of the old hematoma.

Extra-axial Hemorrhage

Acute subarachnoid hemorrhage can be impossible to differentiate from normal CSF on MRI, and CT remains the imaging modality of choice, particularly if the hematoma is only small and not focal. Sensitivity of MRI can be improved by use of FLAIR sequence, particularly if the diagnosis has been delayed, when the CT scan is more likely to be negative. An MR angiogram can be performed whilst the patient is in the scanner.

Extradural and subdural hematomas are very well demonstrated on MRI. Small collections over the surface of the brain and tentorium will be better demonstrated in the coronal plane. The evolving hematoma signal patterns are similar to those of parenchymal hematomas except in the chronic stages, as hemosiderin is not stored. The collection becomes similar to CSF on routine T1 and T2 weighting but remains high signal on proton-density and

Table 2.3. Evolution of hematoma

Phase	Time	Hb Product	T1 weighted	T2 weighted
Hyperacute	0–12 h	Oxy Hb	Gray	White
Acute	2–36 h	Deoxy Hb	Gray	Black
Early subacute	2–7 days	Intracellular met Hb	White	Black
Late subacute	3–14 days	Extracellular met Hb	White	White
Chronic	Weeks to years	Hemosiderin Ferritin	Gray	Very black

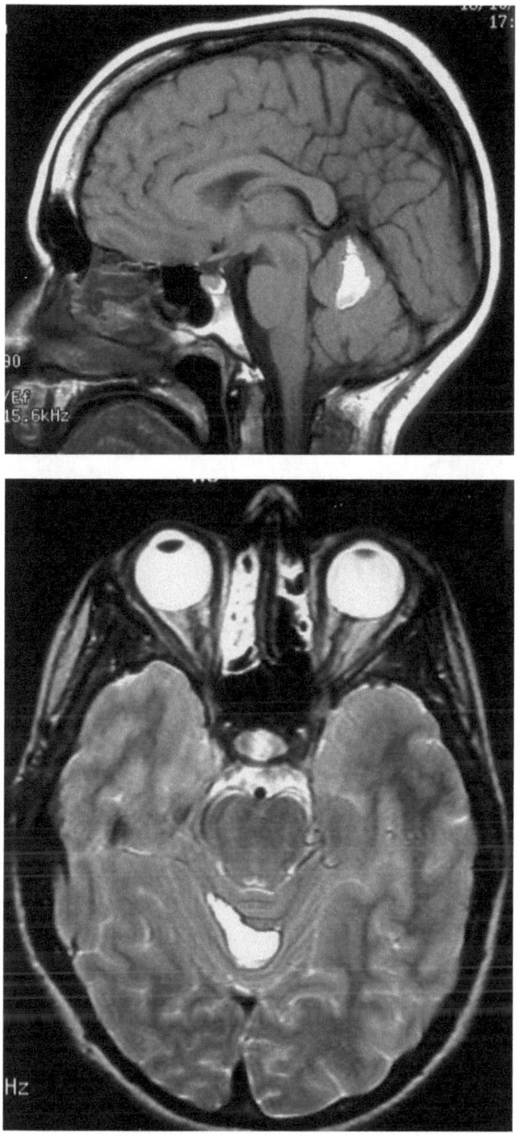

Fig. 2.5. a–b Severe headaches 2 weeks previously, with cerebellar signs. Subacute hematoma is shown with high signal on the T1- and T2-weighted images. **a** Sagittal T1. **b** Transverse T2.

FLAIR sequence (Fig. 2.6). Re-bleeding into an old collection produces characteristic appearances, with loculated areas of different signal and fluid–fluid levels.

The ability of MRI to stage different ages of subdural hematoma has an important role in the diagnosis of child abuse [13].

One recurring question concerning intracranial, and particularly parenchymal, hematomas is: "What is the underlying cause?". Parenchymal hematomas occurring anywhere near the major intracranial arteries can be due to aneurysmal bleed. This is particularly seen with middle cerebral artery aneurysms, which can bleed into the adjacent temporal lobe, producing large hematomas and often surprisingly little SAH. Angiography should be considered for all patients without a clear cause of hemorrhage and who are surgical candidates, particularly young, normotensive patients [14]. Older, hypertensive patients with a hemorrhage in the basal ganglia, thalamus, cerebellum or brainstem do not need to undergo angiography [15]. In a young adult who has negative investigations, drug abuse should then be suspected [5].

MRI is particularly helpful in the diagnosis of hemorrhagic tumor. Although there are no absolute criteria, features such as enhancement with gadolinium, marked heterogeneity of signal, and extent of edema are characteristic of tumor. Multiplicity of lesions is not always helpful as cavernous hemangiomas are multiple in 30% of cases (Fig. 2.7). Delayed scanning will be definitive with persisting edema, delayed and very heterogeneous evolution of the hemoglobin breakdown products being diagnostic of tumor. Hemorrhage tends to occur in the more aggressive tumors, such as glioblastoma multiforme, primitive neuroectodermal tumors, ependymomas, oligodendrogliomas and vascular metastases (most commonly from lung or renal primary tumors or malignant melanoma). An exception to these is pituitary adenomas, with hemorrhage occurring in up to 27% of cases, and many of these will have no clinical features of pituitary apoplexy [16].

Safety Issues of MRI

There are several potential problems with MRI and patient safety, namely the high magnetic field, the radio frequency pulses, the gradient coils and the size of the magnetic bore. Many studies have been performed to investigate the biological effects of MRI, but no biological risk has been found with MR scanners in clinical use. Even so, routine MRI is not performed during the first trimester of pregnancy, but if clinical urgency dictates, it would be used in preference to imaging modalities that use ionizing radiation. Acoustic noise produced by the gradient coils can be a problem, particularly with certain

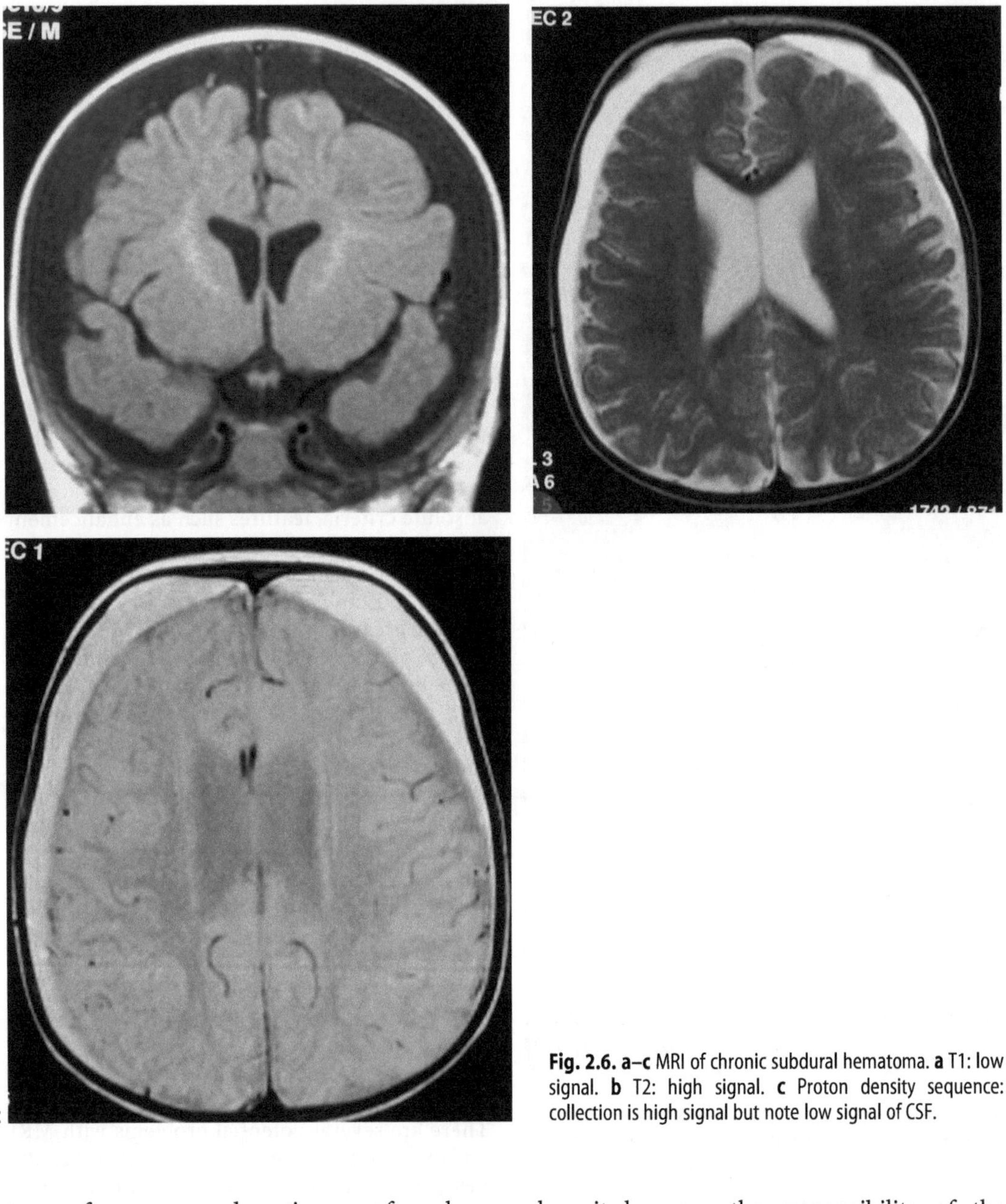

Fig. 2.6. a–c MRI of chronic subdural hematoma. **a** T1: low signal. **b** T2: high signal. **c** Proton density sequence: collection is high signal but note low signal of CSF.

types of sequence, and routine use of earplugs is advisable.

Of most concern regarding patient safety is the presence of metallic implants, materials and foreign bodies. Listed in Table 2.4 are some of the more common contraindications to MRI.

All patients should complete a questionnaire to exclude these contraindications before entering the MR scan room. This may not be possible with the confused and unconscious patient, when it becomes the responsibility of the attending doctor.

The final problem is the size of the magnet bore, which results in significant claustrophobia and anxiety in 5% of patients. Some patients will require sedation, but once inside the scanner, direct observation is not possible and MRI-compatible monitoring equipment is required. Ferro-magnetic objects of certain types should not be brought into the MRI

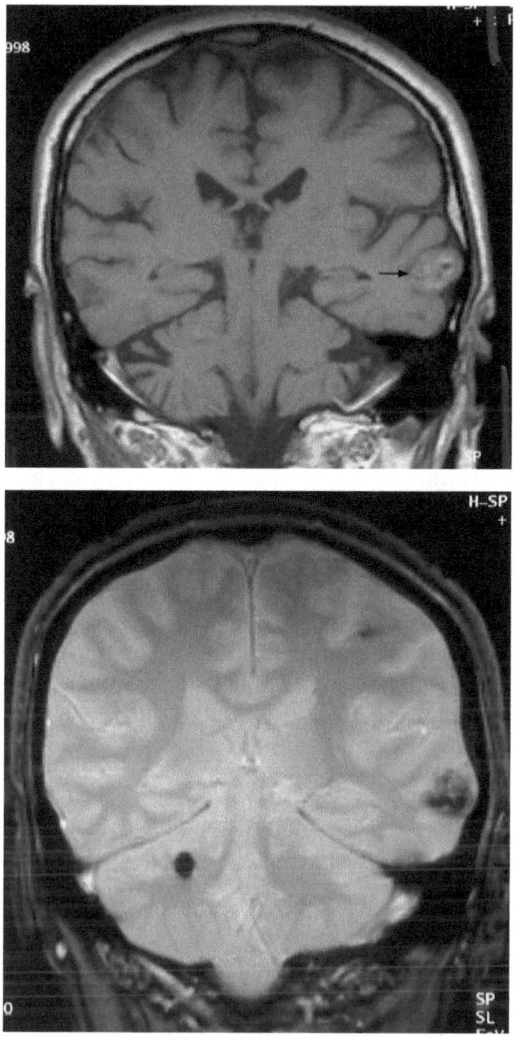

a b

Fig. 2.7. a–b Multiple cavernous hemangiomas. **a** Coronal T1 – subtle lesion in the temporal lobe (arrow). **b** Gradient echo T2. This sequence accentuates the low signal produced by calcium and hemosiderin, demonstrating multiple lesions.

room as they can be rapidly projected into the scanner with the possibility of injury to any adjacent personnel.

A comprehensive list of metallic implants, devices and materials tested for MR safety is listed in Shellock and Kanal's book [17] and up-to-date information is available on the Internet at www. radiology.upmc.edu/mrsafety.

Magnetic Resonance Angiography

Magnetic resonance angiography (MRA) is performed using special sequences based on GE techniques. These sequences produce signal in flowing blood that can be distinguished from adjacent stationary tissue. The basic concepts involve either time of flight (TOF) or phase contrast (PC) techniques. With the TOF technique, stationary tissue is saturated with multiple radio-frequency pulses. The free protons within blood are unsaturated so can be excited and give back signal, i.e. appear white on the scan against a black background. PC techniques rely on change in phase of the transverse spin magnetization that occurs in moving protons (i.e. within moving blood) within the magnetic field.

The TOF technique is more generally used as it produces better spatial resolution and is more easily obtained than the PC technique, which is reserved for special applications such as assessment of velocities of flow and CSF flow studies. The PC technique is also helpful if there is a large amount of hematoma present as high signal from hematoma can interfere with the TOF images and obscure subtle pathology.

Once the acquisition has been performed, the "raw data" are processed by maximum intensity projection techniques, which pick out the high signal in the section (i.e. the flowing blood) and reconstruct it into an image that is similar to

Table 2.4. Some contraindications to MRI (see reference 17 for complete list)

Cardiac pacemakers
Neurostimulators
Intracranial aneurysm clip
Artificial heart valves, e.g. Starr–Edwards valve
Cochlear implants
Shrapnel – if close to vascular structure
Metallic fragments in the globe of the eye

conventional angiography. Reconstruction in multiple planes can be produced and viewed through 360°. Other reconstruction techniques, such as multiple projection reconstruction and volume-rendered or endoluminal views, may be helpful in assessing complex vascular anatomy.

The use of gadolinium enhancement can reduce scanning time and is particularly useful where small vessels are being studied, e.g. spinal MRA. The patient does need to be cooperative and still for up to 10 minutes. This, and the noisy environment, mean that it is not ideal in the investigation of SAH, when CTA is quicker. Arterial digital subtraction angiography (DSA) remains the gold standard for angiography.

MRA is most useful in the detection and evaluation of aneurysms that have no history of SAH or where there has been a significant delay in the diagnosis. Standard MR sequences are also performed at the time of the examination as aneurysms may be seen as low signal. Aneurysms as small as 2 mm can be shown but an accuracy of at least 80% is seen for aneurysms of 5 mm and larger. Aneurysms that present with mass effect and cranial nerve palsy can be very accurately demonstrated (or excluded) by MRI with MRA. The non-invasive nature of MRA makes it very attractive as a screening test for aneurysms. This may be desirable in certain high-risk groups such as polycystic kidney disease or familial aneurysm disease. The implications of aneurysm screening for an incidental aneurysm have to be carefully discussed with the patient. Recent evidence suggests a much lower risk of hemorrhage (0.05%/year in small aneurysms) than have previous studies and also a higher morbidity/mortality (up to 14%) for surgical treatment [18].

Follow-up of aneurysm after endovascular treatment may be performed with MRA. MRA can be helpful in the evaluation of AVMs, particularly when combined with standard MRI. Exact anatomical location and size of the AVM can be obtained from conventional spin-echo techniques, which greatly help management decisions about the possible permutations of surgery, radiosurgery and endovascular treatment.

Vascular stenosis, particularly of the carotid bifurcation, can be assessed by MRA usually as a confirmatory test following ultrasound.

Catheter Angiography

Catheter angiography has been the investigation that is definitive of a neuroradiologist. Whilst it is an invasive technique with significant complications, cerebral angiography has become progressively safer owing to DSA, non-ionic contrast media and improved catheters and guide wires.

Technique

The right femoral artery is punctured using the Seldinger technique. The catheter can then be advanced up to the aortic arch and then selectively into the required artery. The catheters are usually 4F or 5F in size and pre-shaped to facilitate selective catheterization. Once in position in the desired artery, the formal DSA is undertaken with the contrast injection by hand or mechanical pump [19]. Multiple projections are used to demonstrate the vasculature and images are obtained as far as the venous phase in several planes. Commonly, the internal carotid circulation is studied in lateral, posteroanterior 20° and oblique projection, e.g. 30° cranio-caudal, 30° lateral (Fig. 2.8a, b, c). The posterior circulation is studied in lateral and Townes' projection (30° fronto-occipital). Numerous supplementary projections can be performed according to which vessel is to be demonstrated. This is particularly important in the demonstration of aneurysms where a clear demonstration of the neck of the aneurysm is required, especially if endovascular treatment is to be considered. When available, three-dimensional angiography simplifies and improves the definition of this anatomy. In the study of SAH, all vessels need to be studied as multiple aneurysms are reported in up to 45% of cases. Reflux down a contralateral vertebral artery will often demonstrate the posterior inferior cerebellar artery (PICA) so that formal four-vessel angiography is not always necessary.

Complications

Local complications occur in about 5% of cases and range from self-limiting hematoma to fatal retroperitoneal hematoma. Vessel injury can result in pseudo-aneurysm, arteriovenous fistula and distal emboli.

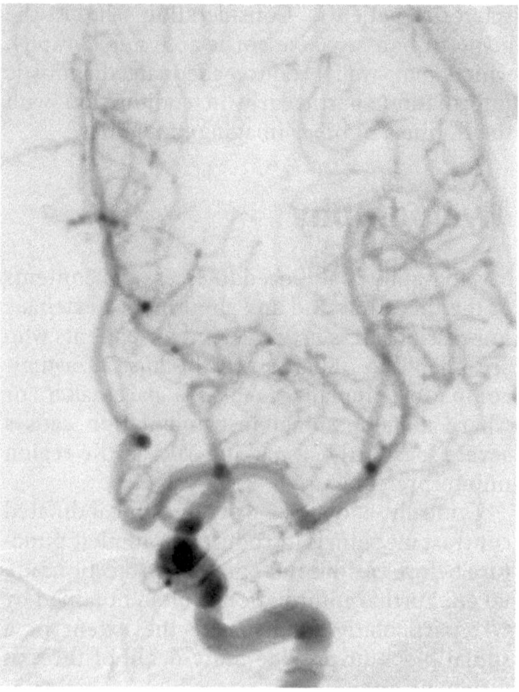
a

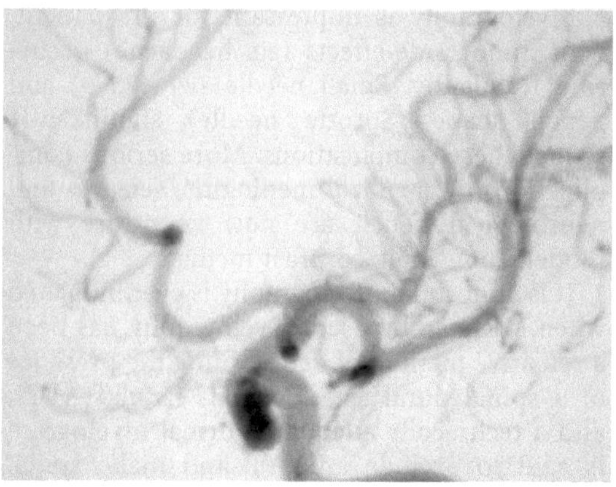
b

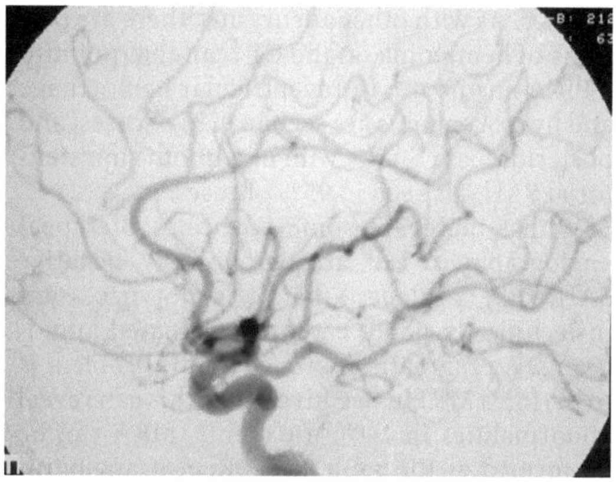
c

Fig. 2.8. **a–c** Internal carotid injection. **a** PA projection. **b** Oblique projection, 30° in both planes. **c** Lateral projection.

Systemic complications are related to the contrast media or, very occasionally, to local anesthetics and sedation. Contrast media reactions are common to all radiological procedures using iodinated contrast. The risk is increased by history of previous reaction and in asthma sufferers, where the risk of severe reaction is about 0.2%.

Neurological complications range from headache to disabling stroke or death. The risks are increased in the older population (over 50 years), particularly if there is atherosclerosis, vasculitis or sickle cell disease. The patient needs to have consented to the procedure in the knowledge of these risks and a reasonable level of risk to quote is 1% for transient neurological deficit, permanent deficit 0.5% and death 0.1% [20].

Current Indications

Cerebral DSA remains the investigation of choice in a number of conditions despite improvements in Doppler ultrasound, MRA and CTA. The most common reason for its use is in the investigation of SAH, where DSA remains the gold standard. Even with good-quality angiography, in up to 20% of patients with SAH, no abnormality will be found and repeat angiography may be required. The peri-mesencephalic pattern of SAH is well recognized [21] in angiographically negative patients. The clinical course of these patients appears to be different from that of aneurysmal SAH. Such patients often appear "too well" to have had a SAH and clinical outcome is typically excellent. Even so, this pattern of hematoma is seen with CT in 10% of posterior fossa aneurysms. The PICA aneurysm can be missed if both distal vertebral arteries are not satisfactorily demonstrated by reflux or selective catheterization of both vertebral arteries. As with other aneurysms, there are patterns of hematoma on the CT scan that point to a PICA aneurysm. Intraventricular hemorrhage and hydrocephalus are seen in 93% of cases, and posterior fossa SAH – with or without supratentorial SAH – is seen in 95% of cases.

Whilst there are some advocates of repeat angiography in all angiographically negative SAH, others suggest that it is not necessary in technically good, carefully evaluated angiograms. A pragmatic approach to this problem is to perform MRI in negative cases; this can reveal abnormalities in 14% of patients. MRA can be performed at the same time. Repeat angiography is reserved for cases where severe spasm, large focal hematoma or brain edema could have obscured the aneurysm or vascular malformation, particularly if the pattern of blood on the CT scan points to a particular site. In patients with repeated SAH and negative investigations, it is worth considering a spinal cause of the SAH as this has been reported with spinal tumors or vascular malformations.

If multiple aneurysms are detected, it is important to decide which has bled. There may be clues on the CT scan such as surrounding hematoma giving rise to a filling defect or localized SAH. The larger aneurysm, the irregular lobulated configuration, and localized spasm may point towards the aneurysm that has bled. If distinction is not possible, then multiple aneurysms will need protecting at the same operation.

Other indications for angiography include: assessment of aneurysms (e.g.fusiform, dissecting, mycotic, giant) that have not presented with SAH; assessment of AVMs and other vascular lesions, such as carotico-cavernous fistula or dural fistula; demonstration of tumor vascularity, particularly if pre-operative embolization is being considered; and investigation of various cerebrovascular disorders, such as vasculitis.

The final indication is to diagnose accurately the degree of stenosis of cervico-cranial atherosclerotic disease. Initial screening and investigation of this should be non-invasive with a combination of ultrasound, MRA and CTA, dependent on local expertise and availability. Angiography should be reserved for patients where the non-invasive investigations indicate stenosis on the borderline between surgical or conservative treatment, as complications of angiography are undoubtedly higher in atherosclerotic patients. Consideration should be given to non-selective aortic arch angiography, which may well produce adequate diagnostic information, particularly in conjunction with the findings of other imaging modalities.

Myelography

Myelography is still used to assess the contents of the thecal sac and any abnormal or extrinsic impressions. It is now reserved for patients who are unable to undergo MRI because of a non-compatible implant, such as a pacemaker, or where metallic spinal instrumentation causes severe local artifact, making MRI of the region uninterpretable.

Typically, a total of 3 g of non-ionic iodinated contrast medium is introduced by lumbar puncture before various radiographic projections are taken. Further information is often obtained by CT, particularly to delineate the extent of a spinal block or provide more detail of the exit foramen.

Myelography is unpleasant for the patient, with minor side-effects (eg. headache) occurring frequently. Small needle size (25 g) and pencil shape (Sprotte needle) significantly reduce these complications. More serious complications of chemical meningitis, seizures and neurological deficit are now very rare with modern non-ionic contrast media.

It is doubtful if myelography is ever indicated when MRI can be used. Myelography has been a sensitive method of determining the presence of a spinal dural arteriovenous fistula (AVF), and a technically adequate normal myelogram is said to exclude an AVF and make spinal angiography unnecessary. Advances in MRI, notably linear-array surface coils and the use of gadolinium, have replaced myelography in this condition. The prominent draining vein of the AVF is enhanced with contrast on T1-weighted images and is seen as low signal on spin-echo T2 weighting. It remains true that if myelography or MRI raises the suspicion of a spinal AVF, then formal spinal angiography becomes necessary. This is a complex and time-consuming procedure that requires selective catheterization of all prospective feeding vessels to the spinal cord and canal.

Nuclear Medicine

Nuclear medicine is used to look at function, physiology and metabolism, and the images are generally of a low spatial resolution. Radioactive elements such as technetium (Tc), which decay to produce gamma-rays, are used. They are labeled to pharmaceutical compounds (e.g. hexamethyl propylene amine oxime, HMPAO), enabling them to enter appropriate body compartments. The radiopharmaceutical can be introduced into the body and the gamma-rays (photons) can be externally recorded to produce an emission image. The recorded image can be a planar single-photon image or it can be produced using single-photon emission computed tomography (SPECT) or positron emission tomography (PET).

PET and SPECT are used to create cross-sectional functional images of the brain. SPECT, which is available in all nuclear medicine departments, can be used to study changes in regional blood flow in the brain. It has been used in the investigation of dementia, where changes in regional blood flow can differentiate between multi-infarction dementia and Alzheimer's disease. It is helpful when considering surgery for intractable complex partial seizure disorder, giving further weight to structural information concerning mesial temporal sclerosis seen on MRI.

PET radiopharmaceuticals are very short lived, requiring close proximity to a cyclotron. Installation and maintenance costs are very high, severely restricting their availability in many countries. PET can produce unique information concerning regional utilization of glucose metabolism as well as oxygen, or even fatty acid, metabolism or neurotransmitter receptor densities. It is mainly a research tool for neurophysiology and neuropharmacology. In a clinical context, it is used to help differentiate recurrent tumor from radiation necrosis and in assessing tumor response to therapy, but has a low accuracy. Applications in the study of psychiatric disease, movement disorders and epilepsy, to name but a few, are reported [22]. To some extent, the rapid developments in MRI have overtaken these applications of a very expensive technique.

Applications of conventional nuclear brain scans, such as diagnosis of cerebral infarction or subdural hematoma, are now historical. CSF rhinorrhea or otorrhea can be investigated with nuclear medicine but CT cisternography (Fig. 2.9), or even MR cisternography [23], are now advocated by many neuroradiologists.

Ultrasound

Ultrasound is a relatively cheap, portable and safe technology. Sound-wave reflection takes place at tissue interfaces within the body, and the depth of reflection is determined by the time taken for the echo to return to the crystal. Tissues with a very high acoustic impedance, such as bone, reflect almost all of the sound waves, producing an acoustic shadow and effectively no useful image in the distal field. This is clearly of paramount importance in neurosurgery when imaging the brain and spine.

Some of the most important applications of ultrasound within neurosurgery are described below.

Transcranial Ultrasound in the Neonate

The first real-time images of the neonatal brain were obtained through the anterior fontanelle of a newborn infant in 1979. The rate of subsequent development has been exponential, with high-quality machines and high-frequency small footprint transducers now able to produce extremely high resolution images of both the normal and abnormal neonatal brain. Doppler studies of the cerebral vasculature allow physiological monitoring of both the normal and abnormal brain with analysis of birth asphyxia, pre-term brain injury and hydrocephalus.

Vascular lesions are common in the brains of immature neonates – so frequently seen on special-care baby units. Subependymal germinal matrix hemorrhage can be reliably demonstrated, as can any subsequent intraventricular or parenchymal extension. The ischemic lesions of periventricular leukomalacia may also be recognized and are important in the differential diagnosis of brain injury. In the mature infant, extra- and intracerebral hemorrhage may result from both traumatic and other pathology and may again be diagnosed with ultrasound.

Ultrasound is the first investigation of choice in a neonate with an enlarging head and will reliably diagnose ventriculomegaly and, frequently,

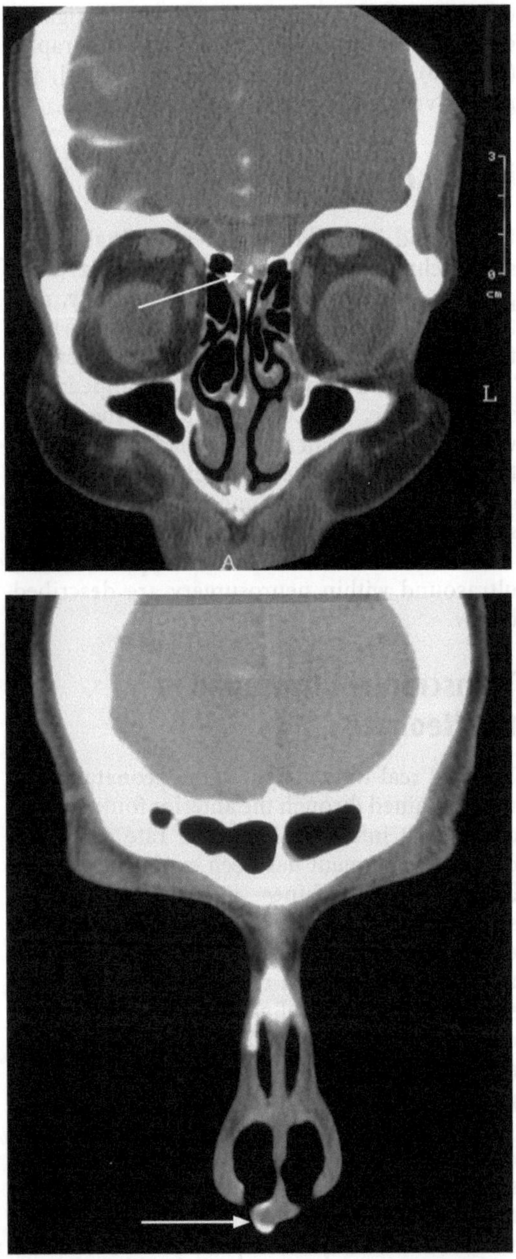

a

b

Fig. 2.9. a–b CSF rhinorrhea following head injury. CT scan post installation of contrast medium by lumbar puncture. **a** Direct coronal CT scan demonstrating defect in the anterior cranial fossa filling with contrast media (arrow). **b** Rhinorrhea with a droplet of radiopaque contrast medium (arrow).

its cause (Fig. 2.10). Differentiation must be made between raised intracranial pressure and cerebral atrophy. Ultrasound may guide neurosurgical shunting procedures, while also monitoring subsequent progress.

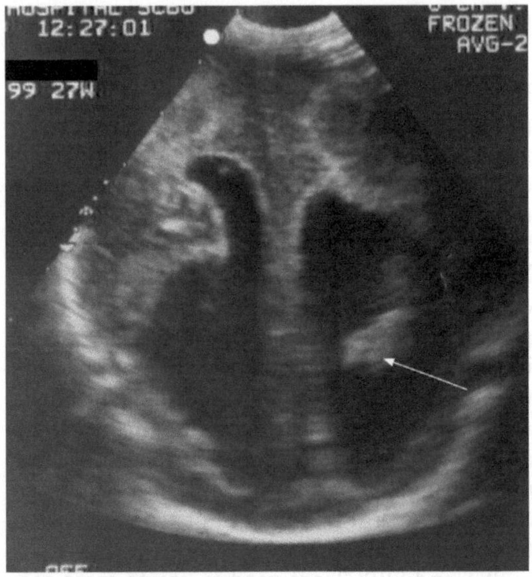

a

Fig. 2.10. Ultrasound scan of premature neonate, showing marked hydrocephalus with intraventricular hematoma (arrow).

Carotid Ultrasound

Multicenter, randomized clinical trials of carotid endarterectomy have shown that the operation significantly reduces the risk of stroke in patients with severe (>70%) internal carotid artery stenosis [24].

Whilst angiography is accepted as the "gold standard" modality for diagnosing a significant stenosis, carotid duplex imaging, in conjunction with color and power imaging, is now recognized as the better initial test and often the only test necessary. Not only does ultrasound have the great advantage of being non-invasive, but it is also in general the most cost effective of the possible relevant investigations. Ultrasound has been shown to be very accurate in assessing the degree of stenosis, as assessed by pathological review of endarterectomy specimens, although it must be noted that the degree of operator skill is of crucial importance. Angiography is required where the duplex study is equivocal or if there is any doubt about total vessel occlusion.

Miscellaneous

Intraoperative ultrasound (IOUS) may be used as a guide in both brain and spinal surgery. In the spine, ultrasound may be used to guide the approach to a tumor, reducing the extent of the laminectomy and dural opening. With intramedullary tumors, the extent of the posterior myelotomy can be defined, together with the presence of syringomyelic cavities and deep tumor extension [25]. In some cases there may be pointers to a histological diagnosis and, where indicated, ultrasonic-guided aspiration and biopsy can be performed. Similarly, IOUS is well able to localize and define the margins of both superficial and deep intracranial tumors, and can subsequently accurately determine the extent of resection.

Finally, IOUS may be of use in the evaluation of both the brain and spinal cord in trauma patients. Localization of hematomas, bone fragments and foreign bodies is possible and ultrasound may subsequently provide dynamic guidance to facilitate their removal.

Conclusions

The future of neuroradiology will see further development of MRI so that it becomes the central, and often only, diagnostic tool needed. MRA and CTA will replace diagnostic angiography. Functional and physiological data will be routinely available although newer techniques, such as magnetoencephalography, may have a limited role in complementing MRI. CT scanning will remain important and even myelography will have a limited role. The neuroradiologist will remain central, being the interface between the application and interpretation of these sophisticated technologies and the clinical problems of the patient.

Self-assessment

- ☐ What are the features of a subdural empyema on a CT scan?
- ☐ What are the MRI appearances of an acute parenchymal hematoma?
- ☐ What are the common hemorrhagic tumors of the brain and what are their characteristic features on MRI?
- ☐ What are the complications of cerebral angiography?
- ☐ A patient presenting with subarachnoid hemorrhage is found to have multiple aneurysms. How do you decide which has bled?

References

1. Osborn AG. Diagnostic neuroradiology. St Louis: Mosby Year Book, 1994.
2. Atlas SW. Magnetic resonance imaging of the brain and spine, 3rd edition, Philadelphia; Lippincott-Williams-Wilkins, 2002.
3. Rankine JJ, Gill KP, Hutchinson CE, Ross ERS, Williamson JB. The therapeutic impact of lumbar spine MRI on patients with low back and leg pain. Clin Radiol 1998;53:688–93.
4. Hounsfield GN. Computerised transverse axial scanning (tomography). Part I. Description of system. Br J Radiol 1973;46:1016–22.
5. Osborn AG. Intracranial haemorrhage. In: Osborn AG, editor. Diagnostic neuroradiology. St Louis: Mosby Year Book, 1994; 154–98.
6. Katayama H, Yamaguchi, Kozuku T et al. Adverse reactions to ionic and non-ionic contrast media: a report from the Japanese Committee on the safety of contrast media. Radiology 1990;175:621.
7. Vieco PT. CT Angiography of the intracranial circulation. Neuroimaging Clin N Am 1998;8(3):577–92.
8. Schild HH. MRI made easy. Berlin/Bergkamen: Schering AG, 1990.
9. Connelly A, Jackson GD, Frackowiak RSJ, Belliveau JW, Vargha-Khadem F, Dadian DG. Functional mapping of activated human primary cortex with a clinical MR imaging system. Radiology 188: 125, 1993.
10. Castillo M, Kwock L, Scatliff J, Mukherji SK. Proton MR spectroscopy in neoplastic and non-neoplastic brain disorders. Magn Reson Imaging Clin N Am 1998; 6(1): 1–21.
11. Moriarty TM, Kikinis R, Jolesz FA, Black PM, Alexander E. Magnetic resonance imaging therapy: intraoperative MR imaging. Neurosurg Clin N Am 1996;7(2):323–31.
12. Le Bihan D. Diffusion and perfusion magnetic resonance imaging. New York: Raven Press, 1995.
13. Sato Y, Yuh WTC, Smith WL et al. Head injury in child abuse. Evaluation with MR imaging. Radiology 1989; 173:653–57.
14. Broderick JP, Adams HP, Barson W et al. Guidelines for the management of spontaneous intracerebral hemorrhage. Stroke 1999;30:905–15.
15. Zhu XL, Chan MS, Poon WS Spontaneous intracranial hemorrhage: which patients need diagnostic cerebral angiography? A prospective study of 206 cases and review of the literature. Stroke 1997;28:1406–9.
16. Lenthall RK, Dean JR, Bartlett JR, Jeffree MA Intrapituitary fluid levels following hemorrhage: MRI appearances in 13 cases. Neuroradiology 1999;41: 167–70.
17. Shellock FG, Kanal E. Magnetic resonance bioeffects, safety and for MR imaging safety and patient management. In: Patient management, 2nd edn. Philadelphia: Lippincott-Raven, 1996.

18. The International Study of Unruptured Intracranial Aneurysms Investigations. Unruptured intracranial aneurysms - risk of rupture and risks of surgical intervention. N Engl J Med 1998; 339:1725–33.
19. Hughes DG, Patel U, Forbes WC, Jones AP. Comparison of hand injection with mechanical injection for digital subtraction selective cerebral angiography. Br J Radiol 1994;67:786–89.
20. Heiserman JE, Dean BL, Hodak JA et al. Neurologic complications of cerebral angiography. Am J Neuroradiol 1994;15:1401–40.
21. Van Gijn J, Van Dongen KJ, Verneulen M, Hijdra A. Perimesencephalic hemorrhage, a non-aneurysmal and benign form of subarachnoid hemorrhage. Neurology 1985;35:493–7.
22. Wagner HN. Clinical applications of positron emission tomography. In: Maissey MN, Britton KE, Gilday DL, editors. Clinical nuclear medicine, 2nd edn. London: Chapman and Hall Medical, 1991; 504–14.
23. Shetty PG, Shroff MM, Sahani DV, Kirtane MV. Evaluation of high-resolution CT and MR cisternography in the diagnosis of cerebrospinal fluid fistula. Am J Neuroradiol 1997;19:633–9.
24. North American Symptomatic Carotid Endarterectomy Trial Collaborators. Beneficial effect of carotid endarterectomy in symptomatic patients with high grade stenosis. N Engl J Med 1991;325:445–53.
25. Maiuri F, Iaconetta G, DeDivitis O. The role of intraoperative sonography in reducing invasiveness during surgery for spinal tumours. Minim Invasive Neurosurg 1997(Mar);40(1):8–12.

3

Neuropathology

Cheng-Mei Shaw and Ellsworth C. Alvord, Jr

Summary

The history of Neuropathology is inseparable from that of Neurosurgery. Since the creation of Cushing's Tumor Registry, it has been apparent that neurosurgeons should understand the elements of diagnostic neuropathology. Over the past few decades, there have been extensive developments in histologic tools requiring lengthy specialized training for neuropathologists. The new diagnostic imaging techniques enable clinicians to discover and locate numerous lesions other than tumors and abscesses. The imaging advances also allow the evolution of the lesions to be studied. This chapter focuses on the neuropathologic approaches that neurosurgical trainees should understand. The following three questions should be answered, (1) How is histo-pathologic diagnosis made? (2) How can one understand the changing diagnostic terminology? (3) What are the limitations of histopathologic diagnosis of surgical specimens?

When the young Harvey Cushing arrived at Johns Hopkins Hospital as an assistant resident in William Halsted's Surgical Service, he knew very little about pathology and bacteriology. However, it was the responsibility of the house officers to carry out all of the clinical bacteriological and pathological studies for every patient under their charge. Years later, Cushing wrote that he owed to this system what little he knew of histological pathology and admitted that his early bacteriological studies, some of which got into print, would otherwise never have been made.

In the early 1900s, Cushing operated unsuccessfully on a 14-year-old girl who presented with headache, failing vision, obesity and lack of secondary sexual development. The patient died several days after examination of the posterior cranial fossa followed by occipital exploration and decompression. Autopsy showed a large pituitary cyst, which William Welch called a "teratoma", but which was probably a "Rathke's cleft cyst" in today's terminology. The importance of this case was not fully appreciated until several years later, when Cushing asked the pathology department for the tissue; it could not be found. From then on, Cushing was insistent that he should be responsible for the pathological study of all specimens from the patients under his care. His insistence rightfully caused some difficulties with his colleagues but was granted because he was fortunate to have understanding friends, such as William Welch and W.G. MacCallum. After he moved to Harvard, he made a similar request and more difficulties were encountered, but he was unyielding. His insistence resulted in the development of his own neuropathological laboratory under the supervision of Percival Bailey, who had had unusual training in the techniques of the microscopic study of the nervous system. The renowned "Cushing Tumor Registry", a historical collection of more than 2,000 cases of verified brain tumors, was thus founded. Through the study of this collection, a classification of brain tumors based on histogenesis was made by Bailey and Cushing [1, 2] – the forerunner of many subsequent and continuously revised classifications of brain tumors.

Cushing and his associates were fortunate because the basic histological techniques were already well developed and the repertoire of neuropathological lesions was limited in those days to expanding lesions, such as tumors and abscesses in the central nervous system (CNS). Thus, neurosurgeons were able to undertake pathological studies of the specimens they dug out between their busy clinical and surgical schedules. However, the extensive developments of new techniques in neurosurgery, neuroradiology and neuropathology over the past few decades make it extremely difficult today for neurosurgeons to assume such studies. The new histological tools include immunocytochemistry and molecular biology, as well as numerous tinctorial staining techniques, and require an expensive set-up for laboratories and lengthy specialized training for neuropathologists. Furthermore, the new diagnostic imaging techniques enable clinicians today to discover and locate numerous lesions other than tumors and abscesses. As a result, the repertoire for neuropathologists has expanded enormously to include many exotic lesions that were hitherto unknown in surgical pathology. The ability to visualize small millimeter-size lesions under sophisticated diagnostic imaging and by stereotactic biopsy now forces neuropathologists to make more and more diagnoses from smaller and smaller specimens, including those that look much larger to the neurosurgeon, who removes them under open microscopic control!

Cushing was able to follow up his patients by requesting them to write to him every year on the anniversary of their operation. By this system he was able to collect data concerning the end results of his operations, ultimately to learn the probable life expectancy of patients with any particular type of tumor. Today, serial imagings give an advantage to the clinician, enabling them to follow the patients postoperatively, to visualize the subsequent evolution of the lesion, to disclose signs of recurrence at an early stage, and even to calculate the growth rate of tumors. The data collected by Cushing and his followers concerning the life expectancy of brain tumors prior to CT–MRI (computed tomography/magnetic resonance imaging) days, however, should be readjusted for today's statistics. The neurosurgeons then were operating on brain tumors that had become so large as to produce papilledema and other signs that increased the morbidity and mortality of those patients. Today's patients are typically operated on after their first seizure, the lesion visualized via CT–MRI. The tumors now are relatively small, sometimes even found incidentally after a head injury, and one would expect the life expectancy of each particular patient to be much longer than that suggested by the data collected in the early days. The fact that the survival period of the patients can be improved by finding diseases earlier is well known as the "Will Rogers' effect": the "Okies" who left Oklahoma for California increased the IQ in both states! And all of this ignores the very valuable contributions of the anesthesiologists, nurses, rehabilitation and other personnel comprising today's neurosurgical team.

As a side-product of CT–MRI, contemporary neuropathologists are given many opportunities to observe the histological sequences in the evolution of tumors and the effects of radiation and chemotherapy. Similarly, many non-neoplastic lesions are seen, such as various stages of inflammatory processes, the early stages of active demyelinating processes, embolized tumors and vascular malformations, and numerous other conditions, which used to be seen only at autopsy and were never considered in the practice of surgical neuropathology.

Thus, the history of neuropathology is inseparable from that of neurosurgery, as if the shadow follows the form. Neuropathology, especially of tumors, was born within Cushing's neurosurgical kingdom by neurosurgeons. It was fortunate for the future of neuropathology that it was founded as a subspecialty of pathology at the same time that neurosurgery was established as a subspecialty of surgery. It has become a tradition in the USA to require trainees in neurosurgery to spend some months in a neuropathology lab in order to learn the elements of diagnostic neuropathology. As it is not possible for neurosurgical trainees to learn all aspects of neuropathology during their short rotation, we have tried to design some limited approaches that will be most beneficial for their future practice of neurosurgery. It is our opinion that the answers to the following three questions should be emphasized:

How is a histopathological diagnosis made?

How can one understand the changing diagnostic terminology?

What are the limitations of the histopathological diagnosis of surgical specimens?

1. How is a Histopathological Diagnosis Made?

Neuropathology can frequently be used simply to confirm or disprove a clinical diagnosis that is made by clinicians based on the clinical presentation and on radiological and laboratory findings. Owing to remarkable advances in diagnostic techniques with high-tech equipment and sophisticated laboratory assays, the clinical diagnosis is probably correct in the great majority of cases. MRI can easily demonstrate neoplasms in the brain and spinal cord and can differentiate extra- or intra-axial site, low or high grade, with or without cyst, calcification and hemorrhage. One can reach a fairly accurate histopathological diagnosis of tumors without a biopsy by combining these factors. Of special note is the fact that MRI is especially sensitive to water, which is notoriously difficult for pathologists primarily because we extract all of the water before embedding the tissue to be stained!

However, there are still groups of pathological processes in which the clinical data cannot be so precise, especially in non-neoplastic lesions, when histopathological study becomes crucial. Students who are trained in particular clinical skills tend to rely on their own clinical experiences and can be prejudiced by their own knowledge. They may be searching for only those signs to support their clinical diagnosis and may overlook other important evidence leading to other diagnoses. On the other hand, those who are trained in basic pathological skills tend to rely on their primary trade and may be caught not only on relatively insignificant artifacts but also on their lack of familiarity with clinical signs and specific neuroanatomical points.

In order to decrease such inevitable bias we encourage students to study the surgical specimens first without any prior demographic and clinical information and to leave the clinicopathological correlation to later, when the final diagnosis can be revised as appropriate. If the histopathological findings were unique and specific in each disease, one should be able to make a diagnosis of a disease solely by histopathological study with total objectivity. Unfortunately, this has proven frequently not to be the case. The definition of a disease is often too arbitrary and there have been too many diseases for the number of conceivable pathogenetic reactions of human tissue. Therefore, pathologists may not be able to form a specific diagnosis when they examine the specimen without other supportive information, although they should be able to form a group of diagnoses to be differentiated from each other by more advanced techniques or by other clinical information.

In order to be an unbiased observer, one should not assume: (1) that all specimens are pathological, or (2) that all surgical specimens represent some kind of tumor. For those who are not very familiar with histopathological diagnoses, we recommend that they consider the following questions when they confront an unknown slide:

What is the origin of the tissue?

Is it normal or abnormal?

If abnormal, is the abnormality specific or non-specific?

If specific, to which of the following categories does it belong:

- Developmental anomalies?
- Inflammatory processes?
- Vascular diseases?
- Degenerative diseases?
- Traumatic lesions?
- Neoplasms?

If it belongs to one of the above processes, can you narrow your diagnosis more specifically as to the type of process?

Does your tentatively final diagnosis make sense clinically and anatomically?

Let us consider each of these in turn.

What is the Origin of the Tissue?

The more abnormal the tissue, the more difficult it may be to identify the origin of the tissue. Frequently, however, some clues can be found at the edge of the specimen. One may see gray matter, recognizable with neurons, but bits of cerebral cortex cannot easily be differentiated from basal ganglia or spinal cord gray unless one sees leptomeninges on the surface. One may see white matter or myelinated fibers, which should differ in CNS or peripheral nervous system (PNS), but bits of CNS white matter in the cerebrum cannot be distinguished from those in the spinal cord or cerebellum unless one sees other landmarks – again, leptomeninges being helpful in non-cortical locations. White matter bundles separated by thin connective tissue septa are a relatively specific architecture of the optic nerve. Other structures, such as the pituitary gland, pineal gland, peripheral nerve, choroid plexus and leptomeninges can usually be identified with little difficulty.

Is the Tissue Normal or Abnormal?

If one can recognize the site, the degree of abnormality becomes relatively easy to determine. Otherwise, the hypercellularity of most neoplasms and inflammation is usually easy to see. But in other diseases, especially in so-called "borderline cases", hypercellularity may be absent or very difficult to see. A mild increase in glial cells and a mild decrease in neurons can also relate to the thickness and plane of the section. In addition, one may have to struggle with artifacts, especially those that can appear during the removal of the tissue or during the preparation of the slides. It should be noted that the presence of nodular clusters of neurons without lamination is abnormal in neocortex but normal in the pyriform cortex – found in the parahippocampal gyrus. The presence of an external granular cell layer in the cerebellar cortex is normal in the infant up to about 18 months of age. Large clusters of immature granular cells in the striato-thalamic junction or over the caudate nucleus, known as the "germinal matrix", are normal components of fetal brains.

If Abnormal, is the Abnormality Specific or Non-specific?

There are certain pathological changes – abnormal but very common, frequently associated with age or derived from old subclinical injuries – that usually pose no clinical significance. These should not delay the investigation too much and include the following: thickening of the leptomeninges, atherosclerosis, fibrosis or hyalinization of blood vessels, mineral deposits in various parts of the nervous system, lipofuscin in neurons, corpora amylacea, mild gliosis without other specific pathological changes, acute (usually operative) and even old (remote) hemorrhages, necrosis without other specific findings, and mild inflammatory changes in the absence of other specific changes.

Among these may be considered the differential diagnosis of gliosis vs low-grade glioma. This is the most frequent problem that neophytes expect to encounter according to their grapevine! Actually, however, for the usual neophyte the boundary lies well up in the scale of hypercellularity simply because the true neophyte has had essentially no experience with the normal, much less the abnormal.

Gliosis is a scar in the CNS analogous to fibrosis in other organs. It only tells us that the tissue is abnormal because something has happened there, or near there, in the remote past and has been repaired. The scar remains but the cause of the scar is no longer present. An old gliosis consists of abundant astrocytic fibers and few cell bodies or nuclei. More recent gliosis contains more cell bodies with plump cytoplasm ("gemistocytes") and less prominent fibers. Such recent or progressive gliosis is difficult to distinguish from a low-grade astrocytoma.

Gliosis vs Glioma

This is a problem on which even expert neuropathologists disagree frequently, especially when the biopsy specimen is either insufficient in quantity or misses the target. There is no single easy criterion to separate the two conditions. Increased density of cells is not always diagnostic of a glioma, since atrophic white matter can be more hypercellular than even a real low-grade glioma. Immune stains for glial fibrillary acidic protein (GFAP) usually show multipolar star-shaped astrocytes distributed at relatively regular intervals in gliosis, compared with a "shoulder-to-shoulder" pattern in gliomas. The most important criterion in gliomas is nuclear pleomorphism. When other criteria, such as vascular changes, mitoses and Ki67 cycling activity are present, the tumor is no longer low grade and poses no problem in being distinguished from gliosis.

When all is said and done, the most important fact for the biopsist to remember is that most lesions are spherical, with a center (which may be actively growing neoplasm, necrotic neoplasm or other tissue, demyelination, etc.), an active edge and an outer surrounding reaction. A radial biopsy is the best, a tangential (or further away) one rarely being helpful. In general, the active edge is pleomorphic, containing a background of normal cells (neurons, blood vessels, glia), reacting cells (microglia in all stages of development, astrocytes in various stages of reaction) and the "cells of the lesion". A low-magnification orientation is at least helpful, if not essential. We have seen experts get lost in the pleomorphism of the edge, not seeing the center as either necrotic or demyelinated, and not seeing the surrounding reaction as it decreases from the active edge of the tumor or the plaque.

If Specific, To Which of the Following Categories Does the Tissue Belong?

Developmental Anomalies

This category includes cerebral dysplasias, tubers, hamartomas, heterotopia, polymicrogyria and cysts of various types. Encephaloceles and meningomyeloceles are readily diagnosable on the external appearance of the patients and usually contain fragments of CNS and PNS tissues, nerves, nests of blood vessels and fibrous connective tissue. Cortical dysplasias, tubers, heterotopia and polymicrogyria are frequently resected for seizure control. "Hamartoma" is included but its diagnosis is difficult because the definition is vague and controversial. We try not to make a diagnosis of hamartoma except for cases of hypothalamic hamartoma, which has become a well established clinicopathological entity. Tubers are relatively unique because of the presence of extremely bizarre neurons and astrocytes and other cells of indeterminate, intermediate or mixed nature. Cysts can be lined by arachnoid cells, glial tissue (Fig. 3.1), epithelial cells and non-specific connective tissue (pial or other) membranes [3]. Epidermoid and dermoid cysts can be considered to be developmental anomalies but are customarily included in the category of neoplasms.

Inflammatory Lesions

Abscesses due to purulent bacteria and granulomas secondary to tuberculosis were common in the old days but their incidence has decreased markedly with the advent of antibiotics. The recent epidemic of AIDS, however, has revived this category. Furthermore, the causative agents are no longer limited to simple staphylococci, streptococci, pneumococci, Hemophilus influenzae and tuberculosis, but have expanded their spectrum enormously to include many that were hitherto unknown to be pathogenetic for humans. The most common opportunistic infections today are probably by Toxoplasma and Aspergillus, but many other exotic bacteria, fungi and viruses can be found in patients with immunodeficiencies. AIDS leucoencephalopathy is an uncommon new entity and should be taken into consideration when one is dealing with AIDS patients. Sarcoidosis and vasculitis of various types may be considered among the differential diagnoses. Progressive multifocal leucoencephalopathy (PML), another opportunistic infection by a papovavirus, reveals demyelinating and partially necrotic white-matter lesions that characteristically show bizarre Alzheimer Type I astrocytes and intranuclear viral inclusions in glial cells.

Demyelinating Diseases vs Gliomas Until the advent of MRI and the culmination of studies of experimental allergic encephalo-myelitis (EAE), both occurring about 30 years ago, the concept of multiple sclerosis (MS) was derived almost entirely from clinical and autopsy studies. The former remained questionable until evidence of "multiple lesions in time and space" provided the clue, but this occurred only after the disease was well established. The latter almost necessarily revealed only the end stage: sharply defined plaques involving the white matter and manifest by loss of myelin and gliosis with

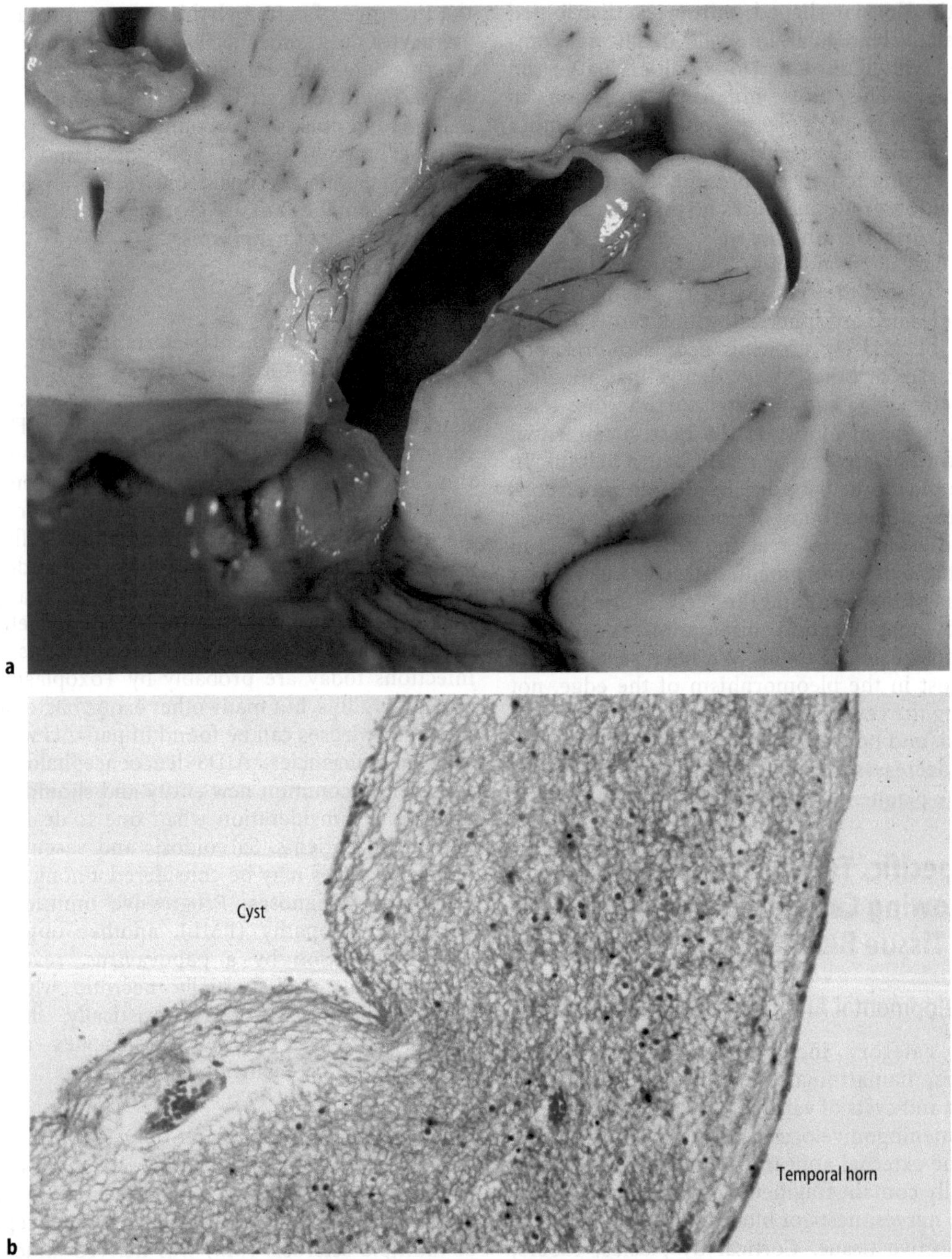

Figa. 3.1. a Incidentally observed at autopsy, this congenital intracerebral cyst is in the region of the hippocampal fissure. **b** Microscopic section shows a glia-lined cyst separated from the ependyma-lined temporal horn by gliotic brain tissue. NP2391, H&E.

preservation of axons. There was a long temporal gap between the two fields of study, so much so that MS was frequently considered to be degenerative rather than inflammatory. The status of "activity" remained speculative. Lesions that contained lipid-filled macrophages ("gitter cells") were thought to be active, forgetting that macrophages can persist for many months, even years. Other lesions were only loose mesh works of astrocytic fibers and were truly old. Mild, focal, perivascular lymphocytic cuffs were also considered "active" but rarely did neuropathologists encounter a really active lesion: a small focus at the circumference where microglia in various stages of phagocytosing and digesting myelin (Fig. 3.2) could be seen as evidence of some process beginning only a few days before death. Neuropathologists did not expect a biopsy of an MS lesion until modern scans began to reveal "solitary" expanding lesions that required a biopsy to differentiate a neoplasm (glioma, lymphoma or metastatic carcinoma) from an abscess or granuloma. MS was just not on the list of differential diagnoses in those days.

When the authors saw their first case of MS at biopsy (Fig. 3.3), their first impression was anaplastic astrocytoma with pleomorphic nuclei (later shown to be both microglia and astrocytes in various stages of evolution), the astrocytes being especially pleomorphic with chromatin patterns that were suggestive of mitoses but which are now recognized as micronuclei. There was only mild perivascular lymphocytic cuffing. The evolving macrophages were not obvious on H&E (hematoxylin & eosin)-stained sections and, indeed, the authors were not sensitized enough even to be looking for macrophages. Only when they saw the CT scan showing what looked like a head full of marbles did they realize that not only were they wrong in their diagnosis of glioma but also that the clinicians were wrong in diagnosing metastatic cancer. The diagnosis had to be MS even though the primary complaint had been an epileptic seizure! Fortunately, although the concept of pleomorphic xantho-astrocytoma (PXA) was not yet popularized in those days, the foamy and spongy stroma of the tissue raised their suspicion of MS. Subsequent special stains revealed that the lesion was packed with foamy macrophages and had a sharply defined loss of myelin and preservation of axons.

They thus learned the hard way that demyelinating disease must be added to their list of differential diagnoses. However, it can still be quite confusing because the edge is not always sharp and the preservation of axons far from perfect. They know of several cases of litigation against pathologists because of the misdiagnosis of neoplasm.

Abscess and Granuloma vs Tumor Hypercellularity is one of the characteristics of most neoplasms but it is not specific. The number of cells increases even more markedly in many inflammatory processes but the types of cells are quite different and should cause only temporary difficulty in differential diagnosis. The granulation tissue in the wall of an organizing abscess or granuloma with abundant, actively proliferating, immature fibroblasts may look quite wild and mimic pleomorphic astrocytomas, especially if the adjacent reactive gliosis is included in the specimen and the more central inflammatory exudate is not. Macrophages are usually present in the granulation tissue and these contribute to the pleomophism as the microglia evolve into macrophages. On the other hand, acute and chronic inflammatory exudates may be seen focally in glioblastomas, probably in response to necrosis. This can cause a differential nightmare when the specimen is small and does not show representative areas of the glioblastoma. Since the treatment for glioblastoma and abscess is so different, rebiopsy has to be requested if the problem cannot be solved.

Vascular Diseases

Hemorrhages, old and recent, usually pose no problem for diagnosis except that the gliosis adjacent to an old hemorrhage can be so disorganized as to raise a question of glioma. Foci of vascular malformation in gliomas, both low and high grade, are not uncommon and oligodendrogliomas are notorious for spontaneously bleeding as their first sign. When a large arteriovenous malformation (AVM) is present adjacent to a glioma, it is difficult to tell whether the AVM is a focal change in the glioma or two independent lesions that just happen to occur in the same location.

Congophilic angiopathy should be considered and the amyloid-containing blood vessels

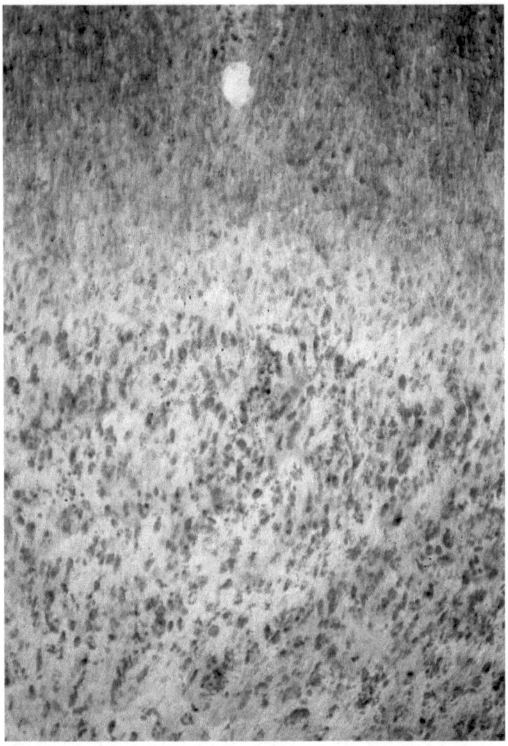
a

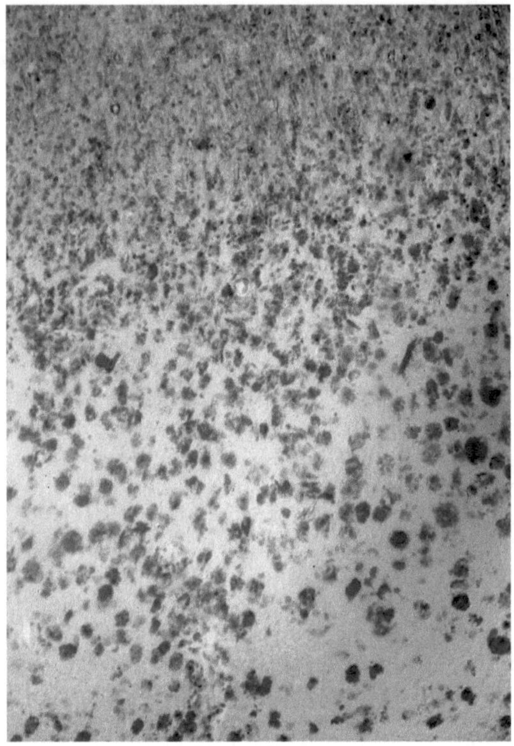
b

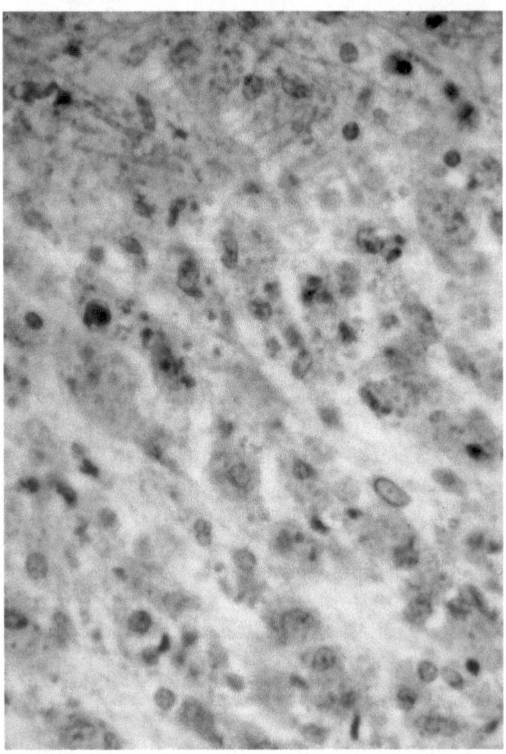
c

Fig. 3.2. a An inactive plaque of MS at autopsy, packed with lipid-filled gitter cells (red in the original), the sharp edge and the uniformly plump macrophages indicating that the lesion is at least many months old. NP4249, oil-red-O-hematoxylin (ORO-H). **b** A small focus of activity at the edge of another old plaque in the same patient, the gradation in size of the microglia as they digest the myelin into ORO-positive droplets indicating that the lesion began less than a few days before death. NP4249, ORO-H. **c** Another small focus of activity in another case of MS, the progressively decreasing sizes of the myelin debris (blue in the original) phagocytosed by microglia and converted into periodic acid–Schiff (PAS)-positive granules (red in the original) paralleling the lipid production in **b**. NP2169, Luxol-fast-blue-PAS-hematoxylin (LFB-PAS-H).

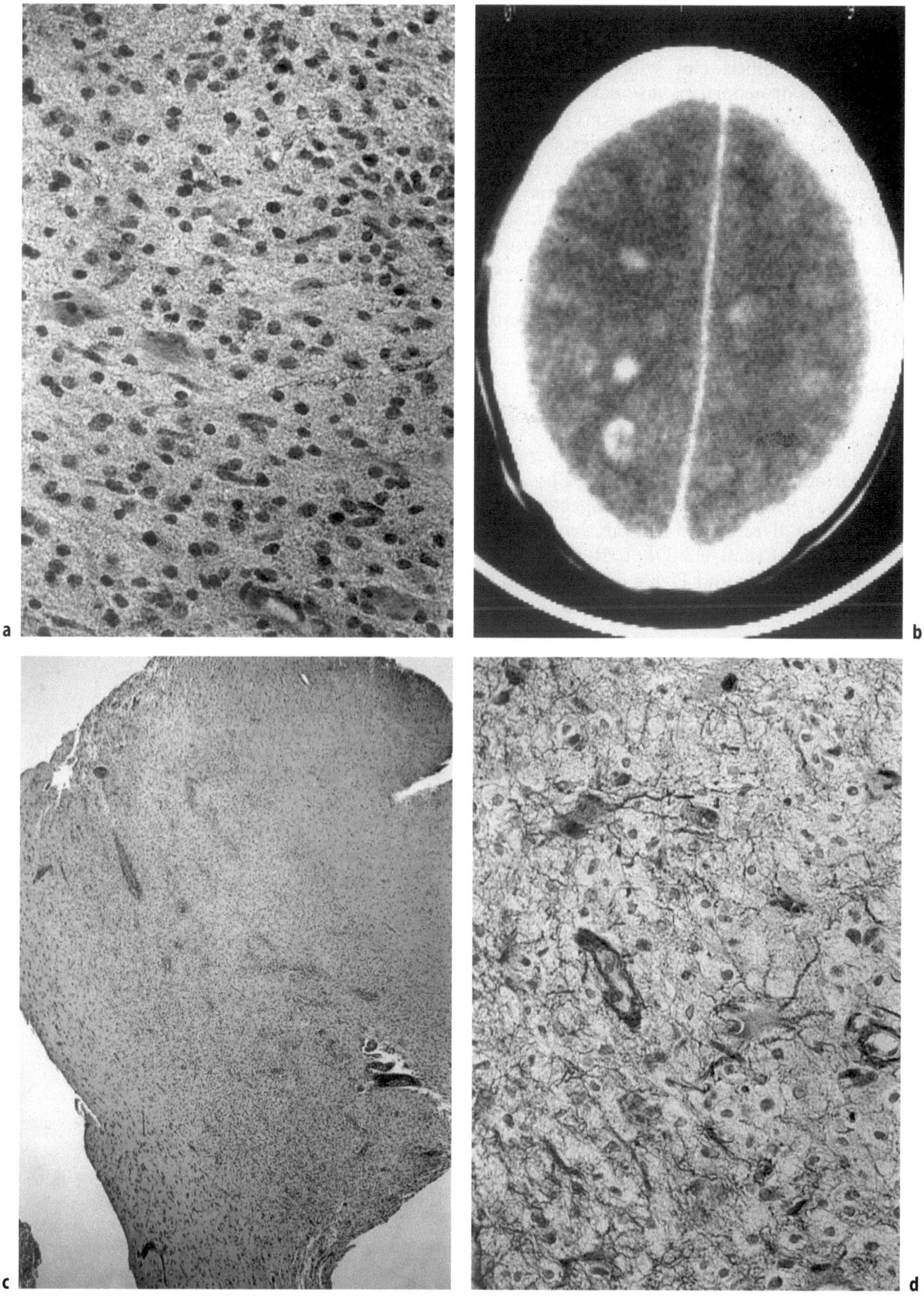

Fig. 3.3. a Pleomorphic nuclei and cytoplasms (H&E), at first suggesting an anaplastic astrocytoma. **b** The CT scan, however, showed multiple lesions that suggested metastatic cancer and prompted the biopsy seen in **a**. The combination of **a** and **b** suggested MS, which was confirmed by the sharp-edged demyelination in **c**, the upper right triangular portion being blue in the original (LFB-PAS-H), even though the astrocytes were quite pleomorphic in **d** (NP8667, Holzer's crystal violet for astrocytes).

should be looked for in hematomas evacuated from anyone over 50 years of age. Other diagnoses include blood clot without abnormal blood vessels or neoplasm, vascular malformations of various types (AVM, cavernous malformation, venous angioma, telangiectasia and aneurysm), and ischemic and hemorrhagic infarcts of various durations. Some may be biopsied when they cannot be differentiated clinically from tumors. Atheromatous plaques removed at carotid endarterectomy may appear as non-specific fibrous tissue with or without calcification, cholesterol clefts or cholesterol granulomas.

Degenerative Diseases

So far, the authors have found it rare to have the final diagnosis be an unexpected degenerative disease. Neurosurgeons may be asked by neurologists to perform a biopsy for suspected neuronal storage diseases and leukodystrophies of different types, Creutzfeld–Jakob disease (CJD), Alzheimer's disease and Pick's disease, as well as for patients who show progressive deterioration that cannot be characterized clinically. The location and amount of the specimen may be critical but we generally recommend a good cubic centimeter of cortex and white matter so that adequate blocks for frozen and paraffin sections and electron microscopy can be performed. Unfortunately, often only non-specific gliotic tissue is obtained in these cases and the disease remains frustratingly undetectable.

Trauma

Occasionally, cases may present as diagnostic problems: (1) Did the patient fall because of an underlying disease or was the trauma primary? (2) Is the necrosis due to the trauma (contusion of the crests of superficial gyri) or to vascular disease (usually deep in the sulci)? Contused cerebral tissue with petechiae; blood clots from epidural, subdural and intracerebral hemorrhages; and organizing subdural membrane usually give little difficulty in diagnosis. One can recognize the relatively slow evolution of the outer membrane of a subdural hematoma (Fig. 3.4) compared with the almost-non-changing

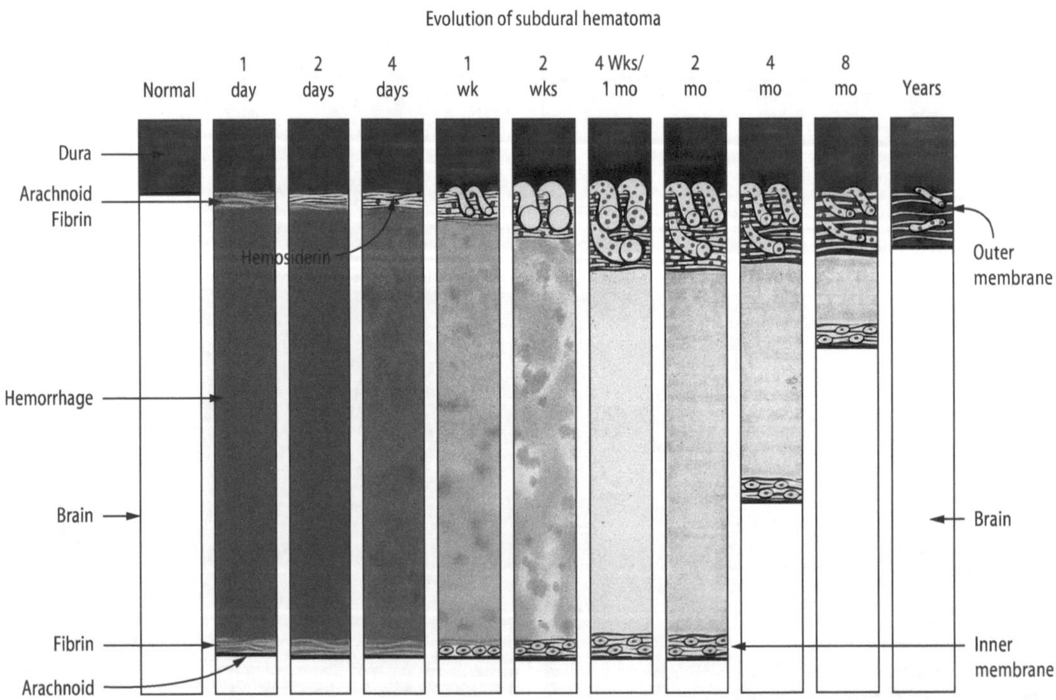

Fig. 3.4. Schematic evolution of a subdural hematoma of moderately large size. Note that most of the reaction is in the outer membrane. Trichrome (green staining dura and fibrous tissue and red staining hemorrhage in the original) and iron (blue staining hemosiderin in the original) stains. Note RBC in dilated sinusoids at 1 month.

inner membrane, and one must also recognize the much more rapid organization of an epidural hemorrhage with its immediate access to the surrounding connective tissue and blood vessels.

Neoplasms

This category is obviously the largest - neurosurgeons' biases historically shaped this direction! - and consists of 70-80% of all neurosurgical specimens, but the distribution depends on the populations served and the strengths of subspecialties of neurosurgeons in any one institute. The magnet effect of individuals - so obvious in Cushing's pituitary tumors, but also involving public, private, academic, large and small institutions - is still in play! There are already many books describing gross and microscopic findings for each type of tumor and there are already too many revisions of classifications of tumors [4,5,6,7,8], so we will not be repetitive in describing each tumor. Books that not only describe the findings of each tumor but also discuss the differential diagnoses more extensively are more helpful [6]. The authors would caution, however, that the types of tumors have changed dramatically, from "wait until the tumor is large enough to be seen by pneumoencephalography" to " biopsy after the MRI after the first fit". They would also suggest that the character of a tumor can be defined biologically (i.e. only the ranges of growth and invasive characteristics can be inferred, not measured histologically, and these ranges are notoriously wide: fast, slow, diffuse, etc.). But this may be a subject for discussion in its own right!

Having reached a tentative conclusion that a given specimen probably represents a neoplasm, one should be able to say whether it is: (1) primary or secondary (metastatic), (2) intrinsic (neural) or extrinsic (non-neural), and (3) its type and grade.

The nature of the edge is very helpful since primary intrinsic neoplasms tend to be infiltrative of the CNS whereas metastatic or extrinsic neoplasms tend to be sharply demarcated from the CNS. Of course, truly extrinsic neoplasms are rarely excised with any CNS but there may be a capsule of fibrous tissue that helps. One must always be aware that rapidly growing primary gliomas may break through the pia, infiltrate the arachnoid and dura and grossly resemble meningiomas. The reverse is also true - that even benign meningiomas and craniopharyngiomas may break through the pia and infiltrate the CNS, craniopharyngiomas especially evoking a remarkable gliosis with many Rosenthal fibers.

In determining the type and grade of neoplasms, one usually relies on the cell morphology, frequently assisted by the pattern of cellular arrangement as well as by stromal and vascular changes. Let us consider each of these below.

Cell Morphology The authors assume familiarity with the neurohistology of normal neurons, astrocytes, oligodendroglia, ependymal cells and microglia, as well as that of blood vessels and meninges. In general, touch or smear preparations of freshly removed specimens stained with H&E generally reveal the structure of individual cells better than frozen or even subsequently prepared paraffin sections, provided, of course, that enough cells stick to the slide. Touch or smear preparations are especially useful with pituitary adenomas as the normal pituitary cells do not come out of their enclosure in small pockets or capsules of connective tissue. In adenomatous tissue, the connective tissue septa diminish and large nodules of adenoma cells are easily squeezed out. Cells with abundant processes that are tightly woven together, as in schwannomas and astrocytomas, come out only as thick chunks. Patterns of cellular arrangement and vascular changes are usually not discerned in touch preparations. Necrotic coagula are easily seen but may be missed as an artifact.

To make a diagnosis of the cell type, one looks for resemblance of tumor cells to normal cells. Sometimes our concept of "normal" may seem a little strange; witness the "fried egg" or " honeycomb" (Fig. 3.5) pattern of oligodendrogliomas. This pattern is really an autolytic artifact that most pathologists find diagnostic, even though the normal oligodendrocyte usually shows much less of this artifact.

Cells showing more deviation away from the norm are said to be less differentiated or more anaplastic. At its maximal end, the cells appear so undifferentiated and uncharacteristic - consisting only of nuclei with little or no cytoplasm or processes - that their identity is lost and they can only be designated as primitive neuroectodermal cells. However, whether they are truly

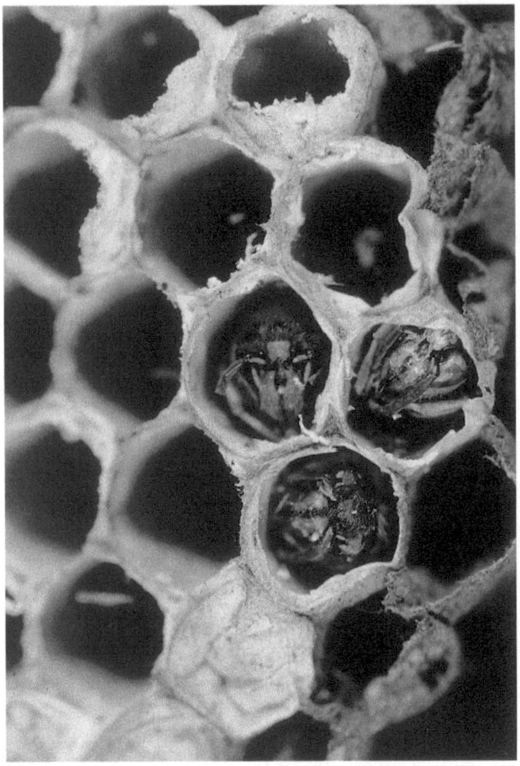
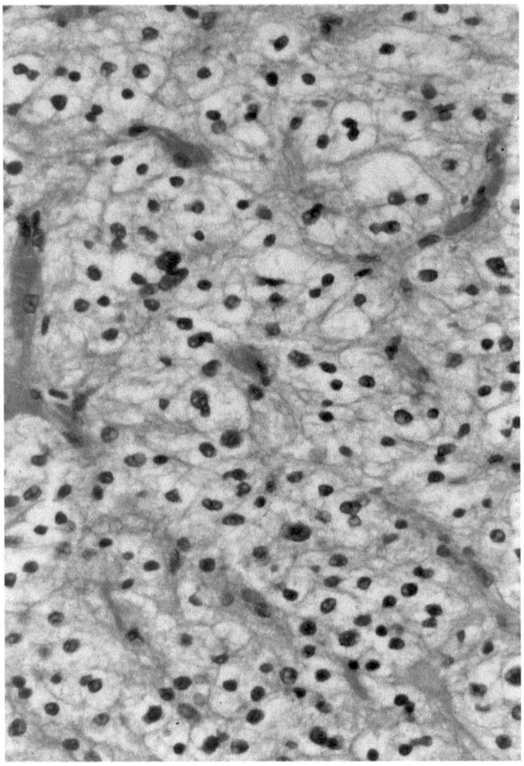

Fig. 3.5. a A honeycomb, some still filled with baby bees, corresponding to the nuclei of an oligodendroglioma. **b** "Honeycomb" pattern of an oligodendroglioma. S-4362-81, H&E.

neuroectodermal or not needs to be proven by other studies.

Many well differentiated tumors frequently consist of more than one type of cell, just as a family contains old and young persons, male and female, tall and short, even skinny and obese. This is especially true in gliomas, as astrocytes (fibrillary, gemistocytic or protoplasmic), oligodendroglia and even ependymocytes share the same progenitor. When a diagnosis of a particular type of glioma is made, it does not necessarily imply a pure culture of that particular type of glia cell, only a majority of that type of cell. When the proportion of other types becomes significant, a diagnosis of mixed glioma can be made, although a determination of the necessary proportion is quite arbitrary and subjective – usually at least 25%. This is another area where controversies arise.

Patterns of Cellular Arrangement

Each tumor appears to be different. In order to classify tumors into groups, one has to find some common denominator for each group. As we mentioned above, we first use the morphology of the tumor cells to estimate the lineage of the cell and tumor. However, although the histological variations on normal cells are very limited, those of tumor cells are quite marked. No matter how we combine the shape, size and degree of staining of the nucleus and cytoplasm and the shape, size and number of cell processes, we can make only a limited number of normal cell types, which can resemble the tumor cells to various degrees. Not all tumors are diffusely infiltrating or consist of randomly arranged or packed cell masses. Tumors belonging to a similar lineage have a tendency to show a particular pattern formed by groups of cells. These patterns are not specific and frequently overlap among different groups but are helpful when combined with cell morphology. The patterns are not necessarily present in the whole tumor but are often found only in small foci, which one has to search for.

Diffusely Infiltrating with No Significant Pattern This type of pattern can be seen in all types of gliomas: gangliogliomas, lymphomas, primitive neuroectodermal tumors (PNETs), germinomas, melanomas, sarcomas and some types of carcinoma. Some show relatively subtle patterns: germinomas can be identified because of the mixture of two distinct cell types: large epithelioid cells and small lymphocytes. Islands of nuclei in a sea of glial fibers are seen in the adult spinal cord (Fig. 3.6a) and are typical of subependymomas (Fig. 3.6b). Lymphoma cells tend to be densely packed around blood vessels, even laminated. Homer Wright pseudorosettes, described below, may be found in PNETs with neuroblastic differentiation but frequently require careful search.

Perineuronal Satellitosis Oligodendrogliomas have a tendency to proliferate close to the cell bodies of neurons in the gray matter, a phenomenon known as "perineuronal satellitosis". Astrocytes and microglia also occur normally and abnormally in a satellite position but oligodendrogliomas seem to be the most common neoplasm to produce this pattern. Two or three glial cells around a neuron are common, indeed normal, but more than that is abnormal. In tumors, there are an increased number of satellite cells, which usually show some nuclear pleomorphism (Fig. 3.7). Often the presence of a neuron in the center is obscure and one sees only a regular scattering of clumps of tumor cells in the gray matter, suggesting the distribution of neurons previously present. Satellitosis is not specific for a neoplasm, but can be seen in reactions to various non-specific infections and intoxications.

Streams and Bundles Most frequently seen in schwannomas, streams of interlacing bundles of elongated spindle-shaped cells are present in Antoni Type A regions (Fig. 3.8); cut in cross-section, the spindle-shaped nuclei become small and round. Meningiomas, especially of the fibrous variant, can also show this pattern, but

a

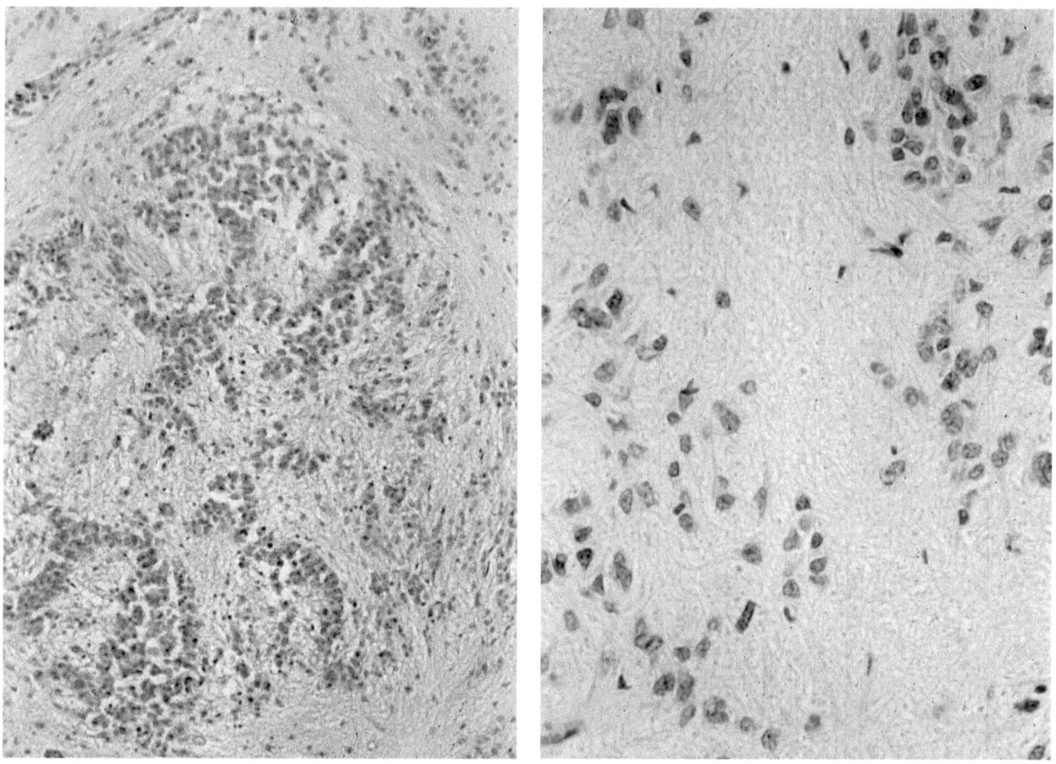

b

Fig. 3.6. a Islands of nuclei in a sea of glial fibers in a normal adult spinal cord. NP282, H&E. **b** Similar islands in a subependymoma. NP171, H&E.

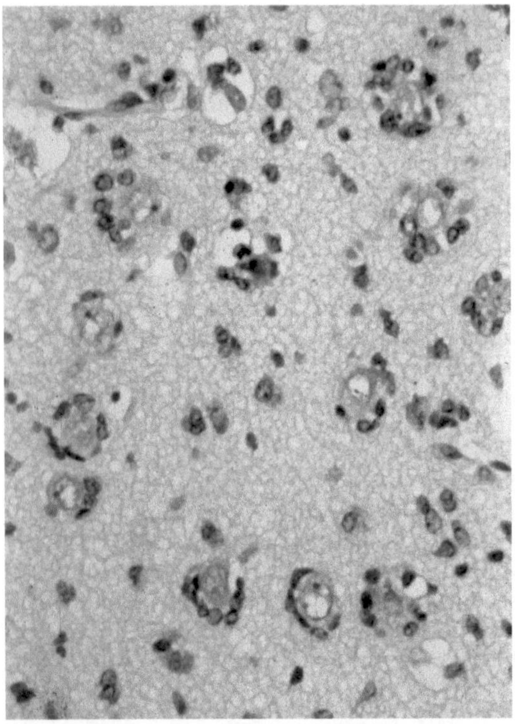

Fig. 3.7. Perineuronal satellitosis in an oligodendroglioma. NP7146, H&E.

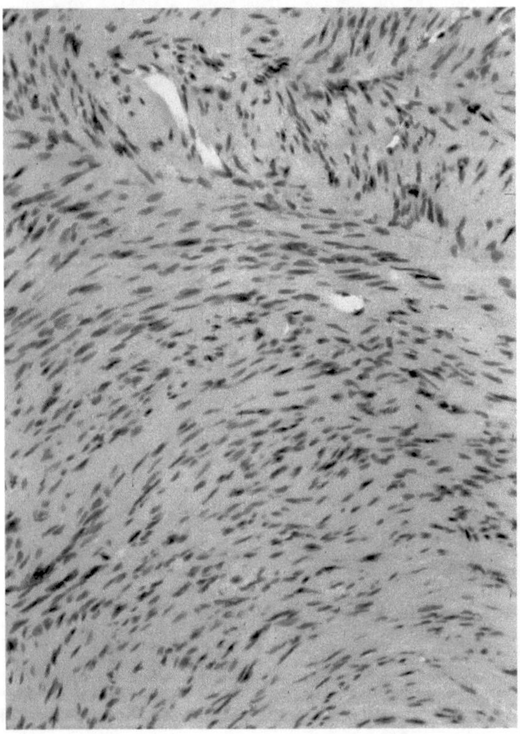

a

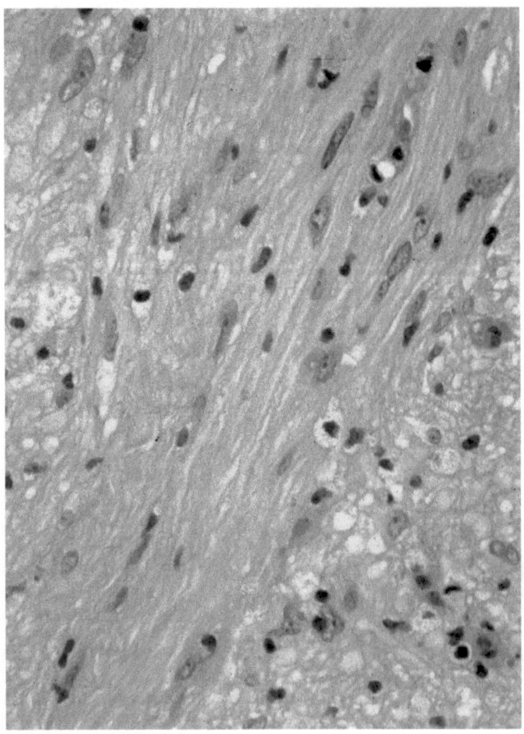

b

Fig. 3.8. a–b Streams or bundles of spindle cells typical of a schwannoma. NP16042, H&E. **a** Low magnification. **b** High magnification.

the nuclei of meningioma cells tend to be less spindle-shaped. In addition, streaming cells forming parallel rows with little interlacing can be seen in pilocytic astrocytomas, fibrillary astrocytomas and oligodendrogliomas.

Whorls, Loops, Onion-skin Pattern and Psammoma Bodies These patterns are characteristic of meningiomas in which there are concentric layers of tumor cells around a center, which may contain no structure or which may show a small blood vessel, a hyaline body or even a calcified granule. Psammoma bodies are calcified granules that are usually laminated and non-specific, unless one can see the whorling meningioma cells around them (Fig. 3.9a, b). Whorls can also be seen in schwannomas but they are not as distinctly outlined by a thin fibrous membrane as in meningiomas and tend to be larger with an indistinct border (Fig. 3.9c). Larger whorls may look more like oval loops. Cross-sections of neurofibromas may show a somewhat similar pattern, known as an "onion skin" or "onion bulb". These structures are more numerous and loosely spaced, typically with a demonstrable axon in the center of the onion bulb.

Nodular, Lobular and Alveolar Patterns Tumors consisting of nodules and lobules of various sizes are numerous. Small nodules and large lobules separated by thin fibrous membranes are typical of meningiomas, separated by capillaries or hypocellular gliotic tissue frequently in oligodendrogliomas and separated by connective tissue septa in pituitary adenomas. Similar lobular patterns are also seen in chordomas, chemodectomas, metastatic carcinomas and alveolar soft-part sarcomas. Alveolar and follicular patterns are more or less synonymous with a lobular pattern (Fig. 3.10).

Palisades and Pseudo-palisades Nuclei that form parallel rows are known as "nuclear palisades". Anuclear eosinophilic cytoplasmic bands between nuclear rows in a schwannoma are known as "Verocay bodies" (Fig. 3.11). The combination of nuclear palisades, Verocay's bodies and interlacing bundles of spindle-shaped cells (see Fig. 3.8) is relatively specific for schwannoma, although an almost identical pattern can be seen in occasional astrocytomas (bipolar spongioblastomas or "central schwannoma"). Palisading of nuclei can also occur in PNET, again as a clone of the rare primitive spongioblastoma. An area of coagulative necrosis surrounded by rows of nuclei is often called "pseudopalisading", more accurately called "perinecrotic palisading", and is often seen in glioblastoma multiforme. Adjacent areas of dense (Antoni A) and loose (Antoni B) tissue is typical of schwannoma (Fig. 3.11).

Rosettes and Pseudo-rosettes There are four types of these patterns: two types of true rosettes and two types of pseudo-rosettes. All show cells radiating around a center. One true rosette is an ependymal rosette that has a small or large lumen in the center, resembling the central canal of the spinal cord with cilia or blephaloplasts around the lumen (Fig. 3.12a). Such rosettes are found in some ependymomas (Fig. 3.12b). Another true rosette is composed of rods and cones and is seen in some retinoblastomas. One type of pseudo-rosette includes a blood vessel in the center, a perivascular pseudo-rosette (Fig. 3.13a, b), the cell processes from the surrounding cells tapering toward the vascular wall. These can be seen with H&E stain but more easily seen with van Gieson (VG) stain (Fig. 3.13c). Perivascular pseudo-rosettes are very common in ependymomas, and are much more common than true rosettes. When the center consists of anuclear eosinophilic cytoplasm (on H&E stain), it is known as a "Homer Wright pseudo-rosette", a pattern typical of neuroblasts growing in culture. They are found in some PNETs but more frequently in neuroblastomas (Fig. 3.14), central neurocytomas and pineocytomas. The eosinophilic amorphous areas tend to be larger and more irregular in pineocytomas and neuroblastomas.

Cartwheels and Perivascular Crowns Difficult to distinguish from perivascular pseudorosettes, a cartwheel formation has been described as characteristic of astroblastomas in which radially arranged tumor cells show cell feet attached to the vascular wall, whereas only tapering cytoplasmic processes are demonstrable in ependymomas. When no cellular processes are present around the blood vessel, the pattern is simply called a "perivascular crown", as seen in numerous types of tumors, including astrocytomas (Fig. 3.15), adenomas and carcinomas .

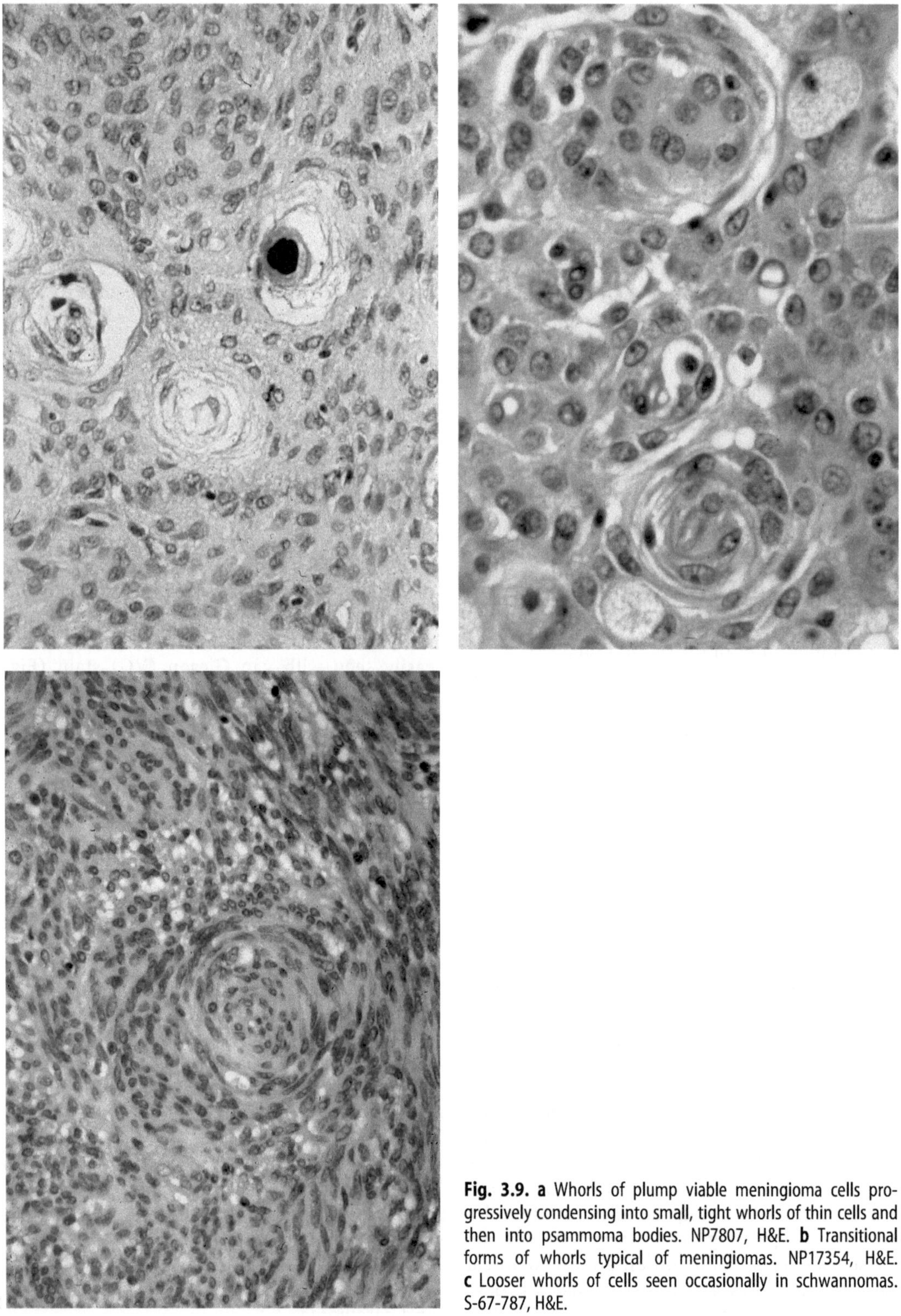

a b c

Fig. 3.9. **a** Whorls of plump viable meningioma cells progressively condensing into small, tight whorls of thin cells and then into psammoma bodies. NP7807, H&E. **b** Transitional forms of whorls typical of meningiomas. NP17354, H&E. **c** Looser whorls of cells seen occasionally in schwannomas. S-67-787, H&E.

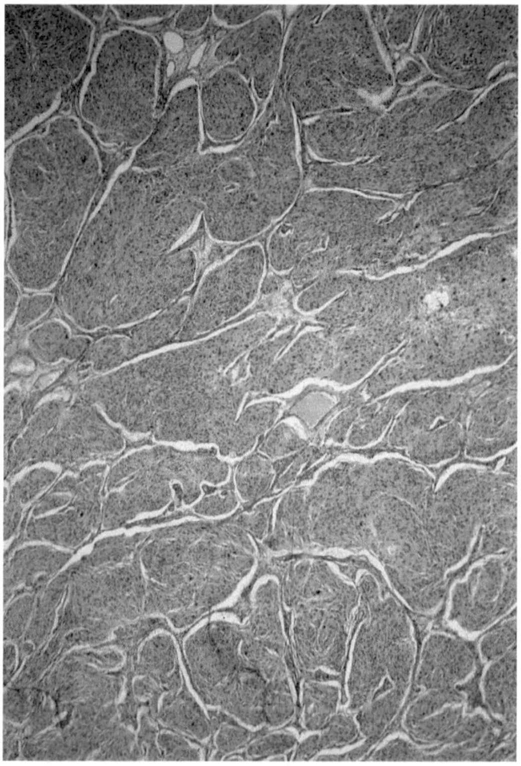

a

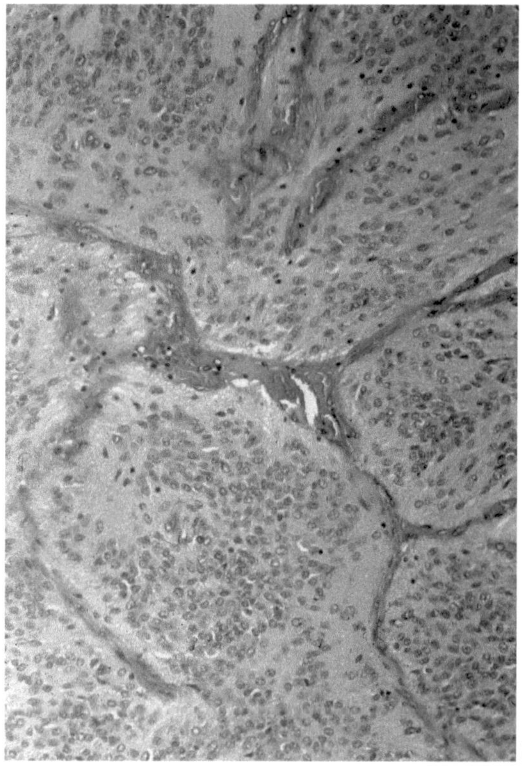

b

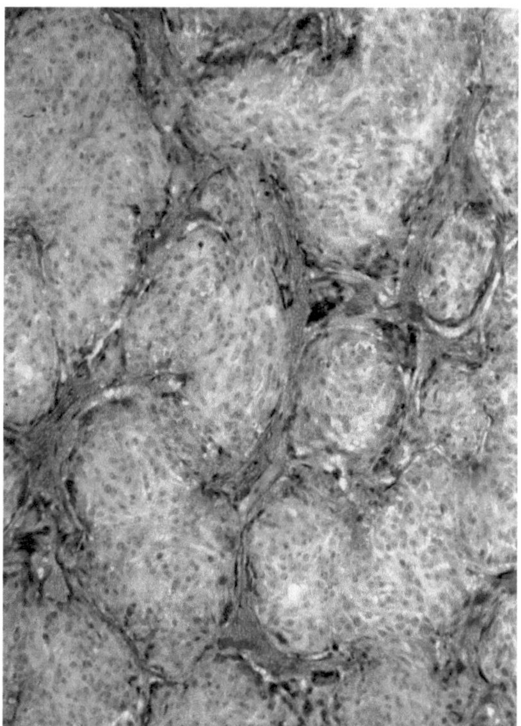

c

Fig. 3.10. a Lobular pattern in a meningioma. N90, H&E. **b** Lobular pattern in an oligodendroglioma produced by "chicken wire" pattern of thick capillaries. Note absence of the autolytic honeycomb pattern shown in Fig. 3.5b. NP10891, H&E. **c** Lobular pattern in a prolactinoma. NP7275, H&E.

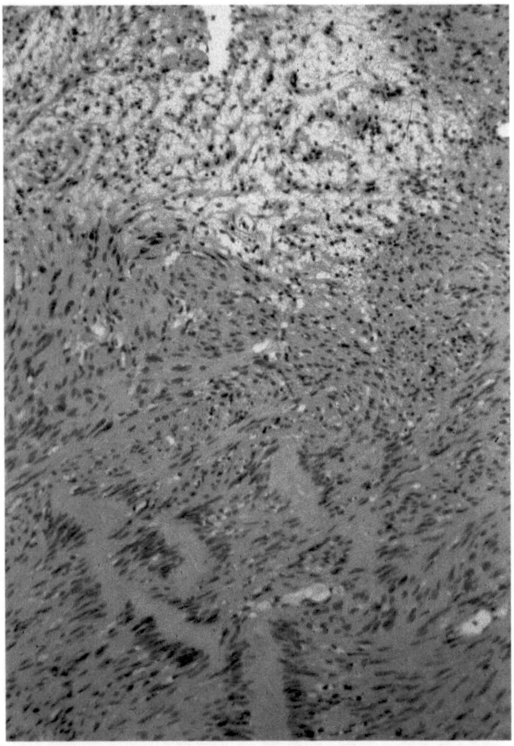

Fig. 3.11. Schwannoma showing nuclear palisades forming Verocay bodies in Antoni A (dense) region next to Antoni B (loose, foamy) region. NP15094, H&E.

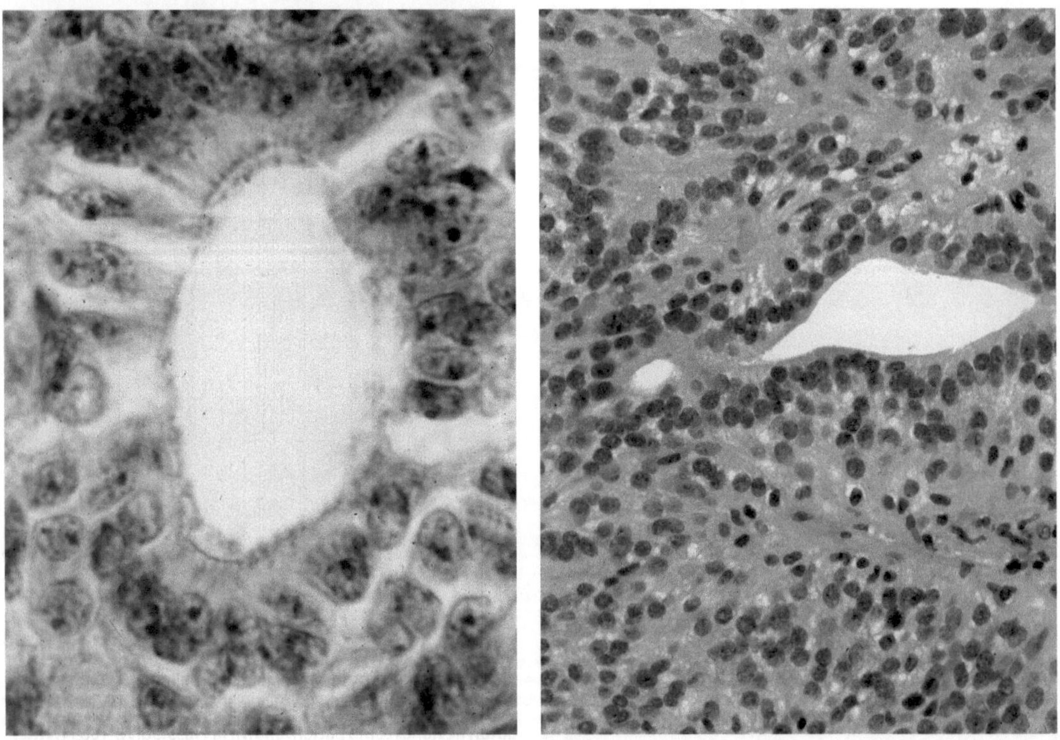

a b

Fig. 3.12. a–b True rosettes. **a** Normal ependymal canal and **b** ependymal rosette in an ependymoma. NP27902, H&E.

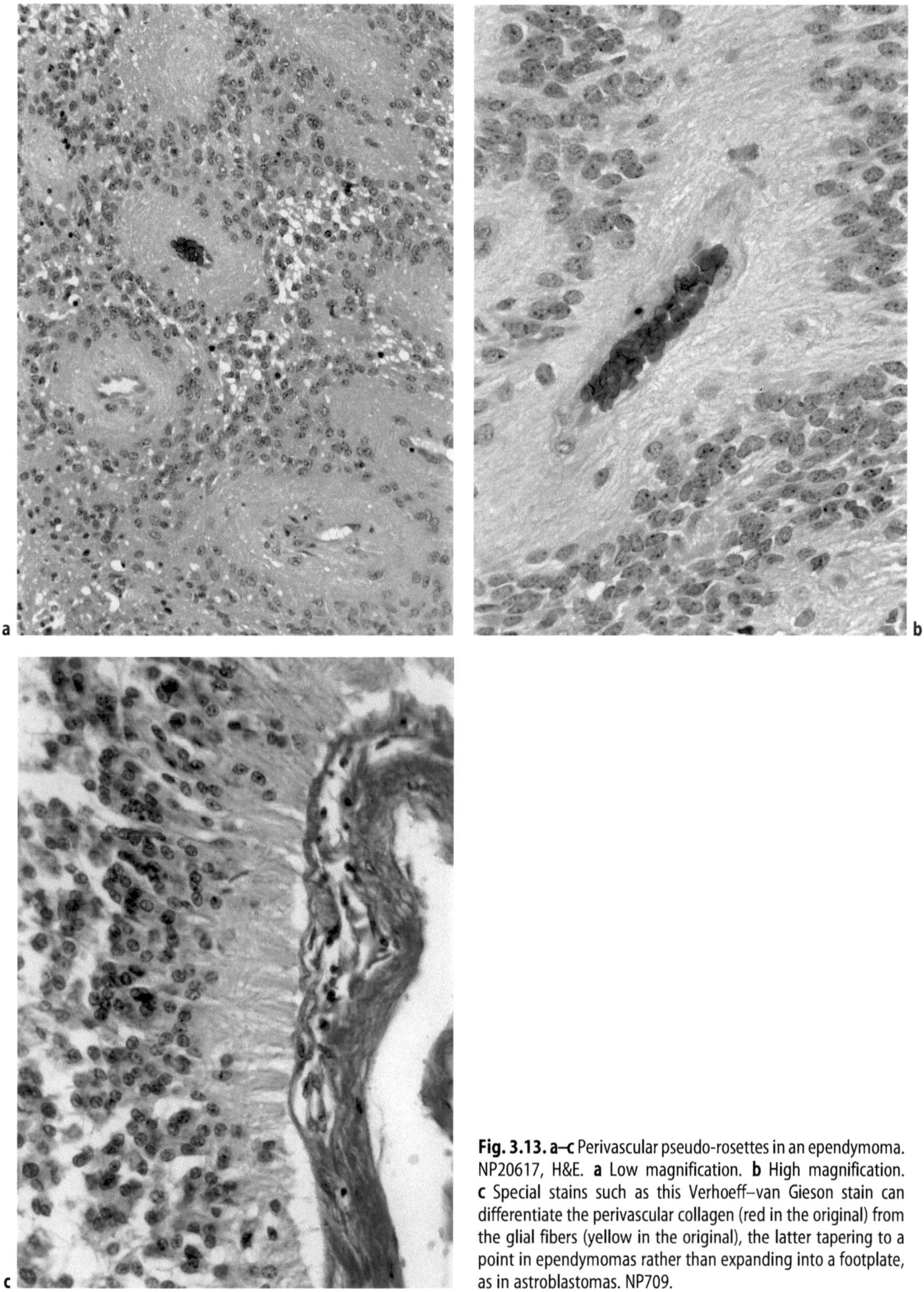

Fig. 3.13. a–c Perivascular pseudo-rosettes in an ependymoma. NP20617, H&E. **a** Low magnification. **b** High magnification. **c** Special stains such as this Verhoeff–van Gieson stain can differentiate the perivascular collagen (red in the original) from the glial fibers (yellow in the original), the latter tapering to a point in ependymomas rather than expanding into a footplate, as in astroblastomas. NP709.

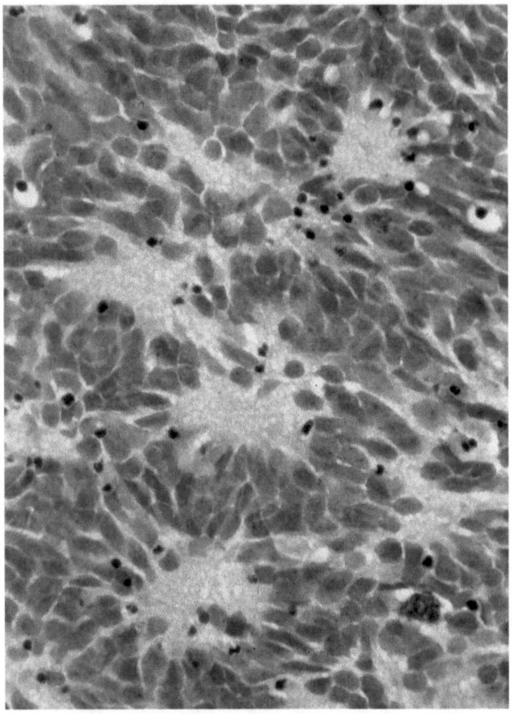

Fig. 3.14. Homer Wright neuroblastic pseudo-rosette in a medulloblastoma (cerebellar PNET). NP25458, H&E.

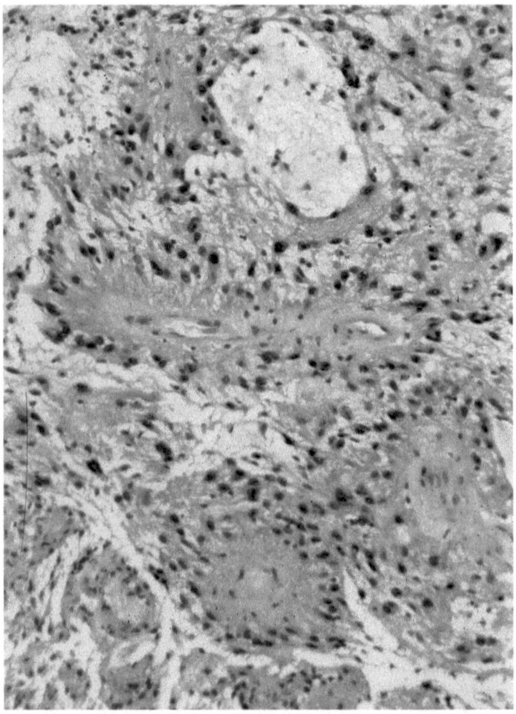

Fig. 3.15. Perivascular crowns in an astrocytoma. NP13936, H&E.

Papillae Papillae are finger-like processes of hyperplastic tumors, each process with a connective tissue stroma, usually with accompanying blood vessels, covered by epithelial cells. The best example is, of course, a choroid plexus papilloma but papillae can also be seen in ependymomas, pituitary adenomas, metastatic adenocarcinomas (Fig. 3.16) and in a rare form of meningiomas known as "papillary meningiomas".

Checkerboard and Lattice Formations This mosaic pattern with alternating dense fibrillary and loose hypocellular areas is typically found in pilocytic astrocytomas (Fig. 3.17a, b). The loose areas represent areas of mucinous degeneration and the beginning of cyst formation. Rosenthal fibers are usually found in the dense part. A similar pattern with tumor nodules partitioned by connective tissue septa is found in optic gliomas (Fig. 3.17c).

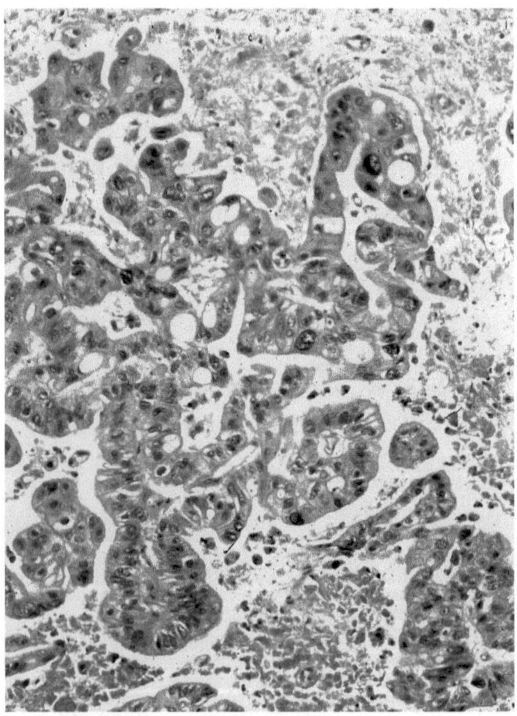

Fig. 3.16. Papillary adenocarcinoma. NP16375, H&E.

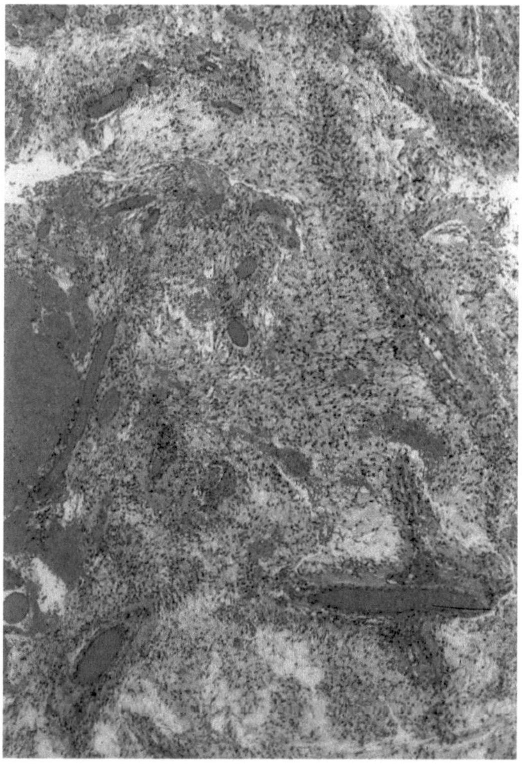
a

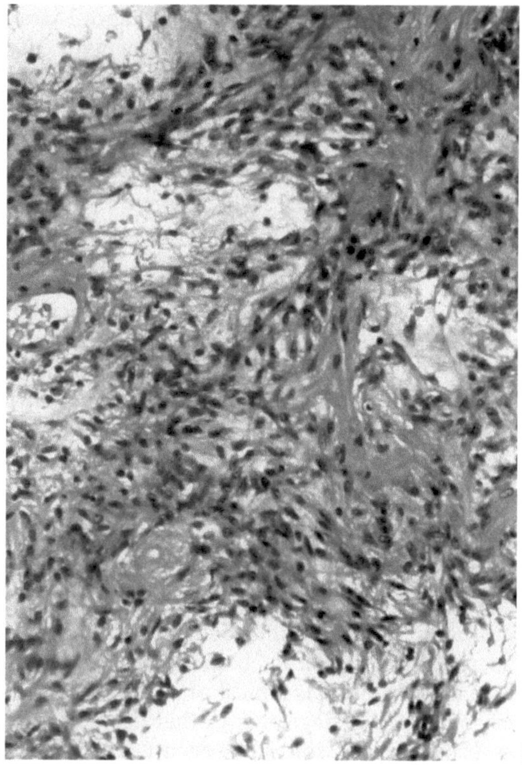
b

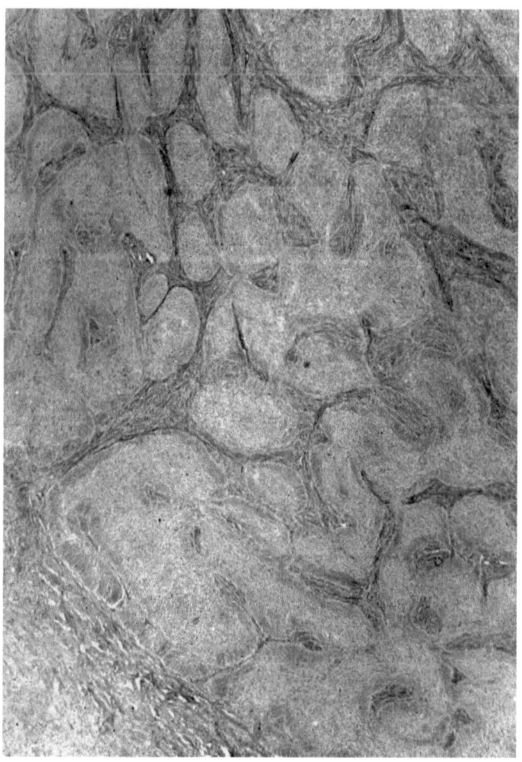
c

Fig. 3.17. a–c Lattice pattern in a pilocytic astrocytoma. NP14609, H&E. **a** Low magnification. **b** High magnification. **c** Septate pattern in an optic glioma. NP4260, H&E.

The various patterns described above are not necessarily specific for any one type of tumor but are useful in beginning to formulate a histological differential diagnosis. When combined with other findings, such as the morphology of the tumor cells and stromal and vascular changes, the particular pattern is very helpful.

Stromal Changes

In addition to the appearance of the principal cells, there are many ancillary changes that occur in tumor tissue. These changes again are not specific and diagnostic by themselves but are helpful in making a diagnosis, especially in determining the degree of anaplasia of the tumors.

Necrosis with or without Palisading Necrosis represents death of tissue. There are two types, liquefactive and coagulative, but most of the latter become liquefactive in time as macrophages digest it. Liquefactive necrosis from the beginning is typical of an abscess with pus, but the later stage of any other necrosis can be progressively soft and eventually liquid. Tumor necrosis and radiation necrosis tend to be coagulative with very little phagocytic activity. Necrosis due to infarction is initially coagulative, although grossly soft, but slowly becomes liquefactive with extensive phagocytosis to digest the dead tissue. Even when tumor necrosis is considered to be due to vascular occlusion within the tumor, the dead tumor tissue does not appear to attract many phagocytic cells. The presence of tumor necrosis with surrounding palisading is indicative of cellular proliferation without concomitant vascular and/or nutrient support and is, therefore, a sign of a rapidly growing tumor. The presence of necrosis is one of critical importance in the diagnosis of glioblastoma. The clinical correlate of necrosis in ependymomas and oligodendrogliomas is not as clear as in astrocytomas [9].

Radiation also induces coagulative necrosis, predominantly in the white matter, frequently almost identical to that of untreated glioblastomas. In cases of a re-operated tumor with a history of previous radiotherapy, it is practically impossible to distinguish the necrosis as being an inherent part of the tumor or secondary to radiation. Some emphasize the presence of pseudo-palisading around the necrosis as specific to tumor necrosis, but the absence is ambiguous since there may not be sufficient numbers of remaining tumor cells necessary to form palisades or their growth rate may have been slowed by the radiotherapy.

Mineralizations (Calcification, Ferrugination and Ossification) Calcification is found in relatively slow growing tumors, including meningiomas, oligodendrogliomas, gangliogliomas, craniopharyngiomas and astrocytomas, but it can also follow irradiation. It can be found in the parenchyma and adjacent cerebral tissue and in the blood vessel walls in oligodendrogliomas. In meningiomas, calcification may be present in the form of psammoma bodies, which may show concentric lamination, and in the form of more amorphous larger calcified masses. In craniopharyngiomas, teratomas, chordomas and dermoid cysts, the calcification appears as masses of various sizes. Scattered calcified granules within coagulative necrosis are typically seen in radiation necrosis.

Cyst Formation and Mucoid Degeneration A cyst is simply a fluid-filled closed cavity and tends to be found in slow-growing tumors. The fluid may be dark brown (so-called "motor oil"), watery (like CSF), xanthochromic of various degrees or hues, milky or mucinous depending on the amount of hemosiderin and protein present, and with or without cholesterol crystals in craniopharyngiomas. The cyst usually arises from liquefactive necrosis or mucoid degeneration of the tumor tissue. In oligodendrogliomas, pilocytic astrocytomas and chordomas, both mucoid degeneration and cyst formation may be present. A large, more or less solitary, cyst is typically found in hemangioblastomas and pilocytic astrocytomas that appear as a mural nodule. Numerous microcysts are common in oligodendrogliomas (Fig. 3.18) and astroblastomas as well as in pilocytic astrocytomas. Cysts in craniopharyngiomas or chordomas are variable in size. Cysts are uncommon in meningiomas and schwannomas and rare in PNETs and germinomas. Glioblastoma has been defined as a multiform glioma, so it should not be surprising to find foci of low-grade glioma with cysts and calcifications, not to forget cysts due to necrosis.

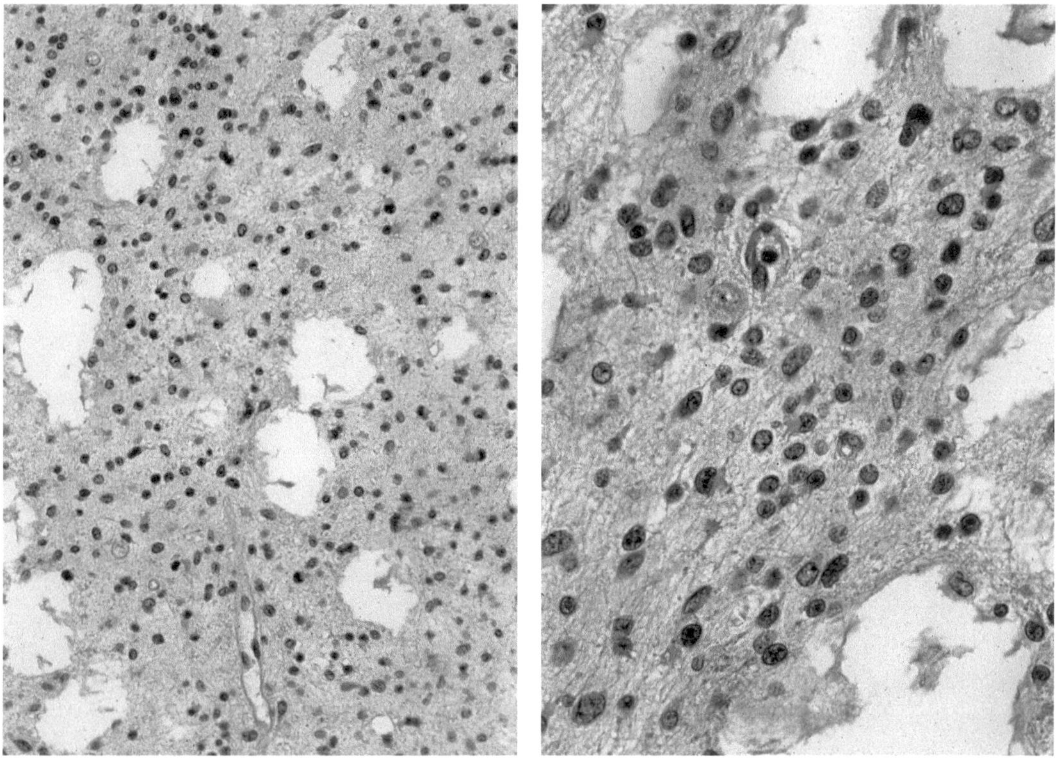
a b

Fig. 3.18. a–b Microcysts are frequently seen in oligodendrogliomas, usually owing to mucinous degeneration, as evidenced by the faintly stained contents. NP19529, H&E. **a** Low magnification. **b** High magnification.

Rosenthal Fibers, Cytoid Bodies and Eosinophilic Hyaline Bodies Eosinophilic hyaline bodies of variable shapes and thicknesses (commas, sausages or just thick bands) are known as "Rosenthal fibers". These structures are usually densely red with a mild purplish tinge and sometimes resemble columns of red blood cells. They are found typically in pilocytic astrocytomas and gliotic white matter surrounding craniopharyngiomas. The origin of Rosenthal fibers has been debated but they probably represent a degenerated form of glial fibers on which crystalline is deposited. They stain variably with GFAP but not so intensely as do the usual astrocytic fibers. Eosinophilic hyaline bodies, cytoid bodies and eosinophilic granular bodies are found in low-grade gliomas, such as pilocytic astrocytomas and oligodendrogliomas, but their origin has not been clarified.

Keratin (Dry Keratin) and Parakeratin (Wet Keratin) Multilaminated desquamated epithelial membranes appear as thin parallel lines to hexagonal plates, depending on the plane of section. They are known as "keratin" or "dry keratin" ("dandruff") and are typically seen in epidermoid and dermoid cysts (Fig. 3.19a), where the dehydrating pattern of maturation is to be expected on exposure to air. By contrast, dead, swollen, mucosal epithelium ("wet keratin", where the swelling represents maturation of cells exposed to moisture) appears as eosinophilic masses with pale membranous septa representing cell walls and ghosts of nuclei (Fig. 3.19b). Wet keratin is characteristic of craniopharyngiomas, which develop from Rathke's duct and nasopharyngeal mucosa.

Desmoplasia and Fibrosis Excessive fibrous connective tissue sometimes forms the stroma of tumors and at times divides tumors into numerous small nodules or cords. This phenomenon is seen especially when a tumor invades and infiltrates the leptomeninges, even

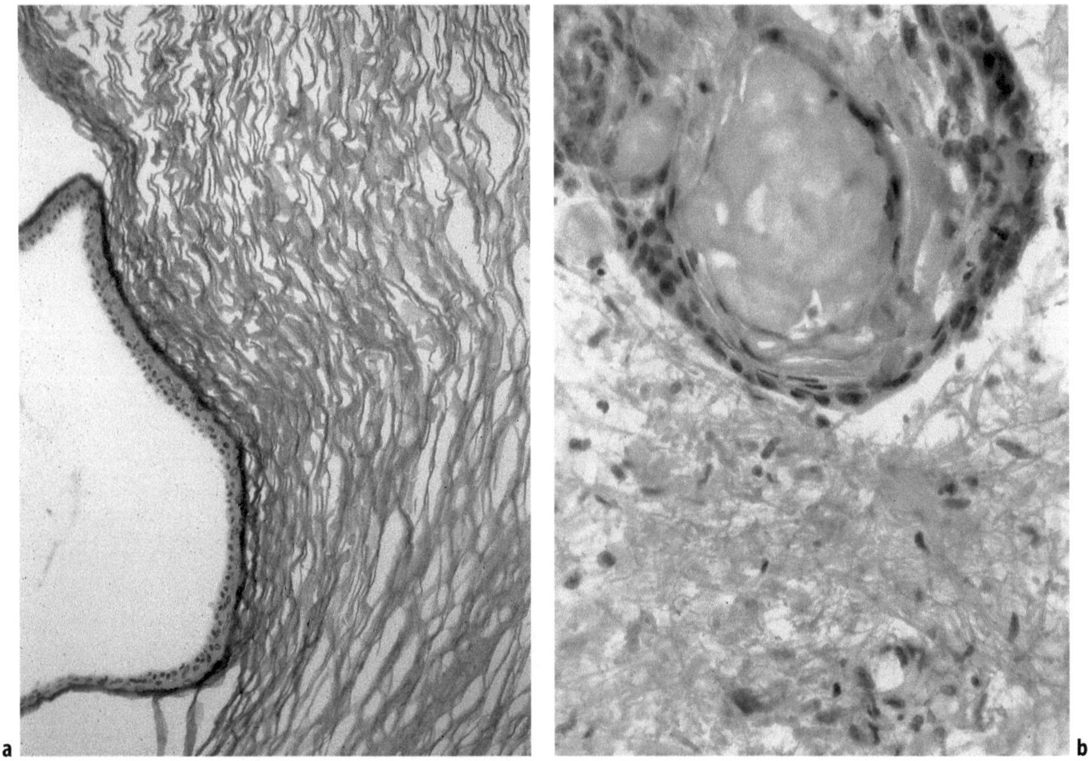

Fig. 3.19. a Dry keratin appears as parallel lines expanding into hexagonal plates depending on the plane of section. NP3880, H&E. b Wet keratin appears as swollen cells with ghosts of nuclei in a craniopharyngioma. NP-02-286, H&E.

more when it invades the dura, or when there is an excessive reaction in the connective tissue portion of the vascular components. Fibrous scar formation is almost always found in cases with previous surgical intervention. Irradiation also induces excessive proliferation of connective tissue. The differentiation from a sarcoma or a mixed glio-sarcoma is difficult unless one can demonstrate neoplastic features in the connective tissue, i.e. mitoses and numerous cycling nuclei in addition to the pleomorphism frequently seen in actively reacting fibrous tissue.

Terminology may be deleted with experience, and the "cerebellar sarcoma" – so diagnosed decades ago because of its rich fibrous connective tissue dividing the tumor into nodules (Fig. 3.20a) – is now known to be a desmoplastic medulloblastoma, but the prognosis remains the same with CSF metastases (Fig. 3.20b, c), just as in other medulloblastomas. Terminology also increases, of course, and both desmoplastic infantile ganglioglioma (DIG) and desmoplastic cerebral astrocytoma of infancy (DCAI) occur in the superficial cerebrum of infants, are rich in collagenous tissue, and tend to have a relatively favorable prognosis.

Inflammation Mild focal perivascular lymphocytic cuffs are common but non-specific in many gliomas and other tumors. Pre-operative diagnostic procedures such as angiography may contribute to a mild inflammation. Foci of neutrophilic reaction are occasionally seen in glioblastomas, causing differential diagnostic problems with other causes of necrosis or inflammation, especially when the specimen is inadequate. Lymphocytes of various types constitute the small cells of germinomas and become of diagnostic importance.

Hemorrhages, Old and Recent Evidences of recent and old hemorrhages may follow various treatments but also occur spontaneously in

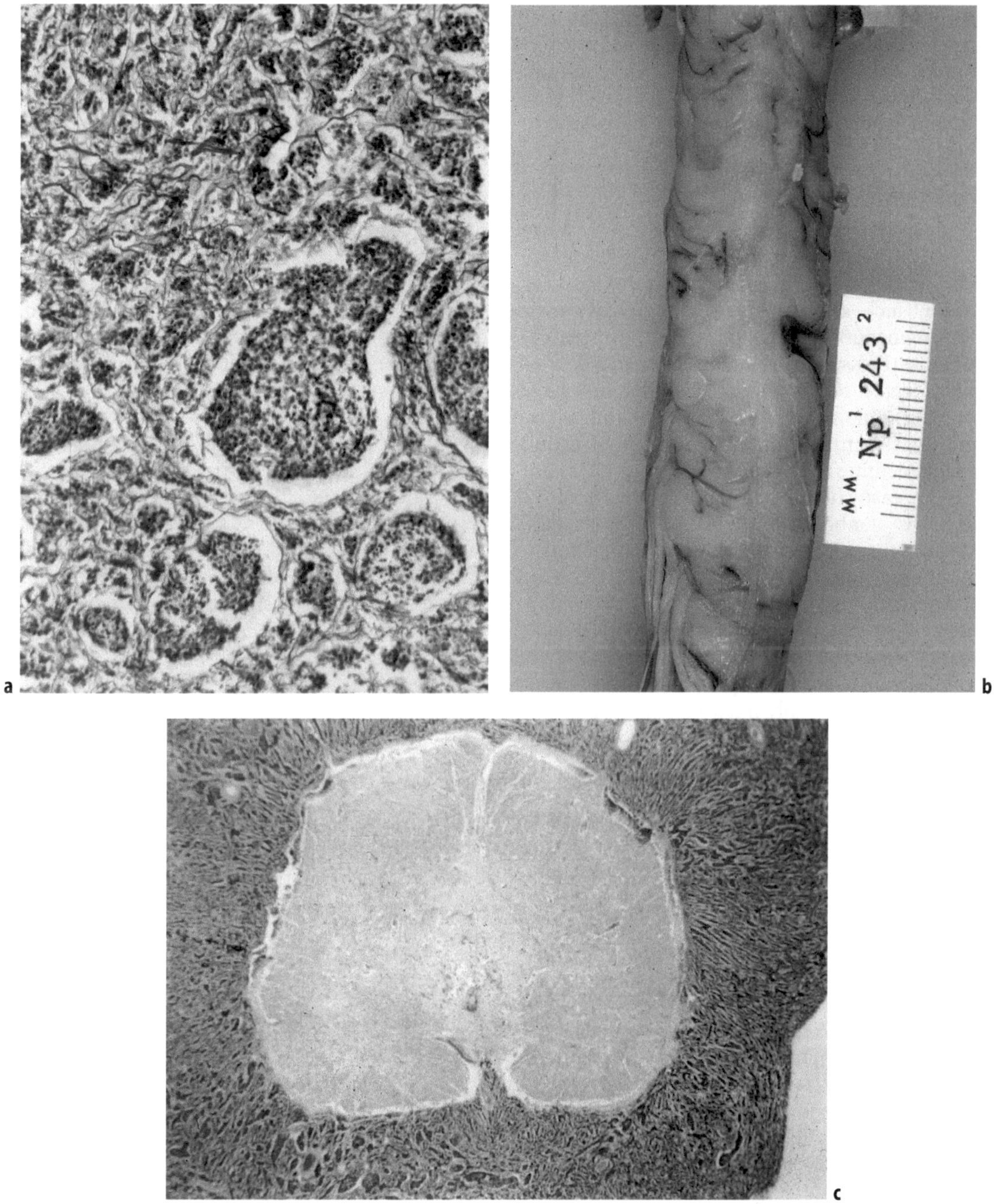

Fig. 3.20. a Medulloblastomas sometimes evoke so much connective tissue reaction as to suggest sarcoma (NP243, reticulin). **b** Although the posterior fossa was irradiated, the failure to appreciate that the tumor was really a medulloblastoma led to the patient's death by metastases through the CSF, surrounding the spinal cord. **c** gross. H&E.

many tumors characterized by hypervascularity: hemangioblastomas, meningiomas, schwannomas, oligodendrogliomas and ependymomas. Melanomas often bleed and the cells may contain both melanin and hemosiderin pigments.

Vascular Changes

In general, high-grade neoplasms are more vascular than low- grade ones, but there are many exceptions. Obviously, tumors of vascular origin, such as capillary hemangioblastomas, hemangioendotheliomas and hemangiopericytomas, are vascular by definition regardless of their degree of anaplasia. Meningiomas have long been known to be vascular, fed both intra- and extra-cranially, and their surgical resection was sometimes disastrous in the old days, but they are easily handled today with pre-operative selective embolization. Among metastatic neoplasms, melanomas, hepatomas and choriocarcinomas are well known to be vascular and to bleed easily. Ependymomas are inherently vascular as part of their perivascular pseudo-rosettes, but an avascular cellular ependymoma without perivascular pseudorosettes can be readily mistaken for an astrocytoma. Oligodendrogliomas can also be very vascular and have spontaneous intracerebral hemorrhages. Pilocytic astrocytomas and schwannomas often show focal areas of hypervascularity, usually markedly hyalinized, but occasionally even with capillary endothelial proliferation.

Capillary Endothelial Proliferation Excessive proliferation of capillary endothelium filling the lumen and/or extending externally to form glomerulus-like masses (Fig. 3.21) or chains is one of the common ancillary "proofs of malignancy" in glioblastomas. However, it is also common in oligodendrogliomas and the walls of cysts of any nature, and is occasionally found in pilocytic astrocytomas and schwannomas without affecting the grading or prognosis.

Telangiectasia and Angioma Formations Foci of telangiectasia and angioma formations are frequently found in high-grade glioblastomas and low-grade oligodendrogliomas, but are not useful as criteria for grading the neoplasm. Spontaneous hemorrhages most frequently occur in these tumors.

Capillary Networks Intersecting the Tumor into Lobules So-called "chicken-wire capillary networks" that intersect the tumor into multiple lobules are one of the characteristic architectural patterns of oligodendrogliomas (see Figs. 3.5b and 3.10b).

Sinusoidal Networks Intersecting the Tumor into Lobules The normal pituitary gland consists of small acini of cells of different types separated by connective tissue septa with sinusoidal vessels. The acini expand in adenomas to destroy the connective tissue septa but the basic pattern may remain, only with enlargement of the acini (see Fig. 3.10c).

Hyalinized Necrosis and Thrombosis of Blood Vessels Hyalinized necrosis of blood vessel walls and recent thrombosis, together with marked proliferation of abnormal blood vessels, including thin-walled and dilated veins and thick-walled fibrous blood vessels of indeterminate nature, may be at least as diagnostic of

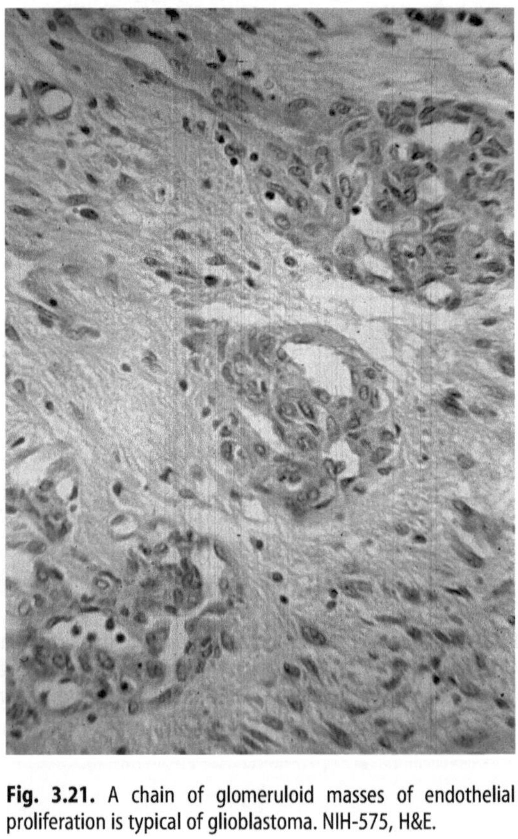

Fig. 3.21. A chain of glomeruloid masses of endothelial proliferation is typical of glioblastoma. NIH-575, H&E.

glioblastoma as the presence of necrosis. Tumor necrosis is most likely the result of these abnormal vascular channels with neovascularization, which inappropriately slows or shunts the blood flow away from the tumor.

Perivascular Fibrosis Perivascular fibrosis is very common and non-diagnostic. With multiple capillary channels it is characteristic of radiation, but it can be found in untreated glioblastomas as a "radio-mimetic effect".

If It Belongs to One of the Above Processes, Can You Narrow Your Diagnosis More Specifically as to the Type of Process?

In narrowing one's list of differential diagnoses, it is frequently necessary to consult textbooks and journals [4,5,6,7,8,10]. Pathology is largely a visual science, so that picture-matching becomes important!

Does Your Tentatively Final Pathological Diagnosis Make Sense Clinically and Anatomically?

There is rarely anything so satisfying as reaching the same diagnosis as did the clinician, both independently using different techniques inherent in each specialty. Even more satisfying is suggesting a better diagnosis that each can then independently confirm by further studies!

2. How Can One Understand the Changing Diagnostic Terminologies?

Time and space do not permit us to answer this question! The only safe method is to ask the other persons what terminology they are using and try to work out a mutually satisfactory translation! One may refer to books already in print on tumors [4,5,6,7,8] and other diseases [10], but one must remember that these were probably out of date before they were published! The classifications and terminologies on tumors are especially numerous, complicated and controversial, particularly when considering gliomas. The logical difficulties are circular: without knowing the histological variations, one cannot tabulate the biological variables. Even though there are some strange compromises that provoke continuing criticisms, the current World Health Organization's classification should be supported as an heroic attempt to standardize terminologies internationally – with all the inherent biases of international relations considered – since this approach is likely to be far more advantageous in the long run. In the mean time, a comment comparing other terminologies is frequently necessary.

As for the future, at least one of us believes that the ultimate resolution lies in actually measuring the growth rates and degree of infiltration to truly define high, intermediate or low grades and to suggest the probable degree of resection that should be attempted. The past behavior should predict the future at least sufficiently accurately to suggest when the next follow-up scans should be obtained and how frequently thereafter, thus providing some estimate of how effective the therapy has been in that particular patient [11,12]. Figure 3.22 illustrates the growth of the average diameter linearly with time, a pattern typical of infiltrating gliomas of low and high grade, the velocities differing by a factor of 10, each extreme being an average of +50%, as estimated by Woodward et al. [13]. By contrast, constant volume-doubling times are typical of the exponential growth of solid tumors (Fig. 3.23). Over short periods of time the proof of one mathematical formula or the other may be difficult clinically, but the difference over long periods of time is really quite striking (Fig. 3.23). The biological difference relates to the subclinical and more or less submicroscopic, invisible, infiltrating cells that convert the "edge" of the detectable tumor into a "travelling wave" that expands linearly with time rather than exponentially, as occurs if there is no external diffusion of cells.

When all is said and done, there are only a few gliomas that are susceptible to total resection: cerebellar astrocytomas and PXAs. In these cases, frozen section studies of the "margins" should be useful, and the surgeon should be tempted into resecting more than the gross may suggest, without, of course, increasing the patient's disability.

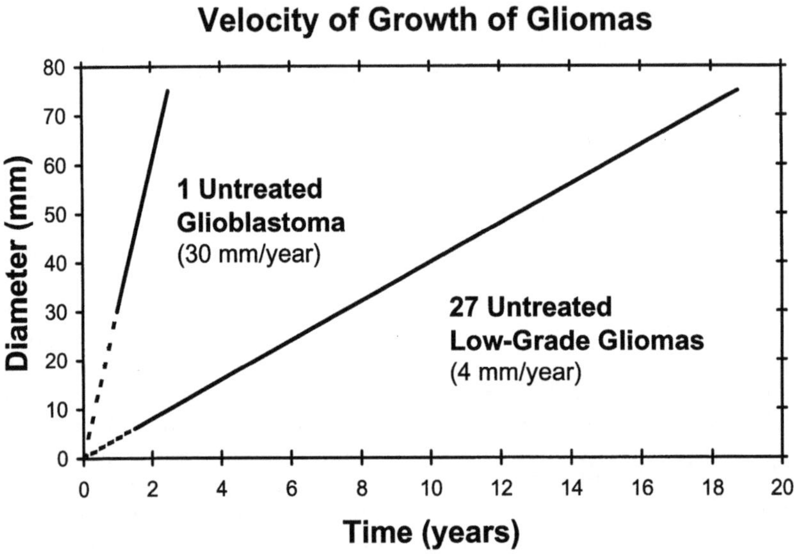

Fig. 3.22. Linear increase in diameter with time: about 4 mm/year as the average of 27 untreated low-grade gliomas (data from Mandonnet et al. [11]) and about 30 mm/year in an untreated glioblastoma (data from Swanson et al. [12]).

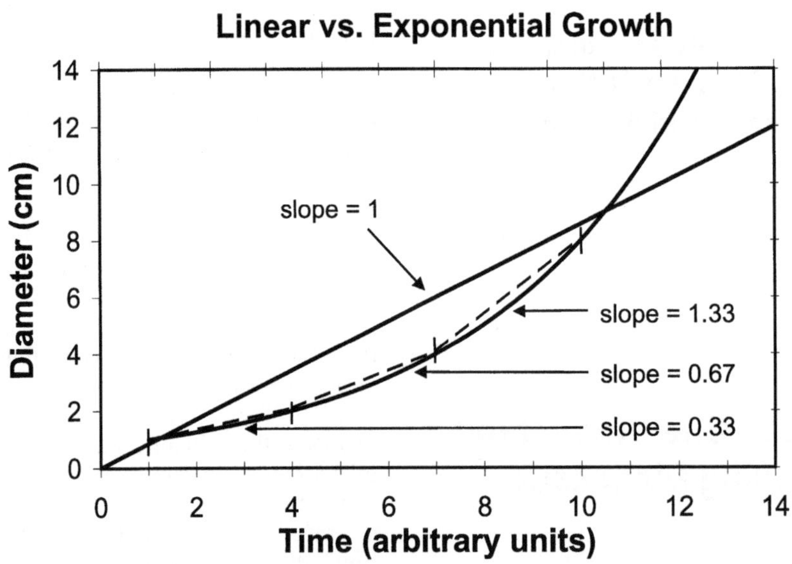

Fig. 3.23. Comparison of linear diametrical growth of infiltrating gliomas and constant volume-doubling time (exponential) growth of solid tumors over the clinically visible portion of most tumors. Time in arbitrary units: years for low-grade and months for high-grade tumors.

3. What are the Limitations of the Histopathological Diagnosis of Surgical Specimens?

The classification and definition of diseases can be purely academic but they also serve two practical purposes: namely interpersonal communication and prediction of a patient's outcome. If the terminologies of all diseases were standard and unified, a patient could carry that diagnosis to any physician anywhere in the world and all physicians would understand the significance of the condition and know the types of treatment that particular patient should receive. Obviously this is only the ideal. The reality is not that simple, as we all know. There are some common diseases that are familiar to most physicians. For instance, most physicians are familiar with meningiomas, which are common adult tumors, and know roughly what types of treatment are useful, even though they may not know that there are double digits of variants that may be descriptively added to the histological diagnosis. By contrast, there are many uncommon or relatively newly described conditions in which the diagnostic terms are not always precise, well established or standardized. Indeed, they are still being modified and changed from time to time as more is learned about their variations in appearance and behavior.

It is always interesting and usually helpful to know the historical transition of the concepts and changes in the terms of particular diseases but it is cumbersome and potentially confusing for neophytes. Thus, it is not uncommon to find many different or similar names given to the same condition. A new disease is usually found and defined by its discoverer. But with time, more cases are described with some variations, resulting in the modification of the definition and expansion of the diagnostic criteria until they overlap with other conditions. The borderlines between these different conditions become obscure. Consequently, arguments start as to whether they should be lumped together under one term or kept as separate entities based on some findings obtained by special diagnostic techniques. Under these conditions the diagnostic terms become ambiguous, even subjective, depending on the different training and experiences of various pathologists.

In addition, some classifications or divisions may be rather artificial, resulting in continuous debates. The best example is seen in the grading of gliomas. The line drawn between grades II and III is still controversial and one first needs to know whether the highest possible grade is grade III or IV! A similar argument concerns the reporting of the degree of cycling activity: Should one report the average (such as might be most accurately measured by flow-cytometry) or the highest percentage of cycling cells that one can find in a high-dry field? What degree of staining should one regard as "positive"? Should one actually count or just "eye-ball" it as a rough approximation? Satisfactory comments explaining the problems are required when reporting these types of results.

Another important role of diagnostic terms is to predict the outcome of a patient, so that both the physician and the patient know what to expect and what treatment would be best for the patient. The long-term outcome and the life expectancy of the average patient with a brain tumor are frequently compared with the pre-scan days, but these are not even a baseline for comparison with today's results since the clinical diagnostic criteria have changed so much. If there is advancement in the timing of diagnosis, say 4 years in the case of the usual oligodendroglioma [14], then there had better be an increase in survival of those same 4 years before improvement in treatment can be claimed! The Will Rogers' effect all over again!

Furthermore, we are making a diagnosis from the specimen that has been removed from the patient, but the outcome of the patient really depends on what remains in the patient's CNS. That variable, plus the variety of individualized treatments, makes it difficult to evaluate the results that are currently being continuously updated. How can one begin to define the histological features that characterize the malignancy of a particular type of neoplasm when one starts with subtotally resected tumors, the residual volumes not measured even if solid and not measurable if infiltrating? Even the most benign such tumor will "recur", i.e. continue to grow!

Contrary to the layman's belief that all answers are there on the slides when neuropathologists look through the powerful microscope with or without special stains and even with electron microscopy, there are many limitations to the histological diagnosis. Another problem is probably fixable: an accurate diagnosis depends on a good specimen. This problem is an everyday affair. A representative site, an adequate quantity and no artifact are three essential requisites from the supplier's side. Good technical and staining techniques are crucial from the preparer's side, to which inquisitive eyes and a brain connected to an effective searching machine containing an appropriate list of differential diagnoses is the final key!

References

1. Fulton J. Harvey Cushing. A biography. Springfield, Ill., Charles C. Thomas, 1946.
2. Bailey P, Cushing H. A classification of the tumors of the glioma group on a histogenetic basis with a correlation study of prognosis. Philadelphia, Lippincott, 1926.
3. Shaw CM, Alvord EC Jr. Congenital arachnoid cysts and their differential diagnosis. In: Vinken PJ, Bruyn GW, editors. Handbook of clinical neurology, vol 31: congenital malformations of the brain and skull, part II. Amsterdam: North-Holland Publishing Co, 1977; 75–135.
4. Zulch KJ. Brain tumors, their biology and pathology. Berlin Heidelberg New York: Springer, 1986.
5. Bigner DD, McLendon RE, Bruner JM. Russell & Rubinstein's pathology of tumors of the nervous system, 6th edn. London Sydney Auckland: Arnold; 1998.
6. Berger PC, Scheithauer BW. Atlas of tumor pathology (vol 10, Tumors of the central nervous system). Washington DC: AFIP, 1994.
7. Asa SL. Atlas of tumor pathology, vol 22: tumors of the pituitary gland. Washington DC: AFIP, 1998.
8. Scheithauer BW, Woodruff JM, Erlandson RA. Atlas of tumor pathology, vol 24: tumors of the peripheral nervous system. Washington DC: AFIP, 1999.
9. Alvord, EC Jr. Is necrosis helpful in the grading of gliomas? Editorial. J Neuropathol Exp Neurol 1992;51: 127–32.
10. Graham DI, Lantos PL (editors). Greenfield's neuropathology, 6th edn. London Sydney Auckland: Arnold, 2002.
11. Mandonnet E, Delattre JY, Tanguy ML, Swanson KR, Carpenter AF, Duffau H et al. Continuous growth of mean tumor diameter in a subset of WHO Grade II gliomas. Ann Neurol 2003;53:524–8.
12. Swanson KR, Alvord EC Jr, Murray JD. Virtual brain tumors (gliomas) enhance the reality of medical imaging and highlight inadequacies of current therapy. Br J Cancer 2002;86:14–18.
13. Woodward DE, Cook J, Tracqui P, Cruywagen GC, Murray JD, Alvord EC Jr. A mathematical model of glioma growth: the effect of extent of surgical resection. Cell Prolif 1996;29:269–88.
14. Mork SJ, Lindegaard K-F, Halvorsen TB, Lehmann EH, Solgaard T, Hatlevoli R et al. Oligodendroglioma: incidence and biological behavior in a defined population. J Neurosurg 1985;63:881–9.

II
Perioperative Care

4

Neuroanesthesia

Maryke Kraayenbrink and Gregory McAnulty

Summary

The basis of general anesthesia is to establish the "triad" of hypnosis, muscle relaxation and suppression of sympathetic reflexes. This, together with manipulation of mechanical ventilation, fluid therapy, temperature and the circulation by the use of anesthetic and vasoactive drugs, can produce the required operating conditions for complex neurosurgery.

Most intravenous anesthetics decrease cerebral metabolism and blood flow and tend to have a cerebral protective effect and decrease intracranial pressure. The inhalational agents are all cerebral vasodilators that can be offset by the induction of hypocapnia through to hyperventilation. The overall effect on cerebral blood flow (CBF) depends on a balance between the concentration of the inhalational agent and the degree of hyperventilation.

Moderate hyperventilation reduces CBF and brain volume. Extreme hyperventilation may be associated with critical reduction in flow to compromised areas and focal ischemia. It is likely that barbiturates offer some protection for the brain against ischemia, but there is evidence that mild hypothermia has a cerebral protective effect that exceeds that of the barbiturates and which is out of proportion to the degree to which the cerebral metabolic rate is lowered.

The induction of general anesthesia depresses normal protective reflexes, and patients are at risk of aspiration of gastric contents. Those with raised intracranial pressure or who have suffered recent trauma causing vomiting are at particular risk.

Manipulation of the blood pressure may facilitate some procedures (e.g. the induction of hypotension during aneurysm surgery). Patients must be appropriately monitored and the risks of the failure of normal autoregulation of the cerebral circulation in patients with cerebral vasospasm must be considered. Careful monitoring control of the arterial pressure is also required where there is potential for cord ischemia.

A significant number of patients suffer moderate or severe pain after craniotomy. Morphine appears to be a safe analgesic and is more effective than codeine in post-craniotomy patients.

Management of the multiply injured patient must initially focus upon the ABC (airway, breathing and circulation) of basic life support.

Introduction

Modern anesthetic drugs, improvements in monitoring, a better understanding of cardiovascular, respiratory and neurological physiology, and advances in intensive care medicine have all contributed to safer neuroanesthesia. It is probably true to say that the development of modern neurosurgery would not have been possible without the advances that have taken place in anesthesia.

Drugs in Neuroanesthesia (see Table 4.1)

The complex interplay between the effects of drugs and physiological variables, such as arterial carbon dioxide (CO_2) tension, body temperature and arterial blood pressure, during clinical neuroanesthesia makes the interpretation of experimental data from the use of particular drugs in isolation difficult. However, in most cases, the administration of a combination of agents, together with manipulation of mechanical ventilation, fluid therapy and temperature, will allow the anesthesiologist to produce the physiological conditions required for optimal surgery. The basis of general anesthesia is to establish the 'triad' of hypnosis (or amnesia), muscle relaxation and suppression of sympathetic reflexes (or analgesia). Each aspect of this triad may be achieved with a variety of drugs and, in order to minimize dose-dependent adverse effects, combinations of agents are generally used. Neuroanesthetic agents will therefore be discussed here under the headings of "sedatives/hypnotics" (including volatile anesthetics), "neuromuscular blocking drugs" (muscle relaxants) and "opioids" (analgesics).

Sedatives/Hypnotics

A diverse group of agents produce sedation at lower doses and hypnosis at higher doses. There is generally also a dose-related suppression of protective reflexes and automatic functions such as respiration and cardiovascular control. The drugs are usually grouped into intravenous and volatile agents. The volatile (or inhalational) agents are administered from a vaporizer via an anesthetic breathing circuit.

Intravenous agents include the barbiturates, propofol, benzodiazepines, etomidate and ketamine. With the exception of ketamine, all intravenous anesthetics decrease cerebral metabolism and blood flow and tend to have a cerebral protective effect and decrease intracranial pressure (ICP). Ketamine, in the spontaneously breathing patient, produces increased cerebral blood flow (CBF) and ICP, but may also have cerebral protective effects as an N-methyl-D-aspartate (NMDA) receptor inhibitor [1].

Unlike the intravenous agents, inhalational agents are all cerebral vasodilators that can be offset by hyperventilation to hypocarbia. They also decrease cerebral metabolism, leading to a coupled decrease in CBF. The overall effect on CBF depends on a balance between the concentration of the inhalational agent and the degree of hyperventilation [2,3]. In addition, nitrous oxide is frequently used in anesthesia of all types as an adjunct to other agents, allowing them to be used in lower doses. Its use in neuroanesthesia is controversial because it increases CBF and may increase ICP in susceptible patients [4]. This effect can also be offset by hyperventilation. Thus, while nitrous oxide has been extensively used in neuroanesthesia without apparent detrimental effect, it is probably prudent to avoid its use in the presence of decreased intracranial compliance.

Neuromuscular Blocking Drugs

Neuromuscular blocking drugs, or muscle relaxants, facilitate intubation of the trachea and mechanical ventilation of the lungs, and prevent movement during surgery. They are charged molecules that do not cross the blood–brain barrier, and so have no direct cerebral effects. However, they may indirectly influence the central nervous system via cardiovascular side-effects, histamine release and active metabolites. These drugs may be depolarizers or non-depolarizers, depending on their mechanism of action at the neuromuscular junction.

Depolarizing drugs (of which succinylcholine – Anectine – is now the only commonly used example) act very rapidly, have a short duration of action and produce excellent intubating conditions. Succinylcholine remains the drug of choice for rapid-sequence intubation to protect at-risk patients against aspiration of stomach contents. It produces initial muscle fasciculation and, frequently, post-anesthetic myalgia. A non-depolarizing-type block may be produced with repeated doses. Vagal stimulation may occur, inducing bradycardia and asystole. Serum potassium concentrations increase

Table 4.1. Drugs used in neuroanesthesia

Drug class	Examples	Beneficial effects	Adverse effects
Barbiturates	Pentobarbitone Methohexitone	Cerebral vasoconstriction (in normo- or hypocapnia) Decrease in $CMRO_2$ **Decrease in CBF** Decrease in ICP Isoelectric EEG with high doses of anticonvulsant	Respiratory depression Myocardial depression (potential for circulatory collapse in hypovolemia or with high doses) Enhanced seizure focus activity (methohexitone)
Isopropyl phenol	Propofol	Rapid recovery Appropriate for total intravenous anesthesia (TIVA) and prolonged sedation Decrease in $CMRO_2$ **Decrease in CBF** Decrease in ICP	Hypotension due to vasodilatation and cardiac depression (may compromise CPP)
Benzodiazepines	Diazepam Midazolam	Anxiolysis Anterograde amnesia Anticonvulsants Decrease in $CMRO_2$ Decrease in CBF Antagonist (flumazenil) available	Active metabolites (prolonged action in renal failure) Respiratory depression
Carboxylated imidazoles	**Etomidate**	Rapid recovery Hemodynamic stability Decrease in $CMRO_2$ Decrease in CBF	Suppression of adrenocortical axis
Phencyclidine derivatives	Ketamine	Analgesic at subhypnotic doses NMDA antagonist Respiratory and cardiovascular stimulation	Increase in CBF and ICP in non-ventilated patients Emergence of delirium and hallucinations
Volatile liquids			
Alkanes	Halothane	Non-irritant	Myocardial depression Cardiac arrhythmias Rare hepatotoxicity
Ethers	Enflurane	Non-irritant	Epileptiform paroxysmal spike EEG activity in high concentrations, accentuated by hypercapnia
	Isoflurane	Minimal metabolism Least cerebral vasodilatation Rapid induction and recovery	Irritant
	Desflurane	Very rapid induction and recovery	Irritant Hypotension Cerebral vasodilatation
	Sevoflurane	Non-irritant, ideal for inhalational induction Very rapid induction and recovery Cerebral pressure autoregulation maintained	
Muscle relaxants			
Depolarizers	Succinylcholine	Rapid onset and recovery Excellent relaxation	Occasional prolonged action May cause increase in ICP in patients with low intracranial compliance Potassium release, especially in burns patients and following denervation Arrhythmias

Table 4.1. continued

Drug class	Examples	Beneficial effects	Adverse effects
Non-depolarizers	Tubocurarine Gallamine Alcuronium Pancuronium Atracurium Vecuronium Doxacurium Mivacurium Pipecuronium Rocuronium	Flaccid paralysis without fasciculation Atracurium, vecuronium, doxacurium, mivacurium, pipecuronium, rocuronium with minimal cardiovascular side-effects Atracurium and mivacurium do not accumulate in renal failure Reversible with neostigmine	Tubocurarine: histamine release, ganglion blockade (hypotension) Gallamine: muscarinic blockade Pancuronium: sympathetic action, muscarinic blockade Atracurium: histamine release
Opioids			
Ultra-short-acting	Remifentanyl	Rapidly metabolized by plasma esterases, rapid termination of effect (minutes)	Depressant effect on blood pressure No residual analgesia
Short-acting	Alfentanil	Short duration (redistributed)	Hypotension ? Increases ICP
	Fentanyl	Short duration (redistributed)	Cardiovascular stability
	Sufentanil	Short duration (redistributed)	Cardiovascular stability (less than fentanyl)
Long-acting	Morphine	Lasting analgesia	Histamine release (hypotension) Active metabolites
	Codeine	Limited analgesic and respiratory effects	Wide variation in efficacy (genetic variation in demethylation ability)

$CMRO_2$, cerebral metabolic rate for oxygen; CBF, cerebral blood flow; ICP, intracranial pressure; CPP, cerebral perfusion pressure

owing to leakage of intracellular potassium. Where sodium–potassium channel populations increase (following burns, denervation, crush injury or tetanus), potassium release may be catastrophic. Approximately 1 : 3,000 of patients given succinylcholine fail to metabolize the drug normally. This may lead to prolonged (several hours) paralysis, the so-called "Anectine apnea". The effect of succinylcholine on ICP and CBF is controversial. There is evidence that succinylcholine can cause an increase in ICP in individuals with compromised intracranial compliance [5]. This may be because the increased muscle spindle activity resulting from fasciculation causes increased cerebral afferent input and increases CBF. Many different stimuli that affect CBF and ICP occur at the time of induction of anesthesia when succinylcholine is given, and it is likely that the effect of succinylcholine on ICP is relatively unimportant in the clinical setting. It can be abolished by pretreatment with a non-depolarizing neuromuscular blocker [6].

Non-depolarizing muscle relaxants competitively block the action of acetylcholine at the neuromuscular junction. They lead to a flaccid paralysis and can be displaced from the acetyl choline receptor by increasing the concentration of acetylcholine by the use of an anticholinesterase (neostigmine). Earlier introduced agents of this group have side-effects such as histamine release or sympathetic stimulation. Atracurium, cisatracurium and mivacurium are broken down to inactive metabolites in the plasma and can be used without prolonged effect in patients with renal failure [7].

Opioids

Drugs of this group are extensively used during neurosurgical anesthesia and for post-operative analgesia. If given in sufficiently large doses, all will cause unconsciousness; however, awareness and recall may occur in the absence of other anesthetics. All are respiratory depressants and, therefore, in the absence of artificial ventilation, can cause CO_2 retention leading to cerebral vasodilatation. All can cause muscle rigidity and some release histamine. The evidence concerning the effects of these drugs on cerebral hemodynamics and ICP is conflicting and depends on their cardiovascular effects as well as the background anesthetic.

The drugs act on specific opioid receptors and their effects can be reversed by specific antagonists. The drugs in this group differ in their onset and duration of action.

Shorter acting drugs fentanyl, alfentanil and sufentanil will allow rapid awakening at the end of the procedure. Remifentanil is an ultra-short-acting opioid. It is broken down in the plasma and can be given as an intravenous infusion [8]. Morphine and codeine are used for post-operative analgesia after neurosurgery.

Naloxone is a specific competitive antagonist that reverses the analgesia and respiratory depression caused by morphine and other opioids. It has no agonist activity. Its duration of action may be shorter than that of the opioid it is intended to reverse, and therefore repeated dosing may be necessary. Naloxone may have deleterious effects in neurosurgical patients, including increased CBF and cerebral metabolic rate (CMR), hypertension and rupture of intracranial aneurysms [9]. Naloxone has been shown to dramatically reverse the lateralizing deficits in patients with cerebral ischemia [10].

Clinical Neuroanesthesia

The selection of anesthetic drugs and techniques is planned so as to provide an optimal environment for the brain and good conditions for surgery, and will vary according to the patient's condition and the planned operation. There is no single correct "recipe" for neuroanesthesia and attention to detail is as important as the choice of drugs.

Pre-operative Assessment and Medication

In all cases, anesthetic care starts with a pre-operative visit and assessment by the anesthesiologist, who will be interested in the patient's general health, comorbidities, current medications and known allergies. For emergency cases, the time of last oral intake of food and fluids is important. The neurological status will be evaluated with particular regard to specific deficits, evidence of raised ICP, brainstem dysfunction and, in the case of cervical spine surgery, stability of the cervical spine.

Investigations will depend on the patient's age, medical condition and the proposed surgery, and institutions will have their own guidelines for investigations as well as for the amount of blood to be cross-matched before specific procedures. The perioperative management of coexisting diseases such as diabetes mellitus and ischemic heart disease is part of the anesthesiologist's responsibility, in consultation with other specialists.

Pre-operative medication is sometimes prescribed in order to provide anxiolysis and sedation, and a drying and vagolytic agent may also be given. Other drugs, such as beta-blockers, may be prescribed for specific indications. Sedative pre-medication is commonly a benzodiazepine or opioid, but sedatives should be used with caution in patients with evidence of raised ICP. Vagolytic drugs, such as atropine, glycopyrrolate and hyoscine, are given to dry oral secretions and to block undesirable vagal reflexes such as bradycardia. A drying agent is particularly important in patients who are to undergo fiberoptic intubation. Glycopyrrolate is preferable to atropine in neurosurgical patients, as it does not cause the same degree of tachycardia. Hyoscine causes sedation and can be associated with delayed recovery, making it unsuitable for craniotomy patients. It can be used before spinal surgery but is best avoided in older patients in whom it can cause post-operative confusion. In general, it is best for patients to take their usual medications, apart, perhaps, from diuretics, on the morning of surgery.

Guidelines for fasting before surgery aim to prevent pulmonary aspiration of gastric contents whilst avoiding dehydration from prolonged fasting. Fasting times of 2 hours for clear fluids, 4 hours for milk and 6 hours for solids have been shown to be safe in patients with normal gastric emptying. Those with raised ICP causing vomiting are at risk of dehydration and may require pre-operative intravenous fluids.

Induction of Anesthesia

Induction of anesthesia is a time when the patient is subjected to the action of several drugs and stimuli that have profound cardiovascular and respiratory effects. These need to be managed carefully in order to avoid adverse effects on intracranial dynamics; therefore good monitoring and venous access must be present from the outset. The aim is to prevent large swings in blood pressure and heart rate, to maintain good oxygenation at all times and to avoid hypercapnia.

The airway must be secured with an endotracheal tube for all intracranial and major spinal surgery. For some non-invasive investigations performed under anesthesia or for minor procedures, a laryngeal mask airway may be used. The endotracheal tube must be carefully positioned and very well secured, as access is difficult once surgery has started. Intubation is carried out after induction of anesthesia when relaxation has been achieved by muscle relaxants, except where there is an indication for awake intubation.

While the induction agents are generally cardiovascular depressants, and the blood pressure often falls on induction, laryngoscopy and intubation are stimulating and cause a rise in heart rate and blood pressure. It is essential to monitor the blood pressure closely throughout the whole period of induction and for the anesthesiologist to be prepared to intervene to treat hyper- or hypotension. A number of drugs have been recommended to obtund the hypertensive response. Commonly used drugs include a small increment of the induction agent, a short-acting opioid such as alfentanil or sufentanil, a short-acting beta-blocker, or lignocaine. There should be no attempts to intubate until muscle relaxation has been achieved in order to avoid coughing, with its attendant effect on ICP.

Some patients are difficult to intubate for anatomical or pathological reasons and special techniques may be needed. Awake fiberoptic intubation may be the preferred approach in such patients as well as for those with an unstable cervical spine.

Monitoring

Monitoring requirements will depend on the nature and extent of the planned surgery and the patient's condition. In all cases, there should be continuous monitoring of the electrocardiogram (ECG), blood pressure, pulse oximetry, inspired oxygen, expired CO_2 and anesthetic gas concentrations. Invasive blood pressure monitoring via an intra-arterial line is required for major intracranial and spinal surgery, but non-invasive blood pressure monitoring may be adequate for less extensive operations such as shunts, burr-hole biopsies and more minor spinal surgery where there is no risk of cord ischemia. The central venous pressure (CVP) should be monitored for vascular cases and where major blood loss is anticipated. More extensive cardiovascular monitoring, such as of pulmonary artery pressures, may be indicated by the patient's condition (e.g. severe ischemic heart disease), but is not routinely necessary. The core temperature should be monitored except in the shortest cases and can be recorded at several sites including the esophagus, where the temperature probe can be combined with an esophageal stethoscope. A peripheral nerve stimulator is mandatory in order to monitor the effects of the neuromuscular blocking drugs, as patient movement or coughing could be disastrous during neurosurgical operations.

For patients in the sitting position, precordial Doppler ultrasonography, transesophageal echocardiography and pulmonary artery pressure monitoring may be used to detect venous air embolism.

Positioning

The position of the patient depends on the site and nature of the surgery and the preference of the surgeon. Serious complications can occur as a result of careless positioning and, because neurosurgical operations may last for many hours, it is particularly important that patients are correctly positioned and pressure or traction on nerves and venous or arterial obstruction are avoided. Spinal cord damage can result from poor positioning and great care must be taken when moving the anesthetized patient with an unstable spine. Pressure on the eye can result in blindness.

Specific problems are associated with the use of the sitting position for operations in the posterior fossa and craniocervical region, including venous air embolism and postural hypotension [11]. Resuscitation may be difficult if cardiac arrest occurs in a patient in an unusual position, but a successful outcome is still possible [12].

Maintenance of Anesthesia

Anesthesia is maintained by inhalational agents or by an infusion of an intravenous agent such as propofol. Rapid awakening is desirable after neurosurgery to allow neurological assessment of the patient, and is best achieved with short-acting drugs. Opioid analgesics and muscle relaxants are given as needed and the patient's lungs are ventilated. Moderate hyperventilation is used for craniotomies in order to reduce CBF and brain volume, thereby providing good operating conditions. However, extreme hyperventilation may be associated with critical reduction in flow to compromised areas and focal ischemia, and is best avoided [13].

Mannitol, frusemide, steroids and CSF drainage can all be used to decrease brain swelling. In patients at risk of cerebral ischemia, mild hypothermia may be achieved by passive cooling. A core temperature of 34°C provides some degree of cerebral protection without exposing the patient to the risks of more severe hypothermia. Patients should be actively warmed to 36°C by the end of surgery if they are to be wakened and extubated.

Cardiovascular parameters are kept as near as possible to physiological in order to ensure good cerebral perfusion. Normovolemia is the ideal, with a hematocrit of about 30%. Normal saline is the intravenous fluid of choice and 5% dextrose should be avoided [14]. Occasionally, deliberate hypotension is indicated for surgical reasons.

In a number of centers, surgery that requires total circulatory arrest is undertaken. In order to minimize ischemic cerebral damage, this is accomplished after the establishment of profound hypothermia by femoral–femoral cardiopulmonary bypass. Barbiturates or propofol are administered beforehand.

Perioperative Brain Protection

The means by which it may be possible to protect the brain from ischemia are pharmacological or physical. Direct pharmacological interventions have focused on drugs that reduce the cerebral metabolic rate (and therefore reduce the demand for oxygen and energy substrate) and on agents that block the cellular mediators of ischemic injury (including calcium influx and the production of destructive protein kinases and free radicals). Physical means include the maintenance of an adequate cerebral perfusion pressure and arterial oxygen carriage and the optimizing of blood viscosity and temperature control.

With the exception of barbiturates [15], direct pharmacological brain protection has been, so far, disappointing. Traditionally, the dose of barbiturate is titrated to achieve burst suppression of the electroencephalogram (EEG). However, this has been questioned and there is evidence from animal studies that lower doses may be equally effective [16]. Barbiturates depress the myocardium, dilate arterioles and interfere with normal baroreflexes and sympathetic tone, and may induce cardiovascular collapse in patients who are hypovolemic or have already impaired cardiovascular systems. Careful monitoring is essential and circulatory support may be required particularly in patients receiving higher doses. The intravenous anesthetic agent propofol may achieve a similar degree of protection with better cardiovascular stability [17].

There is evidence that mild hypothermia has a cerebral protective effect that exceeds that of the barbiturates and which is out of proportion to the degree to which the cerebral metabolic rate is lowered [18]. Profound hypothermia during total circulatory arrest has been shown to be remarkably protective on gross measurement of outcome [19]. Animal studies suggest that prolonged periods of arrest (>70 min) may be associated with damage to Purkinje's cells of the cerebellum [20]; however, the technique may allow procedures to be performed that would be otherwise impossible.

Hypothermia has a number of adverse effects, including poor wound healing, increased susceptibility to infection, alterations in platelet function, changes in drug metabolism and increased oxygen consumption during rewarming. However, with mild hypothermia (brain temperature of 34°C) the benefits seem to outweigh the risks.

Action to increase the mean arterial pressure whilst temporary vascular clips are in place during clipping of cerebral aneurysms is advocated by many authors. Some evidence exists for a beneficial effect of judiciously timed application of hyperbaric oxygen in focal and global ischemia, but the treatment may itself induce oxygen-free radical formation [21].

Despite the many possible avenues for intervention in the face of impending, established or relieved cerebral ischemia, in clinical anesthetic practice, only barbiturates given in anticipation of focal ischemia, and hypothermia before and after focal or global cerebral ischemia, have been shown to be useful in humans [21].

Attention to cerebral perfusion pressure, avoidance of hyperthermia, appropriate levels of anesthesia and maintenance of normoglycemia are probably of greater overall importance.

Emergence

Towards the end of surgery, anesthetic agents are reduced and then discontinued. The residual neuromuscular block is reversed when the operation is finished and, when the patient is able to breathe and protect his airway; the tracheal tube is removed. As with induction, emergence from anesthesia is a time when hemodynamic instability can occur, and the awakening patient may cough on the tracheal tube. Specific medications may be needed to control the blood pressure at this time.

On occasion, immediate extubation is not desirable, for example when there have been serious intraoperative difficulties and the brain is swollen at the end of surgery, or if problems with the airway are anticipated. In such cases a decision may be made to keep the patient sedated and ventilated post-operatively for a period. Decisions of this kind should be made jointly by the anesthesiologist and surgeon. Patients who have had surgery in the posterior fossa or craniocervical region may have inadequate airway protective reflexes post-operatively and should not be extubated until airway reflexes have returned.

Recovery

Patients who have had major intracranial or spinal surgery should be cared for in a high-dependency area where they can receive intensive nursing care post-operatively. Frequent observations of cardiac and respiratory variables as well as neurological observations are mandatory for the early detection and treatment of complications such as bleeding. Post-operative nausea and vomiting are common after anesthesia and surgery, particularly posterior fossa surgery, and are multifactorial in origin [22]. Post-anesthetic shivering may occur, particularly after long operations, and is associated with a number of undesirable effects. Oxygen consumption, CO_2 production and metabolic rate may increase by up to 500% and it is not well tolerated by patients with cardiac or pulmonary disease. Patients should be actively warmed to a core temperature of 36°C. Surface warming with a hot-air mattress is very effective.

Post-operative Analgesia

It is now recognized that a significant number of patients suffer moderate or severe pain after craniotomy. There is a tendency to avoid morphine for post-operative analgesia in craniotomy patients for fear of respiratory depression leading to hypercapnia and excessive sedation and because it may interfere with the assessment of the size and reactivity of the pupils. However, morphine appears to be safe and provides more effective analgesia than codeine in post-craniotomy patients [23]. Patient-controlled analgesia (PCA) with morphine may be better for patients with normal levels of consciousness.

Non-steroidal anti-inflammatory drugs (NSAIDs) can be a useful adjunct for post-operative pain control. However, NSAIDs have some well-known adverse effects, including effects on platelet function and renal function, and may increase CBF [24]. Further studies comparing the efficacy and safety of different analgesic regimens in craniotomy patients are needed.

Neuroanesthesia for Specific Circumstances

Pediatric Neuroanesthesia

Induction of anesthesia in children can be intravenous or inhalational, depending on the child's preference. A smooth, calm induction with avoidance of crying and struggling is more important than which drug is used. Gaining venous access can be made more acceptable to the child by the prior application of local anesthetic preparations to the skin, such as eutectic mixture of local anesthetic ("Emla") cream or amethocaine gel. Maintenance of anesthesia is with controlled moderate hyperventilation, and many pediatric neuroanesthesiologists use nitrous oxide despite evidence that it is a significant cerebral vasodilator in children [25]. Muscle relaxants and analgesics are given as indicated. Good positioning is essential to avoid venous congestion, but positioning can be more difficult in small children as their relatively large heads and short necks can easily give rise to venous obstruction if the head is rotated.

Because of the relatively large size of the head in a child, significant blood loss is to be expected in craniotomies and excellent venous access is essential. Accurate estimation of blood loss can be difficult and the anesthesiologist may be aided by cardiovascular parameters such as heart rate, blood pressure, capillary refill time and core-peripheral temperature difference in maintaining normovolemia. Small children can become hypoglycemic during long procedures and blood glucose levels should be monitored during surgery.

Children, because they have a larger surface-area-to-weight ratio and less subcutaneous fat, can become significantly hypothermic during long operations unless active steps are taken to maintain body temperature. As with adults, the aim is for normo- or mild hypothermia. Hyperthermia is highly detrimental.

Midline posterior fossa tumors account for a significant proportion of brain tumors in children, and some pediatric neurosurgeons prefer to operate on them with the patient in a sitting position. This provides excellent operating conditions and is associated with decreased blood loss [11]. Venous air embolism (VAE) is a serious complication that must be detected and treated immediately. Nitrous oxide will equilibrate rapidly with the air bubbles and, being 30 times more soluble than nitrogen, will cause them to increase in size. If an air embolus is suspected, immediate attempts should be made to aspirate the air via a right atrial catheter. The surgeon should flood the wound with saline and the anesthesiologist should apply digital pressure to the jugular veins. This allows the site of the open vein or sinus to be identified and controlled.

Surgery for tumors in the floor of the fourth ventricle can be associated with cardiovascular instability, usually bradycardia and hypertension, owing to surgical interference with vital areas in the brainstem. This may also lead to bulbar problems post-operatively and such children may need prolonged intubation.

Craniofacial surgery often involves children who have difficult airways, and special techniques and expertise may be needed to gain control of the airway. These operations are frequently prolonged and major blood loss is likely. Post-operatively the airway may be in jeopardy from local edema and it may be safer to keep the child intubated and ventilated until the swelling has abated.

Children who are awake, warm and breathing well with no airway problems can be extubated at the end of surgery.

Sedation

Children may require sedation for procedures that adults are able to tolerate without sedation. Proper supervision and monitoring are essential for the safe provision of sedation to children whether they are under the care of anesthesiologists or other medical personnel.

The aim should be for conscious sedation. However, it is important to realize that the child may lapse into deep sedation once the stimulus of the procedure stops or if drug absorption is delayed. Because of the possibility of respiratory and cardiovascular depression with deeper levels of sedation, it is essential that the attending personnel are trained in life-support techniques and that full resuscitation equipment is immediately available. Pulse oximetry should be monitored as the minimum and should be continued until the child has recovered completely.

Children must be adequately assessed before receiving sedation and the fasting guidelines used for general anesthesia apply equally to patients undergoing sedation. The presence of a parent or carer can often give great comfort to a child undergoing medical procedures. Where procedures are expected to be painful, local anesthetics or analgesics, used as adjuncts, may reduce the necessity for increasing the level of sedation. Drugs commonly used in pediatric sedation include benzodiazepines, opioids, chloral hydrate, ketamine and trimeprazine.

Anesthesia for Neuroradiology and Magnetic Resonance Imaging (MRI)

Absolute patient immobility is often necessary for high-quality images to be obtained in neuroradiology and, as these procedures are often prolonged and uncomfortable, general anesthesia or sedation may be needed. Additional factors reducing patient acceptability of the MRI scanner are claustrophobia and the loud noise during scanning. Patients who need anesthesia or sedation include infants and children and confused or mentally ill adults. Unconscious or critically ill patients will need airway protection and ventilatory and cardiovascular support.

Procedures for which anesthesia may be required include computerized axial tomography (CAT scan), myelography, angiography and interventional radiology. The X-ray department is sometimes considered to be a hostile environment for anesthesia, and patient access may be limited, but exactly the same standards of monitoring and patient care are needed as in the operating room.

The requirements for anesthesia are similar to those for neurosurgery and include avoidance of fluctuations in heart rate and blood pressure, prevention of hypoxia, hypercapnia and raised venous pressure, and rapid recovery to allow for early neurological assessment. In many cases the laryngeal mask airway can be used to maintain the airway and avoid the need for intubation. Angiography in adults under local anesthesia with sedation may provide greater cardiovascular stability than with general anesthesia [26].

Many conditions are now treated by interventional neuroradiology, including arteriovenous malformations (AVMs), vascular tumors and aneurysms. Sometimes frequent neurological assessment is needed during the procedure, e.g. during embolization of AVMs. The patient needs to be awake and able to cooperate with testing but can be sedated for comfort between assessments. Propofol, with its rapid onset and offset of action, is ideal for this purpose. Sedation of this kind should be administered by an anesthesiologist as respiratory depression and even apnea can easily ensue. Adequate monitoring must be used, including pulse oximetry, ECG and blood pressure monitoring, and supplemental oxygen should be available. Equipment and drugs to support the airway, breathing and cardiovascular system must be readily available.

Endovascular obliteration of aneurysm sacs through superselective catheters placed during angiography is an increasingly popular alternative method of treatment to surgical clipping. The procedure can be prolonged in particular with large aneurysms and, as there is less need for patient assessment during the procedure, general anesthesia is often used for patient comfort.

The strong magnetic field of an MRI scanner can interfere with monitoring and anesthetic equipment. At the same time the equipment can cause degradation of the nuclear magnetic signals, leading to poor-quality images. Because of the strength of the magnetic field, ferromagnetic objects can become dangerous missiles in close proximity to the scanner and must be excluded or adequately secured. Special non-ferromagnetic equipment is available but adds significantly to the cost. Metal objects distort the field and result in poor image quality, and can also heat up and cause burns when subjected to radiofrequency electromagnetic fields. Reliable and accurate monitoring is essential in the MRI scanner as the patient cannot be easily seen and is remote from the anesthesiologist. Artifacts can be induced in the ECG by the radiofrequency currents but can be minimized by the use of shielded cables, telemetry or fiberoptics. ECG electrodes must be non-magnetic and should be place carefully to reduce artifacts. Shielded MRI-compatible oximeters are available. Good airway control is important, as the anesthesiologist is not easily able to intervene if airway obstruction develops during the scan. The laryngeal mask airway is ideal for this purpose.

Anesthesia for Posterior Fossa Surgery

Interference with the cardiorespiratory centers in the brainstem can result in cardiovascular instability during surgery and in airway and breathing problems post-operatively. Pressure on the nucleus of the vagus results in profound bradycardia, even cardiac standstill, and other cardiac arrhythmias and hypertension can be caused by brainstem manipulation. Vigilance by the anesthesiologist and close cooperation between surgeon and anesthesiologist are essential.

Respiratory complications can occasionally result from interference with the respiratory centers, giving rise to impaired respiratory drive post-operatively. More commonly, edema around the lower cranial nerve nuclei results in inadequate airway protection with respiratory obstruction, difficulty in swallowing and pulmonary aspiration. As a result, patients occasionally need to remain intubated post-operatively and a few need prolonged respiratory support.

Anesthesia for Aneurysm Surgery

During induction of anesthesia, intubation and the placement of the pin head rest, meticulous attention to the patient's hemodynamics is essential. Mean arterial pressure is the critical determinant of cerebral perfusion but systolic arterial pressure is probably more important in determining the wall stress and tendency to rupture in a cerebral aneurysm [27].

Induced hypotension may be used during aneurysm surgery to reduce aneurysm wall tension and operative bleeding. However, it must be used with caution as autoregulation is disrupted in patients with cerebral vasospasm. Measurement of jugular bulb oxygen saturation can help to determine the minimum level of mean arterial pressure that should be allowed [28]. Vasodilating drugs are used to induce hypotension (isoflurane, sodium nitroprusside, phentolamine), frequently in combination with a beta-adrenergic receptor blocker. Careful monitoring is required and drugs that have a relatively short half-life are preferred to allow restoration of normal perfusion pressures as soon as possible once control has been gained. The advent of temporary aneurysm clips has lessened the requirement for hypotension during clipping of cerebral aneurysms and may result in better patient outcomes. Cerebral vasospasm is less of a problem when AVM is the cause of subarachnoid hemorrhage; therefore induced hypotension can more safely be used during excision of AVM where it may reduce bleeding and the need for blood transfusion.

The surgical exposure of the vessels at the base of the brain by retraction of brain tissue can be aided by positioning of the patient, withdrawal of CSF and dehydration with diuretics. The use of induced hypocapnia by hyperventilation is controversial in aneurysm patients as it may enhance vasoconstriction in those with cerebral vasospasm. It is probably safe to use mild hyperventilation, but in the presence of induced hypotension, normocapnia should be maintained.

Anesthesia and the Cervical Spine

Several anesthetic problems may occur during cervical spine surgery. The pathology for which the patient is receiving surgical treatment may, in itself, render normal techniques for securing the airway difficult or hazardous to the patient. For the anesthesiologist, access to the airway and the tracheal tube is difficult once surgery has started, so the possibility of tube dislodgment or disconnection from the breathing circuit is a real hazard. Trauma to, or ischemia of, the cervical cord or damage to the phrenic nerves may lead to respiratory paralysis or severe compromise post-operatively. Partial or complete airway obstruction may occur post-operatively as a result of edema of the tissues of the airway, recurrent laryngeal nerve palsy, or hemorrhage into the neck.

Many conditions are associated with restricted movement or instability of the cervical spine. The list includes: degenerative osteoarthritis and spinal canal stenosis, ankylosing spondylosis, Down's syndrome, Klippel–Feil syndrome, Arnold–Chiari malformation, other congenital malformations such as dwarfism, type IV Ehlers–Danlos syndrome, metastatic lesions, osteomyelitis and rheumatoid arthritis, as well as trauma with demonstrated or suspected cervical spine injury.

Induction of anesthesia and intubation results in the loss of protective muscle tone as well as the potential for flexion and extension greater than that which would be tolerated by the awake patient. The cervical cord may be at risk if there is a tight stenosis or potential for subluxation from either movement or a fall in the perfusion pressure of the neural tissue owing to hypotension. Potential for cord injury dictates careful immobilization during manipulations to secure the airway and will frequently require special techniques and monitoring. Fixed cervical vertebrae may make conventional intubation very difficult or impossible because conventional laryngoscopy requires a certain amount of flexion of the neck and extension of the head. Awake intubation (most usually with a flexible fiberoptic bronchoscope) may be the safest option in many cases where there is potential risk to the cord or where a secure airway cannot be obtained conventionally. This is carried out with intravenous sedation and local anesthesia of the airway.

Careful control of the arterial pressure during induction and maintenance of anesthesia is clearly critical when there is potential for cord ischemia in order to ensure maintenance of an adequate cord perfusion pressure. Good communication and cooperation between the anesthesiologist and the surgical team is essential during patient transfer and positioning, particularly if the patient is to be turned prone.

At completion of surgery, patients are usually extubated upon return of protective reflexes. However, if there is a risk of upper airway obstruction, for example after transoral procedures, the safest option is elective ventilation with sedation in the intensive care unit until the danger of post-extubation obstruction is past. Emergency re-intubation of patients who have developed upper airway obstruction after cervical spine fixation may be extremely difficult, particularly if the neck has been immobilized in a device that interferes with access and vision. Efforts to maintain oxygenation may result in undesired movement of the unstable neck and damage to the cord. It is therefore imperative that the patient is able to maintain a safe airway before extubation, and in some cases an elective tracheostomy performed at the time of surgery may be advisable.

Post-operative hematoma formation in the neck, although fortunately rare, can severely compromise the airway. Not only does the hematoma compress and distort the airway; it may interfere with venous and lymphatic drainage, resulting in edema of the airway. Decompression of the hematoma may not relieve the obstruction if there is significant airway edema, and re-intubation may be required but may be very difficult due to distortion and swelling of the tissues. A high morbidity may be associated with such cases [29]. Because of the danger of airway obstruction, all patients who have had cervical surgery should be cared for in a high-dependency environment with close nursing supervision and frequent monitoring. Those who have had extensive procedures will need full intensive care.

Emergency Neuroanesthesia

Neurosurgical patients who require emergency anesthetic intervention fall into two groups. There are those who present with, or who have suffered an acute deterioration of, a condition of the brain or spinal cord. These patients may have compromised ventilation or other system failure as a consequence of their primary disease. They have the potential for aspiration of stomach contents if they have lost protective airway reflexes or if they are anesthetized without specific measures to prevent regurgitation. They may be hemodynamically unstable because of dehydration, sepsis or interference with autonomic reflexes. They may have specific effects of a disease process that affects a number of organ systems (e.g. rheumatoid disease, metastatic carcinoma).

The other group of neurosurgical patients are victims of trauma in whom neurological damage may be only one of a number of life- or limb-threatening conditions. In these patients there may be several injuries that compete for intervention, but appropriate management of one may be detrimental to the management of others. A methodical and coordinated approach will minimize the risk of missing serious injuries and will treat life-threatening injuries in appropriate order of priority. Management of the multiply injured patient must initially focus upon the ABC (airway, breathing and circulation) of basic life support. Implicit in management of the airway is avoidance of unnecessary movement of a potentially unstable cervical spine. However, hypoxia and aspiration of gastric contents into the lungs are more certain killers than theoretical cervical instability. Aggressive management to maintain cerebral perfusion pressure in these patients appears to be associated with improved outcome [30]. Novel therapies that may decrease secondary injury may have a place in the future.

Anesthesia for Awake Craniotomy

In these procedures the patient is required to be responsive and cooperative so that immediate assessment of the function of areas such as the motor cortex or speech areas can be made during resection of tissue close to, or involving, these areas. However, until the brain tissue is exposed and after the intended resection is completed, sedation or anesthesia can be administered to improve patient acceptability during such phases of the procedure as scalp incision, drilling of the skull, fashioning of the bone flap and closure. In the past, neurolept techniques (using fentanyl, alfentanil or sufentanil) were generally used, but short-acting opioid and propofol combinations are now the norm. The airway may be secured with the laryngeal mask airway, which is removed for the awake part of the procedure. Additional local anesthetic infiltration is given to reduce the stimulation of insertion of cranial pins and scalp incision. Monitoring must be of the same intensity as for conventional craniotomy as complications such as venous air embolism, airway obstruction and convulsions can occur. The anesthesiologist must have a full understanding of surgical intentions in order to anticipate the need to alter the depth of sedation appropriately. Very close cooperation between the surgeon and the anesthesiologist is absolutely essential to the success of this procedure.

Key Points

- *The complex interplay between the effects of drugs and physiological variables during clinical neuroanesthesia makes the interpretation of experimental data from the use of particular anesthetic drugs in isolation difficult.*
- *Moderate hyperventilation reduces CBF and brain volume. Extreme hyperventilation may be associated with critical reduction in flow to compromised areas and focal ischemia. Intravenous anesthetics generally decrease cerebral metabolism, CBF and ICP. Inhalational agents are all cerebral vasodilators. The overall effect on CBF depends on a balance between the concentration of the inhalational agent and the degree of hyperventilation.*
- *Pharmacological brain protection has been, so far, disappointing.*
- *Adequate monitoring must be used when patients are sedated. Supplemental oxygen, equipment and drugs to support the airway, breathing and cardiovascular system must be readily available.*
- *Close cooperation between the surgeon and the anesthesiologist is absolutely essential.*

Self-assessment

- ☐ What are the three components of general anesthesia? Which of these is most important for neuroanesthesia?
- ☐ How might rapid awakening at the end of surgery be best achieved?
- ☐ Which patients may require post-operative ventilation?
- ☐ How may anesthetic agents and techniques contribute to neuroprotection?
- ☐ Discuss the implications of the use of induced hypotension in aneurysmal surgery.
- ☐ What is the rationale for pre-operative starvation? What precautions are needed for emergency anesthesia?

References

1. Mayberg TS, Lam AM, Matta BF, Domino KB, Winn HR. Ketamine does not increase cerebral blood flow velocity or intracranial pressure during isoflurane/nitrous oxide anesthesia in patients undergoing craniotomy. Anesth Analg 1995;81:84–9.
2. Reinstrup P, Ryding E, Algotsson L, Messeter K, Asgeirsson B, Uski T. Distribution of cerebral blood flow during anesthesia with isoflurane or halothane in humans. Anesthesiology 1995;82:359–66.
3. Cho S, Fujigaki T, Uchiyama Y, Fukusaki M, Shibata O, Sumikawa K. Effects of sevoflurane with and without nitrous oxide on human cerebral circulation. Transcranial Doppler study. Anesthesiology 1996;85:755–60.
4. Algotsson L, Messeter K, Rosen I, Holmin T. Effects of nitrous oxide on cerebral haemodynamics and metabolism during isoflurane anesthesia in man. Acta Anaesthesiol Scand 1992;36:46–52.
5. Marsh ML, Dunlop BJ, Shapiro HM. Succinylcholine: intracranial pressure effects in neurosurgical patients. Anesth Analg 1980;59:550–1.
6. Stirt J, Grosslight K, Bedford R, Vollmer D. 'Defasciculation' with metocurine prevents succinylcholine-induced increases in intracranial pressure. Anesthesiology 1987;53:50–3.
7. Boyd AH, Eastwood NB, Parker CJ, Hunter JM. Comparison of the pharmacodynamics and pharmacokinetics of a cis-atracurium (51W89) or atracurium in critically ill patients undergoing mechanical ventilation in an intensive care unit. Br J Anaesth 1996;76:382–8.
8. Rosow C. Remifentanil: a unique opioid analgesic. Anesthesiology 1993;79:875–6.

9. Estilo A, Cottrell JE. Naloxone hypertension and ruptured cerebral aneurysm. Anesthesiology 1981;54:352.
10. Baskin DS, Hosobuchi Y. Naloxone reversal of ischemic neurological deficits in man. Lancet 1981;2:272.
11. Porter JM, Pidgeon C, Cunningham AJ. The sitting position in neurosurgery: a critical appraisal. Br J Anaesth 1999;82:117–28.
12. Kelleher A, Mackersie A. Cardiac arrest and resuscitation of a six month old achondroplastic baby undergoing neurosurgery in the prone position. Anesth Analg 1995;50:348–50.
13. Tung A. Indications for mechanical ventilation. Int Anesthesiol Clin 1997;35:1–17.
14. Ravussin P, de Tribolet N, Boulard G. Neuroanésthesie. Quelques aspects nouveaux. Neurochirurgie 1993;39: 145–8.
15. Cheng MA, Theard MA, Tempelhof R. Intravenous agents and intraoperative neuroprotection. Beyond barbiturates. Crit Care Clin 1997;13:185–99.
16. Warner DS, Zhou JG, Ramani R, Todd MM. Reversible focal ischemia in the rat: effects of halothane, isoflurane, and methohexital anesthesia. J Cereb Blood Flow Metab 1991;11:794–802.
17. Stone JG, Young WL, Marans ZS, Solomon RA, Smith CR, Jamdar SC et al. Consequences of electroencephalographic-suppressive doses of propofol in conjunction with deep hypothermic circulatory arrest. Anesthesiology 1996;85:497–501.
18. Nemoto EM, Klementavicius R, Melick JA, Yonas H. Suppression of cerebral metabolic rate for oxygen (CMRO2) by mild hypothermia compared with thiopental. J Neurosurg Anesthesiol 1996;8:52–9.
19. Kouchoukos NT, Daily BB, Wareing TH, Murphy SF. Hypothermic circulatory arrest for cerebral protection during combined carotid and cardiac surgery in patients with bilateral carotid artery disease. Ann Surg 1994;21:699–705.
20. Fessatidis IT, Thomas VL, Shore DF, Sedgwick ME, Hunt RH, Weller RO. Brain damage after profoundly hypothermic circulatory arrest: correlations between neurophysiological and neuropathological findings. An experimental study in vertebrates. J Thorac Cardiovasc Surg 1993;106:32–41.
21. Stamford J. Beyond NMDA antagonists: looking to the future of neuroprotection. In: Stamford J, Strunin L, editors. Neuroprotection. London: Baillière Tindall, 1996; 581–98.
22. Rowbotham DJ. Current management of postoperative nausea and vomiting. Br J Anaesth 1992;69:46S–59S.
23. Goldsack C, Scuplak SM, Smith M. A double-blind comparison of codeine and morphine for postoperative analgesia following intracranial surgery. Anesthesia 51:1996;1029–32.
24. Cashman J, McAnulty G. Nonsteroidal anti-inflammatory drugs in perisurgical pain management. Mechanisms of action and rationale for optimum use. Drugs 1995;49:51–70.
25. Leon JE, Bissonnette B. Transcranial Doppler sonography: nitrous oxide and cerebral blood flow velocity in children. Can J Anaesth 1991;38:974–9.
26. Clayton DG, O'Donoghue BM, Stevens JE, Savage PE. Cardiovascular response during cerebral angiography under general and local anesthesia. Anesthesia 1989; 44:599–602.
27. Ferguson GG. The rationale for controlled hypotension. Int Anesthesiol Clin 1982;28:89–93.
28. Moss E, Dearden NM, Berridge JC. Effects of changes in mean arterial pressure on SjO2 during cerebral aneurysm surgery. Br J Anaesth 1995;75:527–30.
29. Bukht D, Lanford R. Airway obstruction after surgery in the neck. Anesthesia 1983;38(4):389-90.
30. Rosner MJ, Rosner SD, Johnson AH. Cerebral perfusion pressure: management protocol and clinical results. J Neurosurg 1995; 83:949-62.

5

Neurosurgical Intensive Care

Tessa L. Whitton and Arthur M. Lam

Summary

Neurological disease frequently has multiple systemic manifestations, and management of patients with critical neurological illness requires a multidisciplinary approach with meticulous attention to organ dysfunctions. Many of these patients will suffer a poor outcome not as a result of the primary neurological disease, but as a result of medical complications. Thus, improvement of the intensive medical care of these patients will lead to an overall improvement of morbidity and mortality.

Introduction

The prevention of secondary insults to the central nervous system and close monitoring of neurological function are mainstays in the treatment of patients requiring neurosurgical care. The neurosurgical intensive care unit provides a setting for an integrated approach to the care of these patients and an organizational framework for delivery of this care. It represents the continuum of care applied to monitoring and treatment modalities instituted prior to or during surgery, which is essential for optimal recovery. Early treatment of complications may reduce morbidity from secondary insults; the intensive care unit should provide conditions for the rapid recognition and management of such complications. This chapter will discuss the theory and practice of intensive care management of the neurosurgical patient, with reference to general principles and specific neurological conditions.

Basic Physiological Concepts

Intracranial Pressure

The skull and vertebral canal form a rigid covering for the brain, spinal cord, cerebrospinal fluid (CSF) and blood. All of these intracranial compartments are non-compressible, thus the intracranial volume is essentially constant (the "Monro–Kellie doctrine"). Volume expansion of any compartment can only occur at the expense of compression of other compartments. The only buffering capacity is secondary to compression of the venous sinuses and the caudal displacement of CSF to the lumbosacral axis. Once this is exhausted, any tendency to increase volume in any of the compartments (as in an expanding mass) will result in an increased intracranial pressure (ICP).

The compliance of the intracranial system is often expressed as the "compliance curve" by plotting ICP against the expanding volume, although it should more accurately be described as the "elastance curve" (Fig. 5.1). A steep curve implies increased elastance or decreased compliance, as occurring with a rapidly expanding mass, as in a subdural or intracranial

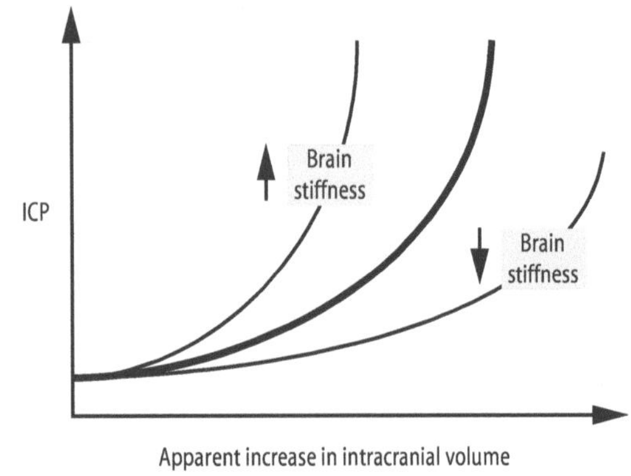

Fig. 5.1. Intracranial compliance curve.

hematoma. This "compliance" can be quantified by adding or withdrawing a known volume of saline to the CSF via a ventriculostomy, and noting the rise in ICP – the volume pressure response.

Elevation of ICP decreases cerebral perfusion, and may result in secondary ischemia, as the net cerebral perfusion pressure (CPP) is determined by the difference between mean arterial blood pressure (MAP) and ICP. (CPP = MAP – ICP or MAP – JVP, where JVP = jugular venous pressure. This applies when the cranium is open and ICP is zero.) In addition to its effect on CPP, an elevated ICP can also result in herniation. Although a clear-cut threshold cannot be determined, an elevated ICP >30 mmHg is associated with an increased risk of transtentorial or brainstem herniation. Thus monitoring and treatment of ICP is of paramount importance in the ICU.

In patients with spinal cord injury, the perfusion pressure to the cord is similarly determined by the difference between MAP and CSF pressure. Although most cord-injured patients present with complete lesions, anatomical disruption is rare, and maintenance of adequate perfusion is important to preserve cord function to ischemic regions proximal to the main site of injury.

Cerebral Blood Flow, CO_2 Reactivity and Cerebral Autoregulation

Reduction in cerebral blood flow (CBF) is one of the major causes of secondary cerebral ischemia in the damaged or edematous brain. Under normal circumstances CBF is tightly controlled by homeostatic mechanisms. Normal CBF is approximately 50 ml/100 g/min, coupled to a cerebral metabolic oxygen consumption rate of 3.2 ml/100 g/min. In patients with brain injury, CBF of 18–20 ml/100 g/min is generally considered to be the ischemic threshold, below which secondary injury may occur, although cellular integrity is usually preserved until CBF is <8–10 ml/100 g/min. Many factors control the cerebrovascular tone, including endothelial factors (nitric oxide, endothelin), cerebral metabolism, neurotransmitter release, systemic blood pressure, blood carbon dioxide content, blood viscosity and humoral substances. In physiological terms the important considerations include flow-metabolism coupling, CO_2 reactivity, and pressure autoregulation. Under normal circumstances, blood flow to the brain is tightly coupled to its metabolism, globally as well as regionally. The cerebral vasculature is exquisitely sensitive to carbon dioxide, changing by 3–4% per mmHg change in P_aCO_2. In contrast, P_aO_2 has a negligible effect on CBF. Although the molecular mechanism of cerebral autoregulation remains unknown, CBF is generally maintained constant between CPP of 50–150 mmHg. Blood flow becomes pressure-dependent at blood pressures outside the normal range, and this flow–pressure curve is shifted to the right in the presence of chronic hypertension. The purported mechanisms of autoregulation control include metabolic feedback and myogenic feedback.

Intracranial pathology may impair one or more of these homeostatic mechanisms [1]. CO_2 reactivity appears to be more robust than autoregulation, and is frequently preserved even with severe brain injury. With the exception of arteriovenous malformation and vasospasm (see below), the loss of CO_2 reactivity is generally associated with a poor prognosis.

Cushing's Response

CBF changes according to the formula:

CBF = CPP / CVR
or (MAP – ICP) / CVR

where CVR is the cerebral vascular resistance.

With elevation of ICP and compression of the brainstem, compensatory changes involving both MAP and CVR may occur. This compensatory rise in MAP, effected by increased sympathetic discharge from the vasomotor center in response to a rise in ICP causing brainstem ischemia, was first documented in 1901 by Cushing and is known as "Cushing's response". While MAP increases as a result of increased systemic vascular resistance, cerebral vasodilation occurs in response to the decrease in CPP as the autoregulatory compensatory response. However, with decreased intracranial compliance (increased intracranial elastance), this vasodilation may lead to further increase in ICP and reduction in CPP.

Critical Closing Pressure

The CPP has traditionally been calculated as the difference between MAP and ICP or JVP and thus may easily be derived when ICP is monitored. Although not a frequent occurrence, regional compartmentalization of ICP may result in regional variation in CPP, and hence in CBF. Moreover, when venous pressure is elevated or higher than ICP, both the arterial inflow from the systemic driving force (MAP) and the venous outflow need to be considered in order to optimize CPP.

On the basis of studies of other organs and the peripheral circulation, it can be demonstrated that the critical closing pressure (CCP), located at the arteriolar level, determines the downstream pressure in the vasculature of that organ. The cerebral CCP is defined as the arterial pressure threshold below which arterial vessels collapse, and is determined by both the ICP and the cerebral arterial tone. Thus CCP is the minimum perfusion pressure necessary to keep the cerebral vessels open. This is influenced by the surrounding extrinsic pressure (ICP) as well as by any distal resistance (e.g. jugular venous obstruction). This is not an easily quantifiable variable, but it represents the overall downstream resistance of the cerebral vasculature, and may be a more important determinant of CPP than ICP (i.e. CPP = MAP – CCP) [2]. Complex relationships therefore exist between ICP, systemic blood pressure, cerebral metabolism and CBF, all of which must be taken into consideration in the intensive care management of neurosurgical patients. These principles apply whether the patients had suffered traumatic brain injury, subarachnoid hemorrhage or ischemic stroke. Recent advances in monitoring modalities, which will be discussed later in the chapter, have made it theoretically possible to manipulate 'real-time' information to optimize treatment of these patients.

Management of Elevated Intracranial Pressure

Intracranial hypertension is defined as an ICP >15 mmHg. A progressive rise from this level, or sustained ICP >20 mmHg, should prompt investigation and treatment. A progressive rise in ICP may indicate the development of hemorrhage/hematoma, edema, hydrocephalus or a combination of these causes, and an immediate CT scan is indicated. A sustained elevated ICP increases the risk of secondary injury from ischemia and/or herniation.

In patients with surgically correctable pathology, such as subdural/epidural/intracerebral hematoma, or hydrocephalus, prompt surgical treatment is indicated. In other patients ICP can be effectively controlled by manipulating the different compartments of the intracranial contents. In patients refractory to medical management, decompressive craniectomy is indicated. These approaches are discussed below and summarized in Table 5.1.

Reduction of Cerebral Blood Volume

Head Elevation

Elevation of the head of the bed to an angle of 20–30° reduces ICP by optimizing cerebral venous return. However, in hypovolemic patients, head elevation may cause a decrease in the CPP. If normovolemia is maintained, elevation to 30° has been shown to decrease ICP without compromising CPP or CBF in head-injured patients.

Care should be taken to avoid obstruction of cerebral venous return by cervical collars or endotracheal tube ties, and to keep the head maintained in the neutral position.

In patients with preserved cerebral autoregulation, elevation of MAP will lead to compensatory vasoconstriction with reduction of ICP.

Table 5.1. Treatment of elevated ICP

Conventional measures
1. Elevation of head and relief of potential venous obstruction
2. Elevation of MAP (if appropriate)
3. P_aCO_2 of 30–35 mmHg, or 25–30 mmHg if there are signs of brain herniation
4. Mannitol 0.5–1.0 g/kg q. 6 h prn and furosemide 20 mg prn. Keep serum osmolality <320.
5. Maintain hypovolemia; monitor CVP, if possible.
6. Ventriculostomy for drainage of CSF, if applicable.
7. Sedation with opiates, benzodiazepines and/or propofol
8. Fine-tune the level of PEEP, if applicable.
9. Maintain normovolemia.
Aggressive measures (in patients refractory to conventional measures)
1. Induction of hypothermia to 33–34°C
2. Maximal EEG suppression with induction of propofol or barbiturate coma
3. Hyperventilation to P_aCO_2 of 20–25 mmHg (monitor $S_{jv}O_2$ or $P_{br}O_2$)
4. Hypertonic saline (3% or 7.5% 25–50 ml/h); monitor serum sodium
Extreme measures
1. Decompressive craniectomy
2. Excision of infarcted tissues ± lobectomy

This can be accomplished with maintenance of normovolemia and infusion of phenylephrine at 1–10 μg/kg/min, or norepinephrine at 0.05–0.2 μg/kg/min.

Hyperventilation

Because of the exquisite sensitivity of CBF to P_aCO_2, hyperventilation will reduce CBF, and concomitantly cerebral blood volume (CBV), resulting in an acute decrease in ICP. Although the acute reduction in ICP and improvement in CPP is theoretically desirable, and hyperventilation has been traditionally used as an effective treatment modality, in recent years the concern for the risk of cerebral ischemia has curtailed its use. CBF studies have demonstrated that even moderate hyperventilation may increase brain regions with CBF below the ischemic threshold [3]. Reduction of jugular venous oxygen concentration ($S_{jv}O_2$) and brain tissue PO_2 ($P_{br}O_2$) have also been repeatedly demonstrated in studies in head-injured patients. Moreover, in the only randomized controlled trial conducted on this therapeutic modality, prophylactic hyperventilation has been shown to be associated with adverse outcome. Thus the Brain Trauma Foundation Guidelines suggest that hyperventilation should not be used for the management of patients with head injury, unless the ability to monitor independently for evidence of cerebral ischemia is available (CBF, $S_{jv}O_2$ or $P_{br}O_2$). In addition, because of normalization of pH in cerebrospinal fluid, the efficacy of hyperventilation on CBF, CBV and ICP declines after 24 hours. However, despite these studies, the issue of hyperventilation remains controversial. Whereas it is clear that a low P_aCO_2 would lead to a reduction in CBF, resulting in regions with CBF approaching or below the ischemic threshold, the definitive evidence of "ischemia" is lacking. Using positron emission tomography, Diringer et al. were unable to demonstrate any decrease in cerebral metabolic rate or change in the pyruvate–lactate ratio with acute hyperventilation, suggesting that the low basal metabolic rate of brain-injured patients paradoxically "protects" these patients from the low CBF [4]. As we await more definitive evidence on hyperventilation, $PaCO_2$ is best maintained at 35-40 mmHg. In acute situations where there is impending or ongoing brain herniation, hyperventilation to P_aCO_2 of 20–30 mmHg is warranted. However, this should be viewed as a temporizing measure while waiting for definitive therapy. For maintenance, P_aCO_2 should be kept at 30–35 mmHg. Xenon CT and SPECT (single-photon emission computed tomography) may be useful in gauging regional CBF response to hyperventilation.

Elevation of Blood Pressure

In patients with intact cerebral autoregulation and decreased intracranial compliance, decrease in systemic blood pressure will lead to compensatory vasodilation and an increase in CBV [5]. This will lead to a further decrease in CPP, with a spiraling downhill effect and progressive decrease in net cerebral perfusion. On the other hand, patients with impaired cerebral autoregulation may exhibit an increase in ICP with increase in blood pressure. Since it is not possible to predict the presence or absence of autoregulation, it is important to maintain an adequate or even elevated systemic blood pressure to delineate the ICP response.

Reduction of Brain Mass

Because of the presence of the blood–brain barrier, which is relatively impermeable to sodium and chloride ions, the movement of water into and out of the brain cells is primarily determined by the osmotic gradient. An effective osmotic diuretic that is frequently used to treat elevated ICP is 20% mannitol. Given as a bolus at 0.5–1.0 g/kg, the action is immediate in onset, but peaks at 30 minutes, lasting for about 90 minutes. The loop diuretic, furosemide, potentiates the actions of mannitol, may also have direct ICP lowering effects, and is often given as an adjunct. The effects of mannitol on systemic hemodynamics are complex, with initial reduction of systemic vascular resistance, followed by intravascular volume expansion, which may be accompanied by systemic hypertension. Patients with poor cardiac function may develop acute pulmonary edema with infusion of mannitol. With the onset of diuresis, contraction of intravascular volume occurs, and this would result in hypotension if fluid replacement is inadequate. The complications from mannitol therapy include fluid overload, dehydration and renal failure.

During mannitol therapy, electrolytes and serum osmolality should be monitored frequently, and serum osmolality should not exceed 320 mOsm. Although the primary mechanism of mannitol is based on the osmotic gradient, it may also cause reflex vasoconstriction and reduce CSF production. Patients who become refractory to mannitol often would respond to hypertonic saline infusion (3% or 7.5%). Despite numerous clinical reports attesting to its efficacy, there have been no randomized clinical trials on the use of hypertonic saline, and rebound intracranial hypertension is a potential complication.

In patients with vasogenic edema associated with tumor, steroids are effective, and dexamethasone 10 mg is generally given every 6 hours. Steroids in general are considered to be contraindicated in patients with traumatic brain injury and ineffective in patients with subarachnoid hemorrhage or ischemic stroke. In patients with spinal cord injury, high-dose methylprednisolone has been shown to improve functions when given within 8 hours. In most centers, when seen within 3 hours, these patients are given methypredisolone 30 mg/kg bolus, followed by 5.4 mg/kg/h for 24 hours, and for 48 hours if seen between 3–8 hours (NACIS III). The improvement is, however, marginal, and many query if the benefits outweigh the risks of pneumonia and infection. Nevertheless, in view of the efficacy of steroid in spinal cord injury, the use of high-dose methylprednisolone in head injury is being re-examined, and a randomized trial aiming to enroll 20,000 patients is currently under way [6].

Reduction of CSF volume

Twenty-five percent of patients with subarachnoid hemorrhage from a ruptured aneurysm will develop acute hydrocephalus with elevation of ICP. Insertion of ventriculostomy with controlled drainage of CSF is an effective treatment of ICP. Some of these patients will eventually require a ventriculo-peritoneal shunt. Placement of a lumbar subarachnoid drain can also reduce CSF volume, but at the increased risk of brain herniation. This is less useful in patients with head injury, as the ventricles are frequently compressed, making them inaccessible and drainage less effective.

Sedation and Paralysis

Adequate sedation is essential in all patients with elevated ICP in order to minimize agitation and movement, and to improve tolerance of the endotracheal tube. Coughing or gagging on the tracheal tube or during tracheobronchial suction can cause rapid, extreme elevations in ICP. Neuromuscular paralysis effectively prevents this but at the expense of eliminating neurological examination as a monitor of the patient's condition. In addition, prolonged pharmacological blockade may result in the development of myopathy and persistent paralysis. Moreover, neuromuscular blocking agents (NMBs) should only be used in patients who are adequately sedated in order to avoid paralysis in an awake patient. Intermittent dosing and periodic discontinuation, coupled with careful monitoring of the degree of neuromuscular blockade, should allow regular neurological assessment.

Propofol

Sedative drugs that decrease ICP via an effect on cerebral metabolism and CBF include most of the intravenous anesthetic agents except ketamine. All have a depressant effect on the central nervous system, resulting in a dose-related decrease in level of consciousness and metabolic rate. Propofol has a similar metabolic and vascular profile to barbiturates, causing a dose-related decrease in cerebral metabolic rate and coupled decrease in CBF, resulting in a reduction in ICP in patients with cerebral metabolic activity. However, in some studies the decrease in CBF exceeded the concomitant decrease in metabolic rate. Its pharmacokinetic profile, with a short half-life, makes it a particularly suitable sedative agent in neurosurgical patients, allowing prompt neurological assessment within 2–3 hours of discontinuation of the infusion in usual doses (50–150 μg/kg/min). In a multicenter trial, propofol was efficacious in reducing ICP although the study failed to show an improvement in neurological outcome. In high doses (>300 μg/kg/min), it can be used to induce pharmacological coma with burst-suppression on electroencephalogram to achieve maximal metabolic suppression for control of ICP. In children, when used as a continuous infusion for a prolonged period, propofol has been reported to be associated with the development of a metabolic syndrome that is characterized by acidosis, rhabdomyolysis, cardiac failure and a high mortality rate [7]. More recently, a similar syndrome has also been reported to occur in head-injured adults treated with propofol >5 mg/kg/h [8]. In both children and adults, the actual incidence of this syndrome is unknown and the pathophysiology remains unclear. However, given the high mortality reported in children, and apparently conclusive data in a clinical trial (as yet unpublished), the use of propofol infusion in children is currently not advised. In adults, where indicated, the benefits of propofol outweigh this potential risk and should not be withheld from patients in the neurointensive care unit. However, prolonged infusion for more than 1 week, at doses greater than 5 mg/kg/h, is not advised, and the infusion should immediately be discontinued should any acidosis or cardiac dysfunction develop. In addition, propofol in high doses will result in systemic hypotension, often necessitating the use of vasopressors for blood pressure support.

Etomidate

Although etomidate had been used in the past as a sedative agent, it should not be given by infusion as it inhibits corticosteroid synthesis by the adrenal glands. It causes less cardiovascular depression than propofol or barbiturates and has been used in intermittent dosage in less stable patients. It reduces ICP by its effects on CBF and CVR.

Dexmedetomidine

Dexmedetomidine is a selective alpha-2-receptor agonist, and has recently been approved for use as a sedative agent for cardiac patients in the intensive care unit. Although not well investigated in neurosurgical patients, its pharmacological profile suggests that it may be a useful sedative in this group of patients. When given as an infusion at 0.6 mg/kg/h, most patients are well sedated but arousable, with minimal respiratory depression. It causes cerebrovasoconstriction and should reduce ICP, although the reduction in CBF is not matched by reduction in cerebral metabolism. Our own studies show that autoregulation and CO_2 reactivity are not affected by sedative doses of dexmedetomidine (unpublished data). In experimental ischemia it has been shown to reduce the number of damaged neurons in transient global ischemia in gerbils, and following focal cerebral ischemia in rats. The mechanism of action is thought to be via a reduction in norepinephrine release. Additionally, it appears to enhance the disposal of glutamine by oxidative metabolism in astrocytes, thus reducing the availability of glutamine as a precursor of neurotoxic glutamates. As yet, there have been no clinical trials on its use as a sedative agent in the neurointensive care unit, but the lack of significant respiratory depression makes it a very appropriate sedative in spontaneously breathing patients with poor intracranial compliance.

Barbiturates

Barbiturates reduce ICP by suppressing cerebral metabolism and, correspondingly, CBF. They do this both directly and by reducing seizure activity. Both pentobarbital and thiopental have been used to induce barbiturate coma. Their use is usually reserved for those patients whose intracranial hypertension has been refractory to other treatments. Similar to other sedatives, thiopental use is associated with systemic hypotension and should only be used in normovolemic patients. Two randomized controlled trials have assessed the efficacy of thiopentone for the treatment of raised ICP in patients with head injury. One trial showed a reduction in ICP that was significantly greater in the group treated with barbiturates, but with no improvement in long-term outcome. The second trial found that the ICP was controlled in approximately one-third of the treatment group, and that in those patients who responded, long-term outcome was also improved. A proportion of patients treated with barbiturates show no decrease in ICP. This may be due to uncoupling of cerebral metabolic rate of oxygen consumption from CBF, and is an indicator of poor prognosis.

Hypothermia

Hypothermia reduces cerebral metabolism and CBF, with resultant reduction in CBV and ICP. It may also be neuroprotective by decreasing the release of excitotoxic amino acids. Despite initial enthusiasm reported with the therapeutic use of moderate hypothermia in a single-center trial, a multicenter, randomized controlled trial could not demonstrate any beneficial effects, although a subset of patients aged less than 45 years, who were admitted hypothermic and randomized to hypothermia, had better results than patients who were rendered normothermic [9]. A new trial focusing on younger patients commenced in 2003. Despite the lack of proof of definitive benefits, most studies demonstrate a favorable ICP response to hypothermia. Moreover, the beneficial effects of therapeutic hypothermia on neurological outcome were recently demonstrated in patients who suffered cardiac arrest from sudden ventricular fibrillation. For now, therapeutic hypothermia should be used as an effective and useful adjunct for the control of ICP.

Decompressive Craniectomy

Decompressive craniectomy is indicated in patients with persistent elevated ICP refractory to medical treatments. In patients with unilateral swelling following hematoma evacuation or tumor resection, hemicraniectomy or removal of a large cranial flap with dural patching has been successful in reducing ICP. In patients with cerebral edema of both hemispheres, bilateral craniectomy may be necessary. Rarely, removal of damaged tissue or lobectomy may be performed as a last-ditch effort to decrease the intracranial contents in the most severe cases of intracranial hypertension. This procedure appears to be effective both for traumatic brain injury as well as for swelling secondary to stroke or subarachnoid hemorrhage. A multicenter trial to assess its efficacy as an early treatment for traumatic brain injury will determine its future role as a definitive treatment for intracranial hypertension [10].

Use of Positive End-expiratory Pressure in Patients with Elevated ICP

Positive end-expiratory pressure (PEEP) is frequently used to improve oxygenation in patients with respiratory distress syndrome or loss of lung volume due to a variety of pulmonary diseases. Theoretically, this can increase intrathoracic pressure, which in turn impedes venous inflow from the head, causing increase in ICP. However, this appears to be only clinically relevant if the patient has good intrathoracic compliance and poor intracranial compliance. Its safety was recently demonstrated in patients with acute stroke [11]. In practical terms, when properly indicated, PEEP up to 10 mmHg seldom causes significant elevation of ICP. However, it remains prudent to monitor the ICP response to PEEP in patients, particularly when PEEP >10 mmHg is used.

Management of Blood Pressure/Cerebral Perfusion Pressure

Head Injury

Optimal CPP–ICP management in the head-injured patient should be predicated on: (1) prevention of secondary injury and (2) promotion of recovery and repair of damaged neurons. Although maintenance of adequate CPP is the obvious and intended goal, there is controversy about the precise level of blood pressure required to achieve this goal. Because of the lack of randomized clinical trials, at least in the context of head injury, several approaches have been suggested, with all reporting improved results in their series. There are currently five approaches to the treatment of severe head injury that have been advocated: (1) guidelines issued by the Brain Trauma Foundation, (2) ICP management (Marshall approach), (3) CPP management (Rosner protocol), (4) "Lund therapy", which maintains low systemic pressures (MAP >50 mmHg) and normal colloid osmotic pressure to avoid vasogenic cerebral edema (prostacyclin to improve microcirculation) [12], and (5) the "cerebral ischemia model" (Robertson option), which relies upon the use of jugular venous oxygen saturation ($S_{jv}O_2$) monitoring to avoid global cerebral ischemia. These different options are summarized in Table 5.2. Although there is not a unified approach, with the exception of the Lund therapy, the consensus appears to be CPP at >60 mmHg [13] and MAP at >80 mmHg. Phenylephrine and norepinephrine are the most common agents used to support blood pressure in these patients. Both agents have negligible direct effects on the cerebral vasculature. Commonly used vasoactive agents are listed in Table 5.3.

Table 5.3. Vasoactive agents

Vasopressors/inotropes
Phenylephrine: 1–10 μg/kg/min
Norepinephrine: 0.05–0.2 μg/kg/min
Dopamine: 1–20 μg/kg/min
Dobutamine: 1–20 μg/kg/min
Vasopressin: 0.01–0.04 units/min
Vasodilators/hypotensive agents
Labetalol: 5-10 mg bolus q. 10 min, infusion at 50–100 mg/h, titrated to BP and HR
Esmolol: 500 μg/kg bolus, 3–15 mg/kg/h
Clonidine: 0.1 mg q. 4 h
Enlapril: 0.625–2.5 mg q. 6 h
Hydralazine: 10–20 mg q. 2 h prn
Sodium nitroprusside: 0.1–10 μg/kg/min

Table 5.2. Comparison of four different approaches and the Brain Trauma Foundation guidelines for the management of acute head injuries

	Approach: ICP	CPP	Threshold for MAP/SBP	Therapy for ↓CPP	Ischemia monitors
BTF guidelines	<20–25	>70	SBP >90	Colloid, dopamine, phenylephrine	$S_{jv}O_2$, CBF, $AVDO_2$ if using hyperventilation
ICP (Marshall approach)	<20	>60	SBP >80	N/A	Not routine
CPP (Rosner protocol)		>70–80	MAP >90	Phenylephrine, norepi, colloid	Not routine
Lund therapy	<20–25	>40–60	N/A	N/A	Not routine
Cerebral ischemia (Robertson option)	<20	>70	MAP >90	Colloid, dopamine, phenylephrine	$S_{jv}O_2$, CBF, $AVDO_2$

ICP, intracranial pressure; CPP, cerebral perfusion pressure; BTF, Brain Trauma Foundation; MAP, mean arterial pressure; SBP, systolic blood pressure; CSF, cerebrospinal fluid; STP, sodium thiopental; norepi, norepinephrine; $S_{jv}O_2$ jugular venous oxygen saturation, CBF cerebral blood flow; $AVDO_2$, arteriovenous oxygen difference.

Subarachnoid Hemorrhage

In patients with ruptured and unsecured aneurysms and in good grade, blood pressure should be controlled and maintained at normal or slightly reduced values to reduce the risk of re-bleeding. Labetalol and beta-blockers have no effect on CBF and are the hypotensive agents of choice. In patients refractory to this treatment, the addition of clonidine or enlapril generally would control the blood pressure. In difficult cases, intravenous sodium nitroprusside may be necessary. Agents such as nitroprusside, hydralazine and nicardipine are cerebral vasodilators, and thus must be used with caution in patients with poor intracranial compliance or increased ICP. Continuous monitoring of ICP will enhance safety in these patients. In patients with elevated ICP and in poor grades, ongoing cerebral ischemia is an important consideration and blood pressure may have to be maintained at normal levels appropriate for the patient, albeit at the expense of increased risk of bleeding. Prompt surgical treatment will minimize this complication.

Patients in vasospasm will require hypertensive therapy to improve cerebral perfusion. The optimal blood pressure should be guided by the patient's clinical conditions and the magnitude of vasospasm. In general, systolic blood pressure of 140–160 mmHg is maintained for patients with mild vasospasm, and 160–180 mmHg for patients with evidence of moderate-to-severe vasospasm. Occasionally, even higher blood pressure may be required. A therapeutic dilemma occurs when vasospasm occurs in patients with unsecured aneurysms. However, therapeutic hypertensive therapy should not be withheld in these patients as the risk of hemorrhage appears to be very small.

Hemorrhagic and Ischemic Stroke

In patients with hemorrhagic stroke, control of blood pressure is important to prevent further hemorrhage. However, it is important to rule out the occurrence of hypertension secondary to increase in ICP (Cushing's response), in which event the mean arterial pressure should be reduced gradually, and not below 130 mmHg in known hypertensive patients, and lower (100 mmHg) in previously normotensive patients. On the other hand, mild-to-moderate hypertension (160–180 systolic and 90–100 diastolic blood pressure) should be left untreated in patients with ischemic stroke. Vasopressors to support blood pressure may be necessary.

Arteriovenous Malformation

Unlike cerebral aneurysms, increase in systemic blood pressure has not been identified as an etiological factor in hemorrhage in patients with arteriovenous malformations (AVMs). Control of blood pressure while the patient is awaiting surgery following hemorrhage is therefore relatively unimportant. However, because of the chronic adaptation of the adjacent blood vessels to a low pressure system, following resection of AVM, patients may develop hyperperfusion syndrome at normal blood pressure. Control of blood pressure at a normal or slightly reduced level is therefore crucial in the post-operative management.

Monitoring in the Intensive Care Unit

Basic Monitoring

Neurological Examination

Physical examination of the neurological system, although a non-parametric and subjective tool, is rapid and easy to perform and is useful in the detection of changes in the patient's neurological status. Its importance should not be overlooked and it should be a basic skill of all staff involved in the care of the neurological patient. Inter-observer variation is common but may be minimized by the use of quantitative examination methods. Mental status, motor/sensory assessment and coordination testing may all be rapidly evaluated in the conscious patient. Both conscious and unconscious patients should be assessed for pupillary size and light response, deep tendon reflexes and response to peripheral noxious stimuli. Pupillary deviation and flexor or extensor posturing may also be present.

The desire for quantification of neurological status has led to the development and wide-

Table 5.4. Glasgow Coma Scale

Eye opening		Verbal response		Motor response	
Spontaneous	4	Oriented	5	Obeys commands	6
To verbal	3	Inappropriate	4	Localizes pain	5
To pain	2	Incomprehensible	3	Flexion/withdrawal	4
None	1	Makes sounds	2	Flexion/abnormal (decorticate)	3
		None	1	Extension (decerebrate)	2
				None	1

spread use of scoring scales, such as the Glasgow Coma Scale (Table 5.4), originally developed for use in the head-injured patient. In addition to establishing a baseline, these scales are most useful when performed regularly in order to give a more objective impression of deterioration or improvement over a period of time.

Sedatives and analgesics given in the intensive care unit should ideally have a short duration of action, and should be allowed to dissipate once a day to facilitate assessment of the neurological status.

Monitoring of Intracranial Pressure

Although there are no data from randomized trials, it is generally accepted that monitoring and aggressive treatment of elevated ICP can minimize secondary ischemia and improve outcome. Thus the use of intracranial devices for the continuous measurement of ICP has become standard practice in the care of neurological patients in whom an elevated ICP is an issue. These devices include intraventricular catheters, subarachnoid bolts, epidural systems and fiberoptic intraparenchymal devices. Ventriculostomy catheters and fiberoptic intraparenchymal devices appear to give comparably accurate measurement of ICP (Fig. 5.2). Ventriculostomy catheters are generally considered to be the gold standard for ICP monitoring. This type of catheter has the additional advantage of allowing drainage of CSF to lower ICP.

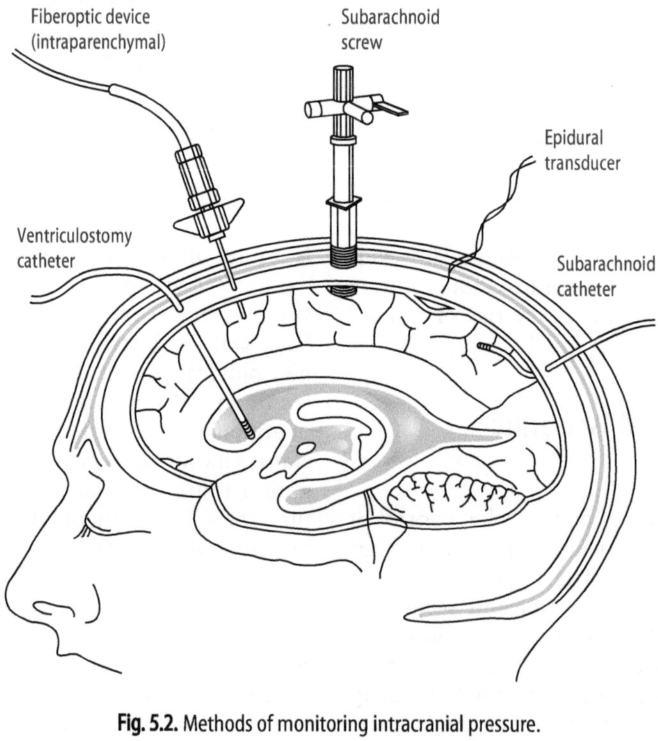

Fig. 5.2. Methods of monitoring intracranial pressure.

However, it is associated with a higher risk of infection compared with the fiberoptic intraparenchymal catheters. Subarachnoid monitors should be placed on the same side as the lesion in order to avoid inaccuracy due to pressure differential between the two hemispheres. Computerized recording and display of the transduced ICP pressure wave is now standard with most multimodal bedside patient monitors: the 'real-time' pressure wave and analysis of any trend in pressure may be viewed and compared with other monitored signs such as systemic blood pressure or central venous pressure (CVP).

Indications for ICP Monitoring

An ICP monitor may be useful in the management of any neurosurgical patient in whom a raised ICP is suspected, although it is in the management of severe head injury that its utility is most established. In those patients with moderate head injury in whom non-neurosurgical surgery is essential, an ICP monitor may also provide the only indication of deterioration of the patient whilst anaesthetized. Maintenance of an adequate CPP is only possible with knowledge of the ICP and systemic blood pressure in order to avoid secondary ischemic insults. ICP measurement also facilitates the ability to gauge response to therapeutic measures and gives early warning of the expansion of mass lesions. In general, ICP monitoring is indicated in all patients who are comatose with brain injury, and in patients with deteriorating neurological status with an abnormal CT scan. As mentioned above, many consider ICP monitoring desirable in patients with moderate head injury requiring prolonged surgical procedure under general anesthesia. In addition, routine post-operative ICP monitoring following major neurosurgical procedures is performed in some centers. The only absolute contraindication for ICP monitoring is the presence of uncorrected coagulopathy.

ICP Tracings

The nature and characteristics of ICP waves were extensively described in 1960 by Lundberg from his observation of ICP monitoring in neurosurgical patients. He described three wave-types: A-waves or plateau waves, B-waves and C-waves.

A-waves, termed "plateau waves" for their characteristic shape, are associated with both an increase in CBV as a result of vasodilation and a decrease in CBF. They manifest in an abrupt rise in the ICP to levels of 60–80 mmHg for a duration of 5–20 minutes and are an indicator of poor prognosis (Fig. 5.3).

Rosner and Becker showed that plateau waves in cats with mild brain trauma are preceded by a decrease in systemic blood pressure to approximately 70–80 mmHg and that CBV increases exponentially with this decrease. In association with poor intracranial compliance, this increase in CBV is accompanied by an exponential rise in ICP, seen as the plateau wave. Plateau waves may be abolished with an increase in CPP or with maneuvers to improve intracranial compliance.

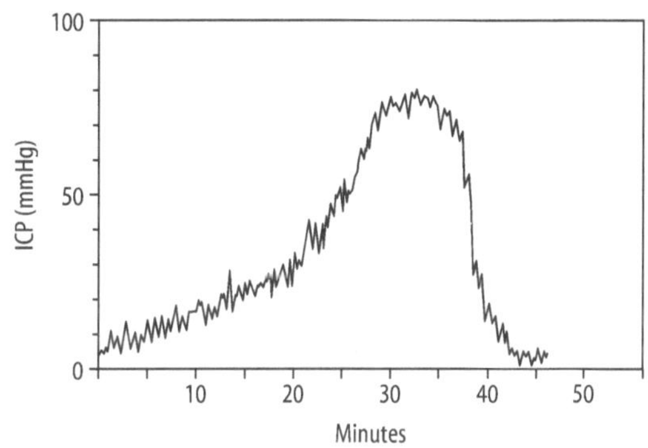

Fig. 5.3. Example of an A-wave.

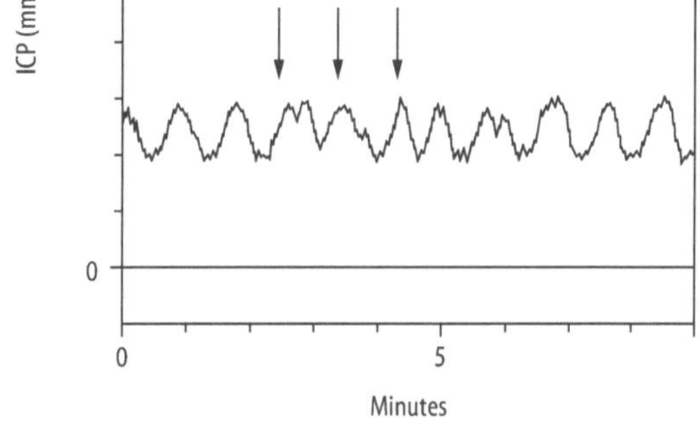

Fig. 5.4 Example of a B-wave.

The B-waves described by Lundberg are repeating waves of usually 10–20 mmHg with a frequency of 0.5–2 waves/min, and reflect fluctuation in CBV owing to vasomotor waves of the regulating vessels. They usually indicate decreased intracranial compliance (Fig. 5.4).

C-waves were considered by Lundberg to reflect arterial Traube–Hering waves and to indicate decreased intracranial compliance.

Advanced Monitoring

Monitoring of Cerebral Oxygenation/Metabolism

Jugular Venous Oximetry, Tissue PO_2, and Near-infrared Spectroscopy

As cerebral ischemia and secondary injury are the common factors leading to deterioration, monitoring of some indices of cerebral oxygenation would provide guide to appropriate therapy. By placing a fiberoptic oximetric catheter into the jugular bulb, cerebral venous oxygenation can be monitored continuously, providing an index of the balance between cerebral blood flow (supply) and cerebral metabolic consumption of oxygen (demand) ($CMRO_2 = CBF \times AVDO_2$, or $AVDO_2 = CMRO_2/CBF$). In essence, it is the arteriovenous oxygen content difference that represents the balance between supply and demand. However, if hemoglobin concentration stays relatively constant, and we ignore the contribution of dissolved oxygen, then the jugular venous saturation ($S_{jv}O_2$) effectively reflects the adequacy of CBF relative to oxygen consumption [$AVDO_2 = Hgb \times 1.39 \times (1- S_{jv}O_2)$]. Thus, a high $S_{jv}O_2$ implies luxury perfusion, and a low value reflects increased extraction, or inadequate delivery relative to the degree of consumption. It has been demonstrated that multiple episodes of desaturation below 50% are associated with poor prognosis in head-injured patients. Paradoxically, a high $S_{jv}O_2$ also indicates a poor prognosis as the brain is no longer extracting oxygen. However, it is a global measurement and does not and cannot reflect regional ischemia. Thus it is a highly specific but very insensitive monitor. Despite these limitations, when used properly it yields information that can help management, and has become a standard monitor in the care of the head-injured patient in many centers. Combining this with lactate measurement enhances its value as a monitor. The potential complications of this technique include bleeding and thrombosis, none of which has proved to be clinically significant. The most predominant cause of jugular venous desaturation is probably excessive hyperventilation. Treatment of a low $S_{jv}O_2$ should include a careful examination of all systemic and cerebral factors (Fig. 5.5).

Tissue PO_2 electrodes are miniature Clark electrodes that can be inserted into brain parenchyma to measure tissue PO_2 ($PbrO_2$). The placement of these electrodes necessitates the drilling of burr holes, and is therefore more invasive than jugular oximetry. However, they provide regional measurement and can be inserted into brain tissues considered to be at risk. There are two types of electrodes that are commercially available: the Neurotrend and the Licox. The Neurotrend monitors PCO_2 and pH in addition to PO_2 (requiring a larger burr hole) whereas the Licox only measures PO_2. Both are combined with ICP and temperature monitors. The normal values of $P_{br}O_2$ are 25–30 mmHg. Values below 15 mmHg are associated with poor prognosis, and values less than 10 mmHg are usually incompatible with survival. It is debatable whether $P_{br}O_2$ truly reflects tissue oxygenation or a balance between the delivery and consumption of oxygen at the local level. Studies with $P_{br}O_2$ have repeatedly demonstrated that increase in F_iO_2 consistently causes an immediate rise in $P_{br}O_2$. Although this is considered beneficial by some, others consider it may be more related to P_aO_2 than to brain tissue oxygenation.

Near-infrared spectroscopy measures tissue oxygenation non-invasively using reflectance oximetry. Briefly, a light source is placed on the scalp, and light reflected from the scalp and brain is measured by optodes placed at a distance from the light source. Theoretically this can monitor not only oxygenation saturation, but also the amount of desaturated hemoglobin, regional CBV and the cytochrome redox state. Although attractive in theory, the many drawbacks, including variable optical path, contamination by scalp and bone, interference by ambient light, and the necessary placement on the forehead, have limited its usefulness as a clinical monitor. Extensive development and refinement are required before it can become a functional monitor.

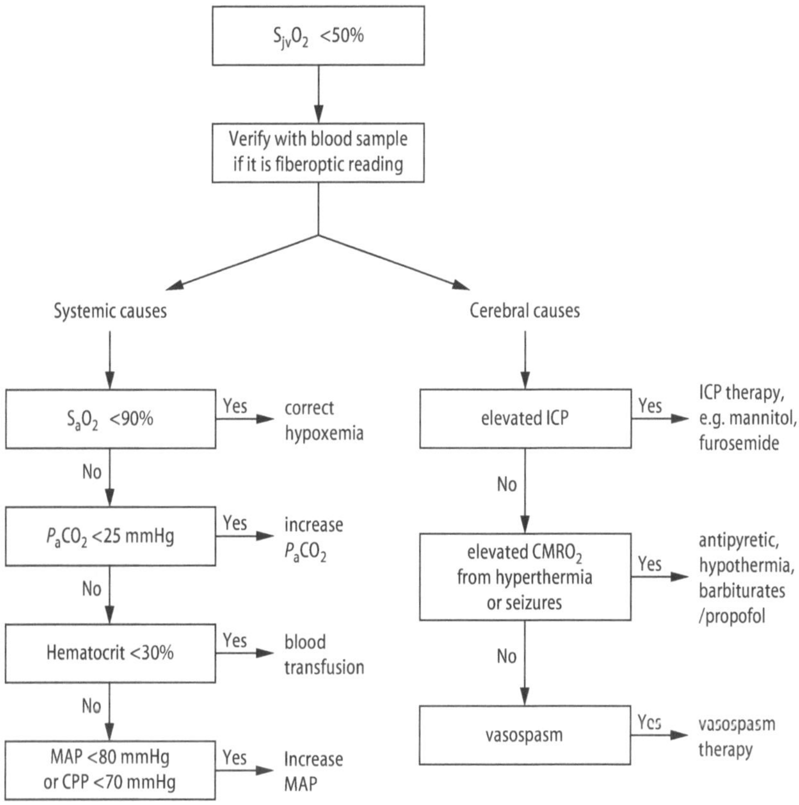

Fig. 5.5 Treatment algorithm for jugular venous desaturation.

Microdialysis

With placement of an intraparenchymal microdialysis catheter, it is now possible to do bedside measurement of local cerebral metabolite/ neurotransmitter, including that of lactate, pyruvate, glucose and glutamate [14]. These microdialysis measurements complement other cerebral monitoring by confirming or refuting the presence of cerebral ischemia.

Positron Emission Tomography (PET)

PET can measure CBF, CBV and oxygen consumption, as well as glucose consumption. It is, however, expensive and remains an investigative tool. Recent PET studies of head injuries show that some patients may develop regional hyperglycolysis during the early stages of head injury.

Monitoring of Cerebral Blood Flow

Numerous methods have been employed to assess both global and regional CBF. This information has been used to evaluate autoregulation and CO_2 reactivity, to ensure adequate CBF, to assess the effect of treatments in modifying CBF, and to assess CBF as an outcome predictor. Although many methods are available, as yet there is no functional bedside method for the measurement of CBF that can be performed repetitively in a clinically useful manner. Several semi-quantitative methods are nevertheless clinically useful.

Quantitative Global and Regional CBF

Kety–Schmidt Technique The gold standard for global CBF measurement is the Kety–Schmidt technique of nitrous oxide washin. Although first described in 1945, the technique remains valid today. It measures global hemispheric blood flow, necessitates cannulation of the jugular bulb, thus allowing derivation of cerebral metabolic rate for oxygen, and can be performed at bedside.

Radioactive Xenon Washout The Xenon133 washout method is derived from the Kety-Schmidt technique, and is probably the most commonly used bedside technique today. Xe133 can be administered by inhalation or intraarterial injection, but is most commonly given by intravenous injection. Multiple detectors placed next to the head allow measurements of regional CBF. Accuracy may be impaired in low-flow conditions, and areas with no flow cannot be detected (the "look-through phenomenon").

Stable Xenon CT Quantitative CBF can also be determined using stable xenon (30%) by inhalation and CT. Flows at multiple regions of interest can be measured. Transportation to the CT suite is necessary, and stable xenon is expensive and, at 30%, has significant cerebral vasodilatory effects. Repetitive measurements are possible and evaluation of therapeutic response to treatments aiming to modify CBF may be carried out with this method.

CT Perfusion Scan Quantitative CBF can also be obtained using contrast CT. The computer algorithm examines the transit time of contrast and derives the regional CBF. Compared with stable xenon, only limited slices can be obtained. This technique also allows repetitive measurements, making it possible to assess the patient's response to therapeutic maneuvers such as hyperventilation or augmentation of blood pressure.

Positron Emission Tomography As mentioned above, PET can measure regional CBF, metabolism and volume. This is, however, expensive and, with limited availability, remains primarily an investigative tool.

Local CBF

Laser Doppler Continuous monitoring of CBF is possible using laser Doppler flow probes. This, however, involves implantation of a probe via a small burr hole directly into the brain parenchyma and can only measure local CBF in a volume of 1 mm^3.

Semiquantitative/Qualitative Cerebral Blood Flow

Single-Photon Emission Computed Tomography (SPECT) Using Technetium[99] isotope administered intravenously, relative regional distribution of blood flow can be quantified. However, absolute CBF cannot be derived. This technique is relatively non-invasive, involves less radiation than a CT scan, and is useful in the assessment of cerebral ischemia secondary to vasospasm.

Transcranial Doppler The transcranial Doppler (TCD) was introduced by Rune Aaslid in 1982. Using a 2 MHz pulsed Doppler, flow velocities of the basal cerebral arteries can be measured in a non-invasive manner. Although actual CBF cannot be derived from the velocities, valuable information can nevertheless be obtained that can aid patient management. When the diameter of the insonated vessel stays constant, changes in flow velocity reflect corresponding change in flow. Under normal conditions, the basal cerebral arteries, being conductance vessels, vary little in diameter with physiological vasodilation or vasoconstriction, conditions that depend on change in resistance vessels. On the other hand, pathological constriction of the conductance vessel will lead to a dichotomy, with increase in flow velocity paradoxically reflecting a decrease in flow, as in the case of vasospasm following subarachnoid hemorrhage. TCD has been found to be useful in the management of vasospasm, allowing early diagnosis and assessment of therapy.

Vasospasm vs Hyperemia

Increase in flow velocity as diagnosed by TCD can be secondary to development of vasospasm or hyperemia, with obvious different clinical implications. This is particularly relevant in patients with traumatic subarachnoid hemorrhage (SAH), since 20–40% may develop vasospasm. To distinguish vasospasm from hyperemia, the ratio of intracranial flow velocity to extracranial internal carotid flow velocity (Lindegard index) is frequently used. Hyperemia is considered to be present when the index is less than 3. Mild vasospasm occurs when the index is greater than 3, moderate vasospasm when the index is 5–7, and severe vasospasm when the index is greater than 7.

Non-invasive Assessment of ICP

Significant elevation of ICP compromising cerebral perfusion results in a characteristic flow pattern on TCD with low diastolic flow velocities. Increasing ICP will result in correspondingly decreasing diastolic velocity, culminating in a "reverberating flow" pattern, with forward flow during systole, and backward flow during diastole, signifying the onset of intracranial circulatory arrest. Based on these considerations, many investigators have proposed using TCD as a non-invasive monitor of ICP, and preliminary results are promising.

Autoregulation Testing

Patients who suffer traumatic brain injury or SAH frequently develop impaired cerebral autoregulation, increasing the risk of brain injury with sudden changes in systemic blood pressure. Elevation of blood pressure may increase the risk of vasogenic edema, whereas decrease in blood pressure may result in cerebral ischemia. Elucidation and quantification of the state of autoregulation would facilitate clinical management of these patients. Furthermore, it has been shown that delayed ischemic deficits are more likely to develop in patients with the combination of vasospasm and impaired cerebral autoregulation, as determined by TCD.

A number of different methods have been investigated. These include:

Spontaneous relationship between blood pressure and flow velocity changes. With intact cerebral autoregulation there is a negative correlation between changes in blood pressure and change in flow velocity, and a positive correlation when autoregulation is impaired. By monitoring both blood pressure and flow velocity simultaneously over multiple time epochs, the state of cerebral autoregulation can be qualitatively determined.

Transient hyperemic response. When autoregulation is intact, compression of the extracranial internal carotid artery for 7–10 seconds will result in a transient hyperemic response in the ipsilateral middle cerebral artery.

Dynamic autoregulation. When autoregulation is intact, a transient decrease in blood pressure effected by sudden deflation of inflated thigh cuffs will cause a very brief decrease in middle cerebral artery flow velocity, rapidly returning to baseline value.

Static autoregulation. Below the upper limit of autoregulation, elevation of systemic blood pressure using a vasopressor (phenylephrine) will not affect cerebral artery flow velocity when autoregulation is intact.

Imaging Modalities

Computed tomography of the brain is the most important diagnostic imaging modality in the care of the critically ill neurological patient. Patients with traumatic head injury may require daily CT during the initial course, and more often if the neurological status is fluctuating. It is important to obtain CT whenever there is sudden deterioration in the neurological status or sudden increase in ICP to rule out surgically correctable causes. Magnetic resonance (MR) imaging is more helpful in delineating infarcts and ischemic lesions, particularly with diffusion-weighted and perfusion-weighted imaging. However, it is time consuming and generally not as available as CT. Angiography is essential in the establishment of vasospasm and institution of interventional treatment.

Monitoring Electrophysiological Functions

EEG and Evoked Potentials

EEG and evoked potentials may be useful for diagnostic purposes. In patients suspected of having seizures, a diagnostic EEG may be helpful. In patients with status epilepticus treated with muscle relaxants, continuous EEG monitoring to guide pharmacological therapy is essential.

In patients with severe head injury, EEG is of relatively little value, whereas somatosensory evoked potentials (SSEPs) can provide important prognostic information. With unilateral or bilateral absence of cortical SSEP, the outcome is uniformly fatal. Preservation or early recovery of normal SSEP is compatible with high degree of recovery. Brainstem evoked potential, in combination with cortical SSEP, may allow assessment of the integrity of brainstem function and the site of injury to be located.

Electrocardiographic and Cardiac Monitoring

Patients with isolated severe neurological injury can develop ECG changes. In patients with aneurysmal SAH, 40–60% of the patients may exhibit ECG abnormalities comprising of ST segment changes or arrhythmia. Acute left ventricular dysfunction can also occur, and in some patients acute pulmonary edema can develop. Frank myocardial necrosis secondary to SAH has been documented, although it is exceedingly rare. Patients with poor clinical grades are more likely to have ECG abnormalities as well as ventricular dysfunction, but there is poor correlation between these two abnormalities. Cardiac enzymes should be measured in patients with ECG changes to rule out myocardial infarction, and echocardiograms should be performed in patients with clinical ventricular dysfunction. Central venous pressure monitoring is indicated in these patients and, despite recent studies questioning the value of pulmonary artery catheter placement, measurement of filling pressures may facilitate the management of patients in vasospasm.

Management of Vasospasm

Angiographic vasospasm occurs in up to 70% of patients after aneurysmal SAH, although only about 30–40% of patients become clinically symptomatic. Although nimodipine prophylaxis improves the neurological outcome of patients, it neither decreases the incidence nor alters the magnitude of vasospasm. Vasospasm typically occurs on day 3 after SAH, peaks on day 7, and generally subsides by the end of 14 days. Vasospasm is the main cause of delayed ischemic deficit, resulting in brain infarction or death. Early vasospasm results in elevated flow velocities, which can be detected by TCD, but the diagnosis must be confirmed with angiography in symptomatic patients. SPECT can detect regional differences in perfusion and facilitate management. Currently, the only medical treatment for symptomatic vasospasm is augmentation of cerebral perfusion by elevation of blood pressure, and cardiac output. Although its value has not been established with randomized clinical trials, triple-H therapy (hemodilution, hypervolemia, hypertension) is a standard management therapy for severe vasospasm in many neurointensive care units. This entails aggressive fluid therapy to maintain pulmonary wedge pressure at 14–16 mmHg, systolic blood pressure at 160–180 mmHg, and hematocrit at 30. Patients not responding to therapy may be candidates for angioplasty with or without papaverine infusion. Patients with vasospasm secondary to traumatic SAH generally respond to the same treatment regimen, although the risk of development of vasogenic edema may be higher.

Fluid and Electrolytes

To maintain adequate cerebral perfusion, it is important to maintain normovolemia. The practice of keeping neurological patients dehydrated to minimize cerebral edema is outdated, and in head-injured patients is associated with poor outcome [15]. Fluid balance tallying total input and output should be monitored daily, and insensible loss of 500–800 ml per day should be allowed. Patients with head injury often suffer multiple injuries that may result in significant blood loss, contributing to hypovolemia and hypotension. On the other hand, patients who suffer SAH can develop acute decrease in circulating blood volume unrelated to blood loss. Patients with hemorrhagic or ischemic stroke may also be hypovolemic, and the volume status cannot be assessed by the presence or absence of systemic hypertension. A thorough history and clinical examination is crucial to the establishment of the correct diagnosis. To ensure normovolemia, isotonic fluids or normal saline should be given, although the latter, when given in large amounts, would inevitably lead to hyperchloremic metabolic acidosis.

In patients with partially disrupted blood–brain barrier (BBB), colloids have a theoretical advantage, and their benefits in reducing edema can be demonstrated in experimental focal cerebral ischemia. However, there is no clinical evidence of its efficacy. Moreover, meta-analysis of clinical trials suggests that the use of colloids for resuscitation of critically ill patients is associated with an increase in mortality. If colloids are to be used, albumin is preferred to hetastarch, as the latter can interfere with coagulation system and may cause bleeding in susceptible neurological patients, despite being given in small amounts. Monitoring of central venous pressure or pulmonary wedge pressure would help to guide fluid therapy, particularly in the management of patients in vasospasm. Anemia should be treated promptly to maintain adequate oxygen delivery. The optimal hemoglobin concentration for patients with brain injury has not been determined. In critically ill patients it has been demonstrated that, with the exception of patients with significant coronary artery disease, a conservative transfusion strategy is associated with better results than a liberal strategy, and transfusion to a hematocrit value of higher than 25–27 is not warranted. However, until data on patients with neurological disease are available, it remains prudent to maintain hemoglobin at about 10 g or hematocrit at 30.

In patients with severe head injury and stroke, as well as SAH, the presence of hyperglycemia is associated with a poor prognosis. Although stress is clearly a contributing factor, hyperglycemia itself can contribute to poor outcome. Thus hyperglycemia should be treated vigorously.

Neurological patients are prone to development of electrolyte disturbances; thus they should be measured daily, and appropriate replacements made. In particular, because of the relative impermeability of the BBB to ions, change in serum sodium and osmolality can have profound influence on movement of water across the BBB into neurons, and can exacerbate brain swelling/dehydration, causing coma and/or seizures.

Hypo- and Hypernatremia

Both hyponatremia and hypernatremia can occur in the neurological patient. The two major causes of sodium disturbances are: (1) iatrogenic and (2) CNS pathology related. Iatrogenic causes include administration of hypotonic fluids and the use of thiazide diuretics. Although normal hemostatic mechanisms will regulate sodium and water balance to maintain serum sodium within the normal range, persistent administration of hypotonic fluids, particularly in patients with poor renal functions or low cardiac output syndrome, will result in hyponatremia. The tonicity and composition of usual intravenous fluids are listed in Table 5.5. Following SAH, hyponatremia is particularly common, although only hypernatremia has been noted to be associated with a poor outcome. Disease-related causes include the development of diabetes insipidus, the syndrome of inappropriate antidiuretic hormone (SIADH), and cerebral salt-wasting syndrome (CSWS). It is extremely important to distinguish between the last two entities as the treatment is vastly different. With SIADH, the patient retains fluid, and excretes urine with high serum sodium and osmolality. Thus the appropriate treatment for SIADH is fluid restriction with or without diuretics, whereas with CSWS the

Table 5.5. Electrolyte composition of crystalloid and colloid fluids

Fluids	Osmolality (mOsm/kg)	Na (mEq/l)	Cl (mEq/l)	K (mEq/l)	Ca (mEq/l)	Mg (mEq/l)	HCO3-* (mEq/l)	Glucose (gm/l)	pH	Oncotic pressure (mmHg)
Crystalloid										
Plasma-lyte	294	140	98	5		3			7.4	
0.9% NS	308	154	154						5.7	0
0.45% NS	154	77	77							0
3% NS	1024	513	513							0
7.5% NS	2566	1283	1283							0
Lactated Ringer's (LR)	273	130	109	4	2.7		28		6.7	0
D5LR	525	130	109	4	2.7		28	50		0
D5W	252							50	4	
D5NS	560	154	154					50		
D5 0.45%NS	406	77	77					50		0
Normosol	295	140	98	5	0	3			7.4	
Mannitol (20%)	1098									0
Colloid										
Hetastarch (6%)in NS	310	154	154						5.5	30
Albumin (5%)	290									20

NS, normal saline
*Lactate in these fluids is converted to bicarbonate.

patient is usually hypovolemic as well as hyponatremic. Release of natriuretic peptides following SAH contributes to the development of CSWS, and the resultant hypovolemia and hyponatremia may exacerbate symptomatic vasospasm. Both atrial natriuretic peptide and B-type natriuretic peptide are acutely elevated after SAH, while the role of C-type natriuretic peptide remains unclear. The appropriate treatment for hyponatremia associated with hypovolemia in patients with SAH is volume replenishment with normal saline and increased salt intake. In symptomatic patients the use of hypertonic saline is warranted, although the rate of correction should not exceed 1–2 mEq/l/h to minimize the risk of development of central pontine myelinolysis. Fludrocortisone is a useful adjunct; it reduces natriuresis and expands intravascular volume.

The use of mannitol can also result in hyponatremia and hypokalemia. In addition, change in serum magnesium and phosphates frequently occur in critically ill patients, necessitating appropriate replacement therapy.

Pneumonia, Antibiotics and Mechanical Ventilation

Pulmonary complications are common and are a major cause of morbidity and mortality for patients requiring neurointensive care. In one study on patients with SAH, half the deaths attributable to medical causes were pulmonary in origin. Risk of pneumonia appears to peak within the first 3 days (early-onset pneumonia or EOP) and has been found to be associated with trauma and, in non-trauma patients, with a Glasgow Coma Scale (GCS) of less than 9. In this cohort of patients, the organisms responsible for EOP were Staphylococcus aureus (33%), Haemophilus (23%), other gram-positive cocci (22%) and other gram-negative bacilli (19%). A second peak occurred on days 5 and 6; in this group, gram-negative bacilli other than Haemophilus spp. accounted for 45.4% of organisms isolated. EOP appears to be related to aspiration of gastric contents occurring at the time of, or soon after, injury or ictus. Late-onset pneumonia is more likely to be ventilator-associated pneumonia, and caused by organisms which have colonized the airways. Appropriate antibiotic therapy should be guided by systemic manifestations, cultures and sensitivity of organisms. Occasionally, empiric therapy with a broad-spectrum antibiotic is indicated. Daily chest X-ray is important in intubated patients, and broncho-alveolar lavage is indicated in patients not responding to antibiotic therapy or spiking a fever while on antibiotic therapy.

Patients with high cervical spinal cord injury frequently develop acute respiratory failure because of the sudden loss of intercostal muscles. Thus it is not surprising that tracheal intubation and mechanical ventilation are frequently indicated in these patients. Other indications include: depressed level of consciousness, inability to maintain or protect airway, respiratory failure, pneumonia, sepsis and pulmonary edema. Unconscious or obtunded patients are at risk of aspiration and development of pneumonia and adult respiratory distress syndrome (ARDS). In addition, many patients may require intubation and ventilation for imaging or angiography procedures. Pulmonary edema can develop from fluid overload and/or cardiac failure. Neurogenic pulmonary edema can develop in patients with acute traumatic brain injury, SAH or acute cervical spinal cord injury, presumably on the basis of severe sympathetic stress, leading to pulmonary vasoconstriction, with increase in pulmonary vascular permeability and disrupted capillary endothelium. Some patients also develop acute ventricular dysfunction. Although diuretics may be helpful, improvement is mainly dependent on dissipation of the sympathetic stress, and recovery of cardiac function, with or without inotropic support. Placement of a pulmonary artery catheter and echocardiographic examination of the heart is indicated in these patients. Weaning off ventilatory support in neurological patients should be no different from that in other patients. When weaning parameters are met using standard criteria (tidal volume, rapid shallow-breathing index, negative inspiratory pressure), the patient should be extubated. There is no standard method of weaning in these patients, and either intermittent mandatory ventilation or spontaneous continuous positive airway pressure can be used. Extubation should not be delayed because of depressed level of consciousness; the delay results in increased rate of nosocomial pneumonia and prolongs hospital stay.

In patients fulfilling the diagnostic criteria of ARDS, protective lung strategy with small tidal volume, high frequency and low airway pressure is indicated. This may lead to CO_2 retention, resulting in cerebral vasodilation and increase in ICP. Optimal management in these patients requires both careful consideration of both organs and a balancing of the relative risks and benefits of protective lung therapy vs high CO_2 to arrive at the appropriate strategy.

Gastrointestinal Complications

Neurological patients are at increased risk of gastrointestinal bleeding or perforation. In one cohort of non-trauma neurosurgical ICU patients, 6.8% had endoscopically or surgically documented evidence of post-operative GI complications. The majority had bleeding, but two patients had both bleeding and perforation. Multivariate analysis suggested five risk factors of independent significance: (1) the presence of SIADH, (2) pre-operative coma, (3) the presence of post-operative complications, (4) age over 60 years, and (5) pyogenic infection of the CNS. Pre-operative coma was the only significant factor to predict the occurrence of life-threatening GI complications. Thus prophylaxis with a proton pump inhibitor or H_2 antagonists is routinely indicated in these patients.

Patients on broad-spectrum antibiotics may also develop pseudomembranous colitis, which usually subsides with discontinuation of antibiotic therapy.

Anticoagulation Prophylaxis

Obtunded neurological patients are at risk of development of deep venous thrombosis (DVT). Unless contraindicated, all patients should be maintained on subcutaneous heparin or low-molecular-weight heparin in addition to compressor stockings. Contraindications include active intracerebral hemorrhage and impending surgery. Post-operatively, it is safe to restart subcutaneous heparin after 48 hours. Doppler ultrasound to rule out DVT in the lower extremities should be performed when indicated.

Pulmonary embolism occurs not infrequently in these patients, and any sudden deterioration in gas exchange or systemic hemodynamics should prompt investigations. Spiral pulmonary CT is a good diagnostic test and, when confirmed, systemic heparinization is indicated. Where this is contraindicated because of intracerebral hemorrhage, placement of a filter in the inferior vena cava is appropriate.

Nutritional Support

Early nutritional support for critically ill patients is considered important. Specific guidelines have been issued for patients with traumatic brain injury (Brain Trauma Foundation, 2000). In general, enteral feeding via a nasogastric or nasoduodenal tube should commence within 24–48 hours of admission into the ICU. For patients who require long-term nutritional support, percutaneous endoscopic gastrostomy should be performed.

Seizure Prophylaxis

The presence of intracranial lesions predispose patients to risk of seizures, although the role of seizure prophylaxis is not established for all conditions. Patients with traumatic head injury should be treated with dilantin for 1 week, as prophylaxis is effective for early but not for late post-traumatic seizure disorders. Patients undergoing aneurysm surgery should be maintained on dilantin during the perioperative period. For acute seizures, intravenous lorazepam 0.1 mg/kg or midazolam 0.1–0.15 mg/kg is generally effective. Propofol and thiopental are also effective agents, but their use would generally necessitate tracheal intubation. Phenobarbital or thiopental can be used to control status epilepticus, and dosage should be guided by electroencephalography monitoring as well as by serum levels.

Temperature Control

Because of the risk of nosocomial infections, fever is very common in patients in the neurointensive care unit. Moreover, patients with neurological illness may have dysfunction of the temperature control mechanism and develop fever without infections. Although the role of hypothermia in neuroprotection remains to be defined, it is generally accepted that hyperthermia is detrimental to neuronal recovery. In addition, it is now recognized that a gradient may exist between body temperature and brain temperature; thus temperature of the brain may be underestimated, increasing the risk of neurological injury. Thus aggressive treatment of fever is warranted.

References

1. Czosnyka M, Smielewski P, Piechnik S, Steiner LA, Pickard JD. Cerebral autoregulation following head injury. J Neurol 2001;95:756–63.
2. Thees C, Scholz M, Schaller MDC, Gass A, Pavlidis C, Weyland A et al. Relationship between intracranial pressure and critical closing pressure in patients with neurotrauma. Anesthesiology 2002;96: 595–9.
3. Coles JP, Minhas PS, Fryer TD, Smielewski P, Aigbirihio F, Donovan T et al. Effect of hyperventilation on cerebral blood flow in traumatic head injury: clinical relevance and monitoring correlates. Crit Care Med 2002;30:1950–9.
4. Diringer MN, Videen TO, Yundt K, Zazulia AR, Aiyagari V, Dacey RG Jr et al. Regional cerebrovascular and metabolic effects of hyperventilation after severe traumatic brain injury. J Neurosurg 2002;96:103–8.
5. Rosengarten B, Ruskes D, Mendes I, Stolz E. A sudden arterial blood pressure decrease is compensated by an increase in intracranial blood volume. J Neurol 2002;249:538–41.
6. Edwards P, Farrell B, Lomas G, Mashru R, Ritchie N, Roberts I et al. The MRC CRASH Trial: study design, baseline data, and outcome in 1000 randomised patients in the pilot phase. Emerg Med J 2002;19:510–14.
7. Bray RJ. Propofol infusion syndrome in children. Paediatr Anaesth 1998;8:491–9.
8. Cremer OL, Moons KG, Bouman EA, Krjijswijk JE, de Smet AM, Kalkman CJ. Long-term propofol infusion and cardiac failure in adult head-injured patients. Lancet 2001;357:117–18.
9. Clifton GL, Miller ER, Choi SC, Levin HS, McCauley S, Smith KR Jr et al. Lack of effect of induction of hypothermia after acute brain injury. N Engl J Med. 2001;344:556–63.
10. Coplin WM. Intracranial pressure and surgical decompression for traumatic brain injury: biological rationale and protocol for a randomized clinical trial. Neurol Res 2001;23:277–90.
11. Georgiadis D, Schwarz S, Baumgartner RW, Veltkamp R, Schwab S. Influence of positive end-expiratory pressure on intracranial pressure and cerebral perfusion pressure in patients with acute stroke. Stroke 2001;32:2088–92.
12. Naredi S, Olivecrona M, Lindgren C, Ostlund AL, Grande PO, Koskinen LO. An outcome study of severe traumatic head injury using the "Lund therapy" with low-dose prostacyclin. Acta Anaesthesiol Scand 2001;45:402–6.
13. Robertson CS. Management of cerebral perfusion pressure after traumatic brain injury. Anesthesiology 2001;95:1513–17.
14. Hutchinson PJ, Gupta AK, Fryer TF, Al-Rawi PG, Chatfield DA, Coles JP et al. Correlation between cerebral blood flow, substrate delivery, and metabolism in head injury: a combined microdialysis and triple oxygen positron emission tomography study. J Cereb Blood Flow Metab 2002;22:735–45.
15. Clifton GL, Miller ER, Choi SC, Levin HS. Fluid thresholds and outcome from severe brain injury. Crit Care Med 2002;30:739–45.

III
Techniques

6

Neuroendoscopy

Jonathan Punt

Summary

Advances in optical technology and in neuroimaging, together with a rising interest in minimally invasive techniques, have resulted in the establishment of modern neuroendoscopy. As with most neurosurgical technologies, there is a regrettable dearth of Class I evidence and, although there are areas in which the benefits appear to be self-evident, this is unsatisfactory. Neuroendoscopic third ventriculostomy is currently the primary treatment of choice for selected cases of non-tumorous and tumorous hydrocephalus; the only demonstrable benefit on present evidence is freedom of complications from implanted devices. There are particular applications in the management of shunt complications, intraventricular and paraventricular tumors, and non-tumorous cysts. The future may bring more sophisticated applications in conjunction with image guidance. Proper training is essential and the technique should probably remain within the hands of a restricted number of specialists. Unstructured propagation is likely to be associated with avoidable morbidity. Prospective studies are required to evaluate the hazards as well as the benefits in comparison with older approaches. Regulatory authorities should monitor morbidity until the position is clear.

Historical Landmarks

It is interesting to reflect that even 'high-tech' neurosurgery has its origins in the versatile skills and open minds of the earliest neurosurgeons in the first two decades of the last millennium, and that more recent technological advances have enabled latter day pioneers of voyages into the intracranial compartments to venture further and more effectively, creating a renaissance in this elegant therapeutic modality. The history of neuroendoscopy has been described elsewhere [1], and is seen to be a study in miniature of the ways in which techniques wax and wane in surgery, more often riding on the ebb and flow of fashion than on the hard facts of evidence-based science.

In 1910, Lespinasse reported to a Chicago medical society that he had employed rigid cystoscopes to perform choroid plexus ablation on two hydrocephalic infants; one child died post-operatively but the other survived for 5 years. Eighty-four years later, the phrase "minimally invasive endoscopic neurosurgery" was coined.

In 1920, at Massachusetts General Hospital, Mixter performed the first endoscopic third ventriculostomy on a 10-month-old baby, using a urethroscope and a sound. Although follow-up was for less than 1 year, he takes credit for obtaining manometric and dye injection proof of patency of the ventriculostomy. Amongst the few neurosurgeons who persisted with endoscopic neurosurgery, the most notable were Putnam, who persevered with endoscopic choroid plexectomy, and Scarff, who also employed endoscopic third ventriculostomy.

The 1950s saw the advent of the first implantable valved shunting systems for the treatment of hydrocephalus, and inevitably the interest in neuroendoscopy waned. However, even before widespread disenchantment with the fickle nature of hydrocephalus shunts had set in, this first era of neuroendoscopy was marked by important papers by Scarff [2], the results of which are summarized in Table 6.1. An interesting observation was that, whereas when 618 patients treated surgically by choroid plexectomy or third ventriculostomy, without an implanted device, were compared with 1,087 patients treated by a shunt, there were equivalent operative mortalities of about 15% and early success of about 65%, the late complication rates were 3–5% without a shunt but 35–100% with a shunt. This early experience still holds true as, although the early mortality of both types of surgery has fallen, it serves to emphasize that, in discussing the optimum treatment for any particular patient with hydrocephalus, one has to consider not only the acute efficacy and hazard, but also the late morbidity.

Major improvements in visibility came with the solid glass rod endoscope and the cohesive fiberoptic bundle. Vries in the USA, followed by Jones in Australia, Sainte-Rose in France, and the present author in the UK, saw the potential for a return to a neuroendoscopic approach to the treatment of hydrocephalus, while Griffith in the UK also perceived a wider application of neuroendoscopy both within and outside of the ventricular system, coining along the way the term "endoneurosurgery" [1].

Instrumentation [3]

Modern neuroendoscopic techniques are enabled by, and are dependent upon, purpose-built neuroendoscopes utilizing high-quality optical systems and dedicated instrumentation. Although there are a number of neuroendoscopes available, there are three basic patterns: rigid, flexible and, more recently, the disposable Channel™ neuroendoscopes. The comparative features are detailed in Table 6.2. Individual surgeons will inevitably have their own preferences based upon the usual range of experiences, prejudices, purchasing opportunities and persuasiveness of sales people. However, it is important in selecting neuroendoscopes to consider the use to which they will be put. The most commonly performed intraventricular procedure will always be third ventriculostomy; for some surgeons that may be the only neuroendoscopic operation that they adopt. The superior visibility, ease of use, and simplicity of orientation make a rigid endoscope or the Channel™ neuroendoscope the most frequently employed devices. Although flexible neuroendoscopes are relatively unpopular, they come into their own when procedures are to be performed at two anatomically distinct sites, such as tumor biopsy coupled with third ventriculostomy. Similarly, if there are unusual anatomical conditions such as those encountered in patients with hydrocephalus associated with the dysraphic states or particularly narrow interventricular foramina, then a flexible neuroendoscope may be the only safe and practical choice. This is particularly the case in pediatric practice.

For tumor biopsy, the size of the specimen is important so as to give the neuropathologist the maximum material for diagnosis and to minimize the effects of crush artifact; the

Table 6.1. Comparison of surgical treatments for hydrocephalus [2]

	CP	NTV	Shunts
n	95	529	1087
Follow-up (years)	up to 27	7.5 (avg)	2 (avg)
Operative mortality	15%	15%	10%
Success	60%	70%	60%
Adverse late effects	–	3%	57%
Alive at 5 years	–	30%	2%

CP, choroid plexectomy; NTV, neuroendoscopic third ventriculostomy

Table 6.2. Features of neuroendoscopes: rigid vs flexible vs disposable

Type of endoscope	Advantages	Disadvantages
Rigid	Excellent optics Ease of use Good instrumentation Durable Relatively inexpensive	Larger size Restricted range of angulation
Flexible	Manoeuverable Smaller size	Disorientation More difficult to use Poorer optics Poorer instrumentation Smaller biopsies Fragile Relatively expensive
Channel™ (disposable)	Very easy to set up Good optics Relatively small caliber Excellent instrumentation Inexpensive Convenient, safe single use	Restricted range of angulation

present author finds the generous caliber of biopsy forceps permitted by the Channel™ neuroendoscope to be superior.

The range and quality of adjunctive instrumentation continue to increase, and currently include monopolar and bipolar diathermy, biopsy and grasping forceps, scissors, dissecting hooks, aspirating needles, catheters and inflatable balloons. The laser has advocates, and the author has found the KTP laser (Laserscope UK) to be particularly appropriate to neuroendoscopy. More specialized viewing endoscopes have been developed for endoscope-assisted ventricular shunt insertion and for endoscope-assisted microneurosurgery. A fine malleable endoscope is the most useful adjunct in aneurysm surgery and in some skull-base procedures. For transnasal endoscopic pituitary surgery, the endoscopes and allied instruments used in endoscopic sinus surgery are the most appropriate. An absolute requirement is a competent irrigation system in order to maintain good visibility. There is no evidence that special 'physiological' irrigating fluids are advantageous. The author's practice is to employ normal saline, irrigated under simple pulsed pressure that is operated by a footswitch and passed through a blood warmer.

A camera, a monitor and a fiberoptic light source are required. Ever since the first endoscopic photographs of the living human cerebral ventricles were taken in Philadelphia in 1922, the value and attraction of a photographic record have been recognized. The ability to make good-quality videocassette recordings cannot be overstated. Not only are they useful for training and teaching purposes, but also they are of great value to the surgeon for self-education and improvement on the rather steep learning curve involved. Recordable DVDs are replacing videocassettes.

Neuroimaging

Cranial ultrasonography can be usefully employed in babies with an open anterior fontanelle. It is extremely operator dependent, but with care, skill and experience it can provide much information on ventricular size and configuration and the relationships between fluid-filled intracranial spaces. Post-operatively, a 5 MHz and color Doppler ultrasonogram can demonstrate CSF flow [4].

Computed tomography (CT) remains the mainstay of much diagnostic imaging in neurosurgery. CT can be used as a satisfactory basis for planning many neuroendoscopic procedures, but there is no doubt that magnetic resonance (MR) is superior because of its multiplanar functionality, the better demonstration of blood vessels, the identification of membranes between fluid-filled spaces, and the ability to detect CSF flow.

A sequence of particular value, which is proprietary to Siemens MR scanners, is "constructive interference in the steady state" (CISS): this is of superior quality in demonstrating structures with one or more interfaces with CSF, such as the floor of the third ventricle, membranes within the ventricular system, and paraventricular cysts and subarachnoid structures [5]. Patients with hydrocephalus in association with the dysraphic states may have very complex ventricular anatomy, which will be best understood if examined by MR with CISS. The avoidance of ionizing radiation, especially in younger patients who may well require repeated imaging, is a further advantage. MR is therefore the modality of choice for pre-operative planning and for post-operative evaluation. Close collaboration and good communication between neurosurgeon, neuroradiologist and neuroradiographer will be rewarded by a more effective analysis of cases and an optimized, and safer, neuroendoscopic approach. Some practitioners have found the employment of intraoperative positive-contrast ventriculography of value in confirming patency of third ventriculostomies.

Neuroendoscopic Procedures and Applications

The operative interventions in which neuroendoscopy can play a definitive or supportive role can be classified by site and disease into: those within the internal cerebrospinal fluid spaces – principally the cerebral ventricles, those within the brain parenchyma, and those outside the brain in the subarachnoid or subdural spaces or extracranial skull base (Table 6.3).

Although most neuroendoscopic operations are minimally invasive, they should not be regarded as "minor procedures". They should only be undertaken in fully staffed and equipped neurosurgical operating rooms by surgeons who are prepared to proceed to an open operation if necessary. Nursing and resident medical staff must be available for post-operative observation and supervision as for any other intracranial neurosurgical operation. The operations most commonly undertaken relate to the management of hydrocephalus.

Table 6.3. Neuroendoscopic indications and procedures

Anatomical site	Condition	Treatment
Intraventricular	Hydrocephalus	Primary treatment
		NTV
		Shunt insertion
		Aqueductaplasty
		Choroid plexectomy
		Shunt complications
		NTV
		Shunt liberation
		Marsupialization
		Shunt removal
	Tumors	Biopsy
		Removal
	Cysts	Marsupialization
		Drainage
Parenchymal	Hematomas	Evacuation
	Abscesses	Drainage
Extracerebral	Subdural collections	Drainage
	Aneurysm	Assisted craniotomy & clipping
	Skull base tumors	Assisted craniotomy & excision
		Microvascular decompression
		Transnasal excision

NTV, neuroendoscopic third ventriculostomy

Neuroendoscopic Third Ventriculostomy (NTV)

NTV can be employed as the primary treatment of hydrocephalus (primary NTV) or as an alternative to shunt revision in the management of shunt complications (secondary NTV). NTV is the most frequently undertaken neuroendoscopic procedure. Ideally, pre-operative MR is acquired to give the necessary anatomical details and to assist in the evaluation for suitability and the operative approach.

Although techniques will differ in detail from one surgeon to another, the principles are fairly constant. The intention is to make an opening in the floor of the third ventricle and thereby create an internal fistula between the ventricular system and the basal subarachnoid spaces. Although the full procedure can best be understood by reference to video clips [3], there are a number of critical technical points that are worthy of attention. Under general orotracheal anaesthesia, the patient is placed supine with mild-to-moderate flexion of the head and neck. A burr hole is placed accurately on, or just anterior to, the coronal suture in the mid-pupillary line. The lateral ventricle is located with a brain cannula, which is then replaced with the neuroendoscope.

Most neuroendoscopes are inserted through a sheath. If a disposable plastic 'peel away' sheath is used, it is best not to peel it apart or fix it to the scalp as the additional mobility afforded by keeping the sheath free can be an advantage. The sheath can be used to direct a flexible neuroendoscope or can be advanced through the interventricular foramen so as to protect its margins. The foramen of Monro is navigated carefully, without damaging the choroid plexus, the thalamo-striate vein or the fornices. The configuration of the foramen of Monro is quite variable. Correct selection of the point at which to incise the floor of the third ventricle is crucial so as to avoid the tip of the basilar artery. Careful attention to this critical vascular relationship on the pre-operative MR is recommended, as there is more anatomical variation than is generally appreciated. The correct site is on the anterior part of the floor of the third ventricle, slightly posterior to the pink vascular area that marks the pituitary infundibulum. Practices and opinions differ as to how best to make the opening. Some surgeons simply perforate the floor with the tip of a rigid endoscope [6]; others use biopsy forceps, diathermy or laser, with or without enlargement of the opening by an inflatable balloon [7]. Beneath the floor of the third ventricle lies Liliequist's membrane; it is variable in extent, and its superior attachment may lie anterior or posterior to the mammillary bodies. In the former case of pre-mammillary attachment, failure to open it may result in ineffective CSF drainage [8].

An opening of at least 4 mm is desirable, and it is advisable to pass the endoscope through the third ventriculostomy into the basal cisterns to confirm that the opening is of adequate proportions and that there is indeed an unencumbered passage into the interpeduncular or prepontine cistern. On withdrawing the endoscope into the third ventricle, an encouraging sign that is likely to presage a successful outcome is a gentle undulation of the margins of the ventriculostomy that is clearly different from the cardiac or respiratory cycle [9]. There is frequently a small amount of bleeding that settles with irrigation. Often, one can observe a progressive spontaneous enlargement of the ventriculostomy over the course of a few minutes. In general it is best to resist the urge to go on a tour of the ventricular system after completing the ventriculostomy, and it is preferable to leave the ventricles fairly plump rather than to aspirate them, so as to encourage flow through the opening.

In patients with neural tube defects, a number of anatomical peculiarities may be encountered. The interventricular foramen is frequently a rather oblique narrow triangle. The massa intermedia may be unusually large, but more significantly there may be an extra commissure running in the sagittal plane above the anterior part of the floor of the third ventricle obscuring the site of the intended ventriculostomy; there may be buckling of the floor of the third ventricle, and there can be multiple basal cistern subarachnoid adhesions. Many of these hurdles can be identified pre-operatively on CISS MR.

In performing a secondary NTV, particular attention should be paid to a variety of anatomical considerations that may make the procedure difficult, more hazardous, or even impossible. The skull can be pathologically thick in those who were shunted primarily in infancy, and can restrict the range of direction of approach when using a rigid neuroendoscope. There may be thick, calcific subdural membranes from past subdural hematomas. The wall of the lateral ventricle may be tough and thick, especially in those patients shunted for perinatal post-hemorrhagic hydrocephalus, those with slit-ventricle syndrome, and those who have suffered ventriculitis. The internal anatomy of the lateral ventricle can be bizarre. There may be synechiae related and unrelated to the presence of a ventricular shunt catheter. The usual landmarks leading to the interventricular foramen may be absent, especially in patients who have suffered intraventricular hemorrhage, or ventriculitis associated with meningitis or serious ventricular shunt infections. On occasion, the lateral ventricles can be subdivided by complete or incomplete septae. The septum pellucidum may be spontaneously perforated or absent. The interventricular foramen may be completely obliterated by gliosis or may have assumed an abnormal configuration. Alternatively, patients with very large lateral ventricles due to chronic shunt malfunction can have very large interventricular foramina that are so huge that the third ventricle is almost assimilated into the lateral ventricle. The third ventricle can also be very abnormal, with gliotic septae obscuring or frankly obstructing the pathways. The cavity of the third ventricle may be narrow.

The usual landmarks on the third ventricle floor may be quite unclear. The anterior part of the floor may be thick and opaque; fortunately, the vascular area that marks the recess of the pituitary infundibulum is usually preserved. The interpeduncular cistern may be densely obliterated by subarachnoid adhesions that may in themselves conceal the basilar artery and its branches and cranial nerves III and VI. Liliequist's membrane may be abnormally thick. The circle of Willis may be in an unusual position. The two most frequent variants are an unusual application of the basilar artery to the dorsum sellae and upper clivus, usually due to subarachnoid scarring, and an abnormal tortuousness of the anterior communicating artery, which may bulge into the anterior part of the third ventricle. Patients with intracranial tumors may have anatomical distortions due to the presence of tumor tissue or the effects of previous surgery and radiation therapy.

Regression of clinical symptoms and avoidance of an implanted diversionary CSF shunt indicate a successful outcome. Routine postoperative imaging is not mandatory. In 60% of cases ventricular size is unchanged despite relief of symptoms; ventricular volume may drop despite ventricular size remaining constant. A flow void through the ventriculostomy on appropriate MR sequences is confirmation of functional patency of the ventriculostomy and correlates with radionuclide studies; flow voids in the interventricular foramina and interpeduncular cistern indicate active CSF flow, but signal in the prepontine cistern alone reflects basilar artery pulsation.

Results of NTV

One of the longest running and largest series is that accumulated in Sydney, Australia, which extends back to 1978. In a mixed series of 103 children and adults, there was an overall success rate of 61%, with no difference between those undergoing primary, as opposed to secondary, NTV [10]. In a purely adult series from Nottingham, UK, followed for a mean of 3 years, 80% of 63 patients were successfully treated by NTV [11]. In both of these series there was no difference between those having primary NTV and those previously shunted patients undergoing secondary NTV. In an earlier, predominantly pediatric, series from Nottingham, with a median age of 16 months, there was a success rate of 62% [1]. Smaller series have reported much higher success rates, but in highly selected cases. For example, a French center reported 33 successes in 35 previously untreated cases [12]; around 60% would seem to be the overall success rate in unselected cases across all ages. Although there is a wider range of experience for secondary NTV, most reported series from experienced operators report success in 60–80% of cases (Table 6.4). This probably reflects a

Table 6.4. Success rate of secondary NTV

Series	[ref]	*n*	Success (%)
Jones, 1992	[6]	27	74
Teo, 1996	[19]	54	72
Nottingham, 1997		47	77
Cinalli, 1998	[20]	23	78
Hopf, 1999	[29]	25	84
Nottingham, 2001		88	61

range of happenstance selection bias. There are, of course, clinical circumstances in which the patient is so dogged by shunt complications that even a relatively low chance of success makes an attempt at secondary NTV justifiable. In general, given the recurrent tendency of shunt complications, it seems reasonable to at least consider secondary NTV in every case of shunt malfunction, as proposed by some practitioners [13]. Such a strategy, adopted by some, does have implications in terms of staff and equipment [1].

Some series have recorded a higher failure rate in the very young (Table 6.5), 16 out of 25 NTVs failing in babies aged under 6 months [10]. This has led some surgeons to regard failure as being age-related to the point that some are most reluctant to use NTV in the first year of life. Although overall success rates of 23% for those undergoing NTV in the first year of life [14], and 32% for those born prematurely [15], have been reported, more recent studies have shown that the outcome relates more to the pathology than to age [1]. For aqueductal stenosis there is no difference in outcome between those aged younger than 6 months and those that are older [16], and success rates of more than 80% for congenital aqueductal stenosis have been achieved [17]. A particularly unfavorable pathology for which primary NTV should probably not be attempted is post-meningitic hydrocephalus. However, the low success rate for this pathology, and also for the unfavorable post-hemorrhagic hydrocephalus, is less marked at a later age, and subsequent secondary NTV for shunt failure is always worth considering [16].

Other patients for whom both primary and secondary NTV is particularly successful are those with midline tumors [18] and those with myelomeningocele [19], with success rates of up to 100% and 80% respectively.

Neuroendoscopy in the Management of Shunt Complications and Complex Hydrocephalus

Apart from secondary NTV, neuroendoscopy has other contributions to make in the management of shunt malfunction. Firstly, it should not be overlooked that secondary NTV can still be used to provide ventricular drainage following treatment of shunt infections. Most neurosurgeons manage shunt infections by the technique of shunt removal, interval external drainage with antibiotics, and then shunt insertion; the last stage can often be replaced by NTV [1, 20].

Loculation of the cerebral ventricles is a serious complication of intraventricular hemorrhage and infection, which can be the cause of much morbidity and mortality and frustrated neurosurgical endeavor. Although the surgery looks seductively easy on viewing the imaging, the reality is very different – neuroendoscopic deloculation can be one of the most challenging procedures. The absence of normal anatomy, the unexpected thickness and the vascularity of the septa, and the tendency for the operative field to become rapidly like a souvenir of the Eiffel tower in a snowstorm all make for great difficulties. Pre-operative planning should always include MR, preferably with CISS or equivalent sequences. Intraoperative guidance by ultrasound may assist if there is an appropriate sonographic window. Fenestrations should be as large as possible, and certainly greater than 1 cm in diameter. Cutting/coagulating diathermy is the tool of choice. Multiple procedures may be required.

The most dangerous variant is the loculated fourth ventricle. Unfortunately a neuroendoscopic approach is only rarely feasible as the cerebral aqueduct is usually densely occluded

Table 6.5. Success rate of NTV in infants

Series	[ref]	*n*	Characteristics	Success (%)
Jones, 1994	[10]	25	Age <2 years	32
Teo, 1996	[19]	11	Myelomeningoceles	9
Buxton, 1998	[14]	27	Age <1 year	23
Buxton, 1998	[15]	19	Prematures	32
Hopf, 1999	[29]	4	Age <1 year	0
Javadpour, 2001	[17]	21	Age <1 year	48

over most of its length. Occasionally there may be a simple membrane, division of which will restore communication between the third and the fourth ventricles. Again, MR with CISS is invaluable in defining the anatomy.

Neuroendoscopy can also be useful for liberating ventricular shunt catheters, either to make their removal safer, or as a definitive procedure if secondary NTV is not feasible [13]. It can be used to retrieve loose shunt components. This is also a situation in which cutting/coagulating diathermy is most useful to cut down on the ventricular catheter, just as would be done in dissecting out the extracranial portion of a shunt.

Slit-ventricle syndrome is another most unpleasant shunt complication in which neuroendoscopy may play a useful role. An initial subtemporal decompression may be effective in promoting sufficient ventricular enlargement to permit secondary NTV. Alternatively, patients may undergo shunt externalization, followed by a period of invasive intracranial pressure monitoring without CSF drainage, with those showing elevated or symptomatic intracranial hypertension then proceeding to NTV. The risk of acute deterioration mandates very careful observation.

The small ventricular size and relatively non-compliant ventricles do bring a risk of life-threatening cardiac dysrhythmias during NTV, so great care needs to be taken when irrigating.

Neuroendoscopy in the Management of Non-tumorous Cysts

Neurodevelopmental arachnoid cysts in suprasellar, quadrigeminal, middle cranial fossa, interhemispheric septum pellucidum, and parenchymal locations have all been approached neuroendoscopically. The guiding principle is to marsupialize the cyst into an adjacent normal cerebrospinal fluid chamber or pathway. Pre-operative MR with CISS is again enormously helpful in planning an approach by displaying the fluid/cyst wall/fluid interfaces in three orthogonal planes. The next important principle is, wherever possible, to approach the lesion via a normal cerebrospinal fluid space or chamber. Even if this space is smaller than the cyst, the advantage of having some normal, and hopefully recognizable, anatomy greatly exceeds the perceived difficulty in entering a space that may not be particularly dilated. Generous fenestrations of 1–2 cm are required, and are best made using cutting/coagulating diathermy. Suprasellar cysts are approached by the right frontal route to the lateral ventricle, and then via the interventricular foramen. The dome of the cyst is widely opened into the ventricular system (cysto-ventriculostomy) and the cyst then usually collapses, exposing the hitherto obstructed posterior third ventricle and aqueduct. There is debate as to whether the base of the cyst should then be opened into the interpeduncular cistern (cysto-cisternostomy) [12].

The author's approach is to perform both cysto-ventriculostomy and cysto-cisternostomy if the latter seems safe. However, if the area is very vascular, such that there is no very apparent safe route, then a generous cysto-ventriculostomy usually suffices. Quadrigeminal plate cysts can usually be opened into the third ventricle by an approach via the lateral ventricle and interventricular foramen, although on occasion there is an interface presenting into a lateral ventricle that can be accessed. Intraparenchymal cysts can often be marsupialized into a lateral ventricle. Other midline cysts may be made to communicate with the ventricular system or the subarachnoid space. Symptomatic cysts of the septum pellucidum may be approached via a lateral ventricle. If the cyst is punctured directly, the very different anatomy will warn the surgeon of the position and, with care regarding the midline vascular structures and the fornices, the cyst can be marsupialized into the third ventricle. Many of these cysts will require unique approaches and directions of attack that are not along straight lines; it is in this type of case that the flexible neuroendoscope really comes into its own and has considerable advantages over a rigid instrument. On occasion, small intraventricular third ventricle cysts of presumed ependymal origin, unsuspected from pre-operative imaging, have come to light in the course of performing a NTV; these can be readily opened up to relieve the hydrocephalus.

The place of neuroendoscopy in the management of colloid cysts of the third ventricle remains uncertain. Early reports concerned diagnostic rather than therapeutic interventions [1]. Subsequently it became clear that some colloid cysts could be dealt with endoscopically, and encouraging single-center reports continue to appear [21]. The debate tends to center on safety issues and the ability to achieve complete resection. Proponents of endoscopy, image-guided stereotactic drainage, and open microsurgical resection continue to maintain their respective corners. These lesions are best tackled with a rigid or disposable Channel™ neuroendoscope because of the superior visualization and better instrumentation. As always, the direction and line of approach is all important; a pre-frontal entry point is required so as to be able to access the roof of the third ventricle and deal with the origin of the cyst. Dense solid cysts will continue to pose problems by any route other than an open transcallosal approach but, happily, are in the minority. The matter is clearly not going to be resolved without a randomized prospective study.

Management of Intracranial Tumors

Certain intraventricular and paraventricular tumors can be approached endoscopically via dilated ventricles. One of the pioneering applications of the flexible neuroendoscope was in this field, and both pineal region and paraventricular tumors were biopsied through custom-made, flexible, fiberoptic neuroendoscopes. Interestingly, the authors of these papers did not consider the possibility of performing a concurrent NTV to relieve hydrocephalus.

The success rate for biopsy was low for those tumors that were not actually in the ventricular system, and this was attributed to the small size of the biopsies. Other problems are that many paraventricular tumors are still separated from the ventricular system by an intact layer of ependyma that must be breached if tumor tissue is to be obtained [3]. The relatively small size of the tissue samples is compounded by crush artifact. This is a particular problem with the flexible neuroendoscope and, wherever possible, a rigid or disposable Channel™ neuroendoscope is preferable because of the larger size of biopsy obtainable. One successful technique is to use a stereotactic biopsy needle passed though the endoscope (J. Firth, personal communication). In view of the age-related predilection for sites on and adjacent to the midline, neuroendoscopy has a considerable role in the management of pediatric brain tumors. The value of neuroendoscopy is not confined to children, and in a Nottingham series of 87 procedures in 77 patients, age ranged from 5 months to 70 years [18]. Relief of hydrocephalus by NTV remains a principal indication with a high level of success: 63 out of 66 cases (95%) in the short term, with durable shunt-free outcome in 55 out of 66 cases (83%). Neuroendoscopic tumor biopsies were successful in providing a tissue diagnosis in 17 out of 29 cases (61%) [18]. A very particular application is in pineal region tumors, in which there is the possibility of delivering "one-stop" neurosurgery that provides relief of hydrocephalus, tumor biopsy and cerebrospinal fluid sampling for tumor cytology and biochemical evaluation of germ-cell tumor markers.

Very high diagnostic accuracy has been documented [22]; under these circumstances there can be no justification in performing an open operation for pineal germ-cell tumors unless committed efforts have first been made to make the diagnosis by these alternative means. It has been stated that NTV is contraindicated in those patients who have undergone radiation therapy, both on the grounds of inefficacy and risk of complications [6]; this has not been the experience of the present author. NTV can be successfully used to relieve hydrocephalus due to posterior fossa tumors [18]. The ideal timing is yet to be defined; in patients with very chronic or massive hydrocephalus, there is a case for leaving an interval of a few days between NTV and definitive posterior fossa exploration. As a relatively small proportion of patients with hydrocephalus in association with a posterior fossa tumor will require a ventricular shunt following tumor resection, it is difficult to justify the routine performance of NTV in such cases, and it might be appropriate to reserve the procedure for those at greatest risk of persistent hydrocephalus, such as children under 5 years of age. The optimum strategy is yet to be established. However, when NTV is performed there is the added value of being able to inspect the ventricular system for possible metastases, to take samples of cerebrospinal fluid for tumor cytology, and, if a flexible neuroendoscope is used, to pass through the cerebral aqueduct and inspect the relationship of the tumor to the floor of the fourth ventricle.

Resection of intraventricular and parenchymal tumors remains a relatively infrequent practice owing to the limiting factors of hemorrhage, deteriorating visibility, length of operation and the limited range of available instruments.

A dual-portal approach has been piloted that uses one channel for illumination and visualization, and the other for the passage of instruments; complete resection was achieved in five out of six patients, one case being abandoned in favor of open operation due to hemorrhage [23]. Although there was no immediate reported morbidity, the potential hazards of multiple cortical punctures were a cause for concern. Extensive endoscopic resection of deep-seated parenchymal brain tumors has remained the practice of a very small number of committed neurosurgeons, often using highly sophisticated image-guided stereotaxy and laser ablation, or ultrasound guidance. Notwithstanding the high level of skill and elegance involved, the absence of any randomized trial data regarding disease-free remission or survival makes it difficult to evaluate and define the role of this technology in tumor management.

Treatment of Non-tumorous Parenchymal Brain Lesions

The marriage of image-guided stereotactic localization with neuroendoscopy can be used to maximize evacuation of pus from intracerebral abscesses. However, a second procedure is often needed [24].

Endoscopic evacuation of intracerebral hematomas is also possible, and although one randomized study of drainage of subcortical hematomas in patients aged under 60 years with preserved consciousness suggested an advantage over best medical treatment, this is yet to be confirmed in larger trials [25].

Endoscope-assisted Procedures

The development of small-caliber rigid endoscopes and malleable endoscopes has facilitated the marriage between neuroendoscopy and microneurosurgery. The overriding principles are to use the endoscope to bring light into the operative field, and to enable alternative lines of sight. Simultaneous images through the microscope and through the endoscope can be displayed on a single monitor. Particular applications are: the improved application of aneurysm clips, access to skull base tumors, microvascular decompression of the trigeminal and facial nerves through very minimal access approaches, and transsphenoidal pituitary surgery [26]. For those surgeons able to cope with the simultaneous integration of so much technology, and who can find space in the operating room for the additional equipment, the rewards do seem substantial in terms of enhanced visualization and accuracy.

Complications

When the author introduced neuroendoscopy into the Nottingham neurosurgical department, he was concerned to register both outcomes and complications, not only for the purposes of scientific inquiry, but also to enable accurate data to be available to inform discussions with patients and colleagues when reaching decisions in management. The resultant purpose-built database "ENDOSPREAD" contained, in anticipation, a list of possible complications plus space for any unique or unexpected ones (Table 6.6)!

There was therefore some concern that, until relatively recently, there was an apparent dearth of reports regarding complications, despite word-of-mouth anecdotes of such momentous events as basilar artery injuries either requiring formal surgical repair or having fatal outcomes. Even stranger was that reports were not appearing of those that were successfully repaired. Following a number of verbal communications at international meetings, at which it became clear that very major complications of NTV – principally of a vascular nature – were not being reported, the ice finally broke [27]. These papers, from an extremely experienced leader in the field, served to acknowledge and define the position. The author's distinction between significant and insignificant complications was a helpful one, in that it provided a matrix and a benchmark for further analysis. In 173 procedures over a 2-year period, there was an incidence of 22 intraoperative events (13%); 7% of the patients suffered a significant complication. Insignificant complications are those such as

Table 6.6. Complications of neuroendoscopy (as coded & recorded in "ENDOSPREAD")

1	Intraoperative hemorrhage – operation abandoned
2	Intraoperative hemorrhage – operation continued
3	Hemorrhage – intraventricular
4	Hemorrhage – intracerebral
5	Hemorrhage – subdural
6	Hemorrhage – extradural
7	Infection – deep
8	Infection – superficial
9	Cranial nerve lesion – transient
10	Cranial nerve lesion – persistent
11	Neurological impairment – transient
12	Neurological impairment – persistent
13	CSF fistula – transient, requiring no more than suture
14	CSF fistula – persistent
15	Novel epilepsy <7 days from operation
16	Novel epilepsy >7 days from operation
17	Exacerbation of epilepsy <7 days from operation
18	Exacerbation of epilepsy >7 days from operation
19	Neuroendocrine – transient
20	Neuroendocrine – persistent
21	Cerebral infarct – asymptomatic
22	Cerebral infarct – symptomatic
23	ICU admission post-operatively
24	Death within 30 days of operation
25	EVD inserted – intraoperatively
26	EVD inserted – post-operatively
27	Intraoperative cardiac event

EVD, external ventricular drain

minor intraoperative bleeding that stops with irrigation and does not compromise the patient or the procedure. Significant ones are those that do, or might, have serious or lasting sequelae for the patient. It must be acknowledged that, whilst defining these categories is useful to the surgeon, in the mind of patients and families even a relatively small event such as a transient leakage of cerebrospinal fluid that resolves with a single suture is a cause for concern. Whereas the incidence of insignificant complications declined with experience, the occurrence of significant ones did not. The most frequent and the most serious complications are listed in Table 6.7.

Of some concern are reports of what appear to be sudden and unexpected deaths in patients who have undergone NTV. It is unclear whether these were truly without prodrome or whether the patients had been lulled into a sense of false security following successful NTV, and simply failed to seek medical attention when headaches

Table 6.7. The frequent or serious complications of neuroendoscopy

Intraoperative complications
Intraoperative hemorrhage causing procedure to be abandoned
Traumatic cerebral artery aneurysm
Intracerebral hematoma
Life-threatening cardiac dysrhythmias
Transient bradycardia
Transient hypertension
Post-operative complications
Death within 6 weeks
Cerebral infarction
New cranial nerve palsy
New neurological deficit
Subdural collections
CSF leak
Meningitis or ventriculitis
Superficial infection
Epilepsy
Hypothalamic damage

or even visual symptoms recurred. They may therefore have been in no different a situation to the patient with a shunt who becomes a victim of failed follow-up.

Strategies for Reducing Complications

The risk of damage to the basilar artery and its branches and to cranial nerves can be minimized by careful attention to: the local anatomy on pre-operative imaging; care in selecting a point on the floor of the third ventricle that is just posterior to the infundibular recess, rather than just anterior to the mammillary bodies; and a cautious technique for opening the floor of the third ventricle. It is worth reiterating that the only constant feature on the anterior third-ventricle floor is the pink, vascular area signaling the infundibular recess. The mammillary bodies in the first few months of life are surprisingly flat, and may only be identified by the very small whisker-like arteries running over them; the surface of the ventricular floor may be featureless or scarred as a result of previous infection or hemorrhage, or distorted by tumor invasion. Although a very fine ultrasound probe has been of value in identifying a 'safe', sonically silent area, the technology is very expensive and has not been generally adopted, even in specialist departments. There are strongly held views regarding the relative safety or otherwise of different instruments and methods for perforating the floor.

The argument against using laser or diathermy is the perceived risk of vascular damage, but no study has demonstrated an advantage in terms of either efficacy or safety for any particular method. The absence of any reporting system for adverse events, beyond individual personal or institutional systems, makes any such opinion difficult to confirm, but it is probably wise to keep any use of diathermy to a minimum, and to ensure that it is always used under direct vision. Similar strictures relate to the methods used for enlarging the opening. The most widely used is probably the balloon catheter, and as long as care is taken, it may well be safer than diathermy. Blunt hooks, as can be used through a disposable Channel™ neuroendoscope, appear to be safe and are most intuitive to the neurosurgeon, especially in the subarachnoid space. A sensible precaution would seem to be the practice of starting with a small, centrally placed opening and then looking through it into the space below the floor to check on position and the presence or absence of second membrane, adhesions, vessels or tumor. This will be easier to accomplish with a flexible neuroendoscope or a Channel™ neuroendoscope than with most rigid neuroendoscopes. The only safe rule is to abandon the procedure if the anatomy is not clear.

Throughout, the surgeon must be mindful regarding the irrigation, ensuring that there is easy egress of irrigate; with flexible and disposable Channel™ neuroendoscopes, the route of escape of the irrigate is between the endoscope and the inner wall of the plastic cannula. It is not difficult to allow the cannula to slip out of the ventricle, under which circumstance there will be no way for irrigate to escape.

At moments of high tension the surgeon may inadvertently pinch the plastic cannula, occluding it, allowing irrigate to accumulate in the ventricles with resultant rise in intracranial pressure. This will be particularly dangerous if the neuroendoscope is within the narrow confines of the third ventricle. Such circumstances can cause cardiac dysrhythmias, especially if the ventricular walls are stiff.

Whereas it is always tempting to take a wander through the ventricular system, especially with a flexible neuroendoscope, the surgeon should avoid the enticement of 'ventricular tourism' (with acknowledgement to Professor Christian Sainte-Rose) and withdraw from the operative scene. The cerebral ventricles should be left full so as to encourage flow through the NTV. Attention to the wound and its closure is worthwhile: in babies and infants with thinner, less well developed scalp tissues, the author now uses a small scalp flap of the size that would be used for insertion of a ventriculostomy reservoir, thus avoiding having a scalp incision directly over the dural incision. Formal closure of the dura is said to help eliminate cerebrospinal fluid leakage (G. Cinalli, personal communication), and the scalp is closed in layers.

The anesthetist must concentrate on the monitoring, and must be alert to the possibility of cardiovascular changes and the need to report them immediately to the surgeon.

A pilot study employing sophisticated statistical analysis failed to show any increased risk of epilepsy in children undergoing NTV [28].

Training

Neuroendoscopy carries a steep learning curve and involves the acquisition of a variety of novel skills, including those relating to: the selection of patients; the imaging; the operating room set-up; the equipment; the practice of operating from a monitor with only two-dimensional images; working in close concert with an assistant; and being alive to a number of parameters that have to be monitored. There are also a number of hard-learned tips that are better assimilated in advance, rather than re-discovered anew.

Neuroendoscopy also lends itself to workshop training. In recognition of this, a number of 'hands-on' courses have been established, such as those in Mainz, Germany; St Louis, USA; and London, England. From the time that the author first established the Nottingham neuroendoscopy course, now held at the Royal College of Surgeons of England, London, it has been apparent from personal feedback that participants have benefited from attendance. It has been of particular significance when some senior neurosurgeons have decided that neuroendoscopy is not for them. Complementary to training workshops and in-service training with an established practitioner is the possibility of gaining experience by proxy from libraries of video clips on CD-ROM [3]. The development of computer 'virtual' surgery training will be of value, and is under development in Aalborg, Denmark (J. Haase, personal communication).

Research and Future Directions

Research Questions in Neuroendoscopy

The modern era of neuroendoscopy encapsulates some of the lessons to be learnt about the introduction of new technology, especially when it is suggested that it may replace existing methods. The natural enthusiasm of the surgeon to be amongst the first to offer the patient an alternative that may be 'better' runs hard on the commercial keenness of the salespeople to sell new and expensive kit. In some cultures and health systems, the ability to provide the latest facility may impact upon the income of the surgeon. In other societies, those who fund the purchase of new equipment may hide behind a pretend shield of "Where's the proof?" as a means of preventing progress. Meanwhile, those who are in a position to introduce the new technology do so, accumulate and present results, and begin to assume fixed positions regarding the value of the "new way". By this time it is probably too late in practical, though not in ethical, economic or scientific terms to run the studies that would be needed to seek the evidence in favor, or against. This is particularly so when existing methods are less than perfect, as is the case with hydrocephalus shunts.

So, is NTV "better" than a shunt? There are many who think so, including the present author, based simply upon the premise that shunts are vicarious, and that to be without the risk, or the actuality, of the misery of their complications is a better position in which to live one's life. Whether NTV is a better treatment per se for the hydrocephalic brain, complications of therapy aside, is not known.

One non-randomized, retrospective study comparing 30 children treated by NTV with 38 treated by ventriculo-peritoneal shunts found no difference between the two groups in neurological, endocrine, behavioral or social outcome [7]. As our aspirations for our patients become greater, it is appropriate that studies should be established to identify which method of treatment is better for the young brain in terms of neurodevelopment, and for the adult brain in terms of neuropsychological function.

For some categories of very young patient the success rate for NTV is low, but the complication rate of shunts is also high; a randomized study here would also be appropriate.

It is not known whether the apparently good results published from centers in which there are acknowledged experts in neuroendoscopy can extend to a whole population of neurosurgeons and their patients, yet this is a crucial point if advice is to be given on a national or international basis. A prospective study capturing all patients treated by NTV needs to look at this wider picture. With the concerns regarding complications, this could be matched with a central registry of adverse events. It is noteworthy, as an observation only, albeit not capable of analysis, that in Nottingham in an early study of 47 children and young people undergoing 51 secondary NTVs, there were only three significant complications (6%) [1]; yet in a series extending into a later epoch, of 63 adults undergoing 66 NTVs, there was a total complication rate of 17.5%, with an 11% serious complication rate [11].

Without any imputation, one operational change that occurred between the earlier study and the one including later patients was that the number of surgeons performing NTV rose from three consultants to six consultants plus a number of supervised trainees. This may mean nothing, but the question still needs to be asked as to whether this is a technique that can be pursued safely by all surgeons, or whether it should be subject to sub-specialization.

There are certain specific applications of NTV that could be addressed in prospective studies, e.g. the value of "routine" NTV in children with posterior fossa tumors, or the efficacy of NTV in treating syringomyelia when that condition is associated with ventriculomegaly.

With regards to other neuroendoscopic procedures, there is a clear place for a randomized study of endoscopic vs open resection of third-ventricle colloid cysts.

These study proposals will require multi-center collaborative studies. An encouraging start was made by Professor Bernhard Bauer (Hanover, Germany) and Professor Shizuo Oi (Tokyo, Japan) when they inaugurated the International Study Group on Neuroendoscopy (ISGNE) in Hyogo, Japan, in October 2001.

Future Developments

The major requirements are in the fields of instrumentation and guidance. The present armamentarium could usefully be expanded to enable better methods of lifting and incising tissues. Methods of image enhancement should be brought to bear so as to increase the information available from images obtained, especially with fiberoptic neuroendoscopes.

Concerns regarding transmissible disease are likely to grow, such that there will be demands for completely disposable instrumentation; the neuroendoscope designers and manufacturers should anticipate this need. Although several surgeons have found a useful dialogue between neuronavigation and neuroendoscopy, the present position is far from ideal, and there is a need for real-time intraoperative neuronavigation that would enable more accurate localization when dealing with complex anatomy. All of these developments will require a closer working relationship between the surgeons and the companies involved.

Acknowledgements

The author wishes to record the generosity of the following, whose fund-raising efforts enabled the establishment of neuroendoscopy at Nottingham University Hospital: the late Anthony Ozolins and his family, the family of the late Helen Ringrose, and the family of the late Emma Clayton.

Copyright Warning

Key Points

- *Advances in optical technology and in neuroimaging have resulted in the establishment of neuroendoscopy – a minimally invasive technique.*
- *There is a dearth of Class I evidence of the benefits and risks of this technique.*
- *Neuroendoscopic third ventriculostomy is currently the primary treatment of choice for selected cases of non-tumorous and tumorous hydrocephalus.*
- *The only demonstrable benefit on present evidence is freedom of complications from implanted devices.*
- *There are particular applications in the management of shunt complications, intraventricular and paraventricular tumors, and non-tumorous cysts.*
- *Proper training is essential and the technique should probably remain within the hands of a restricted number of specialists.*
- *Unstructured propagation is likely to be associated with avoidable morbidity.*
- *Regulatory authorities should monitor morbidity until the position is clear.*
- *Prospective studies are required to evaluate the hazards as well as the benefits in comparison with older approaches.*
- *The future may bring more sophisticated applications in conjunction with image guidance.*

References

1. Punt J, Vloeberghs M. Endoscopy in neurosurgery. Minim Invasive Ther & Allied Technol 1998;7:159–70.
2. Scarff JE. Evaluation of treatment of hydrocephalus. Report of third ventriculostomy and endoscopic

cauterization of choroid plexuses compared with mechanical shunts. Arch Neurol 1966;14:382–91.
3. Punt J, Vloeberghs M, Terrett M. An introduction to neuroendoscopy. A computer based tutorial system on CD-ROM. Nottingham: HyperTech/2nd Messenger, 1996.
4. Wilcock DJ, Jaspan T, Punt J, Kwok BCT. CSF flow through third ventriculostomy demonstrated with colour Doppler ultrasonography. Clin Radiol 1996; 51:127–9.
5. Laitt RD, Mallucci CL, McConachie NS, Jaspan T, Vloeberghs M, Punt J. Constructive interference in steady state 3D Fourier Transform MRI in the management of hydrocephalus and third ventriculostomy. Neuroradiology 1999;41:324–7.
6. Jones RFC, Teo C, Stening WA et al. Neuroendoscopic third ventriculostomy. In: Manwaring KH, Crone KR, Dante MD, editors. Neuroendoscopy, 1st edn New York: Liebert; 1992; 63–77.
7. Sainte-Rose C. Third Ventriculostomy. In: Manwaring KH, Crone KR, Dante MD, editors. Neuroendoscopy. 1st edn. New York: Liebert; 1992; 47-62.
8. Buxton N, Vloeberghs M, Punt J. Liliequist's membrane in minimally invasive endoscopic neurosurgery. Clin Anat 1998;11(3):187–90.
9. Jones RFC, Kwok BC, Stening WA, Vonau M. The current status of endoscopic third ventriculostomy in the management of non-communicating hydrocephalus. Minim Invasive Neurosurg 1994;37(1):28–36.
10. Jones RFC, Kwok BCT, Stening WA, Vonau M. Neuroendoscopic third ventriculostomy. A practical alternative to extracranial shunts in non-communicating hydrocephalus. Acta Neurochir Suppl 1994; 61:79–83.
11. Buxton N, Ho KJ, Vloeberghs M, Macarthur D, Punt J, Robertson I. Neuroendoscopic third ventriculostomy for hydrocephalus in adults: report of a single unit's experience with 63 cases. Surg Neurol 2001;55:74–8.
12. Decq P, Yepes C, Anno Y, Djindjian M, Nguyen JP, Keravel Y. L'endoscopie neurochirurgicale. Indications diagnostiques et therapeutiques. Neurochirurgie 1994; 40(5):313–21.
13. Mallucci C, Vloeberghs M, Punt J. Neuroendoscopic third ventriculostomy: the first-line treatment for blocked ventriculo-peritoneal shunts? Child's Nerv Syst 1997;13:498.
14. Buxton N, Macarthur D, Mallucci C, Punt J, Vloeberghs M. Neuroendoscopic third ventriculostomy in patients less than one year old. Pediatr Neurosurg 1998;29:73–6.
15. Buxton N, Macarthur D, Mallucci C, Punt J, Vloeberghs M. Neuroendoscopy in the premature population. Child's Nerv Syst 1998;14:649–52.
16. Cinalli G, Saint-Rose C, Chumas P, Zerah M, Brunelle F, Lot G et al. Failure of third ventriculostomy in the treatment of aqueductal stenosis in children. J Neurosurg 1999;90:448–54.
17. Javadpour M, Mallucci C, Brodbelt A, Golash A, May P. The impact of endoscopic third ventriculostomy on the management of newly diagnosed hydrocephalus in infants. Pediatr Neurosurg 2001;35:131–5.
18. Macarthur DC, Buxton N, Punt J Vloeberghs M, Robertson IJA. The role of neuroendoscopy in the management of brain tumours. Br J Neurosurg 2002;16:465–70.
19. Teo C, Jones R. Management of hydrocephalus by endoscopic third ventriculostomy in patients with myelomeningocele. Pediatr Neurosurg 1996;25(2): 57–63.
20. Cinalli G, Salazar C, Mallucci C, Yada JZ, Zerah M, Sainte-Rose C. The role of endoscopic third ventriculostomy in the management of shunt malfunction. Neurosurgery 1998;43:1323–9.
21. Longatti P, Martinuzzi A, Moro M, Fiorindi A, Cartieri A. Endoscopic treatment of colloid cysts of the third ventricle: 9 consecutive cases. Minim Invasive Neurosurg 2000;43(3):118–23.
22. Pople IK, Athanasiou TC, Sandeman DR, Coakham HB. The role of endoscopic biopsy and third ventriculostomy in the management of pineal region tumours. Br J Neurosurg 2001;15:305–11.
23. Jallo GI, Morota N, Abbott R. Introduction of a second working portal for neuroendoscopy. A technical note. Pediatr Neurosurg 1996;24:56–60.
24. Hellwig D, Bauer BL, Dauch WA. Endoscopic stereotactic treatment of brain abscesses. Acta Neurochir Suppl 1994;61:102–5.
25. Auer LM, Deinsberger W, Niederkorn K, Gell G, Kleinert R, Schneider G et al. Endoscopic surgery versus medical treatment for spontaneous intracerebral hematoma: a randomized study. J Neurosurg 1989;70: 530–5.
26. Grotenhuis JA. Endoscope-assisted microneurosurgery – a concise guidebook. Nijmegen: Machaon, 1998.
27. Teo C, Rahman S, Boop FA. Complications of neuroendoscopic neurosurgery. Child's Nerv Syst 1996;12(5): 248–53.
28. Svendsen F, Bassi S, Punt J. Seizures after neuroendoscopic third ventriculostomies. Child's Nerv Syst 2002;18:259.
29. Hopf NJ, Grunert P, Fries G, Resch KDM, Perneczky A. Endoscopic third ventriculostomy: outcome analysis of 100 consecutive procedures. Neurosurgery 1999; 44(4):795–806.

7

Principles and Practice of Image-guided Neurosurgery

Kristian Aquilina, Philip Edwards and Anthony Strong

Summary

Image-guided neurosurgery depends on the registration of pre-operatively acquired images with the physical space of the patient on the operating table. With the aid of a computer workstation and a tracking device, the neurosurgeon is able to obtain a three-dimensional, visual, real-time image of a registered probe in relation to the patient's anatomy and pathology. Image guidance facilitates localization of target structures and their anatomical relations and allows the pre-operative planning of the ideal, minimal risk, trajectory. It has become a useful tool in the surgical management of intracranial tumors and has also been applied to arteriovenous malformations, pericallosal aneurysms, epilepsy surgery, intracranial endoscopy and spinal surgery. The principal problem is the system's dependence on pre-operatively acquired images; perioperative updating of these images by perioperative magnetic resonance imaging overcomes this difficulty.

Introduction

No neurosurgeon needs to be reminded of the challenge posed by the need to identify and localize accurately structures on the brain surface and within the brain that are critical for neurological function, and which may be indistinguishable visually from adjacent, non-critical structures. Indeed, perhaps a frequent – but usually unspoken – question from a patient to their surgeon is: "How are you going to find your way around in there?". The practice of safe and effective neurosurgery rightly places increasing emphasis on the need to minimize risk. Reliable navigation in and around the brain, and the localization of surgical targets, are important contributions to the achievement of this goal.

A variety of technical approaches are available to the surgeon, and although much developmental work has taken place in several centers, involving collaborations between physicists, software engineers and surgeons, the commercial market has matured recently. Surgeons have some degree of choice of systems and technical solutions, and have a duty to understand both the nature of the procedures that contribute to neuronavigation, and the factors that determine reliability and accuracy. It is also important that evolution of the technology is driven not by technical advances but by specifications influenced primarily by surgeons.

In this chapter we shall set out the principles and methodological approaches that underlie the concept of image-guided neurosurgery, review and assess the state of development of applications to specific surgical procedures, and briefly consider potential future developments.

We believe that the term "stereotaxy" should be confined strictly to procedures in which a stereotactic frame is used, and that the term "image-guided neurosurgery" is a much more appropriate description of the subject; thus "frameless stereotaxy" is inappropriate, not least because it implies a degree of accuracy that is available only in frame-based systems.

Methodological Approaches

In this section we will describe the standard methodology of alignment of images to the patient on the operating table, and consider the factors affecting accuracy and performance of image-guided surgery systems. Finally we provide a set of principles by which neuronavigation systems can be evaluated and compared.

Statement of the Problem

In conventional surgery pre-operative images are largely used for diagnosis only and are present in theater only as a series of slices on a light-box. The positional relationship between these images and the patient's anatomy is established only in the mind of the surgeon. The three-dimensional nature of modern imaging techniques (e.g. MRI and CT) is under-utilized in such a scenario.

The aim of image-guided surgery is to align the 3D pre-operative images to the patient on the operating table and to present the accurately aligned image data to the surgeon in a manner that aids navigation. The technical problem can be stated as follows. We have accurate 3D information about patient anatomy and pathology from pre-operative scans. We wish to establish a correspondence between the image data and the physical space of the patient in order to present the surgeon with well-aligned anatomical information using a suitable visualization scheme.

Method

In order to align pre-operative images to the patient on the operating table, it is first necessary to define a physical coordinate system with respect to the patient. In frame-based methods, these coordinates are defined by the arc system on the frame itself, whereas in image-guided neurosurgery a coordinate measuring device is used. Various technologies have been proposed for this purpose, including mechanical arms, radiofrequency transmitter/receiver coils, ultrasound spark gaps and optical trackers. We will consider the relative merits of these devices in the next section.

Having defined a physical coordinate system in theater, the problem is now to align the pre-operative images to the patient in order to present the surgeon with image data that correspond to the patient's anatomy. This is achieved by identifying corresponding features in the pre-operative images and on the surface of the patient. These features will generally be landmarks, but may also include the skin surface or, as the operation proceeds, bone surface. The process of establishing correspondence between the image and the patient is termed "registration".

Defining the Patient Coordinates

Stereotactic Frames

Frame-based stereotactic neurosurgery has been an established clinical routine since the 1950s. Here, the patient coordinate system is defined by an arc device that attaches to the frame. The frame carries high-contrast imaging markers and is rigidly bolted to the patient's skull prior to imaging. An entry and target point is defined in the images, and the arc angles are calculated to achieve this trajectory according to the manufacturer's instructions. The bulky and somewhat invasive nature of such frames has limited their application. Since only a target and trajectory can be defined, frames are generally used only for biopsies or placement of electrodes or cannulae. They are widely regarded as highly accurate, though some studies have suggested that the accuracy may be overstated [1].

Mechanical Arms

The first frameless neuronavigation device to be widely used was the "Faro Arm", a mechanical device that attaches to the side of the table. Encoders on each of the axes of the arm enable calculation of the tip position. Problems with such a device are that the range of movement is somewhat limited, that any movement of the head clamp requires re-registration, and that the inherent accuracy was found to be somewhat lower than that of other methods. Marketed as the "ISG wand", this mechanical localizer was a critical component in the first regular applications of image-guided surgery [2].

Ultrasound Localization

The first example of frameless navigation was a system developed by Roberts et al. [3]. This system used a microscope both to register the images to the patient and to provide the guidance information. The localization system was based on ultrasonic spark-gap transducers. These emit a very short ultrasound pulse, which can be detected by three or more microphones in the operating room. The time delay for the sound pulse to reach each microphone gives a measure of distance and hence localizes the spark gap. Others have developed this technology for conventional pointer-based guidance [4]. Some problems have been encountered owing to variations of the speed of sound with temperature and air flow. This localization system was implemented in the Picker Viewpoint system, but was subsequently replaced by optical tracking.

Optical Tracking

With either three linear cameras or two 2D cameras, if a point can be located in each view, the 3D location of the point relative to the cameras can be calculated. This is the basis of a number of tracking systems. The localized points are either active (bright infra-red-emitting diodes, IREDs) or passive (highly reflecting spheres). In smaller camera systems, such as the Polaris or IGT systems, each IRED can be localized with an accuracy of 0.2–0.4 mm. With the Optotrak – a larger and more expensive version – accuracy is 0.1–0.2 mm. The main difficulty with optical tracking is that line-of-sight between the cameras and tracked objects must be maintained. However, the high accuracy and stability of these systems have meant that optical tracking is now the technology of choice for most commercial image-guided surgery systems.

Registration

Having defined a coordinate system for the patient, we now need to align the pre-operative images to this reference space. This is achieved by defining features in the pre-operative images that can also be identified by our localization device on the surface of the patient. Point-like landmarks are the most common type of feature and these are generally referred to as "fiducials". The fiducials may be purely anatomical points on the skin surface, skin-affixed markers or bone-implanted fiducials. The choice of fiducial depends on the accuracy required by the application.

For early pointer-based guidance we have used anatomical landmarks such as the nasion, the medial and lateral canthi, the external angular processes, the tip of the mastoid process and the occipital protuberance. Experience tells us that these can be located at best to within 3–5 mm, achieving a registration error of similar magnitude. Skin markers have been reported to provide a registration accuracy of 2–4 mm when used with great care. Inaccuracies can occur due to movement of the skin surface either with head repositioning, with application of protective eye covers, or with the force of the pointer used for registration. Care must be taken to protect the upper face after registration, and to mark the center of the marker whilst applying as little force as possible to the skin surface.

The only validated and approved method that provides sub-millimetric accuracy is to use bone-implanted markers [5]. Though this is clearly a rather invasive process, it does provide the most accurate registration for neuronavigation.

Patient Immobilization and Tracking

Whatever the technology used, patient tracking is relative to some reference frame; the frame is an array of tracked targets that are locked in constant orientation with the patient's head. This can be the reference frame of the device itself, as is the case with mechanical localization. A more common approach is to attach an optical tracker to a Mayfield or similar clamp. To maintain accuracy it is advisable to keep this tracker as close as possible to the surgical field without hampering the procedure. It has also been proposed to attach a tracker either to the patient's palate or the upper teeth [6]. This allows freer movement of the patient's head for interventions where a head clamp is inappropriate. The use of a reference frame is essential, and permits movement of the head relative to the tracking cameras, or vice versa, without loss of registration.

Accuracy Considerations

When performing point-based registration, there are a number accuracy metrics that can be described. It is very important when talking about the accuracy of a particular system that the measurements used are clear and that their meaning is understood. In a paper by Fitzpatrick et al., the three main error metrics associated with point-based registration are described and a derivation of the most important statistic is given [7]. We will describe their results and the implications thereof for image-directed neurosurgery in this section. It is vital that any surgeon using point landmarks as a means of registration for image guidance understands these results.

Error Metrics

We will call the point landmarks "fiducials". The first statistical measure of error we will describe is the "fiducial localization error" (FLE). This is simply the accuracy with which one can generally locate a given fiducial. An estimate of FLE for a particular fiducial must take into account the accuracy with which the point can be found by the user in the images and on the patient, as well as the intrinsic accuracy of the localization device.

The second metric is the "fiducial registration error" (FRE). This is the root mean square (rms) residual error on the fiducials after transformation. For example, if we have a set of points in image coordinates and their corresponding physical locations, we can calculate a transformation from image to physical space. By transforming the image points, we have two sets of points that should coincide: the transformed image points and their measured physical positions. Because there are errors in our measurements, these points do not coincide exactly and the distances between them provide the FRE. It is common, because it is easy to calculate, for commercial systems to quote FRE either as an rms or as an error on each point. As we shall see, however, FRE is not a good measure of registration accuracy.

The third, and most clinically relevant, metric is the "target registration error" (TRE). This is the accuracy with which a point other than our fiducials can be located. If we are performing an electrode placement heading for a specific target, the TRE is a measure of the accuracy with which we can locate that target given the registration we have obtained from our fiducials. This is clearly the error in which we are most interested.

Fitzpatrick et al. [7] have found a formula relating TRE to FLE and the configuration of the landmarks, as follows:

$$\langle TRE^2(r)\rangle = \frac{\langle FLE^2\rangle}{N}\, 1 + \left(\frac{1}{3}\sum_{k=1}^{3}\frac{d_k^2}{f_k^2}\right)$$

where there are n fiducial points, where fk is the rms distance of the fiducials to the principal axis, k, of the point distribution, and where dk is the distance from this same axis to the target point, r. In image-guided neurosurgery we are interested in reducing the TRE. From this equation we can see that there are two methods of achieving this. One is to increase the number of fiducials used; the other is to increase the spread of these fiducials.

For systems that quote FRE only, there may be a temptation to ignore landmarks that have a high FRE and reduce the set until the mean FRE falls below a given value. This is a very poor method of achieving registration. It will tend to mean that a poor configuration of landmarks will remain, perhaps all being close together or all close to lying along a line. Though a low FRE may result from this process, the associated TRE, especially at a distance from these landmarks, may be very poor indeed. Landmarks with high FRE should only be discarded if there is a good reason for thinking that they are outliers, e.g. if a skin marker has clearly moved.

Manufacturers of IGS systems should be encouraged to incorporate the above equation into accuracy assessments provided to the surgeon. Until this is the case, it is paramount that surgeons are aware of the issues affecting the true target accuracy of navigation.

Clinical Applications

Brain Biopsy

Accurate biopsy of brain lesions has been possible since the introduction of stereotactic frames. The frame, however, restricts access to the surgical field, interferes with instruments, and requires immediate pre-operative imaging. It gives no feedback to the surgeon and requires multiple calculations that are not always intuitive and simple. It is also inconvenient to the patient. Stereotactic biopsy in the lateral temporal lobe is contraindicated with some frames, where the needle track is liable to traverse the Sylvian fissure, placing the middle cerebral artery at risk. The development of frameless image-guided systems was an important step in increasing the user friendliness of localization systems. Light-emitting diodes (LEDs) attached to the biopsy needles allow their precise tracking by the camera within the operating space, and holding arms have been developed to maintain biopsy needles rigidly in the correct position. The ideal trajectory to approach and biopsy the lesion can be worked out preoperatively and stored in the workstation. The development of trajectory and targeting software allows the needle to be advanced according to such a pre-planned pathway, with real-time 3D visualization of the position of the needle tip within the brain.

Brain biopsy procedures require a higher accuracy than is necessary for most other procedures performed under image guidance. The use of scalp-applied or even skull-implantable fiducial markers, as well as the holding of the patient's head in a rigid Mayfield head holder, is important. The accuracy now given by most systems is better than 2 mm, but the limitation imposed by the thickness of the image slices remains.

In a study by Barnett et al. [8], 218 biopsy procedures were performed using scalp-applied fiducial markers. The average minimum lesion diameter was 27.7 mm and the average depth from the scalp was 39.8 mm. Lesions included glial tumors, metastases, lymphomas, meningiomas and demyelination. The procedure yielded a diagnosis that supported the clinical and radiological findings in 96.3% of cases. This was comparable to the accuracy achieved by frame-based stereotactic systems. The most significant complication was intracerebral hemorrhage, which occurred in five cases, two of which required craniotomy. It was noted that the diagnostic accuracy for posterior fossa biopsy, at 70% (7 out of 10 patients), was much lower than that for supratentorial lesions; it was suggested that scanning the patient in the prone position and the application of skull-implantable fiducials would increase the accuracy.

Surface Lesions

For access to lesions on the brain surface, guidance with registered images allows the performance of a small craniotomy, planned to give maximal exposure of the tumor and at the same time decreasing the extent of exposure. The disruption of normal tissue is minimized. Most importantly, an accurate craniotomy decreases the brain retraction required. This is of particular value in convexity meningiomas, where excessive brain retraction leads to postoperative swelling, which may be difficult to control and may lead to significant morbidity. A lower degree of brain manipulation decreases the risk of a post-operative intracerebral hematoma. In meningioma surgery, a smaller bone flap also decreases the intraoperative blood loss. The brain shift associated with surface lesions has been studied [9,10]. It is more predictable than for deeper lesions, and consists of bulging of the lesion and the surrounding brain on opening the dura; this is associated with an outward movement of the deep brain/tumor interface. The cortex at the resection site sinks back on completion of resection.

Skull Base and Pituitary Surgery

Tumors of the skull base have a high propensity to invade osseous boundaries and distort anatomy, obscuring surgical landmarks in a region crowded with critical neurovascular structures. Image-guided surgery is becoming an important tool in the resection of complex skull base tumors, particularly in the petroclival and parasellar regions, as well as in the foramen magnum and the jugular foramen [11].

When compared with other lesions, such as vault meningiomas, cerebral gliomas and non-gliotic intra-axial lesions, skull base lesions are associated with substantially lower degrees of post-imaging, intraoperative brain shift. This implies that the accuracy of frameless image-guided methods is higher for such lesions [9].

Sure et al. [11] evaluated the role of neuronavigation in a series of 10 skull base tumors. The value of pre-operatively acquiring both CT and

MRI scans, with subsequent fusion of the two image sets on the navigation workstation, was described. The CT scan allowed accurate patient-to-image registration on the basis of bony landmarks. The MRI scan allowed detailed evaluation of soft tissue and bony distortion by the tumor. A registration error of less than 2 mm was obtained in each of the 10 cases.

The workstation facilitates selection of the optimal skull base approach for maximal resection of the lesion. Sure et al. [11] found it particularly useful in deciding whether a pterional or an orbitozygomatic approach would give the better access to a given parasellar lesion. In posterior fossa surgery, it allows precise definition of keyhole craniotomies in relationship to the underlying dural venous sinuses. Neuronavigation also allows a clear pre-operative indication of how much tumor can be excised safely, depending on the proximity of the tumor to important structures.

Intraoperatively, early identification of important anatomical landmarks, such as the clinoid processes in anterior fossa surgery, and the petrous apex, the arch of the atlas, the vertebral artery, the occipital condyle and the bone cells in the posterior fossa, is useful. Major vessels and critical neural structures can be identified early during intratumoral decompression, facilitating their preservation when displaced by, or encased within, the tumor mass. It allows the neurosurgeon to calculate the position of the instrument within a large tumor cavity devoid of landmarks. A better understanding of the topography of complex anatomical structures is afforded; this is relevant, for example, when the petrous portion of the carotid artery is being protected during drilling of invaded or eroded petrous temporal bone. Bony infiltration by skull base meningiomas is sometimes not grossly identifiable, even under the microscope, and image guidance then allows a more complete tumor resection.

In one of the few studies that also takes account of the overall cost effectiveness of image guidance, Elias et al. [12] described the role of CT-based neuronavigation in transphenoidal surgery for pituitary tumors. The maintenance of an appropriate midline trajectory is vital in transsphenoidal surgery. Intracranial entries into the anterior fossa floor and through the clivus have been reported. Whereas intraoperative fluoroscopy only provides sagittal guidance, the neuronavigation system gives constant 3D information and allows adjustments in both the sagittal and the coronal planes during the approach to the sella. Attachment of reflective markers to ring curettes and their calibration within the navigation system allow the neurosurgeon to identify the sellar boundaries and to delineate the cavernous sinus and the carotid artery on each side. The system, however, cannot reliably demonstrate soft and potentially mobile tissues within the sella once excision of the adenoma has begun. Use of the image-guidance system to dynamically assist in, or confirm, the complete removal of the adenoma necessitates the incorporation of some form of intraoperative image updating.

The usefulness of such a system in defining and confirming the midline trajectory is particularly evident in re-operations. Disruption of important midline landmarks, such as the vomer, the anterior nasal spine and the rostrum of the sphenoid, renders such operations hazardous. Image guidance allows the neurosurgeon to approach the sella with increased confidence and goes a long way to increase the safety of the procedure.

In an effort to decrease the additional cost ($318 per procedure) and the time requirement in the setting up and registration of the system (mean of an extra 12 minutes per procedure), the same neurosurgical unit has evaluated frameless fluoroscopy-guided transsphenoidal surgery using the FluoroNav Virtual Fluoroscopy System (Medtronic Sofamor Danek Inc., Memphis, TN) [13]. A dynamic reference arc was attached to the headholder fixed to the patient's cranium. A calibration device containing multiple light-emitting diodes was attached to a standard C-arm fluoroscope. This device supplies information regarding the relationship of the C-arm and the reference arc to the computer. Frontal and lateral videofluoroscopic images were then obtained, calibrated and stored in the computer. With a referenced probe, the surgeon was then able to refer to the stored images and visualize its position in real time. The principal advantages of this system are: (1) radiation exposure to the patient is reduced (fluoroscopy is only used once at the beginning of the procedure, and there is no preoperative CT scan); (2) the fluoroscope can be removed from the theater before draping the patient, cutting down on radiology costs;

and (3) as in CT-guided neuronavigation, this system allows more confident maintenance of the midline in re-operations. The cost of each procedure was calculated to be $750 less than for the CT-guided system, primarily because no pre-operative navigation protocol imaging is required; the mean increase in set-up time was only 7.2 minutes.

Intrinsic Brain Tumors and Functional Mapping

Image-guided surgery has become an integral component in the surgical management of brain tumors. The clear advantages include: the possibility of performing a smaller craniotomy centered directly over the pathology; localization of tumors deep within the cortical surface with minimal disturbance of the surrounding brain tissue; definition of the relationships of the tumour to eloquent cortex and other important structures; and definition of the tumor–brain plane, especially when this is poorly visible at surgery, such as in low-grade astrocytomas. The completeness of resection may also be enhanced, although this is controversial unless some form of intraoperative image updating is also used. The opportunity to plan the optimal approach to the tumor pre-operatively is also valuable.

The integration of functional data into the anatomical image data set was the next logical step in the development of image-guided surgery systems. If the function of relevant eloquent brain in the vicinity of a lesion can be mapped onto the MR image on the workstation, maximal resection with minimal neurological morbidity is facilitated. The potential to increase the safety of the procedure is evident. It is not always possible to accurately identify eloquent brain regions perioperatively with reference to standard anatomical landmarks, as tumors may cause significant gyral displacement and distortion of surface cortical anatomy.

Intraoperative, invasive, functional mapping using cortical stimulation techniques is time consuming and requires modification of the anesthetic regimen. Patients need to be awake for assessment of language function, but light anesthesia without muscle relaxation is adequate for motor mapping. Unlike pre-operative non-invasive mapping, this technique does not allow pre-operative planning and risk evaluation.

Magnetoencephalography (MEG) and functional MRI (fMRI) have been successfully used to obtain functional information that was subsequently integrated with the pre-operatively acquired image data set. In the former [14], cortical neuromagnetic signals are generated by repetitive sensory and motor stimulation; in practice, this involves mechanical stimulation of the index finger or repetitive finger-tapping movements. These signals are picked up and localized by a biomagnetometer, consisting of two 37-channel sensors placed over the scalp. Electrical sources can be localized with high spatial and temporal accuracy. The locations of the sensory and motor cortex are therefore identified, and, using a contour-fit algorithm, the MEG results can be overlaid onto the MR images. Lesions close to the motor cortex were successfully removed in 50 patients [14], with procedure-related neurological impairment in only one patient. Perioperative somatosensory evoked potentials agreed with the co-registered MEG localizations to a high level of concordance.

Functional MRI is non-invasive and uses widely available equipment [15]. Unlike MEG, it does not detect neural activation directly, but identifies a region within the cortex that is metabolically activated during the repetitive performance of an activity such as finger tapping. Performance of the task causes a substantial increase in cerebral blood flow in the corresponding brain region, sufficient in fact to lead to a decrease in the level of deoxyhemoglobin in the veins draining that region. This is detected as an increase in the T2-weighted MR signal. The signal-to-noise ratio is low, and many repetitions are required to generate each image slice. The fMRI image is then fused with the anatomical data set. In a study in which 12 patients underwent excision of lesions near the motor cortex, the prediction error ranged from 0 mm to 10 mm. This was considered to be satisfactory, as the target was the precentral gyrus rather than a single point on it. Intraoperative confirmation using somatosensory evoked potentials and phase reversal to identify the sensory and motor cortices respectively showed that fMRI identified the region correctly in each case. All of the tumors were excised without causing new neurological deficits [15]. Interestingly, patients with severe peri-lesional edema consistently showed a higher prediction error. This may be related to impairment of vascular autoregulation with decreased activation-dependent changes in cerebral blood flow in regions of high edema. It was also noted that distortion of the fMRI images could be a problem when the region of interest is closely related to bone, as may occur with the inferior temporal lobe.

Identification and mapping of white matter tracts is now also possible [16]. Image-fusion software then allows the accurate fusion of these maps with the anatomical image data set. The presence of the axonal membrane and the neurofilamentary cytoskeleton restricts the diffusion of water to the long axis of the fiber tracts – anisotropy. Diffusion-anisotropy MRI identifies the restricted diffusion as a hyperintense area, delineating in three dimensions the position and direction of the tract. In four patients presenting with tumors displacing the pyramidal tract, this technique was helpful in the peri-operative identification of the tract. As in fMRI, peri-lesional edema poses a problem, as there is no restriction of diffusion direction in edematous foci; tract identification is then difficult. It has been suggested that this method can also be used to map the optic radiation and the commissural fibers if these structures are relevant to the procedure.

Movement of the Brain During Surgery

A critical limitation of image-guided surgery, particularly relevant to tumor resection, is the reliance on a pre-operatively acquired image data set. Progressive movement or distortion of the brain during the procedure means that the pre-operative image becomes progressively outdated as the surgery proceeds [10]. Reliance on the image-guided system would lead to errors in the intraoperative delineation of tumor location and borders, as well as in the relationship of the tumor to adjacent eloquent cortex. Brain distortion, relative to the pre-operative image, is due to the release of cerebrospinal fluid (CSF), pressure changes on skull opening, unopposed gravity, ventricular compression, brain retraction and tumor resection. Patient positioning, the physiological effects of diuretics and mechanical ventilation are also relevant. Dorward et al. [9] studied the magnitude and direction of post-imaging brain distortion in 48 cases; maximal brain shifts were found to be greater than 1 cm in magnitude. The degree of shift depended on the size of the tumor, the degree of midline shift, and the presence of peritumoral edema; significant differences were identified between meningiomas, gliomas, non-glial intra-axial lesions and skull base lesions.

Nabavi et al. [10] studied post-imaging brain deformation in 25 patients using a 0.5T vertically open bore MR imager. Baseline imaging was performed after positioning; further images were taken after dural opening and initial CSF drainage, after tumor resection, and after dural closure. Software allowed image overlapping on the same coordinates to facilitate comparison between the images. In this study, brain shift was shown to have a high degree of inter-individual variability and was a continuous and dynamic process, evolving separately and differently in distinct brain regions. It was noted that the direction of deformation might even reverse within relatively short time-frames. The occipital and parietal lobes were seen to be less mobile than the frontal and temporal lobes. It is clear that brain biomechanics are still far from understood, and although software may be designed to predict unidirectional surface shifts secondary to gravity and CSF loss associated with small surface lesions, predictions of multi-directional subsurface movements associated with larger lesions are unlikely to be accurate.

The effects of brain shift can be minimized by paying attention to some operative details, such as allowing as little CSF as possible to escape, by delaying aspiration of cystic tumor components, and by removing tumor adjacent to eloquent cortex first. The use of dehydrating agents such as mannitol should be avoided and the positioning of the patient should be such that the craniotomy site lies at the highest point.

Intraoperative MRI

One solution to the problem of intraoperative brain movement is to combine guidance from registered pre-operative images with intraoperative MRI. This allows the acquisition of image updates intraoperatively; these updates are then fused with the pre-operatively acquired image data set. Several centers have reported their experience with such systems [17,18,19]. The difficulties and cost of modifying the usual operating theater set-up to suit the requirements of MR scanning are clear. Several options have been used in various centers:

- The use of a vertical open-bore MRI scanner, allowing two surgeons to operate within the scanner. This avoids the need for patient movement but requires the use of non-ferromagnetic instruments as well as magnetic shielding of the operating room [19].
- The use of a twin operating theater; surgery is performed in a conventional theater and the patient is transported to an adjacent MRI suite for imaging. The scanner can be rendered more cost effective by allowing its use for diagnostic scans unrelated to theater sessions [17].
- The use of a single-shielded operating theater, with the surgery being performed in the fringe field of the magnet. Normal ferromagnetic instruments and microscopes are then allowed [18].

There is a steadily growing volume of literature on intraoperative MRI and it is not possible to discuss this topic in detail here. Its value was demonstrated in a recent study [17] in which 40 patients underwent image-guided resection of gliomas (WHO grades II–IV) using an image-guidance system. An intraoperative MRI scan was obtained after the surgeon felt that the planned extent of tumor resection was achieved. Of these patients, 53% were found on MRI to have had a less than optimal resection. It was noted from this study that patients with a tumor volume higher than 20cm^3 are more likely to have incomplete resections, probably because the degree of brain shift is much higher for larger lesions.

The intraoperative MRI system described by Hadani et al. [18] is characterized by a vertical-bore 0.12T open magnet that can be stored below the operating table when not in use. The patient's head occupies a fixed position relative to the magnet. With the magnet in the scanning position, real-time navigation can be employed using an MRI wand. This is independent of the optical tracking system and the magnet is the only reference point. Alternatively, the magnet can be lowered under the operating table once an image update has been obtained; optical tracking using the standard guidance set-up then allows navigation on the updated image data set. Image updating is independent of fiducials and skin markers, because the same relationship between the magnet and the patient is maintained throughout the procedure. Ferromagnetic instruments are used when the magnet is not in the scanning position.

There are several issues relating to intraoperative MRI that are still unclear. The presence of residual tumor on intraoperative images is ascertained on the basis of contrast enhancement around or within the resection cavity [17]. Increased permeability of the blood–brain barrier also occurs as a direct result of surgical manipulation, and indeed, surgically induced nodular as well as diffuse enhancement has been reported. This is probably more likely after contrast agents have been injected several times during the same procedure. The use of contrast agents that bind the tumor for a longer period of time and that are cleared from the circulation before the operation is begun has been investigated; iron oxide microparticles are phagocytosed by glioblastoma cells. It would then be possible to avoid administration of contrast agents just before or during the procedure. Bohinski et al. found that biopsy of residual enhancing tissue after partial glioma resection yielded tumor in 81% of cases [17]. Comparison with pre-operative contrasted scans is useful to differentiate tumor-induced enhancement from surgery-induced enhancement.

The edema associated with retraction is easily identifiable on T2-weighted imaging. As enhancement in the dependent part of the resection cavity might also be due to blood clot, it is essential that adequate hemostasis be secured prior to imaging. Blood is also identifiable on T2-weighted images. Oxidized cellulose in the cavity is another factor that interferes with the identification of tumor remnants. The debris of a metal drill produces significant artifact on MRI and it is preferable to use only diamond drills [19]. Even when all of these precautions are taken, however, definition of the borders of low-grade astrocytomas is still a challenge.

Other unanswered questions relate to the frequency of intraoperative scanning. Ideally one should obtain enough information to ensure that the image data set used for navigation is not outdated, and also to control resection of the target, without prolonging the operation or moving the patient unnecessarily. Should scanning be tied to critical events, such as the completion of tumor resection or the preservation of a functional region?

Intraoperative Ultrasonography

The use of intraoperative ultrasonography to update the pre-operative image has been considered. Ultrasonography is inexpensive; also, it allows fast multiplanar examination and can reliably detect tumor remnants. Tracking of the ultrasound probe allows 3D reconstruction. However, the overall quality of soft-tissue visualization is not as good as that of MRI, and the fusion of the ultrasonic image with the MR image is still difficult to obtain.

Outcome of Image-guided Surgery for Intrinsic Tumors

A more important question is whether a more complete resection of a high-grade glioma, as is possible with image-guided surgery, leads to a better prognosis. Recurrence of gliomas generally occurs at the site of residual tumor, and therefore gross total resection might increase the progression-free survival and improve the quality of life when compared with subtotal resection or biopsy. There is also evidence to suggest that the immediate complication rate after gross total resection is lower than that after biopsy or subtotal resection [20]. A systematic analysis of survival times, with and without target resection control for matched patients and tumors, is required.

Epilepsy Surgery

Image guidance has been used in several aspects of epilepsy surgery, including the removal of deep lesions, selective amygdalo-hippocampectomy, callosotomy, temporal resection, cortical resection and the placement of depth electrodes [21]. The hippocampus and the corpus callosum are relatively fixed structures, and there is only minimal brain shift along the anteroposterior axis. Once hippocampal resection has begun, however, CSF drainage and the mesial displacement of the brain due to gravity lead to error in the mesio-lateral plane. According to Olivier et al. [21], this did not lead to interference with localization and gross total resection of the mesial structures.

In transylvian selective amygdalo-hippocampectomy, surgical orientation is achieved primarily through the exposure of anatomical landmarks, namely the uncus and the sulcus circularis insulae. This requires a wide opening of the Sylvian fissure with the associated risks of vessel injury and vasospasm. Image guidance allows orientation without the necessity to expose and identify such landmarks. Trajectories to the hippocampus and resection borders can be defined pre-operatively. Image guidance directs trans-sulcal dissection and also ensures complete resection of the relevant hippocampal structures; the outcome of epilepsy surgery has been shown to be closely related to complete hippocampal resection.

The location of focal cortical dysplasia is often difficult to identify macroscopically. Image guidance allows accurate anatomical correlation in cortical resections, and this becomes more accurate if the system is used concurrently with electrocorticography and motor mapping. It also facilitates the confirmation of the length of a callosal section, and in temporal lobectomy it aids a decision on the volumes of lateral temporal cortex and hippocampus that can safely be resected.

Arteriovenous Malformations

Although the importance of neuro-endovascular therapy and radiosurgery in the management of arteriovenous malformations (AVMs) has been increasing steadily over the past 5 years, microsurgical excision still retains a primary role, particularly as it is the only treatment option that immediately eliminates the risk of bleeding. The frequent intimate relationship of AVMs to eloquent brain tissue has rendered neuronavigation techniques useful in surgical management, in an effort to reduce post-operative neurological morbidity.

Image-guided surgery based on a pre-operatively acquired MR scan allows pre-operative planning and identification of the ideal location and size of the skin incision and bone flap. For lesions with minimal gyral representation, it allows precise localization of the AVM through a small, optimally placed craniotomy. More importantly, it allows planning of the optimal surgical trajectory to the AVM, maximally avoiding eloquent brain tissue, particularly for AVMs located close to, or within, motor, sensory, speech or visual areas.

A recent study [22] described image-guided AVM surgery based on CT angiography rather than on MRI. Segmentation and 3D reconstruction of the AVM allowed exact definition of the nidus, as well as the draining veins and feeding arteries, in relation to the underlying brain tissue. Manipulation of the reconstruction through rotation and subtraction allowed multi-angle viewing of the relationships of the AVM vessels. Preliminary image-guided temporary clipping of the sulcal feeding arteries led to decompression of the AVM nidus in most cases, rendering easier the subsequent step of dissection along the previously localized draining veins. However, temporary clipping prior to complete feeder dissection is associated with a low risk of clipping en-passant vessels. Another limitation of this study was that only vessels larger than 3 mm in size could be identified – a direct result of the resolution limit of the segmentation process.

By demonstrating the configuration and margins of the nidus, image guidance decreases the risk of inadvertent surgical entry into the AVM. The plane between the AVM and the surrounding brain tissue can be readily identified, minimizing tissue manipulation and decreasing intraoperative bleeding.

It is still unclear, however, whether image-guided surgery for AVMs does in fact result in a lower morbidity when compared with standard, free-hand techniques.

Surgery for Intracranial Aneurysm

Few surgeons see any indication for image guidance in the approach to the majority of intracranial aneurysms, usually located in the region of the supraclinoid segment of the internal carotid artery. However, aneurysms located more distally, in particular pericallosal aneurysms, can present a significant problem, and localization is facilitated by the use of image guidance.

Endoscopic Surgery

Guidance from registered images has been used extensively in conjunction with endoscopic neurosurgery. Unlike frame-based stereotaxy, it allows free-hand movement of the endoscope with real-time feedback of its tip position. The versatility of the software is such that a 'tool file' is available for each of the various instruments introduced through the sheath. A change of instrument only necessitates a change in the active tool file on the computer workstation. The pre-calibrated parameters and length of the instrument then allow representation of that instrument in the multiplanar views on the screen.

In a study by Schroeder et al. [23], the principal usefulness of guidance from registered images was in the selection of an ideal entry point and trajectory to the lesion with minimal injury to the fornices and eloquent brain. Most procedures were then performed under direct endoscopic visual control. The pre-operative trajectory planning was very useful when the ventricular system was small and when the posterior third ventricle had to be approached through a small foramen of Monro. In the management of arachnoid cysts, a trajectory penetrating as many of the septae as possible, as well as ensuring an optimal fenestration point, would be planned. In such situations, as well as in multi-loculated hydrocephalus, there are few, if any, anatomical landmarks, and there is a real risk of disorientation, particularly if the membranes are thick [23]. The value of image guidance in the maintenance of orientation was clear. In the endoscopic resection of colloid cysts, guidance from registered images facilitated the maintenance of a trajectory leading to the most lateral and anterior aspect of the foramen of Monro, without injury to the fornices or the caudate nucleus; this would, in turn, allow visualization of the roof of the third ventricle, rendering complete dissection of the cyst from its base easier.

The authors did not find pre-operative image guidance useful for endoscopic third ventriculostomy [23]. In this procedure the ventricles tend to be large, and a high degree of endoscope maneuverability is possible. Clear intraventricular landmarks, such as the thalamo-striate vein, the foramen of Monro and the choroid plexus, determine the orientation. The basilar artery can often be seen through the thinned-out floor of the third ventricle, and its position can be scrutinized from the mid-sagittal pre-operative MRI. The optimal position of the stoma is determined via visual information through the endoscope.

The problem of CSF drainage and brain shift remains, however. The authors advise positioning the patient with the cyst at the highest point. Other studies [18,19] have pointed to the value of intraoperative MRI-based updating of the pre-operative image data sets in such situations. The decompression of cystic lesions and multiloculated hydrocephalus under continuous (every 3 seconds) MRI scanning has also been described [24]; the changes of the relationships on drainage and fenestration of the cysts can then be observed in real time. This, of course, requires an intraoperative MRI set-up.

Spinal Surgery

The development of increasingly complex spinal surgical techniques and instrumentation has meant that 2D lateral intraoperative fluoroscopy is now considered to be insufficient for safe and effective insertion of implants. The application of the principles of intracranial neuronavigation to the spine is not straightforward, for several reasons. Registration of the spine cannot reliably depend on skin markers or fiducials, in view of the high mobility of the spinal column and the overlying skin. Indeed, registration needs to be performed intraoperatively on the exposed spinal anatomy of the segment requiring surgery, using points that are easily and accurately identifiable on the exposed spine and on the pre-operatively acquired images. These may include the superior and inferior portions of the spinous processes and the medial and lateral limits of the facet joint in the cervical spine, and the posterolateral aspect of the transverse process tips on each side in the thoracic spine. Problems may arise when the posterior elements of the relevant segment are disrupted by trauma or previous surgery. A minimum of three points is required for the vertebra in question. Because each level in the spine represents a separate and distinct anatomical structure, each vertebra should ideally be registered and tracked individually during surgery. The spine is mobile within the body and therefore the reference arc or LED array must be attached to the spine itself. In practice, this is clamped to a spinous process of the same, or an adjacent, vertebra for posterior approaches, and to a Caspar retractor for anterior approaches [25]. This is essential because the spatial relationships of adjacent spinal segments during pre-operative image acquisition (in the supine position) may be different from those during surgery, often in the prone position, particularly in situations of spinal instability such as high-grade spondylolisthesis and spinal fractures. Frequent perioperative confirmation of registration accuracy is advised; this is readily done by placing the activated probe on an easily identifiable bony point within the operative field and by ensuring that the cursor on the computer points to the corresponding point on the pre-operative image. A significant decrease in accuracy, usually recorded at around 2 mm, should prompt re-registration. The absence of clear bony landmarks and the flat 2D nature of the anterior vertebral bodies imply that accurate registration of the spine for anterior or anterolateral approaches remains difficult.

Virtual fluoroscopy technology (FluoroNav, Medtronic Sofamor Danek Inc., Memphis) does not require a pre-operative image. The C-arm is equipped with an LED attachment and a fiducial display that acts as a calibration target. The bony anatomy is first exposed; a reference arc is then attached to the spine. A lateral or anteroposterior image is taken. The fiducial display is used by the computer to register the anatomy instantaneously. Data from the optical camera allow the computer to identify the spatial relationships between the C-arm and the reference arc attached to the spine. This registered image then forms the basis on which navigation, using LED-marked instruments that appear on the image in real time, can proceed.

Probably the most important spinal application of image-guided surgery is the insertion of pedicle screws [26,27]. Pedicle screws confer high rigidity to a spinal construct, allowing the insertion of a shorter and more reliable construct, with maximal preservation of movement at the adjacent segments. In the lumbosacral spine, using perioperative radiography only, the rate of penetration of the pedicular cortex has been shown to be between 21% and 31%. Poor pedicle screw insertion is associated not only with neural injury, but also with fixation failure, particularly if the pedicle is fractured. Image guidance allows evaluation of the pedicular anatomy, the selection of the appropriate screw entry point, the identification of the optimal trajectory in the axial and sagittal planes, and also the ideal depth of insertion, allowing the longest bone purchase in the best-quality bone.

The surgeon is able to select the ideal screw diameter and length in the pre-operative planning phase; the computer provides a 3D view of the selected screw in the pre-operatively acquired image. It also provides a "target" window to facilitate screw insertion along the predetermined trajectory. In one of the earlier clinical studies in the use of image guidance for the insertion of lumbosacral pedicle screws [26], 137 out of a total of 150 screws were optimally placed. Only one screw was found to be in a significantly unsatisfactory position. No nerve root injuries were reported.

Image guidance is even more valuable in pedicle screw insertion into the thoracic spine [27]. Compared with its lumbar counterpart, the thoracic pedicle is smaller, has a more complex 3D morphology and has a variable cross-section in the coronal plane. There is a high degree of variability in the diameter, shape and angle of the thoracic pedicle. Moreover, its proximity to the pleura, nerve roots and the relatively fixed spinal cord means that inappropriate insertion is less forgiving. From clinical and cadaveric studies, up to 25% of thoracic pedicle screws were found to violate the pedicular cortex when perioperative fluoroscopy alone was used. In a recent study using post-operative CT evaluation, only 5 out of 266 screws inserted at all levels of the thoracic spine in 65 patients showed a structurally significant (defined as more than 2 mm) inadvertent violation of the pedicular cortex. These tended to cluster in the mid-thoracic spine. The majority of these misplacements occurred in severe traumatic fracture subluxations, implying that the increased intersegmental mobility in these situations interferes with the accuracy of registration of the image-guidance system. The authors also advocate an alternative screw trajectory through the rib head into the vertebral body if the pedicle is smaller than 4 mm in its widest coronal diameter, or scaphoid in shape, or laterally directed. This information can only be gleaned through pre-operative pedicle evaluation on the image-guidance system.

Image guidance is also useful when there is a concurrent anterior construct, such as a Kaneda system, for example. Pedicle screw insertion then allows a rigid parallelogram of fixation [25].

Applications to the cervical spine have included anterior cervical diskectomy and vertebrectomy, transoral odontoid resection, and the insertion of C1–C2 transarticular screws and lateral mass plates [25]. In anterior cervical surgery, image guidance allows the identification of the lateral resection margins of osteophytes and their relationships to the transverse foramen, the vertebral artery and the nerve root foramen. The risks of vascular and neurological injury (to the nerve roots and spinal cord) for these procedures have been quoted as up to 5% and 1% respectively. Image guidance also reduces the risk of incomplete osteophyte excision.

Surgical difficulties in the C1–C2 region include the complexity of the anatomy, which may be distorted by inflammatory pannus or tumor, and a limited operative field. Image guidance allows the determination of the position of unexposed structures, minimizing the need for extensive exposures. Insertion of atlanto-axial transarticular screws can then be performed with a higher margin of safety and with increased confidence.

Current Developments

There are a number of issues that remain to be tackled to improve the accuracy and delivery of neurosurgical guidance. An increasing amount of information is available to the surgeon in the operating theater, particularly from intraoperative imaging devices. This may be used to improve registration and provide information about structures beneath the available tissue surface. This becomes particularly important in the presence of tissue deformation, sometimes referred to as "brain shift".

There are several imaging devices that are routinely available to a neurosurgeon. They provide real-time information about the current position and shape of the patient. If these devices are calibrated to relate the image space to physical space, they can then be incorporated into a neuronavigation system. The simplest way that this can be achieved is to show the position of a pointer or tool in the intraoperative image.

X-ray guidance is an important part of the transsphenoidal approach. The use of X-ray images to register pre-operative CT data to the patient has been proposed for use in surgery of the head and spine. X-ray angiography may also provide useful information on current patient position.

Ultrasound is not generally used to guide neurosurgical procedures because of the poor quality of the images and the difficulty in identifying anatomical features. The real-time nature of the technique could prove useful in aligning pre-operative images to the patient, however. Ultrasound has been proposed for use in compensating for brain shift and also in improving rigid registration by finding the bone surface in spinal surgery.

Attention is also being paid to the ergonomics of surgical guidance. The systems have sometimes been seen as a cumbersome addition to an already crowded operating theater, and the interface between the system and the surgeon is often too complicated. Simplicity and ease of use are vital if image-guided neurosurgery is to become standard practice. Visualization of pre-operative images is an important factor in this regard, especially for microscopic procedures. The surgeon often finds that looking away from the operative view is distracting and inconvenient. Visualization of the target lesion and surrounding critical structures directly on the optical view of the patient, sometimes referred to as "augmented reality", is one way of avoiding this problem. In the MAGI (microscope-assisted guided intervention) system [28], this is achieved accurately and in stereo, offering the possibility of 3D perception of structures beneath the viewed surface (Fig. 7.1).

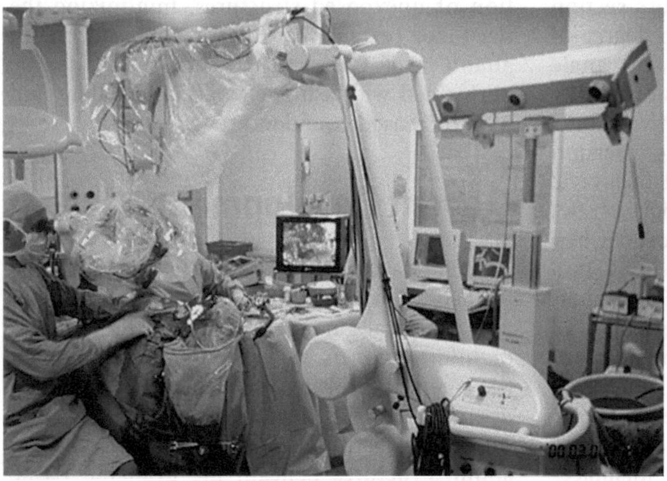
a

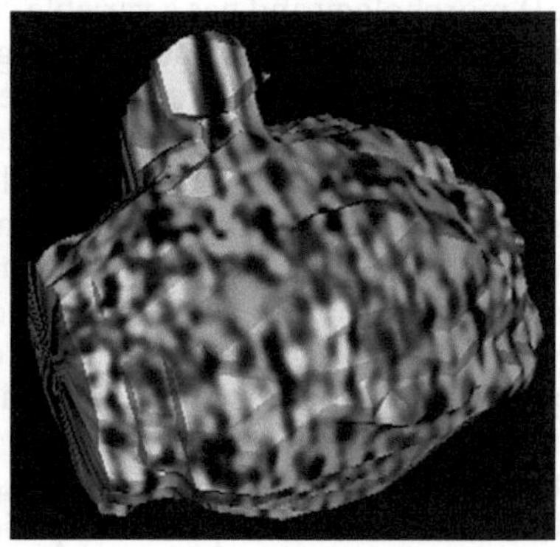
c

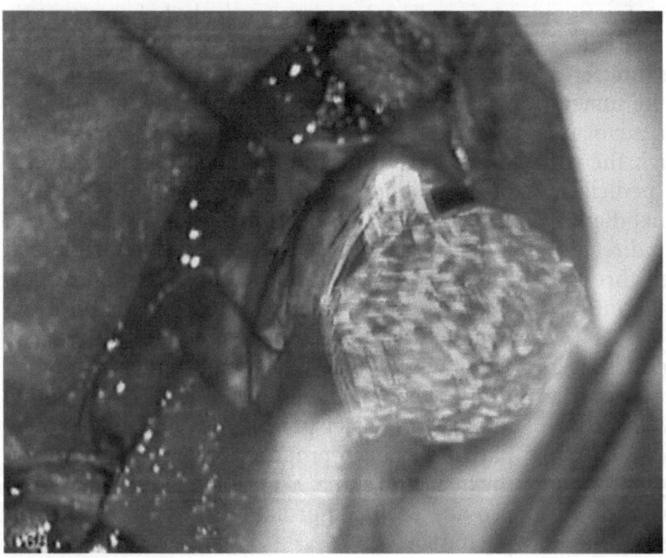
b

Fig. 7.1. The MAGI (microscope-assisted guided intervention) system in the operating theater. (**a**) An example overlay on the operative scene. (**b**) A rendering of the lesion from a similar viewpoint. (**c**) The views in (**b**) and (**c**) are seen by the surgeon in true stereo. The lesion is a vestibular schwannoma seen extending into the internal auditory meatus (IAM).

The Future

In speculating about the future for image-guided neurosurgical interventions, it is interesting to consider whether registration of pre-operative images to the patient will still be important. The advent of interventional MRI has led some to suggest that the quality of intraoperative imaging will provide all the necessary information to carry out a surgical procedure. Visualization and interaction with this data is an important issue, however.

Incorporation of a navigational device into an interventional scanner is important. The surgeon wants to see the location of a pointer or surgical tool in the images without needing to re-scan with the tool in place. This flexibility will enable scans to be performed only when there is significant movement or tissue deformation.

Also, as the scope of intraoperative imaging widens, so does that of pre-operative imaging. There will be more accurate and more functional data available from pre-operative scans that may not be practical to obtain during a procedure. Ideally, the segmentation of relevant features will be done automatically in real time. This process may be more practically achieved by alignment with previously segmented images.

The challenge for future navigation systems will be to incorporate pre-operative and intraoperative data seamlessly into the neurosurgical process, with real time update of the pre-operative model to compensate for both rigid and non-rigid movement of the patient. The relevant features will be visualised by the surgeon without complicated interaction and ideally directly on the operative view of the patient. Advances in imaging, tracking, computational power, algorithms, perception and display devices will be required. Significant research effort is being directed towards all these areas and will hopefully make this a reality.

Key Points

- *Image-guided neurosurgery involves the alignment of the patient in the operating space to a set of pre-operatively acquired images. Although accuracy issues need to be considered, it generally provides the ability to localize a target to within 2 mm.*
- *Image guidance facilitates the accurate localization of the target pathology or structures; the neurosurgeon can plan a smaller and more precise craniotomy and follow the ideal trajectory, minimizing the extent of brain exposure and retraction.*
- *The technique is particularly useful in the management of intracranial tumors, but is also being applied to vascular disease, particularly arteriovenous malformations and some aneurysms, epilepsy surgery, intracranial endoscopy and craniocervical and spinal surgery.*
- *Image guidance is very valuable in the insertion of spinal instrumentation, usually for fusion purposes. It facilitates the appreciation of pedicular anatomy and allows the choice of the ideal screw length and diameter prior to insertion.*
- *Current developments include the fusion of anatomical with functional images using functional MRI technology, and perioperative MRI, which allows the pre-operative images to be updated during surgery.*

Acknowledgement

P. Edwards was supported by EPSRC under the MedLINK program (project M108) in collaboration with Leica, Heerbrugg and BrainLab, Munich.

References

1. Maciunas RJ, Galloway RL, Latimer JW. The application accuracy of stereotactic frames. Neurosurgery 1994; 35(4):682–94.
2. Sandeman DR, Patel N, Chandler C, Nelson RJ, Coakham HB, Griffith HB. Advances in image-directed neurosurgery – preliminary experience with the ISG viewing wand compared with the Leksell-G frame. Br J Neurosurg 1994;8:529–44.
3. Roberts DW, Strohbehn JW, Hatch JF, Murray W, Kettenberger H. A frameless stereotaxic integration of computerised tomographic imaging and the operating microscope. J Neurosurg 1986;65:545–9.
4. Reinhardt HF, Horstmann GA, Gratzl O. Sonic stereometry in microsurgical procedures for deep-seated brain tumors and vascular malformations. Neurosurgery 1993;32(1):51–7.
5. Maurer C, Fitzpatrick MJ, Wang MY, Galloway RL, Maciunas RJ, Allen GS. Registration of head volume images using implantable fiducial markers. IEEE Trans Med Imaging 1997;6(4):447–61.

6. Hauser R, Westermann B, Probst R. Non-invasive tracking of patients' head movements during computer-assisted intranasal microscopic surgery. Laryngoscope 1997;211:491–9.
7. Fitzpatrick MJ, West JB, Maurer C. Predicting error in rigid-body point-based registration. IEEE Trans Med Imaging 1998;17(5):694–702.
8. Barnett GH, Miller DW, Weisenberger J. Frameless stereotaxy with scalp-applied fiducial markers for brain biopsy procedures: experience in 218 cases. J Neurosurg 1999;91:569–76.
9. Dorward NL, Alberti O, Velani B, Gerritsen FA, Harkness WFJ, Kitchen ND et al. Post-imaging brain distortion: magnitude, correlates and impact on neuronavigation. J Neurosurg 1998;88:656–62.
10. Nabavi A, McL Black P, Gering DT, Westin CF, Mehta V, Pergolizzi RS et al. Serial intraoperative magnetic resonance imaging of brain shift. Neurosurgery 2001;48:787–98.
11. Sure U, Alberti O, Petermeyer M, Becker R, Bertalanffy H. Advanced image-guided skull base surgery. Surg Neurol 2000;53:563–72.
12. Elias WJ, Chaddick JB, Alden TD, Laws ER. Frameless stereotaxy for transsphenoidal surgery. Neurosurgery 1999;45:271–7.
13. Jane JA, Thapar K, Alden TD, Laws ER. Fluoroscopic frameless stereotaxy for transsphenoidal surgery. Neurosurgery 2001;48:1302–8.
14. Ganslandt O, Fahlbusch R, Nimsky C, Kober H, Moller M, Steinmeier R et al. Functional neuronavigation with magnetoencephalography:outcome in 50 patients with lesions around the motor cortex. J Neurosurg 1999;91:73–9.
15. Schulder M, Maldjian JA, Liu WC, Holodny AI, Kalnin AT, Mun IK et al. Functional image-guided surgery of intracranial tumours located in or near the sensorimotor cortex. J Neurosurg 1998;89:412–18.
16. Coenen VA, Krings T, Mayfrank L, Polin RS, Reinges MHT, Thron A et al. Three-dimensional visualisation of the pyramidal tract in a neuronavigation system during brain tumour surgery: first experiences and technical note. Neurosurgery 2001;49:86–93.
17. Bohinski RJ, Kokkino AK, Warnick RE, Gaskill-Shipley MF, Kormos DW, Lukin RR et al. Glioma resection in a shared-resource magnetic resonance operating room after optimal image-guided frameless stereotactic resection. Neurosurgery 2001;48:731–44.
18. Hadani M, Spiegelman R, Feldman Z, Berkenstadt H, Ram Z. Novel, compact, intraoperative magnetic resonance image-guided system for conventional neurosurgical operating rooms. Neurosurgery 2001;48: 799–809.
19. Black P McL, Moriarty T, Alexander E III, Steig P, Woodard EJ, Gleason PL et al. The development and implementation of intraoperative magnetic resonance imaging and its neurosurgical applications. Neurosurgery 1997;41:831–45.
20. Fadul C, Wood J, Thaler H, Galicich J, Patterson RHJ, Posner JB. Morbidity and mortality of craniotomy for excision of supratentorial gliomas. Neurology 1988;38:1374–9.
21. Olivier A, Germano IM, Cukiert A, Peters T. Frameless stereotaxy for surgery of the epilepsies: preliminary experience. J Neurosurg 1994;81:629–33.
22. Maucevic A, Steiger HJ. Computer-assisted resection of cerebral arteriovenous malformations. Neurosurgery 1999;45:1164–71.
23. Schroeder HWS, Wagner W, Tschiltschke W, Gaab MR. Frameless neuronavigation in intracranial endoscopic neurosurgery. J Neurosurg 2001;94:72–9.
24. Kollias SS, Bernays RL. Interactive magnetic resonance imaging-guided management of intracranial cystic lesions by using an open magnetic resonance imaging system. J Neurosurg 2001;95:15–23.
25. Bolger C, Wigfield C. Image-guided surgery: applications to the cervical and thoracic spine and a review of the first 120 procedures. J Neurosurg (Spine) 2000;92:175–80.
26. Kalfas IH, Kormos DW, Murphy MA, McKenzie RL, Barnett GH, Bell GR et al. Application of frameless stereotaxy to pedicle screw fixation of the spine. J Neurosurg 1995;83:641–7.
27. Youkilis AS, Quint DJ, McGillicuddy JE, Papadopoulos SM. Stereotactic navigation for placement of pedicle screws in the thoracic spine. Neurosurgery 2001;48(4): 771–9.
28. Edwards PJ, King AP, Maurer CR, de Cunha DA, Hawkes DJ, Hill DLG et al. Design and evaluation of a system for microscope-assisted guided interventions (MAGI). IEEE Trans Med Imaging 2000;19(11):1082–93.

8

Stereotactic Radiosurgery

Andras A. Kemeny, Matthias W.R. Radatz
and Jeremy Rowe

Summary

Stereotactic radiosurgery is a novel method of treating well-defined targets in the brain, causing cell destruction, vascular occlusion or just functional changes within it. It is one of the fastest growing fields within neurosurgery. The range of appropriate indications has not yet crystallized but it is increasingly popular with patients, particularly those with a "high-risk" surgical lesion.

Introduction

Stereotactic radiosurgery is a neurosurgical technique that utilizes focused radiation as a tool. It was introduced for functional neurosurgery but its applications have widened to encompass cerebral arteriovenous malformations and a wide range of well-defined benign and malignant intracranial neoplasms.

Although it may be considered by some to belong to the realm of radiotherapy rather than neurosurgery, neurosurgical trainees must become familiar with the basics of this technique and particularly with its indications and limitations.

The minimally invasive nature and the perceived, and in most cases truly, low risk of this treatment make it popular with patients and ensure that an increasing proportion of conditions traditionally requiring open surgery are treated by this technique.

Historic Notes

The expression "stereotactic radiosurgery" (SRS) was coined by Lars Leksell, the Swedish neurosurgeon who first introduced this technique into neurosurgical practice. The term stands for a single fraction, stereotactically guided, high-dose radiation treatment on a small and well-defined volume of the brain. In this phrase (as in the method) he combined a number of important individual elements. The first, stereotaxy, the coordinate-based guidance technique in the brain, has developed from the initial endeavors of Victor Horsley and Robert Clark in 1908 and the first clinically used apparatus, devised by Spiegel and Wycis in 1947. Using this guidance system Leksell directed ionizing radiation to achieve the desired clinical effect. He included the term "surgery" to try and ensure that, as in open surgery, the selection of patients and targets would be done by neurosurgeons who were trained in neuroanatomy, neurophysiology and neuropathology and who were also familiar with the value and indications of the open surgical alternatives.

As the reader will know, Leksell greatly contributed to stereotaxy by designing his own simple and clinically easy-to-use frame. In order to reduce the invasiveness of even a precision-guided surgical procedure, he introduced ionizing radiation to substitute for the knife or needle. He began with photons from a 300 kV X-ray tube mounted on his stereotactic apparatus. In Berkeley, California, in 1950, Tobias had begun cross-firing the sella turcica with charged particles to suppress pituitary function, and work with proton beams was taken up at the Gustaf Werner Institute, Uppsala, in 1954, tested clinically from 1958 onwards, and subsequently in 1961 by Kjellberg, in Boston. In the late 1950s and 1960s, Leksell and Larsson explored the practicability of protons from the Uppsala synchrocyclotron, as well as the theoretical advantages of other particles, before deciding that gamma rays, from a heavily shielded static array of Co60 sources directed towards a central point by narrow collimators, provided the simplest and most practical system for daily clinical use. The first Leksell "gamma knife" was completed in 1967 and became operational in Stockholm in 1968. It was designed for treating functional targets, and thus intractable pain and movement disorders were the first indications. The introduction of stereotactic radiosurgery was initially received with skepticism. However, since that time, the gamma knife (as the later model became known owing to its ease of use and precision) found its way into the neurosurgical armamentarium in many centers around the world. Indeed, some purists are of the view that the phrase "gamma knife surgery" should be applied in order to emphasize the differences from other delivery methods of radiosurgery on one hand, and the crucial role of neurosurgeons in this intervention on the other. After the initial experience became better known, further "gamma units" were installed in 1984 and 1985 in Buenos Aires, Argentina and Sheffield, England, respectively. The next unit, installed in 1987 in Pittsburgh heralded an increasingly broad acceptance worldwide. According to data held at the manufacturer, by September 2001 more than 170,000 patients had been treated with a gamma knife worldwide.

Colombo and others modified the radiotherapy linear accelerator to provide a similar treatment technique. By virtue of the different technical properties, linear accelerator (Linac) radiosurgery has developed in many ways very differently from gamma knife surgery. In particular, at least in part due to the lesser degree of precision achievable with a Linac, a fractionated delivery of radiation was favored, and thus "stereotactic radiotherapy" (SRT) was born. This technique is a multi-fraction, stereotactically guided radiation therapy. Although it is possible to deliver SRT with the gamma knife, it is usually performed using a Linac.

In parallel with the developments in the radiation delivery technique, the imaging localization of the target has also undergone dramatic developments over the last five decades. The initial treatments were based on plain X-rays and pneumo-encephalography. With the introduction of computed tomography in the 1970s and magnetic resonance imaging in the 1980s, it became possible to properly delineate the pathological substrate of the treatment. Moreover, the precise identification of adjacent normal structures further dramatically improved the safety and efficacy of the technique.

Principles of Radiosurgery

Stereotactic radiosurgery in all its forms consists of the following steps: stereotactic imaging, dose planning and dose delivery.

Stereotactic Imaging

This requires the application of a set of standard reference points, or a "fiducial system", around the head followed by the acquisition of radiological images. The images obtained provide information about the precise spatial position of anatomical and pathological structures in relation to the fiducial system. The highest precision is achieved using a stereotactic frame fixed to the skull before imaging. It is usually carried out under local anesthetic for all adults unless claustrophobia prevents this. Children aged over 12 years are also treated with local rather than general anesthetic. Where the lesion is large, it is acceptable to use a less precise fiducial system, based on a dental imprint and straps to fix to the skull.

With the stereotactic frame in situ, images are taken to demonstrate the pathological lesion. In most patients this consists of a magnetic resonance imaging (MRI) scan. In the case of arteriovenous malformations (AVMs), a high-quality arterial angiogram is used. The recent trend is to combine these modalities in order to enhance the precision of outlining the margins of the lesion. Three-dimensional information is essential for precise delineation of the contours. Unfortunately, MR images, when used alone, contain potential spatial inaccuracies. These arise from non-linearities inherent in MR physics. Some can be improved by careful quality control and choice of sequences. Certain factors, for example metallic foreign bodies, in the patient, which will distort the local magnetic field and create image artifacts, cannot be overcome. In contrast, the physics of CT is linear and allows greater spatial accuracy. Therefore, in the case of smaller targets, a combination (fusion) of MRI scan and CT scan is used. Such image fusion combines the advantages of the superior soft-tissue definition of MRI scanning and the precision of CT scanning. Co-registration of MRI and angiography helps in determining the three-dimensional distribution of an AVM nidus. The added combination of functional imaging with functional MRI (fMRI) and positron emission tomography (PET), etc., is being explored on an experimental basis. Having defined the coordinate system and, within this, the contours of the target, the treatment can be planned.

Dose Planning

The aim of this step is to match the radiation treatment as precisely as possible to the contour of the lesion. Inclusion of adjacent normal tissue would lead to side-effects and complications, whereas omission of part of the lesion reduces efficacy. The precision of this step is measured not only by the precision of hitting the target point but also by the degree of matching to the contour. The most refined indices of radiation conformity take into account both the amount of target, e.g. tumor, not receiving sufficient radiation dose and the proportion of normal tissue outside the target that would be needlessly irradiated [1]. These indices show a superiority of gamma knife planning to the alternative with a Linac [2].

In addition to matching the shape, particular care is taken to avoid passing the radiation beams through eloquent structures adjacent to the lesion or even at a distance (e.g. the lens in the eye). This is achieved by plugging some of the radiation sources in the gamma knife and choosing the entry of the beams in linear accelerator techniques.

Dose Delivery

The Gamma Knife

The gamma knife uses an array of 201 Co60 sources, which are evenly distributed around a hemispherical source core. Each source (together with its associated collimator housing) produces a narrow beam of gamma radiation, and these are all directed towards a common focal spot at the center of the hemisphere ("isocenter"). The cross-firing of 201 radiation beams results in a sharp focus in which the central radiation intensity is high, and the intensity of dose falls rapidly with distance in any direction.

The size of the focal radiation field is controlled by the addition of secondary collimators, which are housed in a "helmet" situated at the head of the patient couch. Four collimator sizes are available, producing fields with nominal sizes of 4 mm, 8 mm, 14 mm and 18 mm.

A simple, single-field treatment requires the target tissue (e.g. entry zone of the trigeminal nerve for trigeminal neuralgia) to be accurately positioned at the center of the helmet collimator system where the fine radiation beams converge. This can be achieved with 0.1mm precision. The couch, helmet system and patient are then moved into the central body of the gamma knife. The treatment begins when the secondary collimators align with the sources.

Typically, the treatment of an intracranial lesion will require the overlapping of a number of foci or fields of radiation. After each field of radiation, the patient couch withdraws from the treatment position, and the position of the patient is adjusted to target an adjacent portion of the tumor. The latest C-model gamma knife offers an automatic positioning system for the head, both reducing human error and increasing precision. The ease with which this latest model affords treatment to many target points in succession encourages the planner to use a larger number of isocenters. This allows more complex plans using more isocenters to be formulated, the increased number of isocenters allowing greater conformity in matching the treatment volume to the tumor whilst sparing the surrounding tissues.

Linear Accelerators

Linear accelerators, used for years in radiotherapy, have been modified by the addition of a secondary collimator system to perform radiosurgery. Single-focus multiple non-coplanar arc and conformal block techniques are the most widely used. These phrases need explanation to the neurosurgery reader. The former technique means that the radiation source is moved along a large arc, while pointing to the same center (the so-called "isocenter"), then a similar arc is drawn tilted a few degrees away from the first one. A series of arcs are being used to maximize the dose to the center (the target) and minimize the exposure of the surrounding tissues. The second technique involves manufacturing an irregularly shaped portal for the radiation, attempting to match the shape of the targeted lesion as if viewed from the direction of that beam. Similar blocks are made for each entry beam (usually five or six). A series of static, shaped beams are then used to irradiate the lesion from a number of angles. In order to improve conformality, in some centers multiple overlapping foci are used (in a similar fashion to that described for the gamma knife). However, the calculations and set-up of numerous fields are much more difficult with the moving source of a linear accelerator than when using a gamma knife, and this deters most centers from using this technique.

More flexibility is incorporated into the system if the linear accelerator is adapted with a micro-multileaf collimator. The device consists of a series of individually motorized tungsten leaves that can be positioned automatically to create any desired beam shape. This is effectively the same principle as the conformal block technique but avoids the need to make up specific blocks for each use. The relatively short collimation length and radiation transmission between the collimator leaves are factors that may degrade the sharpness of the final radiation dose gradient and could result in higher doses to normal adjacent brain tissues. The high cost and complexity of these additions resulted in a slow initial acceptance of this method. In the intensity-modulated radiotherapy (IMRT) technique, the dose is delivered in different intensities across the lesion. The collimator leaves dynamically open and close under computer control to selectively expose or shield portions of the tumor according to predetermined limits. Treatment planning for IMRT is complex. All components of the treatment and planning thus require computer control. This promising technique is in its early stages of development and is still under clinical evaluation.

Suitable Targets

The physical properties of lesions best suited for SRS are:

- small size
- sharply defined margins, and
- favorable shape.

On size, it is customary to quote 3–3.5 cm maximum diameter as the upper limit. In spite of the high precision of targeting ("hitting" the target point: 0.1 mm for gamma knife and 1–2 mm for Linac) and conformal planning, the outer margin of the radiation field is not absolutely sharp. The radiation dose drops very rapidly at the margins but there is a definable penumbra, which receives potentially harmful radiation. The steepness of the margin becomes less with larger lesions. Also, the surface of the lesion increases in proportion to the square of the radius, and thus the volume of adjacent normal brain receiving potentially harmful radiation would become unacceptable for a large target. In these cases single-dose radiation has to be given in lower doses and thus efficacy suffers. This is true whichever equipment one uses.

The margins of the lesion have to be well defined. An infiltrative glioma or a diffuse AVM does not lend itself to precise dose planning. If these lesions are nevertheless treated, the treatment must be considered to be palliative, whereby the aim is to achieve an effect only in the limited volume covered by the treatment plan.

A very flat shape may also pose a dose-planning problem. Examples of these lesions would include "en-plaque" extensions of meningiomas or dural AVMs.

There are many lesions that are adjacent to highly eloquent structures, e.g. the optic chiasm. Good dose planning can minimize the risk to those structures. The precise details of the techniques achieving this are beyond the scope of this review, particularly as they are equipment dependent. However, there is no particular advantage in this respect of any one delivery method. Even the most advanced dose planning would fail to achieve protection of the structure at risk in the situation where the eloquent tissue is in the middle of the tumor and thus in the center of the radiation field, for example an optic nerve meningioma wrapped around the still-functioning optic nerve or an AVM doing the same in Wyburn-Mason's syndrome. These lesions remain a challenge for management.

Single Fraction and Fractionation

Fractionation is a well-established principle of radiotherapy, and describes fractionating or dividing the dose of radiation into many smaller increments. This reduces the effect of the radiation on the surrounding normal tissues. It is most effective when there is a high α/β ratio, i.e. when there is a marked difference between the radiosensitivity of the pathological target tissue and that of the surrounding structures. In conventional radiotherapy this is important, because the lack of localization means that the radiation field includes a large volume of normal tissue. Philosophically, gamma knife radiosurgery uses exactly the opposite approach: it relies on imaging, matching the radiation fields to conform precisely to the target tissue, and spares neighboring structures in this way, the actual radiation dose being given as a single unfractionated treatment. Intuitively, the stereotactic approach may be advantageous when the α/β ratio is not that high, typically the case with benign tumors, and hence the role of SRS in treating acoustic neuromas, meningiomas and AVMs. Conversely, fractionation (either with or without stereotaxy) may be more useful treating flat "en-plaque" tumors, large lesions, and pathology adjacent to radiosensitive structures such as the optic chiasm, where, even with image guidance, there is concern about the radiation delivered to the surrounding area.

Fractionation carries with it the disadvantage of necessitating multiple treatments. When it is used with stereotaxy, relocatable frames are necessary. These are inherently less accurate than the single fixed frame used in SRS. The impact of these concerns in clinical practice, and the relative role of SRS and SRT, are yet to be ascertained.

Pathologies

The gradual broadening of indications for radiosurgery was not driven by scientific considerations. Neurosurgeons, usually in charge of the gamma knife in their respective institutions, were all too aware of the complications encountered in open surgical management of their patients, and so the more "high surgical risk" conditions were referred for the alternative. This was the main explanation for the emergence and rise of AVM radiosurgery. The initial few, tentative, referrals were followed by increasing numbers when the general advantages of radiosurgery and the good results became apparent. The second driving force was the evolution that took place in the hearts and minds of patients who obtain information from the Internet and other sources. This is most apparent in patients with benign conditions, e.g. vestibular schwannomas. These patients have the time to research their condition and to enquire about side-effects and complications and compare those with different interventions. They encounter their brethren through patient organizations. Such personal observations may be biased but often prove decisive. Patients tend to make up their minds based on perception and emotional reasons and not leave to their surgeon or to chance the decision as to whether to have major brain surgery or undergo a day-case procedure. Patient pressure is a very powerful force.

Scientific evidence in the form of prospective randomized controlled trials is lacking for both surgery and radiosurgery for most pathologies. Given the problems in recruiting sufficient numbers for the trials, and problems with patients dropping out and crossing over, such data are unlikely to become available. On the other hand, case series provide useful data. The strength of radiosurgery publications is the easy reproducibility of the results in similar units; quite the opposite would apply to microsurgical results published only from centers of excellence, with average and poorer results never becoming available.

Arteriovenous Malformations

The primary aim in the management of AVMs is to remove the risk of hemorrhage. This risk is 2–4% per annum, with approximately 25–30% mortality rate per bleed. In view of this risk, immediate removal of the lesion is the ideal treatment for those AVMs that can be operated upon with minimal morbidity, and indeed this is the practice in the UK and elsewhere for these lesions. The AVM is characterized by the size, position and venous drainage of the nidus. This allows a classification (Spetzler-Martin grade), which correlates with surgical mortality and morbidity. An AVM in a non-eloquent brain area, less than 3 cm in diameter in size and with superficial venous drainage (Spetzler-Martin grade 1) would be an "operable" lesion.

In emergency situations where a large hematoma requires urgent removal, the AVM is often removed during the same procedure. On the other hand, in these situations it may not be possible to obtain satisfactory angiographic images to plan surgery, and thus many end up with remnants demonstrated on post-operative imaging – requiring further treatment.

In operable, cold cases the risk of neurological complications in the hands of neurosurgeons specializing in this field may be low, and the risks of intracranial surgery (infection, seizures, pneumonia, deep venous thrombosis) and the unavoidable inconvenience (protracted hospital stay, discomfort of a craniotomy, a temporary ban on driving, etc.) may appear worth taking. Thus, surgery is accepted by many patients. However, one has to observe in an increasing proportion of patients the trend to seek less invasive alternatives.

The use of radiosurgery for "operable" AVMs remains controversial; indeed, this group of patients is the only one in which a "surgery vs radiosurgery" debate is still ongoing. Schramm & Schramm [3] performed a meta-analysis of published radiosurgery results for low surgical risk AVMs. His own excellent personal operative results appeared to be better than those for radiosurgery, if the analysis of the latter included the statistical risk of hemorrhage during the latent period, i.e. before radiosurgery would have had its effect. However, the rate of immediate new post-operative neurological deficits or worsening of pre-operative deficits was 27.4% – a figure many times that of gamma-knife-treated patients.

Unfortunately, not all AVMs are ideal or indeed suitable for elective surgery. The resulting problems are incomplete resection and surgical complications. Those with higher Spetzler-Martin grade have a higher neurosurgical risk and surgery has to be more cautious. This leads to not infrequent post-surgical remnants, particularly with AVMs located in the thalamus, basal ganglia and brainstem [4]. Despite the negative reporting bias, the evidence is clear that surgery for these deeply placed AVMs carries a high surgical risk [5].

Endovascular techniques are increasingly used for cerebral AVMs. Analysis of the technique and role of interventional radiology is beyond the scope of this chapter. Suffice it to say that a close cooperation with one's neuroradiologist is an essential factor in the successful management of AVMs.

Since the early reports by Steiner et al. [6], describing successful obliteration of AVMs by radiosurgery, many hundreds of abstracts of proceedings, papers and book chapters have appeared to prove the same [7, 8, 9]. Concerning the mechanism, the main effect of radiation is upon the endothelial cells within the nidus, with an additional effect of myofibroblast development in the connective tissue stroma [10].

It is broadly accepted that about 80–90% of AVMs undergo thrombo-obliteration after single-dose radiation (Fig. 8.1). The efficacy depends on the radiation dose given to the periphery of the lesion. In small ($<1 cm^3$) lesions, this dose is usually 25 Gy, which can achieve close to 100% obliteration rate [11]. In cases of larger AVMs, the dose is kept lower in order to keep complications to around 5%. Series with a significant component of large malformations and utilizing lower doses have lower response rate, but even in those the success rate is around 65–75% [12]. It has to be emphasized that these series largely consist of patients referred for radiosurgery because the surgeon in charge of the patient considered open surgery to be of too high risk, usually owing to the eloquent position of the nidus ("inoperable").

The response shows a latency of 1–3 years, with only minor changes occurring in the third year. The risk of hemorrhage appears to decline

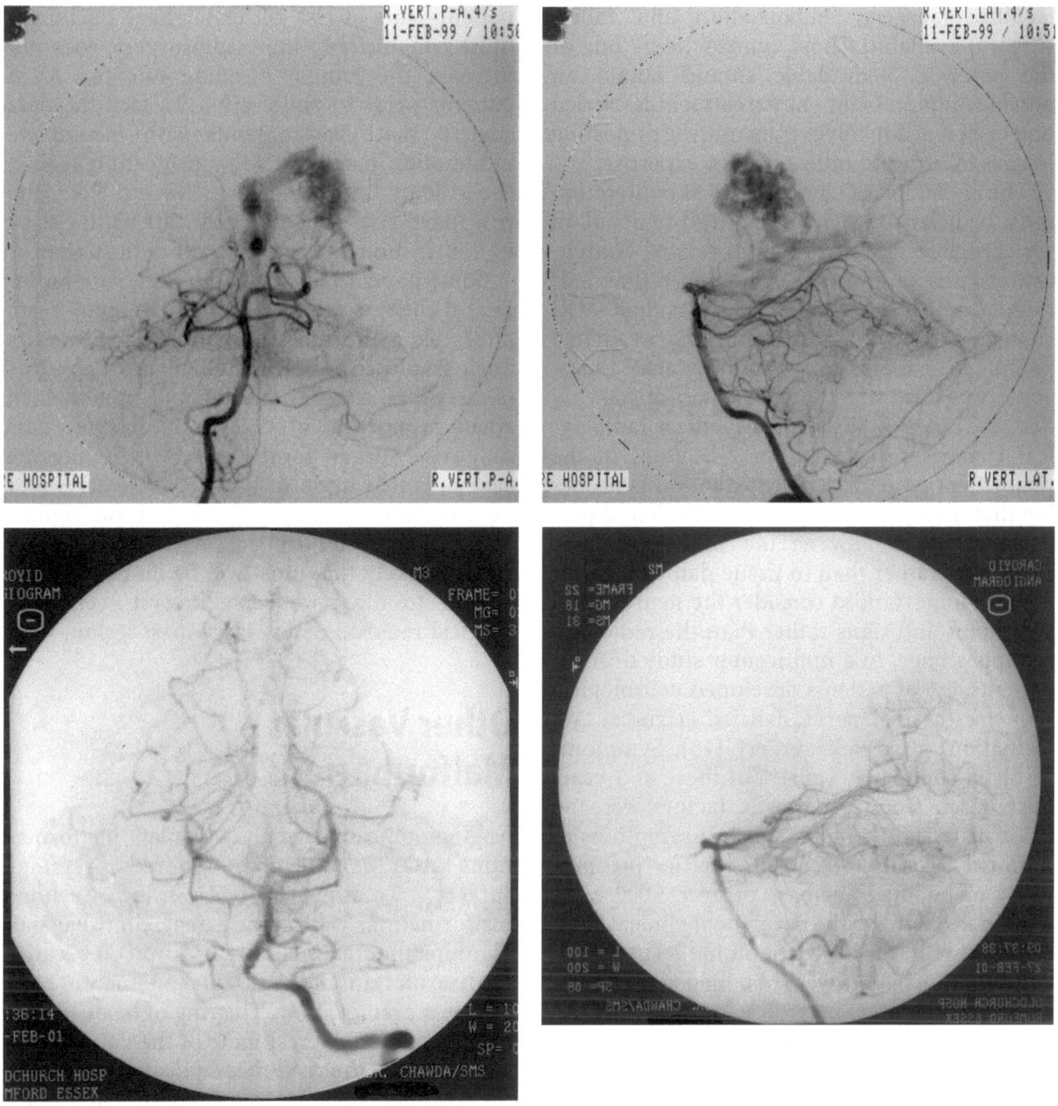

Fig. 8.1. a–d. Obliteration of cerebral AVM 2 years after gamma knife radiosurgery: 25 Gy peripheral dose used. **a** PA view. **b** Lateral view. **c** PA view after radiosurgery. **d** Lateral view after radiosurgery.

slowly after radiation but it is not eliminated fully until obliteration is complete. No doubt, the slow response during the latent period contributes to the safety of the method, avoiding pressure-breakthrough hemorrhage by altering the hemodynamics slowly. A speedier reaction could be achieved by higher radiation doses, but the incidence of permanent untoward neurological sequelae may then rise above 5%. The current dose regimens achieve this while achieving overall obliteration rates of 75%, or considerably better in more favorable cases.

It is not possible to give a strict system of criteria for suitability, as the decision as to which technique to use, or which one to use first, is multifactorial. The site, shape and size of the nidus, the angio-architecture, the patient's age, general health, etc., are all factors in this decision. Each case should be considered in a multidisciplinary fashion by a team that has all facilities (surgery, embolization and radiosurgery) available. Those centers where one or the other is unavailable should obtain an outside opinion before any treatment is carried out, even if this involves transmitting or posting images in order to utilize distant expertise.

The likelihood of complete AVM obliteration must be balanced against the need to avoid an unacceptable rate of radiation-related complications after radiosurgery. Flickinger et al. [13] found that 30% of AVM patients had MRI changes adjacent to or within the irradiated volume at a median of 8 months after radiosurgery. However, though some mistakenly describe this as "radionecrosis", these radiological changes resolve within 2–3 years in the majority of patients. The explanation is probably that the signal change is due to altered perilesional blood flow as the nidus gradually obliterates rather than to tissue damage [14]. It is more important to consider the neurological symptoms and signs rather than the radiological appearance. In a multicenter study of AVM patients, 8% of patients developed neurological sequelae (cranial nerve deficits, seizures, cyst formation) after radiosurgery [15]. Symptoms resolved completely in 54% of these at 3 years post onset. Good prognostic factors were no prior history of hemorrhage and symptoms of minimal severity. According to the prospectively maintained database of over 3,000 cases treated in Sheffield, the permanent clinical complication rate is 3.8% (data on file). These low-complication figures were obtained with gamma knife treatment. Linear-accelerator (LINAC) technology results in somewhat worse statistics [16].

Earlier reports on AVM radiosurgery suggested that the annual hemorrhage rate after radiosurgery prior to obliteration was greater than that occurring in the natural history of untreated AVMs. More recent reports, analyzing radiosurgical hemorrhage rates, found that radiosurgery did not change the annual bleeding rates during the latency interval [17, 18]. Karlsson et al. [19] reported 1,604 patients with a total of 2,340 patient-years at risk of a hemorrhage. They detected a decrease in hemorrhage rates within 6 months after radiosurgery and patients who received higher radiation doses were conferred the greatest protection from bleeding. When considered together, these three reports with 2,000 patients and more than 3,000 patient-years at risk of hemorrhage document quite convincingly that radiosurgery does not increase the annual bleeding rate for AVM patients prior to obliteration. In fact, the data suggest that even patients with incomplete obliteration may have some protection against the risk of future bleeding. Nevertheless, the continued risk of hemorrhage during the delay in obliteration is a drawback of radiosurgery.

Some papers [20] highlighted the late radiological changes seen on MRI, noted many years after the malformations had been shown by angiography to be obliterated. In most cases this is merely an imaging finding, but in a selected small proportion of cases clinical symptoms may arise. Surgery for these cysts (including one case operated upon in our department) found no neoplastic change. The long-term significance of these fluid-filled cavities is uncertain but it is likely that most will be innocuous and similar to the porencephalic cyst seen after surgical removal of any large mass lesion.

Other Vascular Malformations

Angiographically occult vascular malformations (AOVMs) are often referred for radiosurgery. Treatment of cavernous venous malformations is, to some extent, controversial. Planning the treatment may be difficult because the true margins of the vascular anomaly are not obvious, even on MRI. The ring of hemosiderin may lead to an overestimate of the volume and thus increase the risk of complications. Indeed, the treatments planned on CT in the early years were associated with side-effects. The natural history of these lesions is still not clear and many, particularly the incidentally detected ones, are only observed. Those that are in a surgically easily accessible position are usually removed by microsurgery, particularly if they had bled or caused epilepsy. Those in an eloquent site (brainstem, basal ganglia, etc.) may be good radiosurgical targets. There is increasing statistical evidence that the risk of hemorrhage is reduced by radiosurgery. The difficulty in interpretation of the results lies in the fact that obliteration cannot be demonstrated radiologically. Epilepsy may also improve after treatment.

Radiosurgery is ineffective at best and may be harmful if pursued.

Pure vein of Galen malformations are best treated by endovascular methods. However, these should be distinguished from true AVMs with demonstrable nidus; the latter are treatable with radiosurgery.

Vestibular Schwannomas (Acoustic Neurinoma)

The indications for the radiosurgical option evolved over the years. First we considered only the elderly and medically infirm who would not tolerate a long surgical procedure. The next group of patients – those with tumors in their only hearing ear or with bilateral tumors – were referred later as a result of the recognition of a perceived superior hearing preservation with radiosurgery. Similarly, facial nerve preservation may be difficult with surgery for recurrent tumors, so these were considered for radiosurgery. Finally, it became a primary choice for those who refused microsurgery in order to avoid the inconvenience and interruption of their daily life by open surgery. The latter group is undoubtedly influenced by the plethora of information available on the Internet both from other patients and from institutions.

Those patients with brainstem compression symptoms usually benefit from at least partial removal of the mass. Therefore, they should undergo open surgery rather than hoping for a slow decompression by eventual shrinkage of the tumor. The arbitrary upper limit of 3.5 cm maximum diameter is born out of the observation that a larger tumor cannot be irradiated with a therapeutically effective single dose without unacceptable cranial nerve neuropathies. There are, of course, anecdotal successes even amongst these large tumors.

The aim of radiosurgery is different from that of open surgery. It does not aim to remove the lesion, merely to control its growth. This control may be defined as "no growth compared with the pre-treatment size", or the looser definition advocated by some, where the criterion is "the absence of need for further intervention"; the latter is open to biased interpretation. The control rate is reported to be about 97–98%, with an actual reduction in size in 23–55% [21]. Involution of the tumor occurs slowly, through several years (Fig. 8.2). Considering the rates of residual and recurrent tumors seen even in the best published surgical series, not to mention the case material submitted for radiosurgery, tumor control with radiosurgery is at least as good.

Complications of radiosurgery can be immediate and late. In the first 24 hours, nausea and headache were seen, particularly in the early days of radiosurgery when larger radiation doses and less precise dose planning were used. The combination of conformal planning, delivering no more than 12–15 Gy peripheral dose, and perioperative steroid cover eliminated these side-effects. Late cranial neuropathies are dependent on peripheral dose and the size of the tumor. The latter is an important factor, as with larger tumor size a longer section of the nerves receives toxic dose. On the other hand, intracanalicular tumors may also pose a challenge. They are more difficult to delineate precisely, and the relative imprecision of MRI imaging may lead to complications. In these cases fusion with CT scan is particularly helpful.

Hearing preservation is reported in 30–75%, and as the fading of hearing is gradual, the result is dependent on length of follow-up. In our own material (in Sheffield) concerning unilateral vestibular schwannomas (VS), using the Gammaplan planning software, no higher than 15 Gy peripheral dose and at least 5 years' follow-up, hearing preservation was achieved in 75% of patients (submitted for publication). Over-enthusiastic reduction in the delivered dose may be counterproductive: losing tumor control would lead to morbidity through increased tension on the cranial nerves. One must not forget that, after all, most VS are originally diagnosed as a result of progressive hearing loss.

In considering tumor control and the management of patients after radiosurgery, it is important to understand the changes that occur with time after the treatment. Early on, around 1 year, the tumor is frequently larger. It is important not to rush into surgery as subsequently the tumor may well involute and shrink. At that time the cranial nerves may be at their most fragile, rendering the operation higher risk. Failure of tumor control should not be declared until 4–5 years after radiosurgery owing to the slow effect of the treatment.

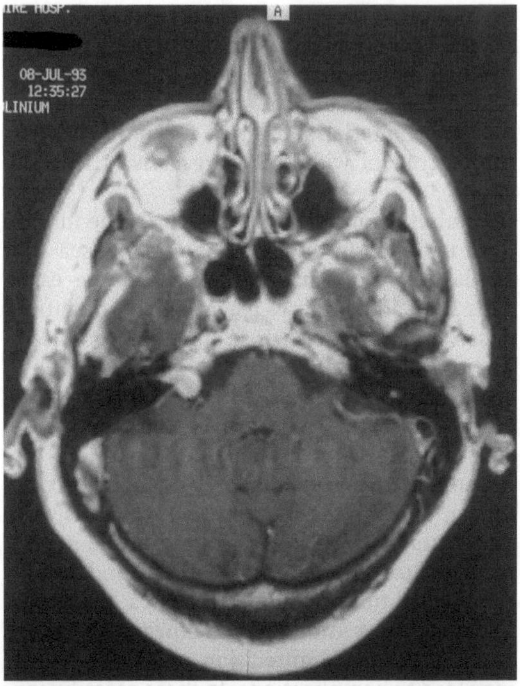

a

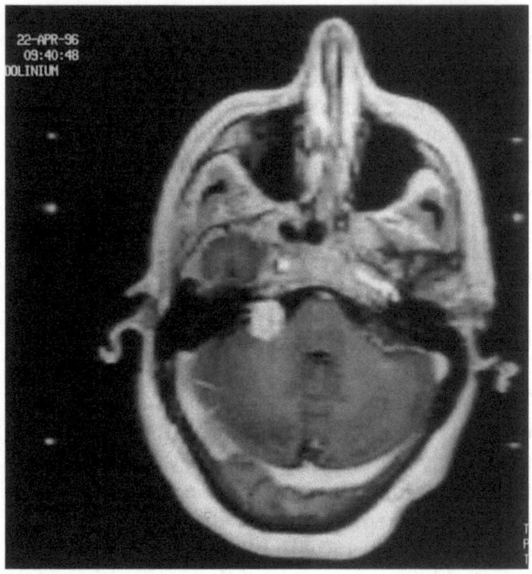

b

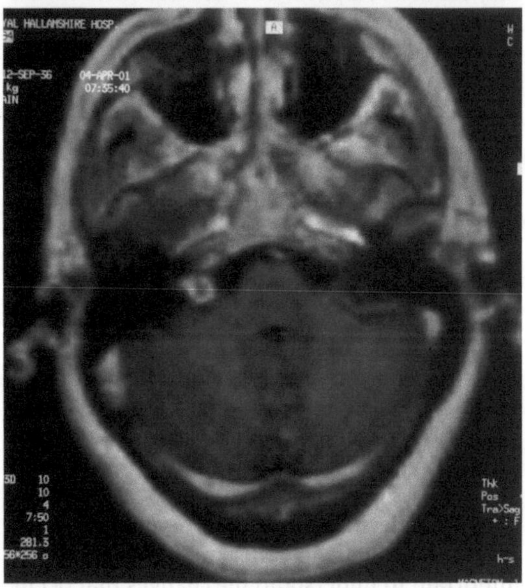

c

Fig. 8.2. a–c. Involution of vestibular schwannoma (VS) after gamma knife treatment with 13 Gy peripheral dose. **a** MRI scan of right VS at presentation. **b** Enlarged tumor at the time of radiosurgery. **c** Typical appearance 5 years after treatment.

There has been concern expressed about the late consequences of radiosurgery. Excision after radiosurgery may be more difficult due to scarring, even in later years, though the evidence for this is very weak and anecdotal. There is a possibility of malignant change in the irradiated schwannomas [22]. So far the statistics suggest that such a change is only a remote possibility, but long-term follow-up of these patients continues.

In summary, radiosurgery is an attractive alternative for patients with small and medium-sized VS, particularly if hearing and/or facial nerve preservation on the affected side is paramount. It is increasingly considered (at least by the patients) to be the primary procedure of choice for those with small tumors. It is often chosen to treat recurrent tumors. There are indications that recurrence after microsurgery may be the result of less radical removal in an attempt to achieve hearing preservation. In our material of over 500 acoustic neuromas referred for radiosurgery, 36% had one or more previous operations on their tumor. This is a particularly important group as, owing to the almost uniformly present post-operative hearing loss, they may not have new symptoms until the tumor is large and causes ataxia. One of the common criticisms of radiosurgery relates to the need for follow-up imaging – true, but the high proportion of post-surgical cases in our material suggests that vigilance is necessary even after excision; the notion that microsurgery is a "definitive treatment", without the risk of recurrence, is a myth. Long-term supervision is warranted after all treatments of these tumors, whether surgery or radiosurgery is applied.

Malignancy

In principle, infiltrative tumors should not be considered to be suitable for a focal treatment. This statement is particularly true for high-grade gliomas that infiltrate far from the main mass. We rarely use this technique in such cases. However, in the case of metastases, local infiltration into the normal tissue is fairly limited and thus both surgery and radiosurgery confer a benefit by local cytoreduction. Furthermore, radiosurgery treatment has a penumbral effect, as opposed to the truly sharp boundary with surgical excision, and this may even result in superior local control compared with surgery alone. A multicenter randomized trial is in progress in Europe, which compares gamma knife radiosurgery alone to surgery with whole-brain radiotherapy.

This pathology is especially important for healthcare planners. During the course of their disease, 20–40% of cancer patients will develop brain metastases, and this predicts almost half a million patients with brain metastases per year in the USA alone. Given the number of cases, the following question arises: "How many of these cases are appropriate for radiosurgery?" Appropriate is defined as "the patient stands a reasonable chance of obtaining a benefit in terms of control of brain disease and retention/improvement in quality of life with treatment". In order to identify a group of patients who might benefit from more aggressive treatment, such as radiosurgery, one can use the experience of the RTOG (Radiation Therapy Oncology Group) protocol 79-16, a radiation therapy protocol on brain metastases. The four factors predictive of improved survival were:

- Karnofsky performance status ≥70%
- Absent or controlled primary disease
- Age <60 years
- Evidence of metastasis to brain only

In our unit we use these criteria to include patients in the radiosurgery program, but also consider the number of metastases visible on MRI. We are reluctant to treat in cases where there are more than three lesions as the benefits of focal treatment are lost when there is an obvious generalized disease. Technically speaking, most metastases are close to ideal for radiosurgery. They are easily visible on imaging, they are rarely beyond the suitable size-range, and they are usually spherical with sharp outlines, therefore the matching of the shape of the lesion is easy. There is published evidence from a multicenter study [23] showing that there was a 2.84 times higher risk of local recurrence after LINAC treatment than after gamma knife treatment. The reason for this finding is controversial but it may question in the future the acceptability of LINAC use, as opposed to gamma knife use, for this indication.

It is particularly important in this patient group to state that the aim of radiosurgery is only to achieve local tumor control. This may be achievable in up to 90% of cases. Prospective randomized trials are needed to properly define the role of radiosurgery for cerebral metastases.

Functional Indications

As mentioned in the introduction, radiosurgery was originally devised to be used for lesion making in functional indications. A wide range of interventions were carried out, including anterior capsulotomy for obsessive–compulsive disorder, thalamotomies for pain and movement disorders, and irradiation of the trigeminal ganglion for neuralgia. Subsequently, the technique became increasingly used for vascular and neoplastic lesions, as discussed above.

However, over the last few years the fastest growing indication for radiosurgery, particularly in the USA, has been trigeminal neuralgia. This revival was made possible by the development of imaging enabling the identification of, and thus targeting the entry zone of, the trigeminal nerve, or indeed the nerve itself. The reader will be familiar with the wide range of treatments and procedures in use for this condition. The reason to add another was the perceived surgical risk of microvascular decompression on one hand, and the recurrence rate with the alternative operations on the other. In practical terms the procedure is particularly straightforward as there is very little shape matching necessary when planning this treatment. Most gamma knife centers use a single 4 mm collimator field, prescribing 70 or 80 Gy to the isocenter. It was observed that irradiation of a longer section of the nerve using two adjacent fields may increase the risk of post-operative facial sensory impairment. In terms of efficacy, gamma knife surgery does live up to the expectations: in primary cases 85–90% pain-free state is achieved. The only drawback is the 3–12 weeks lag period before the cessation of pain. Salvage procedures after previous destructive operations are less effective but may result in good and excellent outcome (pain free with or without continued medication) in 65–70%. The permanency of the results appears to mirror microvascular decompressions rather than the percutaneous rhizotomies. Whether in the long run the recurrence rate remains as low as it appears at present is not yet clear. The risk of facial dysesthesia or numbness is low, and the other risks of surgery (e.g. cerebrospinal fluid rhinorrhea, meningitis, hearing loss, etc.) are avoided. The attraction of a day-case procedure under local anesthetic for an elderly or infirm patient is obvious.

After treating AVMs associated with focal-onset epilepsy, many observed an improvement or cessation of epileptic activity. This prompted treatment of small indolent lesions and good seizure-control results were observed. Since 1995, Regis presented several patients with mesial temporal sclerosis who had been treated using focused radiation with the gamma knife. His results were very convincing, achieving seizure control in a high proportion of cases. Other centers, including the authors of this review, followed suit, treating small series of patients. Our experience showed that seizure control at 3 years following irradiation is very similar to that achieved with temporal lobe resections, and thus this method could be advocated for those who are unable or unwilling to undergo resective surgery. However, our observation was that there was a long, 12–36-month time lag to achieve the seizure-free state. Furthermore, some patients found it difficult to cope with the slow alteration of their seizure pattern and the appearance of frequent auras for some months. In our small series we have not observed permanent neurological deficit, but about 50% of patients required several weeks of dexamethasone treatment owing to focal cerebral swelling after about a year. The method certainly deserves to be exposed to wider scale trials, but its role is not yet established.

Sporadic reports are available concerning the revival of radiosurgery for traditional functional indications. Thalamotomies, anterior corpus callosotomies and even cingulotomies have all been described using radiosurgery. Admittedly, it would be attractive to make the lesions currently made using radiofrequency techniques without the need for a burr hole and physical penetration of the brain. The limitation of radiosurgery for these indications is the lack of feedback obtained by stimulation and recording. Although the need to adjust the target coordinates during open procedures is infrequent, the reassurance before making the lesion is required by most neurosurgeons. An additional problem is the relative variability of the size of the brain lesion made even with a standard radiation dose. These indications should be considered as experimental.

Future Trends

The history of radiosurgery shows that, over the years, the greatest development has occurred in imaging. It is likely that this trend will continue at least for the foreseeable future. MRI techniques are likely to improve within years to allow the AVM nidus to be identified without arterial angiography. New protocols are already being developed (e.g. one in our unit, termed "MR-DSA") to be used for post-radiosurgery assessment of the nidus, although at present an apparent cure would still have to be confirmed by high-quality digital subtraction angiography.

The currently used planning software for the gamma knife technique and for some of the Linac techniques allows protection of adjacent eloquent structures. Automated planning will make these procedures even safer and easier in the future. It will be helpful to include functional information in the planning of treatment near important cortical structures, and a combination of structural MRI with functional MRI will no doubt be increasingly utilized. The role of PET is likely to grow, both in pre-operative work-up and post-radiosurgery assessment of tumors, in the same manner as it is currently used to differentiate between radionecrosis and recurrence after radiotherapy.

Delivery of focused radiation is also likely to change. The precision and reliability of the gamma knife is far superior to LINAC-based systems, but it is hoped that the latter techniques will add flexibility to treat larger lesions and those in extracranial positions. The role of fractionated delivery will be clarified. The potential for malignant changes and other late complications will also be explored in years to come.

Key Points

- *Stereotactic radiosurgery delivers a high dose of radiation to well-defined targets in the brain. In most situations lesions of less than 3.5 cm maximum diameter are considered to be suitable.*
- *Thrombo-obliteration of AVMs is achieved in 60–95%, depending on size, and with 4–9% risk of neurological complications, depending on eloquence of the area.*
- *Vestibular schwannomas can be controlled in over 90% of cases, with 1% risk of permanent facial nerve deficit and 25% risk of hearing loss.*
- *Functional indications are still under evaluation.*

Self-assessment

- ☐ What are the main indications for stereotactic radiosurgery?
- ☐ What are the two principal technologies used in delivery of the radiation?
- ☐ What are the main factors taken into account in the decisions regarding suitability?

References

1. Paddick I. A simple scoring ratio to index the conformity of radiosurgical treatment plans. J Neurosurg 2000;93(suppl 3):219–22.
2. Borden JA, Mahajan A, Tsi JS. A quality factor to compare the dosimetry of gamma knife radiosurgery and intensity-modulated radiation therapy quantitatively as a function of target volume and shape. J Neurosurg 2000;93(suppl 3):228–32.
3. Schaller C, Schramm J. Microsurgical results for small arteriovenous malformations accessible for radiosurgical or embolization treatment. Neurosurgery 1997;40: 664–72.
4. Lawton MT, Hamilton MG, Spetzler RE. Multimodality treatment of deep arteriovenous malformations: thalamus, basal ganglia, and brain stem. Neurosurgery 1995;37:29–36.
5. Morgan MK, Drummond KJ, Grinnel IV, Sorby W. Surgery for cerebral arteriovenous malformation: risks related to lenticulostriate arterial supply. J Neurosurg 1997;86:801–5.
6. Steiner L, Leksell L, Forster DMC, Greitz T, Backlund E. Stereotactic radiosurgery in intracranial arteriovenous malformations. Acta Neurochir (Suppl) 1974; 21:195–209.
7. Lunsford LD, Kondziolka D, Flickinger JC, Bissonette DJ, Jungreis CA, Vincent D et al. Stereotactic radiosurgery for arteriovenous malformations of the brain. J Neurosurg 1991;75:512–24.
8. Steiner L, Lindquist C, Adler JR, Torner JC, Alves W, Steiner M. Clinical outcome of radiosurgery for cerebral arteriovenous malformations. J Neurosurg 1992;77:1–8.
9. Colombo F, Pozza F, Chicrego G, Casentini L, De Luea G, Francescon P. Linear accelerator radiosurgery of cerebral arteriovenous malformations: an update. Neurosurgery 1994;34:14–21.
10. Szeifert G, Kemeny AA, Timperley WR, Forster DMC. The potential role of myofibroblasts in arteriovenous malformation obliteration after radiosurgery. Neurosurgery 1997;39:67–70.
11. Lunsford LD, editor. Stereotactic radiosurgery clinics of North America, vol 3, no. 1. Philadelphia: WB Saunders, 1992.
12. Yamamoto Y et al. Interim report on the radiosurgical treatment of cerebral arteriovenous malformations. The influence of size, dose, time, and technical factors on obliteration rate. J Neurosurg 1995;83:832–7.
13. Flickinger JC, Kondziolka D, Pollock BE, Maitz A, Lunsford LD. Complications from arteriovenous

malformation radiosurgery: multivariate analysis and risk modeling. Int J Radiat Oncol Biol Phys 1997;38: 485–90.
14. Pollock BE. Patient outcomes after arteriovenous malformation radiosurgery. In: Lunsford LD, Kondziolka D, Flickinger JC, editors. Gamma knife brain surgery (Progress in neurological surgery, vol 14). Basel: Karger, 1998; 51–9.
15. Flickinger JC. Kondziolka D. Lunsford LD et al. A multi-institutional analysis of complication outcomes after arteriovenous malformation radiosurgery. Int J Radiat Oncol Biol Phys 1999;44:67–74.
16. Miyawaki L, Dowd C, Wara W et al. Five year results of LINAC radiosurgery for arteriovenous malformations: outcome for large AVMs. Int J Radiat Oncol Biol Phys 1999;44:1089–106.
17. Pollock BE, Flickinger JC, Lunsford LD, Bissonette DJ, Kondziolka D. Hemorrhage risk after stereotactic radiosurgery of cerebral arteriovenous malformations. Neurosurgery 1996;38:652–61.
18. Friedman WA, Blatt DL, Bova FJ, Buatti JM, Mendenhall WM, Kublis PS. The risk of hemorrhage after radiosurgery for arteriovenous malformations. J Neurosurg 1996;84:912–19.
19. Karlsson Lidquist C, Steiner L. The effect of gamma knife surgery on the risk of rupture prior to AVM obliteration. Minim Invasive Neurosurg 1996;39:21–7.
20. Yamamoto M, Jimbo M, Kobayashi M, Toyoda C, Ide M, Tanaka N et al. Long-term results of radiosurgery for arteriovenous malformation: neurodiagnostic imaging and histological studies of angiographically confirmed nidus obliteration. Surg Neurol 1992;37:219–30.
21. Flickinger JC, Lunsford LD, Coffey RJ et al. Radiosurgery for acoustic neurinomas. Cancer 1991;67: 345–53.
22. Hanabusa K, Morikawa A, Murata T, Taki W. Acoustic neuroma with malignant transformation (case report). J Neurosurg 2001;95:518–21.
23. Shaw E, Scott C, Souhami L, Dinapoli R, Kline R, Loeffler J et al. Single dose radiosurgical treatment of previously irradiated primary brain tumours and brain metastases: final report of RTOG protocol 90-05. Int J Radiol Oncol Biol Phys 2000;47:291–8.

IV
Tumors

9

Low-grade Gliomas in Adults

Henry Marsh

Summary

The treatment of low-grade gliomas remains one of the most uncertain and controversial areas of modern neurosurgery. It is an increasingly important area because the widespread availability of MRI scanning has meant that more and more cases are being diagnosed. A small number of patients can be cured by complete surgical resection, and modern neurosurgical techniques, combined with awake craniotomy and intraoperative histology, have probably increased this number. Nevertheless, the majority of patients cannot be cured and the decision as to how best to treat them can be very difficult, especially since low-grade gliomas are very variable in their size, location, histology and biological behavior. Treatment decisions need to be made jointly by neurosurgeons and neuro-oncologists. Careful follow-up and explanation to the patient are often just as important as any treatment undertaken.

Introduction

The term "low-grade gliomas" is used by neurologists and neurosurgeons to describe a group of intrinsic cerebral tumors arising primarily from astrocytes, oligodendrocytes or ependymal cells that are characterized by their relatively slow rate of growth and certain radiological appearances when compared with the commoner malignant or "high-grade" gliomas. The use of the term is often confusing since it is not a precise pathological definition. It is sometimes used to refer only to low-grade astrocytomas, but oligodendrogliomas, ependymomas, gangliogliomas and pleomorphic xanthoastrocytomas will sometimes be included as well. To add to the confusion, the pathology of these various tumors often overlaps, and "mixed oligoastrocytomas" or "ependymal differentiation in an oligodendroglioma", for instance, are quite often reported by pathologists on micro scopic examination of biopsy specimens. Furthermore, there is no precise border between "low grade" and "high grade", and many tumors will be found, on histological examination, to contain cells of differing degrees of malignancy. Although "low-grade" tumors typically grow quite slowly, it is euphemistic to describe them as "benign" since the great majority of adults with these "low-grade" tumors will die from the disease within 10 years of the initial diagnosis, irrespective of any treatment that they might have received [1]. Death most frequently occurs as a result of the tumor eventually transforming into a more malignant form (in up to 80% of tumors, according to Russell and Rubinstein [2]) or occasionally as a result of slow but steady expansion of the tumor without obvious malignant change. Patients with these tumors, therefore, are best seen as suffering from a chronic, usually incurable, illness where treatment is only palliative in the great majority of cases.

Low-grade gliomas of all varieties account for about 15–20% of primary cerebral neoplasms in adults and most commonly present in young adults with epilepsy and without any neurological deficit. In the modern era of widely available and increasingly sensitive CT and MRI scanning, they are diagnosed more frequently, at an earlier stage, when the tumor is smaller, than in the past. Nevertheless, it is remarkable how large some of these tumors can become before they produce any symptoms. Only a small number of patients will have symptoms of raised intracranial pressure or a focal neurological deficit at the time of presentation. Their comparative rarity and long natural history have made it difficult to establish how best to treat them and there have been no controlled trials comparing different methods of treatment. The published literature is largely anecdotal and retrospective (see, for instance, the review by Marantz [3]). If low-grade gliomas as a whole are considered, evidence-based conclusions cannot be drawn as to whether treatment has any significant impact on life expectancy or not.

It must never be forgotten that the diagnosis of a brain tumor is quite devastating for the patient and the patient's family. They will hope for confident and certain advice from the neurosurgeon to whom they are referred. The neurosurgeon's difficulty in knowing what to advise, given the lack of evidence from any controlled trials, is made even more difficult by the fact that treatment is never entirely safe and is often very unpleasant. Most of the patients will be entirely well at the time of presentation, often having only suffered a single epileptic fit. Not surprisingly, therefore, opinions vary as to how best to treat these tumors, ranging from the so-called "conservative treatment" of doing nothing at all (other than treating the epilepsy with anticonvulsants), to minimal biopsy, to radical resection, with or without chemotherapy or radiotherapy. Despite the lack of firm evidence, it is possible, however, to establish certain principles that should guide management and to identify a few subtypes of low-grade glioma in adults where it is reasonably certain what should be done.

The main forms of treatment for these tumors are surgery and radiotherapy, and to a much lesser extent chemotherapy. Because of the uncertainties surrounding the best way to treat patients, it cannot be emphasized strongly enough that patients with these tumors should be treated jointly by neurosurgeons and neurooncologists working in close cooperation, although care must be taken to prevent the "specialist team" turning into an impersonal committee.

Pathological Classification

Varieties

The pathological classification of intrinsic cerebral tumors is various and, at times, confusing. A clear account is to be found in the standard work by Russell and Rubinstein [2]. We are concerned here primarily with the slow-growing gliomas of the cerebral hemispheres that are found in adults, so the list below will not, therefore, include the various astrocytomas found in children, such as optic pathway astrocytomas, brainstem gliomas and pilocytic cerebellar astrocytomas, some of which are truly benign in the sense of being curable by surgical resection. These essentially pediatric tumors can, however, occasionally be found in young adults.

Low-grade gliomas may be classified into the following categories:

Astrocytoma (grades I and II)

Oligodendroglioma

Mixed oligoastrocytoma

Miscellaneous, including ganglioglioma, pleomorphic xanthoastrocytoma and neurocytoma

Presentation

In modern practice, the great majority of low-grade gliomas present with epilepsy. A small number of patients (1% in the author's own series of 160 patients with low-grade gliomas) will present with raised intracranial pressure or a focal neurological deficit. Most patients are relatively young: low-grade gliomas are found only occasionally in patients over the age of 40 years.

Diagnostic Imaging

MRI scanning is the most sensitive means of detecting these tumors and showing the degree of infiltration into the surrounding brain. Good-quality CT (computed tomography) is less effective at delineating the extent of the tumor, and will completely miss some of the smaller tumors that are seen with MRI.

Low-grade gliomas in adults typically do not enhance. If a degree of enhancement is present, however, it is generally considered to mean that anaplastic change is present, that the grade of the tumor will be higher, and that the prognosis will be correspondingly worse than if there was no enhancement. There are some exceptions to this, such as pleomorphic xanthoastrocytomas and pediatric astrocytomas, which occasionally present in young adults and where enhancement is not necessarily an ominous finding. It is important to recognize that CT and MRI scanning are not always a reliable way of determining the histological grade of a tumor [4]. Interpretation of brain scans of patients who have undergone previous treatment can be particularly difficult, with post-operative changes causing enhancement that can mimic recurrent tumor, and radiotherapy producing white matter changes that are very similar to infiltrating tumor or cerebral edema caused by recurrent tumor.

The typical MRI findings for low-grade astrocytomas are of low-signal intensity on T1 spin-echo sequences, and of high-signal intensity on T2 and proton-density sequences, with varying degrees of white matter infiltration and edema around the central part of the tumor. On CT, the tumors appear as areas of low density, sometimes with patchy calcification, which is seen most commonly in oligodendrogliomas.

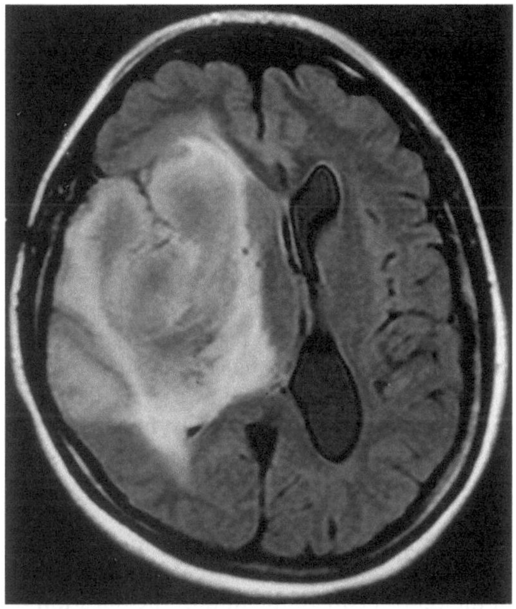

Fig. 9.1. Case HO. Inoperable low-grade astrocytoma (histologically verified).

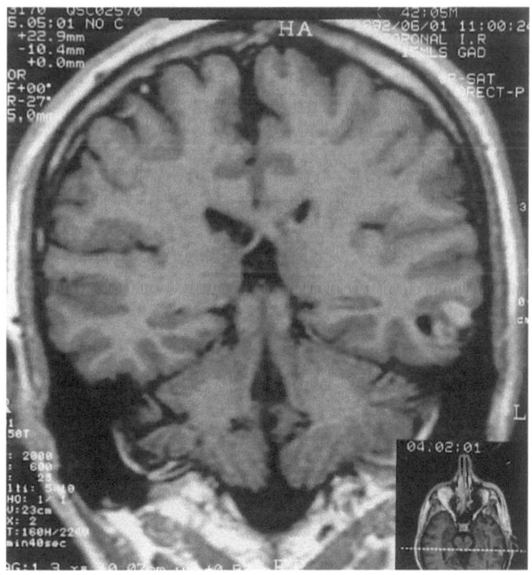

Fig. 9.2. Case MB. A small left temporal tumor that is histologically identical to Case HO.

Pathological Anatomy

The degree of infiltration of the surrounding brain by low-grade gliomas is very variable. Some tumors can appear to occupy much of a cerebral hemisphere, with the patient suffering surprisingly little, if any, neurological impairment (Fig. 9.1). In these cases the differential diagnosis from gliomatosis cerebri can be somewhat arbitrary. Other tumors (Fig. 9.2) can be relatively small and appear well circumscribed, although histologically all of these tumors are infiltrative to a greater or lesser extent. Most of these tumors do not infiltrate or cross the pia arachnoid so that on the scan, and at surgery, one will find quite clear superficial edges to the tumor that are formed by the cerebral sulci. The infiltration occurs in the deep white matter beneath the cortex and it is the lack of a clear tumor–brain interface here that makes radical surgical resection difficult and often impossible. Radical resection can be made even more difficult by the fact that, as Skirboll et al.[5] have shown, tumor cells can infiltrate functioning brain, and histological studies have shown that the MRI scanning can underestimate the depth of tumor infiltration into the brain [6].

At surgery, with superficially placed tumors, one typically finds an area of the brain where the cerebral gyri are widened. Sometimes the surface of the abnormal area of the brain is paler and less vascular than that of the surrounding brain; sometimes it is more vascular. On opening the cortex, one usually finds that the white matter is firmer than normal, and sometimes slightly darker. The author will still often find it very difficult, after opening the dura, to know whether he has found the tumor or not. Usually it is fairly easy to be certain that one is in the central core of the tumor; the question of navigation, mapping and perioperative smear histology will be dealt with later. The problems arise, if one is aiming for radical resection, as one approaches the peripheral areas of the tumor, where it becomes impossible to know, by purely surgical appearances, whether the white matter is still infiltrated by tumor or not.

Although low-grade gliomas in adults can occur in any part of the brain, they are distinctly unusual in the posterior fossa, which is clearly in contrast to what is found in children. They can occur in any of the "lobes" of the cerebral hemispheres (which, it should be remembered, are relatively arbitrary anatomical boundaries), or deep in the basal ganglia. A few patterns of growth seem to be characteristic, such as the tumors that grow in the frontal lobe and root of the temporal lobe, so that they present on both sides of the Sylvian fissure.

Management

The typical case of low-grade glioma is of a young adult who has had an epileptic fit, who has no neurological deficit, and in whom a brain scan has shown an intrinsic cerebral tumor without any contrast enhancement. The tumor may be remarkably large or relatively small. It may appear to be relatively well circumscribed, or it may be diffusely infiltrating. It may be very close to eloquent brain, or it may be located in the tip of one of the frontal, temporal or occipital lobes, or deep within the basal ganglia. It can be appreciated at once that there can be no single treatment policy for a tumor type that can be so variable. This variety of forms also explains why the neurosurgical literature is so unsatisfactory on the subject of low-grade gliomas, since few, if any, of the published papers stratify their results in accordance with the varied macroscopic anatomy.

The question that arises with this "typical" patient is whether any treatment should be offered at all, given the lack of evidence that treatment makes any significant difference to overall survival or median time to progression if patients with low-grade gliomas are taken as a whole. The central problem in the management of low-grade gliomas is whether radical or debulking surgery in patients without raised intracranial pressure makes any difference to long term prognosis. In other words, it is simply not known whether the extent of surgical resection has any impact on prognosis or not in these patients. A further problem is that there is no easy way of defining the extent of surgical resection; surgeons talk about "radical" or "subtotal" removal, or "debulking" of these tumors, but have no way of quantifying this. Post-operative MRI scanning clearly helps to some extent, but for the reasons mentioned earlier, these scans can be hard to interpret. Nevertheless, despite this central uncertainty, the neurosurgeon must make a decision on whether to operate or not, and if so, what form the operation should take.

For practical purposes, the management of low-grade gliomas can be divided into five groups. For the purposes of this discussion, "complete" resection is taken to mean "curative" resection, as shown by subsequent, long-term follow-up scanning, whereas "radical" resection only means that initial follow-up scanning shows no residual tumor. The groups are:

- Large tumors in eloquent areas that, on the basis of the pre-operative scan, are too large for extensive resection to be possible without an unacceptably high risk of producing a major post-operative neurological deficit
- Small tumors where, on the basis of the pre-operative scan, complete or radical resection is anticipated with little risk of neurological damage

Tumors where it is uncertain whether complete or radical resection can be achieved
Tumors that recur after treatment
Tumors that cause intractable epilepsy

1. Tumors that are Too Large for Complete Resection to be Possible Without Unacceptable Risk

Complete resection is clearly impossible in patients where the tumor is bilateral, having crossed the corpus callosum, or involves the basal ganglia and insular cortex. Early involvement of the corpus callosum is not, in itself, a complete contraindication to surgery, since it is possible to resect areas of the corpus callosum without major risk. However, the significance of corpus callosum involvement is that in most cases it is associated with bilateral hemispheric infiltration, and one of the fundamental rules of neurosurgery remains that bilateral hemispheric damage is associated with a high risk of major neurological deficit. In a very small proportion of these cases, at the time of presentation, there will be symptoms of raised intracranial pressure. In these cases standard debulking surgery is indicated. Since there is no evidence that debulking surgery prolongs survival in patients without raised intracranial pressure, some authors [7] have argued that there is little justification in carrying out such surgery in the absence of raised pressure. Others have argued, for instance Berger et al. [8], that aggressive debulking surgery delays recurrence when compared with more conservative resection, but no studies have shown any certain benefit in terms of long-term survival. It is an article of faith for some neurosurgeons that debulking surgery, sometimes described more impressively as "cytoreduction", is beneficial, but the fact remains that this is entirely unproven, and any theoretical benefits must also be balanced against the greater morbidity of aggressive surgery. Even with very large tumors several years can pass before raised pressure develops and palliative surgery becomes indicated. Since there is also no evidence [9] that radiotherapy prolongs life in this group of patients, there is little purpose in carrying out a biopsy (stereotactically or otherwise) unless there is doubt about the interpretation of the scan or unless the neurosurgeon's neuro-oncological colleagues strongly favor adjuvant treatment in such cases.

If it has been decided not to treat a patient in this group, and instead to follow up the patient with repeat scans, the tumor will, sooner or later, be shown to be growing larger, probably before the onset of the symptoms of raised intracranial pressure. A more rational approach might be to postpone repeating the scan until such symptoms have developed. However, most patients will wish to be followed up with scans, in the hope that they will not show any progression, and it is very difficult for the surgeon to refuse to organize follow-up scanning. However, once the scan shows progression – albeit asymptomatic – it is very difficult to continue to withhold treatment even though treatment is, by definition, palliative and there are no new symptoms to palliate.

There are two possible options. Firstly, further conservative treatment may be given with the blunt admission to the patient that there is no convincing evidence that treatment will make a significant difference. Secondly, treatment can be recommended in the hope that it will slow down the rate of progression, even though the evidence is lacking that such treatment works. In the author's experience, most patients will favor the latter policy.

Treatment can take the form of surgery and radiotherapy, or debulking surgery alone.

Biopsy will be required with either policy. Biopsy can be either closed or open, depending on the location of the tumor and the surgeon's preference. Different parts of the tumor can show different histological features and there is an argument either for multiple targets, if biopsied stereotactically, or for removing a reasonable volume of tumor if open biopsy is carried out. With large tumors it must be remembered that biopsy without debulking can precipitate post-operative cerebral herniation. Preoperative steroids are essential and, on occasion, debulking surgery, even in the absence of symptoms of raised intracranial pressure, may need to be carried out as part of the biopsy. Treatment can also be confined to debulking surgery, and radiotherapy postponed until there is further evidence of progression, provided that histology shows that the tumor has not undergone malignant change. Once such malignant change has occurred, the tumor should be treated as a high-grade tumor, and palliative adjuvant treatment is then indicated in the great majority of cases.

Illustrative Example: a 28-year-old woman with frequent focal epileptic fits affecting the left arm but no deficit (Fig. 9.3 and 9.4)

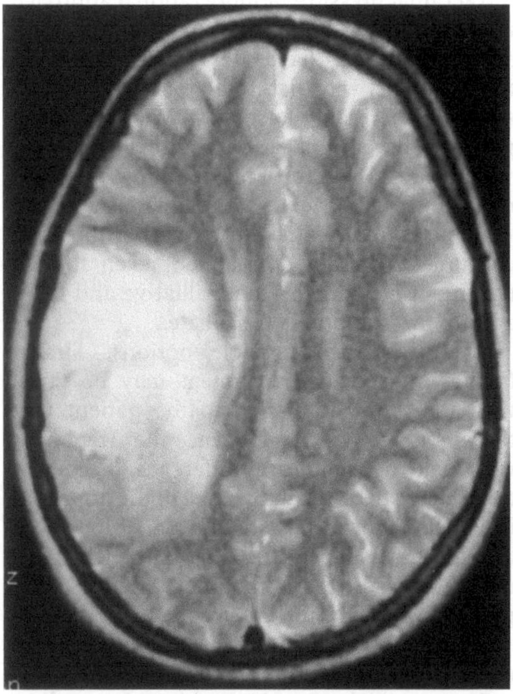

Fig. 9.3. Case CM. Before surgery.

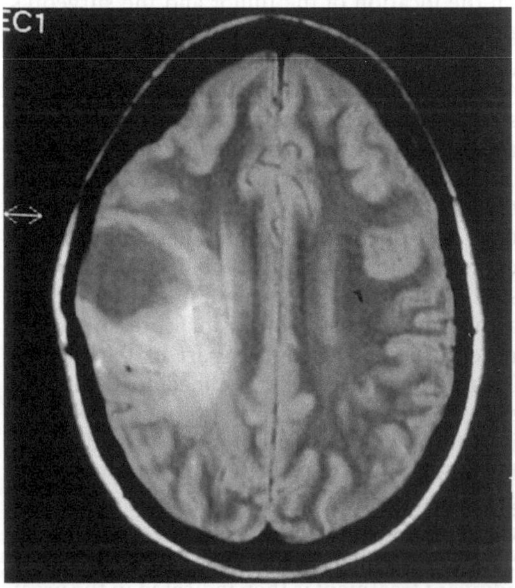

Fig. 9.4. Case CM. After partial resection.

The scan shows an extensive, infiltrating tumor involving both sides of the insular cortex.

A debulking operation under local anesthetic was attempted but abandoned after the patient developed severe weakness of the left arm. This did not get better and the epilepsy remained a major problem. The tumor was shown to be a low-grade astrocytoma. She died 6 years later from tumor progression.

Comment: This operation was carried out before the author's initial enthusiasm for radical surgery for large low-grade gliomas had been tempered by experience. In retrospect, it is easy to see that there was no prospect of obtaining sufficient tumor removal to influence the epilepsy and absolutely no question of "total" excision of the tumor. All that the operation achieved was to add weakness of her left arm to her epileptic fits.

2. Tumours where, on the Basis of the Pre-operative Scan, Complete Resection is Anticipated

These tumors are, unfortunately, in a distinct minority (probably no more than 5%). It is clear to all neurosurgeons that a few small, well-circumscribed, low-grade gliomas can be cured by radical surgery. (The relatively rare pleomorphic xanthoastrocytomas are usually cured by surgery alone but are clearly different from the majority of low-grade tumors.) The question of the suitability of a low-grade glioma for radical surgery is therefore a question of:

- Tumor size and the degree of infiltration of the surrounding brain
- The relationship of the tumor to eloquent structures (in other words, the risk of surgery producing a significant neurological deficit)
- The surgeon's technique and experience.

Illustrative Example: a 35-year-old army officer (Fig. 9.2 and 9.5) with a single epileptic fit

The scan shows a small left inferior temporal tumor, presumed (and ultimately confirmed by surgery) to be a low-grade astrocytoma. An initial neurosurgical opinion advised against surgery on the grounds that it involved some risk of producing dysphasia, and there was no evidence that surgery would make any difference to the 10-year 80% mortality rate.

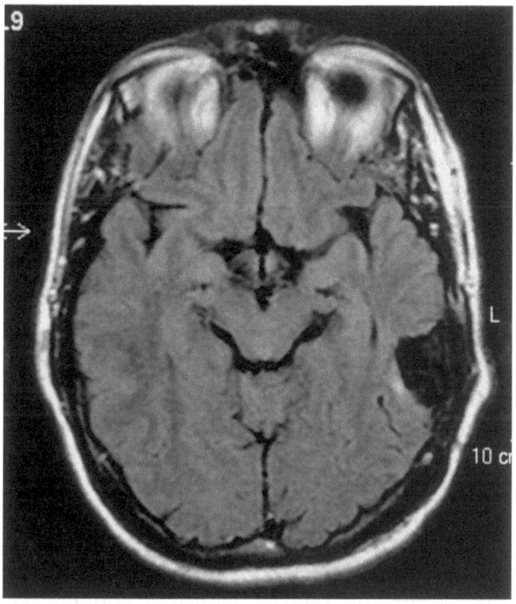

Fig. 9.5. Case MB 9 years after surgery. The small area of high signal on this FLAIR sequence has remained unchanged since surgery and presumably represents gliosis.

Using speech mapping with awake craniotomy and multiple marginal biopsies, what appeared to be complete removal was achieved without producing any neurological deficit. Ten years later, the patient remains free from fits, is off anticonvulsants with no evidence of recurrence on follow-up scanning, and is on active service in the army.

Comment: If the patient had not been operated upon and had been judged to have an effectively "inoperable brain tumor", he would have lost his job as well as remaining at risk of the tumor progressing. He would also have had the psychological burden of "living with" the tumor. Modern techniques have made resection reasonably safe although, from a single case such as this, one cannot know whether surgery has improved his chances of survival or not when compared with conservative treatment.

3. Tumors where it is Uncertain Whether Complete Resection can be Achieved

It is easy to justify an attempt at radical, curative resection of a small tumor, superficially placed in the tip of a lobe, without MRI evidence of extensive infiltration. The risks of such an operation are the risks of any craniotomy – that is, the risks of hemorrhage or infection – and these risks are almost certainly less than the risks of the tumor undergoing malignant change and proving fatal in the future. It can become a question of fine surgical judgement as to the point at which it becomes unrealistic to hope for total resection.

Radical resection depends upon:

- Careful study of a pre-operative MRI scan, supplemented by functional MRI studies and neuronavigation if appropriate and available;
- The use of intraoperative mapping methods combined with smear biopsy analysis (if the surgeon is lucky enough to work with a neuropathologist who is able to carry out smear analysis on many dozens of marginal biopsies as the resection proceeds). In a few centers, intraoperative MRI scanning is now available, but it is not yet clear if this makes a major difference to the surgery of these tumors.

Two principles must guide selection of patients for radical surgery of this sort. Firstly, there must be a realistic chance of "total" excision of the tumor. It will often not prove possible during the operation to achieve such a removal, but there must be a reasonable possibility of achieving this on the basis of examining the pre-operative MRI scan. Secondly, it is not acceptable to produce any degree of permanent neurological impairment since all of these patients are, by definition, in perfect condition and we know that the majority of them will eventually die from the tumor, despite treatment. That having been said, of course, there is bound to be some morbidity, although often temporary, especially when operating in the supplementary motor area. In the author's series of 130 "radical" operations for low-grade gliomas, there has been a 7% incidence of significant, permanent morbidity (although no mortality) and all in patients who ended up having only partial excision of their tumor. The morbidity, in short, probably conferred little benefit on the patients in terms of eventual outcome. Temporary neurological deficits, which resolved completely, occurred in 20% of patients.

By using neuronavigation, magnification, intraoperative mapping under local anesthetic

[9] and intraoperative histology, there can be no doubt that more low-grade gliomas are now suitable for an attempt at surgical cure than in the past. As discussed earlier, most of these tumors do not cross the pia arachnoid and hence are often well demarcated on the surface of the brain. The typical appearance of such a tumor is of an area of expanded, abnormally pale gyri, bounded by sulci. This superficial area can be identified in most cases by the experienced surgeon by eye alone, but others will find neuronavigation helpful. The area that is directly infiltrated is unlikely to be functional, but if eloquent speech or motor cortex is nearby, they should be identified by cortical mapping. The tumor can cause considerable distortion of the surrounding normal gyri, and the conventional anatomical and radiological landmarks for cortical localization no longer apply. In some cases it can be surprisingly difficult to know whether the tumor is in front of, or behind, the central sulcus. If tumors do not present on the cerebral surface, there can be considerable difficulties in finding them without navigation or ultrasound, but since they are more probably in the deep white matter, it is also less likely that they are suitable for an attempt at radical resection.

The reason why most low-grade gliomas are not curable by surgery is because they invade the deep white matter. It is impossible to establish any kind of surgical plane here. The marginal infiltrated areas of the brain adjacent to the central bulk of the tumor will look and feel no different from normal brain to the surgeon. Once one is operating in the deep white matter, there is also the risk of causing extensive neurological deficits from both undercutting the adjacent cerebral cortex and disrupting the association tracts. Neuronavigation will not help in the deep white matter as a result of both brain shift and distortion produced by surgery and the fact that MRI scanning often does not define the true boundaries of the tumor. The surgeon can only be guided by smear marginal biopsies (in some cases the author has sent more than 60 such biopsies during an operation) and by the patients themselves, who will need to be kept awake so that if any relatively deep resection is being carried out and a developing neurological deficit is identified early during resection, any further resection can then be abandoned.

Awake craniotomy allows the surgeon to operate with greater confidence close to eloquent areas of the brain, but "complete" removal of these tumors will often remain impossible. One difficulty with the awake-craniotomy technique is that patients can develop a degree of neurological deficit while the resection proceeds, which subsequently recovers. It can be a question of fine judgement as to when to abandon further resection as a deficit develops. It is only possible to carry out simple neurological testing during awake craniotomy – in particular of limb movements and speech, and sometimes of the visual fields. It is not possible to assess more subtle cognitive functions, but the patient's general alertness and responsiveness can serve as a guide to these to some extent. It is most important that the awake craniotomy is supervised by an anesthetist with experience in this area [9]. In skilled anesthetic hands it is remarkable how relaxed, pain free, cooperative and alert patients can be, despite being subjected to a very extensive craniotomy.

Illustrative Example: a 26-year-old woman with a single generalized epileptic fit (Figs. 9.6, 9.7, 9.8)

The scan shows a large tumor arising in the region of the right primary sensory cortex. This was judged to be potentially resectable. Histology showed the tumor to be an oligodendroglioma, and she remains free from fits and without neurological deficit. Follow-up scanning shows persistent abnormality in the brain adjacent to the resection cavity. The abnormality has become a little smaller over time but it must remain likely that there is residual tumor here.

Comment: The very long natural history of oligodendrogliomas must be remembered when dealing with cases such as this. The author remains undecided as to what to recommend if further follow-up scans suggest tumor recurrence.

4. Tumours that Recur

The interpretation of post-operative scans can be very difficult. Flair MRI sequences are much more sensitive to both post-operative changes and recurrent tumor than are other sequences. Areas of signal change in the brain adjacent to the resection cavity may represent post-operative inflammatory effects or tumor

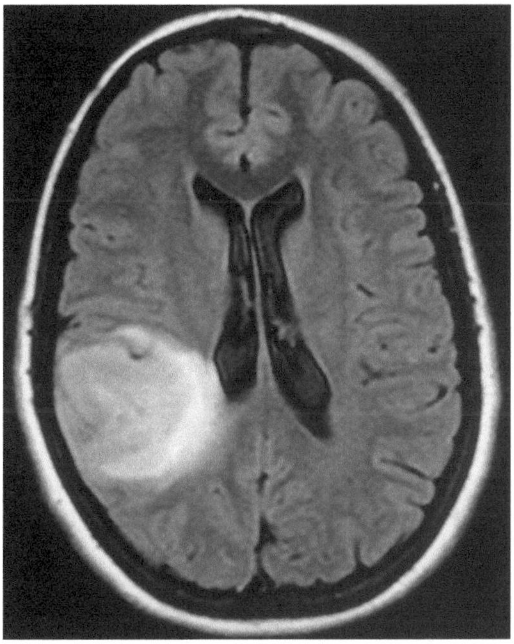

Fig. 9.6. Case LC before surgery.

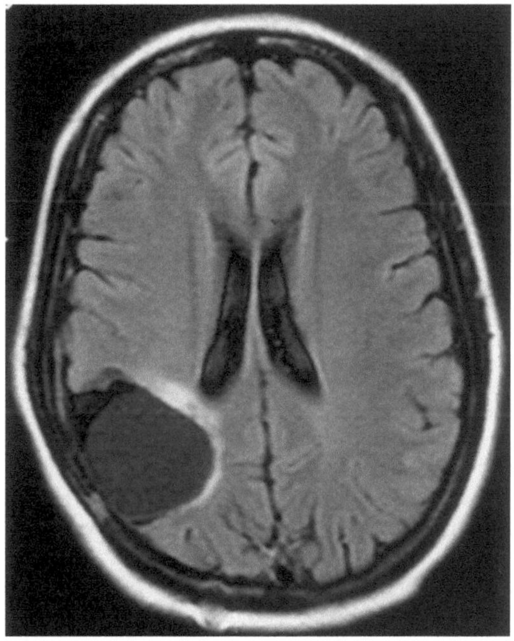

Fig. 9.8. Case LC three years after surgery.

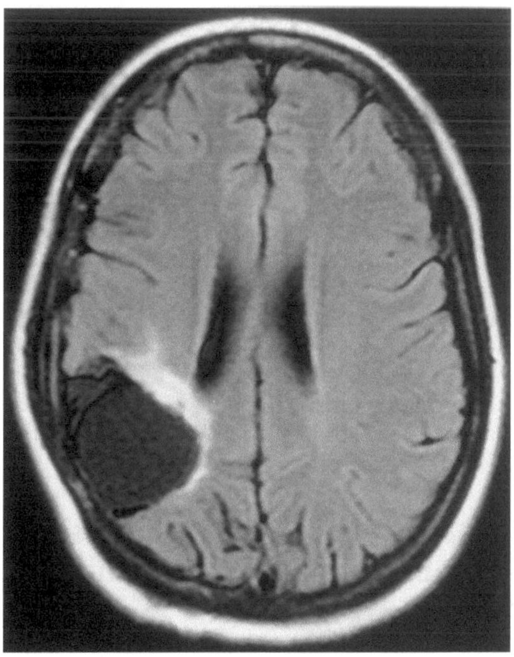

Fig. 9.7. Case LC 1 year after surgery.

recurrence. New contrast enhancement after surgery may reflect malignant change or simply post-operative effects. If there is any doubt, as there often is, about the interpretation, it is best to repeat the scan after a few months. Changes due to recurrent tumor will obviously tend to become more pronounced with time, and post-operative effects less pronounced. As with routine follow-up scanning of large, inoperable tumors, routine follow-up scanning of patients who have undergone what appeared to be "complete" resection will often cause great difficulties for the neurosurgeon and his or her patient when such scans show what is probably residual or recurrent tumor, which is not causing any symptoms.

In some patients it will be clear that the tumor has undergone malignant transformation and treatment is now as for a malignant glioma. Depending on the time interval since initial treatment and the extent of recurrence, further surgery may be indicated as well as adjuvant treatment. If the scans suggest malignant change, biopsy can be required to confirm this if adjuvant treatment is to be considered. If the follow-up scans show only slight progressive change over a number of years, it is reasonable to do nothing, although if the area of recurrence is well circumscribed and not very deep or eloquent, "second-look" surgery can be considered.

The question of how to treat possible or definite recurrence of low-grade gliomas is usually very difficult for both surgeon and patient. As mentioned above, it is most important that decisions about how to manage these cases are made jointly by neurosurgeons and neuro-oncologists working together.

5. Tumors that Cause Intractable Epilepsy

Provided that EEG studies have confirmed the tumor seen on the scan to be the epileptic focus, and provided that complete or near-complete resection of the tumor looks feasible, many patients can expect a significant improvement, with actual cure in some cases, of their epilepsy with surgery. The question of what constitutes "intractable" epilepsy can be difficult, as can the question of whether there are epileptic foci distant from the tumor. Simple, superficial tumors causing epilepsy can be dealt with on their merits, but other cases are probably best managed by surgeons with a particular interest in epilepsy, and are beyond the scope of this chapter.

The Role of Radiotherapy and Chemotherapy

In the past, radiotherapy was used more widely for low-grade tumors than is currently the case. The EORTC controlled trial of adjuvant radiotherapy [10] showed no difference in survival between patients treated with surgery and patients treated with both surgery and postoperative radiotherapy. Whereas there is general agreement that radiotherapy should be used in patients whose tumor has undergone malignant change, its use in patients with low-grade tumors remains controversial. The long-term morbidity of radiotherapy remains a major concern in these patients, especially in view of the fact that so many of them, unlike patients with high-grade tumors, live for many years after treatment, and the known fact that the adverse effects of radiation increase over time. Cognitive impairment can be quite easily missed if not specifically looked for, or mistakenly attributed to the effects of the tumor itself. On the basis of what has been published to date, it is impossible to quantify the nature or degree of these possible long-term adverse effects. In the short term, radiotherapy is well tolerated. Suffice it to say that, given the absence of any good evidence that radiotherapy improves survival in these cases, the author and his neuro-oncological colleagues do not routinely use radiotherapy in asymptomatic patients with low-grade gliomas.

Chemotherapy remains of uncertain value for low-grade astrocytomas that have not undergone anaplastic change. There is no clear evidence of efficacy in the literature and it is not widely used. With oligodendrogliomas [11,12], especially those with anaplastic change, there is an increasing body of evidence that chemotherapy has a role to play. At the present time, opinions vary as to whether it should be considered as first-line or second-line treatment for such tumors.

Management of Oligodendrogliomas

The natural history of low-grade oligodendrogliomas appears to be considerably more indolent than that of astrocytomas, with a median overall survival time reported in one recent series [13] of 16.3 years. The question of whether to offer treatment to asymptomatic patients is therefore all the more important. In the patients reported by Olson et al., 36% of patients who had been treated with radiotherapy developed dementia, 20% treated with chemotherapy suffered toxicity, and 6% of those undergoing surgery suffered permanent neurological impairment. There is little reason to doubt that results in other centres will be similar. It seems reasonable to conclude that treatment should be postponed in these patients, unless the tumour appears amenable to complete and reasonably safe surgical resection, until tumour progression has been documented. Furthermore, there is little, if any, evidence that postponing treatment in this way has an adverse effect on outcome.

Management of Gangliogliomas, Neurocytomas and Pleomorphic Xanthoastrocytomas

These rare tumors tend to have distinctive radiological appearances [14]. Complete resection and surgical cure is more often possible in these tumors than in the other gliomas, although recurrence can occur and the patients should be followed with regular scanning.

Conclusions

Deciding on whether to operate on patients with low-grade gliomas is a particularly difficult area of neurosurgery although, from the purely technical point of view, the surgery itself is often relatively straightforward. It is easy to conclude that small, easily accessible tumors should be removed and that large, infiltrating tumors are best left alone unless they are causing raised intracranial pressure. The problems arise with the great majority of patients whose tumors fall between these two extremes. Using modern neurosurgical techniques, there can be no doubt that more tumors can now be totally excised than was the case in the past. Such patients, however, remain in a small minority. The majority of patients have tumors where there is little prospect of total removal and where is no clear evidence that partial removal improves outcome. It can be very difficult for both the surgeon and the patient to accept that nothing is to be done. Careful and sympathetic explanation is essential whatever treatment is recommended. If surgery is to be undertaken in those cases where total resection is clearly not going to be achieved, it is essential that surgical morbidity should be extremely low. On the other hand, the operation will become a meaningless charade if the morbidity is kept low by merely carrying out a limited biopsy, if it is already known from the pre-operative scan appearances that adjuvant treatment will not be recommended. There is no science in making decisions of this kind: instead the neurosurgeon must be guided by his experience (and, if necessary, by the greater experience of surgical colleagues), by discussion with his oncological colleagues and, above all, by honest and open discussion with the patients and their families.

Finally, it must be stressed that the neurosurgeon's responsibility to his patient does not end once an operation has been carried out, or if a decision has been made to defer treatment of a low-grade tumor, or if a tumor has been deemed inoperable. It is tempting for the surgeon to try to avoid the immense stress and anxiety that many people suffer when a diagnosis of this kind has been made, especially when they will have to live with the knowledge of the tumor, and the patient's probably impending death, for many years. Careful and sympathetic follow-up and explanation will often be just as important as the surgical or oncological treatment in determining the quality of the patient's life.

Key Points

- *There are many varieties of low-grade glioma and few generalizations can be made as to how they are best treated other than that most patients will die of the disease within 10 years of diagnosis, whatever the treatment undertaken.*
- *There is no clear, trial-based evidence that can be used in deciding upon treatment and it is not known whether partial removal of tumors has any significant impact on prognosis.*
- *Small, well-circumscribed tumors can probably be cured by surgical resection, but this only applies to a minority of cases.*
- *Modern microscopic techniques, combined with intraoperative histology and cortical mapping under local anesthetic, increase the number of cases where curative resection is a possibility.*
- *Most patients present with epilepsy and will remain without any significant neurological deficit for several years before they eventually deteriorate. The risks of treatment, and its uncertain benefit in many cases, must be carefully balanced against the relatively benign short-term natural history.*

References

1. Laws E, Taylor W, Clifton M, Okazaki H. Neurosurgical management of low-grade astrocytoma of the cerebral hemispheres. J Neurosurg 1984;61:665–73.
2. Bigner D, McLendon R, Bruner J. Russell and Rubinstein's pathology of tumors of the nervous system, 6th edn. London: Arnold, 1998.
3. Morantz R. Low grade astrocytomas. In: Kaye A, Laws E, editors. Brain tumours. Edinburgh: Churchill Livingstone, 1995;433–48.
4. Kondziolka D, Lunsford LD, Martinez AJ. Unreliability of contemporary neurodiagnostic imaging in evaluating

suspected adult supratentorial (low-grade) astrocytoma. J Neurosurg 1993;79:533–6.
5. Skirboll S, Ojeman G, Berger M, Lettich E, Winn H. Functional cortex and subcortical white matter located within gliomas. Neurosurgery 1996;38:678–85.
6. Lunsford LD, Martinez AJ, Latchaw RE. Magnetic resonance imaging does not define tumor boundaries. Acta Radiol Suppl 1986;369:154–6.
7. Recht L, Lew R, Smith TW. Suspected low-grade glioma: is deferring treatment safe? Ann Neurol 1992;31: 431–6.
8. Berger M, Deliganis B, Dobbins J, Keles G. The effect of extent of resection on recurrence in patients with low grade cerebral hemisphere gliomas. Cancer 1994;74: 1784–91.
9. Sarang A, Dinsmore J. Anaesthesia for awake craniotomy. Evolution of a technique that facilitates neurological testing. Br J Anaesth 2003;90:161–5.
10. Karim AB, Cornu P, Bleehen N et al. Immediate postoperative radiotherapy in low grade glioma improves progression free survival, but not overall survival: preliminary results of an EORTC/MRC randomised phase III study (abstract). Proc Am Soc Clin Oncol 1998;17:400a.
11. Cairncross G, Macdonald D, Ludwin S et al. Chemotherapy for anaplastic oligodendroglioma. J Clin Oncol 1994;12(10):2013–21.
12. Paleologos NA, G CJ. Treatment of oligodendroglioma: an update. Neuro-oncology 1999;1(1):61–8.
13. Olson JD, Riedel E, DeAngelis LM. Long-term outcome of low-grade oligodendroglioma and mixed glioma. Neurology 2000;54:1442–8.
14. Sanders WP,Christoforidis GA. Imaging of low-grade primary brain tumors. In: Rock JP et al., editors. The practical management of low grade primary brain tumours.1999.

10

Neurosurgical Management of High-grade Gliomas

Robert C. Rostomily, Alexander M. Spence
and Daniel L. Silbergeld

Summary

High-grade gliomas include malignant variants of tumors derived from astrocytic and oligodendropheral cell lines. These tumors demonstrate invasive behavior, are rapidly growing and are usually characterized by contrast enhancement and edema on MR or CT neuroimaging. Management includes either biopsy or surgical resection followed by radiotherapy in the majority of cases. Additional adjuvant chemotherapy is also a treatment consideration. Despite advances in management, the prognosis remains poor, with few patients surviving beyond 2–3 years.

Introduction

The term "high-grade glioma" (HGG) refers to a histopathologically defined group of clinically aggressive glial neoplasms, which includes: glioblastoma multiforme (GBM), anaplastic astrocytoma (AA), anaplastic oligodendroglioma (AO), anaplastic oligoastrocytoma or "mixed" glioma, gliosarcoma and, possibly, the gemistocytic astrocytoma (GA). High-grade gliomas are the most common primary cerebral neoplasms in adults, with GBM and AA comprising the vast majority of these neoplasms. HGGs share common hallmarks of varying degrees of glial cell differentiation, an extremely poor prognosis for survival beyond 2–3 years, and a diffuse invasive growth pattern into surrounding brain. The designation HGG distinguishes these aggressive gliomas from their "low-grade" glioma (LGG) counterparts that confer median survival times of 6–10 years. Despite their similarities, the HGGs are biologically heterogeneous and differ significantly in their features of differentiation, presumed histogenesis, treatment responses and prognosis. This heterogeneity must be appreciated when considering management options for a particular patient with a HGG and in the interpretation of clinical trials.

Over the last 25 years, despite a plethora of novel treatment approaches, the prognosis for patients with HGGs has not significantly improved. Limitations imposed by tumor location, intrinsic biological features, and tumor growth patterns complicate the effective management of HGGs. It is now well recognized that HGG is a diffuse disease. While an extensive amount of research has recently targeted the study of HGG cell migration and invasion, we have yet to solve the clinical problem of loco-regional control of HGGs. Ultimately, significant improvement in outcome for HGG patients will require effective loco-regional tumor control, while cure will require novel strategies to address the diffuse invasive component of the tumor. The role of the neurosurgeon in the multidisciplinary management of HGG patients is continually evolving from simply providing tumor resection, to the design and delivery of intratumoral therapy, and adapting new technologies to improve surgical resection. This changing role underscores the need for neurosurgeons managing HGG patients to be versed not only in the technical aspects of HGG surgery but also in the biological principles that underlie these emerging treatments. This chapter reviews surgical management, patient selection and basic biological features of HGG relevant to its surgical management.

Epidemiology

The overall incidence of HGGs in the USA is estimated at about 5/100,000 person-years, with approximately 13,000 new cases per year and 10,000 deaths. There is a direct correlation between age and higher tumor grade or aggressiveness, as well as mortality. Modest 2–4% increases in incidence have been shown in the last 10–20 years, with minimal improvements in 2-year GBM survival from 3 to 6% [1]. The relative incidence of the histological subtypes of HGG is difficult to determine accurately because rare entities such as gliosarcoma (GS) are either not reported separately or, in the case of more controversial diagnostic entities such as anaplastic oligoastrocytoma (AOA), are not uniformly diagnosed and reported. Nevertheless, the Central Brain Tumor Registry of the USA (CBTRUS) database (HYPERLINK http://www.cbtrus.org) reports the incidence of GBM as 2.96/100,000 person-years, anaplastic astrocytoma (AA) as 0.49/100,000 person-years, anaplastic oligodendroglioma (AO) as 0.10/100,000 person-years, and malignant glioma NOS (not otherwise specified) as 0.35/100,000 person-years. Thus, in this database, GBM accounted for 76% of HGGs while AA and AO accounted for 13% and 2.6% of HGGs, respectively.

Histogenesis and Histopathology

The precise histogenesis, or cell of origin, for adult HGGs is not known. Current paradigms invoke either the transformation of resident adult neural stem or glial progenitor cells or the de-differentiation of mature glial cells. The classification and grading of HGG is controversial and has undergone a number of modifications in the last few decades. The World Health Organization (WHO) classification system is currently the most widely used system and was born from an effort to provide a consensus for classifying and grading nervous system tumors [2]. In this chapter, we collectively refer to HGGs as those glial neoplasms that correspond to WHO grade III tumors, including AA, AO, AOA, and grade IV tumors, including GBM, giant-cell GBM, and GS. Of note, the gemistocytic astrocytoma is classified as a grade II tumor in the WHO classification; however, this tumor type has been associated with a more aggressive clinical course that is similar to grade III tumors, and thus these neoplasms are often also considered in the discussion of HGGs.

Molecular Pathogenesis

Patterns of molecular genetic abnormalities have been associated with specific types of HGGs [3] (Fig. 10.1). The high frequency of genetic alterations that inactivate p53 and augment EGFR (epidermal growth factor receptor) activity and its downstream pathways, and their presence in the most common forms of HGG, have led to innovative therapeutic strategies that target these molecules and in some cases directly involve the neurosurgeon. These molecular genetic changes are presumed to underlie gliomagenesis and/or progression to HGG and have been most rigorously studied in glioblastoma. Secondary GBMs arise predominantly in younger patients from pre-existing lower grade tumors, while primary GBMs more commonly occur in older patients and are presumed to arise de novo from a target cell of origin. The former are more likely to have mutations that inactivate p53 function, while the latter typically have overactivation of EGFR-mediated pathways through various mechanisms such as gene amplification or mutation. In GBM, this latter abnormality is often due to the expression of a truncated, and constitutively activated, EGFR called "EGFRvIII", which is being investigated as a target for immunotherapy. In contrast, the molecular genetic changes that lead to the

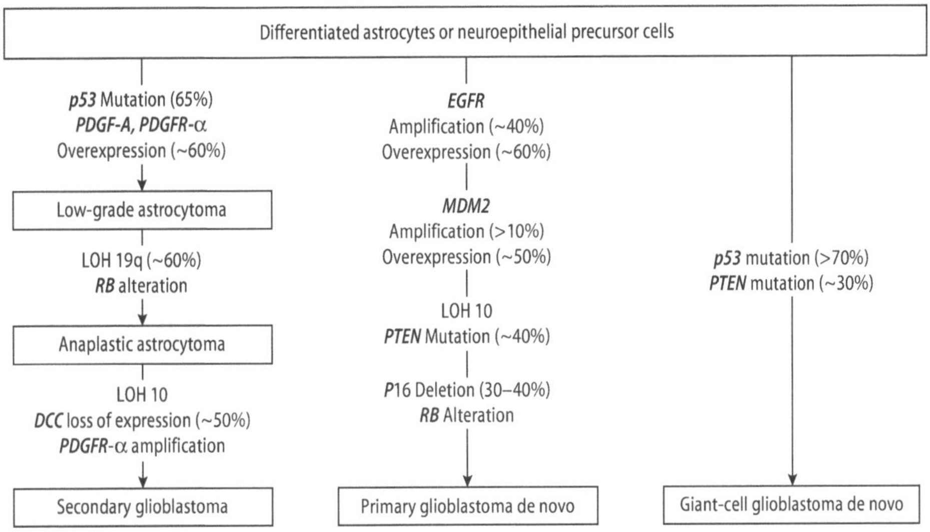

Fig. 10.1. Summary of distinct patterns of molecular genetic changes seen in HGGs that are associated with GBMs arising from lower grade lesions (secondary GBM) vs those arising de novo (primary GBM). Several of the molecular abnormalities noted in this figure have been used as targets for therapy that are delivered intraoperatively by the neurosurgeon (see text). (Courtesy of Kleihues et al. [3].)

formation of AO and AOA are not as well characterized as those that lead to the formation of AA and GBM. The recent description of allelic losses on chromosomes 19q and 1p in most low-grade oligodendrogliomas points to potential early events in their genesis, but candidate tumor suppressors for these loci have not been identified. In a subset of cases, the subsequent molecular changes associated with malignant progression to AO include allelic loss of 9p or homozygous deletion of the cell cycle inhibitor CDKN2A (p16INK4A) gene [4].

HGG Biology

The unique biology of HGGs underlies their dismal prognosis and directly impacts the effectiveness and role of surgery in their management. Those aspects of HGG biology that impact surgical management, or provide targets for therapeutic intervention that potentially involve the neurosurgeon, are reviewed below.

HGG Growth Patterns

HGGs can be modeled as containing distinct anatomical compartments: a central or bulk portion of tumor, which often contains a zone of central necrosis surrounded by regions of solid tumor, and a surrounding zone of infiltrating tumor with isolated migratory tumor cells. These compartments roughly correspond to areas of decreased signal on T1 images (necrosis), gadolinium enhancement (central or bulk tumor) and increased edema-associated T2 signal (infiltrative tumor cells) on MR images (Fig. 10.2). The central regions contribute to mass effect, generally take up intravenous contrast agents, and contain areas of both active metabolism and hypoxic zones that contribute to treatment resistance. The uptake of contrast agents indicates a disruption of the normal blood–brain barrier (BBB) in this tumor region, which is essential for the delivery of effective doses of most systemic chemotherapeutic agents. Although HGG is a diffuse disease process (see discussion below), approximately 80% of HGG tumor recurrences are detected within 2–3 cm of the original resection cavity [5, 6], and only with intense local therapy such as high-activity radiation implants have significant percentages of recurrences been reported outside this zone (45% in one study). Adding to these local problems of tumor control for HGGs is a poorly defined zone that encompasses bulk

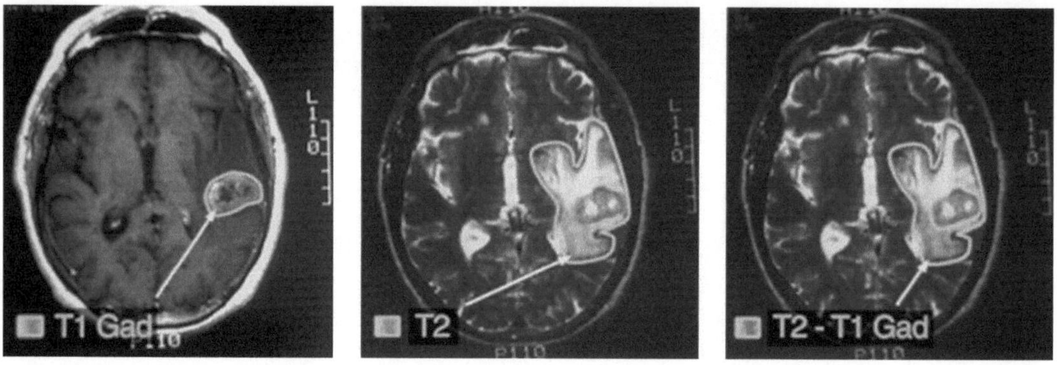

Fig. 10.2. An MR image of a glioblastoma demonstrating the different components of HGGs with central necrosis, surrounding solid tumor delineated by contrast-enhancing tissue and peripheral edema indicating a zone where infiltrative tumor cells reside. Gad, gadolinium.

tumor and is composed of infiltrative and diffuse tumor cells that reside amongst histologically normal brain where the BBB remains intact.

In 1938, Scherer carefully documented the diffusely invasive growth pattern of HGGs and correctly predicted that this biological property of HGGs would limit the ability to surgically cure these tumors [7]. Further confirmation of these studies came with the advent of CT and MR imaging. Histological analysis of stereotactic biopsies taken from radiographically defined regions of HGGs consistently demonstrates the presence of tumor cells beyond areas of contrast enhancement, with infiltration of tumor tissue and/or isolated tumor cells throughout areas of CT hypodensity and prolonged T2 signal on MR images. In a study by Kelly et al., only 18 out of 186 biopsy samples from regions of prolonged T2 signal had no evidence of isolated tumor cells or tissue [8]. Furthermore, isolated tumor cells can be detected histologically or cultured from HGG biopsy samples that are obtained from regions of radiographically *normal* brain [9].

Aside from limiting the ability to effectively resect HGGs, this invasive and diffuse growth pattern likely underlies the demonstration of functional cortex in areas of brain that are infiltrated or grossly involved by tumor [10]. In addition, the presence of an intact BBB in this region limits the ability to deliver many therapeutic agents that rely on its breakdown to achieve cytotoxic doses. While neurosurgical management is generally focused on maximal resection of the central region of necrosis and solid or bulk tumor that contributes primarily to mass effect, emerging treatment modalities that address the invasive tumor component may require neurosurgical expertise as well (see below).

Tumor Cell Invasiveness and Migration

As we achieve better local tumor control, effective therapy for HGGs will ultimately require treatment strategies to address the diffusely infiltrative component of HGGs. Accordingly, intense investigation has recently focused on the cellular and molecular biological characteristics underlying glioma tumor cell migration and invasion. Glioma tumor cell migration and invasion involve the coordination of various cellular processes, which include tumor cell adhesion to specific substrate(s), motility and protease-mediated degradation of extracellular matrix (ECM). Not surprisingly, important roles in this process have been attributed to: proteins that enhance motility (motogens), ECM components and adhesion molecules that provide anchors or permissive substrates for migration, cytoskeletal elements that provide the structural elements for locomotion, and proteases and their regulators that degrade non-permissive elements of the ECM and thus facilitate cellular migration.

Treatment strategies intended to limit tumor cell migration and invasion include agents such as marimistat, which inhibit matrix metalloproteases elaborated by tumor cells that facilitate tumor cell migration by digesting ECM components. Another therapy has used injection of I-131-labeled antibodies into resection cavities after surgery to target the ECM protein tenascin, which is unique to the ECM of HGGs but not normal brain, and appears to promote proliferation and angiogenesis as well as tumor cell migration. Other treatments specifically targeting invasion that require neurosurgical intervention are likely to emerge in the future, such as the use of genetically engineered neural stem cells, which, in animal models, appear to "track down" isolated invasive tumor cells and facilitate localized conversion of prodrugs into cytotoxic compounds [11].

Treatment Resistance

Treatment resistance, a major contributing factor to the dismal prognosis for patients with HGGs, is the result of multiple mechanisms that include, among others, inactivation of drugs, molecular mechanisms of resistance to DNA damage and apoptosis, and attenuation of cytotoxicity imposed by the microenvironment (e.g. hypoxia). Add to these mechanisms the limitations to delivery of therapy imposed by the diffusely invasive growth pattern of HGG tumor cells into brain regions with an intact BBB, and one can begin to understand the daunting problem of designing effective therapies. Through aggressive cytoreduction, the neurosurgeon helps to eliminate a large portion of hypoxic tissue, but the precise impact of cytoreduction on reducing resistance and improving efficacy in adjuvant treatment of residual disease is not known. Targeting one specific mechanism of resistance is unlikely to confer an appreciable improvement in tumor response and the neurosurgeon is likely to be called upon in the future to assist in delivering novel therapies aimed at overcoming multiple mechanisms of treatment resistance.

Prognostic Factors

The prognosis of different subgroups of HGG patients is important to consider when selecting patients for surgery and resection versus biopsy. Prognostic factors are most often determined for overall patient survival, yet the length of an acceptable quality of life is ultimately the most relevant end-point. However, the paucity of prognostic data that specifically analyze quality-of-life issues precludes their general usefulness, and the ensuing discussion will focus on data related primarily to overall survival alone.

Recursive Partition Analysis

Many studies have adopted the Radiation Therapy Oncology Group's prognostic stratification of HGG patients based on a recursive partitioning statistical analysis (RPA) of large numbers of patients enrolled into clinical trials [12]. Tables 10.1 and 10.2 outline these prognostic classes and the median survival for each

Table 10.1. RTOG malignant glioma RPA class definitions (courtesy of Curan et al. [12])

Class	Definition
I	Age <50 years, anaplastic astrocytoma, and normal mental status
II	Age ≥ 50, KPS 70–100, anaplastic astrocytoma, and at least 3 months from time of first symptoms to start of treatment
III	Age <50 years, anaplastic astrocytoma and abnormal mental status
	Age <50 years, glioblastoma multiforme and KPS 90–100
IV	Age <50 years, glioblastoma multiforme and KPS <90
	Age ≥50 years, KPS 70–100, anaplastic astrocytoma, and 3 months or less from time of first symptoms to start of treatment
	Age >50 years, glioblastoma multiforme, surgical resection and good neurological function
V	Age ≥50 years, KPS 70–100, glioblastoma multiforme, either surgical resection and neurological function that inhibits the ability to work, or biopsy only followed by at least 54.4 Gγ of RT
	Age ≥50 years, KPS <70, normal mental status
VI	Age ≥50 years, KPS <70, abnormal mental status
	Age ≥50 years, KPS 70–100, glioblastoma multiforme, biopsy only, receiving less than 54.4 Gγ or radiation therapy

RPA, recursive partition analysis; RTOG, Radiation Therapy Oncology Group; KPS, Kamowski Performance Status

Table 10.2. Survival for HGGs by RTOG RPA (courtesy of Curan et al. [12])

RPA class	Median survival (months)	2-year survival (%)
I	58.6	76
II	37.4	68
III	17.9	35
IV	11.1	15
V	8.9	6
VI	4.6	4

RPA, recursive partition analysis; RTOG, Radiation Therapy Oncology Group

RPA class, respectively. These studies confirmed prognostic factors found in most other studies, including age, Karnofsky performance status (KPS), histological grade, mental status, length and/or presence of neurological symptoms, surgical resection and adequate radiation. The predictors of outcome at the time of HGG recurrence have been evaluated in a large review of 375 patients enrolled on phase II treatment trials, which reported median survival for all recurrent HGGs of 30 weeks, with overall survival rates at 1 year of 47% and 21%, for AA and GBM patients respectively [13]. This study confirmed the prognostic significance of histology (AA vs GBM), KPS and prior intensive therapy, which were found in other previous studies [14]. The appropriate choice of surgical candidates and the aggressiveness of resection for primary and recurrent HGGs, discussed below, must account for these histological and clinical characteristics that dominate clinical outcome.

Tumor Variables

Of all the tumor-related variables that have been analyzed for their prognostic significance, the histopathological grade, which integrates various specific histological features such as mitotic activity and anaplasia, shows the most profound influence on outcome. Other tumor variables, including tumor volume and location, molecular genetic alterations, gene expression patterns, and proliferation and apoptotic indices do not consistently show such an association with outcome. For example, while aberrant p53 function clearly plays an important role in gliomagenesis and malignant progression, the mutational status of p53 has not been convincingly shown to independently predict prognosis. Similarly, indices of tumor proliferation or cell death (apoptosis) alone have not been shown to predict outcome consistently for patients with HGG. However, in a few studies attempting to estimate net cell production, apoptotic/proliferative ratios have shown predictive significance for outcome. Currently, the only example of a molecular genetic abnormality that has been consistently shown to correlate with survival and treatment response is the predictive value of 1p and 19q deletions for anaplastic oligodendroglioma, which, in the most favorable group, showed median survivals from diagnosis of greater than 123 months compared with 16 months for the least favorable group that lacked the 1p deletion (Fig. 10.3) [15]. It is likely that more general variables such as tumor grade and clinical status are better prognostic indicators than are individual tumor features, since they represent the biological summation of individual tumor and molecular variables. However, larger controlled studies may achieve statistical power to identify specific molecular features or profiles that reliably predict patient outcomes or even treatment response.

Treatment Variables

Radiation

Radiation therapy following biopsy or resection for HGGs is the most effective adjuvant treatment modality available. It is generally administered in 180 cGy fractions to a total dose of around 60 Gy when treating the bulk tumor plus a margin that encompasses the area of increased T2 signal. In a randomized trial of anaplastic glioma patients, the overall survival of patients treated with "best conventional care", BCNU alone, radiation alone, and radiation plus BCNU was 17 weeks, 18.5 weeks, 37.5 weeks and 40.5 weeks, respectively [16]. This beneficial effect of radiation on survival applies to other HGGs and GBM as well. The efficacy of radiation has been further validated for HGG by the demonstration of a dose–response relationship. Accordingly, external beam irradiation has become standard therapy for HGG patients after biopsy or resection. In addition, an objective radiographic response to radiation is also an independent predictor of prolonged overall survival for patients with GBM. Thus, the uniformity and adequacy of radiation treatment must

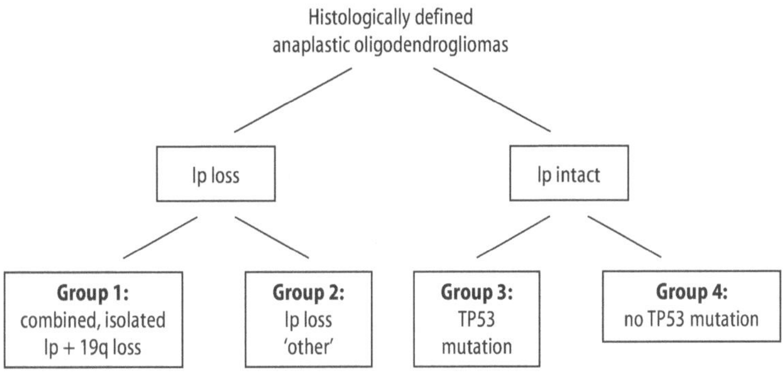

	Group 1	Group 2	Group 3	Group 4
Number of patients	23	5	8	13
Age	43	51	30	52
Response rate	17/17 (100%)	4/4 (100%	2/6 (33%)	2/11 (18%)
Duration response	>31 months	11 months	7 months	5 months
Survival from *dx*	>123 months	71 months	71 months	16 months

Fig. 10.3. Grouping of patients with anaplastic oligodendroglioma by molecular genetic profiles defines specific prognostic groups. Group 2 includes patients with 1p loss and either no 19q loss or "other" molecular genetic changes, including TP53 mutation, PTEN mutation, 10q loss, EGFR amplification or CDKN2A deletion. Group 4 patients have mutations including PTEN, 10q loss, EGFR amplification, CDKN2A deletion, or ring enhancement on CT. (Courtesy of Ino et al. [15]).

be determined when considering the prognostic impact of other treatment variables on outcome for HGGs.

Chemotherapy

A multitude of cytotoxic and cytostatic chemotherapeutic regimens have been used for the treatment of HGGs and, with the exception of PCV therapy (procarbazine, CCNU & vincristine) for AO and AOA, the results have been disappointing. A complete review of the various chemotherapy protocols is beyond the scope of this chapter but a recent meta-analysis, which drew on data from 12 randomized trials of chemotherapy for adult HGGs, demonstrated an increase in 1-year survival from 40% to 46% and an overall 2-month increase in median survival [17]. An important exception is the demonstrated durable response and prolonged survival for AO and AOA associated with deletions of the 1p and 1p+19q chromosomes (see Fig. 10.3 and text above) [15].

Surgical Resection

The impact of extent of surgical resection on survival for HGGs continues to be debated. Clearly, given the biological constraints noted above, a "complete" resection of an HGG is not possible. Extent of surgical resection is best defined based on volumetric analysis [18] of residual contrast-enhancing volume on MR or CT imaging obtained within 24–48 hours of surgery, although non-specific contrast enhancement can be seen after operation for non-neoplastic lesions as soon as 17 hours postoperatively [19]. While contrast enhancement is the most obvious and consistent radiographic indicator of HGG tissue, a small percentage of GBMs do not enhance, and 30–50% of non-GBM HGGs lack contrast enhancement on CT imaging. Conversely, up to 40% of non-enhancing gliomas are anaplastic.

The scientific analysis of cytoreductive surgery for HGG is further confounded by a lack of uniformity in defining and assessing extent of resection and use of subsequent treatment modalities that can prolong survival, and the variable and poorly understood interaction of the multiple patient, treatment and tumor factors that collectively determine patient survival. It is doubtful that a single study could be designed that would definitively address all of these confounding issues and clearly determine the impact of surgical resection on patient outcome. However, in the only study of its kind,

Keles et al. objectively quantified residual post-operative tumor volumes based on MRI, and showed that the volume of residual disease correlated with both time to progression and overall survival [20] (Fig. 10.4). The increasingly frequent demonstration of a significant impact for surgical resection in more recent studies may reflect the routine use of MR or CT imaging post-operatively to objectively quantify residual tumor. The determination of surgical impact on outcome is informative when a study accounts for established prognostic factors and objectively analyzes residual disease rather than percentage of resection or other subjective measures of resection not based on rigorous imaging data [21].

Two subgroups of HGG patients deserve additional mention: the elderly and non-GBM patients. The role of radical surgery for the elderly is controversial. While aggressive treatment strategies have been employed for the elderly (>65 or 70 years of age) and have been shown to provide meaningful periods of survival, the impact of surgical resection has not been adequately analyzed as an independent variable to more definitively define its impact on outcome. Evaluating the impact of surgical resection for grade III lesions is even more problematical than for grade IV lesions because they are more responsive to conventional therapy, display greater biological, clinical and radiological heterogeneity (e.g. less often contrast enhance), are less common than grade IV tumors, and the analysis of their extent of resection is often embedded in generic studies of HGGs. Not surprisingly, studies evaluating the efficacy of resection for grade III HGGs have reported conflicting outcomes.

It is virtually inevitable that HGGs recur or, more correctly, progress. The role of re-operation at the time of recurrence and its impact on outcome have been evaluated in several studies that demonstrate, at best, modest impact on overall survival and, in some cases, prolonged good quality of life compared with patients treated without re-operation [14, 22]. In a recent large study of re-operation in patients enrolled in clinical trials, surgical patients had a median survival of 36 weeks compared with 23 weeks for non-operated patients [22], but the difference was partially attributed to selection bias. Other studies have shown no association between extent of resection and survival at recurrence, with median survival of 33 weeks for GBM patients and 79 weeks for AA patients [14].

If the utility of surgical resection is based primarily on cytoreduction, then it would be important to know what proportion of the tumor burden is represented by the enhancing portion of a tumor versus the diffusely infiltrative component. Accurate assessment of total tumor burden is not possible with current imaging techniques, and problematic even with detailed examination of pathological material.

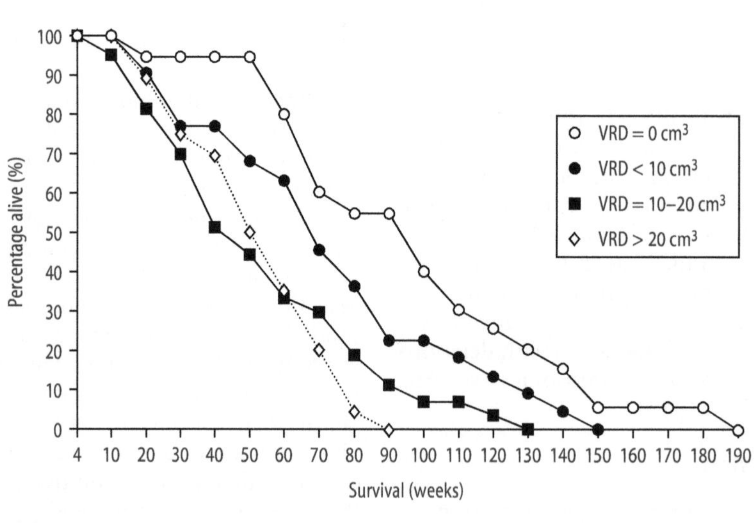

Fig. 10.4. Kaplan–Meier plots showing increasing survival with smaller post-operative tumor volumes in patients with GBM. VRD, post-operative tumor volume. (Courtesy of Keles et al. [20].)

One report estimates that the enhancing component represents as little as 50% of the total cell burden [23]. The fact that recent studies have been able to show any impact of surgical resection based on extent of removal of contrast-enhancing material suggests that this component of the tumor subserves an important biological function that is independent of tumor burden or volume. Recognizing that gross total resection improves outcome but that these benefits were negated by surgically induced neurological deterioration, Shinoda et al. developed a pre-operative MRI-based grading scheme that incorporates tumor size, location and proximity to eloquent cortex to select candidates suitable for gross total resection [24].

Patient Evaluation

Pre-operative evaluation of patients with possible brain lesions requires a careful history and physical examination (including an accurate assessment of the patient's KPS) followed by radiological evaluation. The duration of preoperative symptoms varies greatly, because some patients have harbored lower grade gliomas that have undergone malignant transformation, leading to longer histories than those with HGGs that arise de novo. Patients with HGG often present with headache (approximately 35%), new-onset seizures (approximately 20%), altered mental status (approximately 15%), or focal neurological signs and symptoms. Headaches associated with brain tumors vary in severity, location and quality. However, these headaches are usually different from previous headaches that the patient may have had, and because they may be secondary to elevated intracranial pressure (ICP), they are often associated with nausea and vomiting, and exacerbated by exercise and postural changes. Although drugs, alcohol and metabolic derangement may lead to seizures, new-seizure onset in adults is often associated with structural brain lesions, mandating a brain imaging study. Neurological signs and symptoms vary depending on tumor location and size. While large tumors in the frontal lobes may impart only subtle personality changes, small tumors in the brainstem or eloquent cortical regions may cause significant focal deficits. Patients with HGG rarely present with significant weight loss or pain (other than headache). These problems more often accompany systemic malignancies, which raises the diagnostic probability that the brain lesion may be metastatic or infectious.

Prior to contemplating any form of surgical intervention, the patient's overall medical status must be evaluated. Age, cardiopulmonary status, and medications that hamper coagulation (non-steroidal anti-inflammatory drugs, heparin, coumadin, etc.) may greatly impact the surgical strategy. Elderly patients, those with other life-shortening medical problems, and those with very low KPS may benefit more from biopsy than from an aggressive cytoreductive procedure.

The role of anti-epileptic drugs (AEDs) in patients with gliomas remains somewhat controversial. For those patients who have had seizures, it is clear that AEDs are indicated. Likewise, for patients who are to undergo cortical stimulation mapping during surgery, AEDs offer some protection from iatrogenic seizures. For patients who have never had seizures, the routine use of AEDs is arguable.

Corticosteroids are routinely administered to patients with HGG. Dexamethasone has become the steroid of choice owing to its high glucocorticoid effect and minimal mineralocorticoid effect. Steroids reduce peritumoral edema, often lowering ICP and reducing symptoms. These drugs may also impart some protection from surgical trauma when given prior to surgery. In contradistinction, steroids given following brain trauma do not improve neurological outcome and may increase infectious complications and peptic ulceration. It must be remembered that the normal daily steroid production is less than 1 mg of dexamethasone. Therefore, slow tapers of this medication, while indicated for persistent edema or evolution of neurological deficits, are not rational for hypothalamic-pituitary axis reasons. For HGG patients who are debilitated or elderly or have been on steroids for prolonged periods, dexamethasone should be replaced by prednisone and tapered carefully.

Biopsy vs Resection

As discussed above, the three most important prognostic factors for patients with newly diagnosed HGG are age, KPS and tumor grade. Resection provides an accurate diagnosis, with a smaller chance of sampling error than biopsy. Resection can decrease mass effect, which can cause neurological impairment, steroid dependence and even death. However, the risks of open resection are higher than those of biopsy.

The best predictor of a specific post-operative neurological deficit is the presence of that deficit pre-operatively. Therefore, pre-operative neurological status is an important consideration for surgical strategy. The most important predictor of post-operative hemorrhage and clinically significant post-operative edema is residual tumor. Bilateral tumors and tumors that clearly extend into important functional areas may be best treated with biopsy and post-operative therapies. Patients with significant medical problems, the very elderly and those with a KPS of less than 60 should be offered biopsy. Furthermore, when the diagnosis of tumor vs other lesions (stroke, infection, demyelinating disease, multiple metastases, lymphoma, etc.) is in doubt, biopsy may be a better initial step.

Anesthesia for Biopsy or Resection (see also chapter 4)

The anesthetic must be chosen to lower ICP and minimize seizure risk (especially during cortical stimulation mapping). The patient's hepatic, renal and cardiopulmonary status will also impact on the anesthetic chosen .

Volatile anesthetics are highly halogenated molecules with an unknown mechanism of action. The group includes halothane, enflurane, isoflurane, desflurane and sevoflurane. Halogenated anesthetics provide amnesia, analgesia, and muscle relaxation at higher dosage. The newer agents have a low solubility, permitting rapid adjustment of anesthetic depth and prompt awakening. Halogenated anesthetics decrease cerebral metabolic rate and oxygen consumption ($CMRO_2$) while increasing the CBF, hence producing a metabolic decoupling. They all preserve CO_2 reactivity. Volatile anesthetics can increase ICP, this effect being more prominent with halothane and desflurane, but this rise may be prevented by hyperventilation.

Nitrous oxide (N_2O) is a poorly soluble agent permitting rapid achievement of alveolar and brain partial pressure, and hence has a rapid onset and termination of action. It possesses weak amnestic properties, but provides prominent analgesia with no muscle relaxation. N_2O increases ICP, this effect being completely reversed by hyperventilation. In addition, since N_2O readily diffuses into sealed air pockets, it may cause a severe and rapid increase in ICP in the presence of a pneumocephalus. However, as shown by Domino et al. in craniotomies, it is usually not necessary to discontinue its use prior to dural closure [25]. CO_2 reactivity appears maintained when N_2O is used alone or added to propofol, but may be reduced when used with isoflurane.

The site of action of barbiturates is located on the GABA receptor complex. Thiopental is a fast-onset short-acting drug, producing unconsciousness in 10–20 seconds. The short duration of action is explained by the rapid redistribution half-life of 7 minutes. Thiopental is principally used as an induction agent. Thiopental decreases $CMRO_2$ and CBF and can produce EEG suppression at clinical doses. It also decreases the intracranial pressure (ICP) of patients with intracranial hypertension to a greater extent than it decreases the mean arterial pressure (MAP), thus improving the cerebral perfusion pressure (CPP). CO_2 reactivity of brain vasculature is preserved with thiopental and does not change over time.

Like barbiturates, etomidate possesses a GABA-mimetic activity. Etomidate is a fast-onset drug producing loss of consciousness in 10 seconds. Etomidate is used as an induction drug, but it can also be used as an infusion. Etomidate decreases $CMRO_2$ by 45% and CBF by 35% and can produce a flat EEG. It decreases ICP, while increasing, or at least maintaining, the CPP. CO_2 reactivity of the cerebral vasculature is maintained with etomidate. The brain-protecting effect of etomidate was also shown to be a dose-dependent phenomenon with deleterious effect at higher doses, presumably because of the induction of spiking EEG activity without further depression of $CMRO_2$. In humans, a recent study showed that etomidate may even cause cerebral hypoxia at doses sufficient to induce burst-suppression. Although still widely used for neuroanesthesia, etomidate may not possess the brain-protecting virtues it was once thought to have.

Propofol is administered in an egg-oil-glycerol emulsion, and probably exerts its pharmacological effect by enhancing GABA-activated chloride channel. Propofol is a fast-onset, short-acting drug. Propofol decreases the CBF by 30% to 50%, with a 35% diminution of the $CMRO_2$, preserving CO_2 reactivity. Propofol decreases ICP with a concomitant decrease of MAP.

Narcotics currently used during anesthesia are synthetic phenylpiperidine derivatives and include fentanyl, sufentanil, alfentanil and remifentanil. They are pure opioid receptor agonists, and, unlike morphine, do not liberate histamine. These drugs are all ultrashort- to short-acting drugs. They are used as anesthetic adjuvant, but may be used as the main anesthetic agent. The effect of these drugs on cardiovascular and cerebral dynamics is quite variable. Remifentanil and fentanyl seem to have negligible effect on ICP, while sufentanil and alfentanil may increase it. Mainly because of their effect on MAP, they tend to decrease the CPP, sometimes below the range of autoregulation. Again, of the four drugs, fentanyl has the smallest effect on CPP. Sufentanil may even decrease CBF in a dose-dependent manner under anesthesia. Alfentanil seems to have negligible effects on both CBF and $CMRO_2$. Narcotics maintain CO_2 reactivity. Narcotics are not brain protectants.

Intracranial Pressure Management

Several osmotic diuretic agents have been used to treat elevated ICP, including sucrose, albumin, urea and mannitol. Mannitol appears to be excluded from the CSF to a greater extent than other osmotic agents. Mannitol is a simple unbranched hydrocarbon with a half-life of approximately 0.25–1.7 hours. Its excretion is primarily renal, so its half-life may be extended in cases of impaired renal function. The recommended dose for mannitol is 0.25–2 g/kg intravenously every 4 hours, with a peak decrease in ICP approximately 15 minutes after administration. Use of a loop diuretic 15 minutes after the administration of mannitol has been shown to potentiate its effect. Like all osmotic diuretics, mannitol works primarily by shifting water from the brain parenchyma to the intravascular space, thereby decreasing the volume of the intracranial contents and reducing ICP. Additionally, mannitol reduces intracranial elastance. Mannitol may also affect the reactivity of intracerebral capillaries, leading to an overall vasconstrictive effect and decreased ICP. Finally, mannitol decreases the viscosity of whole blood, thereby decreasing intracerebral resistance. In combination with the increase in intravascular volume and cardiac output, this leads to increased CBF in the setting of decreased ICP, with an overall theoretical increase in CPP. These effects on ICP and CPP appear to be greatest in the setting of intact vascular autoregulation. The effectiveness of mannitol is also highly dependent on the intactness of, and osmotic gradient across, the BBB. Marked disruption of the BBB allows flow of mannitol into the brain parenchyma, thus antagonizing flow of blood into the intravascular compartment. In response to chronic osmotic therapy, the brain also accumulates "idiogenic osmoles", which act to sequester water in the brain compartment.

Barbiturates are a second-line agent for the management of elevated ICP. Their efficacy in this role remains controversial. The mechanism of action is believed to be their ability to modulate cerebral metabolism and therefore CBF. Barbiturates appear to act as cerebral vasoconstrictors, thus reducing intracerebral blood volume and lowering ICP. Barbiturates also appear to preferentially vasoconstrict normal cerebral blood vessels and increase CBF to relatively ischemic areas. Finally, barbiturates decrease $CMRO_2$, i.e. the cerebral metabolic rate and oxygen consumption. Decreases in $CMRO_2$ appear to result in decreased ICP. A burst-suppression EEG pattern (so-called "barbiturate coma") is often required to achieve a maximal decrease in $CMRO_2$. This effect, however, does not come without a significant price. Large doses of barbiturates may cause systemic hypotension and act as negative inotropes, both of which act to decrease cardiac output and, ultimately, CPP in the setting of elevated ICP. Pentobarbital is the most commonly used barbiturate for the management of ICP and has a half-life of 15–50 hours, which may be even further lengthened by the large doses required to achieve a barbiturate-induced coma. This effect is due to perturbation of hepatic-clearance mechanisms and also significantly affects the metabolism of other hepatically cleared drugs. Resolution of pentobarbital coma may take days after cessation of therapy. This side-effect profile mandates the use of frequent monitoring of drug levels, EEG, cardiac output and CBF.

Propofol is now frequently used in the ICU setting for ICP control. In the acute setting, and over relatively short periods of time (hours to days), the agent has an effective half-life of 2–4 minutes. The drug decreases CBF, ICP and $CMRO_2$ and induces less cardiac depression than barbiturates. Because of its short half-life, it has also shown utility for neuroleptic anesthesia. Propofol is also useful for sedation of agitated patients in whom serial neurological exams are necessary. Once the propofol infusion is stopped, within 10–20 minutes effective blood levels have dropped to near zero. Untoward side-effects include negative inotropy, respiratory depression and prolonged clearance after large doses.

Stereotactic Biopsy

The sole goal of stereotactic biopsy of brain lesions is to obtain a diagnosis. Owing to HGG histological heterogeneity, undergrading of the tumor occurs at a rate of approximately 10%. Overall risks from biopsy include anesthesia, bleeding, infection, and obtaining non-diagnostic tissue. The reported complication rates vary from 1% to 5%, while mortality rates are reported as 0–3% [26]. Frameless sterotactic techniques provide the advantage of avoiding the discomfort of frame placement, but the disadvantage of some loss of accuracy. Typically, frame-based techniques offer accuracy within 5 mm.

When using general anesthesia, it is important to simulate the conditions at the time of the scan to maintain accuracy. Therefore, mannitol, hyperventilation and other methods for lowering ICP should not be used (unless they were also used during the time of scan acquisition). Following standard prepping and draping, a small incision is made. The entry site is chosen to provide the shortest, yet safest, course from the cortical surface to the lesion. Obvious regions to avoid include major blood vessels, the Sylvian fissure, and sulci. If the ventricle is entered, it is important not to remove CSF, as this may permit displacement of the target. A target site is chosen that will provide the most accurate diagnosis. Areas of enhancement and necrosis are more likely to yield the diagnosis of HGG. Following tissue acquisition, frozen-section pathology helps to ensure that tumor tissue has been obtained. If this is not the case, a second target site should be sampled. If bleeding occurs with the biopsy, instillation of 0.1–0.3 cm^3 of thrombin solution through the biopsy instrument may be helpful. However, significant hemorrhages may require open intervention. A post-operative CT scan is routinely obtained to verify the target site sampled and confirm that there has been no significant bleeding. It has been our practice to retain biopsy patients in the hospital overnight. Because the wound is small, radiotherapy may commence as soon as a final diagnosis has been provided by the pathologists.

Open Surgical Resection

The objectives of HGG resection are accurate diagnosis, reduction of mass effect and reduction of the tumor burden. Risks from craniotomy for HGG resection vary, with reported morbidity rates ranging from 5% to 15%, and mortality from 1% to 5%. Techniques that minimize these problems and maximize resection will be discussed.

Positioning and Flap Strategies

Patients should be positioned so that all pressure points are well padded, with the neck in a relatively neutral position to assure adequate jugular venous return. The tumor should be located at the highest point, with the patient in moderate reverse Trendelenburg position. Following adequate induction with general anesthesia (as discussed above), hyperventilation and administration of mannitol (1.0 g/kg under general anesthesia, 0.5 g/kg when the patient will undergo awake functional mapping) should commence.

The skin flap should be designed so that it is large enough to permit potential re-operation for recurrence if needed. Although the incision can be extended or "teed", it is best to plan ahead and avoid higher risk scalp flaps. The craniotomy should be large enough to permit adequate tumor exposure and access to potentially functional cortical regions that need to be identified with mapping techniques (see below).

Intraoperative Navigation

Although many HGGs are easily differentiated from surrounding brain, others pose serious problems in this regard. Similarly, resection of tumors that cannot be seen on the cortical surface are best approached with some form(s) of intraoperative navigation (Fig. 10.5). Intraoperative ultrasound (IOUS), which is available at most centers, is helpful when the tumor is not iso-echoic with the brain (Fig. 10.5b). This is often problematic for infiltrating low-grade gliomas, but less often with HGG. IOUS can provide accurate data prior to resection, during resection and at the end of the resection (to determine the completeness of the resection). The accuracy of IOUS is not diminished by brain shifts that occur during resection and subsequent brain relaxation. Frame-based and frameless sterotactic systems are quite useful as well (Fig. 10.5c). They can be used in planning the scalp flap, the craniotomy and the resection. However, the accuracy of these systems relies on concordance between brain position and pre-operative imaging studies. Therefore, alterations in brain volume or shifts of the intracranial contents during resection may render these guidance systems less useful as the resection progresses. Intraoperative imaging systems allow the neurosurgical oncologist to bring the post-operative "gold standard" into the operation. Currently these systems are expensive, often cumbersome and prolong the surgery. However, they combine the advantages of IOUS and stereotaxy.

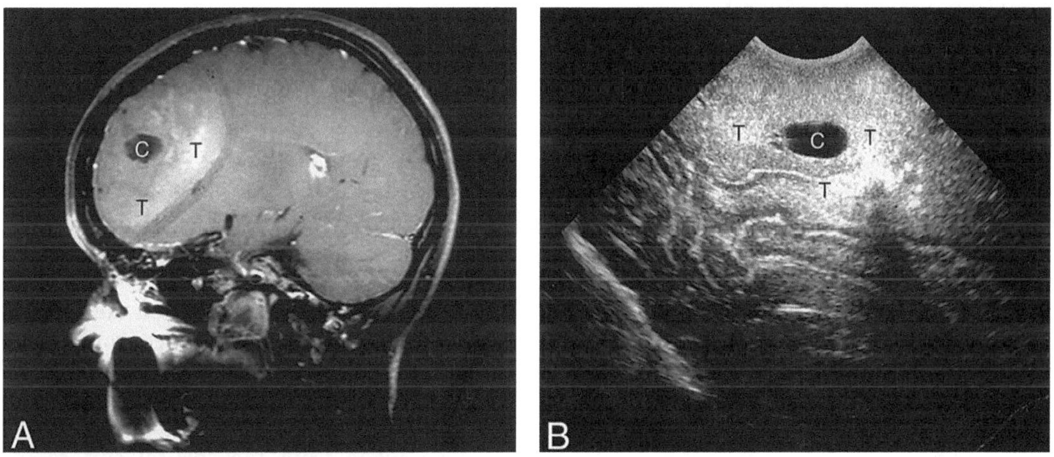

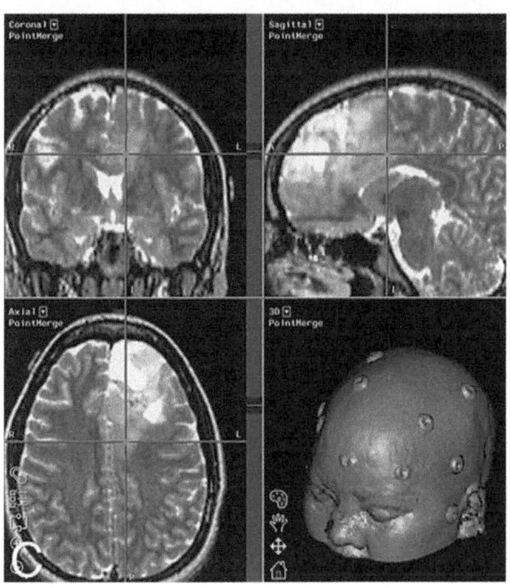

Fig. 10.5. **a** Sagittal MRI (T1-weighted with gadolinium) showing a large left frontal tumor (T) with a small central cystic component (C). **b** Intraoperative ultrasound image obtained in the transverse plane, demonstrating the tumor and tumor cyst. **c** Intraoperative MRI navigational system, demonstrating the posterior extent of the resection (at red crosshair).

Functional Mapping

Identification of functional cortex, including Rolandic cortex and speech cortex, enables the surgeon to avoid these areas when formulating surgical strategy [27]. In addition to preservation of cerebral function during surgery, it is also possible with these techniques to achieve a greater extent of resection with increased safety. While somatosensory evoked potential (SSEP) and cortical stimulation mapping of motor cortex can be performed in patients under either general or local anesthesia, speech mapping requires the cooperation of an awake patient. Although resections in or near functional brain can be made safer by localizing important brain functions, there are a number of pitfalls that the surgeon must be aware of in order to avoid producing functional deficits.

Localization of Somatosensory Cortex Using SSEPs

SSEP mapping to identify the primary somatosensory gyrus provides a quick, reliable means of Rolandic localization in both adult and pediatric populations [28]. SSEPs can be performed under general anesthesia or in awake patients. SSEP mapping has the advantage over stimulation mapping that seizures cannot be evoked because the cortex itself is not stimulated. When performed under general anesthesia, halogenated anesthetic agents should be avoided because they may increase the latency of the cortical SSEPs. High-dose barbiturate or propofol anesthesia may lead to burst-suppression activity, and is therefore contraindicated. Nitrous oxide combined with Pentothal or low-dose propofol provides excellent general anesthetics for these studies.

Techniques for intraoperative SSEP mapping are similar to those used for routine diagnostic studies (Fig. 10.6). A peripheral nerve is stimulated – most often the median nerve at the wrist due to the robust signal that can be recorded at the cortical surface. However, other nerves, such as the tibial nerve, can also be used. Stimulation is performed at a rate of 2–5 Hz with a 0.1–0.3 ms pulse duration, and the current adjusted to produce a minimal (not painful) twitch so that muscle activity can just be visualized. Stimulation can be accomplished with mechanical and thermal stimulation as well. The stimulus generates a signal that is transmitted via the spinothalamic pathways, to the medial lemniscus, then the thalamus, and finally to contralateral somatosensory cortex. Compared with scalp recordings, SSEP recordings made from the cortical surface have much higher voltages (10–100 mV). Recording typically uses a low, cut-off frequency of 1 Hz, a high-frequency filter of 3,000 Hz, and an analysis time of 100 ms. Usually, trials of 100–200 stimuli are needed to elicit well-defined responses from the somatosensory cortex. Cortical responses have a number of different components designated by their positive (P) or negative (N) polarity with respect to the reference electrode, followed by a number representing the typical latency (in ms) of the peaks. For instance, following median nerve stimulation, the contralateral somatosensory gyrus shows an initial N20 component followed by a P25 component.

Following craniotomy and durotomy, an array of electrodes is placed in the axial (transverse) plane on the cortical surface. An eight-contact electrode strip (1 cm center-to-center spacing) is quite adequate. The electrode contacts should extend over areas of the brain anterior and posterior to the presumed somatosensory gyrus. Alternatively, electrodes may be placed on the dura (this is especially helpful for re-operative and post-meningitis cases where the dura is adherent to the underlying cortex rather than directly on the cortical surface). If the craniotomy does not expose Rolandic cortex, an electrode strip can be slid beneath the edge of the craniotomy to reach distant cortical regions. A series of recordings are then made from the cortical surface by moving the electrode to different areas to verify localization of the somatosensory cortex.

Cortical Stimulation Motor and Sensory Mapping

Functional localization by cortical stimulation mapping has been performed for over 40 years. Although this technique is reliable, it is often difficult to elicit responses in children or under general anesthesia. Stimulation mapping of somatosensory cortex requires an awake patient; however, motor cortex can be stimulated with the patient under general anesthesia. It is important to bear in mind during cortical stimulation that repetitive or prolonged stimulation at or

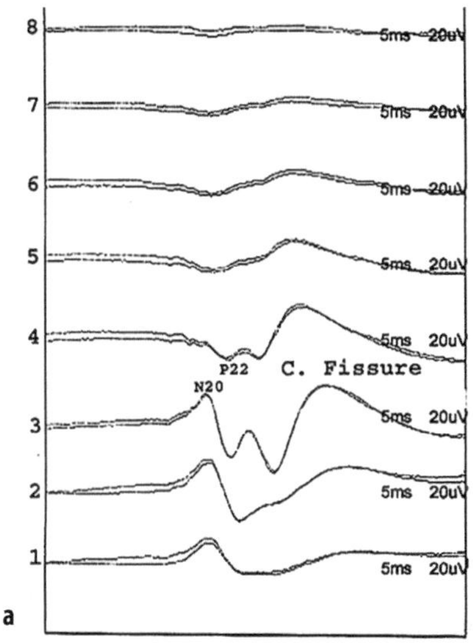

a

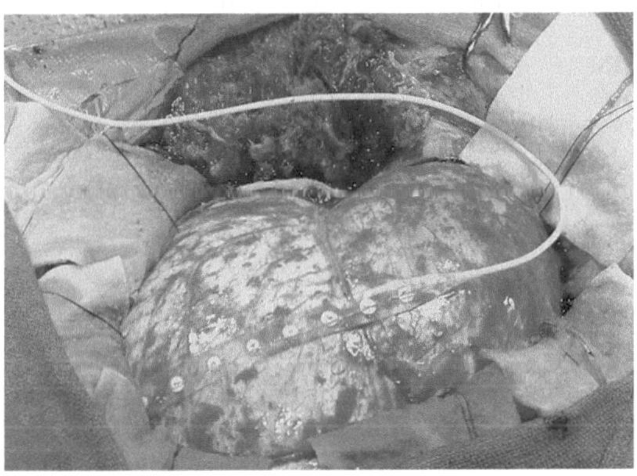

b

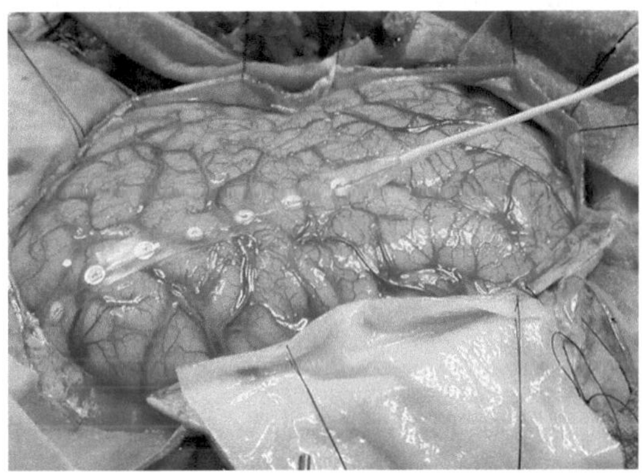

c

Fig. 10.6. **a** Bipolar montage from somatosensory evoked potential (SSEP) recording following stimulation of the right (contralateral) median nerve. The N20, denoting the primary somatosensory cortex is seen in channel "3". The P22, indicating motor cortex, is seen in channel "4". **b** Trans-dural SSEP electrode arrangement with an eight-contact electrode placed on the dura prior to durotomy. **c** SSEP recording directly from the cortical surface.

near the same site, or with higher currents, can elicit local or generalized seizure activity. Therefore, it is important to make sure that the patient has adequate serum anticonvulsant levels pre-operatively and that a short-acting intravenous anticonvulsant is readily available in the event that seizures are elicited.

A constant current, biphasic, square wave, 60 Hz, bipolar stimulator (Ojemann Stimulator, Radionics Sales Corp.; 5 mm between electrodes) set at 2–10 mA is used to elicit movement and/or sensation in the awake patient. Higher current settings may be necessary in younger children, in patients under general anesthesia, or when stimulating through the dura. It is best to start at lower current settings and gradually increase the current until sensation or movement is elicited, as this will help to avoid eliciting seizure activity.

Using this technique, the entire sensory and motor homunculi can be mapped. The technique can also be used to identify descending subcortical motor fibers when resections extend below the cortical surface, such as during supplementary motor area resections and insular resections. When performing subcortical motor mapping, the current needed to elicit movement is the same, or lower than, the current needed at the cortical surface. When the resection is very close to functional cortex, it is helpful to periodically repeat the stimulation mapping procedure to verify that cortical and subcortical functional regions are not damaged.

Mapping of Language Cortex

In contrast to mapping Rolandic cortex, language cortex mapping depends on electrical blockade of cortical function rather than on eliciting function [29]. Most patients, even children as young as 10 years old, have little difficulty with the procedure, especially when propofol anesthesia is used during placement of the field block, cranial opening, the majority of the resection, and during closure. It is important to bear in mind that cortical stimulation mapping of language cortex is used to identify essential language cortex. This is distinctly different from involved language cortex, which is identified by functional imaging techniques such as positron emission tomography (PET) and functional magnetic resonance imaging (fMRI). Furthermore, the specific language task performed by the patient may lead to identification of different language sites.

It is first necessary to determine the after-discharge threshold so that depolarization is not propagated to nearby cortex, which may elicit local seizure phenomena or give false-negative or false-positive results. Therefore, electrocorticography (ECoG) must be performed during stimulation (Fig. 10.7). Using a U-shaped electrode holder, which is attached to the skull at the edge of the craniotomy (Grass model CE1), carbon-tip electrodes are placed over the exposed cortical surface and spaced approximately 10 mm apart. Bipolar stimulation, as described above, is then used, starting with a current of 2 mA. The current is gradually increased (0.5–1.0 mA increments) with successive stimulations until the after-discharge threshold is determined. The current used for language mapping is then set to 0.5–1.0mA below the after-discharge threshold.

Prior to mapping, 15–20 peri-Sylvian sites are selected and marked with small (5 × 5 mm)

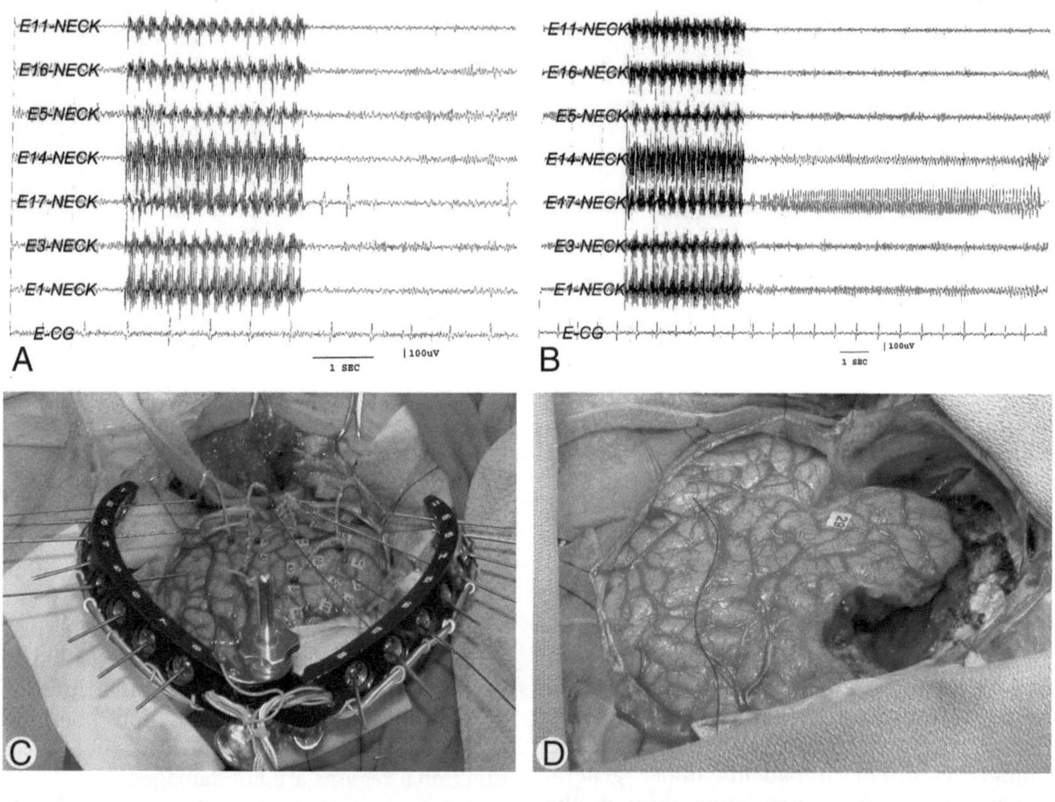

Fig. 10.7. a Intraoperative electrocorticogram showing three afterdischarges following cortical stimulation (in lead E17). The montage is referential to three neck electrodes (balanced neck reference, to minimize ECG interference). **b** A higher current than in a has produced a train of afterdischarges. **c** The cortical electrode arrangement is shown with numbered tickets on the left frontal lobe. **d** Ticket "29" shows the location of motor speech; the suture is on the central sulcus. The frontal lobe tumor resection can be seen.

numbered tags. Sites for stimulation mapping are randomly selected to cover all exposed cortex, including areas where essential language areas are likely to be located and those near or overlying the site of resection. Using a computer, the patient is shown images of simple objects. A new image is shown every 2–4 seconds (depending on the patient's verbal ability). Cortical stimulation is applied prior to the presentation of each image and continued until there is a correct response or the next image is presented. Each pre-selected site is stimulated three to four times, though never twice in succession. Sites where stimulation produces consistent speech arrest or anomia are considered essential to language function. Injury to essential language areas will lead to permanent difficulties.

It is important to remember that the topography of essential language varies from individual to individual. Furthermore, patients who are adept in more than one language will have separate essential language areas for each of their different languages. Standard anatomical temporal lobe resections (e.g. measured resections, resections anterior to the central sulcus, resections anterior to Labbé's vein) do not always spare essential language areas. Ojemann et al. [30] noted that subjects typically have two language areas: one in the posterior inferior frontal gyrus, and one in the posterior temporal lobe. However, individuals displayed a wide variety of language topography and some had three or more sites identified. The basal language area can probably be resected with relative impunity, indicating that, although this site is involved in language function, it is not essential.

As with the other types of mapping described above, language mapping can be performed through the dura or directly on the cortical surface. Furthermore, when the surgeon wishes to stimulate unexposed cortex, this can be accomplished by sliding a strip electrode beneath the edge of the bone flap and then utilizing a device that attaches to the electrode lead wire connection that permits direct bipolar stimulation [27]. When the resection is within 2 cm of the identified language area, it is best to have the patient continue object naming during the part of the resection that is close to the identified language site. The resection can then proceed slowly and be halted if naming errors occur.

Pitfalls of Cortical Mapping

Although cortical mapping is an important tool, potential pitfalls must be recognized so as to use mapping safely and effectively [27]. Below are some of the major difficulties encountered. These have been separated into: (1) inability to identify functional cortex, and (2) injury to functional cortex once it has been identified.

Inability to Identify Functional Cortex

In young patients, stimulation motor mapping is often not possible. SSEPs must be used to localize Rolandic cortex. Under general anesthesia, SSEPs and motor cortex localization may prove difficult. Nitrous/narcotic anesthesia is best for mapping. Inability to identify functional cortex does not prove that one is not in functional cortex. It may be indicative that there was a problem with mapping, not that resection is necessarily safe. During localization of speech cortex, ECoG must be used to determine the after-discharge threshold. This assures that there are no local seizures elicited by stimulation.

Injury to Functional Cortex Following Mapping

There are often two or more essential speech areas within both the temporal and frontal lobes. Therefore, the entire region to be resected should be mapped (i.e. mapping should not be stopped simply because two speech areas have been identified). White matter underlying functional cortex can be injured. For Rolandic cortex, this can be avoided with subcortical mapping. For speech cortex, the patient should continue naming during resection of abutting cortex or white matter. Vascular injury in the neighborhood of functional cortex must be avoided. Lesional distortion of cortex superficially does not indicate that underlying white matter has (or has not) been displaced. Ascending or descending fibers may not travel perpendicular to the gyral crown.

Intratumoral Therapies

Aside from the resection of tumor, neurosurgeons are becoming increasingly involved in the delivery of therapy at the time of resection or the delivery of intralesional therapy. While most of these neurosurgical-based therapies are experimental or undergoing evaluation in phase I or II clinical trials, a few have been approved for general use.

Chemotherapy Impregnated Wafers

The implantation of degradable wafers impregnated with BCNU (Gliadel) has been used extensively at the time of re-operation for recurrent HGGs, and recently has been approved by the FDA for use at the time of initial surgery. In a large phase III trial enrolling 222 patients with recurrent HGGs, the use of Gliadel provided a statistically significant prolongation of survival of 8 weeks (from 23 to 31 weeks) for all HGG patients as well as for the GBM subgroup [31]. A recent multicenter prospective trial evaluated the use of Gliadel at initial surgery and reported median survival times of 13.9 vs 11.6 months for HGG patients receiving Gliadel vs placebo, with median survival of 13.5 vs 11.4 months in the GBM vs placebo group [32].

Complications associated with the use of Gliadel include infection, cerebral edema, wound-healing problems and CSF leak, particularly in patients with recurrent HGG. Careful attention to tissue handling and dural closure, with use of dural patches, helps to reduce these complications.

Brachytherapy

Brachytherapy for HGGs includes the temporary use of high-activity implants and permanent placement of lower-activity sources. Early reports on the use of brachytherapy with temporary high-activity implants were encouraging, but subsequent re-evaluation showed that much of the treatment effect was due to selection bias [33]. Subsequent randomized prospective trials of interstitial, high-activity, temporary I-125 implants, used as a boost at the time of initial treatment, have reported contradictory results. Permanent low-activity I-125 implants placed at initial operation have produced promising results but require additional validation.

Similar brachytherapy strategies using either high-activity I-125 temporary, or low-activity I-125 permanent, implants have been used for HGGs at the time of recurrence. While the efficacy of these approaches is not clearly established, one study reported the survival of patients receiving permanent implants was almost two-fold longer than a comparable group of historical controls treated aggressively with surgery and chemotherapy. One consideration in their use is that treatment-related morbidity appears to be less for permanent low-activity implants than for temporary high-activity implants. One difficulty with any brachytherapy approach is achieving uniform dose distributions to all involved regions of tumor. Dose heterogeneity can lead to under-treated (cold spots) or over-treated areas (hot spots) at risk for rapid progression or radiation injury and necrosis, respectively. While the use of stereotactic radiation techniques provides boosts with more defined dosimetry, it is often difficult to shape the radiation field to the irregular growth patterns of most HGGs.

Future Directions

A host of novel experimental therapies, including gene-based therapy and immunotherapy, have emerged based on our continually evolving understanding of HGG biology. The delivery of many of these newer therapies involves the technical expertise of the neurosurgeon [34]. The following examples of emerging therapeutic approaches emphasize how targeting specific aspects of glioma tumor biology translates into new treatment strategies, and how the delivery of these agents – often with novel techniques – is likely to further involve the neurosurgeon in the future treatment of HGG.

Immunotherapy approaches include the use of antibodies conjugated to radioactive compounds, or toxins directed against tumor-specific antigens (such as transferrin receptors, EGFRvIII, tenascin, and VEGF receptors). Tumor vaccines are being developed, and other means to boost inherent immune responses to tumor antigens, such as dendritic cell therapies, are being actively pursued. Gene therapy encompasses a multitude of different approaches as well. Early clinical trials of gene therapy used the local administration into glioma resection beds of retroviruses engineered with bacterial enzymes (thymidine kinase) capable of converting prodrugs (ganciclovir) into cytotoxic metabolites. Other, newer, gene-based therapies under development include: gene replacement (e.g. p53), production of dominant-negative receptors (e.g. to VEGF receptor) to disrupt signaling pathways, antisense oligonucleotides to knock down expression of specific genes, and administration of cytolytic viral vectors. These approaches are theoretically attractive because they target specific molecular aspects of glial tumors and may reduce toxicity, but none has proven to be particularly efficacious. Thus, their integration into standard therapy will require further investigation.

One of the major impediments to successful treatment of HGGs is the inability to deliver cytotoxic drug concentrations to bulk tumor or to access the diffusely invasive tumor cells that reside within regions of an intact BBB. Not surprisingly, concurrent with the development of new treatment approaches described above has been the introduction of novel techniques for delivery of these therapies and others, which attempt to overcome these limitations. These new approaches to delivery include the use of convection-enhanced delivery and osmotic or pharmacological opening of the BBB and intralesional delivery of high-dose chemotherapy. Convection-enhanced delivery uses intracerebral catheters to infuse therapeutic agents through the brain by bulk flow, such that therapy can be delivered to large areas of brain without reliance on a disrupted BBB. Disruption of the BBB itself by administration of osmotic agents or with drugs that specifically reduce endothelial-cell-tight junctions, such as the bradykinin agonist RMP-7, can be used to achieve higher drug levels within bulk tumor and surrounding diffusely invaded brain tissue with a normally intact BBB. The use of direct intralesional injection of therapeutic agents is also under investigation in an attempt to provide local cytotoxic therapy with minimal systemic toxicity [34].

Perhaps the most intriguing new method for delivery of therapy involves the use of genetically engineered neural stem cells (NSCs). In animal models, NSCs injected intracranially or even intravascularly migrate into the brain and appear to have a unique tropism for isolated invasive tumor cells. NSCs engineered to produce the enzyme cytosine deaminase were shown to be capable of converting systemically administered prodrug 5-FC into the cytotoxic metabolite 5-FU, which led to a significant reduction of implanted brain tumor size in animals [11].

Key Points

- *High-grade gliomas are the most common primary cerebral neoplasms in adults and the majority of these tumors are glioblastoma multiforme and anaplastic astrocytoma.*
- *High-grade gliomas can either arise de novo or arise from malignant degeneration of low grade gliomas.*
- *Treatment of high-grade gliomas includes confirmatory biopsy or surgical resection followed by radiation therapy. Chemotherapy can also be considered.*
- *Important predictors of survival include age, histological grade, Karnofsky performance status and adequacy of treatment.*
- *Despite advances in imaging, surgical techniques to maximize resection, and chemotherapy and radiation therapy techniques, the prognosis for survival beyond 2–3 years remains poor.*

References

1. Legler JM, Ries LA, Smith MA, Warren JL, Heineman EF, Kaplan RS et al. Cancer surveillance series (corrected): brain and other central nervous system cancers: recent trends in incidence and mortality. J Natl Cancer Inst 1999;91(16):1382–90.
2. Kleihues P, Louis DN, Scheithauer BW, Rorke LB, Reifenberger G, Burger PC et al. The WHO classification of tumors of the nervous system. J Neuropathol Exp Neurol 2002;61(3):215–25;discussion:226–9.
3. Kleihues, P, Ohgaki H. Primary and secondary glioblastomas: from concept to clinical diagnosis. Neuro-oncol 1999;1(1):44–51.
4. Bigner SH, Matthews MR, Rasheed BK, Wiltshire RN, Friedman HS, Friedman AH et al. Molecular genetic aspects of oligodendrogliomas including analysis by comparative genomic hybridization. Am J Pathol 1999;155(2):375–86.
5. Chan JL, Lee SW, Fraass BA, Normolle DP, Greenberg HS, Junck LR et al. Survival and failure patterns of high-grade gliomas after three-dimensional conformal radiotherapy. J Clin Oncol 2002;20(6):1635–42.
6. Halligan JB, Stelzer KJ, Rostomily RC, Spence AM, Griffin TW, Berger MS et al. Operation and permanent low activity 125I brachytherapy for recurrent high-grade astrocytomas. Int J Radiat Oncol Biol Phys 1996;35(3):541–7.
7. Scherer HJ. Structural development in gliomas. Am J Cancer 1938;34(3):333–51.

8. Kelly PJ, Daumas-Duport C, Kispert DB, Kall BA, Scheithauer BW, Illig JJ. Imaging-based stereotaxic serial biopsies in untreated intracranial glial neoplasms. J Neurosurg 1987;66(6):865–74.
9. Silbergeld DL, Chicoine MR. Isolation and characterization of human malignant glioma cells from histologically normal brain. J Neurosurg 1997;86(3):525–31.
10. Ojemann JG, Miller JW, Silbergeld DL. Preserved function in brain invaded by tumor. Neurosurgery 1996;39(2):253–8;discussion:258–9.
11. Aboody KS, Brown A, Rainov NG, Bower KA, Liu S, Yang W et al. From the cover: neural stem cells display extensive tropism for pathology in adult brain: evidence from intracranial gliomas. Proc Natl Acad Sci USA 2000;97(23):12846–51.
12. Curran WJ Jr, Scott CB, Horton J, Nelson JS, Weinstein AS, Fischbach AJ et al. Recursive partitioning analysis of prognostic factors in three Radiation Therapy Oncology Group malignant glioma trials. J Natl Cancer Inst 1993;85(9):704–10.
13. Wong ET, Hess KR, Gleason MJ, Jaeckle KA, Kyritsis AP, Prados MD et al. Outcomes and prognostic factors in recurrent glioma patients enrolled onto phase II clinical trials. J Clin Oncol 1999;17(8):2572.
14. Rostomily RC, Spence AM, Duong D, McCormick K, Bland M, Berger MS et al. Multimodality management of recurrent adult malignant gliomas: results of a phase II multiagent chemotherapy study and analysis of cytoreductive surgery. Neurosurgery 1994;35(3): 378–88;discussion:388.
15. Ino Y, Betensky RA, Zlatescu MC, Sasaki H, Macdonald DR, Stemmer-Rachamimov AO et al. Molecular subtypes of anaplastic oligodendroglioma: implications for patient management at diagnosis. Clin Cancer Res 2001;7(4):839–45.
16. Walker MD, Alexander E Jr, Hunt WE, MacCarty CS, Mahaley MS Jr, Mealey J Jr et al. Evaluation of BCNU and/or radiotherapy in the treatment of anaplastic gliomas. A cooperative clinical trial. J Neurosurg 1978;49(3):333–43.
17. Stewart LA. Chemotherapy in adult high-grade glioma: a systematic review and meta-analysis of individual patient data from 12 randomised trials. Lancet 2002;359(9311):1011–18.
18. Duong DH, Rostomily RC, Haynor DR, Keles GE, Berger MS. Measurement of tumor resection volumes from computerized images. Technical note. J Neurosurg 1992;77(1):151–4.
19. Henegar MM, Moran CJ, Silbergeld DL. Early post-operative magnetic resonance imaging following nonneoplastic cortical resection. J Neurosurg 1996;84(2):174–9.
20. Keles GE, Anderson B, and Berger MS. The effect of extent of resection on time to tumor progression and survival in patients with glioblastoma multiforme of the cerebral hemisphere. Surg Neurol 1999;52(4):371–9.
21. Silbergeld DL, Rostomily RC. Resection of glioblastoma. J Neurosurg 2002;96(4):809;discussion:810.
22. Barker FG Jr, Chang SM, Gutin PH, Malec MK, McDermott MW, Prados MD et al. Survival and functional status after resection of recurrent glioblastoma multiforme. Neurosurgery 1998;42(4):709–20; discussion:720–3.
23. Alvord EC Jr. Simple model of recurrent gliomas. J Neurosurg 1991;75(2):337–8.
24. Shinoda J, Sakai N, Murase S, Yano H, Matsuhisa T, Funakoshi T. Selection of eligible patients with supratentorial glioblastoma multiforme for gross total resection. J Neurooncol 2001;52(2):161–71.
25. Domino KB, Hemstad JR, Lam AM, Laohaprasit V, Mayberg TA, Harrison SD et al. Effect of nitrous oxide on intracranial pressure after cranial-dural closure in patients undergoing craniotomy. Anesthesiology 1992;77(3):421–5.
26. Field M, Witham TF, Flickinger JC, Kondziolka D, Lunsford LD. Comprehensive assessment of hemorrhage risks and outcomes after stereotactic brain biopsy. J Neurosurg 2001;94(4):545–51.
27. Silbergeld DL. Cortical mapping. In: Luders HO and Comair YG, editors. Epilepsy surgery. Philadelphia: Lippincott Williams & Wilkins, 2002; 633–5.
28. Silbergeld DL, Miller JW. Intraoperative cerebral mapping and monitoring. Contemp Neurosurg 1996;18(11): 1–6.
29. Silbergeld DL, Ojemann GA. The tailored temporal lobectomy. Neurosurg Clin N Am 1993;4(2):273–81.
30. Ojemann G, Ojemann J, Lettich E, Berger M. Cortical language localization in left, dominant hemisphere. An electrical stimulation mapping investigation in 117 patients. J Neurosurg 1989;71(3):316–26.
31. Brem H, Piantadosi S, Burger PC, Walker M, Selker R, Vick NA et al. Placebo-controlled trial of safety and efficacy of intraoperative controlled delivery by biodegradable polymers of chemotherapy for recurrent gliomas. The Polymer-brain Tumor Treatment Group. Lancet 1995;345(8956):1008–12.
32. Westphal M, Hilt D, Bortey E, Delavault P, Olivares R, Warnke P et al. A phase 3 trial of local chemotherapy with biodegradable carmustine (BCNU) wafers (Gliadel wafers) in patients with primary malignant glioma. Neuro-oncol 2003;5(2):79–88.
33. Florell RC, Macdonald DR, Irish WD, Bernstein M, Leibel SA, Gutin PH et al. Selection bias, survival, and brachytherapy for glioma. J Neurosurg 1992;76(2): 179–83.
34. Broaddus WC, Gillies GT, Kucharczyk J. Minimally invasive procedures. Advances in image-guided delivery of drug and cell therapies into the central nervous system. Neuroimaging Clin N Am 2001;11(4):727–35.

11

Sellar and Parasellar Tumors

Richard J. Stacey and Michael P. Powell

Summary

Pituitary adenomas are by far the most common tumours of the sellar region, comprising 90 to 95% of all such tumours. Meningiomas, craniopharyngiomas(particularly in children), Rathke's cleft cysts and aneurysms are the most likely differential diagnoses. The majority of pituitary tumours are asymptomatic, discovered as "incidentalomas" in the course of investigation for other conditions. The rest, along with other sellar lesions, present with symptoms of endocrine dysfunction, mass effect on surrounding structures, commonly the optic nerves or chiasm, or headache. Apart from Prolactin secreting tumours, which respond to dopamine agonists, the mainstay of treatment is surgery, with or without radiotherapy. Prior to surgery, even as an emergency, all sellar tumour patients should have thyroid function tests, Prolactin levels and adequate imaging. Any patient with a tumour with suprasellar extension should undergo formal visual field assessment. MRI scanning is the imaging modality of choice, with a CT scan for sphenoid septal anatomy if a transphenoidal approach is to be undertaken.

Introduction

Embryology of the Sellar Region

Holding the key position at the center of the skull, the sella turcica ("Turkish saddle") is used as a reference point for many lesions, which may be described as sellar, suprasellar or parasellar. The close proximity of many important structures explains the often striking and characteristic clinical presentation of pathology in this compact region.

The cartilaginous neurocranium is the basal region of the developing skull. In its earliest stage of development, it exists as a narrow condensation of mesenchyme forming a plate that links the anterior rim of the foramen magnum with the most anterior part of the skull. Central to the development of this region is the formation of the body of the sphenoid bone. Subsequently, cartilaginous plates develop on either side of the developing sphenoid body to form the wings and complete the development of the middle cranial fossa.

The greater wings of the sphenoid form the majority of the middle cranial fossa. The lesser wings start at the anterior clinoid processes, passing laterally to become the sphenoid ridge of the pterion. Between the two is the superior orbital fissure. By the middle of the third month of gestation, the skull base is a unified mass of cartilage known as the "chondrocranium".

Subsequent ossification takes place in several centers.

The sella develops as a depression in the body of the sphenoid and is lined with dura and houses the pituitary gland. It is roofed over by the diaphragma, which transmits the infundibulum or pituitary stalk. On either side of the sphenoid bone the cavernous sinuses, made from folded dura, transmit the carotid artery, the maxillary division of the trigeminal nerve, and cranial nerves III, IV and VI.

The cavernous sinuses receive blood from the petrosal and sphenoparietal sinuses in addition to local veins draining the sella. They also interconnect with each other, which explains why petrosal venous sampling seldom localizes the side of a pituitary microadenoma. The posterior articulation of the sphenoid body is with the clivus at the spheno-occipital synchondrosis. Above the sella are situated the optic nerves, chiasm, third ventricle and hypothalamus.

Lesions of the Sellar Region

There are numerous diagnostic possibilities for any lesion in the sellar region (Table 11.1) but the astute clinician or radiologist is aware that there is a high statistical chance of any lesion in the area being a pituitary adenoma. Adenomas in their various forms make up 90–95% of most series. Meningiomas, craniopharyngiomas, Rathke's cleft cysts and internal carotid artery aneurysms make up the commonest of the less frequent lesions. Of the remainder, because their frequency of presentation is considerably less than 1%, it is sufficient to be aware of their existence.

Table 11.1. Differential diagnosis of neoplasms and "tumor-like" lesions of the sellar region

Tumors of adenohypophyseal origin
Pituitary adenoma
Pituitary carcinoma
Tumors of neurohypophyseal origin
Granular cell tumor
Astrocytoma of posterior lobe and/or stalk (rare)
Tumors of non-pituitary origin
Craniopharyngioma
Germ cell tumors
Gliomas (hypothalamic, optic nerve/chiasm, infundibulum)
Meningioma
Hemangiopericytoma
Chordoma
Hemangioblastoma
Lipoma
Giant cell tumor of bone
Chondroma
Fibrous dysplasia
Sarcoma (chondrosarcoma, osteosarcoma, fibrosarcoma)
Post-irradiation sarcomas
Paraganglioma
Schwannoma
Glomangioma
Esthesioneuroblastoma
Primary lymphoma
Melanoma
Cysts, hamartomas and malformations
Rathke's cleft cyst
Arachnoid cyst
Epidermoid cyst
Dermoid cyst
Gangliocytoma
Metastatic tumors
Carcinoma
Plasmacytoma
Lymphoma
Leukemia
Inflammatory conditions
Infection/abscess
Mucocele
Lymphocytic hypophysitis
Sarcoidosis
Langerhans' cell histiocytosis
Giant cell granuloma
Vascular lesions
Internal carotid artery aneurysms
Cavernous angioma

NB. Lesions in italics are discussed in the text.

Pituitary Adenomas

Incidence

The majority of pituitary tumors are asymptomatic, as shown by the discrepancy between the reported prevalence of 200 per million and the post-mortem findings of pituitary tumors in 10–27% of the population [1].

Pathophysiology

The anterior portion (adenohypophysis) of the pituitary gland is thought to develop from endothelium lining the primitive buccal cavity (stomatodeum) passing cranially as Rathke's pouch. This joins a downward projection of the hypothalamus (neurohypophysis), destined to form the posterior lobe and pituitary stalk. This composite gland is distinct and separate from the primitive stomatodeum by the seventh week of gestation and further develops under the influence of the hypothalamus through a series of permissive and specific trans-acting proteins. It is fully functioning by the time of birth but retains considerable plasticity throughout life. Occasionally, cystic remnants of embryological development persist within the pituitary as Rathke's cleft cysts.

The majority of pituitary tumors are benign epithelial neoplasms that develop from adenohypophyseal parenchyma and, as such, resemble normal pituitary histology. In addition to the clinically relevant hormones produced by the pituitary, a number of additional peptides and hypothalamic hormones are known to be produced. These include, amongst many, vasoactive intestinal polypeptide, growth-hormone-releasing hormone (GHRH), somatostatin, substance P and renin. Such findings attest to the functional complexity of the gland.

In addition to the hormone-producing cells, apparently functionally inert or "null" cells are also found in the parenchyma, which also give rise to adenomas. These cells may produce either no hormone or an imperfect form with no biological activity. Multiple-hormone gene and gene receptor products are commonly seen in adenomas; for example, growth hormone (GH) gene expression occurs in 50% of prolactinomas and 30% of corticotrophic adenomas. This functional diversity may explain the occasional response of mixed somatotroph and lactotroph adenomas to dopamine receptor agonists.

The pathogenesis of pituitary adenomas is likely to be multifactorial. As with other neoplasms, the potential mechanisms of oncogenesis fall into three groups:

- Abnormalities of genes regulating growth and development
- Abnormalities of tumor-suppressor genes
- Alterations in the genes controlling programmed cell death

Classification of Pituitary Tumors (Table 11.2)

The new World Health Organization classification divides pituitary tumors simplistically into pituitary adenomas and carcinomas, and the traditional categorization of pituitary adenomas by their tinctorial properties has been abandoned. Ultrastructural appearance, in particular the size of the cytoplasmic granules, also aids in the diagnosis of these tumors. The latter system, however, requires pituitary adenomas to be extensively examined by multiple modalities in specialist centers [2].

Table 11.2. Simplified classification of pituitary adenomas

GH cell adenoma
PRL cell adenoma
Mixed GH cell / PRL cell adenoma
Mammosomatotroph cell adenoma
ACTH cell adenoma
FSH/LH cell adenoma
TSH cell adenoma
Null cell adenoma
Pluri-hormonal adenoma
Unclassified adenoma

The majority of adrenocorticotrophic hormone (ACTH)-producing tumors are microscopic. GH, prolactin (PRL) and ACTH-containing tumors correlate well with endocrinological behavior, whereas the others do not. Pituitary adenomas are also subdivided by virtue of their size into those less than 1 cm in diameter (microadenomas) and those greater than 1 cm (macroadenomas). These divisions usually correlate with presentation – microadenomas presenting with endocrinological manifestations and macroadenomas with compressive effects – although GH-secreting tumors and prolactinomas in males, in particular, may reach substantial size before diagnosis.

Presentation

Pituitary tumors and most other sellar lesions present in four general ways:

- *Endocrinological dysfunction.* This may result from overproduction of the six pituitary hormones: PL, GH, ACTH or, rarely, thyroid-stimulating hormone (TSH) and gonadotrophins, but may also result from underproduction syndromes, such as Addisonian crisis or secondary amenorrheas. Specific endocrinopathy will be covered for each tumor type in turn (see below).

- *Mass effect on adjacent structures* (Fig. 11.1a and b). Tumors usually compress the optic nerves and chiasm, but occasionally they compress the third nerve, particularly in apoplexy [3] (Fig. 11.2). They may also very occasionally cause hydrocephalus by blocking CSF outflow in the third ventricle.
- *Headache.* This may possibly occur as a result of compression or stretching of the dural lining of the sella or of the diaphragmata, which are innervated by branches of the trigeminal nerve. It is this sudden stimulus that is believed to cause the pain of pituitary apoplexy, which may be so severe as to mimic subarachnoid hemorrhage.
- *Incidental finding.* Tumors may be found during investigation for some other condition. They are now officially known as the "incidentalomas".

Endocrine and visual symptoms are the most common forms of presentation, with headache and incidentalomas being infrequent.

Visual Manifestations

The classic bitemporal field loss is found in chiasmatic compression. Early compression may lead to upper quadrantic defects. This results from inferior chiasmal fiber compression. The

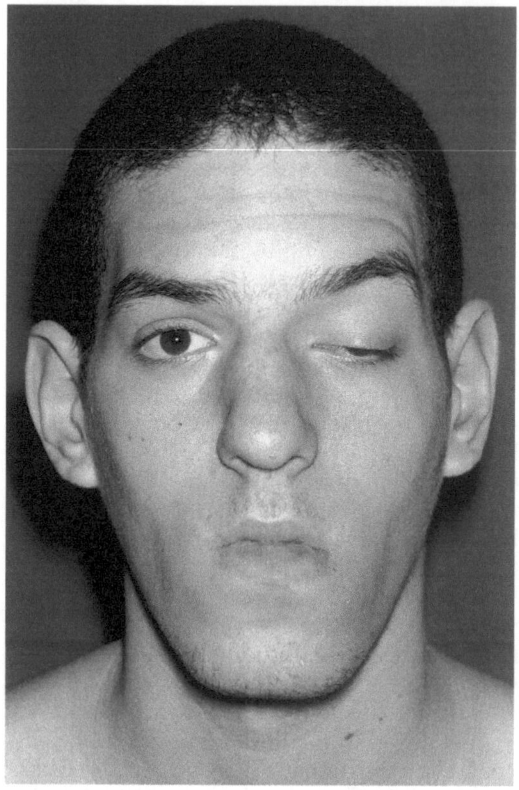

Fig. 11.2. A young man with acromegaly and pituitary apoplexy. The apoplexy has resulted in a left oculomotor nerve palsy.

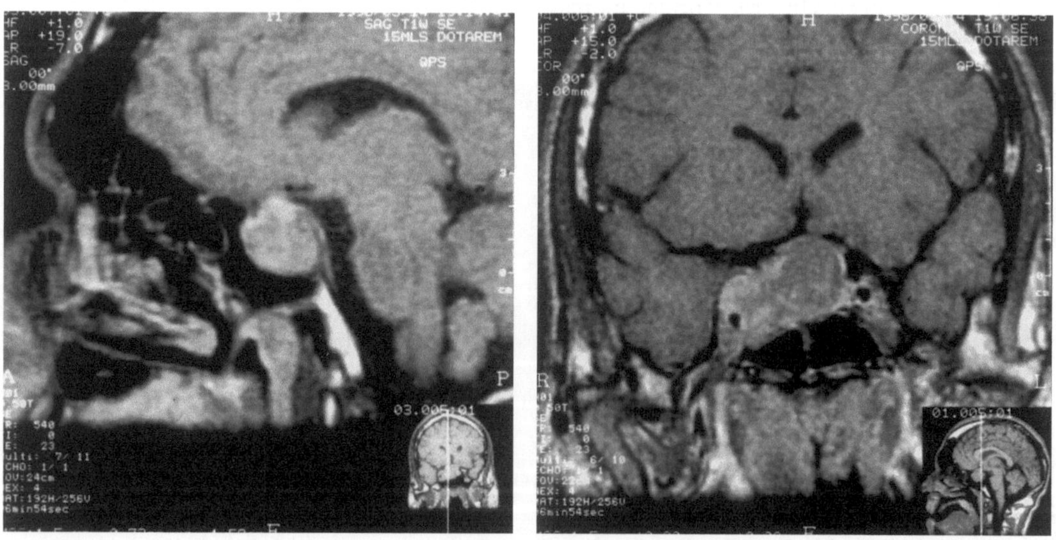

a b

Fig. 11.1. a–b A large pituitary tumor compressing surrounding structures. **a** Sagittal MRI. **b** Coronal MRI.

reverse may occur in lesions compressing the chiasm from above, such as craniopharyngioma. Field loss often begins unilaterally when the intracranial optic nerve is compressed close to its junction with the chiasm. Decussating fibers from the nasal retina of the other eye loop forwards into the optic nerve for a short distance before turning through 180° and passing backwards into the optic tract. Early additional involvement of such decussating fibers is signaled by a small contralateral upper temporal or "junctional" defect. Patients frequently complain of bumping into objects on one or both sides of the contracted visual field, reflecting both unilateral and bitemporal field loss. The affected field is described as absent, or blank, rather than black (blackness is usually a symptom of retinal rather than optic fiber disease). Central vision may be affected by direct compression of the intracranial optic nerve. This may present as a blurring of vision or scotomatous central field defects. This is more common in individuals with a "post-fixed" chiasm - an anatomical variation where the chiasm is situated further back, thus exposing more optic nerve to the compressive effects of an expanding adenoma. If compression has been longstanding, fundoscopy may reveal optic atrophy. Diplopia usually signals lateral compression of the nerves in and around the cavernous sinus either by gradual lateral extension or apoplexy. Optic tract compression in a "pre-fixed" chiasm (the opposite of a post-fixed chiasm) is rare and may produce an homonymous field pattern that may be incongruous.

Visual Testing

All patients with suprasellar extension should have formal eye assessment. This will include:

- *Acuity*, using the Snellen chart.
- *Fields*. For reproducibility, the automated Humphrey field analyzer is the most popular, although in the hands of the expert, the Goldman perimeter is the most accurate and will overcome difficulties of interpretation from true ocular disease.
- *Color vision*, particularly temporal desaturation to red, which will give information on early anterior pathway pathology.

Individual Pituitary Tumor Types, and Related Hormones

Growth-hormone-producing Adenomas

Incidence

This group of tumors includes the somatotroph adenomas, the mammosomatotroph adenomas and the mixed somatotroph–lactotroph adenomas. The prevalence of acromegaly is 30–50 per million and the incidence is five per million.

Clinical Features

Growth hormone, a 191 amino acid protein, is released from the anterior pituitary gland under the stimulatory influence of GHRH. Its release is inhibited by somatostatin, which, in turn, is stimulated by hyperglycaemia. This is useful clinically as somatostatin analogues can be used to suppress GH production and the glucose tolerance test can be used to assess response to surgery (see below). In excess, it causes acromegaly, gigantism or both. Gigantism results from growth hormone excess before epiphyseal closure and frequently it is accompanied by the soft tissue thickening characteristics of acromegaly (Fig. 11.2).

Acromegaly is insidious in onset. The diagnosis may be made coincidentally or because of complications such as carpal tunnel syndrome, diabetes mellitus, hypertension, hypopituitarism or sleep apnea. Chronic hypertension can lead to cerebrovascular disease, coronary artery disease and congestive cardiac failure. Patients with acromegaly also have a higher incidence of malignancy, including colonic polyps, colonic carcinomas and breast carcinoma, than the general population.

Some acromegalic patients have an associated hyperprolactinemia. This has led to the discovery of the mixed monomorphous mammosomatotroph adenomas and the bimorphous somatotroph–lactotroph adenomas mentioned above.

Histology

Grossly the more common macroadenomas are frequently well demarcated. Microadenomas are confined to one of the lateral wings – the principal site of GH-producing cells in the normal gland. Larger tumors often spread outside the sella and invade neighboring tissues. GH levels correlate with tumor size. Mammosomatotroph adenomas are composed of a single cell type that is capable of producing GH and PRL. Mixed lactotroph and somatotroph tumors consist of different, coexisting tumor colonies.

Biochemical Investigations

The biochemical diagnosis is based on the demonstration of a random GH of more than 10 mU/l (5.0 ng/ml), failure of suppression to less than 2.0 mU/l (1.0 ng/ml) following an oral glucose load of 75 g, and an elevated insulin-like growth factor 1 (IGF-1). Very rarely, acromegaly may be due to ectopic GHRH production. Circulating GHRH levels should thus be examined in the case of an acromegalic in whom imaging has failed to demonstrate a pituitary adenoma. Because GH is released in bursts and has a half-life of less than 1 hour, single estimations can be misleading. For this reason some authorities are switching to IGF-1 (somatomedin), with its longer half-life, as a more accurate indication of GH exposure. PRL measurements should always be taken in order to detect cases of mammosomatotroph adenomas, which co-secrete prolactin and which may be sensitive to dopamine agonists such as bromocriptine.

Radiological Investigations

As with most pituitary tumors, MRI is now the investigation of choice. It has excellent spatial resolution and also has the advantage of being able to image in any plane with the acquisition of three-dimensional data sets. These may be used for volumetric analysis and navigational purposes and may be supplemented with MR angiography to assess major vascular relations. The pituitary has no blood–brain barrier, and when gadolinium is given there is an orderly sequence of enhancement of the gland. Within seconds, the infundibulum and posterior pituitary enhance owing to their direct arterial supply. The anterior gland, supplied by the slower portal system, then begins to enhance. Signal intensity becomes homogeneous after about 90s. This is followed by slow washout, which is faster from the posterior pituitary. The cavernous sinuses enhance early, outlining the non-enhancing cranial nerves III and V.

Plain X-rays, in addition to documenting fossa erosion, can give important information about sphenoid pneumatization and septation. This may be of vital importance in transsphenoidal surgery, particularly in adhering to the midline and avoiding lateral structures such as the carotid arteries.

Medical Treatment

The mainstay of treatment is surgery with or without radiotherapy. However, in cases of co-secretion of GH and PRL, 20% will respond to treatment with dopamine agonists. Treatment with the inhibitory somatostatin analogues has been shown to decrease GH secretion. However, its use has been restricted by expense, need for parenteral administration, and tendency to cause cholelithiasis.

Prolactin-secreting Tumors

Incidence

Over half of hormone-producing (functioning) tumors secrete the 198 amino acid lactotroph PRL, the only hormone under inhibitory control by dopamine from the hypothalamus. The clinical syndrome characterized by amenorrhea and galactorrhea was first described by Chiari and colleagues in 1855. PRL was not discovered as a human hormone until 1971.

Clinical Features

Ninety percent of such tumors are in females with secondary amenorrhea as the common presenting feature. Galactorrhea is not always present, perhaps because a permissive level of estrogen may be required for milk production. In men, impotence with decreased sperm count is the endocrinological equivalent. Women, possibly owing to a greater awareness of the effects of hypersecretion, tend to present at a younger age with microadenomas, while men present later in life with visual field disturbances.

Because of the inhibitory control of the hypothalamus, any mass lesion in this area may produce relative hyperprolactinemia. This is termed the “stalk effect”. Generally, when this occurs, the levels are under 3000 mU/l (200 ng/ml). Many physiological events can cause hyperprolactinemia: pregnancy, lactation, stress, physical activity and nipple stimulation. Pharmacological agents such as dopamine receptor agonists (phenothiazines, metoclopramide), tricyclic antidepressants, reserpine and cimetidine may cause increased levels, as may the systemic disorders, hypothyroidism and chronic renal failure.

Histology

Although lactotroph adenomas are recognized as having two variants that are analogous to the two types of somatotroph adenomas (densely and sparsely granulated), sparsely granulated tumors make up the vast majority.

Biochemical Investigations

The diagnosis is made by single blood level measurement and the serum level correlates well with tumor size.

Radiological Investigations

As with all pituitary adenomas, good-quality MRI supplemented with plain films is usually sufficient.

Medical Treatment

First-line treatment of prolactinomas is medical. Dopamine agonists such as bromocriptine and cabergoline will reduce prolactin levels to normal in 85% and 92% respectively and will lead to concomitant shrinkage even in giant tumors, causing visual symptoms. Surgery should be reserved for the dopamine-agonist-intolerant or -resistant patient. Radiotherapy has a disappointing track record in the control of hyperprolactinemia. In patients wishing to conceive, bromocriptine should be continued until a positive pregnancy test, and then stopped. There is no evidence to suggest that bromocriptine is teratogenic. The risk of tumor enlargement in symptomatic patients during pregnancy is 2–5% for treated microadenoma and up to 37% for macroadenoma. Experience would suggest that tumors of less than 5 mm are unlikely to cause problems during pregnancy.

ACTH-producing Tumors

Incidence

ACTH-secreting pituitary tumors are relatively rare, making up only 4% of functioning tumors. It is a dangerous condition with a poor 5-year survival rate if untreated. There is a high female to male ratio of 8:1.

Clinical Features

Lesions associated with excess circulating cortisol produce the manifestations of Cushing's syndrome. This can be due to lesions of the adrenal cortex, to extrapituitary, "ectopic" production of ACTH by neoplasms, to excessive corticotrophin-releasing hormone (CRH) production, and to pituitary-dependent ACTH excess. The latter, termed "Cushing's disease", was recognized and described by Harvey Cushing in 1932. The syndrome is characterized by centripetal obesity, plethoric moon-shaped facies, hirsutism, acne, diabetes, hypertension, muscle weakness, bruising, mental disorders, amenorrhea and osteoporosis, all due to glucocorticoid hypersecretion. Hyperpigmentation is associated with ectopic ACTH production and, in severe cases, with pituitary-dependent ACTH excess. This is because the pro-hormone from which ACTH is eventually cleaved (pro-opiomelanocortin) also contains the amino acid sequences for melanocyte-stimulating hormone. Left untreated, Cushing's disease leads to severe complications.

Histology

The most common cause of pituitary-dependent Cushing's disease is a basophilic microadenoma.

Biochemical Investigations

Loss of diurnal rhythm of plasma (or salivary) cortisol, with increased excretion of urinary free cortisol and lack of overnight suppression of cortisol in response to a low dose (1 mg) of dexamethasone, confirms cortisol overproduction. A combined low-dose and high-dose (8 mg) suppression test usually distinguishes between Cushing's disease and adrenal overproduction. In the former, suppression occurs, but not usually in the case of adrenal adenoma or ectopic production of ACTH. This is because the pituitary adenoma cells still have some susceptibility to negative feedback.

The presence of detectable levels of ACTH suggests ACTH-dependent disease – either pituitary or ectopic. In ectopic ACTH secretion, usually from an oat-cell carcinoma of the bronchus, very high levels of ACTH, pigmentation and hypokalemic alkalosis are found.

If an adenoma is not detected on imaging, then inferior petrosal sinus sampling after CRH injection is justified. With such sampling, peripheral blood ratios of more than 2.0 in the basal state and more than 3.0 following CRH injection are strongly suggestive of a pituitary origin. It does not guarantee the side of the gland where the occult microadenoma may be located because of trans-cavernous sinus veins that allow mixing of the blood from each side. CRH testing can be helpful in differential diagnosis, where a 100 g injection of CRH-41 will produce a normal or exaggerated response in Cushing's disease, but will make no difference in cases of ectopic ACTH secretion and adrenal adenoma.

Radiological Investigations

As with the other pituitary tumors, good-quality MRI and plain films usually suffice, supplemented by petrosal sampling if required.

Medical Treatment

The definitive treatment for Cushing's disease is surgery. For those in whom surgery is not possible or has failed, radiotherapy is usually given. This may be accompanied by adrenalectomy and steroid replacement. Adrenalectomy carries a 20% risk of Nelson's syndrome (pituitary hyperplasia and autonomous production of ACTH) and thus medical rather than surgical adrenalectomy is usually the first choice. The 11β-hydroxylase inhibitor metyrapone is the most commonly used agent. Ketoconazole, which inhibits steroid production and release of ACTH, may also be used, or mitotane, which destroys adrenal tissue. All of these agents have potentially serious side-effects, particularly ketoconazole and mitotane, which my cause liver damage and hypercholesterolemia respectively. Another group of agents acts centrally by enhancing the activity of endogenous inhibitors, or by antagonizing endogenous ACTH stimulators. The most commonly used agents are bromocriptine (dopamine agonist), cyproheptadine (a serotinin antagonist) and the GABA transaminase inhibitor sodium valproate. Responses to these agents are unpredictable and idiosyncratic.

Glycoprotein-secreting Tumors (TSH, FSH and LH)

These hormones are composed of alpha- and beta-chains and differ according to the structure of the latter.

Thyroid-stimulating Hormone (TSH) Adenomas

These are the least common of the overproduction syndromes. There have been only two cases in over 1,000 on the National Hospital pituitary database.

Clinical Features The diagnosis is made on raised TSH in the presence of hyperthyroidism. Pituitary-dependent TSH excess may also be associated with hypothyroidism. These patients have longstanding primary hypothyroidism, which induces hypersecretion of TSH, thyrotroph hyperplasia and even adenoma.

Histology Thyrotroph adenomas are usually large chromophobe tumors with a sinusoidal architecture.

Treatment This is by surgical excision.

Gonadotrophic Adenomas

Although a number of "non-functioning" tumors have gonadotroph expression on immunostaining, the tumors may release only the alpha subunit or have lost the ability to release the hormone. Although it has been suggested that they may be more common in hypogonadal individuals, there is no increase in frequency in menopausal women. Most authorities consider them to be clinically non-functioning tumors.

Clinical Features Although patients with gonadotroph adenomas occasionally present with signs or symptoms of gonadal dysfunction, most present with features of chiasmal compression. Clinically diagnosed gonadotroph tumors occur mainly in middle-aged males. In young women, gonadotrophin-secreting adenomas may masquerade as primary ovarian failure because chronically elevated serum gonadotrophins reversibly inhibit ovarian function.

Histology Gonadotroph adenomas are usually chromophobic tumors with trabecular or papillary architecture and pseudo-rosette formation around blood vessels.

Treatment The treatment is surgical.

Clinically Non-functioning Adenomas

Approximately 25% of pituitary adenomas are clinically non-functioning. Although their presentation is usually visual, they may present with panhypopituitarism or apoplexy. Many of these adenomas may produce excess amounts of the clinically silent alpha subunit unaccompanied by the specific beta unit. Stalk compression may produce a moderate rise in PRL.

Since the tumors are invariably macroadenomas, the most important investigations are of thyroid function and prolactin levels (see below) and visual field and acuity estimation. The treatment is surgical.

Null Cell Adenomas

As their name suggests, these tumors have no specific markers to enable characterization of their cytodifferentiation. Patients are usually older than 40 years and treatment is surgical.

Posterior Pituitary Hormones

ADH overproduction (SIADH) and lack of ADH (diabetes insipidus) are occasionally seen in large pituitary tumors. Diabetes insipidus in the setting of pituitary disease is, however, more usually associated with an inflammatory or infiltrative condition such as lymphocytic hypophysitis or histiocytosis.

Pituitary Carcinomas

Incidence

Primary pituitary carcinoma is extremely rare. Metastatic pituitary deposits, for example from the breast, although rare, are the more common type.

Clinical Presentation

The clinical presentation is usually similar to that of a pituitary adenoma. Although pituitary carcinomas can be associated with acromegaly, hyperprolactinemia or Cushing's disease, they usually present as a pituitary mass.

Investigations

In addition to standard imaging, further investigations should be directed at potential sources of primary tumors such as the breast or lung.

Treatment

This is by surgery to the sella region and other sites, as appropriate, usually followed by radiotherapy.

Pre-operative Investigations and Work-up

Ideally, all pituitary tumors should be managed in specialist centers [4]. In an emergency there are three important tests without which no pituitary surgery should take place. These are:

- *Thyroid function.* Operations on the myxedematous patient severely threaten cardiac function, and also make interpretation of investigation difficult.
- *Prolactin levels.* In macroadenomas with severe visual loss, even short-term dopamine agonist treatment can quickly restore vision, and although tumor shrinkage can lag behind, a better result than with surgery is usually obtained with patience.
- *Adequate imaging.* This should include details of the sphenoid septation if trans-sphenoidal surgery is to be attempted.

Cortisol cover is recommended for all large tumors for safety, as loss of ACTH output is dangerous and may occur postoperatively. Successful surgery for Cushing's tumors demands replacement.

Hydrocortisone 100 mg given with the induc tion of anesthesia is sufficient.

Surgical Aims

Each tumor poses a different problem. Surgery can achieve:

- *Total tumor removal.* This is demanded for true endocrine cure in functioning tumors. Endocrine remission may result from near total removal. For macroadenomas, total tumor removal is probably infrequent.
- *Decompression of the optic chiasm and nerves.* It is surprising how sensitive the chiasm is to small increases in tumor size, but the net result is that vision can recover even when a comparatively small amount of the tumor has been removed.

- *Tumor debulking*. Large invasive tumors are probably best debulked prior to radiotherapy in order to reduce tumor mass.
- *Biopsy*. When radiological diagnosis is uncertain, this may be required to clarify subsequent management.

Surgical Approach

The transsphenoidal approaches are the only rational approaches for microadenomas and usually suffice for tumors with suprasellar extension. They include:

- sub-labial trans-septal approach, as described by Cushing and, later, Hardy
- direct trans-nasal apparoach
- endonasal approach. This approach utilizes elements of both of the above. It was first described by Landolt.
- trans-ethmoidal approach. This approach remains popular in the UK with some otolaryngologists.
- endoscope-assisted surgery.

Transcranial approaches are required for those tumors with complex suprasellar extension, and for those rare tumors with normal fossae but suprasellar extension.

Early Postoperative Management

As the majority of patients will have undergone transsphenoidal surgery, greater detail will be given to these patients [4]. The same principles apply to cranial surgery patients.

General Considerations

Functioning and non-functioning tumors both require rigorous fluid balance, which includes the measurement of urine specific gravity (SG). As a rule, any patient able to concentrate to specific gravity (SG) 1005–1010 does not have diabetes insipidus (DI). DI seldom occurs in the first few hours but should be suspected if the patient is producing more than 1 litre of urine in 4 hours and the serum sodium is above 145 mmol/l. Urinary flow rates alone are insufficient to diagnose the condition, and a number of common perioperative events can produce a relative diuresis. The diagnosis is made on a combination of increased plasma osmolarity >300 mOsmol/kg, hypotonic urine <300 mOsmol/kg and a urine flow of >2 ml/kg/h. If the patient is conscious and has a normal thirst mechanism, DI is seldom dangerous, whereas treatment with DDAVP can lead to hypotonic plasma with all the attendant problems of confusion, epilepsy and even death.

Nasal Packs

These may be removed early. In our unit, they are removed on the first postoperative day.

Antibiotic Prophylaxis

Since two leading authorities with thousands of cases between them do not use them at all, we suggest using the standard local protocol for normal cranial surgery.

Complications

In experienced hands, there should be few complications. Many series have no mortality and many of the complications are both minor and transient. One example, in a series of 67 patients operated on for large tumors causing visual loss, had as complications: five transient CSF leaks, four cases of DI (only one of which persisted for over 3 months), one minor cardiopulmonary event and a period of postoperative confusion. The most serious complications were in three patients who suffered sellar hematomas, one causing temporary worsening of vision and requiring second transsphenoidal surgery.

CSF leaks

Once again, in experienced hands these are relatively rare, even in macroadenoma series. Generally they are dealt with packing and if profuse, a lumbar drain. There continues considerable debate with regard to the need for packing. We use it in cases of obvious leak when fat or fascia lata suffices. For persistent leaks a lumbar drain may be used. It can usually be switched off in 36–48 hours.

Cortisol Replacement

From the postoperative high of 100 mg hydrocortisone twice a day, this may be reduced to 20 mg in the morning and 10 mg in the mid afternoon within 48 hours, and to 15 mg and 5 mg at discharge.

Hyponatremia

This may occasionally occur spontaneously with inappropriate secretion of ADH (SIADH) caused by the non-specific release of ADH from degenerating posterior pituitary neurosecretory terminals 7–14 days following surgery. The condition is managed by fluid restriction.

Specific Postoperative Investigations

Acromegaly

Reduction of growth hormone levels results in an early cessation of sweating. Diabetes mellitus becomes easier to control and many patients can be managed on diet or oral hypoglycemic alone. On the second day, it is useful to carry out a glucose tolerance test with GH levels (i.e. before discharge). GH will fall to below 2 mIU/l, and ideally below 0.5 mIU/l if cured. If the patient is not "cured", early re-exploration is often worthwhile.

Expected cure rates vary between 60% and 80%. If surgery fails, the patient will need to have GH hypersecretion controlled by somatostatin analogues and undergo pituitary irradiation.

Cushing's Tumors

A patient cured of their disease will become dependent on cortisol replacement. If hydrocortisone is not given during the procedure, the cortisol level can be checked the following day, about 24 hours later. If the surgery is successful, cortisol levels will have fallen to below 50, but replacement must start immediately. Surgical failure warrants prompt re-exploration, particularly if an adenoma was found at the first exploration. Most experienced authors in large series report a cure rate of better than 70%. Failed surgical treatment of Cushing's disease requires radiotherapy. Currently, the fashion for bilateral adrenalectomy may be waning in favor of controlling the cortisol hypersecretion with ketoconazole.

Prolactinomas

A single postoperative estimation is sufficient to estimate the success of the procedure. Female patients may regain their menstrual cycle when the level remains a little above normal. Surgical cure rates in prolactinoma series vary between 50–70%. Cure rates for invasive tumours are lower than 20%, with drug treatment and radiotherapy usually required at some stage following surgery.

Long-term Management

This is directed at assessing vision, controlling residual effects of the tumor on endocrine function, and assessing the need for radiation therapy:

Vision is usually improved in about three-quarters of patients [5]. The degree of improvement is related to the severity of the visual loss and, to a lesser extent, the length of the history (as this is notoriously unreliable).

Endocrine function is maintained in the majority (80%) of patients with normal function at the time of surgery, whereas, if this is lost altogether and the patient has panhypopituitarism at the time of surgery, function is not regained.

Because of the ease of imaging, most clinics decide on the need for radiotherapy based on the postoperative MRI approximately 2 months following surgery, when the effects of the surgery in the fossa and sphenoid have lessened. Significant residual tumor usually needs radiotherapy, whereas an empty fossa can be watched. Likewise, most clinicians prefer to leave young patients for as long as possible as radiotherapy leads to pituitary failure in 12–15 years.

Radiotherapy

Conventional radiotherapy will stabilize the majority of large tumors and allow a certain amount of shrinkage. In acromegaly, GH levels usually start to fall within 2–3 years but may only approach normality at 5–8 years. A recent Cushing's series suggests that the response in ACTH-secreting tumors may be better.

Currently, there is a strong pressure to change to conformal techniques – the gamma knife and stereotactic linear accelerator methods (LINAC) – particularly the single dose regimens. The attraction of these techniques is their ability to deliver a higher radiation dose to the tumor, with much greater sparing of normal tissue. Although there is intense interest, their indications, efficacy and complication rates are, to a certain extent, unknown.

Rathke's Cleft Cysts

Incidence

Rathke's cleft cysts (RCCs) are clinically significant but uncommon lesions. They are less common than pituitary tumors. Occasionally they coexist. However, the vast majority must be asymptomatic since they are encountered in 12–33% of normal pituitary glands in routine autopsies [6]. The first symptomatic RCC was reported by Goldzeiher in 1913. By 1977, only 34 cases had been reported. By 1992, this number had more than doubled to 87 cases of histologically confirmed RCC [7]. This recent increase is attributed to the widespread use of MRI.

Pathophysiology

The origin of Rathke's cleft cysts lies in the embryological development of the pituitary gland. During development, a small diverticulum lined with endodermal epithelium – Rathke's pouch – grows from the roof of the primitive buccal cavity or stomatodeum. Simultaneously a small ectodermal process – the infundibulum – grows downwards from the floor of the diencephalon. During the second month of development Rathke's cleft lies in contact with the anterior surface of the infundibulum, and its connection with the oral cavity disappears. Rathke's pouch now flattens itself around the anterior and lateral surface of the infundibulum, forming the pars anterior, pars tuberalis (around the infundibulum) and pars intermedia. These embryological distinctions are rarely seen clinically. The cystic center of Rathke's cleft normally now disappears. It is the persistence and growth of this vesicular space, probably by epithelial proliferation and accumulation of secretions, that give rise to Rathke's cleft cysts. Other theories of RCC formation postulate origin from neuroepithelial tissues or from anterior pituitary cells by reverse metaplasia. The relatively common finding of squamous epithelium in portions of the cyst lining has led to the hypothesis of origin from squamous rests along the craniopharyngeal canal (or hypophyseal-pharyngeal duct). This is a theory that might explain a possible common origin of a spectrum of cystic sellar lesions ranging from RCCs to craniopharyngiomas.

Presentation and Clinical Features

The three main presenting features are similar to pituitary adenomas: endocrine disturbance, headache and visual impairment. In a recent large series of over 28 RCCs [1], the mean age at presentation was 45 years. Clinically, endocrine disturbance was the most common presentation (50%), including amenorrhea (37.5% of female patients), growth retardation, impotence and DI. Biochemically, hypopituitarism, hyperprolactinemia and gonadotrophin deficiencies were the common endocrine findings. Headache was a major feature in 32.1% and visual disturbance in14.3%. Patterns of visual disturbance included central field loss as well as the peripheral field loss expected in sellar region lesions. Four patients had pre-operative DI, a feature that, in the authors' opinion, excludes pituitary adenoma.

Diagnosis

As with other sellar lesions, in addition to the clinical and biochemical features, the mainstay of diagnosis is imaging. CT characteristics include well-defined, homogeneous, non-enhancing sellar lesions without calcification and usually with suprasellar extension. These features, however, are not always specific and can be seen in other sellar lesions such as cystic pituitary adenomas, craniopharyngiomas, epidermoids and arachnoid cysts. The MRI features are also variable, possibly in keeping with the cyst contents, reflecting the number and activity of secretory cells in the wall. Given the variable imaging, the most difficult differential diagnosis remains that between RCCs and craniopharyngiomas. Some would say that the latter is suspected in pre-operative DI, calcification of the cyst wall, and possibly in cases of recurrence, reflecting the behavior of true craniopharyngiomas.

Treatment

The treatment for symptomatic RCCs is surgical. The pre-operative investigations and precautions are similar to those for surgery on pituitary adenomas. The majority can be adequately dealt with via the transsphenoidal route. In this technique the anterior portion of the cyst wall is removed. The remaining cavity is then left to drain into the sphenoid sinus to avoid recurrence. Symptomatic recurrence can be dealt with via a repeat transsphenoidal approach or by using the trans-glabella approach via the frontal sinus.

Postoperative Adjuvant Therapy

Since RCCs are not neoplastic, there is no proven case for either radio- or chemotherapy. Most cases of recurrence are effectively dealt with by repeat surgery.

Outcomes

In our series, recovery of visual acuity and field was seen in 66.6% and 68% of eyes respectively. Postoperative PRL levels declined to normal or near normal in 62.5%, and 20% of those with low pre-operative gonadotrophin levels achieved normal levels after surgery.

Meningiomas

Incidence

The first description of a meningioma was given by a Swiss physician, Felix Plater, in 1664. The first series of "fongueuses de la dure-mère"[8] was described by Antoine Louis in 1774. The term "meningioma" was coined by Cushing in 1922 [9]. Meningiomas comprise 15% of intracranial tumors. They occur predominantly in the fifth and sixth decades, with a peak at around 45 years, and 90% are intracranial. They are more common in females than in males, and, in the case of intracranial tumors, by a ratio of 3:2. Meningiomas are rare tumors in children. Meningiomas of the sellar region comprise approximately 15% of the intracranial total, occurring on the tuberculum sella or planum sphenoidale (suprasellar meningiomas), on the medial sphenoid wing and cavernous sinus (parasellar meningiomas) or, very rarely, within the sella turcica itself. Occasionally they arise from the optic nerve sheath and expand in a dumb-bell fashion, passing from the orbit through the optic canal.

Presentation and Clinical Features of the Sellar Region Meningiomas

Although meningiomas may present with hemorrhage and epilepsy, most exert local pressure effects, and this is especially true of sellar-region tumors.

Tuberculum sellae (suprasellar) meningiomas arise from the meninges of the anterior clinoid or tuberculum sellae. They displace the optic nerves and chiasm upwards or backwards. They present with visual failure involving a central scotoma in conjunction with an asymmetrical bitemporal field loss. Some degree of optic atrophy is usually present and this, in conjunction with lack of papilledema or anosmia, helps to distinguish this tumor from an olfactory groove meningioma. Backward growth of the tumor may impinge upon the hypothalamic-pituitary axis and produce endocrinological deficits.

Cavernous sinus (parasellar) meningiomas present with retro-orbital pain and sixth cranial nerve palsy. The other cranial nerves in the area – III and IV – may also be affected. The first and second division of the fifth cranial nerve may also be involved.

Anterior clinoid and medial third sphenoid wing (parasellar) meningiomas generally present with progressive loss of vision and optic atrophy on examination. There is unilateral loss of acuity due to optic nerve compression; this may be seen in conjunction with an incongruous field loss resulting from an element of chiasmal compression. Tumors growing "en plaque" may invade the cavernous sinus and produce the features mentioned above.

Diagnosis

CT at the base of the skull can be misleading owing to the superimposition of skull density over tumor density and because of artifact. This is particularly true for sellar region tumors. MRI is superior and has the advantage of allowing multiplanar viewing in relation to local structures such as the optic apparatus. MRA and MRV sequences help to assess vascular involvement. This is particularly helpful in sellar region tumors to determine the position of the carotid artery and tributaries in relation to the tumor. Conventional angiography, particularly if pre-operative embolization is envisaged, gives more detailed information and is still the "gold standard".

Treatment

The mainstay of treatment of symptomatic meningiomas is surgery with as complete a resection as possible. In the case of tumors of the sellar region, careful pre-operative planning is essential to assess the extent of possible resection and likelihood of damage to neighboring structures. This is particularly important in the case of cavernous sinus meningiomas, where several questions remain unanswered. Are cavernous sinus meningiomas curable and is the cranial nerve morbidity associated with resection acceptable? Surgeons base these decisions on the degree of involvement of the internal carotid artery. Many authors believe that tumors completely encircling and compressing the artery or invading the cavernous sinus cannot be totally resected without unacceptable morbidity. In such cases a subtotal resection, with or without radiotherapy, may be an effective short-term strategy.

Surgery

Tuberculum Sellae (Suprasellar) Meningiomas

The standard approach is via a frontotemporal or pterional craniotomy, with adequate anterior exposure to allow sufficient subfrontal exposure to gain access to the tumor along the upper part of the sphenoid wing. The side chosen is usually determined by the side on which the optic nerve is most compromised. Another approach, recently adopted in the authors' unit, is via a direct trans-glabella route passing through the frontal sinus. This involves minimal retraction and direct access and is uncomplicated provided that the sinus is adequately repaired. Olfactory tracts are preserved. (This is also suitable for the resection of olfactory groove meningiomas.) The blood supply comes mainly from meningeal vessels over the tuberculum, with little from the carotid. These tuberculum vessels should be taken first as the tumor is undermined. Internal decompression is performed prior to dissection from the vessels and optic apparatus.

Cavernous Sinus and Medial Sphenoid (Parasellar) Meningiomas

The approach for cavernous sinus and medial sphenoid meningiomas is similar to the frontotemporal approach described above, sometimes with orbitozygomatic extension, particularly if the orbit has been invaded. Complete removal of cavernous sinus meningiomas is not usually possible without considerable morbidity. Rather, an aggressive internal decompression is performed in preparation for postoperative radiotherapy should this prove necessary. Medial sphenoid wing meningiomas are more amenable to surgical removal.

Radiotherapy

Reports of tumor response to standard external beam radiotherapy are variable except in the case of malignant tumors and hemangiopericytomas, where there does appear to be some benefit. Recently, attention has been focused on conformal techniques such as stereotactically directed gamma rays ("gamma knife") or X-rays. The object of these techniques is to prevent disease progression while preserving neurological function. Encouraging results have recently been published with progression control in more than 80% [11]. However, the results of studies with longer follow-up times are awaited.

Chemotherapy

Although both estrogen and progesterone receptors have been found in meningiomas, to date attempted hormonal manipulation has met with little success. The observation that hydroxy urea inhibits the growth of meningioma cells in cell culture has led to its use in the treatment of unresectable and recurrent meningiomas of the skull base. In a small study of four patients, three of whom had cavernous sinus meningiomas, the results are encouraging, showing marked regression in three subjects and failure of recurrence of a malignant meningioma in the fourth [12]. The results of larger studies are awaited.

Recurrence

When assessed radiologically, more than 50% of recurrences occur within 5 years and 80% within 10 years. The most important factor in tumor recurrence is the amount of meningioma left behind. Simpson [13] related the recurrence rates to the extent of resection and devised a grading system based upon this (Table 11.3).

Table 11.3. Five-year recurrence rate for meningioma based on the extent of tumor resection

Grade	Description	Recurrence rate at 5 years (%)
1	Complete macroscopic tumor removal with excision of involved dura and bone	9
2	Complete macroscopic tumor removal with coagulation of dura/bone	19
3	Complete macroscopic tumor removal but no treatment of involved dura and bone	29
4	Intracranial tumor left in situ	44
5	Tumor decompression only	–

Hemangiopericytoma

Incidence and Epidemiology

This rare tumor was formerly regarded as a variant of meningioma [14]. However, it has more aggressive behavior and a tendency to recurrence and extraneural metastases.

Unlike meningioma, it occurs more commonly in males.

Pathology

Its macroscopic appearance is that of a red, solitary, firm nodule. It is usually vascular, with a tendency to hemorrhage when cut. Microscopically it is highly cellular, with dense reticulin deposits broken at intervals by "staghorn" vascular spaces. Mitoses are present but, unlike meningiomas, whorls and psammoma bodies are not typical. These features, plus its aggressive behavior, have led it to be classified with the mesenchymal non-meningothelial tumors, such as chondrosarcomas.

Presentation And Clinical Features

Hemangiopericytomas of the sellar region usually present as a suprasellar space-occupying lesion often producing a field defect. Preoperatively they may be mistaken for a pituitary tumor or a suprasellar meningioma. Rarely and confusingly, like the meningiomas, these lesions may also be seen in the ventricular system [15].

Treatment

The diagnosis is not usually made before surgery, but may be suspected at operation owing to its firm consistency and excessive hemorrhage. When the diagnosis is suspected clinically, the lesion is usually approached transcranially. Due to its aggressive behaviour, total excision and radiotherapy is the treatment of choice.

Craniopharyngioma

Incidence and Epidemiology

Craniopharyngiomas comprise approximately 2.5–4% of all intracranial tumors. Although half of these occur in adults, they account for a greater percentage of childhood tumors (5–13%) and are responsible for 54% of sellar region pathology in children. There appears to be a bimodal age distribution, with peaks occurring at ages 5–10 and 55–65 years. There are important differences in clinical presentation, pathology and outcome between children and adults. They remain, whatever the age group, a continuing challenge for the neurosurgeon, endocrinologist and radiotherapist.

Pathophysiology

In common with other sellar region lesions generally and with Rathke's cleft cysts in particular, it seems likely that the origin of these lesions lies, at least in part, in disordered embryogenesis. In 1899, Mott and Barret [16] were the first to appreciate that these sellar and parasellar epithelial tumors might arise from the hypophyseal duct or Rathke's pouch. Subsequently, craniopharyngiomas have been discovered along the path of development of Rathke's pouch from the pharynx to the sella. However, the pathology of RCCs and craniopharyngiomas differs and this might reflect the differing ability of squamous cell rests to undergo neoplastic change and form a craniopharyngioma or to persist as a simple cyst. The pathology is further complicated by the observation that certain craniopharyngiomas, particularly those presenting in childhood, resemble both adamantinomas or tooth bud tumors of the jaw and odontogenic cysts [17]. This raises the possibility of two separate tumor types, with the adult craniopharyngioma arising from squamous metaplasia of pituitary cells later in life. This would help to explain the differences seen in clinical presentation and response to treatment.

Most craniopharyngiomas appear near the infundibular stalk, distorting the surrounding anatomy and eventually obliterating the suprasellar cisterns.

Morphologically these lesions vary from predominantly solid to cystic. Mixed solid and cystic lesions are more common in pediatric series. Predominantly cystic tumors are more common across the age range, with predominantly solid lesions in only 10% of pediatric tumors. Cyst walls may be thin or thick structures impregnated with calcium deposits, and cyst fluid is dark green and laden with birefringent cholesterol crystals. Calcification is found in half of adult tumors and virtually all childhood tumors. Often there is a florid glial reaction around the craniopharyngioma, which is most marked around papillary-like tumor projections into the hypothalamus, making manipulation dangerous. Craniopharyngiomas are often adherent to major vessels, the chiasm and hypothalamus. This may preclude total removal.

Presentation and Clinical Features

The clinical presentation varies between children and adults. Craniopharyngiomas are slow-growing tumors and hence may reach considerable size before diagnosis. Children will often tolerate marked visual deterioration and hydrocephalus before they complain. Non-specific symptoms such as poor school performance, poor memory (hypothalamic compression) and disruptive behavior may go unnoticed. The endocrine features are manifest in short stature, delayed puberty, hyperphagia and obesity (this may be a prominent postoperative feature), and other behavioral problems. DI is less common. Adults present mainly with varying degrees of visual failure. Hydrocephalus at presentation is relatively rare, but neurobehavioral syndromes unrelated to hydrocephalus are relatively common, including confusion, dementia and hypersomnia. The most common endocrinopathy in adults is gonadal failure, presenting as secondary amenorrhea in women and loss of libido in males.

Diagnosis

With its high resolution and multiplanar capabilities, MRI in conjunction with MRA is usually the investigation of choice, particularly when looking at the relationship to surrounding anatomy. This is important in deciding upon an operative approach. Evaluation of endocrine function – particularly cortisol, thyroid function and fluid balance – is, of course, mandatory, as is visual assessment.

Treatment

Total resection can be achieved and offers the best chance of cure, but the degree of tumor removal must be tempered by the degree of difficulty envisaged pre-operatively and encountered intraoperatively if formidable postoperative problems are to be avoided. There is a considerable variation between the surgical "hawks" and "doves" in this difficult disease.

Radiological risk factors include involvement of structures above the chiasm, such as the hypothalamus, as well as extensive lateral spread, particularly through the cavernous sinus and surrounding the carotid arteries. The overall management of the pediatric disease has been reviewed in the excellent paper from the Hospital for Sick Children, Great Ormond St, London [18].

Surgical Approach

Symptomatic hydrocephalus must be controlled and this may require a biventricular shunt if the tumor blocks both foramina of Monro.

When choosing a surgical approach (Table 11.4), there are several factors to consider: firstly the size, secondly whether or not it is cystic, and thirdly, the relationship to surrounding structures, namely the hypothalamus, third ventricle, optic pathways, pituitary and stalk, vessels, brainstem, dura and CSF pathways. In cranial approaches, the position of the chiasm, which is often pre-fixed, and the shape and laterality of the tumor must also be taken into consideration.

If the lesion is confined to the sella, or has moderate suprasellar extension but remains mainly midline, then a transsphenoidal approach may be attempted, particularly if cystic. Equally a subfrontal or pterional approach may be used (with or without orbitozygomatic extension), particularly if there is lateral extension.

In a cooperative study involving 415 patients [19], subfrontal routes were used in 46%, pterional in 27%, transsphenoidal in 8%,

Table 11.4. Operative approaches for craniopharyngioma

Approach	Advantages	Disadvantages
Extra-axial		
Subfrontal	Good visualization of optic nerves and chiasm Below circle of Willis	Poor visualization of third ventricle mass
Pterional	Below circle of Willis Shortest distance to parasellar region Good visualization of retrosellar region	Unilateral Poor view of contralateral optic nerve
Lamina terminalis	Access to mass in anterior third ventricle	Risk of hypothalamic damage
Trans-axial		
Transsphenoidal	No craniotomy Direct sella view and decompression of inferior surface of chiasm	Unable to see supra and parasellar regions Possible pituitary damage
Transcallosal	Direct approach good third ventricle view	Divides corpus callosum Risk of fornix damage Poor view of sella
Transcortical	Good view of ventricular system Risk of postop seizures Poor sella view	Requires hydrocephalus

transventricular in 3%, subtemporal in 2.6% and transcallosal in 0.7%. Anterior approaches allow opening of the lamina terminalis and possible removal of tumors situated wholly or partly within the third ventricle. Transcallosal and transventricular approaches also give good ventricular access, but limited suprasellar access. Some surgeons attempt to solve this with a simultaneous and additional pterional craniotomy. We have also used a trans-glabella approach.

Postoperative Morbidity

Most patients experience anterior and posterior pituitary endocrine deficits postoperatively, with less than 10% having normal endocrine function. Growth hormone deficiency is usually present, as is DI. Hyperphagia and obesity also occur and are attributed to hypothalamic damage. Choux cites the predictive factors in postoperative morbidity as: age less than 5 years, severe hydrocephalus, pre-operative hypothalamic disturbance, large tumors over 3.5 cm and intraoperative complications [19].

Surgical Results

Although total surgical excision gives the best chance for longevity, it can only be achieved in a limited number of cases. Choux quotes 25% in his large cooperative study. However, these results must be set against the appreciable recurrence rate in those having "total" excision of 19.1%.

Other Treatments

Conventional Irradiation

The role of radiation in these tumors remains controversial. The majority of tumors respond and shrink to some extent. Views differ as to the long-term effectiveness in a disease in which the behavior is, in any case, notoriously difficult to predict [20]. Although efficacious, its consequences may be severe, particularly in children.

Stereotactic Radiotherapy

Although its use is becoming more widespread and with some encouraging results [21], the results of large series with longer follow-up are awaited.

Intracavity Brachytherapy and Chemotherapy

Beta emitters have mainly been used, such as gold-198 and yttrium-90. These are implanted stereotactically. Some success is claimed, particularly in the reduction in size of cystic lesions. The cytotoxic bleomycin has also been introduced into cystic craniopharyngiomas via an Ommaya reservoir. This has also produced favorable results, but has yet to become a definitive treatment.

Key Points

- *The majority of sellar and parasellar tumors are pituitary adenomas or meningiomas.*
- *Pituitary tumors usually present with endocrine or visual disturbances, or both.*
- *A PRL estimation is essential prior to surgery since prolactinomas can usually be treated medically.*
- *Sellar region meningiomas present with local pressure effects, and surgical resection is the treatment of choice.*
- *Craniopharyngiomas and Rathke's cleft cysts probably have a common embryological origin.*

References

1. Kontogeorgos G, Kovacs K, Horvath E, Sheithauer BW. Multiple adenomas of the human pituitary: a retrospective autopsy study with clinical implications. J Neurosurg 1991;74:243–7.
2. Wass JAH et al. Pituitary tumours: recommendations for service provision and guidelines for management of patients. J R Coll Physicians Lond 1997;31:628–36.
3. Thompson D, Powell MP, Foster O. Atypical presentation of vascular events in pituitary tumours: "non-apoplectic" pituitary apoplexy. J Neurol Neurosurg Psychiatry 1994;57:1441–2.
4. Powell MP, Lightman SL. The management of pituitary tumours; a handbook. London: Churchill Livingstone, 1996.
5. Powell MP. The recovery of vision following transsphenoidal surgery for pituitary adenomas. Br J Neurosurg 1995;6:367–73.
6. El-Mahady, W Powell M. Transsphenoidal management of 28 symptomatic Rathke's cleft cysts, with special reference to visual and hormonal recovery. Neurosurgery 1998;42(1):7–17.
7. Ross DA, Norman D, Wilson CB. Radiologic characteristics and results of surgical management of Rathke's cleft cysts in 43 patients. Neurosurgery 1992;30:173–9.
8. Louis A. Memoire sur les tumours fongueuses de la dure-mère. Memoires de l'Academie Royale de Chirurgie (Paris), 1774;5:1–59.
9. Cushing H. The meningiomas (dural endotheliomas): their source and favoured seats of origin. Brain 1922;45:282–316.
10. Gordon DE, Olson C. Meningiomas and fibroblastic neoplasia in calves induced with bovine papilloma virus. Cancer Res 1993;28:2423–31.
11. Hakim R, AlexanderE, Loeffler JS et al. Results of linear accelerator based radiosurgery for intracranial meningiomas. Neurosurgery 1998;42:3.
12. Schrell UHM, Rittig MG, Anders M, Koch UH et al. Hydroxyurea for treatment of unresectable and recurrent meningiomas. Decrease in the size of meningiomas in patients treated with hydroxyurea. J Neurosurg 1997;86:840–44.
13. Simpson D. The recurrence of intracranial meningiomas after surgical removal. J Neurol Neurosurg Psychiatry 1957;20:22–39.
14. Kleihues P, Burger PC, Scheithauer BW. The new WHO classification of brain tumours. Brain Pathol 1993; 3:255–68.
15. Abrahams JM, Forman MS, Lavi E, Goldberg H, Flamm ES. Haemangiopericytoma of the third ventricle. Case report. J Neurosurg 1999(Feb);90(2):359–62.
16. Mott FW, Barret JOW. Three cases of tumours of the third ventricle. Arch Neurol (London) 1899;1:417–40.
17. Bernstein ML, Buchino JJ. The histological similarity between craniopharyngeoma and odontogenic lesions: a reappraisal. Oral Surg 1983;56:502–11.
18. De Ville CJ, Grant DB, Kendall BE, Neville BGR, Stanhope R, Watkins KE et al. Management of childhood craniopharyngeoma: can the morbidity of radical surgery be predicted? J Neurosurg 1996;85:73–81.
19. Choux M, Lena G. In: Surgery of the third ventricle, 2nd edn. Appuzo M, editor. William & Williams: Baltimore, 1998.
20. Wara WM, Sneed PK, Larson DA. The role of radiation therapy in the treatment of craniopharyngeoma. Pediatr Neurosurg 1994;(suppl 1):98–100.
21. Kobyashi T, Tanaka T, Kida Y. Stereotactic radiosurgery of craniopharyngiomas. Pediatric Neurosurg 1994; (suppl 1):69–74.

12

Meningiomas

James J. Evans, Joung H. Lee, John Suh
and Mladen Golubic

Summary

The epidemiology, pathology, natural history, and recurrence of meningiomas are reviewed, as are treatment options and their indications. Several important surgical concepts are presented, with an emphasis on general principles that apply to resection of meningiomas at most intracranial locations. The role of therapeutic radiation – including gamma-knife radiosurgery, linear accelerator radiosurgery and intensity-modulated radiation therapy – is discussed. A review of current understanding of meningioma tumor biology is presented, as is the possible direction of future therapy.

Introduction

Surgical management of patients with meningiomas is arguably the most rewarding, challenging and, at times, daunting task for a neurosurgeon: rewarding because of the benign nature of most meningiomas, leading to a possibility of providing cure following total removal; challenging because of the tumor's common sites of involvement in proximity to critical neurovascular structures and/or along the skull base, making surgery difficult and highly risky; daunting because of the associated risks of surgery, the tumor's tendency to recur following incomplete (and at times complete) removal, and its frequent involvement of the surrounding skull-base bone, dura and neurovasculature, making complete removal often impossible.

The term "meningioma" was introduced by Cushing in 1922 to clarify the hitherto confusing and numerous histopathological nomenclatures used to describe the tumor. These names have included: "fongueuses de la dure-mère" (Louis 1774), "epithelial cancer" (Bennett 1858), "tumeurs fibro-plastiques" (Lebert 1854), "cylindroma" (Billroth 1856), "epithelioma" (Bouchard 1864), "sarkome der dura mater" (Virchow 1863), "endothelioma" (Golgi 1869), "villous arachnoid tumor" (Cleland 1864), "arachnoid fibroblastoma" (Mallory 1920) and "meningeal fibroblastoma" (Penfield 1932). Whereas the previous names were descriptive based on the tumor's varying appearances, or based on its presumed histiogenesis, the new term "meningioma" was used to simply convey the meningeal involvement. The first report of this fascinating tumor dates back to 1614, and it is credited to Felix Plater of Switzerland. Although there are earlier reports of partial or failed removal of meningiomas, W.W. Keen is credited with the first successful surgical resection of a meningioma in the USA, in 1887.

Surgery continues to be the treatment of choice for most patients with meningiomas. Recent advances in neuroimaging, anesthesia, microsurgery, surgical instrumentation, radiation oncology and skull-base techniques have improved the overall surgical management of patients with meningiomas and their outcome. However, we are still far from providing optimal care to all patients with meningiomas. Ultimately, the future of meningioma treatment will likely evolve through detailed elucidation of tumorigenic mechanisms at the subcellular level coupled with further advances in molecular therapy that will rely upon the re-classification of these tumors based on their genetic profile yet to be determined.

Comprehensive coverage of meningiomas in a single chapter is utterly impossible. Therefore, in this limited space, the epidemiology, pathology, natural history and recurrence of meningiomas are briefly discussed. Then, treatment options, together with their indications, are briefly outlined. Several important surgical concepts are presented, with an emphasis on general principles that apply to resection of meningiomas at most intracranial locations. The role of therapeutic radiation, including various techniques utilized for treatment of meningiomas such as conventional radiation, gamma-knife and linear accelerator radiosurgery, and intensity-modulated radiation therapy, are delineated. Finally, a review of the current understanding of meningioma tumor biology is presented. Possible directions for future therapy implicated by this basic scientific knowledge are also postulated.

Epidemiology

Incidence

Meningiomas account for 15–20% of all intracranial neoplasms, second only to the incidence of primary gliomas [1,2]. Excluding autopsy data, one study concluded that the most common intracranial tumors are gliomas (43%), meningiomas (21%) and pituitary adenomas (17%) [3]. It should be noted that these incidence data represent only those patients with meningiomas that cause neurological symptoms leading to clinical diagnosis and treatment. With recent advances in neuroimaging, many asymptomatic meningiomas are being detected today, raising the true incidence significantly higher than was previously reported. When autopsy data are included, the proportion of meningiomas among common intracranial tumors changes to 40% for meningiomas, 35% for gliomas, and 17% for pituitary adenomas [3]. The incidence of clinically significant meningiomas is approximately 2.3/100,000 population, and about 5.5/100,000 population when autopsy data are included [3]. Such discrepancy between these incidence rates underscores the fact that the majority of meningiomas actually remain asymptomatic and undetected during life. In fact, Nakasu et al. [4] noted that incidental meningiomas are found in as many as 2.3% of autopsy specimens, and that, among people over the age of 60 years undergoing autopsy, 3% are found to have an incidental meningioma.

The male:female ratio ranges from 1:1.4 to 1:2.1 depending on the series, but it is widely accepted to be approximately 1:2. [1,2]. This finding, however, is not necessarily true among blacks, who have been reported to have a fairly even distribution between males and females [5]. The peak age of clinical presentation for all patients with meningiomas is in the sixth decade.

The intracranial distribution of primary meningiomas has been reported by many authors [1,6]. These reports may vary, depending on the type of neuroimaging used and whether autopsy data are included. DeMonte and Al-Mefty [2] summarized the overall intracranial distribution of meningiomas by combining several large reported series, and concluded the following: parasagittal/falcine 25%, convexity 19%, sphenoid ridge 17%, suprasellar (tuberculum) 9%, posterior fossa 8%, olfactory groove 8%, middle fossa/Meckel's cave 4%, tentorial 3%, peri-torcular 3%, lateral ventricle 1–2%, foramen magnum 1–2%, orbit/optic nerve sheath 1–2%.

Meningiomas occur in children, yet they are exceedingly rare, accounting for only 1–4% of all brain tumors in patients less than 18 years old [7]. Furthermore, pediatric meningiomas account for only 1.5–1.8% of all intracranial meningiomas [8]. In children, the male:female ratio is nearly equal or with a slight male predominance [7]. Intraventricular meningiomas are more common in children than in adults, and make up 11% and 3.9% of all meningiomas in these groups, respectively [6]. In addition to this predilection for unusual locations, children are also more likely than adults to harbor aggressive forms of meningiomas, such as atypical and anaplastic variants. A recent paper, however, suggests that malignant meningiomas in young patients may not be quite as frequent as was previously thought [9]. Meningioangiomatosis, a reactive perivascular proliferation of fibroblasts and meningothelial cells which can trap islands of gliotic cortex, is occasionally associated with meningiomas in younger patients, and may be mistaken for brain invasion [9].

The association of meningiomas and head injury has been addressed by many authors, although the reports are mainly anecdotal [1]. In a rather large review, Inskip et al. [10] did not find a significant increase in the incidence rate of meningiomas, gliomas or neurilemmomas in association with head trauma. It is more likely that a portion of the many asymptomatic meningiomas in the general population is simply detected incidentally by routine neuroimaging following head trauma.

Unlike trauma, radiation as a cause of meningioma development has been well documented [1]. In such cases, the meningiomas must meet certain criteria to be considered radiation-induced, such as the tumor location in the field of radiation, pathology distinct from the original neoplasm or condition under treatment, and occurrence after an appropriately long "latent period" following the radiation exposure [1]. Meningiomas have been reported following low-dose radiation exposure for tinea capitis and following high-dose radiation treatment for other central nervous system (CNS) or head and neck neoplasms. The male:female ratio seems to be more equal for radiation-induced meningiomas, in contrast to the female predominance for sporadic intracranial meningiomas in the general population.

Multiple meningiomas are rare. Only 1–9% of all intracranial meningioma patients have multiple lesions [11]. The patient age and tumor locations do not differ significantly from those with single meningiomas, yet there is a distinction among patients with familial syndromes such as neurofibromatosis (NF) who are prone to developing multiple meningiomas at a much younger age. Intracranial meningiomas are far more common in NF-2 than in NF-1, but they have been reported in both syndromes. It is questionable, however, whether meningiomas occur at a greater rate in NF-1 than in the general population. In NF-2, it has been estimated that 50% of all patients develop meningiomas, and 30% of these patients have multiple meningiomas.

Malignant (i.e. anaplastic) meningiomas account for only approximately 1–3% of all meningiomas. One large series of 936 primary intracranial meningiomas revealed that 94.3% were grade I (benign), 4.7% were grade II (atypical) and 1.0% were grade III (anaplastic). Additionally, anaplastic meningiomas occurred in 12% of males and in only 4% of females in that study. The precise definition of "malignant meningioma", however, has recently been a source of debate. Perry et al. found that frank anaplasia and high mitotic activity (20 or more mitoses per high-powered field) were most closely associated with malignant meningiomas. Extracranial metastases from meningiomas have also been considered to be one of the strong indicators of malignancy and have been shown to occur in 11–23% of patients with frankly anaplastic meningiomas. Interestingly, brain invasion, a traditional criterion of malignant meningiomas, has recently been considered as a diagnostic feature that is more common in atypical meningiomas than in anaplastic types.

Spinal meningiomas occur approximately one-tenth as frequently as intracranial meningiomas. Of all intradural extramedullary spinal tumors, meningiomas account for 25% and are second only to schwannomas, which account for nearly 30%. The peak age of presentation for spinal meningiomas occurs between the 5th and 7th decades, but they may be found in patients of any age. The male:female ratio ranges from 1:3 to 1:6, and 80% of all spinal meningiomas are found in the thoracic region [12].

Ectopic meningiomas are exceedingly rare and likely arise from rests of arachnoid tissue trapped in ectopic locations during development. These must be distinguished from the equally rare extracranial metastases of malignant meningiomas that occur in less than 0.1% of all meningiomas. Primary cutaneous meningiomas are the most common and typically occur in the scalp of frontal and occipital regions. Other reported locations of primary ectopic meningiomas include: paranasal sinuses, eyelids, parotid gland, temporalis muscle, temporal bone and zygoma, as well as some distant sites, such as the lungs, mediastinum and adrenal gland.

Lastly, meningiomas have been found in association with several other types of cancer. Due to the fact that meningiomas are relatively common tumors, and mostly benign with many years' survival, a chance of incidental association with other tumors is possible. However, there have been reports of some tumors that seem to have a "more-than-chance" association with meningiomas. Fox [13] compiled several reported series for a total of 52 cases of (non-NF, non-radiation-induced) meningiomas associated with gliomas of various grades, some of which were juxtaposed and some located at distant intracranial sites. Whether there is some common genetic or environmental factor involved in the concurrent development of meningiomas and gliomas, or whether they are entirely coincidental, remains unclear.

There has also been an association between meningiomas and breast cancer, as suggested by several authors. Studies of hormonal receptors as the link have not been conclusive, although meningiomas have been reported to have an increased incidence and growth rate in women during pregnancy, possibly supporting a hormonal role. Other molecular analyses have placed emphasis on the loss of heterozygosity of the long arm of chromosome 22 and have indicated that a tumor suppressor gene associated with breast cancer may exist at the chromosome locus 22q13 [14]. Interestingly, 22q13 is just slightly distal to the NF-2 tumor suppressor gene locus (22q12) implicated in NF-2-associated meningiomas and in about 50% of sporadic meningiomas.

Pathology

Cellular Origin

John Cleland, an anatomy professor in Glasgow in 1864, made an initial observation of two tumors that seemed to take their origin from the arachnoid, not the dura mater [6]. Schmidt, in 1902, and subsequently Cushing & Weed, in 1915, reported similar findings that these tumors seemed to arise from the arachnoid.

Currently, it is thought that meningiomas originate from specialized cells of the arachnoid granulations, called "arachnoid cap cells", but other possibilities include arachnoidal fibroblasts, or meningoblasts that are theoretical precursor cells of the meninges. Whether arachnoid cap cells are derived from the neural crest or the mesoderm remains unclear as cap cells may exhibit both mesenchymal and epithelial characteristics. Factors supporting the origin of meningiomas from arachnoid cap cells, particularly for the meningothelial variety, include histological and ultrastructural similarities between the tumor and cap cells. These include: the formation of whorls by the cells in-vivo and in-vitro, complex intertwining cell processes, the presence of intracellular junctions, named desmosomes, and an abundance of intracellular intermediate filaments that stain positive for vimentin. Fibroblastic and transitional benign varieties may have additional features that are similar to the fibroblasts found in deeper layers of the arachnoid adjacent to the subarachnoid space.

Classification

It is beyond the scope of this chapter to discuss in detail all the pathological subtypes of meningiomas. Instead, a summary of the latest World Health Organization 2000 classification of meningiomas is presented: grade I (low risk of recurrence and aggressive growth) includes meningothelial, fibrous (fibroblastic), transitional (mixed), psammomatous, angiomatous, microcystic, secretory, lymphoplasmacyte-rich and metaplastic meningiomas; grade II (greater likelihood of recurrence and/or aggressive behavior) includes atypical, clear cell and chordoid meningiomas; grade III includes rhabdoid, papillary and anaplastic (malignant) meningiomas, as well as any subtype named above that has a high proliferation index and/or brain invasion.

Natural History

Understanding the Natural History

Understanding of the natural history of any disease is critical as it forms the basis for treatment. In the case of meningiomas, the natural history has not been well established owing to the fact that most meningioma patients in the past presented with sizable tumors that caused neurological symptoms and deficits, requiring surgical removal. When patients were unable to undergo surgery because of their advanced age, failing health or "inoperable" tumor location, most were treated with radiation and/or not amenable to a long-term "natural" follow-up. Therefore, data on patients diagnosed with a meningioma that were followed clinically, without surgical or radiation treatment, have been very limited and mainly anecdotal.

Autopsy data have revealed that there are a significant number of meningiomas that remain asymptomatic and are undetected during life [3,4]. With recent advances and availability of neuroimaging, asymptomatic meningiomas have been increasingly diagnosed over the past two decades, providing an ample opportunity now to study and understand better the natural history of meningiomas. Patients with asymptomatic meningiomas may not, however, represent a cross-section of all meningioma patients because of a possible selection bias toward tumors that have an inherently more benign course. Nevertheless, important information that is currently unavailable may be derived from such studies. Olivero et al. reported 45 females and 15 males, aged 38–84, who were diagnosed with asymptomatic meningiomas. Forty-five of their patients underwent serial clinical and imaging follow-up. Thirty-five patients (78%) had no change in the tumor size (average follow-up 29 months; range 3–72 months), while 10 patients (22%) showed tumor growth (average follow-up 47 months; range 6 months to 15 years). Among the latter group, tumor growth ranged from 0.2 cm/180 months to 1.0 cm/12 months (average growth rate of 0.24 cm/year). Kuratsu et al. [15] reported on 196 asymptomatic meningiomas out of a total of 504 meningiomas diagnosed in a 6-year period. Sixty-three of the asymptomatic meningiomas were followed conservatively with serial imaging studies. Two-thirds of their patients had no change in the tumor size (average follow-up 36.6 months; range 12–96 months), while one-third of them revealed tumor growth (average follow-up 27.8 months; range 12–87 months). Rates of tumor growth were not included in their report. Although the overall incidence of asymptomatic meningiomas was significantly higher among patients older than 70 years compared with younger patients, there were no significant differences in age, sex or initial tumor size between the group with meningiomas that progressed and the group that did not. Conclusions from both of these studies, in addition to the possible selection bias mentioned above, are certainly limited owing to the short length of follow-up. An update of these cohorts in future years is essential and will be more revealing.

Growth Estimates

Another method of approximating the "natural history" of meningiomas is to estimate the mean doubling time of tumor volume (Td). Jaaskelainen et al. [16] determined the Td in a series of 43 patients with meningiomas by following them for recurrence after resection. Individual and mean Tds for their patients were determined by measuring tumor volume on serial imaging studies. They found that the Td was 415 days (range 138–1045) for benign meningiomas, 178 days (range 34–551) for atypical meningiomas, and 205 days (range 30–472) for anaplastic meningiomas. However, these average estimates are derived from wide-ranging values, and significant overlaps exist among the different groups.

By using bromodeoxyuridine (BUdR) labeling and tumor Td determinations, Cho et al. [17] found Tds ranging from 8 to 440 days in eight tumor samples (two benign, four malignant, two hemangiopericytomas). This group also noted a close inverse correlation between the BUdR labeling index and the tumor doubling time. The implications of these findings were that BUdR labeling may supplement histopathological information in estimating prognosis and may be used to calculate the Td before actual recurrence of the tumor. Clearly, such information would be valuable when formulating plans for any additional treatment of residual tumor following subtotal resection or recurrent meningiomas after complete resection.

Although the Td and BUdR studies have provided some insight toward the growth rates of meningiomas, in clinical practice they require at least an operative biopsy to determine the histology and the BUdR labeling index. A novel approach from Shino et al. [18] was to correlate the MIB-1 staining index (SI) with proton magnetic resonance spectroscopy (MRS) data. They reported that "a significant linear correlation was observed between the increased choline:creatine ratio and the MIB-1 SI" and that a high lactate and/or methylene signal suggested a tumor of higher grade. In this manner, proton MRS data may serve in the future as a non-invasive way of predicting the proliferative rate or malignant potential of meningiomas. Further refinement and availability of MRS will be necessary for this technique to be of value in estimating the growth rate, tumor grade or recurrence in clinical practice.

Recurrence

Recurrence of meningiomas after seemingly complete resection, as well as progression after subtotal resection, has been studied for many decades. In a seminal paper by Simpson [19] in 1957, the rate of recurrence was stratified according to the extent of tumor resection and removal or coagulation of the associated dura: grade I – complete surgical resection of the tumor and its dural attachment; grade II – complete surgical resection of the tumor with coagulation of its dural attachment; grade III – complete surgical resection of the tumor without coagulation of its dural attachment; grade IV – partial tumor removal, leaving the dura in situ; and grade V – simple decompression with or without biopsy. In Simpson's series of 265 meningiomas, 55 (21%) had recurrence. The rates of tumor recurrence according to the extent of resection were: grade I, 9%; grade II, 19%; grade III, 29%; grade IV, 44%. Other studies appearing subsequently, with at least 10 years' follow-up, found similar recurrence rates, which depended on the extent of resection. Using Simpson's classification, Melamed et al. [20] reported recurrence rates of: grade I, 8%; grade II, 15%; grade IV, 29%; and grade V, 33%. Similarly, Chan et al. [21] reported recurrence rates as: grade I, 11%; grade II, 22%; grade IV, 33%; and grade V, 100%. Both of these studies confirmed Simpson's initial finding that the extent of meningioma resection is the single most important prognostic factor for tumor recurrence in benign meningiomas [20,21].

In a study of 225 patients, Mirimanoff et al. [22] reported a recurrence-free rate after total resection of 93%, 80% and 68% at 5, 10 and 15 years, respectively. After subtotal resection, however, the progression-free rates were 63%, 45% and 9% at the same time intervals, respectively. They also evaluated tumor location as a factor for recurrence and found that 96% of their convexity meningiomas were totally resected, with a 3% recurrence rate at 5 years. Fifty-eight percent of the parasellar meningiomas in their study were totally excised, with a 5-year recurrence rate of 19%, while only 28% of the sphenoid ridge meningiomas were totally excised, with a 5-year recurrence rate of 34% [22]. Kallio et al. [23] analyzed the surgical outcome of their series of 935 patients in terms of relative survival rate (RSR) following resection. RSR was defined as the ratio of the observed to the expected survival rate (SR). The expected SR was considered to be that for a population identical to the patient group, except for the meningioma. They found no difference between the observed and expected SR of their patients following resection at 3 months (91%) and at 1 year (89%). At 15 years' follow-up, they found a cumulative observed SR of 63%, which was 78% of the expected SR. The RSR was largely dependent on the degree of resection: the RSR at 15 years was 84% following a complete resection (Simpson grades I & II) and 50% following an incomplete resection (Simpson grades III–V) [23]. Overall, several studies have reached the similar conclusions that surgical outcome and recurrence of meningiomas are dependent on the degree of resection. The degree of resection is, in turn, dependent on the tumor location and, therefore, the accessibility of the tumor and the involved dura and bone [22].

Jaaskelainen observed that the following three factors were significantly associated with meningioma recurrence: (1) coagulation of the involved dura instead of removal, (2) attachment of the tumor to bone, and (3) the soft consistency of the tumor. If none of these criteria were present, the recurrence rate at 20 years was 11%, while if one or two of these criteria were present, the recurrence rates were 15–24% and 34–56%, respectively. Although the histological criteria for grading meningiomas have evolved in recent years, Jaaskelainen et al. [24] reported in 1986 that the 5-year recurrence rates following complete resection were 3% for benign, 38% for atypical, and 78% for anaplastic meningiomas. Pathological features associated with a significantly higher rate of recurrence include histological anaplasia, (20 mitoses per 10 high-powered fields, nuclear atypia, and papillary or rhabdoid cellular features. Kakinuma et al. [25] evaluated 182 meningiomas and found that the Ki-67 SI for recurrent meningiomas (14.78 ± 3.17%) was significantly higher than for non-recurrent meningiomas (4.71 ± 1.96%). Similarly, May et al. [26] noted that a proliferative index of (19% on flow cytometry was associated with meningioma recurrence.

Several authors have attempted to find neuroradiological characteristics that can predict recurrence. Mantle et al. [27] reported that the chance of brain invasion and recurrence increased by 20% with each centimeter of brain edema surrounding the meningioma on computed tomography (CT) scanning. Nakasu et al. showed that the "lobulated" or "mushrooming" appearances of meningiomas noted on pre-operative imaging studies correlated with an increased Ki-67 SI and a higher recurrence rate for these tumors. Lobulated tumors showed higher SI (2.85 ± 3.68%) than round tumors (1.06 ± 0.67%). Three of three "mushrooming" type of tumors and seven of 22 (32%) "lobulated" tumors recurred, while only five of 74 (7%) "round" meningiomas recurred following the similar extent of resection for all three groups. The median interval for recurrence was 10 months for "mushrooming" tumors, 82 months for the "lobulated" ones, and 111 months for "round" meningiomas [28].

Management

Pre-operative Evaluation

Patients with meningiomas are often referred to the neurosurgeon after a primary care physician or neurologist has obtained a CT scan of the head for a variety of neurological symptoms. The radiological appearance of meningiomas with this modality of imaging has been well described. Meningiomas are typically isodense on CT before contrast and homogeneously hyperdense following intravenous iodinated contrast. In addition to being inexpensive and convenient, CT offers the advantages of determining the extent of hyperostosis and the degree of tumor calcification, both of which add to the diagnostic accuracy and help the surgeon with surgical planning.

It is, however, becoming more frequent that the initial head scan performed is magnetic resonance imaging (MRI), due to its increasing availability and decreasing cost. MRI is proven to be the gold standard neuroimaging method of detection for meningiomas. MRI with and without gadolinium contrast is necessary to precisely delineate the full extent of the tumor, particularly in the case of skull base tumors that can involve critical neurovascular structures (such as the optic nerve(s) and major intracranial vessels). On T1-weighted MRI, the majority of meningiomas are isointense, while the remainder is slightly hyperintense to grey matter. Contrast-enhanced T1-weighted images reveal dramatic and usually homogeneous enhancement of meningiomas and, often, their associated "dural-tail". On T2-weighted sequences, nearly 50% of all meningiomas are hyperintense, while the other half are isointense to grey matter. T2-weighted sequence is also highly sensitive in delineating the extent of peritumoral edema. Furthermore, utilization of MRI allows the opportunity to obtain MR-angiography (MRA) and/or MR-venography (MRV) in order to better visualize the extent of vascular involvement, particularly the patency of dural sinuses and the encasement of major arteries. Moreover, the contrast-enhanced MRI is essential in detecting any residual or recurrent tumor following surgery.

For large meningiomas, cerebral angiography may be helpful to determine precisely the extent of involvement of the intracranial arteries and their branches, in addition to providing further information regarding the venous anatomy. Also, large tumors may have significant arterial supply from the external carotid and middle meningeal arteries that may be safely embolized during the angiogram. Many posterior fossa meningiomas are fed by vessels not amenable to catheterization or successful embolization. However, in rare instances of successful embolization of deep-seated, large posterior fossa meningiomas, surgery is dramatically facilitated by embolization. Therefore, in the authors' practice, all supratentorial meningiomas larger than 4–5 cm and infratentorial meningiomas larger than 3–4 cm are routinely evaluated for possible embolization.

When the internal carotid artery (ICA) is noted to be completely encased and/or narrowed by the tumor on pre-operative MRI, ipsilateral ICA test balloon occlusion (TBO) may be performed. Such information is helpful as it allows the surgeon to plan the extent of resection around the ICA. For patients passing the TBO, an aggressive tumor resection may be pursued, and in the rare event of intraoperative ICA injury, the surgeon has the options of direct ICA repair, bypass or ICA sacrifice. If a patient does not pass the TBO, however, tumor resection around the ICA may be more conservative in order to prevent a devastating stroke. Alternatively, an arterial bypass may be performed in preparation for an aggressive tumor resection.

New modalities for imaging meningiomas are emerging. Although MRI is very sensitive and the radiological features of meningiomas have been well described, it can lack specificity and a tissue biopsy, at least, is required for definitive diagnosis. There are numerous reports of other lesions that have mimicked meningiomas on imaging, such as lymphoma, plasmacytoma, primary CNS sarcoidosis and metastases from breast, renal and prostate carcinomas. Highly specific neuroimaging is desirable to definitively diagnose meningiomas, or any other CNS lesions, non-invasively. One example of an advance in this area is MRS, which measures tissue levels of compounds such as choline, phosphocreatine/creatine and N-acetylaspartate. The goal of much ongoing research is to find distinct patterns of these compounds that will provide the ability to non-invasively discern the pathology and the histological grade of a neoplasm. Such information may facilitate therapeutic decisions and prognostic determinations prior to resection, or in place of biopsy.

Another type of imaging - octreotide single-photon emission computed tomography (SPECT) - has proven to be very sensitive for detecting meningiomas. Although virtually all meningiomas have octreotide-binding somatostatin receptors, it must be noted that this technique is not specific for meningiomas alone, as other primary and metastatic CNS tumors often express somatostatin receptors. The non-invasive diagnostic specificity for meningiomas is improved when octreotide-SPECT is used in combination with other neuroimaging modalities. Due to its extreme sensitivity, however, octreotide–SPECT is particularly useful for detecting the recurrence of a meningioma following resection. Some centers are even exploring the utility of combining the information from octreotide-SPECT with F-2-fluoro-2-deoxyglucose positron emission tomograhy (FDG-PET) scanning in an attempt to predict non-invasively which tumors will behave more aggressively, but definitive results are forthcoming.

Pre-operative Medical Therapy

Symptomatic patients with a significant amount of peritumoral edema seen on T2-weighted MRI are started on dexamethasone as an outpatient, and surgery is planned within the following 1–2 weeks. Anticonvulsants are started pre-operatively only for patients who present with seizures. Otherwise, a loading dose of phenytoin is given at induction of anesthesia and then therapeutic levels are maintained post-operatively for 1–6 weeks, depending on the tumor size, brain manipulation required during surgery, and the extent of perioperative swelling.

Treatment Options

In general, management options include observation, surgery, radiation alone, or as an adjuvant therapy following surgery. To date, no definitively effective chemotherapeutic agent has been identified or developed. As meningiomas are mostly benign and slowly progressive tumors, emergency intervention is usually not required. Final treatment plans must be individualized for each patient based on the age, overall condition of the patient, tumor location and size, neurological symptoms and deficits caused by the tumor, and the patient's personal wish after a thorough discussion of all available options.

Observation

Surgery is not necessary for every patient with a meningioma. Observation alone, with periodic (usually yearly) follow-up neurological and MR evaluations, is reasonable for elderly patients, especially if they have minimal or no symptoms caused by the tumor. As people are living healthier and longer lives today, the age at which a person is considered "elderly" is debatable. The patient's absolute age is no longer important in the decision-making process in the management of meningiomas; however, it may be reasonable to consider those with less than

10–15 years of remaining life expectancy to be "elderly". In addition, observation may be an appropriate option for the following people regardless of their age: (1) patients with certain skull base meningiomas with minimal or no symptoms (e.g. cavernous sinus meningioma causing mild facial tingling or numbness), (2) patients with incidental small tumors with no surrounding edema, and (3) patients who insist on non-intervention after a thorough discussion of all treatment options. However, these patients must be compliant with the necessary radiographic and neurological follow-up evaluations.

As with other brain tumors, the risks of surgery may vary in direct proportion to the tumor size, while the chances of total resection vary inversely in proportion to the size of meningiomas of most locations. For example, it is quite obvious that removal of small parasaggital tumors without any involvement of the sagittal sinus would be immensely easier compared to the removal of larger ones which commonly invade the sagittal sinus. The same may be said of small clinoidal or tuberculum sella meningiomas before causing optic nerve and ICA involvement, or petrous meningiomas prior to reaching a large size that would encase the basilar artery and compress the brainstem and cranial nerves. Therefore, the initial recommendation of observation must be decided upon carefully, especially in younger patients, taking into consideration the increased potential risks posed in the future by further growth in the tumor size and involvement of nearby critical neurovascular structures.

Surgery

General Principles

Surgery is the treatment of choice for most patients with meningiomas. In patients with benign meningiomas, which comprise approximately 94% of all meningiomas [24], the tumor location largely dictates the extent of resection, which, in turn, determines the tumor recurrence and, ultimately, the patient's survival [2,19,22,24]. Primary goals of surgery include: (1) total resection of the tumor and the involved surrounding bone and dura when possible, and (2) reversal or improvement in neurological deficits/symptoms caused by the tumor. In meningiomas of certain locations, such as the cavernous sinus or petroclival regions where complete resection is not always possible, additional surgical goals may include confirmation of diagnosis and tumor reduction (to less than 3 cm maximum diameter) in preparation for radiosurgery. Given the benign nature of meningiomas and the established efficacy of adjuvant radiation, the goal of total removal must be balanced by the physician's basic credo to "do no harm". When total removal carries a significant risk of morbidity, a small piece of tumor may be left, with further plans of observation followed by re-operation or radiation when the tumor is noted to be growing or causing new symptoms (Fig. 12.1).

Surgical Technique

Meningiomas of different locations require varying surgical approaches that are primarily dictated by anatomical considerations inherent to each particular location. Surgical procedures of many different anatomical regions are discussed in several other chapters in this book. Furthermore, an abundance of excellent descriptions of "standard" techniques and approaches for meningioma surgery is available [2]. This chapter is written not to replace, but to supplement, those previous important writings on the topic. Several key concepts and principles deemed important are reiterated, and new insights and lessons learned by the senior author, based on his personal surgical experience with over 600 meningioma patients, are summarized and presented.

Surgical approaches may vary in meningioma surgery depending on the tumor location and size and the surgeon's personal experience and preference. However, the following basic principles hold for meningioma surgery of most locations:

- Optimal patient positioning, incision and exposure
- Early tumor devascularization
- Internal decompression or extracapsular dissection
- Early localization and preservation of adherent or adjacent neurovasculature
- Removal of involved bone and dura

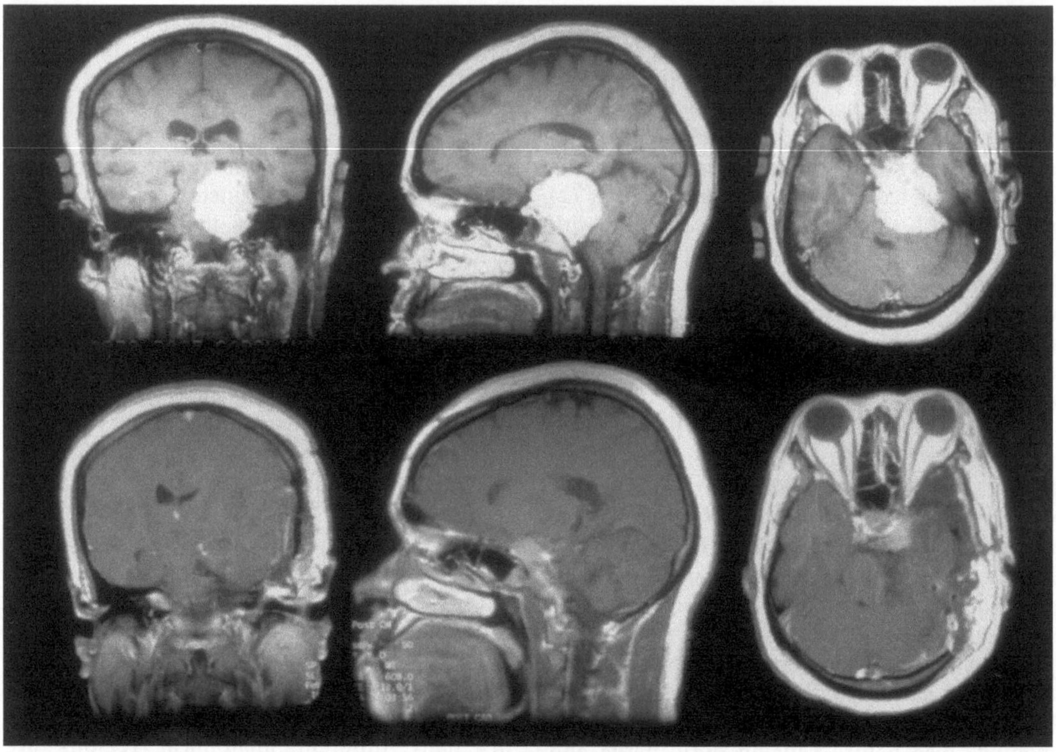

Fig. 12.1. Coronal, sagittal and axial gadolinium-enhanced T1-weighted MR images of a 36-year-old female patient who presented with unsteady gait and cerebellar ataxia (upper left, upper middle and upper right). This large tumor, involving both the petroclival and cavernous sinus regions, was resected in two-staged operations. A small tumor nodule adherent on the intracavernous ICA was left (lower left, lower middle and lower right). Post-operatively, she developed hearing loss and mild hypesthesia in the left V2 and V3 distributions, but her extraocular motility was normal with resolution of her presenting unsteadiness and ataxia. This residual tumor is being observed closely, with plans of gamma knife radiosurgical intervention in the event that the tumor progresses in the future.

Positioning, Incision and Exposure

The patient positioning, appropriate incision placement, and selection of the optimal approach for tumor exposure are the critical elements of successful meningioma surgery. The patient is positioned in such a way that the patient's safety is maximized. Moreover, the ideal position must allow for an approach that provides complete exposure of the tumor and the involved surrounding bone and dura. At the same time, maximal brain relaxation must be achieved by use of gravity and uncompromised venous drainage. The head should be no lower than the level of the heart, regardless of the position selected, and undue severe neck rotation or flexion must be avoided. In addition, surgeon's comfort for the duration of surgery must be maintained. The sitting position, preferred by some neurosurgeons for tumors of the pineal and select posterior fossa locations, places the patient at a higher risk of developing air embolism and the surgeon at an increased level of discomfort. When considering the sitting position for the aforementioned lesions, preoperative sagittal MRI should be reviewed carefully to appreciate the relative size of the posterior fossa and the steepness of the tentorial angle. Patients with a small posterior fossa usually have a low-lying posterior tentorial attachment because of the inferior location of the torcular and inion. This anatomical variation leads to a very steep, nearly vertical tentorial angle, making the infratentorial/supracerebellar approach with the patient seated extremely difficult. Other approaches to be considered in this situation include the transoccipital/transtentorial approach with the patient in the prone position, or the infratentorial/supracerebellar approach with the patient in the modified park-bench (the "Concorde") position (Fig. 12.2).

For superficial tumors (e.g. convexity or parasagittal), the planned scalp flap should contain the tumor in the center, and the patient is positioned so that the tumor is at the highest point. Importantly, the incision must be planned to avoid any visible cosmetic defect or significant compromise to the scalp vascular supply. If a horseshoe-shaped incision is planned, the depth must not exceed the width of the flap. Again, for superficial tumors, the size of the scalp and bone flaps must be sufficiently large so as to allow for maximal exposure of the tumor, the involved bone and dura, as well as the limits of the dural tail as noted on pre-operative MRI scans. With the availability of frameless stereotactic image-guidance systems, the exact extent of the tumor and the dural tail may be fully delineated before surgery. This aids in optimal positioning and placement of incision and craniotomy.

An optimal approach should provide the shortest and most direct route to the tumor without "sacrificing" any normal brain tissue or creating undue brain damage by retraction. The need for retraction is minimized by taking advantage of gravity. For example, for surgery

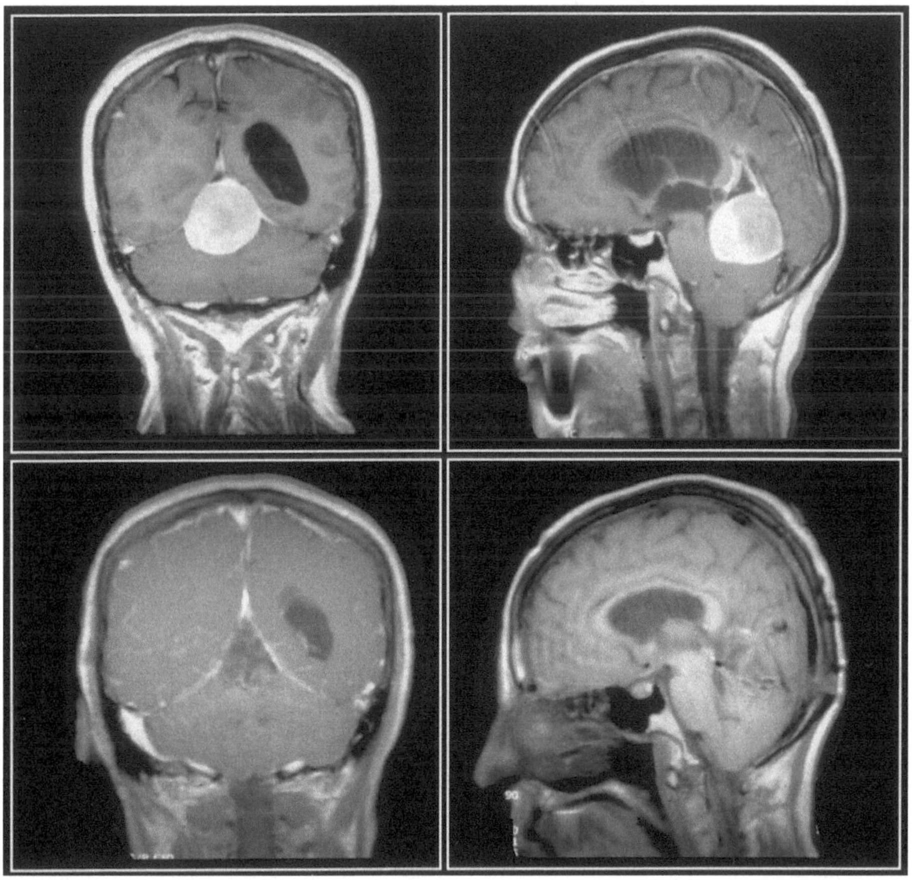

Fig. 12.2. Coronal and sagittal gadolinium-enhanced T1-weighted MR images of a 55-year-old female patient who presented with headache and unsteady gait (upper left and upper right). Because of the small posterior fossa and the near-vertical tentorial angle noted on the sagittal MRI (upper right), the tumor was approached via the occipital interhemispheric/transtentorial route with the patient in the prone position. Following total resection (lower left and lower right), her presenting symptoms resolved completely.

of an olfactory groove meningioma the head can be slightly hyperextended, and for a cerebellopontine-angle lesion the patient may be placed in the lateral position. For large, deep, falcine tumors, the patient's head may be placed with the side of the tumor down and the direction of the sagittal sinus parallel to the operating room floor. In all of these examples, the brain falls away from the tumor and its attachment. In deep-seated tumors, brain retraction may be minimized by use of cerebrospinal fluid (CSF) drainage via either a ventricular drain (in patients with obstructive hydrocephalus) or a lumbar drain. Furthermore, many of the skull base approaches developed over the last two decades, which convert the deep basal meningiomas to more superficial "convexity" lesions by reducing the working distance to the tumor, may reduce the need for brain retraction.

An optimal surgical approach also facilitates surgery by maximizing exposure of the tumor and surrounding structures, thereby minimizing risks of injury to the adjacent neurovascular structures. For example, in surgery of large clinoidal or suprasellar meningiomas, complete removal of the anterior clinoid process (ACP) provides improved access and exposure of the regions surrounding the optic nerve, optic chiasm, ICA and sella. Additionally, by opening the optic sheath as an extension of the dural incision following anterior clinoidectomy, the optic nerve can be decompressed and visualized early, and mobilized safely during surgery, thereby reducing the risk of intraoperative injury to the nerve [29]. This maneuver also expands operative windows, particularly the optico-carotid triangle, facilitating access to tumors in the suprasellar and subchiasmatic regions.

In most situations, there exist a number of options in selecting the patient's position, surgical approach and exposure. The final selection must be based on what is best for the patient and the surgeon, based on the surgeon's knowledge, past experience and preference.

Tumor Devascularization

Many meningiomas can be quite vascular. In addition to utilization of pre-operative embolization when appropriate, early operative devascularization of the tumor reduces blood loss and makes surgery easier. In superficial tumors, upon dural exposure prior to opening the dura, extra time should be expended to coagulate all the dural feeding vessels – most commonly the branches or the main trunk of the middle meningeal artery. In olfactory groove meningiomas, bifrontal craniotomy, preferred by many surgeons, provides early access to the main tumor feeders, i.e. ethmoidal arteries, as they enter the medial anterior fossa floor. In large sphenoid wing meningiomas, which receive significant transdural blood supply, utilizing the extradural skull base technique of orbitosphenoid bone removal obliterates many dural feeders prior to dural opening. Similarly, in petroclival meningiomas, the transpetrosal approach allows the exposed petrous dura and tentorium to be aggressively coagulated and may significantly devascularize the tumor. In falcine or tentorial meningiomas, wide exposure and coagulation of the surrounding falx and tentorium reduce tumor vascularity. Yasargil advocates initial transtumoral devascularization of basal meningiomas by working through a small "window" created in the tumor to reach the blood supply coming through the base. However, this technique may not be suitable for an inexperienced surgeon as there may be a significant risk of injury to unexposed neurovascular structures that may be located on the other side of the tumor.

Internal Decompression and Extracapsular Dissection

Although small meningiomas may be removed "en bloc", internal decompression is a key initial step in actual tumor removal for most meningiomas following adequate exposure and initial devascularization. Internal debulking is carried out until a thin rim of exposed portion of the tumor is remaining. This internal debulking minimizes brain retraction and facilitates extracapsular dissection. Following initial internal decompression, extracapsular dissection is initiated by identifying a layer of arachnoid (maintained in most meningiomas) at the brain–tumor interface. As surgery progresses, rather than increasing brain retraction to expose more of the tumor hidden under the brain, the thinned capsule is pulled towards the center of decompression. Cottonoid patties are placed in the brain–tumor interface as the capsule is being pulled away from the brain, while maintaining the arachnoidal layer intact between the brain and the tumor. As patties are being placed sequentially around the tumor, they are used to gently strip the arachnoid from the tumor capsule, covering the brain and arachnoid together, thereby protecting the brain from surgical trauma. As the remaining tumor capsule is brought into the surgeon's view, any adjacent cranial nerves are carefully dissected, and exposed blood vessels on the capsule surface are thoroughly inspected. Only tumor-feeding vessels are obliterated, preserving and dissecting free those transit vessels that are either passing through the depth of tumor or adherent to the tumor surface. Portions of tumor capsule thus devascularized and completely dissected from the surrounding neurovasculature are further removed in segments. These alternating sequential steps of internal decompression, extracapsular dissection and removal of devascularized capsule are repeated until the entire tumor is removed.

For meningiomas in the clival, petroclival or cerebellopontine-angle regions, the surgeon must analyze the pre-operative MRI scan carefully. First, evidence of surrounding edema in the brainstem noted on T2-weighted scan must be appreciated prior to surgery as this indicates disruption of the arachnoidal layer and the blood–brain barrier. This implies that the surgical plane between the brainstem and tumor may have been obliterated and, therefore, that aggressive resection off the brainstem should be avoided. Second, the basilar artery location in relation to the tumor and brainstem must be noted. Although rare, if the tumor is located between the brainstem and basilar artery or completely encases the artery, this indicates that all the perforating branches of the basilar artery are stretched and course through the tumor. In this situation, an attempt at aggressive tumor removal is likely to result in a brainstem infarct. When the basilar artery is abutting directly on the brainstem, aggressive tumor removal off the brainstem is possible.

During extracapsular dissection, as a rule, no artery or arterial branch is sacrificed except when the vessel is definitely confirmed to be a tumor feeder. Commonly, loops of vessels may be encased by the tumor or may course onto the capsule surface and become adherent. In these situations, the surgeon may initially misinterpret these vessels as tumor feeders. Before concluding that a vessel is a tumor feeder and therefore amenable to obliteration, the afferent and efferent course of the vessel must be fully appreciated. It is very rare for meningiomas to have feeders directly from main intracranial arterial trunks. Therefore, no vessels coming directly off the ICA (in tuberculum sella or clinoidal tumors), basilar artery (in petroclival- and cerebellopontine-angle tumors) or vertebral artery (in foramen magnum meningiomas) should be coagulated. If any appreciable vasospasm occurs while dissecting tumor off arteries, small pieces of gelfoam soaked in papaverine applied directly onto the vessel readily reverse the spasm.

In removing the tumor from cranial nerves, especially the optic nerve, fine vessels feeding the nerves must be preserved. The optic chiasm and intradural optic nerve have main feeders on the inferior surface, and therefore removal of large tumors involving the subchiasmatic and suboptic space must be done carefully so as to preserve these fine vessels. Again, the preserved arachnoid around the cranial nerves facilitates tumor removal and reduces risks of intraoperative neurovascular injury.

Early Localization and Preservation of Adjacent Neurovasculature

Whenever possible, any adjacent or nearby normal neurovasculature (e.g. a cranial nerve or a vessel) should be identified and dissection carried out following this structure into the tumor. For example, in large clinoidal tumors encasing the optic nerve and the ICA, the conventional technique for removal has been first to identify the distal middle cerebral artery branches, and follow these vessels proximally toward the ICA with further tumor removal and dissection. However, until the ICA, and eventually the intradural optic nerve, are located, surgery progresses slowly. More importantly, the risk of intraoperative neurovascular injury persists during surgery as the exact location of the optic nerve and ICA remains unknown to the surgeon, and the optic nerve remains compressed. During this time, any minor surgical trauma caused by retraction, dissection or tumor manipulation may exacerbate compression of the optic nerve, especially against the falciform ligament. To circumvent these critical problems, the optic nerve can be exposed and simultaneously decompressed early in the surgery by unroofing the optic canal, followed by anterior clinoidectomy and opening of the optic sheath [29] (Figs 12.3, 12.4, 12.5). The location of the optic canal, and therefore the intracanalicular segment of the optic nerve, is fairly constant; only the intradural cisternal segment of the optic nerve varies in location, depending on how the tumor causes nerve displacement during its growth. The exposed optic nerve can then be followed from the optic canal proximally, toward the tumor in the intradural location. As tumor resection progresses further, the ICA can be readily found adjacent to the exposed distal intradural segment of the optic nerve. Complete optic sheath opening, along the length of the nerve within the optic canal to the anulus of Zinn, relieves any focal circumferential pressure on the optic nerve contributed by the falciform ligament. Optic nerve decompression thus achieved also leads to reduced intraoperative injury to the nerve, because the force of retraction is then dispersed over a much larger surface area. Moreover, if the tumor eventually recurs, the patient's impending visual deterioration may be delayed as the optic nerve is already decompressed from the surrounding falciform ligament and optic canal. In the senior author's personal experience utilizing the described technique in eight patients presenting with pre-operative visual deterioration from large clinoidal meningiomas, six patients (75%) experienced significant improvement in their vision postoperatively [29].

Whenever possible, no cortical vein or dural sinus is "sacrificed". Although the anterior third of the sagittal sinus is traditionally said to be amenable to obliteration without any significant sequelae, there is a risk of developing significant venous infarcts. Therefore, even in large olfactory groove or planum sphenoidale tumors, rather than routine anterior sagittal sinus obliteration following a bifrontal craniotomy, either a unilateral pterional or a bilateral interhemispheric approach with preservation of sagittal sinus is used whenever possible in the authors' practice. In parasagittal meningiomas, the tumor is removed aggressively, along with the involved segment of sagittal sinus, only when the sinus is completely occluded by the tumor. Otherwise, every effort is made to preserve the sagittal sinus integrity and patency while removing as much tumor as possible. Nearby prominent cortical veins, especially in the posterior two-thirds along the sinus, are preserved as well.

Removal of the Involved Bone and Dura

Following complete tumor removal, the site of tumor origin is carefully inspected. If possible, the involved dura and bone are removed. In tumors of basal locations, the involved bone is drilled using a small diamond burr, which is also quite effective in achieving hemostasis from tumor feeders arising directly from the base of the skull. Involved bone adjacent to paranasal sinuses is aggressively drilled, short of entering the sinus space. Inadvertent opening into paranasal sinuses or mastoid air cells must be recognized and appropriately sealed with muscle/fat graft or bone wax.

In 1983, Dolenc introduced an extensive extradural skull base technique to gain safe entry into the cavernous sinus. The critical steps of this technique, following a routine frontotemporal craniotomy and drilling of the lateral sphenoid wing, include complete bone removal around the superior orbital fissure (SOF), posterior orbitotomy, optic canal unroofing, extradural removal of the ACP, and removal of bone around the foramen rotundum and ovale. Meningiomas of the posterior orbital roof, cavernous sinus (CS), sphenoid wing or orbitosphenoid regions frequently cause hyperostosis of the orbital roof, and the greater and lesser sphenoid wing, including the ACP. For these tumors, the Dolenc approach, with modifications tailored to removal of only the involved bone, is an ideal technique.

In addition, the extensive sphenoid bone removal of the Dolenc approach, when coupled with the extradural exposure of the CS, facilitates removal of the involved dura, especially the portion of temporal dura covering the medial greater sphenoid wing, which simultaneously forms the outer lateral wall of CS. Following extradural bone removal as summarized above, the dural fold at the superolateral aspect of the SOF is sharply cut with microscissors tangential to the temporal dura. The temporal dura forming the outer lateral CS wall is then "peeled" off the underlying inner CS lateral wall. This process of separating the two-layered CS lateral wall is continued laterally and posteriorly until all three divisions of the trigeminal

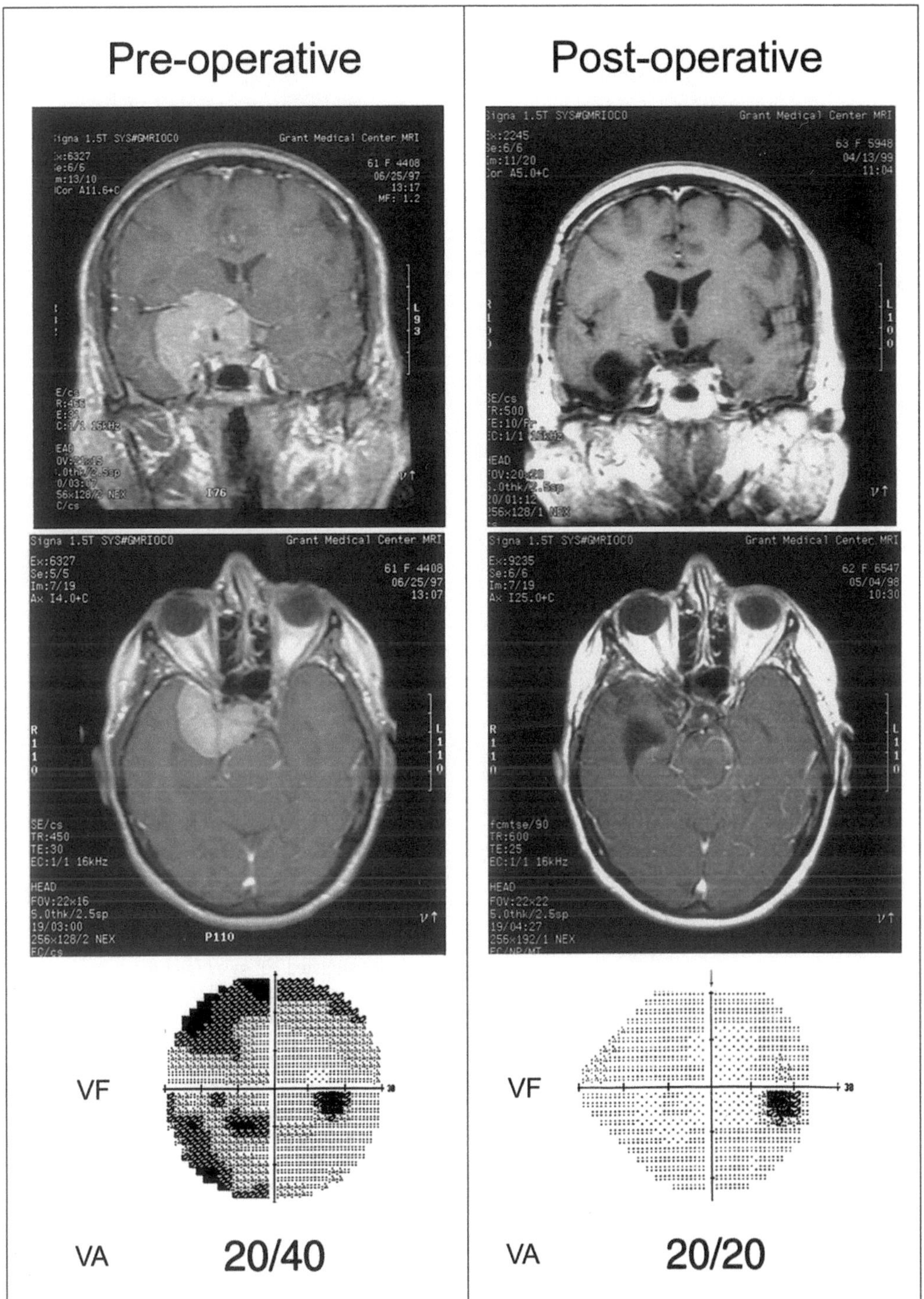

Fig. 12.3. Coronal and axial gadolinium-enhanced T1-weighted MR images of a 61-year-old patient (left upper and left middle) presenting with decreased visual acuity (20/40) and visual field (superior and inferior arcuate defects) (left lower). Following total resection (right upper and right middle), her vision returned to normal (right lower). VA, visual acuity; VF, visual field.

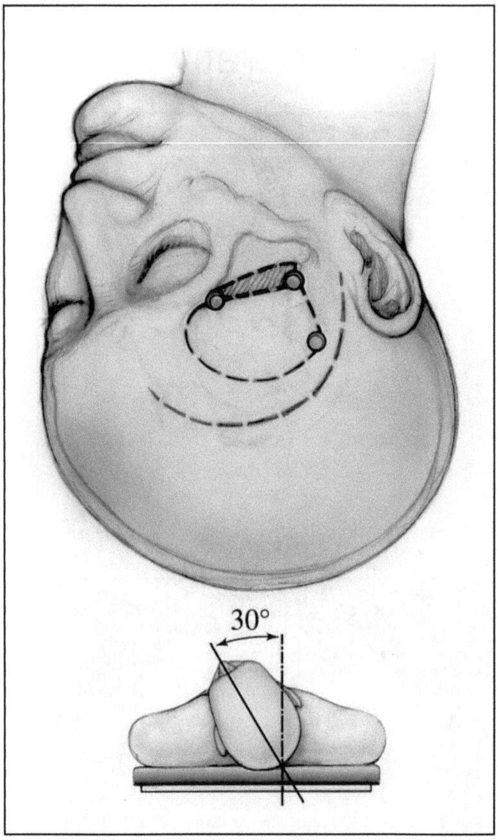

a

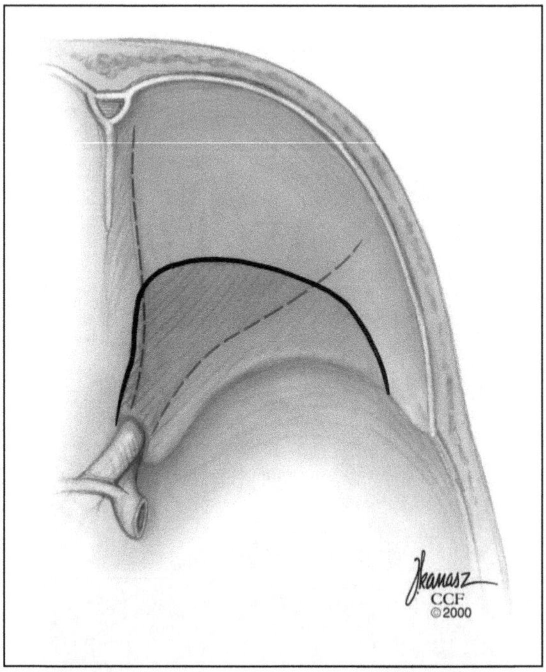

b

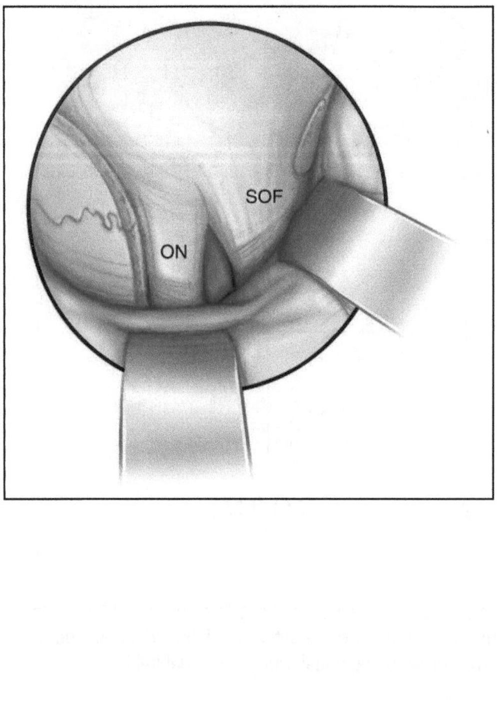

c

Fig. 12.4. **a** Operative position of the patient's head (Mayfield head-clamp not shown). The head of the bed is raised 20° and the patient's head is rotated 30° away from the side of surgery. A standard curvilinear frontotemporal skin incision is made behind the hairline (broken line). A frontotemporal craniotomy is turned (broken line connecting the three burr holes), following which the lateral sphenoid wing is drilled (shaded area). **b** The shaded area depicts the bone removed during the right-sided extradural skull base technique. The removed bone includes the lateral sphenoid wing, posterolateral orbital wall, posterior orbital roof, optic canal roof and ACP. The broken lines outline the orbit. **c** Extradural operative view of the exposed intracanalicular optic nerve and the opened SOF following complete removal of the ACP. ACP, anterior clinoid process;ON, optic nerve; SOF, superior orbital fissure.

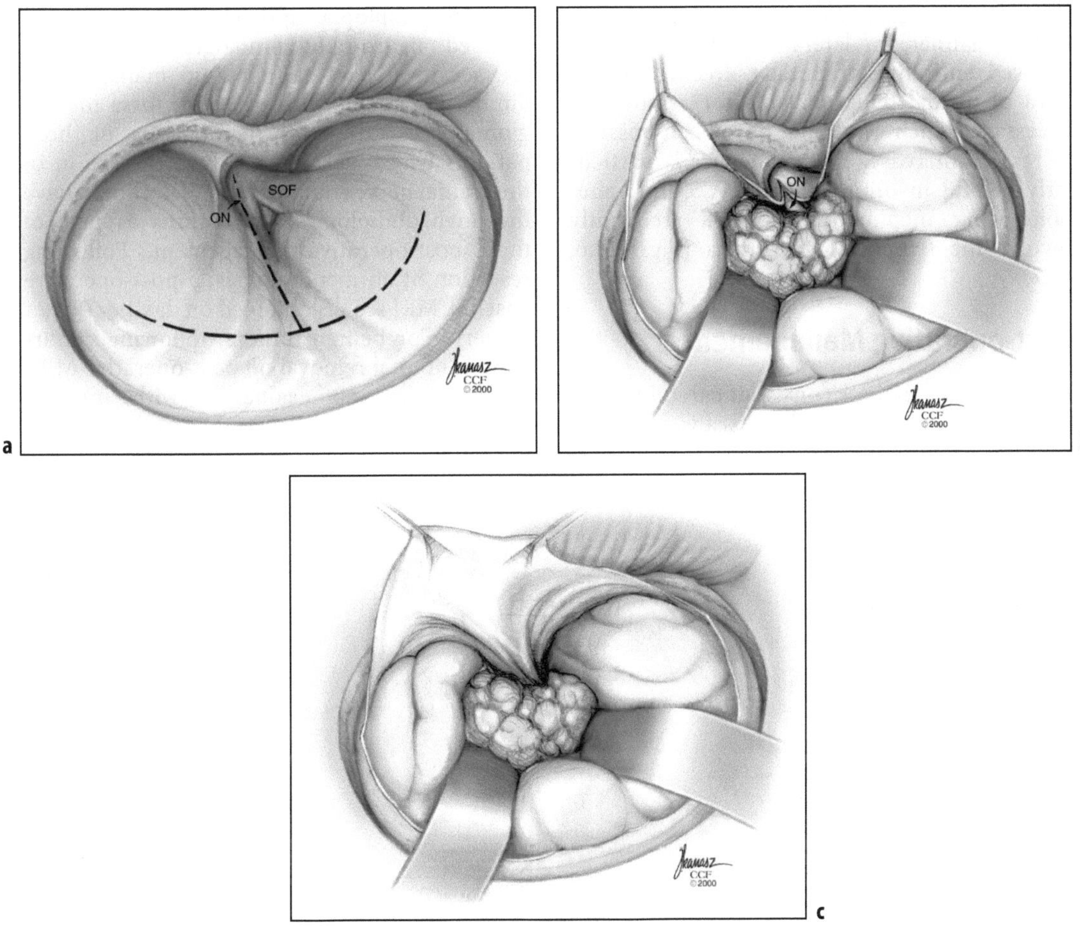

Fig. 12.5. a Extradural view after completion of the skull base technique, including: (1) frontotemporal craniotomy, (2) lateral sphenoid wing removal, (3) posterior orbitotomy, (4) SOF decompression, (5) optic canal unroofing, and (6) extradural anterior clinoidectomy. The dural incision (broken line) is made in two steps: First, a frontotemporal curvilinear opening is created, centered on the Sylvian fissure, followed by a bi-section of the dural flap toward the optic sheath and extending across the falciform ligament and to the anulus of Zinn. **b** The same clinoidal meningioma as depicted in c, following completion of the extradural skull base technique and extending the dural incision into the optic sheath. The optic nerve is readily identified in the exposed optic canal and completely decompressed at the onset of tumor removal. Tumor resection progresses by following the exposed optic nerve proximally. The combination of early optic nerve identification and decompression leads to prevention of intraoperative optic nerve injury. **c** The view of an exposed large clinoidal meningioma after the initial dural opening, using pterional craniotomy and standard frontotemporal dural opening only. Upon tumor exposure, it is noted to be covering the critical neurovascular structures (the optic and oculomotor nerves, ICA). The exact locations of the optic nerve and ICA are unknown to the surgeon, and the optic nerve remains in a compressed state. Tumor resection progresses slowly until the optic nerve and ICA are eventually identified. FL, frontal lobe; ON, optic nerve; SOF, superior orbital fissure; TL, temporal lobe.

nerve and the gasserian ganglion are exposed. In this manner, the lateral aspect of the CS is exposed entirely extradurally, freeing up the dura of medial temporal pole for removal as necessary, which would not have been possible to resect otherwise. This maneuver is particularly helpful in orbitosphenoid, CS and sphenoid wing meningiomas, which frequently involve the temporal polar dura (Figs. 12.6, 12.7).

Post-operative Management

Follow-up evaluations consist of careful neurological examination and MRI scans with and without gadolinium. For patients with pre-operative diplopia and changes in vision, detailed neuro-ophthalmological evaluations are a critical part of follow-up management. Similarly, patients with posterior fossa meningiomas presenting with hearing loss, or those patients whose surgery involved dissection of the cranial nerve complex VII–VIII, should have thorough audiological evaluations as part of their post-operative management. Following resection of all meningiomas, a post-operative baseline MRI scan is obtained on day 1 or 2 after surgery. For benign tumors, following confirmation of total removal on post-operative MRI, further follow-up evaluation with imaging studies are performed every 1–3 years, depending on whether Simpson grade I or II removal

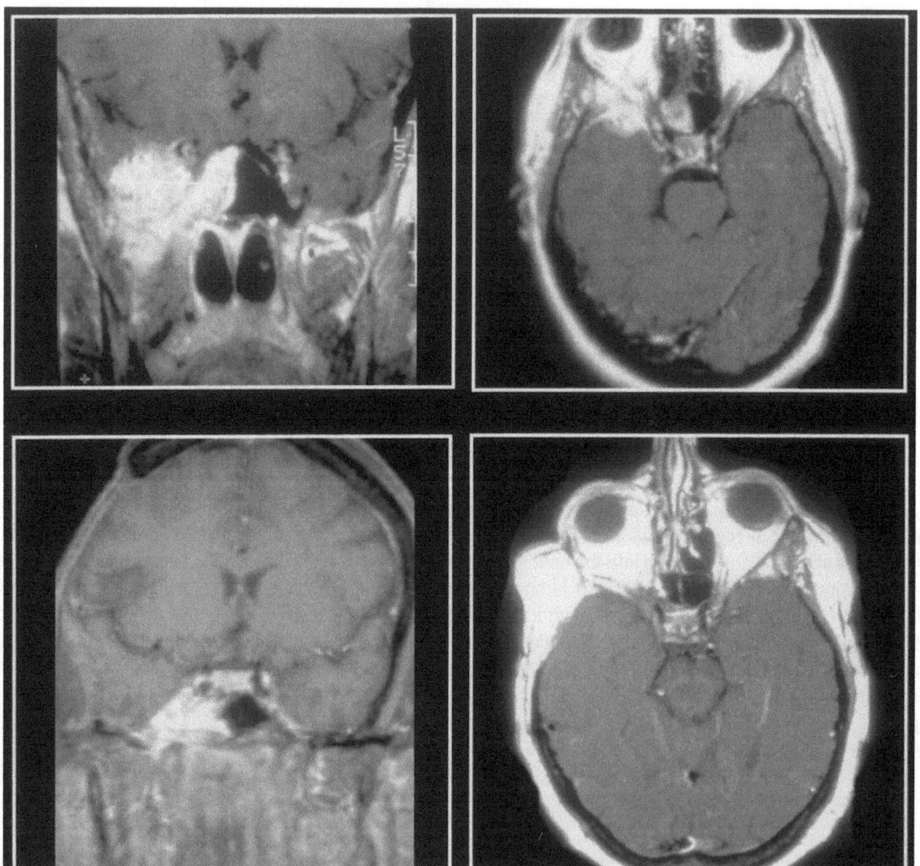

Fig. 12.6. Coronal and axial gadolinium-enhanced T1-weighted MR images obtained in a 47-year-old female patient presenting with a 3-year history of right-sided V2 numbness and mild proptosis (left upper and right upper). This large orbitosphenoid meningioma also extends into the infratemporal fossa and the nasal sinuses. Aggressive subtotal resection was achieved, with the residual tumor in the nasal sinuses only (left lower and right lower).

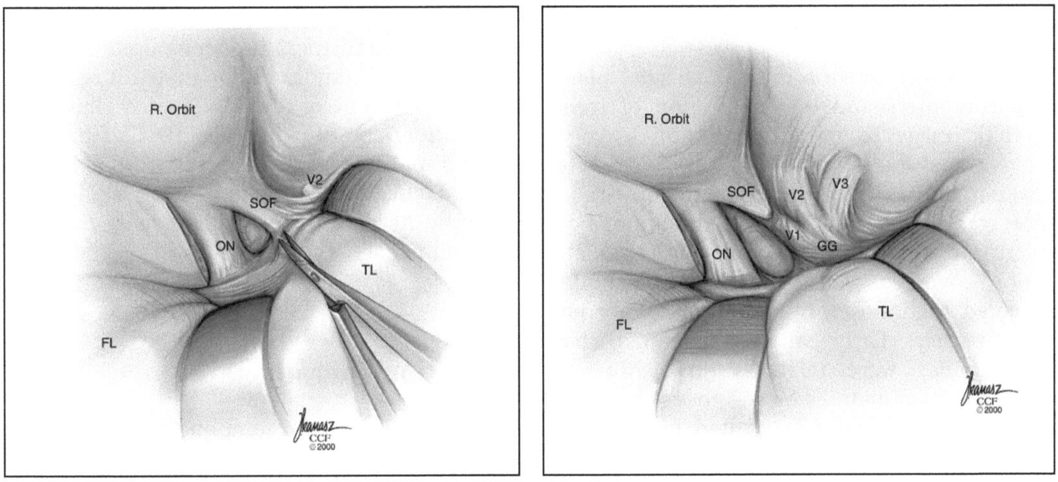

a b

Fig. 12.7. a Following completion of the extradural skull base technique described in Figures 12.4 and 12.5, the process that allows for removal of the sphenoid bone involved by the tumor; the temporal dura forming the outer portion of the two-layered CS wall is "peeled off" the inner CS wall. This is best started by sharply and tangentially cutting the dural fold at the superiolateral aspect of the completely exposed SOF. **b** This "peeling" process is continued posteriorly and laterally until all three divisions of the trigeminal nerve and the gasserian ganglion are exposed. In this manner, the lateral aspect of the CS is exposed entirely extradurally, freeing up the anterior and medial temporal dura, commonly involved by CS or sphenoid wing/orbitosphenoid meningiomas, for aggressive removal along with the rest of the tumor. GG, gasserian ganglion; R, right.

was achieved. Following a subtotal removal, subsequent follow-up with MRI is done every year, with plans of adjuvant radiation if and when there is clinical or radiographic progression of the residual tumor. If the tumor is noted to be clinically and radiographically stable for a few years after initial surgery, the frequency of follow-up may be decreased to every 2–3 years. For atypical meningiomas, after initial post-operative MRI following either subtotal or total removal, subsequent evaluations with MRI are performed every 6 months for the first 2 years. As with benign tumors, radiation is considered in the presence of documented clinical or radiographic progression of the residual tumor. With malignant meningiomas, adjuvant radiation is administered shortly after surgery regardless of the extent of resection. However, if there is any reversible post-operative neurological deficit from brain swelling or cranial nerve manipulation, the timing of radiation therapy should be delayed to allow for adequate recovery. Depending on the extent of resection, follow-up MRI scans are performed every 3–6 months.

Therapeutic Radiation

Role of Radiation Therapy: an Overview

Radiation therapy (RT) represents an important treatment option for patients with benign and malignant brain tumors. Recent advances in computer and imaging technology as well as radiation delivery have greatly improved the radiation oncologist's ability to deliver high doses of radiation to the tumor bed while sparing the surrounding normal tissues. This should decrease complications and perhaps increase control of local disease. Despite these advances, however, the use of radiation therapy in the management of meningiomas remains controversial, partly because these tumors grow slowly and in an unpredictable pattern. Moreover, no randomized clinical trials have been performed to test the optimal timing and effectiveness of radiotherapy in the management of patients with meningiomas. In this section, the currently available radiation-therapy techniques and their results are presented.

Conventional Radiation

Before the introduction of sophisticated planning computers and the integration of radiographic images to optimize radiation delivery, conventional radiation therapy was used to treat patients. With conventional therapy, radiation was delivered not only to the tumor bed but also to a margin (2 cm) to ensure adequate tumor coverage. This approach potentially delivered high doses of radiation to normal brain tissues. Early studies suggested that meningiomas were relatively insensitive to conventional radiation. More modern reports, however, found that RT resulted in excellent local control. Recently, Nutting et al. [30] reported a 5-year progression-free survival rate of 92%, and a 10-year progression-free survival rate of 83%, in 82 patients with benign meningiomas who were treated by surgery followed by external-beam RT.

Despite these impressive results, some have questioned the safety of conventional RT out of a concern over its potential long-term effects, including the induction of malignancies. Thus, researchers have been investigating ways to improve local control and minimize toxicities. This has led to the development of conformal radiation techniques, which enable radiation oncologists to increase the dose and minimize damage to the normal surrounding tissues and structures.

Three-dimensional Conformal Radiotherapy (3D-CRT)

With this type of treatment, three-dimensional computer planning systems are used to deliver radiation that conforms to the shape of the tumor. During the initial planning phase (simulation), a thermoplastic mask is used to immobilize the patient to ensure reproducible, accurate set-ups. CT or MRI is used to localize the tumor. These images are then transferred to a high-speed computer. This allows the physician to contour the normal structures and tumor. A dosimetrist or physicist will then plan the field orientation and optimize the dose distribution. The beams may be shaped using custom-made blocks or collimators. A beam's eye view can be created to determine the orientation of the radiation beams, which helps to tailor the radiation dose around the tumor. Dose–volume histograms can be used to calculate a defined tumor volume that will receive a given percentage of the dose, which allows for the comparison of plans. The 3D-CRT has two main limitations: the accuracy of the results depends heavily on the planner's skills, and multiple iterations are required to develop an optimal plan.

Intensity-modulated Radiation Therapy

Intensity-modulated radiation therapy (IMRT) extends the benefits of 3D-CRT by enabling radiation oncologists to deliver non-uniform beams of radiation. This allows for more conformal delivery of radiation to the tumor and possible dose escalation. The technique uses a computer optimization process that is based on prescribed doses to the target and constraints on normal, sensitive structures. Radiation delivery is further optimized by the use of a multileaf collimator (MLC) or complex compensators, which automatically shape the radiation beam. These two concepts – inverse treatment planning with computer optimization and computer-controlled intensity modulation of the radiation beam – form the basis of IMRT.

One of the more commonly used collimators for IMRT is the multivane intensity-modulating collimator (MIMiC), which attaches to the accessory tray of the linear accelerator (Peacock system, NOMOS Corp., Sewickley, PA). The MIMiC contains 40 small vanes, each of which can alter the intensity of the radiation beam during treatment. The system delivers the radiation dose using arc therapy and segmented fields. The beam can also be modified by using a dynamic MLC that passes across the treatment field or by superimposing a number of static fields. The patient's head can be affixed to the immobilization device either invasively or non-invasively.

Some radiation centers, including the authors' at the Cleveland Clinic, are using IMRT to treat meningiomas in the hopes of achieving excellent local control and minimizing acute and long-term side-effects. No large clinical experiences that have used IMRT to treat meningioma have been reported thus far.

Brachytherapy

Brachytherapy is the implantation of radioactive isotopes into a tumor. This method delivers a high dose of radiation to the tumor while sparing most of the surrounding normal tissue. It may be a good choice for patients with poor health, advanced age, or unresectable or recurrent tumors. The most commonly used brachytherapy method for treating meningiomas is permanent implantation of I-125 seeds. These seeds deliver high levels of radiation for a period of months, which is a potential advantage for treating slow-growing tumors like meningiomas. The seeds can be placed stereotactically or directly sewed or glued into the tumor cavity.

The clinical results of brachytherapy for meningiomas are limited. Patil et al. reported on 26 patients with meningiomas undergoing I-125 seed implant [31]. All 26 patients experienced tumor regression. The authors have treated 14 patients with intracranial meningiomas at the Cleveland Clinic using stereotactic wand guidance. One to five I-125 seeds were placed in each tumor to provide a minimum peripheral dose of 10,000 centigray (cGy) total decay. Overall, the procedure has been well tolerated with encouraging initial results. However, the interest in using brachytherapy as a treatment for meningiomas has waned given the development of radiosurgical and conformal radiation techniques.

Stereotactic Radiosurgery

In 1951, Dr Lars Leksell coined the term "stereotactic radiosurgery" (SRS), which is the delivery of a single, high dose of radiation via stereotactically directed beams into a small target. Presently, three main types of SRS techniques are used: heavy charged particles (proton beam), gamma irradiation from cobalt-60 sources (gamma knife), and high-energy photons from linear accelerators (LINACs). With all of these methods, a stereotactic headframe is used for patient positioning and target determination.

In the past 10 years, SRS has become an increasingly popular option in managing meningioma patients with tumors that are less than 3 cm in diameter. This technique is more advantageous than surgery for a number of reasons. It is minimally invasive, does not require general anesthesia, and can be performed as an outpatient procedure. In addition, it carries a minimal risk of bleeding and infection, and recovery time is minimal. Stereotactic radiosurgery also costs less than conventional surgery.

The gamma knife (Elekta Instruments, Atlanta, GA) is a dedicated machine that performs SRS. The machine uses 201 cobalt-60 sources arranged in a hemispheric dome around the patient's head. Since 1968, more than 100,000 patients with various tumors, vascular malformations and functional disorders have been treated with this device. The goal is to encompass the target area using multiple isocenters or shots to maximize conformality and to minimize the radiation dose to normal surrounding structures. The initial results from gamma knife radiosurgery have been encouraging. Kondziolka et al. reviewed the long-term results of 99 consecutive patients (89% had skull base tumors) who underwent gamma knife radiosurgery for meningiomas between 1987 and 1992 [32]. The patients were assessed using follow-up scans, patient survey, and physician-based evaluations. Using an average tumor dose of 16 Gy (range 9–25 Gy), the authors achieved clinical tumor control in 92 of the patients (93%). Sixty-one (63%) of the tumors decreased in size. Two factors seemed to predict local tumor progression: history of prior resection ($P = 0.02$) and history of multiple meningiomas ($P<0.00001$). The mean actuarial rate of post-radiosurgery complications was 4.85% at 31–120 months. Overall, 96% of the surveyed patients were satisfied with their outcome. Morita et al. [33] reviewed the results of a prospective study of 88 skull base meningiomas treated by gamma knife radiosurgery. With a median follow-up time of 35 months, the progression-free survival rate was 95% [33]. Follow-up scans showed that 68% of the tumors had decreased in size.

Modified and dedicated LINAC-based systems are also commonly used for SRS. To achieve multiple, convergent beams of radiation, the couch and gantry of the LINAC are rotated around the isocenter or target. This achieves the sharp, dose-gradient characteristic of SRS. The results of LINAC radiosurgery seem comparable to those of gamma knife SRS. Shafron [34] reported on 70 patients with 76 meningiomas. After a median follow-up of 23 months, no lesion had enlarged, and 21 out of 48 (44%) had decreased in size after at least 1 year of follow-up. Hakim et al. [35] reported on 106 benign meningiomas that were treated with LINAC radiosurgery. The 5-year actuarial tumor control rate was 89.3%.

Fractionated Radiosurgery (Stereotactic Radiotherapy)

Based on the encouraging results of SRS and the concern about potential normal tissue toxicity from SRS, researchers developed a technique called "fractionated stereotactic radiosurgery" (FSR) or "stereotactic radiotherapy" (SRT). It combines the high-precision technology of SRS with the potential radiobiological benefits of fractionation. Examples of SRT systems include the Gill–Thomas–Cosman frame with a dental plate and strapping system and the bite plate with infrared light-emitting diodes.

Unlike the other methods, which require the use of a minimally invasive head frame, patients can be positioned with a frame that is non-invasive and re-locatable. The initial results of studies that have used SRT to treat meningiomas have been encouraging.

Timing of Radiation Therapy

Although studies have shown that radiation therapy reduces the likelihood for tumor recurrence following subtotal resection and produces results similar to those of complete resection, the timing of radiation therapy is controversial. Given the potential side-effects of radiation and long natural history of this disease, some believe it is reasonable to use radiation therapy only when tumors recur [21]. Others believe that immediate treatment is warranted because any delay may shorten survival, decrease the interval between recurrences, increase the risk of malignant transformation, and decrease the likelihood of salvage with radiation as a result of increasing tumor burden.

For malignant histology, many oncologists recommend immediate radiation treatment (6000 cGy) following surgery, regardless of the extent of resection, owing to the very high rates of local recurrence [21]. For patients with atypical histology, the role of radiation therapy is not as clear, although patients who undergo gross total resection may not require adjuvant radiation. Patients with benign meningiomas who undergo complete resection do not benefit from radiation.

The Gamma Knife Meningioma Study Group evaluated 203 patients with histologically benign parasagittal meningiomas [36]. Based on their results, the authors recommended that patients should receive radiosurgery soon after surgical resection if the procedure leaves behind a residual tumor nodule or neoplastic dural remnant. No prospective, randomized trial has evaluated the timing (immediate vs delayed) of radiation therapy for meningiomas.

In conclusion, radiation therapy seems to play an important role in the overall management of patients with meningiomas. Its use as an adjunctive or primary therapy has thus far been valuable in the multi-modality approach for these patients. Innovative approaches with stereotactic radiosurgery, intensity-modulated radiation therapy, fractionated radiosurgery, and brachytherapy represent promising options. However, because some of these treatments do not have mature results, long-term follow-up is needed before we can make any definitive statements about their effectiveness.

Tumor Biology

Mechanisms of Tumorigenesis

Similar to tumorigenesis in other tissues, development of meningiomas is likely to result from complex interactions between genes and environment. The etiological role of environmental factors in meningioma development has been suggested for ionizing radiation, diet, smoking, head trauma, and occupational exposures to carcinogenic substances. Of these factors, the evidence is convincing only for an association between ionizing radiation and meningiomas. Elevated risk of meningioma development was shown in studies involving patients who received a low-dose radiation therapy for childhood tinea capitis. Meningiomas were also found to occur years after any type of therapeutic cranial irradiation. Moreover, an increased incidence of meningiomas has been recently reported in survivors of atomic bomb explosions. Radiation-induced meningiomas are often aggressive or malignant. They are also likely to be multiple, and they have a high recurrence rate following treatment. Furthermore, it is suggested that they display a distinct pattern of molecular genetic aberrations compared with sporadic meningiomas.

Inherited Susceptibility Factors

In general, germline mutations and metabolic mutations (polymorphisms) are the two groups of genetic alterations that are associated with increased constitutional cancer risk. Both of these groups of inherited susceptibility factors have been implicated in meningioma development. The first group consists of genes that exhibit high penetrance but are present in a low frequency in human populations. The familial occurrence of meningiomas, usually multiple, occurs often in association with NF-2. Overall, more than 50% of NF-2 patients develop meningiomas. The phylogenetically conserved gene that is the target for NF-2 resides on chromosome 22q12 and was cloned in its entirety in 1993. Studies of both meningiomas from NF-2 patients and sporadically occurring meningiomas firmly place the NF-2 tumor suppressor gene in a causal role for tumorigenesis of meningiomas. It was recently shown that NF-2-associated and sporadic meningiomas share a common spectrum and frequency of allelic losses and similar proliferative activity. The NF-2 gene encodes for a protein of 595 amino acids termed "schwannomin" or "merlin". Schwannomin/merlin is a member of the band 4.1 superfamily of proteins that are thought to play crucial roles in linking cell membrane proteins with cytoskeleton, a previously unknown site of activation of tumor suppressor genes in humans.

Werner's syndrome (WS) is one of several rare genetic disorders characterized by genetic instability and premature onset of age-related diseases, such as atherosclerosis and an unusual spectrum of tumors that includes soft-tissue sarcomas, thyroid cancers and meningiomas. The gene mutated in WS patients – WRN gene – encodes for a DNA helicase, an enzyme that helps DNA unwind [37]. The WRN gene appears to function as a key element in resolving aberrant DNA structures that arise from DNA metabolic processes, such as replication, recombination and/or DNA repair, to preserve the genetic integrity of cells. The role of WRN gene product in tumorigenesis of WS-related and sporadic meningiomas, as well as in radiation-induced meningiomas, is unknown.

The second group of inherited susceptibility factors for meningioma consists of genes that exhibit low penetrance but appear in human populations with a high frequency. Glutathione S-transferase and cytochrome P450 are examples of genetic polymorphisms that affect the ability of the body to detoxify carcinogens, including those that can induce meningiomas in laboratory animals. Both GST-T1 null and P450 CYP2D6 poor metabolizer alleles are associated with a significantly elevated risk for meningioma development. Clearly, GST and P450 genes, as well as other polymorphic genes that are involved in the metabolism of carcinogenic compounds found in diet, cigarette smoke and some industrial chemicals, may be promising candidates to explain the gene–environment interactions in meningioma development.

Somatic Alterations in Meningiomas

Cytogenetic studies and analyses of loss of heterozygosity of certain DNA markers in meningiomas suggested the existence of genes that play a role in meningioma development. In spite of the fact that meningiomas are cytogenetically among the best characterized solid tumors in humans, the responsible genes residing in the frequently affected chromosomes remain unidentified. Alterations of the chromosome 22 occur in about 60% of meningiomas, while other cytogenetic alterations such as loss of genetic material on chromosomes 1p, 14q, 10 and 18q, as well as gains on 20q, 12q, 15q and 1q, are less frequent. Some of these changes were associated with progression of meningiomas to more aggressive forms. To date, only the importance of a chromosome 22 deletion in meningioma tumorigenesis has been clearly demonstrated with the cloning of the NF-2 gene.

Tumor Suppressor Genes

NF-2 Tumor Suppressor

Mutational analyses of the NF-2 gene and studies of the NF-2 protein show that the NF-2 protein is often dramatically reduced or absent in about 50% of sporadic meningiomas, including those tumors that do not harbor mutations in the NF-2 gene. Interestingly, alterations in NF-2 gene and protein expression were rarely found in the meningothelial meningioma variant, suggesting the existence of other meningioma susceptibility gene(s).

In spite of intense study of NF-2 gene functions, the molecular mechanisms that enable the NF-2 protein to function as a tumor suppressor are largely unknown. As a member of the band-4.1 superfamily of proteins, the NF-2 protein is considered important in the regulation of actin cytoskeleton and in interactions between cytoplasmic proteins and membranes. A possible physiological role of the NF-2 protein was suggested by its antiproliferative effect on some cell types, including meningioma cells. The NF-2 protein has also been shown to modulate cellular adhesion [38]. Further clues about NF-2 protein functions come from identification of cellular proteins that physically interact with the NF-2 protein. The list of NF-2 protein-interacting molecules includes:

II-spectrin, an actin-binding protein, extracellular matrix receptor β1-integrin, and regulatory cofactor for an Na^+/H^+ exchanger. It is, therefore, possible that mutated/inactivated NF-2 protein contributes to meningioma tumorigenesis by impairing signal transduction from the extracellular matrix and/or ion channels to the cytoskeleton, and thus deleteriously alters molecular pathways that control cell differentiation, growth and survival. In addition, naturally occurring mutant forms of NF-2 protein, but not the full-length NF-2 protein that exhibits growth-suppressive activity, physically interact with a novel coiled-coil protein of unknown function, termed "SCHIP-1" [39]. Clearly, the NF-2 protein is a tumor suppressor that is regulated in a complex manner to control diverse biological functions.

Other Tumor Suppressor Genes

Besides the loss of NF-2 tumor suppressor expression in about 50% of sporadic menigiomas, the expression of another member of the band-4.1 family of proteins was found to be lost in about 60% of these tumors [40]. This novel tumor suppressor gene, DAL-1 (differentially expressed in adenocarcinoma of the lung) from chromosome 18p11.3, appears to be important in the early stages of meningioma tumorigenesis. Recently, a gene from human chromosome 22 that belongs to the glycosyltransferase gene family has been isolated. Abnormal function of that gene may be involved in meningioma tumorigenesis by altering the composition of gangliosides and other glycosylated molecules.

Because of a higher incidence of meningiomas in patients with a history of breast cancer, breast cancer genes BRCA1 and BRCA2 were examined for loss of heterozygosity in meningiomas. However, alterations of these tumor suppressor genes were not detected in meningiomas [41]. Similarly, another tumor suppressor gene, PTEN, was initially suspected as a meningioma tumor suppressor gene because of the gene's location on chromosome 10q, the region with allelic loss commonly associated with malignant progression of meningiomas. The PTEN gene was recently found to be unaltered in meningiomas, and it was therefore ruled out as a meningioma tumor suppressor gene.

Because the loss of p53 tumor suppressor functions is the most common genetic alteration in human cancer, several studies carried out mutational analysis of p53 gene and p53 protein expression levels in meningioma. While the frequency of p53 alterations in meningiomas varies among studies [42], the common finding is that accumulation of p53 protein is associated with meningiomas with a high proliferative potential, i.e. the anaplastic and recurrent tumors [42]. Mutational analysis of tumors with high level of p53 protein expression suggests that overexpressed p53 protein is often not a mutant, but rather a wild-type p53 protein. It was suggested, therefore, that the accumulation of p53 protein and mutations in p53 gene could be used as a potential marker to detect the progression of meningiomas.

Loss of heterozygosity at chromosome 1p, particularly in the 1p36 and 1p34-p32 regions, is frequently detected in meningiomas. Interestingly, the loss of chromosome 1p was shown to be associated with NF-2 gene alterations and more frequent tumor recurrence following surgery. Because of the large size of chromosome 1p, loss of many genes could account for the more aggressive behavior of meningiomas with monosomy of chromosome 1p. Because the tumor suppressor gene p18 resides on chromosome 1p32, its locus was analyzed for loss of heterozygosity in meningioma and excluded as a candidate meningioma gene [43]. Interestingly, the loss of tissue non-specific alkaline phosphatase protein encoded by gene that maps to 1p36.1-p34 was demonstrated in areas of meningioma with monosomy 1p, suggesting its possible role as a candidate tumor suppressor gene in meningiomas [44]. Further genetic research is likely to result in the discovery of novel meningioma-related tumor suppressor gene(s) residing on chromosome 1p and other chromosomes implicated in meningioma tumorigenesis.

Growth Factors and Ras Signal Transduction Pathway

Besides loss of tumor suppressor functions, an enhanced signal transduction through the polypeptide growth factors and protein tyrosine kinase (PTK) receptors is the best-characterized group of molecular alterations that are associated with meningioma tumorigenesis. Growth factors and their receptors, which transduce their signals through Ras GTPase proteins, are overexpressed on the same population of tumor cells compared with normal, precursor leptomeningeal cells. The Ras proto-oncogene family encodes four closely related plasma membrane proteins of 21 kDa that are essential for entry into the mitotic cell cycle, for maintenance of proliferation, and for regulation of differentiation, adhesion molecule expression and cytoskeletal actin organization. Therefore, overexpression of growth factors and their receptors enhances signal transduction through the Ras pathway with a consequent aberration of cellular functions that are considered critically important in meningioma tumorigenesis.

The list of aberrantly overexpressed molecules is long and includes epidermal, platelet-derived, fibroblastic, insulin-like and vascular endothelial growth factors (EGF, PDGF, FGF, IGF, VEGF, respectively) and their PTK receptors. At present, it is not known which growth factors and/or receptors are the most critical in meningioma tumorigenesis. Nevertheless, the expression of VEGF by tumor cells appears to be prognostically relevant. Elevated expression of VEGF is found in most meningiomas, and it correlates with the development of meningioma blood supply from cerebral arteries and emergence of peritumoral brain edema. Further-more, high levels of VEGF expression were recently identified as the most powerful predictor of meningioma recurrence.

The clinical importance of frequent expression of the hepatocyte growth factor (HGF) and c-met, a proto-oncogene that encodes receptor for HGF by meningioma cells, is not known, but HGF and c-met may represent an important link with the NF-2 tumor suppressor pathway. It was recently shown that the HGF-regulated tyrosine kinase substrate physically interacts in vivo and in vitro with NF-2 tumor suppressor protein [45]. At present, it is not clear exactly how the HGF and NF-2 molecular pathways cross-talk. Another line of evidence suggests that the NF-2 protein antiproliferative action may occur downstream of Ras proteins. Overexpression of the NF-2 protein is able to reverse some aspects of the Ras-protein-induced malignant phenotype, such as anchorage-independent growth in a soft agar, and to restore contact inhibition of cell growth.

Sex Hormones

One of the most consistent findings in epidemiological studies of meningiomas is that these tumors are about twice as common in women as in men. The proposed role of sex hormones in meningioma tumorigenesis is further supported by an observation that breast cancer and meningiomas appear to occur together more frequently than would be expected by chance, and by detection of estrogen and progesterone receptors in meningiomas. While it is well recognized that human meningiomas express progesterone receptors, there is still uncertainty about the presence of estrogen receptors in these tumors. However, the use of polymerase chain reaction method, which is more sensitive than the immunohistochemical or ligand binding assays, reveals that both receptors may be present in most meningiomas. At present, it is not clear whether these receptors are functional in meningioma and whether the therapeutic use of progesterone and/or estrogen inhibitors is beneficial. Nevertheless, the presence/absence of progesterone receptors in meningiomas may have prognostic and therapeutic implications. For example, proliferating meningioma cells do not express progesterone receptors, and tumors with a high proliferative index are more likely to express no or low levels of progesterone receptors. In addition, meningiomas that are progesterone-receptor-negative appear to be more likely to recur. Further investigations are required to delineate the definitive significance of sex hormones in meningiomas.

Future Therapy

A more detailed understanding of molecular mechanisms involved in meningioma tumorigenesis has opened the door for new anticancer treatment approaches that are based on the concept of target-specific therapies. Molecular-based treatment strategies targeting the precise molecular abnormalities that create and drive the neoplastic phenotype offer a great hope as future meningioma treatments. These approaches include gene therapy to restore the functions of inactivated NF-2 gene and other meningioma-associated tumor suppressors, and the use of gene therapy or several promising small molecule agents that inhibit signal transduction molecules responsible for overactivation of the growth factor/Ras signaling pathway.

Besides trying to replace a defective tumor suppressor gene with a functional allele, or to deliver genes that can help kill tumor cells, gene therapy technology encompasses many additional applications, such as adoptive immunotherapy, anti-angiogenesis, and anti-telomerase approaches to cancer treatment. For example, virus-mediated delivery was successfully used to introduce functional NF-2 tumor suppressor gene into NF-2-gene-deficient meningioma cell lines. It is likely that such an approach can be used to deliver other meningioma-associated tumor suppressor genes, such as DAL-1 and p53, to target early and late stages of meningioma progression, respectively.

The elevated expression of a large number of polypeptide growth factors and their tyrosine kinase receptors is a hallmark of meningioma tumorigenesis. Many polypeptide growth factors implicated in meningioma tumorigenesis transduce their proliferative signal through Ras proteins. As expected, inhibition of Ras proteins by the adenovirus-mediated transfer of the dominant negative Ras mutant potently suppressed proliferation of exponentially growing and growth-arrested meningioma cells stimulated with serum. As shown in several models, another anti-cancer gene therapy approach to specifically target Ras proteins is to use antisense oligonucleotide inhibitors or antisense ribozymes, catalytic RNA molecules [46,47]. Another attractive molecular target of the growth factor activated Ras pathway is the Raf-1 protein. The application of the antisense oligonucleotide directed against the human Raf-1 kinase (ISIS 3521) has now reached the phase II stage of anti-cancer therapy development. If the evidence for anti-tumor effect is provided, this therapeutic approach may be applied to meningioma treatment in the future.

Anti-angiogenic gene therapy approaches are particularly attractive for meningioma treatment because of the well-documented role of VEGF in meningioma tumorigenesis and tumor recurrence. Targeting of telomerase represents an exciting new approach to cancer therapy. Because telomerase activation occurs frequently in atypical and anaplastic meningiomas, and anti-telomerase gene therapy approaches have been successfully used in animal and tissue culture models for treatment of malignant gliomas and other malignancies, there is no reason to question the applicability of this gene therapy approach to the treatment of meningiomas. The major limiting factor of successful clinical use of gene therapy for treatment of cancer, including meningiomas, is the lack of selectivity and low efficiency of the currently available vector delivery systems. Improved vectors and anti-sense oligonucleotides, and new formulations for enhanced delivery, are likely to circumvent degradation and delivery difficulties and thus improve the clinical application of gene therapy technology.

At present, however, treatment of meningiomas by small molecule compounds that target molecular abnormalities can be a more promising approach to treat meningiomas in humans. For example, recently developed selective kinase inhibitors of PDGF, EGF and VEGF receptors may one day serve as novel therapeutic agents for the treatment of meningiomas [48]. Unfortunately, it is not clear which PTK receptors are the most critical in meningioma tumorigenesis, and therefore, simultaneous specific targeting of several PTK receptors, or use of broad-spectrum PTK inhibitors, is likely to be required to achieve therapeutic response in humans.

A better approach, however, may be to target Ras proteins or molecules downstream of Ras proteins through which meningioma-associated growth factors transduce their signals. These include small molecule inhibitors of the enzyme farnesyl-protein transferase (FPTase) and mevalonate pathway inhibitors that suppress those enzymes that are involved in production of farnesyl diphosphate, the substrate for FPTase. Because farnesylation is critical for converting a cytoplasmic and biologically inactive precursor Ras protein into a functional membrane-associated protein, several pharmaceutical companies are currently assessing anticancer activities of FPTase inhibitors in clinical trials.

Considering the nature of molecular alterations in meningiomas, one can hypothesize that inhibition of proteins that function downstream of the growth factor/Ras pathway by small molecule compounds can also be therapeutically useful. For example, a novel inhibitor drug, PD 184352, was recently discovered to directly and specifically inhibit the Mek-1 kinase, a protein that acts downstream of Ras proteins to activate extracellular signal-regulated kinases Erk-1 and Erk-2. This Mek-1 inhibitor significantly suppressed the growth of human colon and ovarian xenograft tumors in mice without unacceptable side-effects [49].

It is well established that activation of the growth factor/Ras pathway causes increased turnover of the arachidonic acid metabolism, including production of prostaglandins and leukotrienes, by regulating the activity of cytosolic phospholipase A2, cyclooxygenases (COX-1 and COX-2) and 5-lipoxygenase (5-LO), respectively. Dramatically elevated concentrations of arachidonic acid, prostaglandins and leukotrienes have been reported to occur in meningiomas compared with normal brain tissue, and are believed to be important mediators of peritumoral brain edema. One can therefore speculate that inhibitors of these lipid enzymes, such as COX-2-specific and 5-LO inhibitors, may be of use to prevent or treat meningiomas and peritumoral edema. At least six cancer trials with a COX-2-specific inhibitor, celecoxib, are currently underway [50]. Boswellic acids, naturally occurring compounds isolated from the gum-resin exudate from the stem of the tree Boswellia serrata (frankincense), are potent inhibitors of 5-LO. At low micromolar, physiologically achievable concentrations, boswellic acids are cytotoxic for meningioma and glioma cells [51]. A phase I/II clinical trial to establish the effects of boswellic acids on peritumoral edema in glioblastoma patients is currently in progress (at www.medizin.uni-tuebingen.de/~webnonk/clinical.html).

Clearly, an improved understanding of the biological functions of known genes that play a critical role in meningioma development, as well as identification of novel molecular abnormalities, will provide potential targets for new therapeutic approaches that are both more effective and better tolerated than the traditional therapies.

Key Points

- *Surgical approaches may vary in meningioma surgery depending upon the tumor location and size.*
- *The amount of residual tumor after surgery is a major determinant of the rate of recurrence.*
- *Radiation therapy often plays an important role in the overall management of patients with meningiomas.*
- *Radiosurgery is playing an increasingly important role in skull base meningiomas.*
- *The treatment of meningiomas will continue to advance through continued research at the subcellular level coupled with advances in molecular therapy.*

References

1. Rachlin JR, Rosenblum ML. Etiology and biology of meningiomas. In: Al-Mefty O, editor. Meningiomas. New York: Raven Press, 1991; 27–35.
2. DeMonte F, Al Mefty O. Meningiomas. In: Kaye AH, Laws ER Jr, editors. Brain Tumors. New York: Churchill Livingstone, 1995; 675–704.
3. Kurland LT, Schoenberg BS, Annegers JF et al. The incidence of primary intracranial neoplasms in Rochester, Minnesota. Ann N Y Acad Sci 1982;381:6–16.
4. Nakasu S, Hirano A, Shimura T et al. Incidental meningiomas in autopsy study. Surg Neurol 1987;27:319–22.
5. Fan KJ, Pezeshkpour GH. Ethnic distribution of primary central nervous system tumors in Washington DC, 1971–1985. J Natl Med Assoc 1992;84:858–63.
6. Haddad G, AL-Mefty O. Meningiomas: an overview. In: Wilkins RH, Rengachary SS, editors. Neurosurgery. New York: McGraw-Hill, 1996; 833–41.

7. Drake JM, Hoffman HJ. Meningiomas in children. In: Al-Mefty O, editor. Meningiomas. New York: Raven Press, 1991; 145–52.
8. Ersahin A, Ozdamar N, Demirtas E, Karabiyikoglu M. Meningioma of the cavernous sinus in a child. Childs Nerv Syst 1999;15(1):8–10.
9. Giangaspero F, Guiducci A, Lenz FA, Mastronardi L, Burger PC. Meningioma with meningoangiomatosis: a condition mimicking invasive meningiomas in children and young adults: report of two cases and review of the literature. Am J Surg Pathol 1999;23:872–5.
10. Inskip PD, Mellelkjaer L, Gridley G, Olsen JH. Incidence of intracranial tumors following hospitalization for head injuries (Denmark). Cancer Causes Control 1998;9(1):109–16.
11. Parent AD. Multiple meningiomas. In: Al-Mefty O, editor. Meningiomas. New York: Raven Press, 1991;161–8.
12. Levy WJ Jr, Bay J, Dohn D. Spinal cord meningiomas. J Neurosurg 1982;57:804–12.
13. Fox J. Meningiomas and associated lesions. In: Al-Mefty O, editor. Meningiomas. New York: Raven Press, 1991;129–36.
14. Iida A, Kurose K, Isobe R, Akiyama F, Sakamoto G, Yoshimoto M et al. Mapping of a new target region of allelic loss to a 2-cM interval at 22q13.1 in primary breast cancer. Genes Chromosomes Cancer 1998;21(2): 108–12.
15. Kuratsu JI, Kochi M, Ushio Y. Incidence and clinical features of asymptomatic meningiomas. J Neurosurg 2000;92:766–70.
16. Jaaskelainen J, Haltia M, Laasonen E, Wahlstrom T, Valtonen S. The growth rate of intracranial meningiomas in its relation to histology. An analysis of 43 patients. Surg Neurol 1985;24:165–72.
17. Cho K, Hoshiro T, Nagashima T, Murovic J, Wilson C. Predication of tumor doubling time in recurrent meningiomas. J Neurosurg 1986;65:790–4.
18. Shino A, Nakasu S, Matsuda M, Handa J, Morikawa S, Inubushi T. Noninvasive evaluation of the malignant potential of intracranial meningiomas performed using proton magnetic resonance spectroscopy. J Neurosurg 1999;91:928–34.
19. Simpson D. The recurrence of intracranial meningiomas after surgical treatment. Neurol Nerosurg Psychiat 1957;20:22–39.
20. Melamed S, Sahar A, Beller AJ. The recurrence of intracranial meningiomas. Neurochirurgie 1979;22: 47–51.
21. Chan R, Thompson G. Morbidity, mortality, and quality of life following surgery for intracranial meningiomas. A retrospective study in 257 cases. J Neurosurg 1984;60:52–60.
22. Mirimanoff RO, Dosoretz DE, Linggood RM, Ojemann RG, Martuza RL. Meningioma: analysis of recurrence and progression following neurosurgical resection. J Neurosurg 1985;62:18–24.
23. Kallio M, Sankila R, Hakulinen T, Jaaskelainen J. Factors affecting operative and excess long-term mortality in 935 patients with intracranial meningiomas. Neurosurgery 1992;31:2–12.
24. Jaaskelainen J, Haltia M, Servo A. Atypical and anaplastic menigiomas: radiology surgery, radiotherapy, and outcome. Surg Neurol 1986;25:233–42.
25. Kakinuma K, Tanaka R, Onda K, Takahashi H. Proliferative potential of recurrent intracranial meningiomas as evaluated by labeling indices of BUdR and KI-67, and tumor doubling time. Acta Neurochir (Wien) 1998; 140:26–31.
26. May P, Broome J, Lawry J, Buxton R, Battersby R. A flow cytometric study of paraffin-embedded archival material. J Neurosurg 1989;71:347–51.
27. Mantle R, Lach B, Delgado M, Baeesa S, Belanger G. Predicting the probability of meningioma recurrence based on the quality of peritumoral brain edema on computerized tomography scanning. J Neurosurg 1999;91:375–83.
28. Nakasu S, Nakasu Y, Nakajima M, Matsuda M, Handa J. Preoperative identification of meningiomas that are highly likely to recur. J Neurosurg 1999;90:455–62.
29. Lee JH, Evans JJ, Kosmorsky G. Surgical management of clinoidal meningiomas. Neurosurgery 2001;48:1012–21.
30. Nutting C, Brada M, Brazil L et al. Radiotherapy in the treatment of benign meningiomas of the skull base. J Neurosurg 1999;90:823–7.
31. Patil AA, Kumar P, Leibrock LG. Response to extra-axial tumors to stereotactically implanted high-activity I-125 seeds. Stereotactic Funct Neurosurg 1995;64: 139–52..
32. Kondziolka D, Levy EI, Niranjan A, Flickinger JC, Lunsford LD. Long-term outcomes after meningioma radiosurgery: physician and patient perspectives. J Neurosurg 1999;91:44–50.
33. Morita A, Coffey RJ, Foote RL, Schiff D, Gorman D. Risk of injury to cranial nerves after gamma knife radiosurgery for skull base meningiomas: experience in 88 patients. J Neurosurg 1999;90:42–9.
34. Shafron DH, Friedman WA, Buatti JM, Bova FJ, Mendenhall WM. Linac radiosurgery for benign meningiomas. Int J Radiat Oncol Biol Phys 1999;43:321–7.
35. Hakim R, Alexander E 3rd, Loeffler JS et al. Results of linear accelerator-basedradiosurgery for intracranial meningiomas. Neurosurgery 1998;42:446–53.
36. Kondziolka D, Flickinger JC, Perez B. Judicious resection and/or radiosurgery for parasagittal meningiomas: outcomes from a multicenter review. Gamma Knife Meningioma Study Group. Neurosurgery 1998;43: 405–13.
37. Shen J-L, Loeb LA. The Werner syndrome gene: the molecular basis of RecQ helicase-deficiency diseases. Trends Genet 2000;16:213–20.
38. Huynh DP, Pulst SM. Neurofibromatosis 2 antisense oligodeoxynucleotides induce reversible inhibition of schwannomin synthesis and cell adhesion in STS26T and T98G cells. Oncogene 1996;13:73–84.
39. Goutebroze L, Brault E, Muchardt C, Camonis J, Thomas G. Cloning and characterization of SCHIP-1, a novel protein interacting specifically with spliced isoforms and naturally occurring mutant NF2 proteins. Mol Cell Biol 2000;20:1699–1712.
40. Gutmann DH, Donahoe J, Perry A, Lemke N, Gorse K, Kittiniyom K et al. Loss of DAL-1, a protein 4.1-related tumor suppressor, is an important early event in the pathogenesis of meningiomas. Hum Mol Genet 2000;9:1495–1500.
41. Kirsch M, Zhu JJ, Black PM. Analysis of the BRCA1 and BRCA2 genes in sporadic meningiomas. Genes Chromosomes Cancer 1997;20:53–9.

42. Cho H, Ha SY, Park SH, Park K, Chae YS. Role of p53 gene mutation in tumor aggressiveness of intracranial meningiomas. J Korean Med Sci 1999;14:199–205.
43. Santarius T, Kirsch M, Nikas DC, Imitoal J, Black PM. Molecular analysis of alteration of the p18INK4c gene in human meningiomas. Neuropathol Appl Neurobiol 2000;26:67–75.
44. Mueller P, Henn W, Niedermayer I, Ketter R, Feiden W, Steudel WI et al. Deletion of chromosome 1p and loss of expression of alkaline phosphatase indicate progression of meningiomas. Clin Cancer Res 1999;5:3569–77.
45. Scoles DR, Huynh DP, Chen MS, Burke SP, Gutmann DH, Pulst S-M. The neurofibromatosis 2 tumor suppressor protein interacts with hepatocyte growth-factor regulated tyrosine kinase substrate. Hum Mol Genet 2000;9:1567–74.
46. Cooper C, Jones HG, Weller RO et al. Production of prostaglandins and thromoboxane by isolated cells from intracranial tumors. J Neurol Neurosurg Psychiatry 1984;47:579–84.
47. Scanlon KJ, Kashani-Sabet M. Ribozymes as therapeutic agents: are we getting closer? J Natl Cancer Inst 1998;90:558–9.
48. Levitzki A. Protein tyrosine kinase inhibitors as novel therapeutic agents. Pharmacol Ther 1999;82:231–9.
49. Sebolt-Leopold JS, Dudley DT, Herrera R et al. Blockade of the MAP kinase pathway suppresses growth of colon tumors in vivo. Nat Med 1999;5:810–16.
50. Smigel K. Arthritis drug approved for polyp prevention blazes trail for other prevention trials. J Natl Cancer Inst 2000;92:297–9.
51. Park YS, Lee JH, Harwalkar JA, Bondar J, Safayhi H, Golubic M. Acetyl-11B-Boswellic Acid (AKBA) is cytotoxic for meningioma cells and inhibits phosphorylation of the extracellular-signal regulated kinase 1 and 2. In: Honn KV, Nigam S, Marnett IJ, Dennis E, editors. Proceedings of the 6th International Conference on Eicosanoids and Other Bioactive Lipids in Cancer, Inflammation and Related Diseases. New York: Plenum Publishing, 2000.

13

Intraventricular and Pineal Region Tumors

Sandeep Kunwar, G. Evren Keles, Mitchell S. Berger

Summary

Intraventricular and pineal region tumors represent 2% of all primary central nervous system tumors but have many unique features. Because many patients present with symptomatic hydrocephalus, urgent treatment of the tumor or hydrocephalus is often needed. Both benign and malignant tumors can arise in these regions, and often radiographic imaging is non-diagnostic. Surgery remains the main therapeutic approach for these tumors but is complicated by the central location of these lesions. A successful resection of intraventricular and pineal region tumors is based on a thorough knowledge of the relevant cerebral anatomy and the deep vascular system, avoidance of functionally eloquent areas and use of limited retraction.

Intraventricular Tumors

Brain tumors located in the ventricles constitute 1.4% of all primary central nervous system tumors, and 5.4% of all central nervous tumors in the pediatric age group [1]. The most common primary neoplasms of the third ventricle are neuroepithelial tumors [2]. These tumors include juvenile pilocytic astrocytoma, astrocytoma, subependymal giant cell astrocytoma, ependymoma and glioblastoma multiforme. Although juvenile pilocytic astrocytomas most often originate from the floor of the third ventricle, they may arise from the posterior pituitary or optic system and extend into the ventricle. Low-grade astrocytomas, as well as anaplastic astrocytoma and glioblastoma multiforme, typically originate from the thalamic region. Ependymomas, and less frequently subependymomas, originate from the ventricular wall. These lesions are more common in the lateral ventricles. Subependymal giant cell astrocytoma, which may be associated with tuberous sclerosis, often originates at the foramen of Monro and is more frequently seen in the lateral ventricle. Colloid cysts are the most common lesions located in the third ventricle [3]. Although rare, epidermoid and dermoid tumors may occur in the third ventricle, and usually are solid rather than cystic at this location. Meningiomas originating from the velum interpositum and choroid plexus papillomas are also seen in the third ventricle. Craniopharyngioma and suprasellar germinomas can invade the floor of the third ventricle. Another main group of tumors that may grow into the third ventricle originate from the pineal gland and will be discussed in detail later in this chapter. In addition to these primary neoplasms, metastatic tumors may occur in the third ventricle and invade its floor or lateral walls.

Regarding lateral ventricle tumors, in a study excluding tumors that originated in the brain parenchyma with secondary extension into the ventricles, the authors found that the most common histologic diagnosis in adults was astrocytoma, followed by meningioma [2]. In the pediatric age group, the most common diagnosis was subependymal giant cell astrocytoma. In another series [4], the most frequent tumor types were subependymal giant cell astrocytoma, choroid plexus tumors, ependymoma and astrocytoma. The most common location for lateral ventricular tumors was the trigone (38%), followed by the cella media (33%) and the frontal horn (27%) [2].

Intraventricular meningioma, although rare, is a well circumscribed tumor, most often located in the trigone, and constitutes approximately 0.5–2% of all intracranial meningiomas [3] (Figure 13.1). Approximately 80% occur in the lateral ventricles, more commonly in the left trigone, but can occur in the third ventricle, and less frequently in the fourth ventricle. Most patients present in the fourth to the sixth decades, and these tumors are more common in women. The intraventricular location of these slow-growing tumors provides a compensatory mechanism in the form of reserve space, which contributes to the delay in clinical demonstration of symptoms and signs. They may either arise from the choroid plexus and grow within the ventricle, or arise from the tela choroidea and grow partly within the ventricle and partly into the surrounding brain tissue. Imaging characteristics are similar to those of other meningiomas, being sharply defined and globular.

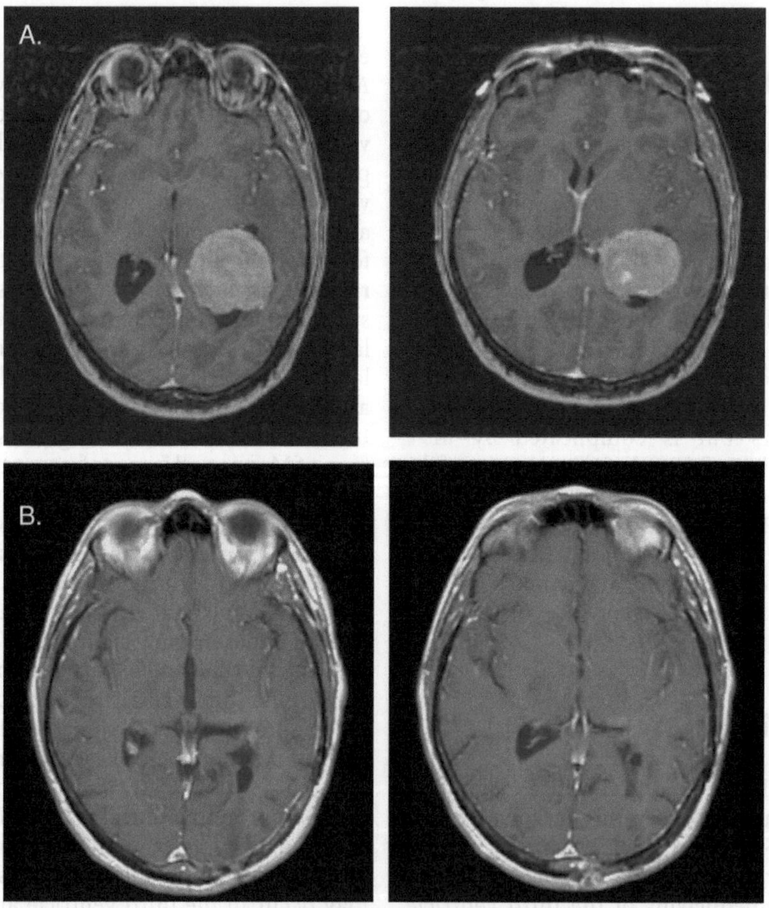

Fig. 13.1. a Despite the large size of the tumor, the patient had minimum symptoms and presented with headaches. **b** Postoperative images after resection via the superior parietal lobule. Because of the location within the dominant hemisphere, a posterior middle temporal gyrus approach would carry risk of speech impairment.

Intracranial ependymomas represent about 2% of brain tumors in adults, and 5.2–6.9% of all tumors in the pediatric population [1]. Approximately one-third of childhood ependymomas arise from the supratentorial ventricular system, and supratentorial lesions are more common in children over the age of 3 years. Adult patients tend to be relatively young, with most series reporting median ages under 45 years [5–7]. Although controversial, age, tumor location, tumor grade and extent of surgical resection have been suggested to be of prognostic significance. Subependymomas are benign, usually asymptomatic, nodules on the ventricular wall and are most commonly detected as an incidental autopsy finding.

Subependymal giant cell astrocytomas are seen in 6–19% of patients with tuberous sclerosis, and may also occur in the absence of this autosomal dominant phakomatosis [8,9]. Despite the benign nature of these tumors, they mostly arise near the foramen of Monro and may grow large enough to obstruct the foramen and cause obstructive hydrocephalus. Intratumoral hemorrhage and malignant differentiation have also been reported.

Choroid plexus tumors are more common in the lateral ventricles when compared with the third ventricle. In contrast to adults, in whom the majority of choroid plexus tumors are located in the fourth ventricle and the cerebellopontine angle, approximately 75% of choroid plexus tumors in children are found in the lateral ventricles, mostly located in the atrium. In a recent meta-analysis including 566 well documented choroid plexus tumors, histology was the most important prognostic factor, as 5- and 10-year projected survival rates were 81 and 77% for choroid plexus papillomas (n = 353) compared to 41 and 35% in choroid plexus carcinomas, respectively ($P < 0.0005$) [10]. Surgery was also a statistically significant prognostic factor for both choroid plexus papillomas and choroid plexus carcinomas.

Relevant Anatomy

As a variety of eloquent structures surround the third and lateral ventricles, a thorough knowledge of the related anatomy, including neural and vascular structures, is essential in evaluating neuroimaging studies and in planning surgery.

The roof of the third ventricle is formed by the tela choroidea and the forniceal body. The anterior wall is formed by the lamina terminalis, forniceal columns, optic recess and the foramen of Monro. Medial surface of the thalamus forms the posterosuperior aspect of the lateral wall of the third ventricle. Separated by the hypothalamic sulcus, the hypothalamus constitutes the antero-inferior aspect of the lateral wall. The third ventricle floor consists of the optic chiasm, the tuber cinerum and infundibulum, mammillary bodies, posterior perforated substance and the superior aspect of the tegmentum. Pericallosal arteries, medial posterior choroidal arteries, internal cerebral veins and the branches of the circle of Willis inferiorly are vascular structures of critical importance in this region.

The lateral ventricles extend from the foramen of Monro anteriorly into the frontal lobe as the frontal horn. The walls of each frontal horn are formed by the genu of the corpus callosum anteriorly; by the septum pellucidum, the foramen of Monro and the forniceal column medially; and by the head of the caudate nucleus laterally. The floor is formed by the rostrum of the corpus callosum. The choroid plexus passes through the foramen of Monro and curves posteriorly to line the roof of the third ventricle. The anteromedially located septal vein joins the posterolaterally located thalamostriate vein at the foramen of Monro to form the inferior cerebral vein. The body of each lateral ventricle extends from the posterior aspect of the foramen of Monro to the junction of the corpus callosum with the fornix. The body is surrounded by the body of the caudate nucleus laterally and by the corpus callosum superiorly. The striothalamic sulcus divides the thalamus from the caudate nucleus and houses the thalamostriate vein and the stria terminalis. Tumors located in the body of the lateral ventricles derive most of their blood supply from the posterior lateral choroidal arteries. Caudal to the thalamus, the lateral ventricle curves laterally and anteriorly forming the temporal horn. Posteriorly from the junction of the body and the temporal horn extends the occipital horn. The triangular expansion of the ventricle between the occipital and temporal horns is the atrium, i.e. the trigone. The visual projection fibers are located laterally to the atrium. Tumors located in the atrium are supplied from the anterior choroidal and posterior lateral choroidal arteries.

Pre-operative Evaluation

Intraventricular tumors are often slow-growing and benign. These lesions frequently grow large before clinical manifestations and, ultimately, produce symptoms secondary to hydrocephalus, either by obstruction of the normal pathways of cerebrospinal fluid flow or by its overproduction. Most patients present with headaches [2]. Colloid cysts, which typically occur anteriorly and superiorly within the third ventricle, have a tendency to intermittently obstruct the foramen of Monro, resulting in acute lateral ventricular hydrocephalus with symptoms of intracranial hypertension. Visual loss, impotence and diabetes insipidus may be caused by tumors invading the floor of the third ventricle. Asymmetric bitemporal hemianopia, starting with inferior temporal field loss, may occur due to dilatation of the third ventricle with pressure on the optic chiasm from above. The extension of the tumor may cause a variety of visual field defects, including homonymous hemianopia, binasal field defects, arcuate defects and central scotoma [11].

The standard preoperative imaging study is MRI. An MR scan provides information regarding the size of the tumor, its degree of invasion, its relationship with the surrounding anatomical structures and the extent of hydrocephalus. Information regarding the relationship of the tumor with surrounding venous structures is also critical in planning surgery. The exact location of the tumor, e.g. posterior third ventricle versus pineal or quadrigeminal, is of crucial importance in planning the surgical approach.

Neuroendocrinologic evaluation may be necessary, depending on the degree of hypothalamic involvement. Germ cell markers that will be detailed later in this chapter should be obtained if the tumor is suspected of being of germ cell origin. Visual field testing is obtained if the visual pathways are affected, and for patients undergoing a posterior approach to a tumor of the occipital horn or atrium.

Any lesion that appears to be highly vascular on MRI may be studied angiographically. Although not routine, angiography is important for large tumors and when the deep venous system should be visualized. Angiography will also provide information regarding the status of the bridging veins between the cerebral hemisphere and the sagittal sinus, useful for surgical planning. Less detailed information regarding the status of vascular structures may be obtained with MR angiography/venography in a non-invasive manner.

In addition to neoplasms covered in this chapter, differential diagnosis should include histiocytosis, sarcoidosis, neurocysticercosis, fungal and indolent bacterial infections and, although very rare, abscesses.

Outcome

Although the main therapeutic approach is surgical resection, the decision to operate on an intraventricular tumor should be based on several factors, including the patient's age, neurological and medical status and expected survival, as well as tumor-related factors such as documented progression and resectability. The surgical approach to be selected must take into account the vital anatomical structures encountered in reaching them and the potential neurologic sequelae. The use of preoperative angiography and embolization, together with intraoperative neuronavigational guidance, may significantly facilitate the operation. A successful resection of intraventricular tumors is based on a thorough knowledge of the relevant anatomy, avoidance of functionally eloquent areas, use of limited retraction and early control of the main blood supply. For patients with no significant surgical morbidity, survival is directly linked to the histopathological characteristics of the tumor. Unlike a patient with a totally resected meningioma, survival for a patient with a totally resected glioblastoma multiforme is not favorable.

Pineal Region Tumors

Tumors of the pineal region can be divided into germ cell tumors, pineal cell tumors and other tumors (including astrocytoma, ependymoma and meningioma) (Figure 13.2). The true incidence of pineal region tumors from historical data is difficult to extrapolate because of the variety of histopathology and often confusing nomenclature associated with them. In the most comprehensive series analyzing "pineolomas" in 4,865 cases of brain tumors, these tumors make up 0.6% of all adult brain tumors and 1–3% of pediatric brain tumors [1,12]. Several

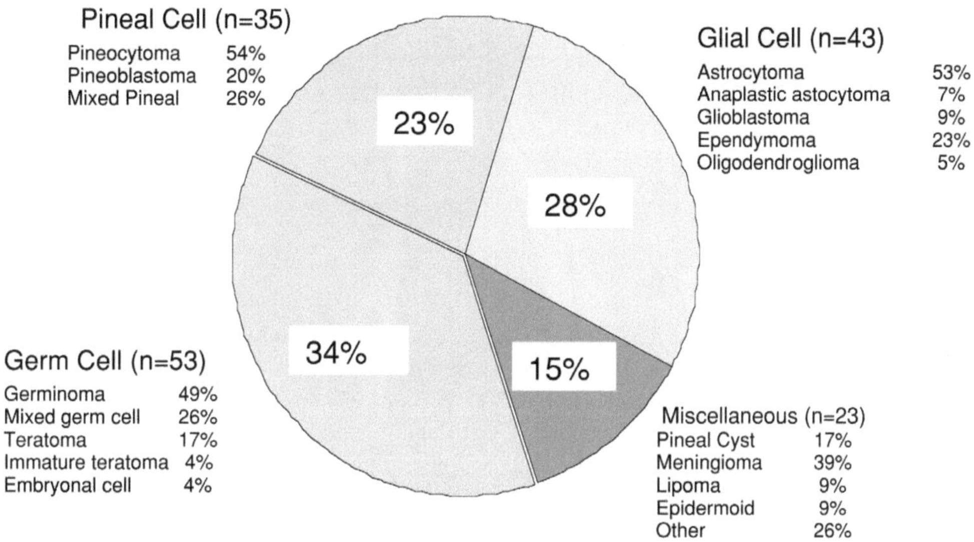

Fig. 13.2. Pathological summary of 154 patients surgically treated for pineal region tumors reviewed by Bruce et al. (1995).

studies have suggested a greater incidence in Japan, ranging from 4 to 6% [13,14]. However, a prospective study of actual population-based incidence between the number of pineal region tumors seen in Niigata, Japan and Western Australia failed to show a statistically significant difference (0.07 vs 0.06 per 100,000 person-years, respectively) [15].

Epidemiology

The most common location of extragonadal germ cell tumors occurs in two midline sites: the mediastinum (thymus) and the diencephalopineal (pineal and infundibulum) region. The origin of these non-neuroectodermal tumors remains unknown but may be related to the persistence of primordial germ cells which disseminate widely throughout many tissues and organs in the early embryo. These extra-gonadal germ cells typically have an ephemeral existence and undergo an apoptotic death. It is possible that some of these cells may survive and, over time, transform into a neoplasm. This is in contrast to the theory that the presence of these cells is related to a migrational defect. The pineal gland is the most common site of intracranial germ cell tumors (37–45%), followed by the suprasellar region (27–35%), with 10% of tumors involving both regions at presentation [16,17] (Figure 13.3). Intracranial germ cell tumors occur most frequently between ages 10 and 21 years (70%) and 95% occur before age 33 [16]. These tumors have a marked predominance in males. Jennings et al. (1985) showed that males are 2.2 times more likely to be affected, while Bruce et al. (1995) showed a stronger male preponderance of 8.5:1. Interestingly, there is an equal sex distribution, or perhaps a bias towards females, among suprasellar germ cell tumors [12,16].

Intracranial germ cell tumors represent a heterogeneous group of tumors, divided into germinomas and non-germinomatous germ cell tumors (NGGCT). NGGCT include teratomas, embryonal cell tumors, choriocarcinomas and endodermal sinus tumors (yolk sac carcinoma). Germinomas are the most common intracranial germ cell tumor, comprising between 40 and 65% of all germ cell tumors [16,18]. Teratomas (18–20%), endodermal sinus tumors (5–7%), embryonal cell tumors (3–5%), and choriocarcinomas (3–4%) are less frequent [16,18]. Furthermore, large series with extensive tissue sampling have shown mixed germ cell histology in up to 25% of germ cell tumors [17]. Thus, it is imperative to establish an adequate histological diagnosis prior to proceeding with radiation or chemotherapy because the management and prognosis of patients with germ cell tumors vary

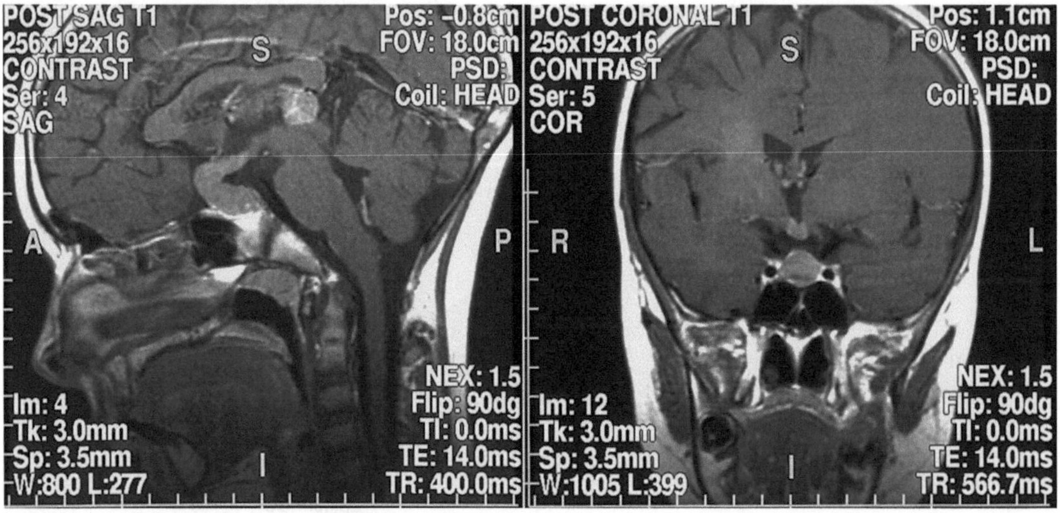

Fig. 13.3. Eight-year-old child with a pineal and suprasellar germinoma. Involvement of the suprasellar and pineal region is most consistent with a germ cell tumor.

greatly on histology. Germinomas, for example, can be cured by radiotherapy alone or in combination with chemotherapy in the majority of cases. NGGCT, however, do not have as good prognosis but, with aggressive surgical resection, high-dose chemotherapy and radiotherapy, long-term control can be achieved. Mature teratomas, which are the least common, are slow-growing and can be cured with surgery alone [16,18].

Parenchymal pineal tumors are neoplasms arising from pinealocytes and account for 0.4–1.0% of the 17,000 primary brain tumors diagnosed each year [19]. These tumors have been categorized as pineocytoma (low-grade), pineoblastoma (high-grade) and mixed [17,19]. Approximately 30–57% of pineal parenchymal tumors are pineocytomas, 23–50% are pineoblastomas and 20% are mixed tumors [17]. The mean age of presentation for all pineal cell tumors was 22 years, ranging from 11 months to 77 years. Pineoblastoma, the more malignant variety, has been found to occur in younger populations with a mean age of 18 years [17,19]. There is no gender preference for these tumors, although a slight male predominance has been suggested in the Japanese literature [14]. Pineoblastoma is associated with bilateral retinoblastomas (trilateral retinoblastoma) and, in such, arise from germ line mutations in the retinoblastoma (Rb) gene. Pineoblastomas have similar histological and clinical behavior as PNETs [17,20] (Figure 13.4).

Other tumors that involve the pineal region include glial cell tumors (astrocytoma, ependymoma, oligodendroglioma), choroid plexus tumors, pineal cysts, meningiomas and metastases, which are rare in this region.

Pathological Appearance

Macroscopically, germinomas are usually soft, grayish pink and friable; some may have a granular consistency. Focal hemorrhages and small cysts may be present. Smaller tumors can appear encapsulated, confined to the pineal region, whereas larger tumors tend to be poorly defined and infiltrate the adjacent structures, including the quadrigeminal plate, the posterior commissure, thalamus and the roof of the third ventricle [17]. Suprasellar germinomas tend to infiltrate the lamina terminalis, the optic chiasm, the septum pellucidum and the hypothalamus. Sometimes, these tumors can appear highly infiltrative without a definite mass, and may mimic an infiltrating glioma. Occasionally, suprasellar growth may extend into the sella turcica and compress the anterior lobe anteriorly or cause compression of the optic chiasm.

Embryonal carcinomas and endodermal sinus tumors have variable gross appearances

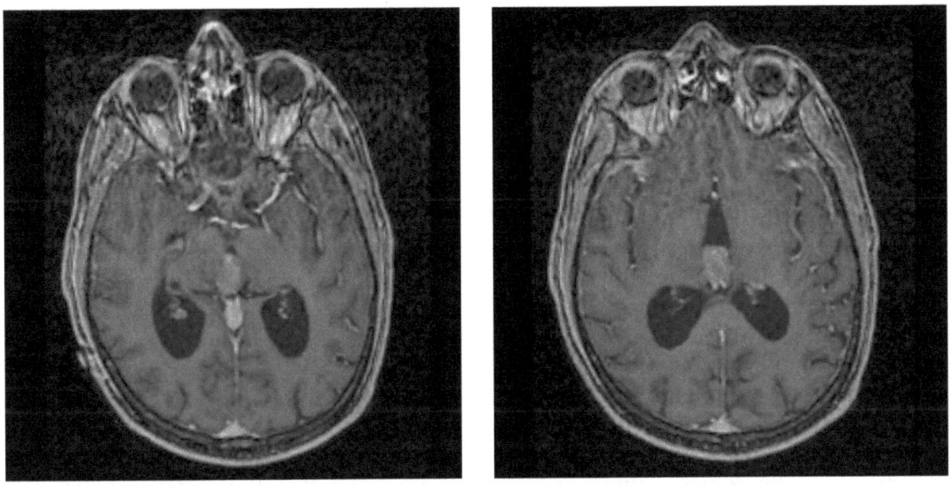

Fig. 13.4. Pineal region tumor presenting with progressive hydrocephalus from aqueductal obstruction. Pathology showed pineoblastoma.

depending on the degree of mixed cell types. Choriocarcinoma is often well demarcated and may contain regions of hemorrhage and necrosis. Teratomas are usually well defined, with an irregular or lobulated outer surface. These tumors may contain cartilage, bone and hair (rarely, teeth) [17]. Typically, the tumor has multiple cysts containing whitish fluid from the desquamation of the dermoid cell lining. Immature teratomas contain hemorrhage and central necrosis and have more invasive features.

Microscopically, germinoma is composed of two clearly distinguishable cell types: large germ cells and small lymphocytes [17]. The germ cells are large, polygonal or spheroidal cells with well defined cell boundaries and an eosinophilic, sometimes vacuolated, cytoplasm with large central spherical nuclei and pale nucleoplasm containing a central nucleolus. Mitotic figures and microscopic mineralization can be present. The second cell type consists of infiltrating lymphocytes clustered around tumor blood vessels. This is thought to represent a granulomatous reaction, although the significance of the immunological reaction is unknown, particularly since this cellular reaction may be completely absent in some cases. The immunological reaction has been found to be primarily a T-cell infiltrate. Occasionally, the local T-cell response predominates the histology, with the germinoma cells being few and difficult to identify. In these cases, confusion with primary cerebral lymphoma may occur. Occasionally, multinucleated syncytiotrophoblast giant cells can be seen, which stain for human chorionic gonadotropin (bHCG). Immunohistochemical stains are useful, since germinomas will stain positive for placental alkaline phosphatase and may show variable staining for cytokeratins, the epithelial membrane antigen or vimentin [17].

Embryonal carcinoma is the least differentiated, having a monotonous pattern with aggregates of primitive epithelial cells in sheets and ribbons [17]. These tumors have the potential to differentiate toward embryonal structures, forming yolk sac or trophoblastic structures. Thus, embryonal carcinoma may give rise to mixed tumors and pure CNS embryonal carcinomas are exceedingly rare. Endodermal sinus tumor is histologically quite close to embryonal carcinomas. The key distinction is the predominance of retiform arrangements, papillary structures, PAS-positive alpha-fetoprotein (AFP)-containing hyaline globules and Schiller–Duvall bodies. Endodermal sinus tumor forms papillary projections constructed of low cuboidal epithelium.

Choriocarcinoma features two predominant cell types: cytotrophoblast and multinucleated syncytiotrophoblast. The cytotrophoblast is recognized by its epithelioid appearance, with clear cytoplasm and a single nucleus. The syncytiotrophoblasts have a very basophilic, vacuolated cytoplasm and multiple hyperchromatic nuclei which stain positive for HCG. Hemorrhage and necrosis are common.

Teratoma is composed of well differentiated tissues from all three germ cell layers (endoderm, mesoderm and endoderm). Mature teratoma may contain solid or cystic foci of squamous epithelium, cartilage or glandular or tubular structures, lined by tall columnar mucus-secreting cells. Teratoma will often contain neuroepithelial tissue showing varying degrees of glial and neuronal differentiation. It is important to differentiate any primitive features, typically in only one of the three germinal layers, which define an immature teratoma. Immature teratomas contain poorly differentiated non-neuroepithelial cells in high density, often staining positive for CEA, cytokeratins or epithelial membrane antigen (EMA) [17].

Pineoblastoma macroscopically is a soft tumor that is pinkish-gray in color and may contain hemorrhagic, necrotic or cystic components. It can be relatively well circumscribed or ill defined and invasive into local surrounding structures, often destroying the pineal gland with growth. By contrast, pineocytoma is well defined and has a pale gray color and lobulated surface. Necrosis, hemorrhage and invasion into adjacent structures are rare findings in pineocytomas. Calcification may be grossly obvious on inspection or on imaging.

Microscopically, pineoblastoma cells are highly cellular, with small, round nuclei resembling cerebellar medulloblastomas. Mitotic figures may be numerous and the tumor cell cytoplasm is scanty. The cells are usually in amorphous sheets, but ill defined Homer-Wright rosettes may be present. Occasionally, perivascular orientation of the cells may be seen. Pineoblastomas also have a propensity to seed the subarachnoid space. Pineocytoma, on the other hand, can be cellular but less so than pineoblastoma. There is a strong resemblance to normal pineocytes, with tumor cells arranged in sheets or diffuse lobules. Giant cells may be present, but mitotic figures are uncommon. Pineocytoma cells may differentiate into mature astrocytes or neurons, or both [17]. Mixed tumors may contain features of both pineocytoma and pineoblastoma, although no consensus exists on where the transition from well differentiated pineoctyoma to undifferentiated pineoblastoma occurs. Some mixed tumors have been designated when divergent differentiation exists along neuronal, glial or both lines; however, more recent designation of mixed tumors relates to the presence of pineoblastoma and pineocytoma elements [19].

The pathological appearances of other tumors (astrocytoma, ependymoma and meningioma) in the pineal region are not site-specific and are histologically similar when found within other areas of the brain.

Relevant Anatomy

The pineal gland has a central location in the brain, such that the distance between it and the surface of any portion of the scalp is almost the same, regardless of which surgical approach is taken to this region. The anatomy of the parenchymal tissue and, more importantly, the vascular structures are critically important in considering the most appropriate approach to these tumors. Pineal tumors occupy the posterior aspect of the third ventricle and the quadrigeminal cistern. They may involve the quadrigeminal plate inferiorly, the posterior commissure and thalamus anterolaterally and the roof of the third ventricle and splenium superiorly. The arterial supply to the pineal gland is from the medial posterior choroidal artery. The draining veins from the pineal body and habenular trigone are the superior and inferior pineal veins that flow into the vein of Galen or the internal cerebral veins. The veins for the superior and inferior colliculi, the superior and inferior quadrigeminal or tectal veins also flow into the vein of Galen or the superior vermian vein. The basal veins of Rosenthal are lateral to the pineal gland and drain into the vein of Galen or the internal cerebral veins. Immediately superior to the pineal gland are the internal cerebral veins, converging and draining into the vein of Galen, sitting superior and posterior to the gland. The superior vermian vein and precentral cerebellar vein lie posterior and inferior to the pineal gland and drain into the vein of Galen as well. From a supratentorial approach, the posterior pericallosal vein and internal occipital vein can also be visualized draining into the vein of Galen.

Pre-operative Evaluation

Patients with primary pineal region tumors present with signs and symptoms of hydrocephalus secondary to compression or involvement of the tectum, occluding the Sylvian aqueduct, including headaches, diplopia, lethargy and ataxia. Compression of the tectum may also cause Parinaud's syndrome, resulting in vertical gaze paresis, impaired pupillary light reflex and convergence nystagmus. The clinical presentation for germ cell tumors is dependent upon the sites of involvement. Suprasellar involvement, particularly with germinomas, may be associated with a long prodrome (month to several years) of signs and symptoms of hypopituitarism. Diabetes insipidus is most common because of the involvement of the infundibulum, but growth failure and hypothyroidism or precocious puberty can also be seen. Children with diabetes insipidus or hypopituitarism may harbor germ cell tumors and should be followed expectantly with MRI scans at regular intervals. Visual field or acuity impairments may occur related to compression of the optic chiasm or direct involvement of the optic nerve. Germinomas can spread directly along the floor and walls of the third ventricle or via CSF pathways. NGGCT have a higher incidence of metastatic dissemination than germinomas, with estimates ranging from 5 to 57%. Etraneural metastasis has been reported in up to 3% of all germ cell tumors, with lung and bone being the most common sites [16].

MRI is the radiographic imaging of choice in evaluating patients with pineal region tumors. CT, however, can be helpful in looking for calcification of the pineal region, which can be seen in the normal gland, germinomas, pineocytomas and teratomas, or for assessing hemorrhage and degree of ventriculomegaly. On MRI scans, germinomas are often isointense to gray matter, and slightly hyperintense on T2-weighted images. These tumors have homogeneous and dramatic contrast enhancement. Cystic areas can occasionally be seen. It is important to assess the suprasellar region and lateral and third ventricles for tumor involvement. There are no typical radiographic features of NGGCT, but they are often heterogeneous on MRI scans and tend to have infiltrating borders with variable degrees of enhancement. Teratomas, in particular, have marked heterogeneity, loculations and irregular enhancement related to lipid, soft tissue and cystic components as well as calcification. Malignant teratomas have similar features but demonstrate invasion into the surrounding structures [21]. Pineoblastomas are often heterogeneous on T1-weighted sequences and tend to be hyperintense on T2-weighted sequences. There is usually strong enhancement with some heterogeneous areas within the tumor (Figure 13.4). These tumors are aggressive and frequently disseminate in the neuraxis. There may be regions of necrosis or hemorrhage contributing to the heterogeneity. Pineocytomas are typically iso or hypointense on T1-weighted imaging with homogeneous and intense enhancement. However, pineocytomas can have variable appearance and can be associated with a hypointense cyst on T1-weighted images, similar to pineal cysts. MRI also provides critical anatomic information when considering surgical approach, extension of the tumor, the degree of brainstem involvement and the relationship of the deep venous system to the tumor.

All patients with pineal region tumors should undergo a high-resolution MRI scan with gadolinium of the head and screening MRI of the spinal axis (post-contrast sagittal view). Patients also require CSF and serum measurements of AFP, human chorionic gonadotropin (HCG) and CEA levels. CSF should also be sent for cytology. Evaluation of pituitary function should be performed if endocrine abnormalities are suspected and formal visual field examination in patients with evidence of suprasellar involvement.

Management and Outcome

Surgery has assumed an important role in the management of pineal region tumors. Radiographic features are not diagnostic and therapy and outcome are dependent on tumor type. Management of hydrocephalus requires urgent attention, since patients can develop acute obstruction and a herniation syndrome. Nearly all patients with pineal region tumors present with symptomatic hydrocephalus. The standard of care has been placement of a ventriculoperitoneal shunt (VPS), at which time CSF can be collected. More recently, endoscopic management of obstructive hydrocephalus with a ventriculostomy, CSF sampling and biopsy of the tumor has gained popularity. Disadvantages of a permanent VPS for the initial management of hydrocephalus in these patients include shunt malfunction, infection and, rarely, peritoneal seeding of tumors. In many cases, if the tumor can be removed, the patient may not need the shunt at all. Endoscopic third ventriculostomy allows for successful treatment of the obstructive hydrocephalus, collection of CSF for markers and cytology and allows for multiple biopsies under direct endoscopic vision as a one-step procedure [22]. We have utilized this approach in the initial management of all patients with pineal region tumors presenting with hydrocephalus. If the biopsy is adequate and demonstrates a germinoma or primary malignant glioma without significant mass effect, the patient is managed with radiation and chemotherapy. For NGGCT, pineal cell tumors and large glial tumors, the patient can then undergo a more elective craniotomy appropriate for the location and size of tumor. Stereotactic biopsy of tumors of this region has also gained popularity but still carries a risk of damage to the complex venous anatomy. A concern with either endoscopic or stereotactic biopsy is sampling error. Germinomas can contain nests of malignant germ cell tumor that would significantly alter therapy and outcome. Likewise, a glial tumor may contain mixed cell types or focal areas of a higher-grade neoplasm, although this is less of a problem since radiographic appearance can help in choosing the most appropriate region to biopsy.

There are many surgical approaches to the pineal region (Figure 13.5). Three surgical approaches are most commonly used: infratentorial supracerebellar, suboccipital transtentorial and paramedian transcallosal. The surgeon's degree of comfort and experience with the procedure and the size and extension of the tumor should determine the most appropriate approach chosen in order to minimize complications.

Surgical results depend more on the tumor's invasiveness and relationship with surrounding structures than on which approach is utilized. The deep location of these tumors makes surgery risky, with possible damage to the tectum, thalamus or deep venous system. The supratentorial approaches are best suited for large tumors that have a significant lateral or supratentorial component. Supratentorial approaches have the disadvantage of requiring retraction of the occipital lobe, resulting in a hemianopsia and an obstructed view of the tumor by the deep venous system. In most cases, we prefer the infratentorial, supracerebellar approach because it allows the most direct access to these midline tumors. Typically, the deep venous anatomy is displaced superiorly, facilitating tumor resection. In the past, the sitting approach was utilized, which allows gravity to help in retracting the cerebellar hemispheres and facilitating dissection [18]. However, because of the risks of air embolism and cortical collapse, we prefer a modified "Concorde" position in which the surgeon operates over the patient's left shoulder. There is a growing appreciation of the value of aggressive tumor removal for improving the prognosis of patients; however, this is dependent on tumor type. With benign tumors, complete resection is usually curative [18]. With malignant tumors, radical debulking is thought to improve the outcome and response to adjuvant therapy [12,13,18].

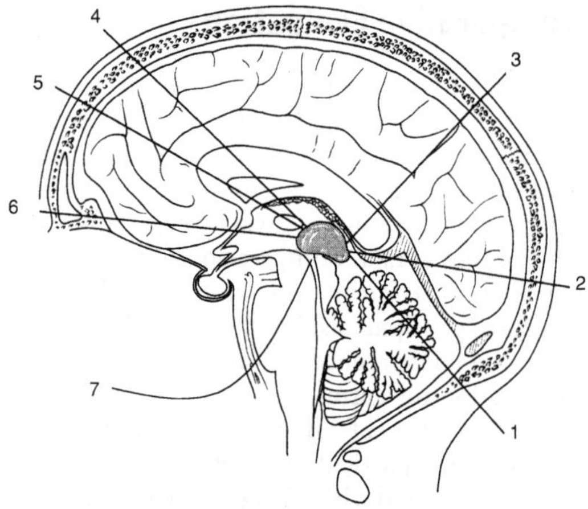

Fig. 13.5. Approaches to the pineal region and tumors of the posterior third ventricle. 1. Infratentorial, supracerebellar. 2. Suboccipital, transtentorial. 3. Posterior interhemispheric, transcallosal. 4. Anterior transcallosal, subchoroidal/transvelum interpositum. 5. Transcortical or interhemispheric transforaminal. 6. Translamina terminalis. 7. Posterior transventricular.

All patients with malignant germ cell or pineal cell tumors require radiation therapy.

The concomitant use of chemotherapy, the extent of tumor involvement and the presence of dissemination have impacted on the field of radiation therapy. For certain tumors, such as ependymoma and malignant astrocytoma, focal radiotherapy is indicated. For pineoblastomas and some germ cell tumors, craniospinal radiotherapy is more appropriate. Radiotherapy has been the primary curative treatment for germinomas arising in the pineal and suprasellar regions. Long-term control rates of 65–90% are well documented for germinomas [23,24]. The control of NGGCT and pineoblastomas with radiotherapy alone is poor, necessitating multimodality therapy. Radiosurgery has been used in boosting the primary site of tumor or in the primary management of low-grade pineal tumors (pineocytomas) [25].

Chemotherapy is being evaluated with increasing enthusiasm for germinoma and certain NGGCT. For germinomas, attempts have been made to reduce or defer radiotherapy after a trial of adjuvant chemotherapy. Recurrence rates as high as 49% for germinomas treated with chemotherapy alone support the continued need for radiotherapy in these tumors [26]. Multimodal therapy for patients with NGGCT with radiotherapy and chemotherapy (bleomycin, vinblastine, carboplatin and etoposide) have shown a 4-year progression-free survival of 67% [27]. Multimodality therapy is also utilized for patients with pineoblastoma, similar to medulloblastomas. In the Childrens Cancer Group protocol, there was a 3-year progression free survival rate of 61% with combined surgery, radiotherapy and chemotherapy [28]. In adults, a review of 11 patients treated at our facility with multimodality therapy showed a median survival of 30 months for patients with positive staging, with all five patients with negative staging having progression-free survival at 26 months [20].

Treatment for patients with primary glial tumors of the pineal region are similar to tumors in other locations and are not specific to this region. However, these patients need to be monitored closely for evidence of CSF dissemination.

Key Points

- *Intraventricular and pineal region tumors often present with hydrocephalus.*
- *Diagnosis is usually based on characteristic imaging features. Serum or CSF markers can add additional diagnostic information in some tumors.*
- *Surgical approaches to anterior intraventricular tumors are accomplished using open surgery or endoscopic techniques.*
- *Pineal region tumors comprise a number of histologic subtypes, some of which are exquisitely sensitive to radiotherapy.*
- *Posterior surgical approaches to pineal tumors are effective in safely resecting these tumors and establishing the diagnosis. Additional chemotherapy and/or radiotherapy is indicated for some tumors.*

References

1. CBTRUS Statistical Report. Primary brain tumors in the United States, 1995–1999. Hinsdale, Illinois: Central Brain Tumor Registry of the United States, 2002.
2. Pendl G, Ozturk E, Haselsberger K. Surgery of tumours of the lateral ventricle. Acta Neurochir (Wien) 1992;116:128–36.
3. Morrison G, Sobel DF, Kelley WM, Norman D. Intraventricular mass lesions. Radiology 1984;153:435–42.
4. Zuccaro G, Sosa F, Cuccia V, Lubieniecky F, Monges J. Lateral ventricle tumors in children: a series of 54 cases. Childs Nerv Syst 1999;15:774–85.
5. Shaw EG, Evans RG, Scheithauer BW, Ilstrup DM, Earle JD. Postoperative radiotherapy of intracranial ependymoma in pediatric and adult patients. Int J Radiat Oncol Biol Phys 1987;13:1457–62.
6. Donahue B, Steinfeld A. Intracranial ependymoma in the adult patient: successful treatment with surgery and radiotherapy. J Neurooncol 1998;37:131–3.
7. Schwartz TH, Kim S, Glick RS, Bagiella E, Balmaceda C, Fetell MR, Stein BM, Sisti MB, Bruce JN. Supratentorial ependymomas in adult patients. Neurosurgery 1999;44:721–31.
8. Shepherd CW, Scheithauer BW, Gomez MR, Altermatt HJ, Katzmann JA. Subependymal giant cell astrocytoma: a clinical, pathological, and flow cytometric study. Neurosurgery 1991;28:864–8.
9. Kingsley DP, Kendall BE, Fitz CR. Tuberous sclerosis: a clinicoradiological evaluation of 110 cases with particular reference to atypical presentation. Neuroradiology 1986;28:38–46.
10. Wolff JE, Sajedi M, Brant R, Coppes MJ, Egeler RM. Choroid plexus tumours. Br J Cancer 2002;87:1086–91.
11. Gradin WC, Taylon C, Fruin AH. Choroid plexus papilloma of the third ventricle: case report and review of the literature. Neurosurgery 1983;12:217–20.

12. Hoffman HJ, Yoshida M, Becker LE, Hendrick EB, Humphreys RP. Pineal region tumors in childhood: experience at the Hospital for Sick Children. Pediatr Neurosurg 1983;21:91–103, 1994;discussion 104.
13. Sano K. Pineal region tumors: problems in pathology and treatment. Clin Neurosurg 1983;30:59–91.
14. Koide O, Watanabe Y, Sato K. Pathological survey of intracranial germinoma and pinealoma in Japan. Cancer 1980;45:2119–30.
15. Ojeda VJ, Ohama E, English DR. Pineal neoplasms and third-ventricular teratomas in Niigata (Japan) and Western Australia: a comparative study of their incidence and clinicopathological features. Med J Aust 1987;146:357–9.
16. Jennings MT, Gelman R, Hochberg F. Intracranial germ-cell tumors: natural history and pathogenesis. J Neurosurg 1985;63:155–67.
17. Russell D S, RLJ. Tumors of specialized tissues of central neuroepithelial origin. In: Russell D S, RLJ, editor Pathology of tumors of the nervous system. Baltimore: Williams & Wilkins, 1989;351–420.
18. Bruce JN, Stein BM. Surgical management of pineal region tumors. Acta Neurochir (Wien) 1995;134:130–5.
19. Schild SE, Scheithauer BW, Schomberg PJ, Hook CC, Kelly PJ, Frick L, Robinow JS, Buskirk SJ. Pineal parenchymal tumors: clinical, pathologic, and therapeutic aspects. Cancer 1993;72:870–80.
20. Chang SM, Lillis-Hearne PK, Larson DA, Wara WM, Bollen AW, Prados MD. Pineoblastoma in adults. Neurosurgery 1995;37:383–90, discussion 390–1.
21. Tien RD, Barkovich AJ, Edwards MS. MR imaging of pineal tumors. AJR Am J Roentgenol 1990;155:143–51.
22. Pople IK, Athanasiou TC, Sandeman DR, Coakham HB. The role of endoscopic biopsy and third ventriculostomy in the management of pineal region tumours. Br J Neurosurg 2001;15:305–11.
23. Jenkin D, Berry M, Chan H, Greenberg M, Hendrick B, Hoffman H, Humphreys R, Sonley M, Weitzman S. Pineal region germinomas in childhood treatment considerations. Int J Radiat Oncol Biol Phys 1990;18:541–5.
24. Linstadt D, Wara WM, Edwards MS, Hudgins RJ, Sheline GE. Radiotherapy of primary intracranial germinomas: the case against routine craniospinal irradiation. Int J Radiat Oncol Biol Phys 1988;15:291–7.
25. Kondziolka D, Hadjipanayis CG, Flickinger JC, Lunsford LD. The role of radiosurgery for the treatment of pineal parenchymal tumors. Neurosurgery 2002;51:880–9.
26. Balmaceda C, Heller G, Rosenblum M, Diez B, Villablanca JG, Kellie S, Maher P, Vlamis V, Walker RW, Leibel S, Finlay JL. Chemotherapy without irradiation: a novel approach for newly diagnosed CNS germ cell tumors: results of an international cooperative trial. The First International Central Nervous System Germ Cell Tumor Study. J Clin Oncol 1996;14:2908–15.
27. Robertson PL, DaRosso RC, Allen JC. Improved prognosis of intracranial non-germinoma germ cell tumors with multimodality therapy. J Neurooncol 1997;32:71–80.
28. Jakacki RI, Zeltzer PM, Boyett JM, Albright AL, Allen JC, Geyer JR, Rorke LB, Stanley P, Stevens KR, Wisoff J, et al. Survival and prognostic factors following radiation and/or chemotherapy for primitive neuroectodermal tumors of the pineal region in infants and children: a report of the Childrens Cancer Group. J Clin Oncol 1995;13:1377–83.

14

Cerebello-pontine Angle Tumors

Peter C. Whitfield and David G. Hardy

Summary

This chapter describes the clinical and radiological features of cerebellopontine angle (CPA) tumors. A detailed account of the management of these lesions is provided, with particular reference to the details of microsurgical treatments. The complications of CPA surgery are protean and may significantly impair the quality of a patient's life. A multidisciplinary approach to the management of these problems is advocated.

Introduction

CPA tumors comprise about 8–10% of all intracranial neoplasms. About 80–85% of CPA tumors are acoustic neuromas, with meningiomas and a wide variety of other lesions accounting for the remainder [1]. This chapter describes the anatomy, pathology and management of these lesions.

Anatomy

The CPA is the wedge-shaped space formed anteriorly by the dural-coated face of the petrous temporal bone, and posteriorly by the ventral surfaces of the pons and cerebellum. It contains the superior CSF cistern, which is traversed by the trigeminal, abducens, facial and vestibulocochlear nerves, the anterior inferior cerebellar artery (AICA) and the superior petrosal vein with its tributaries. The CPA has important relationships with surrounding structures. The cisterna ambiens, containing the trochlear nerve and the superior cerebellar artery, is located superiorly. Inferiorly lies the cerebellomedullary (inferior cerebellopontine) cistern containing the glossopharyngeal, vagal, accessory and hypoglossal nerves, along with the vertebral artery, origin of the PICA and the inferior petrosal vein. Medially lies the prepontine cistern which invests the basilar artery and the origin of the abducens nerve.

The cerebellar hemisphere wraps itself around the postero-lateral aspect of the pons forming the V-shaped cerebellopontine fissure. The middle cerebellar peduncle, flocculus and foramen of Luschka lie in the floor of the apex of the cerebellopontine fissure. The latter, with its tuft of protruding choroid plexus, is an important landmark for the emergence of the VII and VIII cranial nerves in CPA surgery.

Cranial Nerves

The trigeminal nerve, comprising a small motor root and a larger sensory root, arises from the lateral aspect of the rostral pons. It courses, in an anterior, lateral and slightly superior direction, towards the porus trigeminus at the entrance to Meckel's cave. The IX, X and XI nerves arise in the longitudinal sulcus lateral to the olive. They course through the inferior cerebellopontine cistern to the jugular foramen. The facial nerve arises 2 or 3 mm superior to the rostral rootlets of the glossopharyngeal nerve, from the lateral aspect of the pontomedullary sulcus. The VIII nerve leaves the pontomedullary sulcus about 1 mm lateral to the facial nerve. The nervus intermedius is usually closely applied to the VIII nerve at this point. The VII and VIII nerves then become apposed as they course toward the porus acousticus (internal auditory meatus). The presence of transverse and vertical (Bill's bar) crests of bone within the internal auditory canal enable the surgeon to identify with certainty the location of the facial nerve and the subdivisions of the vestibulo-cochlear nerve. The superior and inferior vestibular nerves occupy the postero-superior and postero-inferior quadrants of the canal, respectively. The antero–superior quadrant is occupied by the facial nerve and nervus intermedius, whilst the cochlear nerve lies antero–inferiorly. Since most acoustic neuromas arise from one of the vestibular nerves, the cochlear and facial nerves are usually displaced anteriorly.

Clinical Presentation

Lesions within the CPA may present with symptoms and signs of:

- cranial nerve dysfunction: unilateral hearing loss; tinnitus; dysequilibrium and vertigo; diplopia due to an abducens palsy; facial paraesthesia, anaesthesia, or pain. Facial weakness or spasms are unusual at presentation. Large lesions may lead to dysphonia, dysarthria and dysphagia due to involvement of the IX and X cranial nerves.
- cerebellar and/or brainstem compression: impaired co-ordination, upper motor neurone signs in the limbs.
- raised intracranial pressure secondary to associated hydrocephalus, or occasionally to the mass of the lesion itself.
- pain localized to the ear/mastoid regions, or sometimes non-localizing headache.

With the widespread availability of MRI, an increasing number of patients present relatively early. Unilateral hearing loss frequently presents as impaired speech discrimination noted during the use of a telephone by patients with small acoustic neuromas. However, hearing loss may be sudden and profound in 12–15% of patients with CPA tumors, suggesting a vascular basis for the symptom in some cases [2].

Clinicopathological Correlates

Table 14.1 details the relative incidence of the different tumor types found in the CPA.

Table 14.1. Relative incidence of cerebellopontine angle masses. This table represents 438 patients with CPA lesions operated on in Cambridge, UK between 1981 and 1994 [1].

Pathology		Patients (n)	Percentage of CPA lesions
Acoustic schwannoma		369	84
Meningioma		31	7.1
Other schwannoma	V	2	
	VII	6	3.2
	VIII, IX, X	6	
Primary epidermoid (cholesteatoma)		10	2.3
Glomus jugulare (Fisch Type D)		5	1.1
Metastasis		1	0.2
Cerebellar astrocytoma		1	0.2
Lymphoma		1	0.2
Dermoid cyst of the fourth ventricle		1	0.2

Acoustic Neuromas

Acoustic neuromas arise from Schwann cells at the Schwann cell–glial junction, which is usually found in the internal auditory canal. Around 40% of patients with sporadic acoustic neuromas show loss of heterozygosity in the region of the tumor suppressor NF-2 gene on chromosome 22, suggesting that an underlying genetic predisposition exists in many patients [3]. Indeed the presence of bilateral acoustic neuromas is diagnostic for neurofibromatosis-2, further implicating dysfunction of this gene in the pathogenesis of these tumors.

Acoustic neuromas arise almost exclusively from the vestibular branches of the VIII nerve complex; hence, they are more correctly referred to as vestibular schwannomas. They expand the porus acousticus forming a cone-shaped mass with a canalicular and CPA component in 61% of patients. In 21% of cases, the canalicular component becomes sausage-shaped and "mushrooms" out of the porus into the CPA, leading to a dumbbell appearance. In the remainder (18%), the tumors appear to be largely confined to the CPA with no significant intracanalicular component [4]. The laterally arising tumors tend to present earlier with audiovestibular symptoms. Those arising within the CPA are more likely to present with signs of trigeminal compression, cerebellar dysfunction and raised intracranial pressure. A recent analysis of 473 patients with acoustic neuromas treated in Cambridge shows that 89.3% presented with typical audiovestibular symptoms. Of the 10.7% with an atypical presenting symptom, facial numbness (6.4%), headache (2.1%), otalgia (1%), visual changes (0.6%), taste disturbance (0.2%) and facial weakness (0.2%) were all recorded. A high degree of clinical acumen is required to avoid inadvertent delays in the diagnosis of the lesion in this group of patients.

Macroscopically, the superior cerebellopontine cistern is invaginated by the tumor, forming a double arachnoid plane around the lesion. Whilst many tumors are homogeneous in texture, macrocyst formation occurs.

Histological examination reveals regions characterized by spindle-shaped cells with hyperchromatic, elongated nuclei (Antoni A type) and other regions where vacuolated cells with pleomorphic nuclei are embedded in a loose eosinophilic matrix in which microcystic change may be prominent (Antoni B). Malignant change in acoustic neuromas is exceptional, with few cases reported in the world literature.

Meningiomas

Meningiomas of the petrous face comprise around 7% of all CPA lesions. They present in patients aged 30–70 years and are five times more common in women. Most patients have symptoms of vestibulocochlear nerve dysfunction. About 80% complain of hearing loss, with a dead ear being evident in 19%. Tinnitus (60%), impaired balance (26%), trigeminal signs (45%) and facial weakness (10%) may also occur. Imaging investigations show that the mean tumor size is 3.5 cm at the time of diagnosis [1]. Risk factors probably include previous radiotherapy, e.g. for childhood leukaemia. Inactivation of the NF-2 tumor suppressor gene appears to be important in the pathogenesis of sporadic meningioma in up to 60% of cases.

Meningiomas of the CPA can arise in close proximity to the porus acousticus, or from a separate origin on the face of the petrous bone. Meningiomas of the CPA possess similar pathological features to those found at other, more common intracranial sites. The World Health Organisation classifies meningothelial cell tumors into many subtypes. Anaplastic and atypical meningiomas have a higher propensity for local recurrence, and complete local resection, along with dural attachments and any abnormal bone, are mandatory to minimize the risk of tumor recurrence.

Epidermoid Tumor (Cholesteatomas)

Primary epidermoid tumors, or cholesteatomas, are non-neoplastic, cystic lesions lined with a simple stratified squamous epithelium. They are considered to be congenital, arising from misplaced epidermal cell rests [5]. Cholesteatomas of the CPA must be differentiated from the acquired lesions that occur secondary to middle-ear suppurative disease. The latter are usually restricted to the tympano-mastoid region, but erosion of the petrous bone may occur, with the appearance of a petrous apex cholesteatoma. These acquired lesions are about 1.5 times more frequent in our experience. CPA cholesteatomas present in adults of either sex with a mean age of 43 years. They contain lamellae of desquamated keratin, cell debris and a variable number of cholesterol crystals. Macroscopically, the lesions resemble clusters of pearls. They grow slowly, by a process of desquamation, and infiltrate the cisternal spaces. Cranial nerve palsies dominate the clinical presentation [1].

Glomus Tumors

Glomus tumors result from neoplastic transformation in paraganglionic "jugular bodies". Since spread of these tumors follows the path of least resistance, large tumors may present within the CPA [6]. The presenting symptoms include hearing loss, pulsatile tinnitus, dysequilibrium, dysphonia, dysphagia and aural bleeding.

Other CPA Lesions

Schwannomas may occur on any of the lower cranial nerves. The facial and trigeminal nerves are more frequently affected than the bulbar nerves [1]. These lesions may occur entirely within the CPA but, in the case of trigeminal schwannomas, dumbbell extension through Meckel's cave into the middle cranial fossa is usual.

Cerebellopontine angle arachnoid cysts are rare and often present with headache and ataxia, rather than cranial nerve compression syndromes. If symptoms are few, observation is advocated. However, symptomatic lesions require treatment. This is most safely met through a wide fenestration procedure rather than excision or shunting [7].

Basilar artery ectasia and posterior circulation aneurysms can present as a mass in the CPA. With modern imaging techniques and careful history taking these lesions should be recognised at a stage that enables appropriate neurovascular management to be directed at them.

The foramen of Luschka provides a communication between the fourth ventricle and the CPA. In view of this, lesions of the ventricular system, such as ependymomas, choroid plexus tumors and dermoid tumors, may protrude into the CPA. Presentation may be related to cranial nerve compression, mass effect or hydrocephalus. Other rare tumors of the CPA include chordomas, haemangioblastomas, metastases and lipomas. Whilst MRI findings may provide diagnostic information, an accurate pre-operative diagnosis is often not possible.

Management of CPA Tumors

Since 80–85% of CPA lesions are acoustic neuromas, much of this discussion concerns the management of these lesions.

Investigations

MRI Scanning

Contrast-enhanced MRI is the investigation of choice in patients with symptoms and/or signs of CPA disease. Thin sections in axial and coronal planes can detect acoustic neuromas as small as 2 mm in diameter. CT scans provide complementary information on bone anatomy, but the beam-hardening artefact caused by the petrous bone reduces the resolution of the technique within the CPA. Typical MRI appearances of CPA lesions are shown in Fig. 14.1. Acoustic neuromas and meningiomas may both appear isointense on T2-weighted images and enhance with paramagnetic contrast. Cystic appearances can be present in either lesion. However, meningiomas appear broad-based and form an obtuse angle with the petrous dura. A tail of dural enhancement is frequently present and is a pathognomic sign. Acoustic neuromas characteristically expand the porus acousticus but, if hyperostosis is associated with a meningioma, the porus may be narrowed.

Otoneurological Findings

Otoneurological investigations are indicated when a patient presents with symptoms suggestive of vestibulocochlear nerve dysfunction. Using pure tone audiometry, four patterns of sensorineural hearing loss are recognized in patients with acoustic neuromas. High-frequency loss is seen in 65% of patients. In 22% of patients, hearing loss is depressed equally

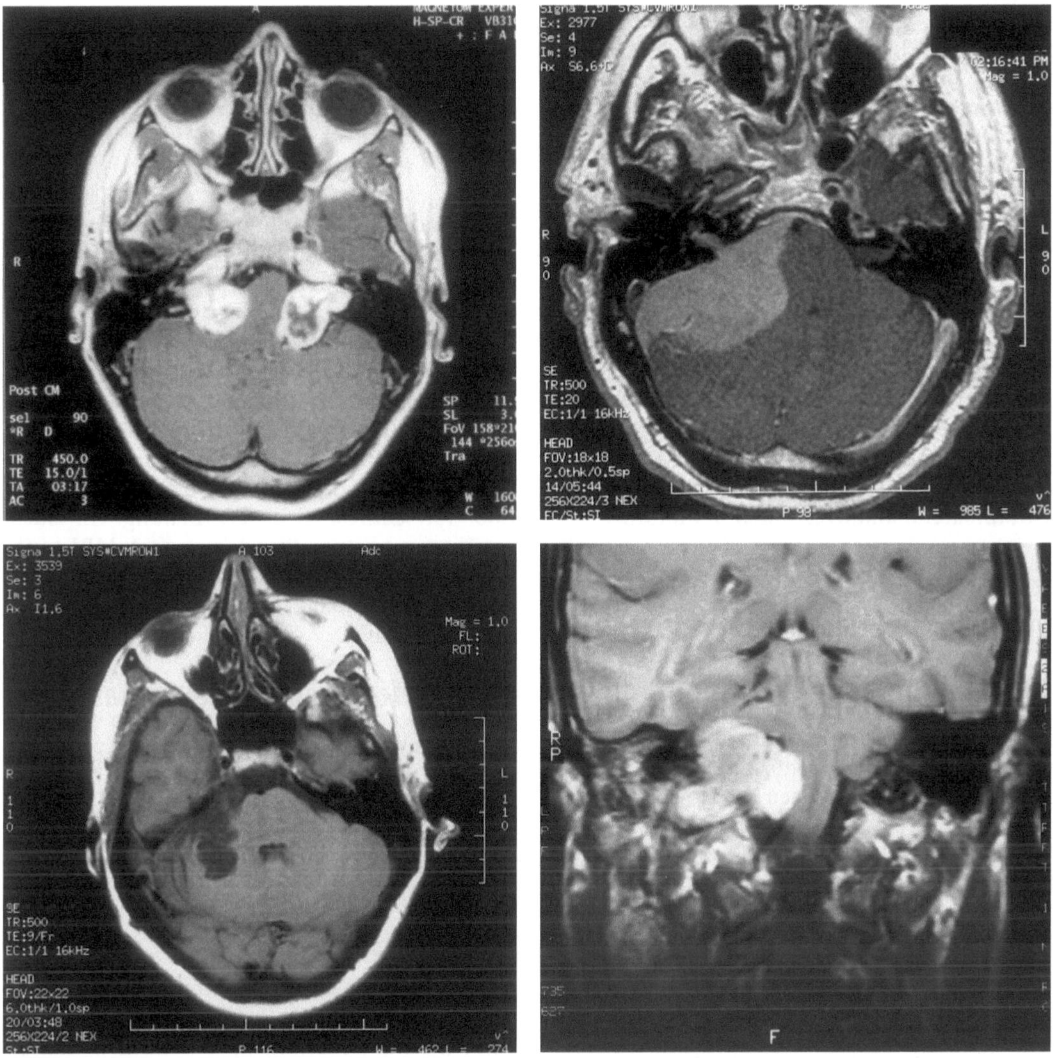

Fig. 14.1. Radiological appearances of CPA lesions. **a** T1-weighted axial image with contrast. Bilateral acoustic neuromas in a patient with NF-2. **b** T1-weighted axial image with contrast showing a CPA meningioma. Notice the normal appearance of the internal auditory meatus and the broad origin of the tumor. The T2-weighted image showed increased signal in the compressed cerebellar hemisphere. **c** T1-weighted axial image showing a CPA cholesteatoma. This lesion did not enhance following contrast injection. **d** T1-weighted coronal image with contrast showing a large CPA glomus jugulare tumor.

across all frequencies. In 7%, low tone loss is evident whilst, in 6%, a trough-shaped loss is seen, with relative preservation of hearing at high and low frequencies [8].

Speech discrimination tests determine the ability of the patient to identify a taped series of words presented at 40 dB above the speech threshold. The quality of hearing can be classified according to the speech discrimination score combined with the pure tone audiogram loss [9]. Hearing is described as excellent if there is a pure tone loss of 0–30 dB with 70–100% speech discrimination. Other grades (serviceable, non-serviceable, poor and absent) represent increasingly poor auditory function. Poor speech discrimination that is out of proportion to the degree of pure-tone loss is a feature of acoustic neuromas. This is attributed to the finding that up to 75% of cochlear fibers may be damaged before the pure-tone deficit is evident. The ability to discriminate speech is of importance when considering the appropriate management strategies, such as hearing preservation surgery, for an individual patient.

Although widely used, the specificity and sensitivity of caloric tests, brainstem auditory evoked responses and acoustic decay reflexes are inferior to MRI as screening tests in patients with symptoms and/or signs of CPA pathology. A recent retrospective analysis has shown that pure tone audiometry was normal in 25% of patients with CPA meningiomas, further supporting the use of MRI as the investigation of choice in patients with symptoms indicative of CPA disease, including patients presenting with unilateral audiovestibular symptoms.

Treatment Strategies in Patients with Acoustic Neuromas

When considering the management of a patient with an acoustic neuroma, several factors preside. The size of the tumor is of paramount importance. In the Cambridge series of 473 patients presenting between 1983 and 1995, 47% of tumors were large (more than 2.5 cm), 32% medium (1.5–2.5 cm) and 21% small (less than 1.5 cm). Large tumors may cause the life-threatening complications of symptomatic hydrocephalus, and direct mass effect. We advocate initial insertion of a ventriculoperitoneal shunt, or, in suitable cases, a third ventriculostomy, to alleviate hydrocephalus. If mass symptoms are evident, early surgery to remove the tumor should be considered. The initial presentation of these tumors in this way is now rare.

At presentation, most acoustic neuromas present with audiovestibular symptoms and do not constitute a threat to life at that time. A complete understanding of the natural history, surgical morbidity and success of radiosurgery is of importance in deciding the appropriate management of patients with these tumors.

Natural History

Intracanalicular acoustic neuromas frequently present early with audiovestibular symptoms, and may be very small at presentation. Imaging studies show that the rate of growth of these tumors varies both between individual tumors and within a specific lesion. Whilst a growth rate of around 2 mm per year is usual, tumors can grow by as much as 17 mm per annum [10]. This information, combined with the fact that quality of life is reduced after surgery for very large tumors, make a strong case for treatment in the young patient with a small acoustic neuroma. A "wait and see" policy condemns the patient to indefinite follow-up, an uncertain future and substantial costs for regular MR scans. However, in the elderly patient with co-morbidity, a conservative approach with careful clinical and radiological follow-up is a reasonable alternative strategy. Although assessment of growth and volumetric estimation of tumor size are complex, repeat imaging for comparative studies usually provides sufficient information for clinical decision making. In such patients, we recommend a repeat MRI scan 6 months after diagnosis, annually for 4 years and then bi-annually, provided tumor growth is not progressive.

Surgery for Acoustic Neuromas

Much has been written about the relative merits of the translabyrinthine, retrosigmoid and middle fossa approaches in the treatment of acoustic neuromas. A synopsis of the historical milestones in acoustic neuroma surgery is shown in Table 14.2.

Intraoperative Monitoring

Intraoperative facial nerve monitoring is useful and widely practiced. A pre-requisite for electromyographic monitoring is that the patient is

Table 14.2. Historical milestones in acoustic neuroma surgery.

Year	Event
1891	McBurney attempts removal of an acoustic neuroma
1894	Charles Ballance successfully removes an acoustic neuroma
1903	Krause describes the sub-occipital approach
1904	Panse describes the translabyrinthine approach
1917	Cushing's acoustic neuroma monograph is published
1931	Cairns successfully preserves the facial nerve
1964	House describes microsurgical translabyrinthine approach
1979	Mortality is reduced to 2.6% in a series of 500 patients

not paralyzed with neuromuscular agents when assessing facial nerve responses. A bipolar stimulating electrode provides a spatially precise means of stimulating the facial nerve, enabling EMG potentials to be recorded using needle electrodes in facial muscles (e.g. orbicularis oculi and oris). The signals are amplified and made audible to the surgeon. Although a randomized study of this technique has not been performed, few surgeons now operate without such monitoring. For large CPA lesions and other skull base tumors, the technique can be adapted to monitor the motor components of other cranial nerves. The trigeminal nerve can be assessed by inserting electrodes into the masseter and/or temporalis muscles. The lower motor cranial nerves can be monitored by inserting electrodes into the soft palate (IX), taping electrodes to the endotracheal tube to assess laryngeal muscle function (X), or inserting electrodes in the sternocleidomastoid and trapezius muscles (XI) or the tongue (XII). Other monitoring systems have been developed based upon mechanotransducers, the stimulus for development being the artifact caused in EMG recording by electrocoagulation. However, newer generation multichannel EMG monitoring devices are likely to become the monitoring tools of choice.

A variety of techniques may be used to monitor intraoperative cochlear nerve function. These include brainstem auditory evoked responses (BAERs) and auditory compound action potentials (CAPs) [11]. BAERs are recorded from vertex and upper cervical electrodes. Sound stimuli at 20 pulses per second at 65 dB above normal threshold are used via earphones. A continuous waveform can be displayed to show the effects of surgery upon cochlear nerve function. The principal drawback of this technique is the time delay between anatomical or physiological disruption of the cochlear nerve and a change in the BAER. This limits the clinical utility of the method. To overcome this problem, direct recording of CAPs from either the cochlear nerve or the cochlear nucleus have been used. Whilst this form of monitoring may reduce intraoperative trauma to the cochlear nerve, an effect upon the outcome of hearing preservation surgery has not been demonstrated.

Translabyrinthine Approach

This approach provides the shortest, most direct route to the CPA. Cerebellar retraction is minimized and the lateral end of the facial nerve is clearly visualized. William House popularized this approach, and we advocate its use in patients with hearing loss and in virtually all patients with large neuromas.

The patient is placed supine with the head turned 70° away from the side of the lesion. The head is flexed, but the chin must remain clear of the contralateral clavicle. The head is tilted so the malar is uppermost. A sandbag is placed beneath the ipsilateral shoulder. The thigh is also prepared to enable fascia lata and fat to be harvested in preparation for wound closure. We use a "hockey stick" incision, curving from just above the posterior-superior aspect of the auricle, descending to a point 1 cm behind and below the mastoid tip. Careful attention is given to opening the scalp in two layers. The periosteum is then reflected anteriorly, exposing the posterior aspect of the external auditory canal and the spine of Henle. Care must be taken not to perforate the skin of the canal during placement of the self-retaining retractor. The temporal bone is then drilled in a systematic fashion to provide a corridor of access to the CPA.

Drilling of the temporal bone is performed in four phases:

- Extended mastoidectomy with exposure of the facial nerve.
- Removal of the semicircular canals.
- Exposure of the bony internal auditory canal. To improve access the jugular bulb can be uncovered and retracted inferiorly.
- Removal of bone around the lateral 270° of the canal.

The dura is then opened longitudinally in the inferior half of the internal auditory canal. The canalicular portion of the tumor is readily evident and the facial nerve identified. The posterior fossa dura is then opened in continuity with the already exposed internal auditory canal, increasing access into the CPA.

The tumor usually displaces the facial nerve anteriorly. This relationship needs to be clarified during resection of the tumor. The superior and inferior poles of the tumor are sequentially inspected, enabling the lateral aspect of the brainstem to be identified. Care must be taken to preserve all blood vessels passing over the surface of the tumor. Many of the arteries looping over the tumor will supply the brainstem. The trigeminal nerve and superior petrosal vein can usually be identified superiorly. Lintine strips are eased into the plane around the tumor capsule to protect the brainstem. Inferiorly, the lower cranial nerves and posterior inferior cerebellar artery are protected from the tumor. Care must be taken in larger tumors not to over-retract either the neuraxis or the tumor. In such tumors, early attention to CSF drainage helps, but exposure of the tumor margins must be performed in an incremental fashion. The surface of the tumor is diathermied to reduce vascularity during this phase of exposure. The canalicular and anterior aspects of the tumor are left undisturbed at this point.

The tumor surface is then incised and the tumor debulked from within using an ultrasonic aspirator. Care is taken not to perforate the tumor during this maneuver. After debulking the tumor, further exposure of the capsule can be made taking care to protect the brainstem structures. Sequential exposure and debulking can then be performed. The brainstem end of the facial nerve requires exposure. Essential landmarks are the choroid plexus of the Foramen of Luschka, the line of the glossopharyngeal nerve and the pontomedullary sulcus. Once the facial nerve has been identified the cochlear and vestibular nerves are sacrificed at the brainstem end. The tumor is then rolled laterally towards the internal auditory canal. The position of the facial nerve is carefully observed. The tumor is then dissected from the facial nerve using microscissors under a modestly irrigated operating field. The tumor may be adherent to the dural margins of the porus acousticus. The ring of dura enveloping the tumor needs to be opened at both shoulders of the tumor. The facial nerve is often very thin and splayed at this point. At times, the facial nerve can be followed from lateral to medial, gently retracting the tumor into the CPA whilst dissecting the tumor from the nerve. Eventually, the tumor will be removed. After ensuring resection is complete, hemostasis is secured, using irrigation and application of a monolayer of oxidized cellulose patches to the brainstem.

The principal objective during closure of the wound is to ensure that CSF leakage cannot occur. The eustachian tube and middle ear are sealed with small pieces of fat and fibrin glue (Tisseel, Immuno IG, Vienna, Austria). A patch of fascia lata (2 × 2.5 cm), secured with fibrin glue, is then placed over the drilled surface of the petrous bone to cover the middle ear. Three finger-sized strips of fat are then placed just into the CPA and anchored superficially with fibrin glue. The mastoid air cells are sealed with bone wax. The pericranium is then closed. The galea, reinforced with a fascia lata patch, is sutured. Finally, the scalp is closed in two layers.

To minimize the risk of CSF leak, we recommend daily lumbar punctures, reducing the CSF pressure to +5 cm on the first three post-operative days. These are performed in preference to leaving a lumbar drain in situ to encourage early ambulation. The post-operative hospital stay is variable, but is around 5 or 6 days in healthy ambulant patients.

Retrosigmoid Approach

Historically, this approach was favored for the removal of acoustic neuromas. However, cerebellar retraction, which in large lesions may be considerable, and difficult access to the lateral internal auditory canal have reduced the utility of the approach in favor of the translabyrinthine exposure in the majority of patients. Furthermore, headache appears to be more persistent than after a translabyrinthine approach. We use the retrosigmoid approach in an attempt to preserve hearing in patients with socially useful hearing (Gardner–Robertson Grade I). We also use this approach in patients with Grade II hearing accompanied by contralateral hearing loss.

The patient is positioned supine with the head turned 80° to the contralateral side, with the neck flexed and the ear uppermost. Brain relaxation is achieved by inducing an osmotic diuresis during exposure. A curvilinear incision commencing posterior to the auricle and descending 2 cm behind and below the mastoid process is used. The sub-occipital muscles and fascia are divided in the line of the incision in separate layers. Care is taken to avoid cutting the occipital artery. The periosteum is then retracted to expose the mastoid tip and the superior nuchal line. A sub-occipital, retrosigmoid craniectomy is performed, exposing the transverse and sigmoid sinuses. The latter is followed inferiorly for about 4 cm. The foramen magnum is not opened. The dura is then opened in a cruciate fashion. A self-retaining retractor is introduced to retract the cerebellum posteriorly. Early drainage of CSF facilitates the exposure, minimizing neuraxis retraction. This is performed by identifying the lower cranial nerves and opening the inferior cerebellopontine cistern. These cranial nerves are then protected with a cottonoid pattie. The tumor is then examined and the arachnoidal plane around the superior and posterior poles opened. If the tumor is small, the proximal VII and VIII nerve complex will be seen at this early stage. Care must be taken to ensure that the facial nerve passes anterior to the tumor rather than taking an aberrant course over the posterior or superior aspects of the tumor. With larger tumors internal debulking, preferentially performed with the cavitating ultrasonic surgical aspirator, will be required prior to identification of the neural structures. Careful dissection of the tumor is then performed, with the objective of preserving the facial and auditory nerves. The vestibular nerves are divided.

Rather than follow the tumor mass along the internal auditory canal, the safest approach is to drill off the posterior wall of the internal auditory canal. The petrous dura is incised and retracted, enabling the posterior lip of the porus and the opening for the endolymphatic sac to be identified. Radical removal of the porus acousticus can inadvertently fenestrate the inner ear, destroying auditory function. After opening the internal auditory canal, the dura is incised, exposing the intracanalicular tumor and the distal nerves. The facial and cochlear nerves are preserved, whilst the vestibular nerves are divided. The tumor is then dissected towards the porus acousticus. With meticulous attention, this most adherent part of the tumor can be removed. Hemostasis is secured, and the drilled petrous bone is sealed with bone wax and covered with a piece of fascia lata (2 × 2 cm) secured with fibrin glue. The dura is closed in a watertight fashion with fascia lata to bridge any defects. Fat patches are placed over the dura. The pericranium, muscles, fascia, subcutaneous fat and skin are closed in separate layers.

Middle Fossa Approach

This approach is utilized for intracanalicular tumors in which an attempt at hearing preservation is desirable. The drawbacks of the approach are temporal lobe retraction, which can result in seizures and focal neurological signs, limited access if the tumor has extended beyond the porus into the CPA and the difficulty in identifying landmarks on the petrous ridge.

The patient is positioned supine with the head turned to the contralateral side, with the ear uppermost. Brain relaxation using osmotic diuretics and/or lumbar CSF drainage is mandatory. A pre-auricular incision is used and a middle fossa free flap craniotomy performed. This must be made as low as possible to minimize the amount of bone that needs to be removed with ronguers. The petrous bone is then exposed extradurally. The arcuate eminence and greater petrosal nerve are useful landmarks to localize the internal auditory canal. Once located, the internal auditory canal must be opened widely. The dural sleeve is opened along the long axis of the canal. The position of the facial nerve is confirmed. The tumor is then excised, with careful dissection from the nerves and vessels in the canal. The cochlear nerve is usually only revealed once the tumor has been resected. A small plug of fat is placed in the tumor bed. The dura is repaired and the craniotomy closed in standard fashion.

Results of Acoustic Neuroma Surgery

The objective of acoustic neuroma surgery is the total removal of the neoplasm with minimal morbidity and mortality. Objective recording of cranial nerve function, CSF leak rates, meningitis incidence and quality-of-life assessments can assess morbidity. Extent of tumor removal can be determined intraoperatively, and recurrence can be monitored with MRI scans.

In the modern era, total tumor removal should be achieved. This was the case in 99.6% of patients with unilateral tumors in Cambridge. Recurrence of acoustic neuromas is exceptional, and has only been seen in two patients in our center between 1982 and 1998. In one of these cases (a patient with NF-2), the tumor was histologically malignant. We perform MRI scans 2 and 5 years post-operatively to ensure recurrence has not occurred.

The mortality of surgery for acoustic neuromas has reduced dramatically over the course of this century. Whilst Cushing's overall operative mortality was 11.4% [12], mortality figures of around 20% were reported in other historical series. However, microsurgical advances have reduced death rates, initially to 5%, then to around 2–3%. In the total Cambridge series of 660 acoustic neuroma operations, we have encountered eight deaths (1.2%). The causes of death include hematomas in the CPA or cerebellum, brainstem infarction and post-operative meningitis, in addition to concomitant medical complications.

Facial Nerve Outcome

Facial nerve function can be assessed using the House–Brackmann scale [13]. This grades facial weakness as normal (Grade I) through mild (II), moderate (III), moderately severe (IV), severe (V) and total paralysis (VI). This method of assessment has a high degree of interobserver reliability and has become widely adopted.

In the Cambridge series (1982–1998), the facial nerve was anatomically intact following tumor resection in 94% of cases. Loss of the facial nerve in patients with small tumors was exceptional. In the 372 patients with long-term facial nerve follow-up, 76% of patients undergoing translabyrinthine surgery achieved a Grade I–III result. Retrosigmoid resection results were slightly better, with 79% achieving a Grade I–III result at 12 months. Table 14.3 shows results for facial nerve function related to tumor size. When the series is analyzed in 5-year time-blocks the Grade I–III facial nerve results improved from 56% (1982–1987), through 81% (1988–1992) to 85% (1993–1997). This indicates that the experience of the surgical team is critical in facial nerve preservation surgery [14].

Multivariate analysis has shown that the most important independent risk factors for poor facial nerve outcome (House–Brackmann Grade IV–VI) are increasing patient age, tumor size greater than 2.4 cm, the translabyrinthine approach and lack of intraoperative facial nerve monitoring [15]. The explanations behind these findings are largely speculative. With increasing age, the vascularity of the facial nerve may become compromized. Risk factors implicating the translabyrinthine route may include thermal injury generated during drilling of the temporal bone, and post-operative facial nerve oedema.

Management of Facial Nerve Palsy

Although Ballance successfully performed the first removal of an acoustic neuroma nearly 100 years ago, the patient required subsequent enucleation of the eye due to trigeminal and facial nerve complications. Exposure keratitis can occur in patients with severe facial palsy due to decreased lacrimation and reduced closure, particularly if associated with trigeminal sensory loss and a poor Bell's phenomenon. Decreased lacrimation can be treated with methyl cellulose eye drops and liquid paraffin eye ointment. The eye should be protected, particularly at night. If eye closure is deficient 1 week post-operatively, botulinum toxin injection or a lateral tarsorrhaphy should be performed. If a facial nerve palsy persists, static (e.g. gold weight in eye lid, fascial slings) or dynamic procedures (e.g. muscle transfers) can be used to protect the eye and improve the cosmetic appearance. If the nerve remained in continuity at operation, spontaneous regeneration offers a better prospect of a good result compared with a reanimation procedure [16].

Table 14.3. Post-operative facial nerve function at 1 year after surgery for small, medium and large acoustic neuromas: Cambridge results.

House Grade	Percentage of patients in each group		
	Small (<1.5 cm)	Medium (1.5–3 cm)	Large (>3 cm)
I	58	42.5	18
II	16.5	19.5	19
III	15	22	26
IV	1.5	4.5	22
V	4.5	4.5	5
VI	4.5	7	21

The latter should therefore be delayed 1 year from the time of surgery unless the facial nerve has been severed. Post-operative electroneuronography 1 week post-operatively has been shown to be of prognostic value. Incomplete degeneration is associated with a Grade I or II outcome whereas complete degeneration forecasts a protracted, incomplete recovery [17].

If the facial nerve is divided at operation a primary repair is the procedure of choice. This may be feasible due to stretching of the nerve by the tumor and by mobilization of the nerve within the petrous bone. A posterior auricular or sural nerve cable graft is useful if a primary repair is technically not possible. Where a reanimation procedure is subsequently performed, a variety of options exist. Several groups currently favor hypoglossal–facial nerve anastomosis. The principal drawback of this operation, namely hemiatrophy of the tongue, is small compared with other potential donor nerves such as the glossopharyngeal, spinal accessory and phrenic. A hypoglossal–facial anastomosis can either be performed by complete division of the hypoglossal nerve, or by fashioning a bifurcation in the nerve at the level of the descendens hypoglossi, leaving some innervation to the tongue intact. In a meta-analysis, good results were reported in 65% of more than 500 cases. After nerve transfer procedures, motor activity takes 6 months to commence and may improve over a few years. The patient needs to learn that manipulating the tongue results in facial movements.

Involuntary and emotional movements of the face do not occur as a result of hypoglossal–facial anastomosis. Such movements require innervation from the facial nerve nucleus in the brainstem. A cross-facial nerve transfer consists of a peripheral nerve interposition graft (usually sural nerve) between a distal facial branch on the normal side to a complementary branch on the affected side. This procedure can improve expressive movements of selected facial muscle groups.

Nerve transfer procedures require relatively lengthy surgery with uncertain, often disappointing, results that take months or even years to achieve a desirable result. A careful selection process is pertinent in performing these procedures. We reserve reanimation surgery for young, well motivated patients with a robust psychological approach to their disease. Static and dynamic cosmetic procedures are more suitable for the majority of patients with severe permanent facial nerve palsy.

Hearing Preservation

What constitutes useful hearing is debatable. Whilst many consider Gardner–Robertson Grade II hearing useful, the distortion and imbalance may be annoying and distracting to many patients. However, if the contralateral ear is damaged, Grade II hearing preservation is highly desirable. Generally, we consider hearing preservation surgery in patients with 70% speech discrimination and a pure tone audiogram within 30 dB of the non-affected side (Grade I). We consider severe pre-operative tinnitus a relative contraindication to hearing preservation surgery. In selected patients the results of attempts at hearing preservation are variable. A recent analysis of 50 hearing preservation operations performed in Cambridge via the retrosigmoid approach has shown that only 4.8% of patients had normal post-operative hearing and 8% had serviceable hearing. A further 18% had some hearing at post-operative assessment [18]. Hearing was preserved in 24% of patients treated at the Mayo Clinic via the retrosigmoid approach [19]. In contrast, of 25 patients with serviceable hearing (Grade I or II) operated upon via the middle fossa approach, 18 (72%) retained hearing post-operatively; however, in only seven (28%) was the post-operative hearing of Grade I quality [20]. The success of hearing preservation is dependent upon tumor size, with dismal results in patients with large tumors.

Nervus Intermedius Function

Although pre-operative symptoms related to dysfunction of this nerve are uncommon, post-operative symptoms are frequent. The nervus intermedius carries secretomotor fibers to the submandibular, sublingual and minor salivary glands, the nasal and palatine mucus glands and the lacrimal gland. It also carries taste from the anterior two-thirds of the tongue and hard palate, and some somatic afferent fibers from the external auditory meatus. Damage to the nervus intermedius is common in CPA surgery. Reinnervation or transephaptic transmission probably accounts for the onset of lacrimation during eating ("crocodile tears") which is present in 44% of patients post-operatively. A reduction in tear production is present in 72% of patients, whilst 48% admit to changes in taste sensation post-operatively [21]. To reduce the distress caused by these symptoms all patients should be adequately counselled pre-operatively.

CSF Leakage and Meningitis

Excluding facial nerve damage, CSF leakage is the most common complication after translabyrinthine or retrosigmoid acoustic neuroma surgery. Most authors report a rate of 10–15%, although meticulous refinement of closure techniques can reduce the incidence to 5% or less [22]. The principal complication of post-operative CSF leakage is meningitis, which occurs in around 2–5% in the major series. This may present some weeks after discharge from hospital, and diligence is required not to overlook the diagnosis. In the Cambridge series, CSF leakage occurred in 5% of patients, although a subset of 188 consecutive patients were operated upon with a leak rate of only 1.6%. CSF leakage usually settles with a period of lumbar CSF drainage. However, 2% of the whole series required re-exploration and wound re-closure.

Quality of Life

Whilst the past four decades have seen a reduction in the mortality rates from 16 to 2–3% and an increase in normal facial nerve function from 3 to 50–60%, a significant hidden morbidity exists in patients undergoing acoustic neuroma surgery. This has been measured in 227 patients using an acoustic neuroma specific questionnaire coupled with the European Organisation for Research into the Treatment of Cancer (EORTC) core questionnaire. This showed that life quality was reduced to 85% (normal = 100%) in patients with acoustic neuromas. In patients with tumors of more than 1.5 cm in diameter, life quality was significantly reduced further to 77%. However, the post-operative life quality did not differ between patients with tumors 1.5–2.5 cm in diameter compared with tumors of more than 2.5 cm. This information carries the implication that surgery in patients with small tumors is justified to prevent the tumor reaching a larger size where quality of life after surgery is reduced further. Despite the findings of this sensitive quality-of-life analysis, only 3% of patients were dependent upon others for important daily activities, with 79% of patients returning to their normal lifestyle. This apparent discrepancy illustrates the difficulties involved in measuring quality of life.

Stereotactic Radiosurgery in the Treatment of Acoustic Neuromas

Stereotactic radiosurgery is increasingly being used in the treatment of small and medium acoustic neuromas. The rapid return to normal activity and avoidance of an open procedure are attractive alternatives to microsurgery. The treatment aims to prevent further tumor growth, maintain neurological function and minimize the risk of new neurological deficits. Worldwide experience with the technique is increasing and long-term results require careful scrutiny. Treatment protocols are evolving as experience with the technique increases [23]. Careful planning using stereotactic MRI enables precise isodose curves with steep radiation fall-off outside the tumor margin to be used in the treatment of small and medium acoustic neuromas. Doses of between 12 and 16 Gy at the treatment margin and 16–24 Gy at the tumor core are being used. If hearing preservation is sought, doses are at the lower limits of these ranges.

Of 162 consecutive patients followed up for a minimum of 5 years in Pittsburgh, tumor size diminished in 62%, remained static in 33% and showed slow growth in 6%. Normal facial and trigeminal nerve function was evident in 79 and 73%, respectively, at follow-up [24]. Preservation of useful hearing was reported in 50% of the 18 patients with useful pre-treatment hearing treated in Sheffield [25]. In the small number of patients we have operated upon following failed radiosurgery, dissection of the tumor from the facial nerve is more difficult due to increased adherence, particularly at the porus acousticus.

To date, no randomized trial has been performed to compare the treatment options in patients with acoustic neuromas. The indications for radiosurgery are relative and are evolving. Patients with co-existing medical ailments, recurrent tumors, which are very rare in our experience, and neurofibromatosis-2 are all suitable. Patients in whom microsurgery is an option need to be counselled, bearing in mind the resources and outcome information currently available.

Bilateral Acoustic Neuromas

Bilateral acoustic neuromas are diagnostic of neurofibromatosis-2. This disease is caused by mutations in the NF-2 tumor suppressor gene on chromosome 22, and follows an autosomal dominant pattern of inheritance. Treating these patients is always difficult. Bilateral facial palsies, deafness and the prospect of other CNS tumors developing point to a miserable existence. Management options include observation or subcapsular removal to minimize risk to the audiovestibular nerves and stereotactic radiosurgery. Both require careful consideration. Other options include early treatment of the smaller neuroma to maximise the chance of hearing preservation or treatment of the larger tumor first, with the aim of delaying surgery on the contralateral side if it remains the only source of useful hearing after the first procedure. The treatments in each of these unfortunate patients require individualization and supportive aftercare. The development of brainstem implant technology to augment auditory function may prove useful in these cases in the future.

Management of Other CPA Tumors

Pre-operative imaging can provide information that is of diagnostic value in many patients with CPA tumors. Most CPA masses require surgical removal, although, increasingly, stereotactic radiosurgery provides an alternative treatment, and may become more important as long-term cohort studies are reported. The surgical approach to CPA is dependent upon the exact location of the tumor, and the presence of associated pre-operative cranial nerve lesions.

Meningiomas

The treatment of choice for meningiomas is complete surgical excision of the tumor, its dural attachments and any abnormal bone. For CPA meningiomas, this may be accomplished by any of the standard approaches described for acoustic neuroma excision, depending upon the hearing status and the precise location of the tumor. Complete macroscopic surgical excision is usually achieved in this group of patients. This objective is only accomplished in about 70% of patients with "non-acoustic neuroma like" meningiomas – a group that includes clival and petrous apex tumors. In the Cambridge series of 31 patients (1981–1994) with CPA meningiomas, the retrosigmoid approach was used in 16 cases. Grade I hearing was present in nine of these patients and Grade II in two patients pre-operatively. Grade I hearing was preserved in six patients (67%) and Grade II in two patients. Other groups have reported similar results. Furthermore, a case has been reported of a patient in whom meningioma excision resulted in a dramatic improvement in hearing. Serious consideration should be given to the retrosigmoid approach rather than the translabyrinthine approach in patients in whom the pre-operative imaging suggests a meningioma. In the Cambridge series normal facial nerve function was present in 65% post-operatively, with 84% having a House Grade I–III result. Other cranial nerve palsies observed in small numbers of post-operative patients involved the IV, V, VI, IX, X and XI cranial nerves [1].

Alternative treatments for meningiomas are not evidence based. Whilst stereotactic radiosurgery may be applicable in some selected patients, the relatively large tumor size at presentation (3.5 cm mean) mitigates against this approach in the majority of patients.

Other Schwannomas

Facial nerve neuromas are usually indistinguishable from acoustic lesions until the tumor is encountered at surgery [1]. Surgery is therefore performed either by the translabyrinthine or retrosigmoid approach according to the patient's pre-operative hearing. Neuromas of the trigeminal nerve often present with a dumbbell mass present in both the posterior and middle cranial fossae. We usually remove such lesions via a pre-sigmoid combined posterior fossa/middle fossa approach. The otic capsule is left intact during drilling of the temporal bone. The petrous face dura is opened to gain access to the posterior fossa. If the tumor is large, the dura in the retrosigmoid region should be exposed and opened. If necessary, the sigmoid sinus is divided to improve access. If this is contemplated, pre-operative venous angiography is advised. A low, middle fossa craniotomy is performed to enable the middle fossa component of the tumor to be adequately exposed. The tentorium cerebelli is divided to greatly enhance simultaneous access into the middle and posterior fossae. The line of division should be parallel to the petrous apex, but just posterior to where the trochlear nerve pierces the dura at the medial edge of the tentorium.

Neuromas of the vagus, glossopharyngeal and spinal accessory nerve are exceedingly rare. Total resection was achieved in all five patients reported in the Cambridge series. All patients had at least one cranial nerve palsy, but only one required phonosurgery (teflon injection to vocal cord), and all swallow satisfactorily.

Primary Cholesteatomas of the CPA

Cholesteatomas usually present with features of audiovestibular nerve dysfunction. The surgical approach is determined by the clinical presentation. If hearing is preserved, a retrosigmoid approach is favored (6/10 in the Cambridge series), whereas a transpetrous approach is used if useful hearing has been lost pre-operatively [1]. Despite this, the chance of preserving hearing is low, with only one of the six patients operated on via the retrosigmoid approach retaining hearing. If the lesion extends far medially, the cochlea may require removal to provide sufficient access. Cholesteatomas usually envelop a multitude of cranial nerves and vascular structures. Whilst the soft contents of the lesion can readily be removed, the capsule, which is usually adherent to vascular and neural structures, needs to be excized to avoid recurrence. Although the mortality from surgery to remove these lesions is low, neurological morbidity in the form of post-operative cranial nerve lesions is frequent. This is most commonly the facial nerve, and is most frequently confined to a House–Brackmann Grade II weakness, but complete lesions can occur. Lower cranial nerve lesions were also present in around 30–40% of cases in the Cambridge series [1].

Glomus Tumors

Historical studies have shown only 29% surviving 10 years in patients with glomus jugulare tumors managed with a variety of modalities ranging from no treatment to craniotomy with radiotherapy. Surgical excision offers a potential cure in the treatment of these patients. We advocate a combined trans and infratemporal approach to Type C (tympanomastoid with infralabyrinthine or petrous apex destruction) and D (intradural extension) tumors as described by Fisch. Pre-operative angiography with tumor embolization, where possible, is mandatory. Preliminary control of the internal carotid artery, the sigmoid sinus and the cavernous sinus is necessary to avoid a vascular catastrophe. Blind sac closure of the external auditory canal is performed, followed by a radical mastoidectomy. This exposes the middle and posterior fossa dura and the venous sinuses. The facial nerve distal to the geniculate ganglion is fully skeletonized and transposed anteriorly when necessary. A wide dural opening, sometimes in combination with transection of the sigmoid sinus and the tentorium cerebelli, is performed. The infralabyrinthine petrous bone needs to be removed to expose the petrous portion of the carotid artery and the jugular bulb. The intradural tumor is dissected using a technique of capsular diathermy and sharp dissection. The lower cranial nerves are frequently inseparable from the tumor in the region of the posterior lacerate canal (jugular foramen). The jugular vein is divided and the attachment of the tumor to the carotid artery is removed. This portion of the dissection may be quite hemorrhagic because of the contribution of caroticotympanic vessels to the tumor circulation. Once the tumor has been removed, time needs to be spent effecting a watertight closure.

One or more of the lower cranial nerves were sacrificed in 40% of patients in the Cambridge series. However, patients showed a remarkable ability to accommodate to the neurological deficit [6]. Whilst dysphonia was initially a problem in 6/15 patients, Teflon injection or thyroplasty significantly alleviated symptoms such that it was a persisting problem in only one patient. Persistent dysphagia was a feature in only two patients. Both were treated with a feeding gastrostomy. The remarkable tolerance of these patients to cranial nerve sacrifice may be related to the presence of mild pre-operative cranial nerve deficits present in most patients. Pre-existing cranial nerve dysfunction appears to lead to an increased capacity for functional adaptation. Traditionally, facial nerve transposition has been considered to lead to a permanent House–Brackmann Grade III palsy in the post-operative phase. However, a permanent facial nerve palsy was evident in only 6/15 of our cases at long-term follow-up. A quality of life assessment showed that 70% of patients had an "excellent", 10% a "good" and 20% a "poor" outcome from surgery for large glomus tumors. Long-term follow-up has shown that a small number of patients may develop local tumor recurrence (3/15). We therefore advocate early post-operative MRI to assess residual disease and provide a baseline for future reference. If tumor recurrence occurs, further surgery and/or radiotherapy needs to be considered.

Conclusion

Acoustic neuromas are relatively common neoplasms of the CPA. Surgical approaches are well described, and the treatment outcomes, namely complete tumor removal with minimum mortality and morbidity, well established. Other tumors of the CPA are very rare. These tumors may have very complex relationships with cranial nerves, blood vessels and the skull base. Whilst surgery remains the mainstay in the treatment of all of these lesions, technical difficulties abound. Extended routes of access are frequently used to achieve maximal excision with minimal morbidity. Considerable experience at treating CPA acoustic neuromas is therefore highly desirable before embarking upon surgery for CPA rarities. Due to the large number of problems that these patients may present, a multi-faceted-team approach is advocated at all stages of treatment. In view of the rarity of these tumors, we strongly advocate a tertiary referral system to allow patients to benefit from the pooling of both experience and resources.

Key Points

- *MRI scans can usually provide the surgeon with an accurate pre-treatment diagnosis for lesions in the CPA.*
- *Microsurgical excision, stereotactic radiosurgery and a "watch, wait and re-scan" policy all have merits in different patients with CPA lesions.*
- *Attention to detail, coupled with operator experience, minimize surgical complications.*
- *A multi-faceted-team approach is required to manage post-operative cranial nerve palsies optimally.*

Self-assessment Questions (based on genuine patients)

- ☐ Discuss the management of a 30-year-old lady presenting with tinnitus in whom an MRI scan revealed a 2-cm acoustic neuroma.
- ☐ A 13-year-old girl presented with dizzy turns and life-long facial asymmetry. An MRI scan of the brain demonstrated bilateral intracanalicular acoustic neuromas, a 2.5-cm trigeminal neuroma, a 1-cm intraventricular tumor and a 1-cm cervico-medullary meningioma. Discuss the management of the child and her family.
- ☐ Describe the anatomical basis for the features of a complete facial nerve palsy.
- ☐ Describe the management of a patient with a House Grade IV facial nerve palsy after acoustic neuroma excision.

References

1. Grey PL, Moffat DA, Hardy DG. Surgical results in unusual cerebellopontine angle tumors. Clin Otolaryngol 1996;21:237–43.
2. Pensak ML, Glasscock ME, Josey AF, Jackson CG, Gulya AJ. Sudden hearing loss and cerebellopontine angle tumors. Laryngoscope 1985;95:1188–93.
3. Irving RM, Moffat DA, Hardy DG et al. A molecular, clinical, and immunohistochemical study of vestibular schwannoma. Otolaryngol Head Neck Surg 1997;116:426–30.
4. Moffat DA, Golledge J, Baguley DM, Hardy DG. Clinical correlates of acoustic neuroma morphology. J Laryngol Otol 1993;107:290–4.
5. Michaels L. Origin of congenital cholesteatoma from a normally occurring epidermoid rest in the developing middle ear. International Journal of Pediatric Otorhinolarngology 1988;15:51–65.
6. Whitfield PC, Grey P, Hardy DG, Moffat DA. The surgical management of patients with glomus tumors of the skull base. Br J Neurosurg 1996;10:343–50.

7. Jallo GI, Woo HH, Meshki C, Epstein FJ, Wisoff JH. Arachnoid cysts of the cerebellopontine angle: diagnosis and surgery. Neurosurgery 1997;40:31–8.
8. Maceri DR, Fox CM. Audiological assessment of the acoustic neuroma patient. Techniques in Neurosurgery 1997;3:89–94.
9. Gardner G, Robertson JH. Hearing preservation in unilateral acoustic neuroma surgery. Ann Otol Rhinol Laryngol 1988;97:55–66.
10. Bederson JB, von Ammon K, Wichmann WW, Yarsagil MG. Conservative treatment of patients with acoustic neuromas. Neurosurgery 1991;28:646–51.
11. Møller AR. Intraoperative monitoring in acoustic neuroma operations. Techniques in Neurosurgery 1997;3: 109–21.
12. Cushing H. Intracranial Tumors. Springfield, Illinois: Charles C. Thomas, 1932.
13. House JW, Brackmann DE. Facial nerve grading system. Otolaryngol Head Neck Surg 1985;93:146–7.
14. Moffat DA, Hardy DG, Grey PL, Baguley DM. The operative learning curve and its effect on facial nerve outcome in vestibular schwannoma surgery. Am J Otol 1996;17:643–7.
15. Grey PL, Moffat DA, Palmer CR, Hardy DG, Baguley DM. Factors which influence the facial nerve outcome in vestibular schwannoma surgery. Clin Otolaryngol 1996;21:409–13.
16. Erickson DL, Ausman JI, Chou SN. Prognosis of seventh nerve palsy following removal of large acoustic tumors. J Neurosurg 1977;47:31–?
17. Croxson GR, Moffat DA, Hardy DG, Baguley DM. Role of post-operative electroneuronography in predicting facial nerve recovery after acoustic neuroma removal: a pilot study. J Laryngol Otol 1989;103:60–2.
18. Moffat DA, da Cruz MJ, Baguley DM, Beynon GJ, Hardy DG. Hearing preservation in solitary vestibular schwannoma surgery using the retrosigmoid approach. Otolaryngol Head Neck Surg 1999 (In Press).
19. Ebersold MJ, Yamamoto Y, Harner SG, Beatty CW, Quast LM. The retrosigmoid approach for acoustic neuromas: the Mayo Clinic experience. Techniques in Neurosurgery 1997;3:122–30.
20. Haines SJ, Levine S. Middle fossa approach for acoustic neuroma. Techniques in Neurosurgery 1997;3:143–9.
21. Irving RM, Viani L, Hardy DG, Baguley DM, Moffat DA. Nervus intermedius function after vestibular schwannoma removal: clinical features and pathophysiological mechanisms. Laryngoscope 1995;105:809–13.
22. Hardy DG, MacFarlane R, Moffat DA. Wound closure after acoustic neuroma surgery. B J Neurosurg 1993; 7:171–4.
23. Kondziolka D, Lunsford LD, Flickinger JC. Stereotactic radiosurgery for acoustic tumors: Technique and results. Techniques in Neurosurgery 1997;3:154–61.
24. Kondziolka D, Lunsford LD, McLaughlin MR, Flickinger JC. Long-term outcomes after radiosurgery for acoustic neuromas. New Eng J Med 1998;339:1471–3.
25. Forster DMC, Kemeny AA, Pathak A, Walton L. Radiosurgery: a minimally interventional alternative to microsurgery in the management of acoustic neuroma. Br J Neurosurg 1996;10:169–74.

15

Skull Base Tumors

R.S.C. Kerr and C.A. Milford

Summary

Skull base tumors are rare, accounting for less than 1% of intracranial tumors. Management options include a conservative approach with serial scans, conventional surgery or radiotherapy/stereotactic radiosurgery. Surgery is difficult because of problems with access, involvement of basal blood vessels/cranial nerves and the potential for post-operative cerebrospinal fluid leakage.

This book contains other chapters that deal specifically with the management of:

- Sellar and parasellar tumors.
- Meningiomas.
- Cerebellopontine angle tumors.

Clearly, these tumors comprise a large number of the cases that a skull base team will see. Readers are therefore referred to other chapters for those specific lesions, and we will deal only with those tumors of the skull base not included in the above.

In the past, the skull base has been a surgical "no-man's land", and the discipline of skull base surgery owes its development to individuals in many disciplines who were prepared to tackle the almost impossible problems confronting them at the time. It began near the turn of the century, with resections of acoustic tumors and approaches to the pituitary. It was not until the pioneering work of Ketcham et al. [1], whose first report appeared in 1963, that co-ordinated efforts between surgical disciplines produced the first series of skull base procedures.

The modern skull base unit comprises a multidisciplinary team, which will include (as a minimum) a neuroradiologist, neurosurgeon, otolaryngologist, plastic and reconstructive surgeon, neuroanaesthetist and intensive care specialist. Nursing and ancillary staff with an interest in neurosurgical/neurological rehabilitation is also mandatory. No one surgeon can obtain, much less sustain, all the skills required to deal with all lesions in this area. Multidisciplinary management is the only approach that is likely to lead to improved outcomes for patients with these difficult problems – successful skull base surgery is a team effort!

The surgery involved in skull base tumors is often lengthy. The teamwork helps not only in bringing together expertise from different specialties but also provides an opportunity for intermittent relaxation during a prolonged surgical procedure.

Whatever the make up of the skull base team, the neurosurgeon often assumes a major responsibility for the patients in the post-operative period, as the majority of the major complications are related to the brain and its coverings.

Presentation of Patients with Skull Base Lesions

Lesions at the skull base are often occult and not easily diagnosed early. Symptomatology varies greatly, depending on the size, site and nature of the tumor.

Lesions of the Anterior Cranial Fossa

Localizing symptoms of lesions in the anterior fossa often include nasal or visual dysfunction. Symptoms may include nasal obstruction as well as pain, epistaxis and hyposmia/anosmia. Optic problems may include visual loss (acuity or visual field), diplopia and proptosis. For lesions involving the frontal lobes, alteration in personality, memory and concentration may also be apparent, especially with bi-frontal changes.

Examination should include endoscopy of the nose/nasopharynx, as well as a full neurological examination.

Lesions of the Middle Cranial Fossa

These may be divided into sphenoid/parasellar mid-line lesions (including nasopharyngeal lesions), and pathologies affecting the true middle cranial fossae on either side of the mid-line structures. The sphenoid lesions may present with endocrine abnormalities through effects on the pituitary and/or cranial neuropathies of nerves II, III, IV, V and VI through effects on the cavernous sinus. Nasopharyngeal lesions may present with nasal symptoms or otologic problems related to secondary Eustachian tube dysfunction, as well as a trigeminal neuropathy. Finally, if more laterally placed, symptoms due to temporal lobe involvement may be apparent, including seizures and visual field defects.

Lesions of the Posterior Fossa

Symptoms and signs of pathology in the posterior fossa are related primarily to dysfunction in cranial nerves V–XII, changes due to brain stem compression and cerebellar ataxia. Symptoms may include facial nerve weakness/spasm, hearing loss, tinnitus and imbalance, dysphonia and dysphagia. In association with larger tumors, patients may develop symptoms of raised intracranial pressure due to hydrocephalus.

In many instances, the pathological diagnosis of a skull base tumor has rested entirely on its imaging characteristics, unless it arises from a site accessible to biopsy, e.g. a paranasal sinus tumor with a nasal component. Increasingly, pathology involving the anterior and middle fossa is amenable to endoscopic biopsy via the nose/nasopharynx/paranasal sinuses. Reliance on imaging characteristics alone is therefore becoming less common. (In our unit, endoscopic biopsy via the paranasal sinuses has led to the pre-operative histologic diagnosis of trigeminal neuroma, lymphoma, meningioma, fibrous dysplasia, ossifying fibroma, plasmacytoma, chordoma and secondary renal carcinoma.)

Imaging of the Skull Base

The skull base represents a bony partition between the intracranial cavity and the orbits, nose, paranasal sinuses, nasopharynx and ear. Imaging characteristics are important in establishing:

- The anatomic location and identity of the tumor.
- The extent of the tumor, especially in relation to the major vessels and cranial nerves, dura and intracranial structures.

MRI and CT are complementary in most areas of evaluation of skull base lesions.

CT is better at detecting calcification and at evaluating the effect of tumors on the bone of the skull base. It can be particularly helpful as part of the assessment of the paranasal sinuses and the temporal bone, and where the tumor is itself calcified. Its disadvantages consist mainly of the inadequately detailed display of intracranial structures.

MRI is superior in demonstrating the relationship of a skull base tumor to soft tissue structures, the carotid artery, sigmoid sinus/internal jugular vein, dura and brain. As far as the carotid artery is concerned, MRA is helpful for assessing patency and its relationship to the tumor. However, conventional angiography probably remains the "gold standard" if there is debate regarding its involvement and for demonstrating small vessel detail. It may also be required in:

- Embolization of the tumor pre-operatively. This is indicated in the case of juvenile angiofibroma, jugulotympanic paragangliomas, vagal paragangliomas and vascular meningiomas.
- Balloon test occlusion of the ICA. This is important if the carotid artery appears to be invaded by tumor, a temporary trial occlusion of the ICA can be used to identify those patients with no flow reserve who are at high risk of developing neurologic sequelae if the carotid is permanently occluded.

General Principles of Skull Base Surgery

It is clearly important that any patient with a skull base tumor should be told the long-term outlook of the tumor itself, i.e. the natural history of the pathology. They also need to be informed of all the management options available and these would usually include:

- Conservative management – monitoring the tumor with serial imaging.
- Conventional surgery – again, patients need information regarding outcomes, surgical morbidity and mortality. The figures one quotes need to relate to your own experience, as well as figures taken from the literature.
- Radiotherapy/stereotactic radiosurgery.

There will be occasions when combinations of the above are appropriate, e.g. where partial removal and post-operative radiotherapy may be the most suitable option.

The choice of management option will rely on such factors as the age of the patient and their general medical status, the natural history of the tumor, the location and size of the tumor, the potential risks of the surgery/radiotherapy/radiosurgery and, importantly, the skill and experience of the skull base team.

As far as the operation is concerned, the surgeon should be guided by one overriding principle: removal of adequate amounts of bone from the cranial base should provide sufficient access without the necessity to retract dura/brain. Remove bone before considering retracting brain, dura or the cranial nerves.

Even though many neoplasms involving the skull base are benign or locally confined malignant lesions, radical resection of extensive lesions remains difficult. The reasons for this include:

- The necessity to retract the brain to achieve tumor exposure (even when adequate bone removal has occurred), with the possibility of retraction-related cerebral injury.
- The involvement by tumor of basal blood vessels, injury to which may lead to stroke and/or death.
- The involvement of the cranial nerves, injury to which may result in significant functional deficits. In any surgical procedure which involves risk to the facial nerve, use of intraoperative electro-physiologic monitoring of the nerve is mandatory.
- The potential for CSF leakage through the skin, paranasal sinuses or nasopharynx, which may be followed by meningitis and death. In any case where the risk of post-operative CSF leak is high, use of a lumbar drain in the post-operative period should be considered.

In the past, the surgical treatment of skull base tumors has been associated with a high rate of local recurrence (related to the problems of gaining good surgical access and the involvement/close proximity of vital structures). Post-operative monitoring is therefore an extremely important part of their management and this will involve serial imaging. A 'base line' scan would usually be performed about 3 months following the surgery and then at regular intervals (often between 6 and 12 months). The choice of imaging may vary occasionally, although MRI will be the modality of choice in the majority of instances.

In some areas of the skull base, e.g. the nose/paranasal sinuses, imaging may be supplemented by endoscopic follow-up. Certainly, in extracranial skull base tumors in this area, endoscopic examination and biopsy will provide a more sensitive follow-up than any imaging modality currently available. The follow-up period varies according to the pathology, but often would be for a minimum of 5 years.

Workload of the Oxford Skull Base Unit

Skull base tumors are rare, probably accounting for less than 1% of intracranial tumors [2], and it is difficult to obtain accurate figures regarding their incidence. Looking at our workload in Oxford does provide some insight into the incidence of these rare problems and their relative incidence in terms of benign and malignant tumors. During the 7-year period up to 2000, we have together seen 501 cases.

Their management involved the following:

- Surgery in 255 cases (51%).
- Conservative management with serial scans in 205 cases (41%).
- Radiotherapy/stereotactic radiosurgery in 41 cases (8%).

This workload represents approximately 71 new cases per year. As our unit serves a population of approximately 3 million, the 71 new cases per year represent an incidence of approximately 1:40,000 population per year. Our figures seem to compare to the few groups who have published details of workload. Sekhar and Janecka (1993) in Pittsburgh, USA, saw a total of 780 cases in a 7-year period, and these patients included 605 with neoplasms who underwent surgery, 487 (76%) with benign tumors and 118 (24%) with malignant tumors. This surgical workload represented approximately 69 surgical procedures per year. Donald (1998), in Sacramento, USA, saw a higher percentage of malignant lesions (37% malignant and 63% benign) and had a surgical workload of 27 cases per year.

Pathology of Skull Base Tumors

Primary tumors of the skull base are rare. It is more common for involvement to occur consequent upon spread from either a primary intracranial or an extracranial neoplastic process. Whether arising primarily from the skull base or involving it secondarily, these tumors are uncommon.

Tumors may be classified as:

- Primary skull base lesions – those arising from the bone and/or cartilage.
- Intracranial – those that arise at the base of the brain, with a tendency to invade the basicranium. They may arise from the neural, vascular or meningeal tissues within the cranium.
- Extracranial – those originating from tissues just below the cranium and invading the skull base secondarily. They often involve the paranasal sinuses, the infratemporal fossa, or the parapharyngeal space.

Primary Skull Base Lesions

Benign Primary Skull Base Lesions

Osteoma

This is a slowly growing, benign tumor that may affect any area of the skull base, most commonly the frontal and ethmoid sinuses. Osteomata may require surgical treatment if they produce orbital or cosmetic problems. They are rarely associated with leakage of CSF or a pneumatocele through involvement of the anterior cranial fossa.

Fibro-osseous Lesions/Fibrous Dysplasia

The term "fibro-osseous lesion" has been used as a general description for a group of tumors and proliferative disorders that may involve any of the cranial fossae. They comprise a number of specific clinical entities, in which the clinical, radiological and histological features often overlap, resulting in confusion for both pathologists and clinicians concerned with diagnosis and management.

The common denominator is the replacement of normal bone architecture by tissue composed of collagen, fibroblasts and varying amounts of osteoid or bone. The two most common conditions falling within this group are ossifying fibroma and fibrous dysplasia.

- Ossifying fibroma is an encapsulated benign neoplasm consisting of fibrous tissue and containing varied amounts of metaplastic bone and mineralized masses. It mainly affects bones which are ossified in membrane, usually presenting as a painless mass. Radiological changes are of a discrete mass with a distinct boundary and thinning of the cortical bone, resulting in an eggshell appearance. In most instances, the mass is surrounded by smooth, well defined cortical bone, which differentiates it from fibrous dysplasia where "blending" into the surrounding bone is universal. Its behaviour is that of a benign neoplasm and hence it continues to grow after skeletal maturity is reached. It normally, therefore, warrants surgical treatment at some point.
- Fibrous dysplasia is a benign, localized bone disorder of unknown aetiology that results in extreme thickening of bone owing to the presence of intraosseous proliferating connective tissue. It may be monostotic (affecting one bone) or polyostotic (affecting several bones). It is a self-limiting process that starts in childhood but, due to a very slow growth rate, may not cause symptoms until adulthood. Growth can be expected to slow or stop after puberty in monostotic disease. The most characteristic radiologic feature is a diffusely blending margin in marked contrast to the sharply demarcated ossifying fibroma (although the features are non-specific, they depend upon the age of the lesion and degree of metaplastic bone formation).

Differential diagnosis of these conditions relies on the correlation of histopathologic and radiologic findings. Both are usually required to provide a definitive diagnosis.

The most common presentation would be with a slow-growing, asymmetrical, painless swelling (see Fig. 15.1). It manifests craniofacial involvement in about 10% of cases and gives rise to cosmetic deformity, proptosis and, more seriously, compression of the optic nerve in the optic canal. Cosmetic concerns of the patient may give rise to pressure for consideration of surgical treatment but, on the whole, the management would be conservative in view of the slow natural history. However, signs of optic nerve compression are an absolute indication for surgery, as is the development of other intracranial complications, e.g. cerebrospinal fluid rhinorrhea.

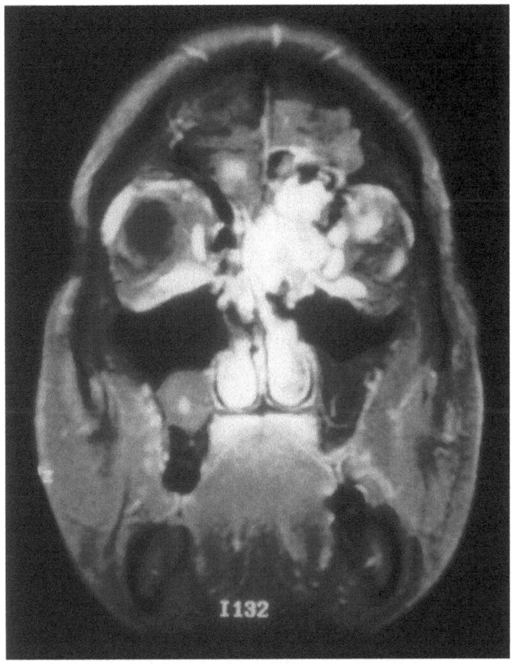

Fig. 15.1. Coronal MRI of patient with extensive fibrous dysplasia involving the anterior cranial fossa.

Malignant Primary Skull Base Lesions

Chondrosarcoma

These are malignant tumors of cartilage that may arise in bone or soft tissues. They comprise 6% of skull base neoplasms [5]. Approximately 75% of all cranial chondrosarcomas occur at the base of the skull, and most of these are found in the middle cranial fossa.

These tumors affect both sexes equally and occur over a broad age range, with a peak distribution at between 30 and 50 years of age. Symptoms vary according to the site of origin but the most common include headaches, visual disturbance, cranial neuropathies, hearing loss and disturbances of gait. Imaging shows mottled calcification within the soft tissue mass on CT scanning.

Chondrosarcoma tends to act less aggressively than other sarcomas but nevertheless pursues a slow and intractably progressive course, which ultimately kills the patient in many cases. The history therefore tends to be long and is punctuated by multiple local recurrences. Distant metastases are relatively rare, occurring in only about 8% of cases [6].

Surgery is the primary treatment modality. Conventional radiotherapy has been used as an adjunct. More recently, some workers have advocated proton beam radiation therapy as the adjuvant radiation modality of choice. This form of irradiation is of interest to the radiation oncologist because of its improved dose localization capabilities in comparison to high-energy X-rays (photons). It is suggested [7] that proton radiation therapy after maximal surgical resection represents the best management policy currently available for patients with chondrosarcomas (and chordomas) of the skull base.

Chordoma

These are slow-growing, locally aggressive malignant neoplasms, derived from vestigial remnants of the notochord found along the axial skeleton. They account for less than 1% of all intracranial neoplasms [8]. They can be divided into three main groups, depending upon the site of origin: cranial (35%), sacrococcygeal (50%) or vertebral (15%). Cranial lesions tend to affect a younger age group (range 20–40 years) compared to the sacrococcygeal group (40–60 years). Men are more commonly affected than women (3:1).

The location of a chordoma within the clivus determines the nature and path of its growth, the associated anatomic structures involved, the clinical symptomatology, and the approach for surgical management. However, whatever their position within the clivus and their symptoms, presentation is usually late after intracranial extension has occurred.

Lesions arising near the inferior tip of the clivus, the basion, usually produce lower brain stem compression as they expand and present clinically with hypoglossal nerve lesions. Tumors arising from the body of the clivus are the most common. They may expand ventrally and produce a nasopharyngeal mass with obstruction, or they may expand dorsally and stretch the sixth cranial nerve as it runs along and penetrates the clival dura, leading to diplopia. Tumors arising at the rostral end of the clivus involve the sella turcica and may present with hypopituitarism. With suprasellar extension, a chiasmal syndrome with bitemporal hemianopia may result. Lateral extension of rostral clival chordomas may produce a parasellar mass or extend into the cavernous sinus, affecting cranial nerves III–VI. Postero-lateral extension of mid-clival chordomas can produce otologic symptoms of deafness, vertigo and tinnitus, with risk of facial weakness through involvement of the petrous temporal bone.

The position of the tumor rarely allows complete surgical resection and thus recurrence rate after surgery remains high. In view of the high local recurrence rate, conventional radiotherapy has been used, with varying success. As mentioned above, it is suggested that proton radiation therapy after maximal surgical resection seems to represent the best management policy currently available for patients with chordomas of the skull base.

Intracranial Skull Base Tumors

Benign Intracranial Skull Base Tumors

Schwannoma (Neurilemmoma)

Clearly, the VIII cranial nerve is the most common site for this tumor. However, other cranial nerves may be affected.

Trigeminal Schwannoma

These tumors account for 2% of intracranial schwannomata. They may originate in any section of the fifth cranial nerve, from the root to the distal extracranial branches; as a result, a variety of symptoms and signs may develop, depending on the direction and extent of tumor growth. Fifty percent of all intracranial trigeminal schwannomata arise from the trigeminal ganglion and remain predominantly localized to the middle fossa. Patients typically present with pain/paraesthesia in a trigeminal distribution, which may spread from one to all three divisions, often followed by progressive sensory loss and, less commonly, by wasting of the muscles of mastication (most easily seen in temporalis).

Approximately 20% arise from the trigeminal root and remain primarily infratentorial within the posterior fossa. They present with ataxia, hearing loss, tinnitus and facial nerve dysfunction, together with trigeminal symptoms. Approximately 25% grow above and below the tentorium ("hourglass tumors") and produce a combination of clinical findings reflecting involvement of both the middle and posterior fossae. Finally, there are a small group of patients where the tumor arises from the distal intracranial branches of the V nerve and extend extracranially, e.g. producing a mass in the pterygopalatine/infratemporal fossa.

On CT, these tumors are usually isodense or slightly hyperdense in comparison to surrounding brain and enhance homogeneously after administration of intravenous contrast. On MRI, they are generally well circumscribed, show decreased signal intensity on T1-weighted images, increased signal on T2-weighted images and show homogeneous enhancement after administration of gadolinium.

Trigeminal schwannomas displace rather than invade adjacent structures and tumor removal can therefore often be accomplished without significant neurological injury (other than anaesthesia in the distribution of the affected branch of the nerve), provided an appropriate operative approach is chosen.

Facial Nerve Schwannoma

Primary tumors of the facial nerve are rare. When they do occur, they can be found along the entire course of the nerve, but most frequently either within the temporal bone or extracranially. As they originate from the Schwann cells of the nerve sheath, their finding within the internal auditory canal or intracranially must be explained on the basis of embryonic rests of ganglionic cells from the geniculate ganglion.

Clinical presentation varies, depending on the site of tumor origin. Schwannomas found along the extracranial course of the nerve present primarily as a parotid mass, with facial nerve weakness being an unusual presenting complaint. If the tumor originates within the temporal bone (and that may be anywhere from the geniculate ganglion to the stylomastoid foramen), it usually produces otologic symptoms and is commonly associated with facial weakness (presumably related to compression within a tight bony canal). Intracranially, these tumors will give rise to the symptoms associated with most other lesions of the cerebellopontine angle.

Both CT and MRI may be helpful in localizing the lesion. They may detect widening of the fallopian canal or bone erosion/soft tissue mass in relation to the intratemporal course of the facial nerve.

The aims of management include:

- Establishing a diagnosis.
- Attempting to preserve continuity of the facial nerve.
- Completing tumor resection.
- Facial nerve reconstruction/facial paralysis rehabilitation.

Because the cell of origin lies within the nerve sheath, it is theoretically possible to consider tumor removal without a nerve transection. In practice, it rarely proves possible and, hence, surgery results in complete facial nerve palsy in the vast majority of cases. There is therefore often a case for a period of conservative management whilst the facial nerve function remains normal or near normal, unless it gives rise to some more serious problems. When surgery is eventually undertaken, complete tumor removal should be confirmed by frozen section examination of the proximal and distal nerve margin. Reconstruction will usually involve an interposition nerve graft (the greater auricular nerve is a convenient local source of a cable graft). The quality of recovery following such a procedure would be between Grades III and V (House–Brackman) at best.

Jugular Foramen Schwannoma

As with trigeminal and facial schwannomas, these are rare. The patient usually presents with a unilateral lesion of cranial nerves IX, X or XI or a combination of the three nerves. When the majority of the tumor is below the skull base, there is rarely a neuropathy and presentation, in our experience, is with the non-specific features of a parapharyngeal mass.

Diagnosis is made from CT and/or MRI. The CT scan demonstrates a smooth-edged enlargement of the jugular foramen, with extension inferiorly into the neck, posteriorly into the posterior fossa or directly into the skull base. MRI may be useful regarding soft tissue relations, particularly in the neck. Carotid angiography may be indicated for assessing cerebral cross-circulation if there is any question that surgery might compromise the internal carotid artery.

Management lies between a conservative approach with the use of serial imaging or surgery. Recommendations for treatment relies on the age of the patient and their general medical health, the size of the tumor, whether it is creating any mass effect in the posterior fossa and the presence or absence of cranial neuropathies. Certainly, older patients do not tolerate the rapid change in lower cranial nerve function that surgery may produce, and are therefore at risk of developing serious pulmonary complications from laryngeal aspiration. In this age group, patients are more likely to adapt to these lower cranial neuropathies if they occur slowly as the disease progresses; a conservative policy may therefore be the most appropriate.

Malignant Intracranial Skull Base Tumors

Olfactory Neuroblastoma (Esthesioneuroblastoma)

An uncommon neuroectodermal tumor that arises from the olfactory nasal epithelium, high up in the nasal roof within the olfactory cleft (the space between the superior nasal septum and the middle and superior turbinates on the lateral wall of the nose), attached to the cribriform plate. It affects both sexes equally and occurs in all age groups. Presentation is often non-specific, with nasal obstruction, epistaxis and, less commonly, anosmia and visual problems.

Although the diagnosis relies on biopsy and histology, imaging allows assessment of the extent of the tumor. Woodhead and Lloyd (1988) reviewed imaging in a series of 24 patients and concluded that there were no specific features to identify this tumor. However, a tumor within the ethmoid and upper nasal airway, expanding into the orbit and eroding the roof of the fronto-ethmoid complex or cribriform plate unilaterally in a young patient, is likely to be an olfactory neuroblastoma (see Fig. 15.2).

The natural history of this malignancy is both variable and unpredictable. Metastasis to cervical lymph nodes occurs in 10–30% of patients during the course of the disease and systemic metastasis (lung and bone) in 8–46% of cases [10–13]. Although often slow-growing, it must be considered as a highly malignant neoplasm, requiring radical initial treatment.

Treatment normally involves a combination of radical surgery and radiotherapy. Survival rates of 60% at 3 years and 40% at 5 years are

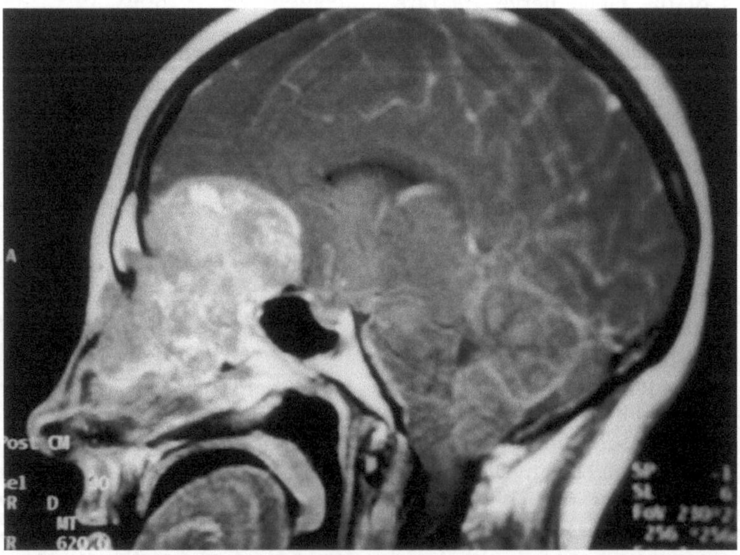

Fig. 15.2. Sagittal MRI of patient with large olfactory neuroblastoma.

quoted [14] for those patients having surgically accessible lesions treated with combinations of excisional surgery and radiotherapy.

Extracranial Skull Base Tumors

Benign Extracranial Skull Base Tumors

Juvenile Angiofibroma

Highly vascular and locally invasive, juvenile angiofibromas occur almost exclusively in adolescent males. Although morphologically benign, these tumors can exhibit aggressive local growth, extending along planes of least resistance or pre-formed pathways and, when large, can invade directly by bone erosion.

Juvenile angiofibromas represent less than 0.05% of all head and neck tumors, with a median age at presentation of around 13 years. It is thought the hormonal changes at puberty are the primary influence on the growth of this tumor. The site of origin is unclear but is likely to be from the sphenopalatine foramen. The tumor spreads laterally into the pterygopalatine fossa, thereby gaining access into the infratemporal fossa as well as the nasal cavity/paranasal sinuses and nasopharynx posteriorly, and the orbit superiorly. Intracranial spread into the anterior cranial fossa may occur, but more likely is invasion into the middle cranial fossa (although it usually remains extradural). Early symptoms of nasal obstruction and intermittent epistaxis are found in over 80% of patients. Nasendoscopy invariably confirms the presence of a mass obstructing the posterior nares. At diagnosis, approximately two thirds of patients have localized disease, and 20% have intracranial involvement [15]. Erosion of the medial pterygoid plate associated with enlargement of the sphenopalatine foramen is a constant feature on CT scan. Involvement of the sphenoid sinus, infratemporal fossa, orbit or middle cranial fossa may be demonstrated but is more easily demonstrated on MRI. The distinction between the mass and fluid in an obstructed sinus and the vascularity of the lesion (signal voids from the vessels within the tumor) can also be made on MRI.

There is little factual evidence to support a common belief that, with increasing age, angiofibromas will show spontaneous involution. It must be assumed that all untreated angiofibromas possess potential for aggressive growth.

Management usually involves surgery (rarely radiotherapy may be indicated in extremely extensive tumors where surgery may carry a high risk of operative mortality). In view of its vascularity, the majority of surgeons would seek the help of the interventional neuroradiologist, with pre-operative angiography and embolization. About 10% of cases recur after surgical resection (probably a reflection upon the difficulty of gaining good surgical access to this area).

Glomus Tumors (Paraganglioma) of the Temporal Bone

Paragangliomas are a group of histologically similar benign neoplasms that arise from neuroectodermally derived paraganglionic cells associated with autonomic ganglia. Two sites of these extra-adrenal paraganglia include:

- Intravagal – these are at the level of the jugular or nodose ganglion. Tumors arising here give rise to glomus vagale tumors.
- Jugulotympanic – these occur along Jacobson's nerve (tympanic branch of IX) and Arnold's nerve (tympanic branch of X), but the majority are found in the adventitia of the jugular bulb in the jugular fossa. Tumors arising from these sites give rise to glomus tympanicum (arising within the tympanic, or middle ear, cavity) and glomus jugulare tumors (arising from the jugular bulb).

Glomus vagale tumors usually present as a parapharyngeal mass, with no obvious neurologic problems. Their involvement of the jugular foramen and possible spread along the internal carotid artery towards the cavernous sinus can make their management difficult.

Jugulotympanic paragangliomas usually present with a unilateral hearing loss and pulsatile tinnitus. More rarely, they present with neuropathy involving the lower cranial (IX,X, XI,XII) or facial nerves. On examination, a vascular mass is seen behind the tympanic membrane or, in larger tumors, the mass may have eroded though the drum and floor of the bony ear canal to present within the ear canal itself.

Multiple or synchronous tumors occur in 3–10% of patients [16], and there is a familial incidence with an autosomal dominant mode of transmission (these patients have a higher incidence of synchronous paragangliomas).

These tumors demonstrate a slow and insidious pattern of growth. They tend to migrate through the temporal bone by vascular channels, naturally occurring fissures and foramina and, most importantly, along air cell tracts. Intracranial extension into the posterior and middle fossae does occur and increases potential morbidity and mortality. Rarely, these tumors may metastasize, usually to cervical lymph nodes.

The clinical picture of jugulotympanic paragangliomas is characteristic, but the clinical findings non-diagnostic. The mainstay of tumor diagnosis is radiological and the main diagnostic objectives are:

- Determine the site and extent of the tumor.
- Determine the presence of synchronous lesions.
- Determine the degree of major vascular involvement.
- Identify any intracranial extension.
- Determine central nervous system collateral circulation.

High-resolution CT scanning or MRI may assess the site and extent of tumor. MRI is superior in assessing intracranial extension and is useful for identifying synchronous tumors. Bilateral carotid angiography is used to determine involvement of the internal carotid artery (ICA) in larger tumors and the degree of collateral blood flow. It will also identify an aberrant ICA/intrapetrous carotid artery aneurysm (both are included in the differential diagnosis of a vascular lesion behind the tympanic membrane), as well as the rare case of anomalous venous drainage, where all intracranial venous return occurs via a single sigmoid sinus/internal jugular vein on the involved side (a contraindication to surgery). If performed pre-operatively, it also allows embolization of the lesion.

The management options for these tumors once again include:

- Conservative management.
- Surgery.
- Radiotherapy (or possibly stereotactic radiosurgery in some cases). This may have a place as a primary form of treatment in some cases, and may be the treatment modality of choice in recurrent/residual disease. The aim of treatment is to prevent further growth rather than to eradicate the disease.

The intricate temporal bone anatomy, the extent of tumor invasion and tumor vascularity combine to make these tumors difficult to manage by any mode of therapy. The critical question to be asked is whether the disease is likely to cause the patient serious problems in the natural course of his/her remaining years. At one end of the spectrum, a large tumor in a young, fit patient almost certainly warrants surgical treatment, whereas a small tumor in an elderly patient probably needs nothing more than careful review. Unfortunately, there is a "gray area" between these two ends of the spectrum although, currently, many would consider surgery as the first-line treatment. The judicious use of surgery is imperative, since an iatrogenic deficit involving the last four cranial nerves may pose life-threatening complications to an older patient with poor respiratory reserve.

Contraindications to surgical treatment include:

- Carotid involvement in the presence of poor collateral circulation.
- Contralateral vagus lesion – surgery that compromises the only functional vagus is a relative contraindication.
- Unresectable tumor – a neurosurgically unresectable intracranial extension is a relative contraindication.
- Anomalous venous drainage – where all intracranial venous return occurs via a single sigmoid sinus on the involved side. In this situation, it may be better to await complete occlusion of the jugular bulb (which allows progressive opening of collateral venous channels) before operating.

Malignant Extracranial Skull Base Tumors

Carcinoma of the Paranasal Sinuses

Virtually all types of malignancy may present in this area but the most frequent are forms of squamous cell carcinoma (the most common malignancy of the head and neck) and adenocarcinoma. Reports on the association between adenocarcinoma of the ethmoid and the woodworking trade (especially hardwood exposure) began in 1965 in the UK [17,18]. The increased relative risk is similar to that for carcinoma of the bronchus in smokers, with a cumulative life-time risk of 1 in 120 and a 500–1,000 times greater risk than the general population of developing the condition. It became a recognized industrial disease in the UK in 1969.

Patients present with nasal symptoms, such as nasal obstruction and epistaxis. Orbital symptoms include swelling, diplopia and proptosis (see Fig. 15.3).

It is well recognized that, in the past, the poor prognosis associated with these tumors was a consequence of local recurrence engendered by inadequate resection. The realization that these tumors affect the inferior surface of the cribriform plate and roof of ethmoid (and hence are likely to have an intracranial component) led to the development of the combined skull base approach. This offered access and more rational, yet radical, resection choices, dependent on anatomic considerations. Many patients with these tumors would be treated with a combination of craniofacial resection and radiotherapy.

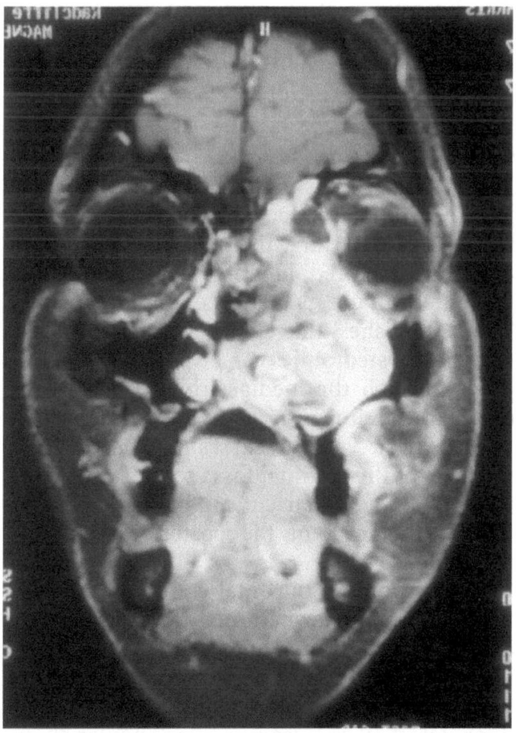

Fig. 15.3. Coronal MRI of patient with carcinoma of paranasal sinuses with involvement of the anterior cranial fossa.

In 1998, Lund et al. [19] published the results of a series of 209 patients undergoing craniofacial resection for sino-nasal neoplasia. The 5-year actuarial survival was 44%, falling to 32% at 10 years for malignant tumors. In the analysis of their results, it became clear that when disease affects the frontal lobe itself (as opposed to dural involvement alone), then there was a uniformly bad prognosis.

Malignant Tumors of the Temporal Bone

Malignant tumors affecting the temporal bone account for only 0.05% of head and neck cancers [20]. Most are squamous cell carcinomas, arising in the external auditory canal and invading inward. Those arising within the middle ear/mastoid are often associated with the long-standing inflammation of chronic middle ear disease.

Patients present with discharge from the ear and associated bleeding and pain. In addition, alteration of facial nerve function should alert the clinician to the possibility of malignancy. In these circumstances, biopsy of any polyp or ulcer is mandatory.

Diagnosis is often made late. CT scan and MRI are used to assess the extent of the primary, and its relationship to the dura, brain, facial nerve and carotid artery. CT is more useful for detailing the intratemporal anatomy and showing the presence of bone erosion (and hence, by inference, presence of tumor). MRI is more useful to define tumor from brain and from the reactive/inflammatory changes that may occur, and gives information regarding ICA or sigmoid sinus patency by the presence or absence of flow void signals. Carotid angiography may, however, be necessary to establish unequivocally involvement of the carotid artery.

No coherent staging system exists and the lack of such a staging system means that comparing various treatment options described in the literature is impossible. Hence, there is great debate regarding an optimum treatment strategy.

In general, surgery and radiotherapy in combination are considered the treatment of choice. A number of surgical approaches are feasible that largely depend on the extent of the tumor.

Complete surgical resection with a clear microscopic margin is the preferred initial treatment objective. For small tumors, radiotherapy is an alternative.

The most widely accepted operative concept is to free the involved temporal bone from its surrounding venous sinuses, protect the internal carotid artery and brainstem and avoid injury to cranial nerves, if they are still functioning. Typically, the patient would also receive adjuvant radiotherapy. Although this approach has probably resulted in an improved quality of life for patients, the impact on survival is unknown.

Surgical Approaches to the Skull Base

Careful planning, consideration of the aims of the surgery, detailed review of the radiology and an in-depth discussion with the patient and family are mandatory before any skull base approach is undertaken. The aim is to help, but this is invariably high-risk surgery and it is vital that the patient and the family understand what is being undertaken and why.

The surgical exposure of skull base lesions commonly involves extensive bone work. Exposure must be adequate and yet not excessive. Adequate exposure reduces the operating distance of deep lesions from the surgeon, reduces the need for brain retraction and provides space for manoeuvring. An adequately planned incision should take into account any previously existing incisions, the vascularity of the flap, cosmetic appearances and the course of the facial nerve. The exposure should also take into consideration proximal and distal control of major vessels. We would utilize electrophysiologic monitoring of the facial nerve in any case where its function could be compromised.

As in every other branch of surgery, there are a vast number of surgical approaches described for different areas of the skull base. We are limited to describing a small number of procedures and will therefore describe only techniques we have used and found "practical".

Anterior Fossa

Anterior and anterolateral craniofacial resections (CFR) are designed to encompass tumors along the anterior and middle cranial fossae. The interorbital compartment, limited by the medial walls of the orbits, the cribriform plate/roof of ethmoid sinuses and the dura encompass the usual specimen removed during anterior CFR. Any lateral extension of the perimeter of excision would then constitute anterolateral CFR.

Anterior Craniofacial Resection

Anterior CFR encompasses structures of the anterior mid-line and paramedian skull base (see Fig. 15.4). The ethmoid sinuses superiorly, the anterior wall of the sphenoid posteriorly, the frontal sinus anteriorly, and the nasopharynx inferiorly are included in the surgical perimeter of the anterior craniofacial resection.

Indications

- Resection of malignant tumors of the paranasal sinuses involving the ethmoid/frontal sinus with proximity to or involvement of the ethmoid roof/cribriform plate.
- Resection of benign tumors of the paranasal sinuses, meninges or skull base with involvement of, or extension through, the skull base.

Surgical Steps

The anterior CFR is performed through bicoronal and paranasal facial incisions. Following facial bone exposure, the medial walls of both orbits are explored, identifying and cauterising the anterior and posterior ethmoidal vessels. This establishes the lateral perimeter of the resection. Osteotomies can be performed at this point through the medial orbital wall of each orbit at the junction with the orbital floor. Anteriorly, a vertical cut can be made from the level of the lacrimal fossa to the level of the nasion, and a similar cut can be made posteriorly at the level of the posterior ethmoidal foramina.

At this point, a bifrontal craniotomy is performed. The bicoronal incision allows wide access to the frontal bone and, most importantly, preservation of pericranium [21] for use as a vascularized flap to repair the anterior fossa floor defect (it is raised in a rectangular shape with its base at the supraorbital region and receives its blood supply from supraorbital and

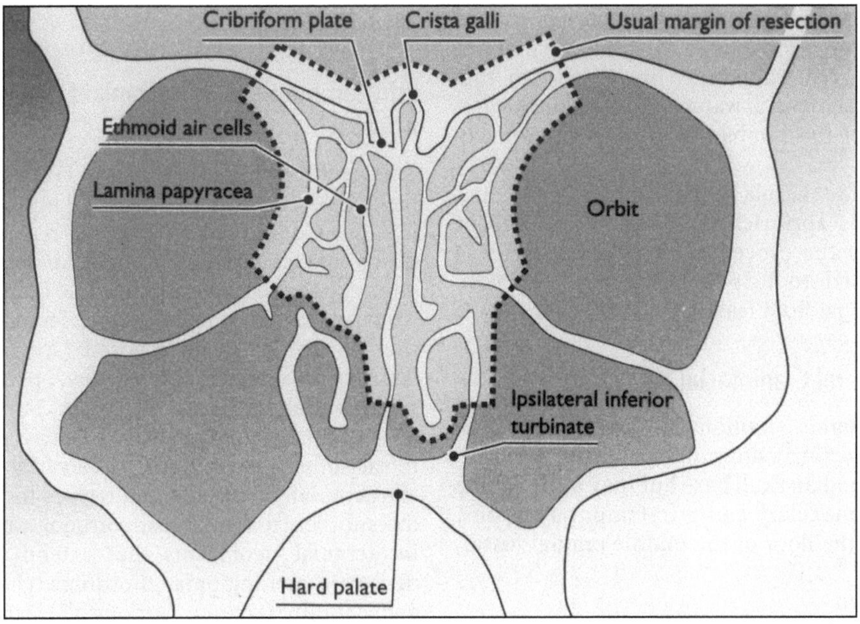

Fig. 15.4. Coronal anatomy, showing area of resection in anterior craniofacial resection.

supratrochlear vessels). A bi-frontal bone flap is then raised, either as a free flap or pedicled on temporalis. Care should be taken to keep the dura intact whilst opening the bone.

Exposure of the floor of the anterior fossa is best achieved by opening the dura on either side of the superior sagittal sinus as far anteriorly as possible. The sinus and underlying falx can then be divided between stay sutures. If a lumbar drain has been inserted, this can now be opened to allow CSF to drain. Diuretics may help provide good exposure without retraction of the frontal lobes.

Full exposure of the anterior cranial fossa floor invariably requires division of the olfactory tracts. Of course, if one or both can be protected, so much the better but, usually, patients with tumors requiring such an approach are anosmic.

The basal dura is reflected along the cribriform plate to the planum sphenoidale (if dura is involved, then it is mobilized more laterally and involved dura is resected with the tumor). Further cuts can then be made into the bone outside the tumor margins through the roof of the ethmoid/orbit laterally, through the planum sphenoidale into the sphenoid sinus posteriorly and through the floor of the frontal sinus into the anterior ethmoid anteriorly (these cuts are often made from both above and below). The tumor specimen is then only attached by the perpendicular plate of the ethmoid (which forms the postero-superior part of the nasal septum), and this is divided using heavy scissors. The specimen can then be "rocked out" through the transfacial exposure, dividing any mucosal attachments that might still remain.

The resultant defect has as its anterior margin the anterior wall of the frontal sinus/nasion, posteriorly the remaining portion of the sphenoid sinus and optic nerves, and the periorbita laterally. Inferiorly, the defect is open to the nasopharynx. Reconstruction of the defect in the anterior cranial fossa floor involves use of the pericranial flap – it is "posted" back into the anterior fossa over the supraorbital bar of bone (and beneath the frontal bone when it is replaced at the end of the procedure). This vascularized graft is then sutured to the basal dura (and if sutures are too difficult to place, tissue glue is used) to provide a carpet-like resurfacing of the anterior cranial fossa. A second layer of free pericranium, placed intradurally, can then be used, again, glued into position. We have not found it necessary to replace bone and have had no problems with brain herniation. However, great care must be taken with this repair to achieve a water (CSF)-tight closure. The use of the lumbar drain post-operatively helps.

Often, the nasolacrimal duct is transected during this approach, and can be stented at the end of the procedure. The nasal cavity is then packed to help avoid a post-operative cerebrospinal fluid leak.

Anterolateral Craniofacial Resection

Antero-lateral craniofacial resection also encompasses structures of the anterior mid-line and paramedian skull base but may also include the orbitomaxillary and infratemporal regions, as well as the floor of the middle cranial fossa.

Indications

- As for anterior CFR, but with orbital involvement.
- Extensive maxillary tumors with orbital/ethmoidal involvement.
- Extensive transcranial middle fossa tumors, e.g. meningiomas.

Surgical Steps

This approach can be performed through a bicoronal scalp flap, especially if a dural graft is required to effect a repair. Alternatively, an extended pterional flap may be used.

The facial incisions are usually paranasal, with possible lip splitting and eyelid incisions. The precise shape of the craniotomy and the extent of any facial osteotomies depend on the size and site of the tumor. For a purely intra-orbital tumor, a pterional approach with extra-dural removal of lateral and superior orbital walls provides good access to the posterior part of the orbital cavity. Clearly, this would be inadequate for an extensive maxillary or ethmoidal lesion with orbital involvement, when a bi-frontal flap will allow far better access. As regards the facial osteotomies, in general, they are made within the orbit along the medial and lateral wall as well as across the zygoma.

For reconstruction, following dural repair, soft tissue may be brought into the area using either temporalis muscle or a free microvascular flap, depending upon the size of the defect.

Middle Fossa

Infratemporal–Middle Cranial Fossa Approach

This technique, pioneered by Fisch [22] and further developed by Sekhar [23] and Schramm [24], provides excellent access to regions previously characterized by difficult dissection and poor exposure. The entire middle cranial fossa, from the petrous ridge to the lesser wing of the sphenoid, can be exposed (see Fig. 15.5). Patients who require this approach present with a wide variety of disease processes. Tumors may be benign or malignant, and may originate intracranially from dura or calvarial bone or extracranially from the soft tissues that occupy the subcranial area. Most common among the intracranial neoplasms that extend extracranially are meningioma, chordoma, chondroma and chondrosarcoma. Among the extracranial tumors that extend intracranially are schwannoma (often of the trigeminal nerve); parotid tumors, especially of the deep lobe; and squamous cell carcinomas from the paranasal sinuses, nasopharynx and temporal bone.

Surgical Steps

The approach is attained through a long incision, extending from the calvarial vertex to in front of the ear, then curving posteriorly under the lobule and into the neck, similar to the modified Blair incision for parotidectomy. The cutaneous flap is elevated anteriorly to a point from

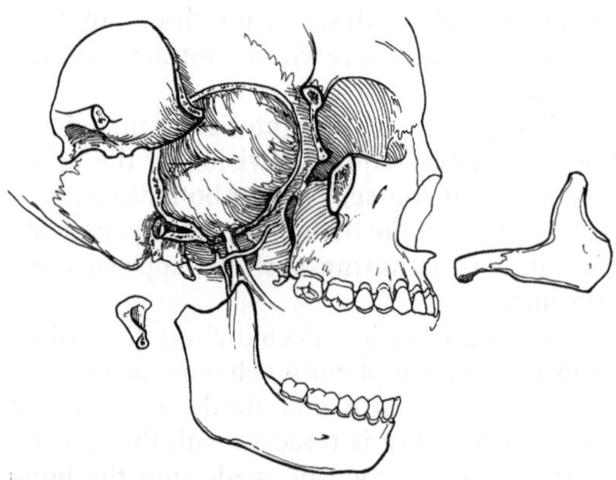

Fig. 15.5. Infratemporal fossa/middle cranial fossa approach. Removal of zygomatic arch (and possibly mandibular condylectomy), allowing access for craniotomy.

the angle of the mandible to the lateral orbital rim. The internal jugular vein and internal carotid artery are isolated in the neck and controlled with vascular loops.

The temporalis muscle, with a cuff of pericranium, is elevated to the zygomatic arch. Having fashioned a fronto-temporal craniotomy, the lateral orbital rim and zygomatic arch are removed in a single piece and stored for later reconstruction. This allows access to the infratemporal fossa, and this access can be improved, if required, by removing the mandibular condyle.

Once the zygomatic arch is removed, the temporalis muscle can be dissected down to its insertion on the coronoid process. This allows an exposure of the undersurface of the sphenoid and temporal bones. A subperiosteal dissection of the subcranial part of the middle cranial fossa is performed from the glenoid fossa posteriorly, to the base of the pterygoid plates anteriorly and is carried medially to the foramen spinosum and foramen ovale. These are the medial landmarks for the subsequent extension of the craniotomy.

The key to the exposure of the middle fossa and its immediate subcranial structures is an L-shaped craniotomy. This has a vertical component comprising the greater wing of the sphenoid and squamous part of the temporal bone, and a short horizontal component that ends at the foramen ovale and spinosum. The size of the craniotomy is determined by the extent of intracranial tumor. If exposure of the intrapetrous internal carotid is required, the craniotomy needs to be extended into the anterior part of the bony external auditory canal.

Extracranial and intracranial tumor can be removed simultaneously or in sequence. Closure of smaller resections may be achieved using the available temporalis muscle, but larger resections may once again require a microvascular free flap.

Posterior Fossa

There are several posterior fossa craniotomies/craniectomies used to access the CPA. The retrosigmoid approach uses an opening in the suboccipital bone posterior to the sigmoid sinus, with dural exposure over the lateral cerebellar hemisphere; for details of this approach, see the section on cerebello-pontine tumors.

The three transtemporal approaches (retrolabyrinthine, translabyrinthine and transcochlear) expose the posterior fossa dura anterior to the sigmoid sinus, but through the posterior aspect of the petrous pyramid. The transtemporal craniotomies require removal of bone, 1–2 cm behind the sigmoid sinus, to allow posterior displacement of the sinus. In the retrolabyrinthine approach, bone is removed up to the semicircular canals. This provides a limited view of the posterior aspect of the CPA. In the translabyrinthine approach, the canals are also removed – a maneuvre that provides access to the IAC and enhances CPA exposure. In the transcochlear approach, the entire inner ear (i.e. semicircular canals and cochlea) is removed and the facial nerve is re-routed posteriorly from its intratemporal course, thus providing access to the anterior aspect of the CPA and the space ventral to the brainstem.

Temporal Bone Resection

This procedure is employed for malignant disease of the external auditory canal and middle-ear cleft (this is most common squamous cell carcinoma). If the tumor has not involved more medial structures, a lateral temporal bone resection is employed (see Fig. 15.6) that removes the ear canal en bloc, with the tympanic membrane and lateral ossicles. A parotidectomy and/or neck dissection often supplements this procedure.

Surgical Steps

At the beginning of this procedure, the ear canal is transected and closed. This closure is different from that used during lateral skull base surgery – simply sewing the tragal skin to the conchal margin permits resection of the skin of the entire ear canal.

After transection of the cartilaginous ear canal just beneath the meatus, an intact canal wall mastoidectomy is performed. The middle ear is opened by performing a posterior tympanotomy (opening into the middle ear from the mastoid between the upper vertical portion of the facial nerve and the chorda tympani). The incus is then removed and the descending portion of the facial nerve is skeletonized.

In order to isolate the ear canal as an en bloc specimen, bone must be removed from 360°

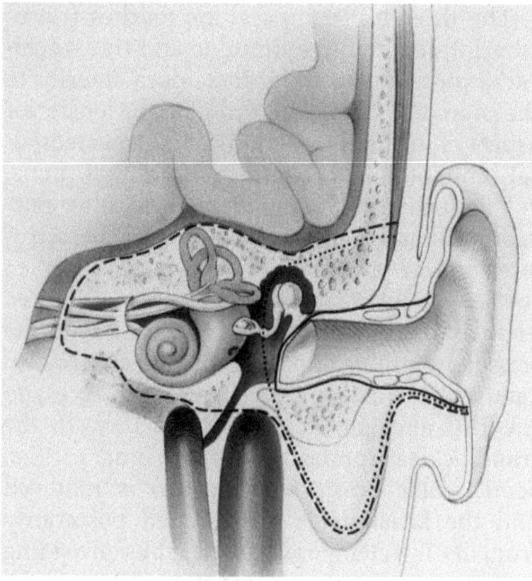

Fig. 15.6. Anatomy of the temporal bone in the coronal plane, showing the extent of the resection in a lateral temporal bone resection (outlined by the dotted line) and total petrosectomy (outlined by the dashed line).

around the ear canal. The posterior tympanotomy is extended to the posterior and inferior aspects of the middle ear. The front of the mastoid is removed between the inferior margin of the bony ear canal and the stylomastoid foramen. Superiorly, the root of zygoma and the posterior aspect of the glenoid fossa are removed.

Working between the floor of the middle cranial fossa and the roof of the ear canal, the root of zygoma is drilled away until the anterior middle ear has been opened into the glenoid fossa. After the ear canal has been isolated from above, behind and below, it remains attached only anteriorly. This bony attachment can then be "cracked" using an osteotome and the specimen removed. This specimen includes both the cartilaginous and bony ear canal, together with the tympanic membrane with the malleus attached.

Approaches to the Clivus

Whether trying to access the upper, mid or lower clivus, careful planning of the approach is paramount. That said, for success, it is important that the approach is familiar and practiced.

In our unit, we have used, in principle, two routes to gain entry to this most difficult of areas:

- Extended pre-sigmoid translabyrinthine approach: this has been used for lesions involving the inner third of the petrous bone and upper half of the clivus.
- Far lateral approach: for access to the lower half of the clivus and the anterior aspect of the foramen magnum.

We shall now consider each of these routes in turn.

Extended Presigmoid Translabyrinthine Approach

Space, or the lack of it, always seems to be the problem here. Certainly, at the beginning of most procedures, visualization of the important structures is difficult.

The principle of the approach is similar to the translabyrinthine route, but combined with a temporal craniotomy and division of the tentorium all the way down to the tentorial hiatus.

The procedure starts, therefore, with the patient in a park-bench position. Diuretics, antibiotics and anticonvulsants should be given. A question-mark-shaped incision is made, extending from just above the zygomatic process of the temporal bone down to below the mastoid process. The skin flap is reflected, leaving the temporalis fascia intact and extended all the way forward to the external auditory meatus.

Incisions are then made to elevate the temporalis muscle forwards on its blood supply, and to reflect the sub-occipital muscles inferiorly. This then allows a posterior fossa craniotomy to expose the straight and sigmoid sinuses, and a temporal craniotomy to expose the temporal lobe above the straight sinus and above the petrous bone. Great care must be taken to avoid injury to the sinuses.

The translabyrinthine exposure is then performed as previously described (see chapter on cerebellopontine angle tumors). This should be taken as far forward as possible and as low as possible towards the jugular bulb, to expose as much of the presigmoid dura as can be achieved. The exposure must include the undersurface of the temporal dura. Clearly, the amount of bone removed can be adapted to the specific requirements of the case.

Now, the dural cuts are performed to expose the surface of the temporal lobe and of the cerebellum. Usually, the posterior fossa dura is opened first. It may be possible to release some CSF early, which will slacken things off. The dural opening is T-shaped, crossing the superior petrosal sinus that always bleeds but is easily controlled. The secret to this is the opening of the dura over the temporal lobe. This must be long enough to allow safe access to the undersurface of the temporal lobe, so that the sinus can be approached from above and below. The vein of Labbe is at risk and must be protected at all times.

The final part of this approach is to divide the tentorium. Again, visualization both above and below allows this to be performed safely. Vessels coursing within the tentorium must be coagulated, the division being done using the microscope. Be careful not to lose direction and watch out for the fourth cranial nerve and the posterior cerebral artery. Division of the tentorium must be complete or access will always be restricted. Once complete, access to the upper clivus and inner petrous bone is possible with minimal retraction.

Closure must focus upon achieving a watertight seal. Meticulous attention to the petrous bone is the secret, with closure of the middle ear, if appropriate, by removal of the ossicles. Fibrin glue is a great help, as is the use of a lumbar drain for several days following the surgery.

Far Lateral Approach

Again, the park-bench position is used. The usual preparations are made, the approach being made through an extended incision to allow access to the upper lateral aspect of the cervical spine. Exposure of the posterior fossa dura is like a retro-mastoid craniotomy for a CPA lesion. However, the sub-occipital muscles are reflected like the leaves of a book to define the transverse process and lamina of C1 and the upper aspect of C2. The vertebral artery courses over the arch of C1 before it enters the posterior fossa via the foramen magnum. Depending upon the extent of the exposure, the artery can be transposed to widen the amount of C1 arch that can be removed and, following that, the amount of the foramen magnum that is removed. Clearly, the further forward this is taken, the more of the condylar joint is removed and thus the greater the requirement for post-operative stabilization. However, failure to remove sufficient amounts of the joint will restrict visibility and access to the anterior part of the foramen magnum and the lower clivus. If exposure is limited, more bone can always be removed.

Once the bone work is completed, dural opening will allow exposure of the area. Within the dura at the foramen magnum lies a dural sinus that has to be divided. The dura is remarkably thick in this area, and the use of stitches to retract the dura may assist the opening process. Be prepared to use artery clips to stop the bleeding whilst completing the dural opening – getting haemostasis is then easier.

Closure of the dura will not be possible without insertion of a dural patch. Again, using a lumbar drain may reduce the incidence of CSF leakage.

Conclusion

Skull base surgery is a challenging and exciting area that can offer hope to patients previously considered "inoperable". Any young neurosurgeon interested in this field needs to recognize that it requires a multi-disciplinary approach – one that can only be developed through mutual trust and respect for your colleagues. It is truly a "team effort" and, if you are going to go into the surgical "no man's land", you want to go with some good friends!

Key Points

- *Skull base tumors are rare, probably accounting for less than 1% of intracranial tumors.*
- *Management options include a conservative approach with serial scans, conventional surgery or radiotherapy/stereotactic radiosurgery.*
- *Removal of adequate amounts of bone from the cranial base should provide sufficient access without the necessity to retract dura/brain.*
- *Surgery for these tumors is difficult because of problems with access, involvement of basal*

blood vessels/cranial nerves and the potential for post-operative cerebrospinal fluid leakage.

- *Skull base surgery requires a true multidisciplinary approach.*

Self-assessment Questions

- ☐ Discuss the surgical difficulties of skull base surgery and how they may be overcome.
- ☐ Discuss the management of a 25-year-old woman presenting with unilateral proptosis and a diagnosis of fibrous dysplasia involving her anterior cranial fossa.
- ☐ A 30-year-old man presents with a 3-year history of anosmia. Nasal endoscopic examination reveals a right-sided nasal polyp and biopsy shows it to be an olfactory neuroblastoma. Describe his further management, including the surgical approach.
- ☐ A 77-year-old lady presents with left pulsatile tinnitus. Imaging confirms the diagnosis of a type B glomus jugulare. What are the management options available?
- ☐ Describe the surgical approaches to the clivus.

References

1. Ketcham AS, Wilkins RH, Van Buren JM et al. A combined intracranial facial approach to the paranasal sinuses. Am J Surg 1963;103:698–703.
2. Uttley D, Moore A, Archer J. Surgical management of mid-line skull base tumors: a new approach. J Neurosurg 1989;71:705–10.
3. Sekhar LN, Janecka IP. Surgery of cranial base tumors. New York: Raven Press Ltd, 1993.
4. Donald PJ. Surgery of the skull base. Philadelphia: Lippincott-Raven Publishers, 1998.
5. Kveton JF, Brackman DE, Glasscock ME et al. Chondrosarcoma of the skull base. Otolaryngol Head Neck Surg 1986;94:23.
6. Robinson PJ, Woodhead P. Primary hyperparathyroidism presenting with a maxillary tumor and hydrocephalus. Journal of Laryngology & Otology 1988;162: 1164–7.
7. Hug EB, Slater JD. Proton radiation therapy for chordomas and chondrosarcomas of the skull base. Neurosurgery Clinics of North America 2000;11(4):627–38.
8. Barnes L. Pathobiology of selected tumors of the skull base. Skull Base Surgery 1991;1:207.
9. Woodhead P, Lloyd GAS. Olfactory neuroblastoma, imaging by magnetic resonance, CT and conventional techniques. Clinical Otolaryngology 1988;13:387–94.
10. DulgerovP, Calcaterra T. Esthesioneuroblastoma: the UCLA experience 1970–1990. Laryngoscope 1992;102: 843.
11. Eden BV, Debo RF, Larner JM. Esthesioneuroblastoma: long-term outcome and patterns of failure – the University of Virginia experience. Cancer 1994;73:2556.
12. Hirose T, Scheitauer BW, Lopes MDB et al. Olfactory neuroblastoma: an immunohistochemical, ultrastructural and flow cytometric study. Cancer 1995;76:4.
13. Schwaab G, Micheau C, LeGuillou C et al. Olfactory esthesioneuroma: a report of 40 cases. Laryngoscope 1988;98:872.
14. Harrison D, Lund VJ. Tumors of the upper jaw. Edinburgh: Churchill Livingstone, 1993.
15. Barnes L, Weber PC, Krause JR et al. Angiofibroma: a flow cytometric evaluation of 31 cases. Skull Base Surgery 1992;2:195.
16. Spector GJ, Ciralsky R, Maisel RH et al. Multiple glomus tumors in the head and neck. Laryngoscope 1975; 85:1066.
17. Macbeth RG. Malignant disease of the paranasal sinuses. Journal of Laryngology & Otology 1965;79: 592–612.
18. Hadfield EH. A studies of adenocarcinoma of the paranasal sinuses in woodworkers in the furniture industry. Annals of Royal College of Surgeons of England 1970;46:301–9.
19. Lund VJ, Howard DJ, Weui WI et al. Craniofacial resection for tumors of the nasal cavity and paranasal sinuses: a 17-year experience. Head Neck 1998;20:97–105.
20. Arena S, Keen M. Carcinoma of the middle ear and temporal bone. Am J Otolaryngol 1988;9:351–6.
21. Snyderman CH, Kanecka IV, Sekhar LN et al. Anterior cranial base reconstruction: role of galeal and pericranial flaps. Laryngoscope 1990;100:607–14.
22. Fisch U. Infratemporal fossa approach for extensive tumors of the temporal bone and base of the skull. In Silverstein H, Norrell H, editors. Neurological surgery of the ear. Birmingham, Alabama: Aesculapiul, 1977; 34–53.
23. Sekhar LN. Operative management of tumors involving the cavernous sinus. In Schramm VL, Sekhar LN, editors. Tumors of the cranial base. New York: Futura, 1987; 393–419.
24. Scramm VL. Infratemporal fossa surgery. In Schramm VL, Sekhar LN, editors. Tumors of the cranial base. New York: Futura, 1987; 421–37.
25. Browne JD, Fisch U. Transotic approach to the cerebellopontine angle. Otolaryngol Clin North Am 1992;25: 331–47.

16

Tumors: Cerebral Metastases and Lymphoma

Sepideh Amin-Hanjani and Griffith R. Harsh, IV

Summary

This chapter focuses on two intracranial neoplasms: cerebral metastases and lymphoma. Cerebral metastases are the most common form of intracranial tumor and often require treatment with surgery and/or radiation. Improvement of neurological function occurs in 50–75% of patients. Primary lymphoma represents about 1% of intracranial tumors and is highly responsive to chemotherapy and whole brain radiotherapy.

Introduction

This chapter will focus on two intracranial neoplasms of increasing prominence: cerebral metastases and lymphoma.

Cerebral metastases are the most common form of intracranial tumor. Although metastases usually convey a poor prognosis, their timely diagnosis and treatment can often palliate neurologic symptoms, prevent progression of brain disease and, less frequently, prolong patient survival. As the efficacy of treatment of systemic disease improves, cerebral metastases will become more prevalent and therapy for cerebral metastases will have an increasing impact on patient survival.

CNS lymphoma occurs either as metastatic disease from systemic primary tumor or as primary CNS lymphoma. Primary CNS lymphoma has become much more prevalent over the past two decades, as a result of an increase in the number of patients with immunosuppression arising from HIV infection or immunosuppressive therapy following organ transplantation. Vigilant surveillance of these two at risk populations is important to early detection and effective treatment of primary CNS lymphoma.

Cerebral Metastases

Cerebral metastases represent the secondary involvement of the brain by neoplasms originating outside the central nervous system (CNS). Currently, cerebral metastases are the most common type of intracranial tumor [1]. The predilection for spread of systemic tumor to the CNS is highly dependent on its histologic type [1].

Epidemiology

Improved neuroimaging has revealed that patients with cerebral metastases outnumber those with primary brain tumors. At autopsy,

25% of cancer patients harbor intracranial metastases [2]. Cerebral metastases - those involving the brain parenchyma itself - occur in about 15% of patients with solid systemic tumors [2]. This prevalence is likely to increase as the proportion of elderly in the population increases, as diagnostic neuroimaging becomes even more sensitive and as patients with cancer live longer.

The pattern of metastasis to the CNS varies with tumor type. Intracranial metastases include those to the skull, meningeal spaces and brain parenchyma. Many skull metastases originate from breast and prostate cancer [3]. Metastases to the pituitary gland are often from breast cancer.

Lung and breast cancer, followed by melanoma, genitourinary cancer and gastrointestinal cancer, are the most common histological types of cerebral metastasis (Table 16.1). The risk of developing cerebral metastasis is highest with malignant melanoma, followed by lung and breast cancer (Table 16.2). Among the types of lung cancer, small cell carcinoma and adenocarcinoma more frequently spread to the brain than does squamous cell carcinoma.

Most cerebral metastases spread to the brain hematogenously. Tumor cells distributed arterially commonly originate from the lung, either from a primary lung tumor or from an extrapulmonary primary that has metastasized to the lung. Less commonly, venous routes are taken. The anastomotic pelvic–vertebral venous plexus described by Batson (termed Batson's plexus) is a potential path of spread of pelvic and retroperitoneal tumors. Tumors from these areas have a predilection for the posterior fossa.

Tumor cells carried arterially are commonly deposited at the junction of gray and white matter of the brain, particularly within watershed zones. Tumor cells are readily lodged within the end vessels of these regions, where vessel caliber changes rapidly. Otherwise, the likelihood of a particular brain region

Table 16.1. Primary sites of cancer in patients with cerebral metastases.

Primary tumor	% of cases (total n = 210)
Lung	40
Breast	19
Melanoma	10
Genitourinary*	7
Gastrointestinal*	7
Female genital tract*	5
Sarcoma	3
Lymphoma	1
Other	6
Unknown	2

* Gastrointestinal: colorectal, esophagus, gastric, pancreas.
Genitourinary: renal, testis, bladder, prostate.
Female genital tract: ovary, uterus, cervix, choriocarcinoma.

Adapted from Posner JB. Neurologic complications of cancer. Contemporary Neurology series. Volume 45. Phildelphia: Davis, 1995.

Table 16.2. Frequency of intracranial metastases from systemic cancers.

Primary tumor	Intracranial tumor at autopsy (%)	Intracerebral tumor at autopsy (%)
All sites	24	15
Melanoma	72	40
Lung	34	21
Breast	30	10
Leukemia	23	3
Lymphoma	16	1
Gastrointestinal*	7	3
Colon	8	5
Pancreas	7	2
Genitourinary*	19	11
Renal	27	21
Prostate	31	0
Ovary	5	5

*Gastrointestinal includes colon, gastric and pancreatic tumors. Genitourinary includes renal, prostate, testis, cervix and ovarian tumors.

Adapted from Posner JB, Chernik NL. Intracranial metastases from systemic cancer. Advances In Neurology 1978; 19:579–92.

developing a metastasis reflects its tissue volume and rate of blood flow. Consequently, almost 90% of metatases are supratentorial and the frontal and parietal lobes are most commonly affected.

Approximately 50% of patients with secondary cerebral tumor have more than one lesion. This incidence of multiple metastasis is likely to increase as neuroimaging becomes more sensitive. Multiple lesions are common with melanoma and lung cancer, whereas patients with breast, abdominal and pelvic cancer more often have a single brain metastasis [3].

Cerebral metastases occur with equal frequency in men and women. The incidence of brain metastasis is the same for all races. Brain metastases are most likely to appear in people between 50 and 70 years of age. In children, CNS metastases are most commonly from leukemia, followed by lymphoma, sarcoma and germ cell tumor.

Clinical Presentation

Brain metastases are most commonly discovered after a diagnosis of the primary tumor has been established; more than 80% of cerebral metastases present after discovery of the systemic source. Most appear at a late stage in the dissemination of the tumor. One exception is lung cancer, in which metastases often occur in the early stages of the disease and neurological symptoms secondary to metastases frequently antedate discovery of the primary tumor [3].

The clinical presentation of a metastasis reflects the location and size of the tumor [4]. The most frequent presenting symptoms are headache, focal deficits and behavioral or cognitive changes (Table 16.3). Headache, although non-specific, is the most common single symptom. In a patient with known cancer, new onset of headaches, especially those occurring in the early morning, warrants radiologic investigation. Behavioral changes are more common with multiple than with single metastases. They may be as subtle and non-specific as mild confusion, memory loss, depression or emotional lability. Symptoms such as headache, behavioral change and focal deficits are usually subtle in onset and slowly progress as the mass effect from the tumor increases.

Seizures, hemorrhage and infarction bring a more acute presentation. Seizures, focal or generalized, are the presenting symptom in about 10% of patients. They, too, are more frequent in patients with multiple metastases [3]. Hemorrhage or infarction from a tumor embolus occurs in 5–10% of cases [3]. Hemorrhage is more common with metastases from melanoma, choriocarcinoma, renal cell carcinoma and bronchogenic carcinoma.

Table 16.3. Presenting symptoms and signs of cerebral metastases.

Symptom/sign	% of cases (total n = 284)
Headache	24
Focal weakness	20
Behavioral and cognitive changes	14
Seizures	12
Ataxia	7
Asymptomatic*	7

Asymptomatic lesions discovered in the course of staging patients with known systemic cancer.

Adapted from Posner JB. Brain metastases: 1995. A brief review. J Neuro-oncol 1996;27:287–93.

The differential diagnosis of the clinical presentation of metastasis includes other mass lesions (abscess, granuloma, resolving hematoma, radiation necrosis) demyelination and infarction (non-bacterial thrombotic endocarditis, cerebral venous occlusion) [4].

Diagnosis

Imaging

Thorough and accurate radiographic imaging is an essential aspect of managing patients with cerebral metastases. CT has been superceded by MRI with gadolinium contrast as the modality of choice [5].

CT is useful for screening for large or hemorrhagic metastases with acute presentations and for skull tumors. Most metastases are hypodense or isodense, well circumscribed masses on non-contrast images. Those with necrotic centers have hypodense interiors. Hyperdensity is seen with acute intratumoral hemorrhage, some melanomas, some densely cellular tumors (adenocarcinoma and small cell lung carcinoma) and rare calcified lesions [5]. Most metastases enhance brightly with intravenous contrast, particularly when given in double dose. CT is relatively insensitive in detecting very small lesions, particularly those in the posterior fossa, and leptomeningeal spread.

Diagnostic screening and treatment planning benefit greatly from the sensitivity, specificity and anatomic resolution (particularly in the posterior fossa) of MRI. Most metastases are isointense on T1-weighted images and hyperintense on T2-weighted images. Central necrosis, cysts and peripheral edema are all hypointense on T1 images and hyperintense on T2 images. The intensity pattern of hemorrhagic metastases varies with the age of the hematoma. Anomalies include melanomas that may be hyperintense on T1 images and adenocarcinomas, highly cellular tumors, and calcified lesions that may be hypointense on T2 images.

Metastases usually enhance brightly and homogeneously with gadolinium, except in their necrotic, cystic or hemorrhagic portions. Rim-enhancing metastases have a center of fluid or necrosis; the rim is more irregular than that of benign cysts, abscesses and resolving hematomas [6]. Metastases may sometimes be distinguished from malignant gliomas that also have nodular rim-enhancement by multiplicity and a circumferential pattern of T1 hypointense, T2 hyperintense edema that is less likely to involve the cortex or corpus callosum [5]. Higher doses of contrast (0.3 mmol/kg) significantly increase the sensitivity of detecting small lesions. Diffuse leptomeningeal disease, carcinomatous meningitis, appears as sulcal enhancement on post-gadolinium T1 scans and as hyperintense linearities on flair sequences.

Biopsy

Biopsy of a brain mass to obtain histologic verification of metastasis is rarely required when there are multiple parenchymal brain lesions in a patient with known active systemic malignancy, particularly if there are metastases to other organs. In contrast, biopsy is almost always indicated when the brain lesion is solitary (the patient's only known tumor) and nonsurgical treatment is planned. The need for biopsy of a single brain lesion in a patient with known systemic cancer depends on several factors. Although one study of biopsy results found that 11% of single brain lesions thought to be metastases based upon enhanced CT were a different pathology [7], current high resolution MRI is often quite specific. Systemic disease in recession (a primary histology that infrequently spreads to the brain) and an atypical radiographic appearance favor biopsy. Active systemic disease, a primary histology that commonly spreads to the brain and a typical radiographic appearance mitigate the need for biopsy. Current stereotactic biopsy techniques permit retrieval of diagnostic tissue in approximately 95% of cases, with a morbidity from hemorrhage, seizure, worsened neurologic deficit and infection of 3% and a mortality of 0.6% [8]. A highly vascular appearance on neuroimaging and a primary histology associated with a tendency for brain metastases to bleed is a relative contraindication to biopsy.

Treatment

Cerebral metastases generally carry a very poor prognosis when not treated. The median survival for patients with symptomatic brain metastases that are not treated is 4–6 weeks. The optimal treatment of brain metastases must consider several factors, including the patient's neurologic and general medical condition, the number, location and size of the lesions, and the histology, the extent, the prior treatment and the response to treatment of the systemic disease. Two current trends in the approach to cerebral metastasis are evident: a shift from mere palliation of symptoms to tumor eradication, in an effort to improve survival, and an increased emphasis on the patient's quality of life. Three main modalities of treatment are used for brain metastases: radiation, surgery and chemotherapy.

Medical Therapy

Corticosteroids often markedly improve neurologic symptoms by reducing peritumoral vasogenic edema. Generalized symptoms, such as headache and lethargy, respond more consistently than do focal symptoms and signs. The clinical response is usually apparent within a day and peaks by 7 days. Dexamethasone, which has the benefit of lacking mineralocorticoid effect, is the steroid used most frequently. Steroids are considered palliative treatment that is used transiently, while other, more definitive therapy is planned or delivered. Treatment with steroids alone results in a median survival of

8–10 weeks. The dose of steroid medication should be tapered and discontinued when clinically possible, to avoid side effects such as myopathy, psychiatric change (agitation, delirium, and psychosis), gastric disturbances (ulceration with bleeding or perforation) and opportunistic infections.

Prophylactic anticonvulsants are not indicated unless there is a history of seizure.

Radiation

Radiotherapy is indicated for almost all patients with cerebral metastasis. The optimal method of delivery, dose and regimen varies with the individual patient. In many cases, these are controversial. Radiation can be administered either as fractionated external radiotherapy to the whole brain (WBRT), the region of the tumor (local fractionated radiotherapy) or both (WBRT with a local boost), as single exposure radiosurgery or as interstitial brachytherapy.

Fractionated whole-brain radiotherapy has been the standard treatment for brain metastases for almost half a century. WBRT increases the median duration of survival of patients to 3–6 months from 1–2 months (10–15% survive for at least 1 year) [7,9]. Treatment improves neurologic function in 50–75% of patients [9]. Large retrospective studies reveal that 50% of the patients treated with WBRT die from systemic cancer, rather than from progressive brain disease. The dosing regimen most commonly employed is 30 Gy over 2 weeks in ten daily 3.0 Gy fractions. This regimen is as effective as those with higher doses or more extended fractionation.

Prognostic factors favoring survival include age less than 60 years, Karnofsky performance score of at least 70, control of the primary tumor and absence of extracranial metastases. Radiation cell sensitizers such as nitroimidazoles are not beneficial. Although certain types of tumor, such as renal cell carcinoma and melanoma, are relatively radioresistant, the duration of patient survival following radiotherapy of cerebral metastases is similar for most tumor types [9].

Radiation therapy has significant risk of acute and long-term complications. Acutely, fatigue, headache, nausea and vomiting may occur during and shortly after treatment and neurologic deficits may be exacerbated. Steroid therapy is often required. Chronically, side effects, such as dementia, ataxia and urinary incontinence, occur in at least 5% of patients who survive longer than 1 year [10]. In one study, 50% of patients surviving for more than 2 years after surgical resection and WBRT developed leukoencephalopathy or atrophy-induced hydrocephalus ex vacuo. More prolonged fractionation schemes and more focal treatment are strategies designed to decrease the risk of dementia. Patients expected to survive longer than 6–12 months are often treated with 40 Gy in 2 -Gy fractions over 4 weeks. In an attempt to spare normal brain, fractionated local radiotherapy has been used for single metastases, but the relative effectiveness of focal and whole-brain therapy has not been studied. Additional local dose can also be administered as a boost to the lesion following WBRT.

Radiosurgery involves single-session high-dose irradiation of a stereotactically defined target. In that radiosurgery intends inactivation of all tissue within a targeted volume, it is a non-invasive alternative to surgical excision. Multiple techniques (Linac, Gamma Knife, Cyber Knife, and Proton Beam) are able to deliver the conformal radiation required. Since the likelihood of controlling tumor growth and the risk of radiation injury to surrounding tissue both increase with increasing dose and the risk of radiation injury increases with increasing target volume, there is an interdependence of tumor volume, dose, tumor control rate and complication rate. Empirically defined relationships specify an inverse relationship between two variables (e.g. tumor size and dose) after two parameters have been established (e.g. minimal acceptable rate of tumor control and maximal acceptable rate of complication). For example, if one posits that at least 15 Gy is required to achieve a 90% rate of tumor control at 1 year and that the acceptable risk of complication is 1%, then the maximal tumor volume that can be safely and effectively treated is 10 cm^3. In other words, given such specifications for safety and efficacy, there is an ideal dose for each tumor volume. In general, stereotactic radiosurgery is an effective treatment for intracranial metastases of less than 10 cm^3 in volume (2.5–3.0 cm in diameter).

Radiosurgery is indicated for surgically inaccessible lesions and is an acceptable alternative to surgery for many accessible ones. Although it is occasionally used in the patient with more than three lesions, it is usually reserved for patients with single or, at most, several metastases. Median duration of patient survival following radiosurgery for an intracranial metastasis is 7–12 months, similar to that for surgical resection [11]. Randomized studies comparing radiosurgical and surgical treatments for single brain metastases have not yet been completed.

Whether WBRT is needed in addition to radiosurgery for single metastases is controversial. Much of the radiosurgical data was accumulated in patients who also received WBRT and, given the conformal nature of the radiosurgical treatment volume, it is unlikely that the addition of WBRT to radiosurgery significantly increases the risk of radiosurgery. Nonetheless, given the inefficacy and toxicity of WBRT and the ability to detect and to treat new lesions conformally with radiosurgery, radiosurgery alone may be appropriate initial treatment for most metastases of appropriate size. Essentially, stereotactic radiosurgery and WBRT can be viewed as complementary: radiosurgery focally targets one to three tumors of 1–10 cm^3 in volume, whereas WBRT intends to control higher numbers of small tumors or microscopic spread throughout the brain. Radiosurgery alone is most strongly indicated for a single metastasis from systemic tumor that is indolent or well controlled (and thus not an immediate threat to survival) and of a histologic type prone to single brain metastases (e.g. breast and non-small cell lung carcinoma) or relatively refractory to fractionated radiotherapy (e.g. melanoma, renal cell carcinoma and sarcoma). WBRT is likely needed in addition to radiosurgery when there are multiple cerebral tumors, especially those with histologies prone to disseminated brain metastases and high sensitivity to fractionated radiation (e.g. small cell lung carcinoma, testicular carcinoma and lymphoma). In many patients with these histologies, WBRT is given first and radiosurgery is reserved for tumors that subsequently resume growth. When brain metastases are multiple and systemic disease is refractory to treatment, WBRT alone is given as palliation.

Interstitial brachytherapy (the temporary or permanent placement of radioactive seeds within a tumor) and interstitial radiosurgery (the transient stereotactic placement of the tip of a miniature generator of X-rays within a tumor) also achieve high-dose focal irradiation of brain metastases. Their invasiveness, with the concomitant risks of infection and hemorrhage, and their limited conformity are disadvantages relative to radiosurgery. However, they do offer an additional treatment option for single, surgically inaccessible tumors that are too large to be treated safely and effectively with radiosurgery.

Surgery

In patients with cerebral metastases and well controlled systemic disease, the former becomes a more significant determinant of survival. It is within this subgroup of patients that aggressive treatment, including surgery, is considered. Resection of single brain metastases was initially advocated for patients with good prognoses because of the low rates of long-term tumor control (40% at 1 year) with conventional WBRT [6]. Prospective randomized trials have firmly established the superiority of surgical resection followed by WBRT to WBRT alone for a single cerebral metastasis [6]. The median duration of survival is 10–14 months rather than 4–6 months. As noted above, although direct comparisons of surgery and radiosurgery for a single metastasis have not yet been completed, radiosurgery is often an acceptable alternative to craniotomy. Also, a surgically inaccessible location, multiple brain metastases or extensive systemic disease usually contraindicate resection. An exception is the need to resect a tumor from a location, such as the posterior fossa, in which it is immediately life threatening, even if the patient has multiple metastases and significant systemic disease.

The utility of surgery for multiple cerebral metastases is controversial. Modern surgical series show that early post-operative mortality and morbidity following resection of multiple metastases is comparable to those following resection of a single metastasis. One study found a significantly shorter duration of survival (5 vs 12 months) of patients who had multiple metastases resected compared to those undergoing surgery for a single metastasis. However, gross resection of all tumors was not achieved in the majority of patients with multiple lesions. Another study reported a median duration of survival of 14 months for patients with two or three metastases that were totally resected - a result similar to that achieved for patients with single metastases. These studies support surgical removal of one to three metastases, particularly those too large to be treated by radiosurgery [12].

Historically, most patients have received WBRT post-operatively - even those whose tumors were totally removed. Currently, however, many consider WBRT to be relatively contraindicated by its chronic sequelae in patients expected to live longer than 6 months. Although some studies have found that post-operative WBRT lengthens median survival, several others have found no significant difference between patients treated with surgical resection alone and those receiving resection and post-operative WBRT. Post-operative WBRT, however, did yield other benefits: improved control of local tumor, decreased risk of distant tumor, increased time to neurological recurrence and decrease in the percentage of patients dying of neurologic disease [13]. Post-operative radiosurgery, in addition to WBRT, may be indicated in cases of incomplete removal of a metastasis. As an alternative to post-operative WBRT, it is likely to improve control of local tumor but not affect the incidence of distant metastases.

Chemotherapy

Unfortunately, chemotherapeutic agents which are effective against primary solid tumors are seldom as effective against brain metastases. The blood–brain barrier is partly responsible but other factors are likely to contribute, as lipid soluble agents are also ineffective, the blood–brain barrier around most metastastic lesions is deficient and intrathecal or intraventricular injection does not significantly improve outcome. However, chemotherapy of cerebral metastases of some histologies, including breast cancer, small cell lung carcinoma and choriocarcinoma, can effect remission, stabilize neurologic deficits and prolong median survival. The current role for chemotherapy of cerebral metastases is limited to adjuvant treatment of such chemosensitive tumors. Improvements in the delivery of drugs to the CNS and new multi-agent regimens may broaden the role of chemotherapy in the future.

Recurrent Metastases

Many of the principles of treating brain metastases at their original presentation apply to treatment of recurrent disease, with the proviso that the effects of the previous therapy must be considered. Local recurrence of a previously treated tumor has different implications from the appearance of distant failure. Surgery, stereotactic radiosurgery, focal radiotherapy, interstitial radiosurgery and brachytherapy are options for local recurrences, depending on the size and location of the lesion. In one study, among patients with a single recurrent tumor and well controlled systemic disease, two-thirds improved neurologically after tumor resection and the median duration of survival was 9 months [14].

Diffuse distant metastases probably warrant WBRT if it has not been given. For tumors recurrent after WBRT, an additional 20 Gy of fractionated radiation may improve the neurologic function of selected patients but does not significantly lengthen survival [15]. In one study, among patients with well controlled systemic disease and a good response to their initial radiation, fewer than half had neurologic improvement after additional radiotherapy and the median duration of survival was 5 months [15].

Summary

The selection of a treatment plan for an individual patient must consider multiple factors. These include the number, location and size of the metastases, the histology, extent and prior treatment of the systemic disease, and the patient's neurologic status, medical condition and personal preference. In general, radiosurgery is the treatment of choice for most patients with one to three brain metastases. Surgical resection is indicated for one or two accessible lesions larger than 2–3 cm in diameter and for those threatening cerebral herniation; adjuvant radiosurgery to any residual tumor or the resection bed is likely warranted. WBRT is indicated when there are more than a few metastases, when the histology predicts disseminated metastasis or radiosensitivity or when the patient has a particularly poor prognosis. Table 16.4 summarizes general recommendations for the treatment of metastases, taking these factors into consideration. The

Table 16.4. Recommendations for management of cerebral metastases.

Systemic disease (median survival)	1–3 (< 10 cc) accessible	1–3 (< 10 cc) inaccessible	1–3 (> 10 cc) accessible	1–3 (> 10 cc) inaccessible	> 3
Absent/Stable (> 6 months)	Surgery or radiosurgery +/- WBRT*	Radiosurgery +/- WBRT*	Surgery +/- WBRT	Fractionated focal radiation	WBRT
Slowly progressive (4–6 months)	Surgery or radiosurgery + WBRT	Radiosurgery + WBRT	Surgery + WBRT	**WBRT + fractionated boost**	**WBRT**
Moderately progressive (2–4 months)	WBRT	WBRT	WBRT	WBRT	WBRT
Rapidly progressive (< 2 months)	None	None	None	None	None

*Given the potential for long-term complications in patients with prolonged survival, noncomitant WBRT is less desirable in these groups of patients.

guidelines propose treating patients with well controlled systemic disease aggressively, by offering treatments that are effective for one to three lesions.

Lymphoma

Lymphoma is a malignant lymphocytic neoplasm that can occur in the central nervous system (CNS), either primarily or as a secondary manifestation of systemic disease. Lymphoma of the brain or spinal cord not involving other areas, except for ocular structures, is termed "primary CNS lymphoma" (PCNSL). The incidence of CNS lymphoma has increased significantly over the last two decades.

PCNSL

PCNSL has been referred to within the literature as reticulum cell sarcoma, perivascular sarcoma, immunoblastic sarcoma, microgliomatosis and malignant reticulosis. The disease most frequently appears as solitary or multi-focal lesions of the cerebrum of middle-aged adults. The immunologic competency of the patient affects the neurologic presentation. Immunodeficiency is a well recognized risk factor for the disease.

Epidemiology

Primary CNS lymphoma represents about 1% of intracranial tumors. The incidence of primary CNS lymphoma has been increasing steadily for the past two decades [16]. This increase is partially attributable to an increased prevalence of immunodeficient patients secondary to acquired immune deficiency syndrome (AIDS) and immunosuppressive treatment after organ transplantation. However, the incidence of the disease among immunocompetent persons has also increased. According to surveillance by the National Cancer Institute, the annual incidence of PCNSL increased from 2.7 cases/ten million persons in 1973–75 to 7.5 cases/ten million persons in 1982–84, even after exclusion of never married men as a relatively high-risk group for AIDS. Continuation of this trend produced an incidence of 30 cases/ten million persons in 1991–92 [17]. Although some of the increase may result from improved radiographic and immunologic detection, the trend antedates the widespread use of such technologies. Other etiologies for the observed increase in incidence of primary CNS lymphoma, such as environmental factors, remain speculative.

For immunocompetent patients, the sixth decade of life is the most common age of diagnosis of PCNSL [16,18]. The median age for presentation in the immunocompromised population falls within the fourth decade. Childhood disease is rare and is usually associated with congenital or acquired immunodeficiency.

In the immunocompetent population with primary CNS lymphoma, 60% of patients are male and 40% are female [16]. This is similar to the gender distribution of patients with systemic lymphoma. The immunocompromised population with PCNSL is even more disproportionately male because of the male predominance in the AIDS epidemic.

Several risk factors for developing PCNSL have been identified (Table 16.5). Given its etiologic role in other lymphoproliferative disorders among immunosuppressed patients, the Epstein–Barr virus (EBV) may contribute to the development of primary CNS lymphoma in immunocompromised patients. EBV RNA has been found in CNS lymphoma tissue obtained from immunocompromised patients. Primary CNS lymphoma also occurs as a second malignancy after treatment of other malignancies, such as Hodgkin's lymphoma, non-Hodgkin's lymphoma and colon, breast and thyroid cancer. It is unclear whether this phenomenon reflects an underlying predisposition to cancer among these patients or it results from exposure to agents used to treat the initial malignancy.

Pathology

Primary CNS lymphoma, like systemic lymphoma, arises from lymphocytes. The source of the pre-malignant lymphocytes is controversial as the CNS lacks lymphoid tissue and lymphatics. The perivascular distribution of cerebral tumor suggests that it may originate from systemic neoplastic lymphocytes that selectively infiltrate CNS tissue. This selectivity may depend on adhesion molecules within the CNS vasculature and parenchyma specific for the malignant cells.

The macroscopic appearance of deposits of PCNSL within the brain varies. They may be leptomeningeal, parenchymal, subependymal or a combination of these. Primary CNS lymphoma may be unifocal or multicentric. In either case, it can appear to be relatively well circumscribed or irregularly margined. In the leptomeningeal variant of PCNL, tumor exclusively infiltrates the leptomeninges, cranial nerves and spinal nerve roots. Primary parenchymal CNS lymphoma softens affected brain tissue and turns it yellow–brown. There may be areas of focal hemorrhage or necrosis.

Microscopically, diffuse infiltration of tumor into brain parenchyma well beyond the macroscopic borders of the tumor is common. Neoplastic lymphocytes aggregate perivascularly and infiltrate the walls of small blood vessels (Fig. 16.1). This perivascular cuffing is most prominent at the tumor margins. Tumor cells also commonly extend in the subpial plane or in the subarachnoid space. An astrocytic reaction can be prominent, especially in the peripheral parts of the tumor. An infiltrate of T lymphocytes is typically present at the tumor margins and occasionally within the tumor itself.

The tumor has histological features similar to those of systemic non-Hodgkin's lymphoma. Hodgkin's lymphoma is almost never seen as a primary CNS tumor. The great majority of PCNSLs are monoclonal B cell lymphomas. T cell lymphomas of the CNS are exceptionally rare and must be differentiated from B cell lymphomas with a prominent reactive T-cell

Table 16.5. Risk factors for primary CNS lymphoma.

Acquired immunodeficiency	AIDS
	Immunosuppressive therapy for transplant or autoimmune conditions
Congenital immunodeficiency	Wiskott–Aldrich syndrome
	Severe combined immunodeficiency syndrome
	IgA deficiency
	Ataxia–telangiectasia
	X-linked lymphoproliferative syndrome
	Chediak–Higashi syndrome
Autoimmune diseases	Rheumatoid arthritis
	Sjögren's syndrome
	Idiopathic thrombocytopenic purpura
	Systemic lupus erythematosis
	Sarcoidosis
Viral infections	Epstein–Barr virus

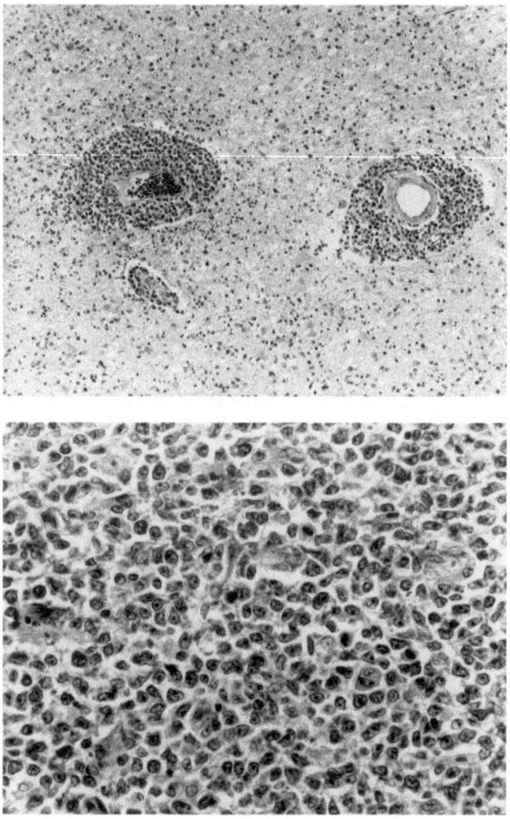

Fig. 16.1. a Perivascular aggregation of neoplastic lymphoid cells typical for primary CNS lymphoma. **b** Malignant lymphoid cells with cytologically atypical nuclei.

component. The relative incidences of B-cell subtypes among PCNSLs differ from those found systemically. Unlike systemic lymphomas, which are typically follicular B cell lymphomas, most PCNSLs are diffuse large cell or large cell immunoblastic in type [18]. Immunological markers help to distinguish B cell lymphomas from other tumors such, as gliomas and small cell carcinomas (antibody against CD45, a leukocyte marker), and from T-cell lymphomas (antibodies against CD20 and CD79a, both B cell markers).

Clinical Features

Primary CNS lymphoma typically presents with symptoms and signs of increased intracranial pressure or cortical dysfunction, depending upon the location of the lesions. Personality changes and altered affect are relatively common modes of presentation, given the relatively frequent involvement of the frontal lobes (Table 16.6). Seizure was a first presenting symptom in 13% of one series of 66 patients [16]. The time elapsing between onset of symptoms and diagnosis is often short – on the order of 2–3 months. The constellation of symptoms is not noticeably different between immunocompetent and immunocompromised patients.

Table 16.6. Frequency of presenting symptoms.

Symptom	% of cases
Personality change	24
Cerebellar signs	21
Headache	15
Seizures	13
Motor dysfunction	11
Visual changes	8

Adapted from Hochberg FH, Miller DC. Primary central nervous system lymphoma. J Neurosurg 1988; 68:835–53.

Murray et al. found the majority of lesions to be solitary and supratentorial (52.1%), with the most frequent sites of involvement being frontal (26%), temporal (15%) and parietal (14%) [18]. Diencephalic and infratentorial lesions, particularly in the cerebellum (11%), were also seen. The tumor is solitary almost twice as often as it is multifocal. Diffuse meningeal disease has also been described and accounted for 12% of cases in the Massachusetts General Hospital (MGH) series of 66 patients [16].

Diagnosis

Imaging

CT reveals an isodense or moderately hyperdense lesion that enhances strongly and homogeneously with contrast. Mild or moderate edema is typical. Tumors in immunocompromised patients in particular may show a ring enhancing pattern. The periventricular area is a common location; most tumors abut the ependyma.

Primary CNS lymphomas are usually isointense or slightly hypointense on T1-weighted MR images and isointense or slightly hyperintense on T2-weighted images (Fig. 16.2). The enhancement pattern in immunocompetent patients is usually dense and homogeneous, but can be heterogeneous (Figs 16.2 and 16.3).

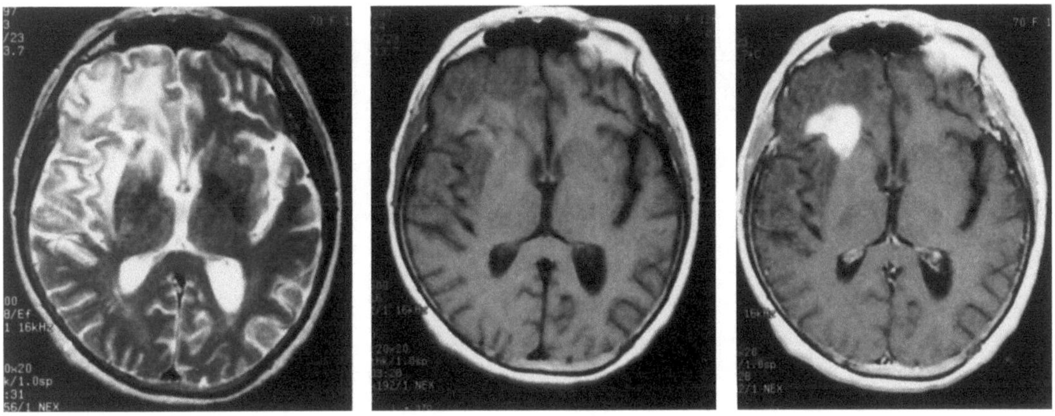

Fig. 16.2. Axial T2-weighted images (left) and T1-weighted images without (center) and with (right) gadolinium enhancement in an immunocompetent patient with primary CNS lymphoma. The right frontal mass appears heterogeneously isointense and hyperintense on T2-weighted images, with surrounding hyperintense edema . On T1-weighted images, the isointense mass enhances densely and homogeneously, following contrast administration.

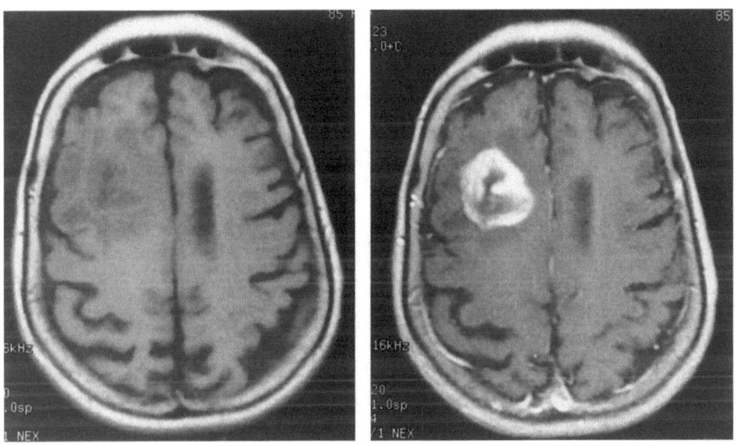

Fig. 16.3. Axial T1-weighted images without (left) and with (right) gadolinium enhancement in an immunocompetent patient with primary CNS lymphoma. The ring enhancing lesion could also be metastasis, malignant glioma or even abscess.

Non-enhancing tumors have been seen, but are rare. In patients with AIDS-associated PCNSL, enhancement may be heterogeneous and is frequently rim-enhancing (Fig. 16.4). Radiographic evidence of hemorrhage and necrosis may be seen.

In patients with AIDS, CNS lymphoma may be very difficult to distinguish radiographically from other common intracranial pathologies, such as toxoplasmosis. Positron emission tomography and thallium SPECT have been proposed as more sensitive imaging modalities for distinguishing lymphoma from infectious lesions. Some authors claim that the combination of increased uptake on thallium SPECT and EBV DNA in CSF has 100% sensitivity and specificity for CNS lymphoma and obviates the need for biopsy [19].

The typical CSF profile with primary CNS lymphoma is elevated protein, low glucose and pleocytosis. CSF cytology showing a monomorphic population of abnormal lymphocytes is diagnostic, but only 10% of patients undergoing CSF analysis at the time of presentation have positive cytologic findings. Furthermore, lumbar puncture may be contraindicated by

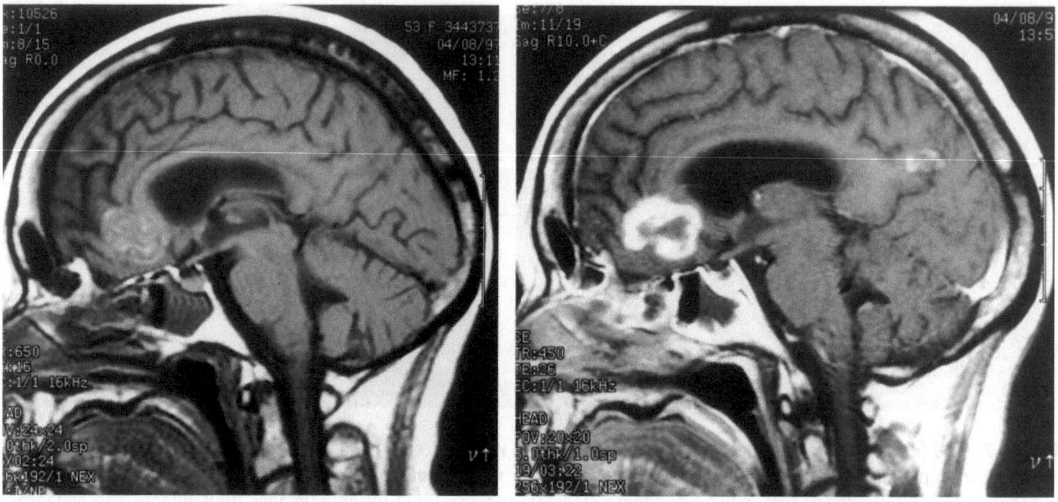

Fig. 16.4. Sagittal T1-weighted images without (left) and with (right) gadolinium enhancement in a patient with AIDS, demonstrating the typical heterogeneous rim enhancement seen with primary CNS lymphoma in this population of patients.

increased intracranial pressure in many patients. Definitive diagnosis usually requires tissue. Biopsy is more likely to yield diagnostic tissue if it is performed prior to the administration of corticosteroids, which, by lysing the malignant tumor cells, may obscure the diagnosis [16].

Once a diagnosis of CNS lymphoma is established, the need for investigations to exclude systemic lymphoma with secondary cerebral involvement is controversial. In immunocompetent patients, spread of systemic lymphoma to the CNS is uncommon. When it does occur, it is usually late in the course of the disease and the leptomeninges are predominantly affected. In general, investigations should be limited to determining the extent of disease within the CNS [20]: cranial MRI with contrast, ophthalmologic examination, spinal MRI with contrast (for patients with neck or back pain or myelopathy) and lumbar puncture (if not contraindicated). For patients with AIDS, systemic lymphoma has a greater propensity to involve the CNS secondarily. In these patients, screening for systemic disease with bone marrow aspiration and chest, abdominal and pelvic imaging is advisable. Because of the association between PCNSL and AIDS, testing for HIV is also indicated for patients first found to have primary CNS lymphoma.

Treatment and Outcome

The options for treating PCNSL have evolved significantly during the last decade (Table 16.7). Radiotherapy and chemotherapy, separately and in combination, have significantly increased the survival of many immunocompetent patients with PCNSL. The prognosis for AIDS-related primary CNS lymphoma, however, remains poor, with a median duration of survival of less than 3 months, despite treatment [21].

Radiotherapy

Primary CNS lymphoma is highly radiosensitive. Early reports indicated an increase in median survival from 3.3 to 15.2 months for patients receiving radiotherapy. Subsequent reports confirmed this benefit to survival. Despite a high initial response rate, radiotherapy alone rarely leads to long-term survival; only 7% of patients are alive 5 years after treatment [22].

The optimal dose of radiation is controversial. Retrospective data suggest that total doses of 40–50 Gy to the primary tumor improve survival [6]. No additional survival benefit follows higher doses. The Radiation Therapy Oncology Group (RTOG) failed to improve outcome with

Table 16.7. Recent trials of combined therapy for primary CNS lymphoma.

Reference	No. of pts	Chemotherapy	Radiotherapy	Median survival	Median survival RT only [d]	Major toxicities
Pre-irradiation chemotherapy						
Bessell, 1991	10	BVAM (MTX 1.5 g/m^2)	WBRT 45 Gy Boost 10 Gy Spine 35 Gy*	10	–	Myelosuppression
Liang, 1993	9	CHOP MTX IT (12 mg)	WBRT 36 Gy Boost 18 Gy	30	–	Leukoencephalopathy
LaChance, 1994	6	CHOP	WBRT 45 Gy Boost 10.8 Gy Spine 30 Gy	8.5	–	–
Glass, 1994	25	MTX (3.5 g/m^2)	WBRT 30–44 Gy Boost 0- 23.4 Gy	33	–	Mucositis Myelosuppression Leukoencephalopathy
Glass, 1996	18	MCHOD (MTX 3.5g /m^2)	WBRT 30 Gy Boost +/-	25.5	–	Myelosuppression Leukoencephalopathy
Schultz, 1996	52	CHOD	WBRT 41.4 Gy Boost 18Gy	16.1	11.6	Myelosuppression
Brada, 1998	31	MACOP B (MTX 0.4–2 g/m^2)	WBRT 30–45 Gy, Boost 15–25 Gy Spine 30–35 Gy*	23	16**	Myelosuppression Mucositis Hepato/nephrotoxicity
Abrey, 1998	31	MTX IV (1 g/m^2) MTX IT (12 mg) Ara-C (post-RT)	WBRT 40 Gy Boost 14.4 Gy	42	21.7***	Leukoencephalopathy
Hiraga, 1999	29	MTX (0.1 g/kg)	WBRT 30 Gy Boost 10–20 Gy	39.3	–	Myelosuppression Leukoencephalopathy
Post-irradiation chemotherapy						
Shibamato, 1990	10	VEPA	WBRT 30–40 Gy Boost 20–30 Gy	16+	7	Leukoencephalopathy/necrosis
Chamberlain, 1992	16	Hydroxyurea, PCV	WBRT 55–62 Gy	41	13****	Myelosuppression
Rosenthal, 1993	6	CHOP	WBRT 45 Gy Boost 10 Gy	25+	18	Myelosuppression
No initial irradiation						
Neuwelt, 1991	17	CMPD (MTX 2.5 g IA) BBB disruption	None (at relapse)	44.5	–	Seizure Myelosuppression
Cher, 1996	19	MTX (3.5–8 d/m^2), or MCHOD	None (at relapse)	51	–	Nephrotoxicity
Freilich, 1996	13	MTX (1–3.5 g/m^2), P +/- V,T,ara-C	None (at relapse)	30.5	–	Leukoencephalopathy
Sandor, 1998	14	MTX (1.5 g/m^2), V,T	None (at relapse)	30+	–	Myelosuppression Neurocognitive decline

MTX, methotrexate; BVAM, BCNU, vincristine, cytosine arabinoside, methotrexate; IT, intrathecal;;CHOP, cyclophosphamide, doxorubicin, vincristine, prednisone; MCHOD, methotrexate, cyclophosphamide, doxorubicin, vincristine, dexamethasone; CHOD, cyclophosphamide, doxorubicin, vincristine, dexamethasone; MACOP-B, methotrexate, doxorubicin, cyclophosphamide, vincristine, prednisone, bleomycin; IV, intravenous; Ara-C, cytosine arabinoside; VEPA vincristine, doxorubicin, cyclophosphamide, prednisolone; PCV, procarbazine, CCNU, vincristine; CMPD, cyclophosphamide, methotrexate, procarbazine, dexamethasone; IA, intra-arterial; BBB, blood–brain barrier; P, procarbazine; V, vincristine; T, thiotepa.

[d] Historical controls.

*Only patients with proven CSF disease treated with full craniospinal irradiation. ** From Brada, 1990.

*** From DeAngelis , 1992. ****From Chamberlain, 1990.

Note: median survival times not supplied by the reference were calculated from Kaplan–Meier analysis of individual survival times reported within the text.

60 Gy (40 Gy to the whole brain, 20 Gy boost to the tumor and its margin) [23].

The optimal extent of radiation is also controversial. Radiation may be administered to the involved field, the whole brain or the entire cranio–spinal axis. Historically, whole-brain irradiation has been the standard treatment, even though its advantage relative to other protocols has never been definitively established [6,22]. In fact, one review reports a median survival of 40 months for local treatment and 25.3 months for whole-brain irradiation, although this difference may merely reflect selection bias [22]. Radiating the entire cranio–spinal axis prophylactically is not warranted. The potential for radiation toxicity and the fact that the survival of most patients with spinal disease is determined by control of cerebral tumor argue against using prophylactic spinal radiation. Spinal irradiation is reserved for patients with spinal disease, demonstrated radiographically or by CSF cytology.

Radiation therapy yields both clinical and radiographic response in AIDS-related primary CNS lymphoma, but the median survival in this population remains poor, ranging from 2 to 5.5 months [24]. Younger age and higher Karnofsky performance status at the time of treatment correlate with better outcome.

The complications of radiation therapy for primary CNS lymphoma are the same as those seen with radiation in any setting. The acute toxicities include headaches, nausea/vomiting and local skin reactions. Chronic complications include cognitive impairment and radiation necrosis of brain tissue. The risk of late neurologic sequelae increases with higher radiation dose and with age.

Chemotherapy

The use of chemotherapy for PCNSL is expanding [26–41] (Table 16.7). Patients receiving chemotherapy and radiotherapy live longer than those receiving radiotherapy alone [36, 41–44]. The median survival following combinations of radiation and chemotherapy has ranged from 16 to 44.5 months; the 5-year survival rate is 20–30%. Long-term follow-up in one group of 31 patients revealed frequent relapse (15 of 29 patients) and a high rate of late neurologic toxicity, especially in patients older than 60 years [32]. Patients with AIDS-associated disease, selected for good performance status, lack of active comorbid disease and high CD4 counts, may also benefit from chemotherapy [45].

Differences among chemotherapy regimens for primary CNS lymphoma are numerous: the agents used, the timing of administration (before or after radiotherapy) and the method of delivery (intravenous, intrathecal, or intra-arterial). The chemotherapeutic agents used are those with demonstrated efficacy against systemic lymphomas: corticosteroids, methotrexate, vinca alkaloids and alkylating agents. Corticosteroids lyse tumor cells and induce radiographic and clinical remission, but their effects are often brief. Methotrexate penetrates the intact blood brain barrier. It has demonstrated impressive efficacy against primary CNS lymphoma [46]. Although agents such as cyclophosphamide have been used with success against systemic lymphomas, they have not proven as efficacious against CNS disease, probably because of poor penetration of the blood–brain barrier.

Toxicity depends on the drug used. In general, acute systemic effects include mucositis, myelosuppression, nausea, vomiting and alopecia. Cognitive impairment is the feared late complication. Methotrexate administered after radiotherapy has been implicated in a higher incidence of this problem.

The rationale for administering chemotherapy before radiotherapy is twofold: (1) since radiotherapy often results in complete radiographic remission, administering it first prevents assessment of the effect of chemotherapy on measurable disease, and (2) the neurologic toxicity of some chemotherapeutic agents, including methotrexate, is less frequent and less severe when the drug is given prior to, rather than after, radiation. Intrathecal injection and intra-arterial delivery following blood–brain barrier disruption have been used to improve the penetration of these agents into the brain parenchyma [37].

Chemotherapy alone, with radiotherapy reserved for failure, has shown promise in uncontrolled trials [38–40]. The high initial response rates and the avoidance of radiation induced toxicity of this strategy warrant its further study.

Surgery

The role of surgery in the management of primary CNS lymphoma is limited. Surgical management is usually restricted to tumor biopsy for diagnosis. Rarely, shunting is needed for obstructive hydrocephalus. Craniotomy for tumor resection does not confer a survival benefit [6, 41].

Recurrent Disease

Relapse eventually occurs in almost all cases of primary CNS lymphoma, even despite newer and more aggressive multimodality treatment [37, 44]. Relapse can be intracerebral, spinal, ocular or even systemic. Approximately 90% of relapses occur within the brain [23]. Treatment is primarily palliative, although additional chemotherapy, usually with different agents, is often appropriate for younger patients, with good performance status.

Secondary CNS Lymphoma

Systemic lymphoma spreads to the CNS in about 10% of cases, most commonly in the setting of advanced or relapsing disease [47]. Certain sites of systemic disease are more likely to seed the CNS: the testis, bone marrow, bone, orbit, peripheral blood and paranasal sinuses. Propensity to spread to the CNS also varies with histologic subtype. Low-grade lymphomas rarely metastasize to the brain. Most metastases are diffuse large-cell or high-grade lymphomas. High-grade histology, elevated LDH levels, advanced disease and symptoms such as fever, sweats and weight loss are predictive of CNS relapse.

CNS involvement by secondary lymphoma is usually leptomeningeal; the parenchyma is rarely involved. The clinical presentation of secondary CNS lymphoma reflects the predominantly leptomeningeal disease. Symptoms and signs typically include headache, altered mental status, meningismus and cranial or spinal neuropathy.

Leptomeningeal involvement by lymphoma is best visualized with contrast-enhanced MRI. Given the common meningeal involvement in secondary CNS lymphoma, CSF cytology is more frequently positive than in primary CNS lymphoma. CSF may be positive in up to 70% of cases [47]. The combination of abnormal brain imaging and CSF findings in the setting of progressive or relapsing systemic lymphoma makes biopsy for diagnosis unnecessary.

Choice of therapy for secondary cerebral lymphoma must consider both the systemic and cerebral disease. Frequently, the combination of systemic and intrathecal chemotherapy is chosen. Whole-brain radiation and the drugs given for primary CNS lymphoma are also used frequently. Response to therapy, as reflected by clinical remission of CNS disease, is a favorable prognostic sign [47].

The prognosis for patients with secondary cerebral lymphoma is poor. Fewer than 15% survive for 1 year. Progressive systemic disease is the usual cause of death. Cerebral involvement is often used as an indicator of the extent of systemic disease. It rarely independently worsens the outcome.

Patients at high risk for CNS involvement, such as those with high-grade lymphomas, warrant prophylactic treatment. Intrathecal methotrexate (the agent most frequently used) reduces the incidence of cerebral metastasis [48].

Conclusion

Cerebral lymphoma, specifically PCNSL, is increasing in incidence. The role of surgery is usually limited to stereotactic biopsy for diagnosis. Multimodality therapy, combining chemotherapy and whole-brain radiotherapy, has improved the survival of patients with primary CNS lymphoma, but long-term relapse-free survival is still rare. Currently, a number of clinical trials are evaluating single-modality treatment protocols, in an effort to lengthen patient survival without incurring late neurologic toxicity.

Key Points

- *Cerebral metastases represent the most common intracranial tumour.*
- *The selection of a treatment plan for an individual patient must consider multiple factors.*
- *Radiotherapy is indicated for almost all patients with cerebral metastases, with the*

method of delivery, dose and regimen individual to each patient.

- *Lymphoma can occur as either metastatic to the brain or as primary CNS lymphoma.*
- *The majority of primary CNS lymphomas are monoclonal B-cell lymphomas.*

References

1. Johnson JD, Young B. Demographics of brain metastasis. Neurosurg Clin N Am 1996;7:337–44.
2. Posner JB, Chernik NL. Intracranial metastasis from systemic cancer. Advances in Neurology 1978;19: 579–92.
3. Posner JB. Neurologic complications of cancer. Contemporary Neurology series. Volume 45. Phildelphia: Davis, 1995.
4. Das A, Hochberg FH. Clinical presentation of intracranial metastases. Neurosurg Clin N Am 1996;7:377–91.
5. Schaefer PW, Budzik RF, Gonzalez GG. Imaging of cerebral metastases. Neurosurg Clin N Am 1996;7:393–423.
6. Murray K, Kun L, Cox J. Primary malignant lymphoma of the central nervous system: results of treatment of 11 cases and review of the literature. J Neurosurg 1987;65:600–7.
7. Patchell RA, Tibbs PA, Walsh JW et al. A randomized trial of surgery in the treatment of single metastases to the brain. NEJM 1990;322:494–500.
8. Chin L, Zee C, Apuzzo M. Special considerations in point stereotactic procedures. In: Apuzzo M, editor. Brain surgery. New York: Churchill Livingstone, 1993;414–25.
9. Cairncross JG, Kim J, Posner JB. Radiation therapy for brain metastases. Ann Neurol 1980;7:529–41.
10. Paleologos NA, Imperatu JP, Vick NA. Brain metastasis: effects of radiotherapy on longterm survivors. Neurology 1991;41(Suppl. 1):129.
11. Alexander E III, Moriarity TM, Davis RB, Wen PY, Fine HA, Black PM et al. Stereotactic radiosurgery for the definitive nininvasive treatment of brain metastases. J Natl Cancer Institute 1995;87:34–40.
12. Lang FF, Sawaya R. Surgical management of cerebral metastases. Neurosurg Clin N Am 1996;7:459–84.
13. Patchell RA, Tibbs PA, Regine WF, Dempsey RJ, Mohiuddin M, Kryscio RJ et al. Postoperative radiotherapy in the treatment of single metastases to the brain: a randomized trial. JAMA 1998;280:1485–9.
14. Sundaresan N, Sachdev VP, DiGiacinto GV, Hughes JEO. Reoperation for brain metastases. J Clin Oncol 1988;6:1625–9.
15. Cooper JS, Steinfeld AD, Lerch IA. Cerebral metastases: value of reirradiation in selected patients. Radiology 1990;174:883–5.
16. Hochberg FH, Miller DC. Primary central nervous system lymphoma. J Neurosurg 1988;68:835–53.
17. Corn BW, Marcus SM, Topham A et al. Will primary central nervous system lymphoma be the most frequent brain tumor diagnosed in the year 2000? Cancer 1997;79:2409–13.
18. Miller DC, Hochberg FH, Harris NL et al. Pathology with clinical correlations of primary central nervous system non-Hodgkin's lymphoma: the Massachusetts General Hospital experience 1958–1989. Cancer 1994;74: 1383–97.
19. Antoniri A, De Rossi G, Ammassari A. Value of combined approach with thallium-201 single-photon emission computed tomography and Epstein–Barr virus DNA polymerase chain reaction in CSF for the diagnosis of AIDS-related primary CNS lymphoma. J Clin Onc 1999;17:554–60.
20. DeAngelis LM. Current management of primary central nervous system lymphoma. Oncology 1995;9:63–71.
21. Remick SC, Diamond C, Migliozzi JA et al. Primary central nervous system lymphoma in patients with and without the acquired immune deficiency syndrome: a retrospective analysis and review of the literature. Medicine 1990;69:345–60.
22. Leibel SA, Sheline GE. Radiation therapy for neoplasms of the brain. J Neurosurg 1987;66:1–22.
23. Nelson DF, Martz KL, Bonner H et al. Non-Hodgkin's lymphoma of the brain: can high dose, large volume radiation therapy improve survival? Report on a prospective trial by the Radiation Therapy Oncology Group (RTOG): RTOG 8315. Int J Radiat Oncol Biol Phys 1992;23:9–17.
24. Goldstein JD, Dickson DW, Moser FG et al. Primary central nervous system lymphoma in acquired immune deficiency syndrome: a clinical and pathologic study with results of treatment with radiation. Cancer 1991;67:2756–65.
25. Bessell EM, Punt J, Firth J et al. Primary Non-Hodgkin's lymphoma of the central nervous system: Phase II study of chemotherapy (BVAM) prior to radiotherapy. Clin Oncol 1991;3:193–8.
26. Liang BC, Grant R, Junck L et al. Primary central nervous system lymphoma: treatment with multiagent systemic and intrathecal chemotherapy with radiation therapy. Int J Oncol 1993;3:1001–4.
27. LaChanceDH, Brizel DM, Gockerman JP et al. Cyclophosphamide, doxorubicin, vincristine, and prednisone for primary central nervous system lymphoma: short duration response and multifocal intracerebral recurrence preceding radiotherapy. Neurology 1994;44:1721–7.
28. Glass J, Gruber ML, Cher L, et al. Preirradiation methotrexate chemotherapy of primary central nervous system lymphoma: long term outcome. J Neurosurg 1994;81:188–95.
29. Glass J, Shustik C, Hochberg FH, et al. Therapy of primary central nervous system lymphoma with pre-irradiation methotrexate, cyclophosphamide, doxorubicin, vincristine, and dexamethasone (MCHOD). J Neurooncol 1996;30:257–65.
30. Schultz C, Scott C, Sherman W, et al. Preirradiation chemotherapy with cyclophosphamide, doxorubicin, vincristine, and dexamethasone for primary CNS lymphomas: intial report of radiation therapy oncology group protocol 88–06. J Clin Onc 1996;14:556–64.
31. Brada M, Hjiyiannakis D, Hines F, et al. Short intensive primary chemotherapy and radiotherapy in sporadic primary CNS lymphoma (PCL). Int J Radiat Oncol Biol Phys 1998;40:1157–62.
32. Abrey LE, DeAngelis LM, Yahalom J. Long-term survival in primary CNS lymphoma. J Clin Onc 1998;16: 859–63.

33. Hiraga S, Arita N, Ohnishi T, et al. Rapid infusion of high-dose methotrexate resulting in enhanced penetration into cerebrospinal fluid and intensified tumor response in primary central nervous system lymphomas. J Neurosurg 1999;91:221–30.
34. Shibamoto Y, Tsutsui K, Dodo Y, et al. Improved survival rate in primary intracranial lymphoma treated by high-dose radiation and systemic vincristine-doxorubicin-cyclophosphamide-prednisolone chemotherapy. Cancer 1990;65:1907–12.
35. Chamberlain MC, Levin VA. Primary central nervous system lymphoma: a role for adjuvant chemotherapy. J Neuro-oncol 1992;14:271–5.
36. Rosenthal MA, Sheridan WP, Green MD et al. Primary cerebral lymphoma: an argument for the use of adjunctive systemic chemotherapy. Aust N Z J Surg 1993;63:30–2.
37. Neuwelt EA, Goldman DL, Dahlborg SA et al. Primary CNS lymphoma treated with osmotic blood-brain barrier disruption: prolonged survival and preservation of cognitive function. J Clin Onc 1991;9:1580–90.
38. Cher L, Glass J, Harsh GR et al. Therapy of primary CNS lymphoma with methotrexate-based chemotherapy and deferred radiotherapy: preliminary results. Neurology 196;46:1757–9.
39. Freilich RJ, Delattre JY, Monjour A et al. Chemotherapy without radiation mtherapy as initial treatment for primary CNS lymphoma in older patients. Neurology 1996;46:435–9.
40. Sandor V, Stark-Vancs V, Pearson D et al. Phase II trial of chemotherapy alone for primary CNS and intraocular lymphoma. J Clin Oncol 1998;16:3000–6.
41. Pollack IF, Lunsford LD, Flickinger JC et al:. Prognostic factors in the diagnosis and treatment of primary central nervous system lymphoma. Cancer 1989;63: 939–47.
42. Brada M, Dearnaley D, Horwich A et al. Management of primary cerebral lymphoma with initial chemotherapy: preliminary results and comparison with patients treated with radiotherapy alone. Int J Radiat Oncol Biol Phys 1990;18:787–92.
43. Chamberlain MC, Levin VA. Adjuvant chemotherapy for primary lymphoma of the central nervous systyem. Arch Neurol 1990;97:1113–6.
44. DeAngelis LM, Yahalom J, Thaler H et al. Combined modality therapy for primary CNs lymphoma. J Clin Onc 1992;10:635–43.
45. Chamberlain MC. Long survival in patients with acquired immune deficiency syndrome related primary central nervous system lymphoma. Cancer 1994;73: 1728–30.
46. Blay J-Y, Conroy T, Chevreau C et al. High-dose methotrexate for the treatment of primary cerebral lymphomas: an analysis of survival and late neurologic toxicity in a retrospective series. J Clin Onc 1998;16:864–71.
47. Liang RH S, Woo EKW, Yu Y et al. Central nervous system involvement in non-Hodgkin's lymphoma. Eur J Clin Onc 1989;25:703–10.
48. Perez-Soler R, Smith TL, Cabanillas F. Central nervous system prophylaxis with combined intravenous and intrathecal methotrexate in diffuse lymphoma of aggressive histologic type. Cancer 1986;57:971–7.

V
Vascular

17

Cerebral Blood Flow: Physiology and Measurement Techniques

Jonathan A. Friedman, Vini G. Khurana, Robert E. Anderson and Fredric B. Meyer

Summary

Cerebral blood flow (CBF) physiology is important to neurosurgeons who manage patients with cerebrovascular disease. The techniques to measure CBF and mathematical methods to calculate CBF have evolved over the past 50 years. These techniques have been refined to enable perioperative and intraoperative measurement of cerebral blood flow qualitatively and quantitatively. Some of the measurement techniques discussed in this chapter include PET, EEG, TCD, Xenon and thermal fusion.

Introduction

Under physiologic conditions, the brain employs aerobic metabolism exclusively for energy production. Accordingly, the brain is critically dependent on the near continuous delivery of oxygen and glucose to sustain cellular energy production. Although the brain accounts for only 2% of total body weight, it requires 20% of the cardiac output, 20% of inspired molecular oxygen at rest and consumes the liver's entire production of glucose in the fasting state.

Depending on the measurement technique, resting CBF in the awake patient is approximately 50–55 ml/100 g brain tissue/min. As CBF decreases, neuronal dysfunction and injury occur. At levels of 16–18 ml/100 g/min, cortical electrical function fails, as evidenced by attenuation in electroencephalographic and somatosensory evoked potential recordings. At levels of 10–12 ml/100 g/min or less, rapid changes in intracellular and extracellular ion concentrations occur, along with the development of intracellular acidosis. Persistence of CBF at levels below this threshold of maintaining ionic balance will result in membrane disruption, irreversible neuronal injury and cell death.

Understanding cerebral blood flow physiology is of great importance to neurosurgeons engaged in the management of patients with cerebrovascular disease. Over the past 50 years, techniques to measure CBF and mathematical methods to calculate CBF have evolved substantially. Intraoperative measurement of cerebral blood flow, both qualitatively and quantitatively, has contributed to improved outcomes from cerebrovascular procedures. In patients undergoing carotid endarterectomy, the use of intraoperative CBF measurements has proven to be effective in reducing operative morbidity. Intraoperative CBF monitoring has also been a useful adjunct in the treatment of complex intracranial aneurysms and arteriovenous malformations, particularly when temporary or permanent vessel occlusion is employed.

Cerebral Blood Flow Physiology

Fundamental Concepts

In the brain, CBF varies directly with cerebral perfusion pressure (CPP; defined as the difference between mean arterial pressure and intracranial pressure) and inversely with cerebrovascular resistance (which is the sum of the resistance to flow generated by the vasculature, particularly at the level of the small pial arteries and penetrating pre-capillary arterioles). In general, the contribution of any given cerebral vessel to overall CBF is defined by factors such as its radius and length, and the viscosity and pressure of blood flowing through it.

The average rate of blood flow in the brain is approximately 50–55 ml/100 g/min. In pathological states, this global flow rate may decrease, leading to rate-dependent neurological manifestations. The link between flow rate and electrophysiological and clinical findings underlies the concept of "flow thresholds". Remarkably, clinical evidence for a neurological deficit may not appear until average flow has fallen to 50% or below of normal levels (i.e. to approximately 25–30 ml/100 g/min). At this threshold, global neurological impairment is noted and, below this, the margin between reversible and irreversible ischemic damage becomes narrow. Brain "electrical failure" begins at rates of about 16–18 ml/100 g/min, while cytotoxic edema from failure of ionic pumps, particularly Na^+K^+ATPases, develops at 10–12 ml/100 g/min. Finally, metabolic failure with gross disturbance of cellular energy homeostasis occur at rates of less than 10 ml/100 g/min.

In 1783, Alexander Monro proposed that the incompressibility of the cranial vault mandated a relatively constant intracranial blood volume at all times – a notion supported by George Kellie at the turn of the century. However, this proposal was later challenged by Sir George Burrows, who postulated that any variation in the volume of one of the three principal intracranial contents, namely brain parenchyma (1200–1600 ml), blood (100–150 ml) and cerebrospinal fluid (CSF, 100–150 ml), was accompanied by a compensatory change in the volume of the other two. In fact, this latter notion forms the basis of the relationship between intracranial pressure and cerebral blood volume (CBV). This pressure–volume relationship implies that in order to maintain a constant intracranial pressure in the face of rising CSF volume, blood volume must fall and when this can no longer occur, the brain will herniate caudally. Importantly, as intracranial pressure rises there is a fall in CBF in association with reduced CBV, most likely from structural compression of the vasculature.

Nitric Oxide

Vascular nitric oxide (NO) plays a key role in the regulation of blood pressure and tissue perfusion. There is considerable evidence supporting the presence of NO-mediated signaling in cerebral arteries, where it contributes particularly to the maintenance of basal CBF. Although a wide variety of modulators of cerebral vasomotor function exist in addition to NO (e.g. endogenous peptides such as bradykinin and endothelins; and molecules related to the enzymatic activity of cyclooxygenase, hemeoxygenase, and superoxide dismutase), the actions of most of these are linked in one way or another to NO itself [1]. Therefore, an understanding of NO-mediated signalling is essential to the study of cerebrovascular physiology and pathophysiology.

Vascular NO signal transduction involves the following: (1) a principal mediator, i.e. molecular NO; (2) a well defined biosynthetic apparatus for NO, i.e. the enzyme nitric oxide synthase (NOS); (3) and an effector pathway and cellular target, namely the NO-activated enzyme guanylate cyclase and the second messenger molecule cyclic 3'5'-guanosine monophosphate (cGMP), located within vascular smooth muscle cells (Figs 17.1 and 17.2).

Nitric Oxide

Endogenous production of oxides of nitrogen by mammals was first suggested by Mitchell and colleagues in 1916 [2]. However, it was not until

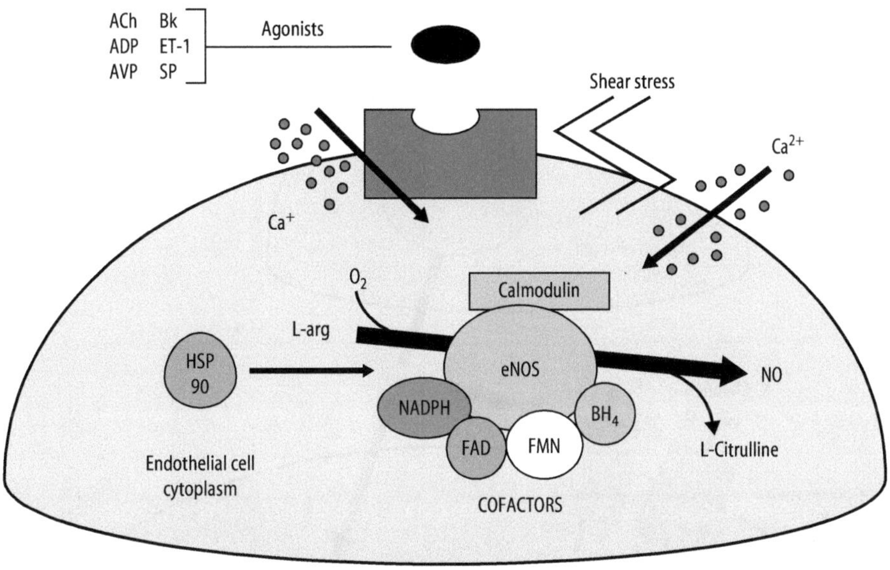

Fig. 17.1. Biosynthesis of nitric oxide. The (constitutive) endothelial isoform of NOS is activated by the influx of calcium induced by shear stress or the binding of agonists to their receptors on the surfaces of endothelial cells. Endothelial NOS uses molecular oxygen and several cofactors to convert the amino acid L-arginine to NO, forming L-citrulline as a by-product. The molecular chaperone HSP90 is known to facilitate this reaction. Abbreviations for Figs 17.1 and 17.2 (see text for cofactor abbreviations): Ach, acetylcholine; ADP, adenosine diphosphate; AVP, arginine vasopressin; BK, bradykinin; cGMP, cyclic-3'5'-guanosine monophosphate; eNOS, endothelial nitric oxide synthase; ET-1, endothelin-1; GC, guanylate cyclase; GTP, guanosine triphosphate; HSP90, heat shock protein 90; L-arg, L-arginine; MLC, myosin light-chains; NO, nitric oxide; PKG, protein kinase G; SP, substance P.

1980 that evidence for an endothelium-derived substance required for relaxation of blood vessels first emerged [3]. Seven years later, Palmer and colleagues and Ignarro and colleagues independently proposed that this substance, initially referred to as Endothelium-Derived Relaxing Factor (EDRF), was in fact NO – a short-lived, highly diffusible molecule whose biosynthesis, rapid diffusion and stimulation of guanylate cyclase are now known to underlie a spectrum of physiological responses in the body [4,5]. In the cerebrovascular system, NO can be synthesized by endothelial cells, smooth muscle cells and adventitial neurons (nervi vasorum), although activated macrophages, neutrophils, astrocytes and adventitial fibroblasts may also participate in NO biosynthesis under certain conditions (Fig. 17.3). It is important to note that oxyhemoglobin and oxygen-derived free radicals (both implicated in the pathogenesis of post-subarachnoid hemorrhage cerebral vasospasm) can chemically react with NO to inactivate it, while nitrovasodilators, such as glyceryl trinitrate, sodium nitroprusside and amyl nitrite, are "nitrergic" in that they result in the release of NO, either directly or indirectly [1].

Nitric Oxide Synthase

The enzyme responsible for the biosynthesis of NO is the heme-containing protein, NOS (Fig. 17.1). The substrate for this enzyme, L-arginine, can be obtained from the diet or from intracellular protein degradation or endogenous synthesis involving the urea cycle. Molecular oxygen is also required by NOS to produce NO, as are calmodulin and four important cofactors: protonated nicotine adenine dinucleotide phosphate (NADPH), tetrahydrobiopterin (BH4), flavin mononucleotide (FMN) and flavin adenine dinucleotide (FAD). Molecular oxygen is incorporated into the two products of this reaction – NO and L-citrulline. Further work has shown that the molecular chaperone heat shock protein 90 (HSP90) can modulate the activity of NOS in peripheral endothelial cells, where it is rapidly recruited to the NOS complex

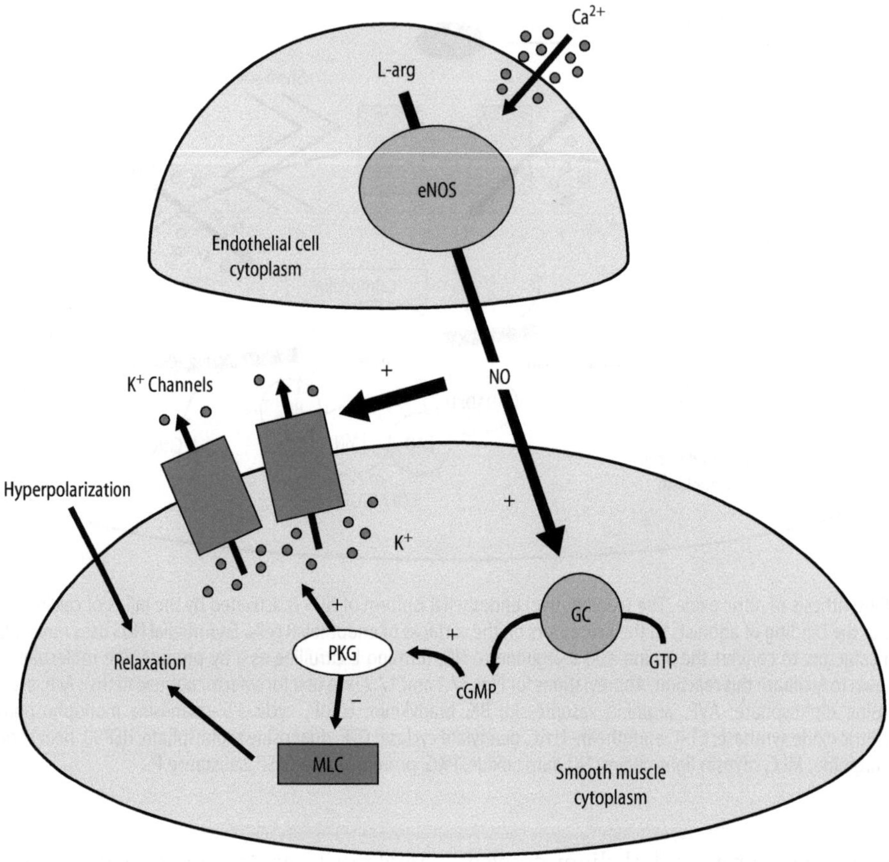

Fig. 17.2. Diffusion and action of nitric oxide. Following its biosynthesis, NO rapidly diffuses to neighbouring cells. In vascular smooth muscle cells, NO activates guanylate cyclase which converts GTP to cGMP, thereby activating protein kinase G. This latter enzyme facilitates vasorelaxation both by facilitating the dephosphorylation of myosin light-chains and activating cell membrane potassium channels. Alternatively, NO can activate potassium channels directly, leading to membrane hyperpolarization and muscle relaxation. See Fig. 17.1 for abbreviations.

by agonists or shear stress, or both (Fig. 17.1). In this light, important functional and spatial associations between NOS and HSP90 have recently been demonstrated in the cerebral vasculature.

Three isoforms of NOS have now been identified, and their cDNAs isolated and sequenced. The nomenclature for any given isoform varies according to: (1) its order of discovery and characterization (i.e. Types I–III); (2) whether it is expressed by the cell type basally (i.e. at rest; "constitutive" cNOS) or inducibly under certain conditions (i.e. "inducible" iNOS); and (3) its tissue localization (i.e. endothelial eNOS vs smooth muscle inducible iNOS vs neuronal nNOS). For the purposes of this chapter, however, the last of these three nomenclatures will be used. Although these isoenzymes share a similar overall catalytic scheme as described above (Fig. 17.1), there are some important differences. First, eNOS and nNOS are constitutively active, unlike iNOS, whose expression and activity are induced (e.g. by bacterial lipopolysaccharide or proinflammatory cytokines such as interleukin-10). Second, although all three isoforms bind calmodulin, iNOS does not require the presence of intracellular calcium and is not modulated by it. Third, unlike the other two isoforms, iNOS, once activated, will continuously produce NO for the remainder of its enzymatic life – a feature likely to be important in the antimicrobial-cytotoxic role of NO

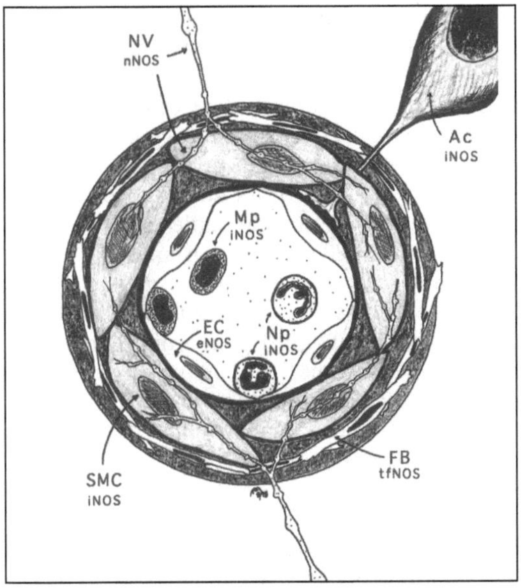

Fig. 17.3. Cross-section of a cerebral blood vessel. NO can be synthesized by the constitutive NOS isoforms present in endothelial cells (EC; eNOS) and (perivascular) nervi vasorum (NV; nNOS). In pathological conditions, the biosynthesis of NO by the inducible isoform of NOS (iNOS) can occur in smooth muscle cells (SMC), astrocytes (Ac) and activated macrophages (Mp) and neutrophils (Np). Finally, NOS isoforms such as eNOS may be transferred (tf) into adventitial fibroblasts (FB) under experimental conditions. See Fig. 17.1 for abbreviations.

from macrophage iNOS and in the pathogenesis of toxic-septic shock. Fourth, the amount of iNOS expression not only varies between different cell types, but may also vary between similar cell types, e.g. microvascular vs macrovascular endothelial cells. Last, although beyond the scope of this review, it should be noted that knockout (gene-deleted) mice have been generated for the NOS isoforms in order to study their individual roles and the effects of their targeted deletions on physiological functions (including regulation of cerebroarterial tone) in intact animals.

Guanylate Cyclase, cGMP and Vascular Smooth Muscle

It is known that, once synthesized, gaseous NO readily diffuses in a heterotopic manner for "cellular" distances limited by its short half-life. A recent study using a photon counting camera reported actual visualization of NO release from electrically stimulated neurons [6]. Interestingly, NO was found to be released along the entire lengths of the neurons studied, confirming its ability to affect putative target cells in the three-dimensional space surrounding all parts of the releasing cell. In the vascular system, NO is released constitutively from endothelial cells and nervi vasorum, exerting its relaxant effect on neighbouring smooth muscle cells. Here, the principal molecular target for NO is the enzyme guanylate cyclase which, when activated by NO, converts guanosine triphosphate (GTP) into cGMP. This so-called second messenger facilitates smooth muscle relaxation through hyperpolarization of the sarcolemma, involving activation of potassium channels and/or closure of voltage-dependent calcium channels, both of which are known to be modulated by NO in a variety of cell types. Although several mechanisms have been proposed to explain cGMP-evoked relaxation, the most likely mechanism may involve activation of cGMP-dependent protein kinase (protein kinase G; G-kinase; PKG), which leads to dephosphorylation of myosin light-chains (MLC) as well as activation of calcium- and voltage-dependent potassium channels in several cell types (Fig. 17.2). It should be noted that besides activating guanylate cyclase, NO can directly (i.e. independently of cGMP) modulate a variety of proteins, including potassium channels – an event which, when occurring in smooth muscle, leads to hyperpolarization and relaxation (Fig. 17.2).

Nitric Oxide in the Cerebral Vasculature

Evidence for the presence of a NO-mediated signalling in the cerebral vasculature has come from several lines of study. First, using antibodies raised against purified NOS, Bredt and colleagues have shown that the enzyme is, among other sites in the rat brain, localized to the endothelial layer of large cerebral blood vessels and nerve fibers in their adventitia; the origin of these perivascular "nitrergic" nerve fibers is the pterygo/sphenopalatine ganglion [7]. While NOS has not been demonstrated histologically in resting vascular smooth muscle cells, treatment with endotoxin and proinflammatory cytokines has been shown to induce its expression in these cells, including those found in the cerebral vasculature. Further, other immunohistochemical studies have also detected NOS immunoreactivity in cerebral microvessels, while Pluta and colleagues have found a marked loss of nNOS immunoreactivity in vasospastic cerebral arteries [8]. Second, several pharmacological studies using inhibitors of NOS, such as L-NMMA, have reported endothelium-dependent contractions to these agents in resting cerebral blood vessels – effects reversed by the NOS substrate L-arginine [9,10]. Endothelium-independent contractions to L-NMMA have also been observed in cerebral blood vessels, indicating that the inhibition of non-endothelial sources of NOS, i.e. constitutive in perivascular nerve fibers or induced in vascular smooth muscle, may also be involved. Third, physiological studies involving transmural electrical nerve stimulation of isolated cerebral arteries have also shown that vasorelaxation produced by this means is abolished by L-NMMA, hemoglobin and extracellular calcium depletion – findings consistent with the active presence of NOS here [11]. Last, recent advances in molecular biology have facilitated a greater understanding of the cerebrovascular NO system through, on the one hand, selective NOS isoform deletions in otherwise intact animals and, on the other hand, transgenic overexpression of recombinant NOS isoforms in hosts, using genetically engineered viral vectors [12]. In this light, Khurana and colleagues have recently carried out the first genetic modification of intact human cerebral arteries, demonstrating the functional benefit of adenovirus-mediated overexpression of eNOS in these vessels [13]. Taken together, these findings not only unequivocally establish the presence of a NO system in the cerebral vasculature, but also indicate that NO is a prime active modulator of CBF.

Cerebral Autoregulation

From a functional perspective, the term cerebral autoregulation refers to the ability of cerebral arteries to maintain CBF (and therefore brain perfusion) at a relatively constant level despite fluctuations in CPP. From a physical perspective, autoregulation involves relatively rapid changes in the caliber of cerebral resistance vessels, principally the pre-capillary arterioles, in response to changes in transmural pressure as CPP varies. As a result of this phenomenon, CBF is relatively independent of CPP between the physiological limits of autoregulation, typically taken to be perfusion pressures of 50–60 mmHg for the lower limit and 150–160 mmHg for the upper. In normal subjects, CPP varies directly with MAP (due to constant ICP), which in turn varies directly with systolic blood pressure. Across the autoregulatory range of approximately 100 mmHg, in order to maintain a relatively constant CBF, cerebral arteries constrict as CPP rises and dilate as CPP falls. As a result, CPP and CBV are inversely related through this phenomenon.

The phenomenon of cerebral autoregulation, first reported in feline pial vessels observed through a cranial window by Fog in the 1930s, has undoubtedly evolved to preserve cerebral homeostasis and protect against the development of cerebral ischemia and edema [14]. Its precise mechanism, however, is not known. It is likely that the mechanism includes intrinsic changes in vascular smooth muscle tone (myogenic hypothesis) modulated by the release of a variety of vasoactive substances from the endothelium (endothelial hypothesis) and periadventitial nerves (neurogenic hypothesis) in response to changes in transmural pressure. A "metabolic" or "humoral" hypothesis has also been proposed to aid in the explanation of cerebral autoregulation; however, for several reasons, is better suited to a description of metabolic regulation of cerebral vasomotor function rather than cerebral autoregulation, which is a pressure-dependent response. First, as measured by microdialysis, the extracellular and perivascular concentrations of H^+ and K^+ (key mediators in metabolic vasoregulation) normally do not change in response to CPP alterations in the autoregulatory range. Second, as reported in studies measuring changes in cerebroarterial diameter or tone in response to variations in perfusion or transmural pressure, autoregulation begins within a few seconds of the pressure change, and is typically complete within 15–30 s. Although not precluding their involvement in this process, this relatively rapid time course suggests that metabolic factors are less likely to be involved. Third, it has been reported that the brain's interstitial concentration of adenosine (another key mediator in the metabolic hypothesis) may be increased at the lower limit of autoregulation. However, despite the possibility of adenosine contributing to autoregulation at this extreme, its concentrations are known not to vary across the bulk of the autoregulatory range. Fourth, the autoregulatory response has been observed in isolated, perfused vessels in vitro (i.e. not subject to alterations in neuroglial metabolism), providing further evidence against a metabolic hypothesis. Taken together, these findings suggest that metabolic factors, despite being capable of strong regulation of cerebral vasomotor function, are unlikely to play a major role in autoregulation.

In 1902, Bayliss reported direct contraction and relaxation of canine hindlimb arteries in response to increase and decrease, respectively, of intravascular pressure [15]. This phenomenon, referred to as the "Bayliss effect", was attributed to intrinsic properties of vascular smooth muscle cells, and formed the basis of the "myogenic hypothesis" of autoregulation. Importantly, contraction occurs in response to an increase in transmural pressure rather than intraluminal pressure alone and, as such, can be thought of as a vascular "stretch response". The single most important piece of evidence supporting the myogenic hypothesis is the presence of stretch-activated cation channels (SACCs) in myocytes. These channels have been shown to be present in a wide variety of cells, including all three types of muscle cells, in addition to epithelial and endothelial cells. Experimentally, SACCs are studied by the patch clamp technique, their minute currents recorded via a cell-attached microelectrode following their gentle suction-induced activation. The characteristic and reproducible pattern of ionic conductance through these channels precludes their currents from being attributable to passive "leak", instead suggesting that they are specific ionic responses to cell stretch. It has been postulated that suction may stress the cytoskeleton, thereby activating SACCs by a relatively rapid but as yet undetermined mechanism. In smooth muscle cells, these channels are non-selective and readily permeable to monovalent cations such as Na+ and K+ and divalent cations such as Ca2+. SACC activation is associated with an influx of cations, leading to cell membrane depolarization. This, in turn, results in the opening of membrane voltage-gated calcium channels (VGCCs), and the heightened influx of Ca2+ into the smooth muscle cell facilitates "calcium-induced calcium release" from the sarcoplasmic reticulum; the end result is smooth muscle contraction. Davis and colleagues have recorded SACC activity in vascular smooth muscle cells, and have shown that it is sufficient to cause contraction, even in the presence of nifedipine (a dihydropyridine inhibitor of VGCCs), suggesting that the non-specific Ca2+ influx through SACCs is adequate to trigger sarcoplasmic Ca2+ release [16]. That the myogenic response is abolished in Ca2+-free media to which Ca2+ buffer has been added provides further evidence for the pivotal role of Ca2+ in its mediation. However, as suggested by the work of Nelson and colleagues, it is likely that the extent of smooth muscle contraction is eventually limited by membrane hyperpolarization following Ca2+-induced activation of Ca2+-dependent K+ (KCa) channels [17]. Finally, it should be noted that there is increasing evidence that the myogenic response, classically thought of as the principal basis of cerebral autoregulation and an intrinsic property of vascular myocytes, is in fact modulated by endothelium-derived vasoactive substances such as nitric oxide, prostacyclin, endothelin-1 and thromboxane A2, as well as perivascular nerve-derived vasoactive substances, including acetylcholine, nitric oxide, calcitonin gene-related peptide (CGRP), norepinephrine, serotonin, bradykinin and substance P.

Pre-operative Assessment

Xenon Computed Tomography

Xenon-enhanced computed tomography (Xe-CT) measurements of CBF have been in clinical use for over a decade and, more recently, have become easier and safer to use [18]. The technique is based on the radiodensity of xenon and its ability to freely cross the blood–brain barrier. CT scanning of the brain is performed before and during a short period of inhalation of 33% xenon gas. CBF is then calculated based on the relative density of areas of interest on the CT scan. The technique has been shown to have an accuracy of greater than 90%.

Xe-CT is used clinically to assess cerebrovascular reserve in occlusive cerebrovascular disease, tolerance of trial balloon occlusion and focal ischemia due to vasospasm after subarachnoid hemorrhage. The most significant disadvantage of the technique is the altered sensorium associated with inhaled xenon at this concentration. While earlier concerns of apnea and oversedation have largely abated, some patients cannot tolerate the sensation of motion and dysphoria associated with xenon inhalation. Patients undergoing Xe-CT examination should be given supplemental oxygen and have continuous monitoring of oxygen saturation.

Single Photon Emission Computed Tomography

Single photon emission computed tomography (SPECT) is the most commonly employed nuclear medicine technique in use for imaging the brain. The SPECT assessment of CBF is based on the rapid diffusion of 99Tc-ECD across the blood–brain barrier, where it is rapidly hydrolyzed from a highly lipophilic form to a water-soluble acid. The water-soluble form is too polar to diffuse rapidly out of the intracellular compartment of the brain. Imaging is then performed with a conventional planar gamma camera, which is rotated at various angles about the head. A typical image might involve acquisition of 60–120 planar images over a 360° rotation of the gamma camera. Frequently, the acquired SPECT scan is then co-registered with MRI of the same patient to provide anatomic correlation to the functional image provided by the SPECT. In two large prospective studies of ischemic stroke, SPECT had a sensitivity of 61–74% and a specificity of 88–98% [19]. The sensitivity is somewhat higher for lacunar strokes.

The central clinical role of SPECT examination is to assess cerebrovascular reserve, both in the setting of cerebro-occlusive disease and prior to planned sacrifice of a major cerebral artery (Fig. 17.4). In some institutions, SPECT is used to diagnose and/or confirm brain death in patients in whom the neurologic examination is unreliable, such as the setting of barbiturate coma. SPECT is also used at many institutions in the evaluation of epilepsy: in the epilepsy-monitoring unit, 99Tc-ECD is injected during the ictal phase, within 40 s of onset of seizure activity. Subsequent SPECT examination demonstrates a pattern of markedly increased cerebral blood flow in the epileptogenic region. In temporal lobe epilepsy, the increased blood flow is seen within the mesial structures of the temporal lobe and often within the anterolateral neocortex. SPECT has been of substantial experimental use for the study of stroke, subarachnoid hemorrhage, arteriovenous malformations, head injury and vascular dementias. However, the clinical utility of the study for these disorders has thus far been limited.

Positron Emission Tomography

Positron emission tomography (PET) uses 15O-labeled carbon dioxide, carbon monoxide and oxygen to obtain quantitative maps of CBF, cerebral blood volume, oxygen extraction fraction and cerebral metabolic rate. PET has been used extensively in experimental studies of stroke, to define the ischemic penumbra and the effects of early reperfusion/hyperperfusion. Clinical uses are less common. Recently, a study of patients with carotid occlusion demonstrated that patients with high oxygen extraction fractions as determined by PET were at significantly higher risk of future ipsilateral stroke [20]. This may potentially identify a subset of patients who would benefit from extracranial–intracranial bypass surgery, and could imply an increased clinical role for PET scanning in the future.

Magnetic Resonance Imaging

Techniques to measure CBF using phase-contrast cine magnetic resonance imaging remain largely experimental. The technique has been used to quantify blood flow in each major cerebral artery and within the circle of Willis. The technique has also been used to document decreased regional CBF – the "steal phenomenon" – in normal brain parenchyma adjacent to arteriovenous malformations. Magnetic resonance techniques of measuring CBF require meticulous attention to technical details to obtain accurate data. As the technique is further refined, it may gain increasing acceptance in the clinical setting.

Trial Balloon Occlusion

Some surgical or endovascular interventions carry a relatively high likelihood of carotid

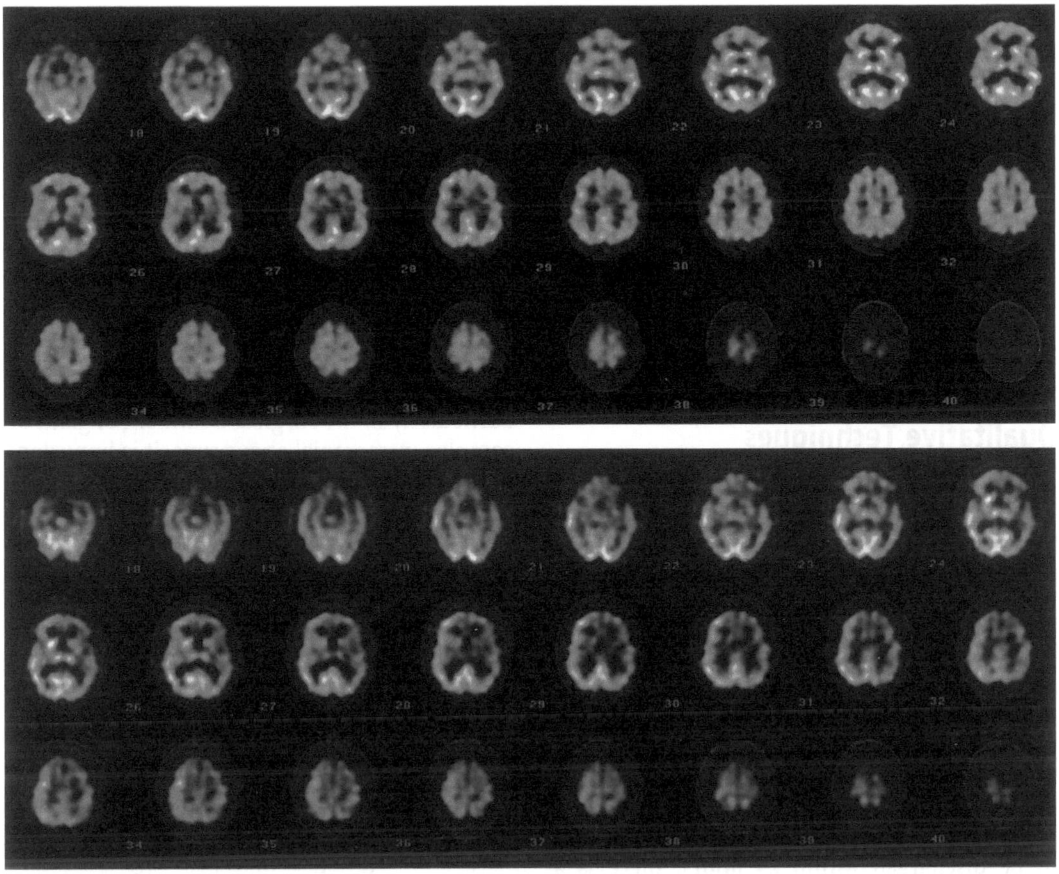

Fig. 17.4. Baseline SPECT imaging in a patient with bilateral carotid occlusions and symptomatic left hemispheric ischemic spells, demonstrating normal and symmetric uptake bilaterally. SPECT imaging in the same patient after acetazolamide administration, demonstrating decreased left hemispheric uptake. The patient was treated with left-sided STA–MCA bypass surgery. SPECT, single photon emission computed tomography; STA, superficial temporal artery; MCA, middle cerebral artery.

sacrifice, such as the repair of giant aneurysms of the cavernous internal carotid artery. In these instances, pre-operative trial balloon occlusion is a useful qualitative tool in assessment of adequacy of collateral cerebral blood flow. We perform trial balloon occlusion in the interventional neuroradiology suite, according to the following protocol: A baseline activated clotting time (ACT) is determined, and the patient receives 5,000–8,000 units of intravenously administered heparin. Serial ACTs are obtained throughout the procedure, and additional heparin is given as needed to maintain the ACT approximately two-and-a-half times the baseline value. A 5.0 French double lumen balloon catheter is placed in the cervical segment of the internal carotid artery and slowly inflated until the artery is occluded. Occlusion is maintained for 30 minutes, during which time the patient is closely monitored for any change in neurologic function. During the period of trial occlusion, the patient's blood pressure is lowered pharmacologically to decrease the mean arterial pressure 20 mmHg from baseline. The collateral circulation through the circle of Willis to the vascular territory to be occluded is assessed during the period of balloon occlusion by obtaining digital subtraction angiograms of the contralateral carotid artery, the ipsilateral external carotid artery and the dominant vertebral artery. Pre- and post-balloon occlusion radioactive xenon CBF measurements are also obtained (see details below in section on 133Xe intraoperative monitoring). In addition, 99Tc-ECD is injected intravenously during the period of trial occlusion, and a cerebral perfusion SPECT scan is obtained after the patient leaves the angiography suite. Development of a neurological deficit, a CBF decline of approximately 30%, or a CBF measurement of less than 25 ml/100 g/min is considered a failed trial balloon occlusion.

Intraoperative Assessment

Qualitative Techniques

Neurologic Exam

The neurologic exam is a sensitive, qualitative technique to assess adequacy of cerebral blood flow during cerebrovascular procedures. The primary limitation is that the patient must be awake during the procedure. For carotid endarterectomy, this generally poses no major difficulties. Using a cervical ganglion block, the procedure is performed with ongoing neurologic and language examination. Since an awake carotid endarterectomy obviates the need for EEG monitoring and allows the patient to be discharged within 24 hours, there is a clear benefit in cost. Furthermore, it is likely that cardiac complications are reduced using regional anesthesia as compared to general anesthesia for carotid endarterectomy. Some patients, however, will not tolerate undergoing an awake procedure.

Electroencephalography and Somatosensory Evoked Potentials

Electroencephalography (EEG) is an indirect, qualitative measurement of cerebral blood flow in patients undergoing cerebrovascular surgery. EEG is a highly sensitive marker of cerebral blood flow, with a strong correlation between alterations in the EEG and diminished cerebral blood flow. The technique has become commonplace for monitoring CBF in patients undergoing carotid endarterectomy. For intracranial procedures, surface EEG strips can be used. Techniques for intraoperative cerebral protection, such as barbiturate administration or hypothermia, may limit the sensitivity of EEG for the detection of cerebral ischemia, yet the EEG is useful in titration of the protective effect when burst suppression is desired. Measurement of somatosensory evoked potentials is another neurophysiologic monitoring technique currently used by some centers during extracranial vascular surgery. Of note is that SSEP monitoring may be valuable when reconstructing the vertebral circulation, as SSEP may be more sensitive in detecting brain stem ischemia than EEG.

Intraoperative Angiography

Particularly in the surgical treatment of giant or complex intracranial aneurysms, it is important to have the option of performing an intraoperative angiogram as a qualitative assessment of the presence and adequacy of cerebral blood flow as pertaining to the patency of specific cerebral blood vessels following aneurysm repair. Routine use of intraoperative angiography for aneurysm surgery has been employed more frequently of late. Intraoperative angiography may lead to clip repositioning in as many as 10% of cases. Accordingly, in all cases in which intraoperative angiography may be required, the head should be fixed with a radiolucent head-holder. It is important to position the patient high up on the operating room table to the extent that the shoulders are hanging over the edge. This will facilitate adequate positioning of the image intensifier. Furthermore, it is advantageous to limit the use of self-retaining retractors, as the retractor bars will obscure good visualization on the intraoperative angiogram. If the cervical carotid artery has been exposed, it provides an easy route to perform an intraoperative angiogram through a direct carotid puncture. Alternatively, the femoral artery can be cannulated for vascular access.

Quantitative Techniques

Transcranial Doppler Ultrasonography

Transcranial Doppler ultrasonography (TCD) has been used to measure CBF velocity in the ipsilateral middle cerebral artery during carotid endarterectomy. Although the technique is well established, due to variations in normal vessel diameter and operator technique, TCD can provide only a relative index of CBF based on normal ranges. As equipment and operator experience have developed, the technique has been used more frequently in intraoperative monitoring. TCD variables may accurately predict stroke during or immediately following carotid endarterectomy. Furthermore, TCD may identify patients at risk for post-endarterectomy hyperperfusion syndrome and hemorrhage with high sensitivity. While the technique has the advantage of being noninvasive, the cost-effectiveness of TCD monitoring during carotid endarterectomy remains unknown.

Ultrasonic Perivascular Flow Probe

An ultrasound-based device previously used in vascular and cardiac surgery, the ultrasonic perivascular flow probe, has recently been used in cerebrovascular procedures - typically, aneurysm surgery [21]. This probe uses ultrasound transit time to measure blood flow, using a small pencil-like device with a semicircular tip. The tip is positioned such that the vessel of interest is contained within the diameter of the semicircle. A quantitative measure of cerebral blood flow is obtained and the accuracy of the technique has been convincingly validated. With this device, blood flow in individual cerebral vessels can be quantified immediately following aneurysm clipping, to verify sufficiency of flow in the parent artery or nearby perforating arteries [21]. The technique is fast, easy to perform and can be repeated with multiple clip applications. We have found it extremely useful in the surgical repair of complex aneurysms, alone or as a quantitative adjunct to intraoperative angiography.

133Xenon

The most widely used method of intraoperative cerebral blood flow measurement, and the technique used at our institution, is the intraarterial injection of 133Xe into the internal carotid artery with extracranial detection of the clearance curve using highly collimated scintillation detectors. 133Xe is a low-energy gamma emitter that diffuses freely through the brain, and thus is an ideal agent for measurement of cerebral blood flow. This radionuclide has an unstable nucleus, continuously emitting beta, gamma, and X-ray photons. The emitted photons are of low energy and, as such, can be absorbed by 0.1 mm of lead to reduce exposure by 90%. It is distributed as a 5% concentration mixed with 95% carbon dioxide, which is then dissolved in 0.9% sodium chloride for injection [22]. 133Xe freely passes through cell membranes, crosses the blood–brain barrier and is not metabolized anywhere in the body. After injection into the internal carotid artery, it is retained momentarily in brain tissue and is then released through normal venous outflow channels. Ninety percent of 133Xe is expelled through the lungs on first-pass, thereby minimizing recirculation of the radionuclide through the cerebral vasculature [22].

It is important to obtain baseline measurements of 133Xe for each patient intraoperatively. Accuracy of instrumentation and measurement devices must also be verified. The main components of the 133Xe CBF measurement system are a scintillation detector, pulse height amplifier, count-rate meter, power supplies and a strip chart recorder (Fig. 17.5). The two types of scintillation detectors in use today

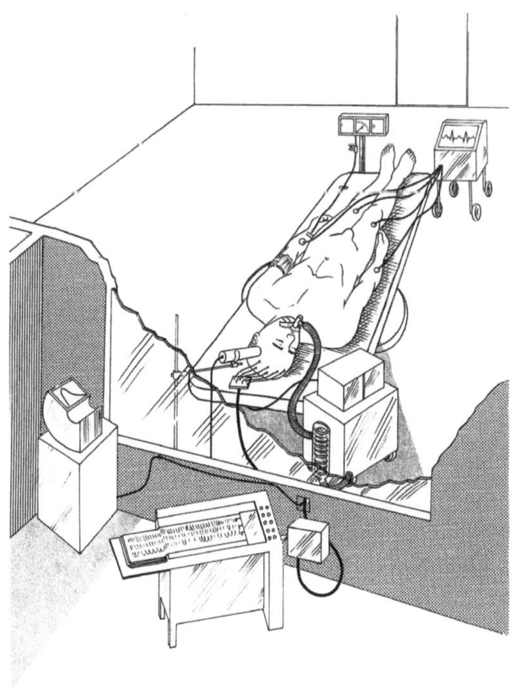

Fig. 17.5. Operating and control room layout for 133Xe cerebral blood flow measurement and electroencephalographic monitoring (by permission of Mayo Foundation. Sundt TM Jr, editor. Occlusive cerebrovascular disease: diagnosis and surgical management. W.B. Saunders, 1987; 182–90).

are thallium-activated sodium iodide crystal (NaI(TL)) and cadmium telluride (CdTe). The NaI(TL) detector uses a scintillation crystal that converts the energy of the incoming photons into visible light and is coupled to a photomultiplier tube, which then converts these scintillations into electrical pulses. The crystal thickness is usually 6 mm, to provide maximum counting efficacy, which is about 90–99% for 133Xe. The crystal is mounted behind a lead collimator that is 25 mm thick and has a tapered opening from 30 mm at the surface of the crystal to 22 mm at the front end. This detector assembly, consisting of the collimator, crystal, photomultiplier tube and pre-amplifier, is mounted on a stand that can be moved up to the patient's head. The CdTe crystal is 16 mm in diameter × 2 mm thick, mounted inside a lead collimator that is packaged in a metal cylinder. This unit is attached to the patient's head by means of a strap. The counting efficiency of this unit with 133Xe is 96%. The detector is lighter in weight and operates at a lower voltage than the NaI(TL) system, but is more expensive.

Signal processing of the electrical pulses generated by the detector assembly requires a pre-amplifier, amplifier, pulse height analyzer and count-rate meter. The pre-amplifier and amplifier function to match the impedance level between the scintillation detector and the pre-amplifier, and amplify the low-voltage pulses from the pre-amplifier to a sufficient level to drive the pulse height analyzer. The pulse height analyzer is used to select only those pulses that coincide to the energy level of 133Xe (81 keV) and discriminate against background noise and scattered radiation outside the selected energy range (75–200 keV). The count-rate meter is used to determine the average number of counts per unit time and is recorded on a strip chart recorder.

Ultimately, the measurements obtained by the scintillation detectors and processed as described above yield clearance curves representing the washout of 133Xe (Figs 17.6 and 17.7). These clearance curves can be analyzed by one of several methods for curve analysis to calculate the value of CBF: initial slope index, determined from the slope of the first minute of the clearance curve; stochastic method; and two-compartmental analysis to yield both gray- and white-matter CBF values. The initial slope index is most commonly used, while the other

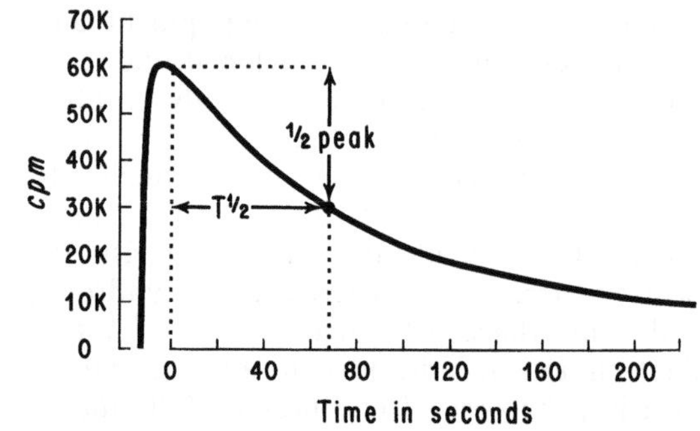

Fig. 17.6. Cerebral blood flow curve following intra-arterial 133Xe injection into the internal carotid artery. Cerebral blood flow in ml/100 g/minute is calculated by dividing 3,600 by the half-peak value in seconds, in this example 55.5 ml/100 g/minute. Cpm, counts per minute (by permission of Mayo Foundation. Sundt TM Jr, editor. Occlusive cerebrovascular disease: diagnosis and surgical management. W.B. Saunders, 1987; 182–90).

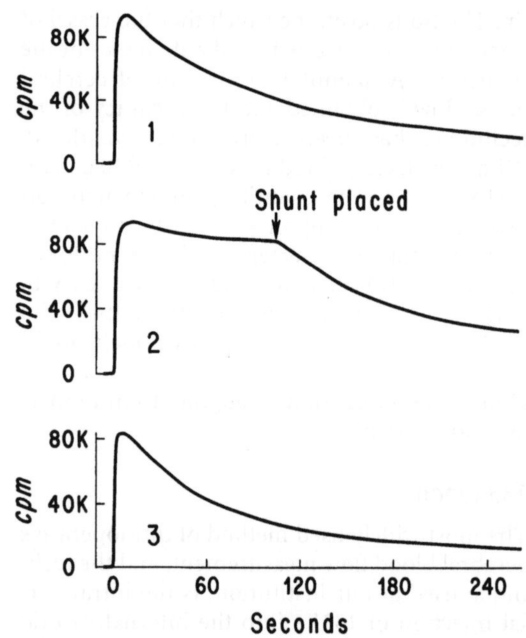

Fig. 17.7. Sequential CBF curves during carotid endarterectomy. Top graph depicts baseline CBF value of 46 ml/100 g/min. Middle graph shows initial occlusion CBF of less than 5 ml/100 g/min, increasing to 44 ml/100 g/min with shunt placement. Lower graph shows CBF value on restoration of flow of 67 ml/100 g/min. CBF, cerebral blood flow (by permission of Mayo Foundation. Sundt TM Jr, editor. Occlusive cerebrovascular disease: diagnosis and surgical management. W.B. Saunders, 1987; 182–90).

two analytic methods require an online computer to determine results.

A primary limitation of CBF measurement using 133Xe is the "look-through" phenomenon. This is the failure to indicate areas of low- or no-flow regions because the detector can see only areas of perfused tissue. In other words, the detector sees the under and/or overlying tissue and also tissue peripheral to the area in the field of view. A second limitation is that performing fast serial measurements introduces error into the measurement. The time interval between CBF measurements at 5 and 10 minutes will result in overestimation of CBF by 10 and 5%, respectively. Therefore, a wait period is recommended between measurements to minimize errors due to a greater-than-normal background. A third limitation is Compton scattering, which may introduce considerable error in the determination of the volume and severity of focal ischemia. Compton-scattered photons can be minimized by setting the lower level of the pulse height analyzer to 75 keV.

Thermal Diffusion Flowmetry

Cerebral blood flow measurement by thermal diffusion technique was originally conceived by Gibbs in 1933 [23]. He used a heated thermocoupler to measure flow though the internal jugular vein. However, by nature of its design, it could accurately reflect relative changes but not absolute values. Brawley extended the technique by incorporating a Peltier stack to improve the stability of the recording probe, thereby making it possible to measure cerebral blood flow over extended periods of time, and the measurements were quantitative [24]. Carter eliminated the Peltier stack to miniaturize the recording probe so that it could more easily used post-operatively in a wide variety of cases [25].

The probe has two gold plates in a thin 3-mm Silastic sheath, one heated and one non-heated. The temperature difference between these plates is monitored constantly, measured by computer, and the resultant difference is converted to CBF in ml/100 g/min. The following is the mathematical formula, derived to quantify cerebral flow by thermal diffusion:

$$CBF = K(1/V - 1/Vo),$$

where CBF is the cortical blood flow in ml/100 g/min, K is the conductivity constant of brain tissue, V is the voltage difference between the two plates and Vo is the voltage difference between the two plates at zero flow. The depth range of the measurement of CBF by thermal diffusion in brain tissue is about 1.5 mm. Care must be taken not to place the probe on any major surface vessel. The probe must be in contact with the tissue surface in order to provide valid temperature measurements. Because the placement of the probe must be visually inspected in relation to the cortex, it may be difficult to install the probe at a bedside setting.

The measurement of CBF by thermal diffusion has been used post-operatively to monitor patients following aneurysm clipping and resection of cerebral arteriovenous malformations. It has also been used to monitor patients with temporal lobe epilepsy and after severe head injury. The advantage of measuring CBF by thermal diffusion is to be able to continuously monitor cerebral blood flow in real time. The disadvantage is that this technique measures small volumes of tissue, resulting in possible inaccuracies because of the heterogeneity of blood flow distribution.

Key Points

- *There has been a recent increase in understanding of the mechanisms of vascular control.*
- *Vascular NO plays a key role in the regulation of blood pressure and tissue perfusion.*
- *CBF can be evaluated clinically using a variety of quantitative and non-quantitative techniques.*
- *Familiarity with vascular control mechanisms and CBF measurement techniques are essential for the modern management of patients with cerebrovascular disease*

References

1. Khurana V, Besser M. Pathophysiological basis of cerebral vasospasm following aneurysmal subarachnoid haemorrhage. J Clin Neurosci 1997;4:122–31.
2. Mitchell H, Shonle HA, Grndley HS. The origin of nitrate in the urine. J Biol Chem 1916;24:461.
3. Furchgott R, Zawadzki JV. The obligatory role of endothelial cells in the relaxation of arterial smooth muscle by acetylcholine. Nature 1980;288:373–6.
4. Ignarro L, Buga GM, Wood KS, Byrns RE, Chaudhuri G. Endothelium-derived relaxing factor produced and

released from artery and vein is nitric oxide. Proc Natl Acad Sci USA 1987;84:9265–9.
5. Palmer R, Ferrige AG, Moncada S. Nitric oxide release accounts for the biological activity of endothelium-derived relaxing factor. Nature 1987;327:524–6.
6. Wiklund NP, Iversen HH, Leone AM, Cellek S, Brundin L, Gustafsson LE, Moncada S. Visualisation of nitric oxide released by nerve stimulation. J Neurosci Res 1997;47:224–32.
7. Bredt D, Hwang PM, Snyder SH. Localization of nitric oxide synthase indicating a neural role for nitric oxide. Nature 1990;347:768–70.
8. Pluta R, Thompson BG, Dawson TM, Snyder SH, Boock RJ, Oldfield EH. Loss of nitric oxide synthase immunoreactivity in cerebral vasospasm. J Neurosurg 1996;84:648–54.
9. Faraci F, Brian JE. Nitric oxide and the cerebral circulation. Stroke 1994;25:692–703.
10. Katusic Z. Endothelium-independent contractions to NG-monomethyl-L-arginine in canine basilar artery. Stroke 1991;22:1399–1404.
11. Toda N, Okamura T. Nitroxidergic nerve: regulation of vascular tone and blood flow in the brain. J Hypertens 1996;14:423–34.
12. Chen A, O'Brien T, Katusic ZS. Transfer and expression of recombinant nitric oxide synthase genes in the cardiovascular system. Trends Pharmacol Sci 1998;19: 276–86.
13. Khurana V, Smith LA, Wieler DA, Springett MJ, Parisi JE, Meyer FB et al. Adenovirus-mediated gene transfer to human cerebral arteries. J Cereb Blood Flow Metab 2000;20:1360–71.
14. Fog M. Cerebral circulation: the reaction of the pial arteries to a fall in blood pressure. Arch Neurol Psuch 1937;37:351–64.
15. Bayliss N. On the local reactions of the arterial wall to changes of internal pressure. J Physiol 1902;28:220–31.
16. Davis M, Donovitz JA, Hood JD. Stretch-activated single-channel and whole cell currents in vascular smooth muscle cells. Am J Physiol 1992;262:C1083–8.
17. Nelson M, Quayle JM. Physiological roles and properties of potassium channels in arterial smooth muscle. Am J Physiol 1995;268:C799–822.
18. Yonas H, Pindzola RR, Johnson DW. Xenon/computed tomography cerebral blood flow and its use in clinical management. Neurosurgery Clinics of North America 1996;7:605–16.
19. Brass L, Walovitch RC. Two prospective, blinded, controlled trials of Tc-99m bicisate brain SPECT and standard neurological evaluation for identifying and localizing ischemic strokes. Journal of Stroke and Cerebrovascular Diseases 1992;1:S59.
20. Grubb R, Derdeyn CP, Fritsch SM, Carpenter DA, Yundt KD, Videen TO et al. Importance of hemodynamic factors in the prognosis of symptomatic carotid occlusion. JAMA 1998;280:1055–60.
21. Charbel F, Gonzales-Portillo G, Hoffman WE et al. Quantitative assesment of vessel flow integrity for aneurysm surgery. J Neurosurg 1999;91:1050–4.
22. Anderson R. Cerebral blood flow: Xenon-133. Neurosurgery Clinics of North America 1996;7:703–8.
23. Gibbs F. A thermoelectric blood flow recorder in the form of a needle. In Proceedings of the Society for Experimental Biology and Medicine. San Francisco, 1933, 141–6.
24. Brawley B. The pathophysiology of intracerebral steal following carbon dioxide inhalation, an experimental study. Scand J Clin Lab Invest 1968;22 (Suppl.):XII.
25. Carter L, Weinland ME, Oommen KJ. Cerebral blood flow monitoring in intensive care by thermal diffusion. Acta Neurochir Supple 1993;59:43–6.

18

Aneurysmal Subarachnoid Hemorrhage

Joan P. Grieve and Neil D. Kitchen

Summary

Subarachnoid hemorrhage (SAH) is a complex pathophysiological process following which secondary cerebral insults are common. A multidisciplinary approach from resuscitation through rehabilitation is needed in order to optimize survival and recovery. During the last decade, advances in SAH management, including early surgery, imaging techniques, hypervolemia, calcium channel blockers, endovascular treatment and aggressive intensive care have provided an opportunity to improve overall outcome. Despite these improvements, the mortality and morbidity associated with SAH remain high.

One third of all neurosurgical literature is about neurovascular diseases and, although this is sometimes conflicting, continued efforts need to be made in order to understand more about the etiological and pathogenetic processes at work in SAH. The roles of endovascular treatment and screening require particular attention.

Introduction

Intracranial vessels lie within the subarachnoid space, giving off small perforating vessels. Hemorrhage from these vessels or from an associated aneurysm occurs primarily into this space, resulting in SAH. Cerebral aneurysms are the most frequent cause of spontaneous SAH, with arteriovenous malformations accounting for approximately 6%, although other causes include trauma and tumors.

Epidemiology

Incidence

Aneurysmal SAH has an annual incidence of 10–20 per 100,000 [1], increasing consistently with age until the sixth decade, with the peak incidence at 55–60 years. There are marked variations in the incidence of SAH worldwide, ranging from 1.1 to 92.3 per 100,000 person years. The incidence is lowest in the Middle East and highest in Japan, Australia and Scandinavia, especially Finland, where the incidence is as much as three times that of the rest of the world. The age-specific rates for SAH appear to be higher in those of Afro-Caribbean origin than Caucasians. There appears to be a female preponderance, with reported male-to-female ratios of 1:1.8 [2].

Prevalence of Cerebral Aneurysms

As few as 0.2% of all aneurysms actually rupture, causing SAH. The number of unruptured intracranial aneurysms (UIAs) coming to medical attention is on the increase due to the widespread availability of non-invasive imaging. As a result, quoted prevalence figures vary greatly. Autopsy studies suggest an aneurysm prevalence of 0.2–7.9% in the general population [2]. This prevalence shows a female and increasing age preponderance [2]. Aneurysms are multiple in 19% of cases [2]. Risk factors for multiple aneurysms include age, female gender, smoking, co-existing arteriovenous malformations (AVMs) and familial cases, where they are present in up to 30%.

Etiology and Pathogenesis of Aneurysm Formation

No hypothesis of saccular aneurysm formation and rupture has been uniformly accepted and the pathogenesis of aneurysms remains uncertain. The main controversy is whether they are congenital or acquired lesions and to what extent environmental factors influence development. The congenital argument suggests that there is a genetic pre-disposition to the development of medial wall or internal elastic lamina defects, supported by the high frequency of multiple aneurysms, familial tendency and their association with AVMs and inherited diseases. The degenerative theory describes an acquired defect in the arterial wall as a result of hemodynamic shear forces, supported by the increasing frequency of aneurysms seen with age, hypertension, smoking and atherosclerosis. They also commonly develop at bifurcations or on high-flow feeding vessels of AVMs, where vascular stresses are maximal.

Aneurysm formation is probably a multifactorial process in which a genetic pre-disposition combines with secondary risk factors to create the lesion. Identification of those factors contributing to this process can focus future screening strategies and enhance screening yield.

Risk Factors for SAH

Heritable Risk Factors

Familial

Most cases of SAH are sporadic. However, there are family cohorts of affected individuals. Segregation analysis has revealed several patterns of inheritance consistent with compiled pedigrees, but no single mendelian model has the overall best fit, suggesting genetic heterogeneity.

Familial IAs are not rare, accounting for 7–20% of patients with aneurysmal SAH. In one study of 8,680 individuals, the prevalence of asymptomatic aneurysms in the subgroups with and without a family history was 10.5 and 6.8%, respectively [3]. Approximately one-third of asymptomatic members of affected families will have evidence of UIA on angiography. The relative risk of siblings of SAH patients suffering a hemorrhage is six times that of the general population, with a threefold increased risk in the parents - an overall fourfold increased risk in first-degree relatives.

Familial aneurysms tend to rupture at a smaller size and at a younger age than sporadic cases and often display genetic anticipation, with hemorrhage occurring at progressively younger ages in each successive generation. The occurrence of aneurysms at identical and "mirror" sites is more frequent in familial cases and appears to be a function of the degree of kinship between affected individuals.

Heritable Connective Tissue Disorders

There are many heritable connective tissue disorders that have been associated with IAs. It is not known to what degree they contribute to total prevalence of UIAs, although it is probably small, at approximately 5%. Recognition of an underlying generalized connective tissue disorder is of considerable importance, although marked phenotypic heterogeneity often complicates the diagnosis of these disorders.

The most commonly inherited disorders that have been reported to be associated with IAs include autosomal dominant polycystic kidney disease, Marfan's syndrome, pseudoxanthoma elasticum, Ehlers–Danlos syndrome and alpha-1 antitrypsin deficiency.

Modifiable Risk Factors

Of the various environmental factors that may confer a pre-disposition to aneurysmal SAH, cigarette smoking is the only factor that has been consistently identified in all populations.

Smoking is associated with SAH in nearly half of cases and increases the risk of SAH by 2–10 times, with a dose-related effect. The SAH risk decreases with the number of years since giving up smoking, with the excess risk largely disappearing 2–4 years after cessation of smoking.

Hypertension is a common comorbid condition and, as a result, there is conflicting evidence regarding the role it plays as an independent risk factor for SAH. Some authors have found that hypertension is not a risk factor for SAH, with no notable excess over an age- and sex-matched control autopsy population, whilst others have found that hypertension does appear to be related to an increased risk of SAH.

Hypertension and smoking act as synergistic risk factors. The risk of SAH in hypertensive individuals who smoke is nearly 15 times that in the non-smoking, non-hypertensive population, although smoking poses a greater risk than hypertension to the population as a whole.

There is a strong temporal association between cocaine use and both ischemic and hemorrhagic cerebrovascular events. The use of sympathomimetic drugs, such as cocaine or metamphetamine, tends to increase the incidence and decrease the age at which rupture occurs in patients harboring aneurysms; aneurysmal size at rupture also tends to be smaller.

Many authors have suggested that hormonal status may have a role to play in the formation of IAs, given the female preponderance in most series of SAH. Use of the combined oral contraceptive (COC) may increase the risk of SAH, particularly in hypertensive smokers. More recent studies have failed to show any significant increased risk with new low-dose COC in individuals less than 35–40 years old, although, again, there may be an increased relative risk of 2.5 in older individuals.

The role of pregnancy as a risk factor for SAH remains unclear. Older studies have shown a 1 in 10,000 pregnancies risk of SAH – a fivefold increase over the expected incidence in a population based study. This may be as a result of growth of cerebral aneurysms caused by increased laxity of vascular walls during pregnancy, although changes in blood pressure, stroke volume and blood volume may also have a role. More recent studies, however, show no significantly increased risk of SAH during pregnancy, although, as maternal mortality from other causes decreases, intracranial hemorrhage may become a more common cause of maternal mortality. Ruptured aneurysms are currently responsible for approximately 5% of maternal deaths. Mortality and morbidity of aneurysmal SAH in pregnancy are high: maternal mortality is 13–35%, whilst that of the fetus is 7–25%.

Hemorrhage Risk

Unruptured Aneurysms

The annual incidence of aneurysmal rupture in patients with known aneurysms has previously been accepted as 1–2.3%. However, the recently published results of the International Study of Unruptured Intracranial Aneurysms (ISUIA) have shown a considerably lower annual incidence of rupture in certain situations [4]. ISUIA followed 1,449 patients with 1,937 aneurysms. In the patients who had no history of SAH, the cumulative rate of rupture of aneurysms that were less than 10 mm in diameter at diagnosis was less than 0.05% per year, whilst in those who had suffered a SAH from a different aneurysm that had been repaired successfully, the rate was approximately 11 times higher (0.5% per year). The rupture rate of aneurysms that were 10 mm or more in diameter was less than 1% per year in both groups, except in patients with giant aneurysms (greater than 25 mm in diameter) who had not suffered a SAH, when the rupture rate was 6% in the first year. Other authors have confirmed that aneurysmal size is a major predictive factor for the risk of future rupture, although many aneurysms are documented as being considerably smaller than 10 mm when they rupture.

The ISUIA study also found that location was important. Among patients with no previous history of SAH, aneurysms situated at the basilar tip, vertebrobasilar, posterior cerebral or posterior communicating (PCOM) arteries were more likely to rupture, whilst in patients who had suffered an earlier SAH from a different aneurysm that had been repaired successfully, only the basilar tip location was predictive of rupture [4]. SAH is rare in cavernous carotid aneurysms: if they rupture, they usually cause carotico-cavernous fistulae (CCF). Most authors would recommend treatment only of those projecting into the subarachnoid space and of those symptomatic with progressive ophthalmoplegia, facial pain or progressive visual loss. Hemorrhage risk is greater in symptomatic patients who represent one-third of all UIA patients but account for nearly three-quarters of those that bleed during observation. Multiple aneurysms increase long-term risk of rupture, with a 6.8% annual risk vs 1.9% for single aneurysms. This may be because the affected individuals are more susceptible to both aneurysmal formation and rupture.

Ruptured Aneurysms

The re-hemorrhage rate is highest during the first 24 hours following SAH. This is occasionally related to early angiography. Fifty percent of patients will go on to re-bleed within the first 6 months, unless the aneurysms are treated, with an annual re-bleed rate of 3%. Early surgery clearly decreases the risk of re-bleed, although a small risk remains from incomplete clipping or the presence of multiple aneurysms.

Risk factors for re-bleeding include time between ictus and angiography, and between ictus and definitive management of the aneurysm. Also of importance are the neurological grade and conscious level of the patient and the presence of hypertension or an intracerebral hematoma (ICH). In the long term, factors influencing the re-bleed rate include aneurysm size and location and the presence of hypertension.

Presentation

Clinical Features

The classic presentation for SAH is of a sudden-onset severe headache. Headache is present in up to 97% of patients and is commonly associated with nausea and vomiting (77%) or nuchal rigidity (up to 50%). Many studies have reported a seasonal variation in SAH. The incidence of SAH in both men and women is lowest in the summer. The peak season for women suffering SAH is winter, whilst those for men are autumn and spring.

Consciousness is frequently altered, with confusion and lethargy in 30%, transient loss of consciousness in one-third and coma in 17%. Neurological abnormalities are seen in 64% of cases with focal signs, such as hemiparesis, IIIrd or VIth nerve palsies in 21%.

Symptoms occasionally help to localize the aneurysm. Anterior communicating (ACOM) artery aneurysms may present with frontal symptoms, and electrolyte disturbance is common. Both anterior choroidal (although uncommon) and middle cerebral artery (MCA) aneurysms may present with a hemiparesis, whilst pericallosal artery and distal anterior cerebral artery (ACA) aneurysms tend to present with a contralateral lower-limb monoparesis, incontinence and frontal symptoms. The classic symptom for PCOM artery aneurysms is a painful IIIrd nerve palsy, seen in 30% of cases at presentation.

Presentation with a painful pupil-involving IIIrd nerve palsy is usually taken to imply imminent rupture of the aneurysm and should therefore be dealt with promptly. Ophthalmic artery aneurysms present with visual field defects in 25% of cases or, rarely, endocrine disturbances. They are often large and commonly present prior to rupture.

Eye Symptoms and Signs

Retinal and pre-retinal hemorrhages are seen in 25% of SAH patients. There are, classically, three types of hemorrhage that can occur alone or in combination. First, retinal hemorrhage which may surround the fovea; second, subhyaloid pre-retinal hemorrhage, seen fundoscopically in 11–33% of cases as bright-red blood near the optic disc, which may be associated with a higher mortality rate and, finally, Terson's syndrome, consisting of hemorrhage within the vitreous humor in SAH patients occurring in approximately 4% of cases and usually bilaterally.

The prognosis for spontaneous visual recovery in 6–12 months is good, but patients should be monitored for complications such as elevated intra-ocular pressure, retinal membrane formation and even retinal detachment.

"Warning Leaks"

Many retrospective studies, which probably overestimate the incidence, suggest that up to 40% of patients have "warning leaks". In one prospective study examining 148 patients with suspected warning leaks, 25% were found to have had SAH[5]. Most occur 1–8 weeks before a major SAH and may not necessarily be seen on CT or lumbar puncture. Headache is usually milder but of similar nature and sudden-onset, lasting several days, and can be associated with nausea and vomiting, although meningism and photophobia are rare.

Grading

The single, most important independent predictor of outcome after aneurysmal rupture is the clinical status at admission of the patient. A number of grading systems have been proposed and are used to guide treatment or predict morbidity and mortality.

Clinical

Hunt and Hess

The Hunt and Hess grading system stratifies patients according to clinical signs and symptoms at time of presentation and is predictive of outcome (Table 18.1) [6]. Any serious systemic illness, such as hypertension, diabetes, severe atherosclerosis, chronic pulmonary disease or vasospasm on angiography, increases the grade by one level.

World Federation of Neurosurgical Societies

Analysis of data from the International Cooperative Aneurysm Study revealed that with normal consciousness, Hunt and Hess Grades I and II had identical outcomes and that hemiparesis and/or aphasia had no effect on mortality. As a result, the World Federation of Neurosurgical Societies (WFNS) proposed further modification to improve reliability (Table 18.1) [7].

Radiological

Fisher

A CT grading system proposed by Fisher et al. [8] is frequently used to predict the likelihood of developing angiographic vasospasm (Table 18.2). When the subarachnoid blood was not detected or was distributed diffusely, severe vasospasm was almost never encountered. In the presence of subarachnoid blood, clots or thick layers of hemorrhage, severe spasm followed almost invariably.

Table 18.1. Hunt and Hess Scale and World Federation of Neurosurgical Societies Scale.

Grade	Hunt and Hess scale	WFNS scale
0	Incidental aneurysm, no subarachnoid hemorrhage	GCS 15 Unruptured aneurysm
1	Asymptomatic or mild headache, slight nuchal rigidity	GCS 15 Absent motor deficit
2	Moderate to severe headache, nuchal rigidity, but no other neurological deficit (except cranial nerve palsy)	GCS 13–14 Absent motor deficit
3	Mild focal deficit, drowsiness or confusion	GCS 13–14 Motor deficit present
4	Stupor, moderate to severe hemiparesis, possible early decerebrate rigidity and vegetative disturbances	GCS 7–12 Motor deficit absent or present
5	Deep coma, decerebrate rigidity, moribund	GCS 3–6 Motor deficit absent or present

Table 18.2. Fisher grade.

Fisher grade	Blood on CT
1	No subarachnoid blood detected
2	Diffuse or vertical layers less than 1 mm thick
3	Localized clot and/or vertical layer more than 1 mm
4	Intracerebral or intraventricular clot with diffuse or no subarachnoid blood

Investigations

Computerized Tomography

CT is the first-line investigation for SAH. It has a high sensitivity, generally revealing diffuse blood of a symmetrical distribution around the basal cisterns, sylvian fissures and cortical sulci (Fig. 18.1). It detects acute SAH in 95% of patients within 48 hours and in 57% of cases at 5 days [9]. When asymmetrical or localized, the distribution of blood may suggest the location of the aneurysm in up to 70% of cases. Intraventricular hemorrhage (IVH) is characteristic of ruptured ACOM artery aneurysms; ICH is most commonly seen with PCOM artery and MCA aneurysms. Following diagnosis, CT is particularly useful for demonstrating ventricular size, cerebral ischemia or infarction, mid-line shift or re-bleed.

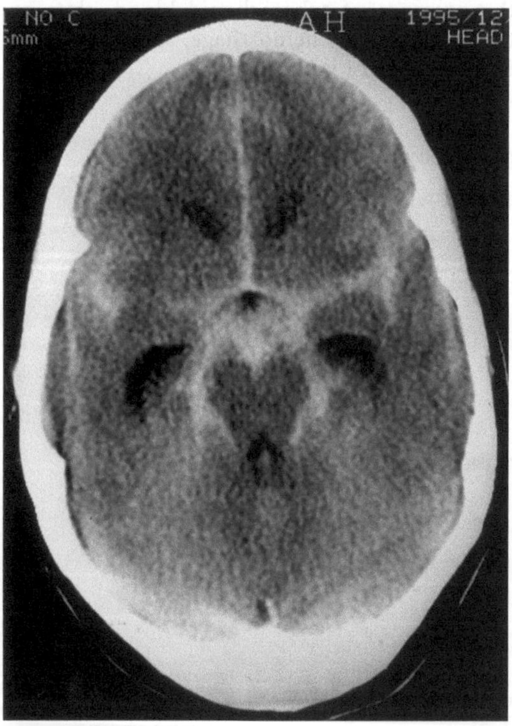

Fig. 18.1. CT scan demonstrating an aneurysmal subarachnoid hemorrhage.

Lumbar Puncture

Two percent of patients will have a negative CT, despite having suffered a SAH, particularly if they are of good grade. Lumbar puncture (LP), in this situation, is indicated to detect hemorrhagic or xanthochromic cerebrospinal fluid (CSF). LP commonly reveals an elevated opening pressure with release of bloody CSF that does not clear on sequential sampling. Xanthochromia may take 24–48 hours to develop but can be present at 6 hours and, rarely, at less than 2 hours. It is present in 70% of cases at 6 hours and 90% at 12 hours following SAH.

Angiography (see also Chapter 2)

Digital subtraction angiography (DSA) is the definitive investigation for the identification of aneurysms and for surgical planning. It should demonstrate the aneurysmal site, type, size, orientation and neck, intraluminal calcification and thrombus, the relationship between aneurysm and parent vessels, collateral flow through the circle of Willis, the presence of adjacent perforators and the state of the cerebral vasculature, including other aneurysms. It also allows visualization of the osseous anatomy surrounding the aneurysm on non-subtracted films, necessary for planning of the surgical approach and decisions regarding operability.

In the case of multiple aneurysms, identification of the ruptured lesion may be difficult. Most useful for identification are the distribution of SAH and the location of any ICH. In situations where the CT reveals diffuse SAH or the SAH has been diagnosed on LP, the aneurysm most likely to have ruptured is larger, has a greater irregularity, mass effect or associated local vasospasm.

Angiogram-negative SAH

Fifteen to 20% of cases will have a normal angiogram [9]. Of these, up to 65% will have a distinctive pattern of subarachnoid blood lying in the prepontine or perimesencephalic cisterns (Fig. 18.2). They tend to be younger, non-hypertensive, of better grade and more often male than SAH patients with positive angiograms. The etiology in these cases is unclear but may be due to venous hemorrhage. The overall

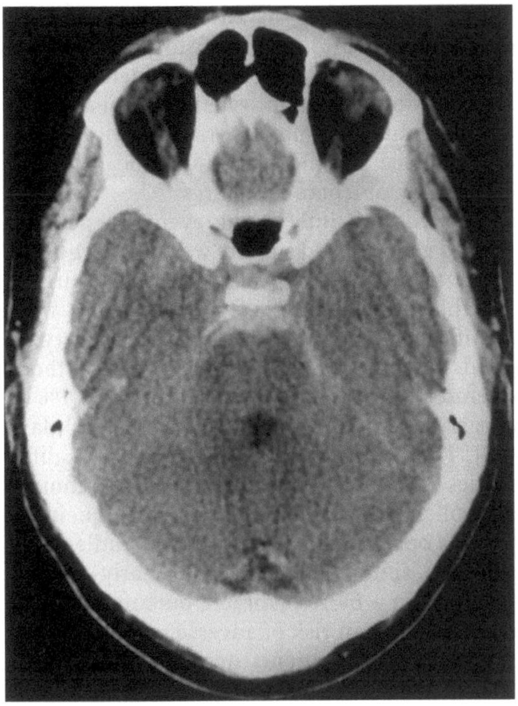

Fig. 18.2. CT scan demonstrating a perimesencephalic subarachnoid hemorrhage.

prognosis tends to be good, partly because re-bleeding is rare and few patients develop delayed ischemic deficit (DID). However, this diagnosis should only be entertained with caution as 10% of vertebrobasilar aneurysms present with a similar distribution of blood. Repeat angiography should be considered carefully as aneurysms may be obscured by vasospasm, hypoperfusion, poor angiographic technique or thrombosis. Undetected aneurysms are found in an additional 2–5% of cases at 2–4 weeks.

Magnetic Resonance Imaging

Acute subarachnoid blood is difficult to differentiate from CSF on most MRI sequences and therefore MRI is not as good as CT for the initial diagnosis. Within 24-48 hours of SAH, there is too little methemoglobin for hemorrhage to be obvious, especially with the small amount of blood often involved. Visualization of blood on MRI is, however, better after 4–7 days and is therefore excellent at demonstrating subacute to remote SAH at 10–20 days, when CT sensitivity decreases.

Magnetic resonance angiography reveals most aneurysms that are greater than 3 mm in diameter. The sensitivity for identification of aneurysms is 85–90%, with a specificity of greater than 90% when compared with DSA [10], with an excellent intra-observer consistency and good-to-excellent inter-observer reproducibility.

Computerized Tomography Angiography

Although not currently used in routine clinical practice, computerized tomography angiography (CTA) can resolve aneurysms as small as 2–3 mm, with sensitivities of 77–97% and specificities of 87–100% [11]. The use of helical CT scanners has dramatically reduced imaging times, as well as patient movement artefact allowing acquisition of the entire CT volume in 30–45 s during first arterial pass of an intravenous contrast injection. Although helpful in demonstrating aneurysms, reformats can be difficult and time-consuming.

The most compelling indication for CTA is in the unstable patient requiring craniotomy for aneurysmal ICH before a cerebral angiogram can be performed, although there may be difficulties in visualizing small perforators. There may be a role for CTA in the follow-up of surgical remnants, unruptured aneurysms and partially coiled lesions.

Aneurysmal Distribution

Most aneurysms arise from the anterior circulation (85–95%), whilst 5–15% arise from the posterior circulation.

ACOM artery aneurysms are the commonest lesion, particularly in men (46 vs 27% in women). Also common are aneurysms arising from the ICA, especially in women (36.8% compared with 18% in men). PCOM artery aneurysms are found in 20–25% of individuals, whilst MCA aneurysms are found in 15–20%.

Within the posterior circulation, 10% arise from the basilar artery, the basilar tip being the most common site, followed by the superior cerebellar junction. Five percent arise from the vertebral artery, the posterior–inferior cerebellar artery being the most common site.

Management of SAH

Initial Management

The main aim in the early management of SAH is stabilization of the patient, with optimization for aneurysm obliteration, together with the prevention of secondary cerebral insults. Initial priorities include adequate ventilation and oxygenation, normovolemia and hemodynamic stability and control of intracranial pressure (ICP).

In all patients, bedrest is recommended until aneurysm obliteration can be undertaken. Frequent neurological examination is required in order to identify any neurological deterioration requiring further investigation or management. The prophylactic use of nimodipine, at a dose of 60 mg 4-hourly, is used in most centers, as it has been shown to improve outcome [12]. With an unsecured aneurysm, gentle volume expansion with slight hemodilution may help to return the circulating volume to normal and prevent or minimize the effects of vasospasm; however, hypertension should be avoided. Some authors recommend central venous pressure measurement in all SAH patients to allow accurate assessment of the hydration of the patient, although this is not routine practice in all units.

Aggressive peri- and post-operative intensive care may be associated with improved outcome, with a decrease in the incidence of medical complications and secondary cerebral insults. SAH is a complex pathophysiological event, which results in a number of systemic and intracranial alterations. These changes are more prevalent in poor-grade patients and are often associated with subsequent DID.

Surgical Treatment

Clipping of Aneurysms

Craniotomy and aneurysm obliteration by clipping has, until now, been the most effective treatment known. Timing of surgery, however, is still an important and controversial consideration in the management of the patient with a ruptured aneurysm.

Until the 1980s, late surgery was generally practiced. With improvements in microsurgical techniques and intensive care of patients, the Cooperative Study on the Timing of Aneurysm Surgery was set up in an effort to establish outcome related to timing of surgery. This was a prospective, observational, epidemiological survey using the patient's neurological and disability status at 6 months, rates of vasospasm and re-bleed and medical and surgical complications as outcome measures. The mortality associated with intervening events in patients treated with delayed surgery was nearly equal to the post-operative mortality after early surgery [9,13]. However, rates of good recovery were significantly improved with early surgery, a good outcome being seen in 70.9% of those operated on at 0–3 days but only 61.7% if surgery was performed at greater than 10 days [13]. There tended to be similar technical difficulties in early and delayed surgery, although a swollen, tight brain was more frequent in patents operated on acutely. Other studies have shown a similar tendency, with early surgery resulting in a more favorable outcome with an equally common risk of adverse intra-operative events in those patients operated on early or late.

Early surgery, with manipulation of the basal cerebral blood vessels, was initially thought to increase the risk of vasospasm. This is probably untrue, as there appears to be no specific relationship between the timing of surgery and the onset of spasm or the development of cerebral infarction, as long as hypervolemia is initiated early. However, patients with surgery planned at days 7–10 (the time of greatest vasospasm) do have the least favorable outcome, with the highest mortality and incidence of focal deficits secondary to vasospasm [14].

Basilar trunk aneurysms are traditionally treated at 10–14 days following SAH, although recent studies have shown good results with early surgery. In addition, aneurysms greater than 2.5 cm are also best treated in a delayed manner, as technical difficulties increase in these individuals, with intraluminal clot, wide neck and prolonged periods of vessel occlusion.

Neurological grade and age of the patient are the most important patient-related factors.

The Cooperative Study showed that if patients were alert at admission, outcome was favorable in 75% at 6 months, while only 11% who were admitted in coma made a good recovery [9]. Traditionally, poor-grade patients are treated in a delayed manner, although they do not appear to tolerate surgery any worse than better-grade patients [9]. Poor-grade patients generally have more blood on CT and are therefore more prone to developing worse vasospasm. Early clipping in this situation allows aggressive hypervolaemic hypertensive treatment. Another argument for early surgery is that transluminal angioplasty for the treatment of refractory vasospasm can be employed more safely.

Age of the patient tends to be inversely related to favorable outcome, particularly in those aged 60 years or over [9]. For this reason, elderly patients also tend to be treated more conservatively. When feasible, however, early surgery in the elderly is reasonable because they do not fare worse with early surgery [14], the re-bleed rate increases with age, they are more likely to suffer IVH or ICH, both of which may be amenable to early surgery, and they often have decreased cerebrovascular reserve and may therefore be more prone to DID. Elderly patients treated conservatively have a mortality of 50% and aggressive management, including surgery, remains their best chance of returning to an independent existence.

Hunterian Ligation

Hunterian ligation (parent vessel occlusion) is generally only considered if occlusion of the aneurysm neck is dangerous or impossible. It reduces flow past the aneurysm, often reducing the size of the lesion and even occasionally causing spontaneous thrombosis.

This can be an excellent option for some giant proximal ICA aneurysms (particularly when presenting with cavernous sinus syndrome), fusiform aneurysms, serpentine MCA aneurysms, wide-necked basilar artery aneurysms and certain vertebral lesions.

A pre-operative test occlusion with or without a hypotensive challenge and CBF measurements is often performed endovascularly. This can be combined with semi-quantitative measures of CBF, such as positron emission tomography, single photon emission computerized tomography (SPECT) scans or transcranial doppler (TCD) ultrasound monitoring to increase reliability. If collateral circulation is adequate, parent vessel occlusion alone is appropriate. Even with experience, there is a 5% risk of delayed stroke in patients who initially tolerate the balloon occlusion.

Wrapping

As an isolated procedure, wrapping with muslin, Surgicel((Ethicon, Belgium), or muscle has fallen out of fashion although is still used in the treatment of some unclippable or fusiform aneurysms. It provides some degree of protection from re-hemorrhage but is not as effective as clipping. One series showed a 8.6% re-bleed rate in the first 6 months and, thereafter, a 1.5% per year re-bleed rate vs 50% if left untreated [15]. It is more commonly used as an adjunct to clipping where a small remnant of neck would otherwise be left unprotected.

Rate of Obliteration

Residual aneurysm is seen in 1–10% of aneurysms clipped. Perfect reconstruction tends to be better for MCA rather than ACOM artery aneurysms, whilst basilar tip aneurysms are notoriously difficult to completely obliterate, particularly if they are pointing posteriorly. Giant aneurysms, those with a wide neck or with calcifications within the wall are often difficult to clip completely and remnants or compromised vessels are common. Giant aneurysms are completely occluded in only 60% of cases compared with 85 and 93% in aneurysms measuring greater than 10 mm and less than 10 mm, respectively.

Complete occlusion of the aneurysm is important, as there is a small but definite chance of aneurysmal regrowth from the unprotected remnant, although, occasionally, this undergoes thrombosis. The management of residual aneurysmal necks differs between units. Some surgeons recommend immediate re-operation to allow complete occlusion, whilst others prefer to watch the remnant with repeat DSA to document any change in size. The risk of hemorrhage from incompletely occluded necks is less than 0.5–1% per year at an average of 10.5 years.

Outcome and Complications

Figures for surgical morbidity and mortality are very dependent on case selection and can be difficult to separate from general outcome figures. Mortality and morbidity following aneurysm surgery are, in the main, related to perforator or large vessel occlusion, brain retraction and cranial nerve traction injury. Five to 10% of cases are complicated by a major vessel occlusion and 50% of those who die following aneurysmal surgery have an infarct at post mortem. Intraoperative rupture, seen in 15–20% of cases, is associated with increased neurological morbidity and mortality.

The influence of aneurysmal location varies between series. Complications following anterior circulation aneurysm surgery are seen in 5% of PCOM artery cases, MCA 8%, ophthalmic 12%, ACOM 16% and ICA 17%. In expert hands, the overall mortality for posterior circulation aneurysms is about 5% and permanent morbidity about 12%. Complications are seen in 2% of aneurysms less than 5 mm, 7% if 6–15 mm and 14% if 16–25 mms in diameter [16]. Giant aneurysms particularly are associated with poor outcome and operative complications.

The operative mortality ranges from 0% in Hunt and Hess Grades I and II to 28% in Grades III and IV, although other studies show no significant difference in surgical outcome between poor- and good-grade survivors. Increasing age also tends to be a poor prognostic indicator for surgery, although good results can be achieved in patients older than 60 years. Mortality is 3% in the third decade, rising to 11% in the eighth decade, with a good outcome in only 50% of those aged 59 years and over.

Results of surgery for unruptured aneurysms have always been thought to be excellent, with a generally quoted risk of 1% mortality and 5% morbidity. More recently, the results of the ISUIA have challenged these figures, suggesting mortality (2.7%) and specifically morbidity (11.7%) associated with surgery for UIA may be considerably higher than first appreciated [4].

Endovascular Treatment (see also Chapter 19)

Coiling

The Guglielmi Detachable Coil (GDC) has been available since 1991 and has been increasingly used in clinical practice [17]. Many radiologists and neurosurgeons have shown that it is possible to exclude an aneurysm from the circulation by their use. The recently published results of the International Sub-arachnoid Aneurysm Trial (ISAT) suggest that patients treated by endovascular means have a better survival, free of disability, at 1 year than those treated surgically, although there was no significant difference in the 1-year fatality rates [18]. Preliminary data suggest that the long-term risk of further bleeding from the treated aneurysm is low with either treatment, but somewhat more frequent with endovascular coiling.

The indications for coiling and results of long-term follow-up need to be examined further before their role in the management of sub-arachnoid patients can be fully delineated. It is an attractive, minimally invasive alternative to surgical clipping that can be carried out at the same time as diagnostic angiography. Current indications for coiling include posterior circulation aneurysms and selected poor-grade patients, dependent on aneurysm morphology, whilst limitations include giant aneurysms, those with a wide neck and more distally placed aneurysms. However, with improvements in technology and the introduction of newer coils and substances (such as ONYX), the role of endovascular treatment may continue to evolve.

Balloon Occlusion

Endovascular occlusion of vessels, most commonly the ICA, offers several advantages over surgical ligation. It can be performed as a single procedure with simultaneous test balloon occlusion on an awake patient, before permanent sacrifice of the vessel is undertaken. Collateral supply can be assessed angiographically at the same time and any residual filling of the aneurysm can be demonstrated. For cavernous segment aneurysms, a trapping technique is usually employed, where the two balloons are placed one just distal to and the second just proximal to the aneurysmal neck, thus trapping the aneurysm. More distal aneurysmal lesions increase the risks of test balloon occlusion, particularly of vessel rupture. In addition, collateral adequacy can be more difficult to assess.

Rate of Obliteration

Complete obliteration is achieved in only 50% of cases coiled; however, rupture typically occurs from the dome or fundus of the aneurysm and therefore partial occlusion may be adequate to prevent re-bleed. One particular problem with coiled aneurysms is that the limited long-term studies available suggest that neck remnants can lead to recurrent aneurysms. Recurrence rates of 16–32% within 2–3 years have been seen.

Clipped aneurysm necks appear to be more stable than a coiled rest. Post-mortem studies have shown endothelialization of the thrombus at the neck of a clipped aneurysm. Although this has been demonstrated in some aneurysms that have been coiled, it appears that the neck walls of a coiled aneurysm are held open, rather than being closely applied by the clip, which may prevent or slow the process of endothelialization. This leaves thrombus open to the circulation and may allow enough time for the flow past the aneurysm to compact the coils, with the development of a recurrent aneurysm.

Complications of Subarachnoid Hemorrhage

Of those reaching neurosurgical care, vasospasm and re-hemorrhage are the two most common causes of death or neurological deficit in SAH patients. The prevention of secondary cerebral insults needs to addressed aggressively, as more than half of patients will develop systemic complications that may compromise outcome.

Vasospasm and Delayed Ischemic Deficit

Definitions and Incidence

Vasospasm, synonymous with angiographic vasospasm, is defined as a delayed focal or diffuse, radiologically detectable narrowing of cerebral arteries and is present in 40–70% of patients following aneurysmal SAH. It has a relatively consistent course, typically appearing at 3–4 days following the hemorrhage, with a peak incidence and severity at 7–10 days. There is a gradual resolution, with normal vessel diameter at 3–4 weeks.

DID or symptomatic vasospasm is the development of a new neurological deficit that is not explained by any post-operative hematoma, hydrocephalus, seizure activity or metabolic disturbance. It occurs in 20–30% of patients following SAH, although, more recently, its incidence has been quoted to be as low as 10% and is clinically at its worst 3–14 days following the hemorrhage.

The mechanism by which vasospasm is effected is poorly understood. A multi-factorial origin is most probable, with the liberation of spasmogenic metabolites during clot lysis in the basal cisterns and the impairment of cerebral vasodilatation related to endothelial dysfunction and structural changes in the arterial wall.

Pre-disposing Factors

The severity and distribution of vasospasm are related to the amount and site of sub-arachnoid blood [8]. It may be focal or diffuse, but is commonly worse in the vessels feeding the ruptured aneurysm and in those surrounded by significant clot. Other risk factors include increasing age of patient, high systolic blood pressure, poor clinical grade, decreased conscious level, the presence of a motor deficit and the presence of hydrocephalus, whilst patients with vertebral aneurysms, predominantly IVH or a negative CT, have a lower risk of developing symptomatic vasospasm.

Clinical Features

Patients commonly present with an insidious onset of confusion, decreasing level of consciousness and focal deficit which may resolve or progress to infarction, coma or death. Patients often have a mild leucocytosis and low-grade pyrexia. More focal symptoms depend on the extent and distribution of angiographic spasm, age and clinical condition of the patient, presence of complicating factors and collateral circulation.

Diagnosis

Effective treatment is dependent on early recognition and diagnosis and requires a high index of suspicion; however, diagnosis can be difficult and is often made by exclusion of other causes of neurological deterioration such as hydrocephalus, electrolyte imbalance, seizures, rebleed or edema. Although the diagnosis of DID is largely clinical, it can be confirmed both invasively by angiography and non-invasively by TCD and, increasingly, xenon CT.

Transcranial Doppler

TCD was first described as a technique in 1981 and its use in the diagnosis of vasospasm in 1982 by Aaslid [19]. It uses a low-frequency

2-MHz range-gated pulsed Doppler insonation through thinner parts of skull to determine blood velocity in the basal cerebral arteries. TCD measures the velocity and direction of blood flow, but does not measure flow rate or perfusion directly. However, elevated cerebral arterial blood velocity correlates well with angiographic vasospasm.

The MCA is the vessel best suited to TCD evaluation because of its location, size and orientation. In addition, MCA is an end artery with relatively limited leptomeningeal collateral supply. Sensitivity and specificity of TCD in demonstrating spasm in the MCA are 60–85 and 89–98%, respectively. Baseline MCA blood flow velocities range from 50 to 74 cm/s, with an average of 62 cm/s [19]. Blood flow velocity increases with progressive narrowing of vessels and, when critical narrowing occurs, blood flow is actually reduced, with the development of neurological deficits. Velocities greater than 120 cm/s indicate mild-to-moderate vasospasm, as seen by angiography, often with impending symptomatology, whereas velocities greater than 200 cm/s correlate with severe spasm. Infarction rarely occurs if the velocity is less than 140 cm/s, whilst velocities of greater than 200 cm/s are frequently associated with ischemia and infarction.

Xenon CT

Stable xenon CT is a relatively new technique, which is being increasingly used to demonstrate quantitative CBF measurements superimposed on anatomical information gained from plain CT. The patient undergoes CT scanning at limited levels through the brain (slices can be chosen to demonstrate anterior, middle and posterior cerebral vascular territories) before, during and after inhalation of non-radioactive xenon in oxygen. Patients with moderate or severe angiographic spasm have been shown to have globally reduced CBF and a poorer outcome than patients without angiographic vasospasm. However, there is often no direct relationship between vessel calibre on angiography and the corresponding regional cerebral blood flow (rCBF) on xenon CT.

Treatment

"Triple" Therapy

Once symptomatic vasospasm has developed, treatment is often ineffective. Moderate hypervolemia and hemodilution are commonly encouraged and instigated at the time of diagnosis of SAH, partly to reverse the usual decreased circulating blood volume associated with SAH and also in an effort to prevent or limit the development of DID. More aggressive, therapeutic "triple H" management, consisting of hypervolemia, hypertension and hemodilution, is usually commenced at the onset of symptoms of DID. The induction of hypertension pharmacologically has been shown to reverse ischemic deficits and may be necessary if hypervolaemic hemodilution is insufficient to improve symptomatology. Caution must be used in "triple H" therapy, as it may aggravate cerebral edema (reducing cerebral compliance), pulmonary edema (reducing the oxygen exchange) or dilutional hyponatremia and, therefore, accurate and often invasive monitoring is required. There is also an increased risk of re-hemorrhage in unsecured aneurysms, which occur in up to 50% of individuals. "Triple H" therapy was previously thought to increase CBF. It is more likely that hemodilution actually increases collateral blood flow to ischemic penumbra, minimizing the size of any infarction.

Nimodipine

Nimodipine, a 1,4 dihydropyridine lipid-soluble calcium antagonist, has been studied in several large prospective randomized–controlled trials [12]. It crosses the blood–brain barrier and selectively blocks the L-type voltage-dependent channels, inhibiting the calcium overload of neurons and smooth muscle cells. It has consistently been shown to improve outcome after spasm in all grades, although, in all but one trial, the incidence of symptomatic spasm was not affected. Angiographically, the calibre of the vessels remains unchanged and there appears to be no obvious effect on CBF. The mechanism by which nimodipine is effective is unclear, but a brain-protective effect is likely, possibly by limitation of calcium influx in marginally ischemic neurons or by increasing pial collateral dilatation. Although the benefit of nimodipine in prophylaxis has been clearly established, its role in the treatment of ischemia is far less clear.

Angioplasty

Angioplasty is being increasingly used in the management of clinical vasospasm refractory to medical treatment. There is significant improvement in 60–80% of patients within minutes of the procedure, with evidence of improved rCBF on TCD and SPECT, correlating with reversal of ischemic deficits. Normal angiographic calibre is achieved in 66% of cases, which persists without recurrent spasm. Most reports recommend intervention as soon as it is apparent that a patient is progressing or failing to improve despite maximal medical treatment and before the development of infarction, as ultimate outcome is dependent on the clinical grade of the patient at the time of angioplasty.

Papaverine

Direct intra-arterial papaverine, using superselective catheters, results in clinical improvement in 50–80% and angiographic improvement in 65–95% of patients with vasospasm [20]. This again correlates with rCBF changes on SPECT, although SPECT shows a greater and more sustained improvement in rCBF with angioplasty than papaverine. Spasm is commonly recurrent following intra-arterial papaverine, but is often successfully reversed with a second treatment.

A combined approach, using both angioplasty and intra-arterial papaverine, has been suggested. Papaverine can be used to dilate up vessels temporarily, to allow the passage of the angioplasty balloon; alternatively, angioplasty can be used to treat proximal vasospasm, whilst papaverine deals with the smaller, more distal vessels that are inaccessible to angioplasty.

Outcome

Death and disability from spasm have decreased from 25–30% in the 1970s to 15–20% in the 1980s [9], to less than 10% currently. These improvements are attributed in part to changes in perioperative fluid and blood pressure management that accompanied the shift in the timing of surgery. However, DID still remains a major source of morbidity and mortality.

Re-hemorrhage

At one time, re-hemorrhage was considered a major cause of morbidity and mortality in patients who had survived the initial hemorrhage; however, a shift to early surgical management has minimized the importance of this complication. If unprotected, 15–20% of patients will re-bleed in the first 2 weeks [21], carrying with it significant mortality and morbidity. In most studies, there is an initial peak of re-hemorrhage in the first 48 hours of approximately 4%, which rapidly plateaus to 1–2% per day until 40 days post-hemorrhage [21]. After 6 months, there is a long-term risk of further hemorrhage of 3% per year. Approximately half to three-quarters of individuals suffering a re-bleed will die as a direct result and, in the Cooperative Study, re-bleeding was responsible for 25% of all deaths [9,14]. The risk of re-bleed is increased with poor clinical grade, posterior circulation lesions, hypertension, elderly patients and abnormal hemostatic parameters.

Control of blood pressure in order to minimize the risk of re-hemorrhage is a controversial topic. No controlled trial has ever shown that lowering of blood pressure reduces the risk of re-bleeding, although the Cooperative Study revealed that re-bleeds occurred in 16% of patients who had a systolic blood pressure of 170–240 mmHg but only 9% of those with a systolic of 94–169 mmHg. Most clinicians would suggest that extremes of blood pressure should be avoided, high blood pressure being more likely to cause a re-bleed and low blood pressure exacerbating hypoxic or ischemic cerebral damage from vasospasm.

Hydrocephalus

Hydrocephalus secondary to SAH may be obstructive, caused by direct intraventricular obstruction, or communicating, caused by an interference with the absorption of CSF through the arachnoid villi. It is seen in 10–35% of patients presenting with SAH, with 25–35% of individuals requiring external ventricular drainage [22]. Approximately 50–60% of individuals requiring external ventricular drainage will ultimately require ventriculo-peritoneal shunts [22]. Disadvantages of external ventricular drainage include an increased risk of re-bleed (14%), parenchymal hemorrhage, infection and ventriculitis. The rate of infection varies according to the series but is approximately 10%. Some authors believe that premature drainage of CSF may increase the likelihood of the patient ultimately requiring a ventriculo-peritoneal shunt. Factors associated with the development of chronic hydrocephalus include IVH, hydrocephalus present on admission CT scan, older age, poor grade at admission, pre-morbid hypertension and Fisher grade.

Intracerebral, Intraventricular and Subdural Hemorrhage

Only 20% of ICHs are aneurysmal in origin, although 30% of SAHs are complicated by ICH. They are most frequently seen with MCA and ACOM artery aneurysms. Their presence in SAH patients increases mortality, in part because they are most commonly associated with a poor presenting clinical grade. There is a tendency to improved outcome with emergency evacuation of the clot, particularly if simultaneous clipping of the aneurysm and aggressive management of spasm are undertaken. Patients with a small-volume hematoma, with little sub-arachnoid blood, who are young and are of good grade have the best prognosis. Subdural hematomas are associated with SAH in 1–2% of cases, whilst IVH complicates SAH in one out of six individuals.

Seizures

The highest risk of seizures is within the first 24 hours of ictus, occurring at presentation in 3–18% of individuals. Long-term seizures occur in 6–15% of survivors – a 20 times greater risk than the general population. Most present within the first 18 months, but 6% develop seizures at more than 2 years following their SAH. Early seizures do not necessarily predict long-term seizures. More recent studies have shown a general decline in the incidence of seizures compared with older series. This may reflect technical advances in neurosurgery and neuroanesthesia aimed at minimizing brain manipulation and optimization of cerebral perfusion and neuronal protection during aneurysm surgery. Risk factors include intraparenchymal hematoma, vasospasm and ischemia, MCA aneurysms, poor neurological grade, systemic hypertension, perioperative complications, re-bleed, pre-operative seizures, shunt-dependent hydrocephalus, thick cisternal blood and neurological deficit. Up to 30% of individuals with MCA aneurysms develop seizures, which is likely to be due to a higher incidence of parenchymal involvement. Thirty-three percent of patients with a poor grade compared with 2.5% good-grade individuals will suffer seizures, whilst 16% of individuals who suffer infarction following SAH will develop epilepsy.

The use of prophylactic anticonvulsants is controversial but there has been little prospective study of their use. The incidence of seizures in those receiving anticonvulsants is similar to that in those not receiving prophylaxis, with most studies showing no benefit in preventing early or late seizures. However, seizures can be devastating in SAH patients, with a significant morbidity in the perioperative period. Status epilepticus occurs in 10% of individuals, with an associated mortality of greater than 10%. Seizure activity increases CBF and blood pressure, with the associated risk of re-bleed. Re-hemorrhage, hypoxia and hyperthermia all contribute to secondary brain injury. Short-term usage of anti-convulsants has few risks and most side effects are reversible and, as a result, many authors suggest a short 7–10-day course of perioperative cover, increasing to 3–12 months in those who are most at risk of developing delayed seizures. Phenytoin is generally the first-line treatment. It can be given intravenously, has a lower incidence of skin reactions (compared with carbamazepine) and is less sedative (compared with phenobarbitone).

Volume and Electrolyte Imbalance

Hyponatremia, a serum sodium of less than 135 mmol l^{-1} for more than 2 days, is seen in 10–34% of individuals and, if left untreated, has high associated morbidity and mortality. Cerebral salt-wasting and syndrome of inappropriate anti-diuretic hormone (SIADH) are the two commonest causes, occasionally co-existing. Their distinction is important, as cerebral salt-wasting has an associated depleted circulating volume, making the patient at higher risk for vasospasm.

Cerebral salt wasting is the most common cause of primary natriuresis, negative sodium balance and concurrent diuresis, resulting in hyponatremia and hypovolemia. Natriuresis is stimulated by the release of Atrial Natriuretic Factor (ANF) from the hypothalamus or a digoxin-like substance, which is thought to be released in response to sympathetic nervous system activation or ventricular distension and normally lasts for 4–5 days. These patients should not be fluid restricted. They usually need treatment with intravenous fluid and sodium supplements, although it does not appear to improve outcome in patients with symptomatic spasm. Fludrocortisone acetate can help volume depletion by reducing natriuresis and sodium loss.

SIADH involves the release of ADH, despite a low serum osmolality. It has an average onset at 8 days and lasts 3–9 days. Patients have a normal skin turgor and blood pressure, a normal or decreased hematocrit, hyponatremia with serum hyposmolality and a urine osmolality greater than serum osmolality. Renal and adrenal functions are normal, as is urinary excretion of sodium. Hyponatremia of SIADH is generally associated with normovolemia from ADH-induced free water retention in the kidney.

Diabetes insipidus complicates 2% of SAHs. It results from a failure of the pituitary to release ADH, despite an adequate osmotic stimulus to brain. Urine becomes inappropriately dilute, leading to depleted intravascular volume. This should be managed aggressively with fluid replacement and vasopressin or DDAVP to prevent the onset of symptomatic vasospasm.

Cardiac Considerations

Cardiac effects of SAH are common and form any part of the spectrum of cardiac disease, from asymptomatic ECG abnormalities to profound myocardial depression. ECG abnormalities are identified in up to 50% of patients and are more prevalent in poor-grade patients and, as a result, the prognosis of patients with ECG abnormalities and especially arrhythmias is often worse. These complications are attributed to sympathetic catecholamine release and posterior hypothalamic injury.

Pulmonary Complications

Pulmonary complications are the commonest medical complication, seen in 15% of SAH patients, and are responsible for half the deaths due to medical complications [9].

Pulmonary edema may be of cardiogenic or neurogenic origin. Neurogenic pulmonary edema consists of an irregular respiratory pattern, with pink frothy airway secretions high in protein content. It is seen in 2–6% of individuals, especially those in coma, and in 13% of cases of fatal SAH [9]. It is caused by disruption of the pulmonary capillary endothelium and increased pulmonary vascular permeability, thought to be caused by SAH-induced vasoconstriction, with a resultant shift of intravascular fluid from the systemic to pulmonary circulation. Cardiogenic pulmonary edema may result from SAH-induced cardiac failure, iatrogenically from fluid treatment for spasm (seen in up to 35% patients treated with "triple H" therapy for spasm) or myocardial infarction secondary to hypertensive therapy.

Screening

Screening for UIAs has major implications for both the individual at risk and the population as a whole. The financial cost of treatment on a per-case basis of aneurysmal SAH has been shown to be significantly greater than that of elective treatment of an UIA. Studies suggest that elective patients have a shorter length of stay and less associated morbidity and mortality, except Hunt and Hess Group V, where early mortality limits medical expenditure. This suggests that early detection and prophylactic occlusion of cerebral aneurysms may significantly reduce treatment costs. Any saving made, however, has to be balanced against the cost of treating lesions that, if left untreated, would never rupture and the cost of implementing such a screening programme.

In any screening programme, it is detection rather than characterization that is the goal. Until recently, DSA has been the only investigation with a satisfactory sensitivity and specificity for detecting aneurysms but it is costly, invasive and has associated risks and is therefore not suitable as a widely used mass screening tool. With neuroradiological advances, the use of MRA and CTA as screening investigations has been increasing. MRA involves no radiation or contrast and has no known risk to the patient, other than those associated with ferromagnetic implants. MRA is therefore preferred, particularly for patients with a history of adverse contrast reactions or at an increased risk of contrast toxicity. CTA, on the other hand, may prove to be better at screening for de-novo aneurysms in the presence of aneurysm clips. Any aneurysm identified by non-invasive methods can be further characterized by DSA.

The effectiveness of screening also depends on the temporal profile of aneurysm formation. If indeed aneurysms do arise over a relatively short time period, during which they are most likely to rupture, a single aneurysm screen may fail to identify the most hazardous lesions, resulting in a wholly ineffective screening program. Neurosurgeons and radiologists may then be left to treat a large number of stable aneurysms, many of which would never have ruptured.

Craniotomy for UIA has until recently been uniformly reported to yield excellent outcomes. These figures have recently been disputed by the ISUIA study results suggesting that mortality and morbidity may be as high as 14.4% [4]. This means that the impact of screening on aneurysm-related death and disability may be disappointing, particularly if the ISUIA results are shown to be nearer the truth.

It is currently less expensive to screen and treat any population of patients that has a minimum aneurysm prevalence of 5% and life expectancy of at least 20 years, assuming a 2% annual rupture rate for UIA, a screening cost of $500 for MRA and a combined mortality and morbidity of treatment of 5% or less. Endovascular treatment may reduce costs further if it is able to shorten hospital stay and therefore reduce costs. However, with its associated longer-term follow-up and higher risk of recurrence, the cost of repeat DSA and endovascular procedures means that this is not currently the case.

Schievink [23] currently recommends screening first-degree relatives aged 18–65 years once a familial aggregation has been established, as 10% of these individuals will have IAs and one-third of these lesions will be greater than 5 mm. In those who have a negative MRA, screening is undertaken 5-yearly to detect de-novo aneurysm formation. Those with affected siblings are screened biannually during the corresponding decade of life at which their sibling was diagnosed. Screening is only considered for children if family members aged less than 18 years have been affected and all monozygotic twins are screened. Screening for IAs in families with only one affected member is not recommended. These individuals have only a modest SAH risk and screening identifies UIAs in only 2–4%.

We currently need a better understanding of the natural history of aneurysm formation and results of treatment before firmer recommendations can be made.

Outcome

Mortality

Overall mortality of those reaching hospital has declined from 30% in the 1960s [24], to 20% in the 1980s [9,24], to its present level of 5–10% [25]. With it there has been a corresponding improvement in reported favorable outcome of 50% in the 1970s, to 70% in the 1980s [9,25], to 80% in the most recent series [25]. This trend has been seen in all age groups except the elderly. A population-based study showed no change in survival rates but an increase in the number of individuals making an independent outcome to 82% in 1980–7 compared to 64% in 1976–8. This improvement has been attributed to the early referral of patients to specialist units, advances in medical treatment and aggressive management to minimize the risks of re-bleeding and spasm, and particularly the practice of early surgery in good-grade patients.

Pre-hospital mortality is 3–26%, with an overall mortality of 45–60% in the first 30 days after SAH. The fatality rate decreases sharply after the hemorrhage: of all the deaths occurring during the first 3 months, the fatality rate is 61% in the first 2 days, 65% in the first week, 12% during the second week and 4% during the third week. Thereafter, the weekly fatalities up to 3 months average out at 1.6%[1]. Most deaths in the first 2 days (58%) are due to the initial ictus, whilst, after 3 days, 22–38% are due to a repeat bleed and a further significant proportion (23%) due to vasospasm [1]. Survival at 1 year is 52–62%.

Morbidity

Overall morbidity is quoted as 25–33%, caused in the majority of patients by spasm, although initial deficits and surgery also contribute [14]. A good outcome is seen in 50–83% of survivors and 23–52% of all patients suffering SAH [25]. Sixty-six percent of those individuals who have undergone aneurysm clipping never return to the same quality of life and only 23% of those with a good neurological outcome are employed at 1 year. These statistics have changed little over the last three decades. Results from clinical series are more optimistic, with 58% having a complete recovery [9] and 86% surviving with a Glasgow Outcome Score (GOS) of 1 or 2.

Predictors of Outcome

The most important predictive factor for ultimate outcome is the impact of the initial hemorrhage [1]. Approximately 40% of individuals die or are left disabled as a result of the initial hemorrhage; the remainder reaching hospital have the potential to go on to make a complete recovery.

Age and grade at hospital admission are uncontrollable factors but are good predictors of outcome. Although age alone should not be used as a basis for denial of treatment, mortality does appear to be higher in the elderly population, with a less favorable outcome and higher complication rate. Studies have shown a 7% mortality and 86% favorable outcome in ages 18–29 years but a 50% mortality and 26% favorable outcome in those over 70 [9,14], with a 5-year survival of 20% in the elderly. Survival is also related to blood pressure, days to admission from SAH, aneurysmal size, volume of blood on CT including ICH or IVH and vasospasm at admission. These are indicators of the severity of hemorrhage and of the presence of medical conditions that predict poor outcome. Patients with basilar aneurysms are three times more likely to die before medical attention and within the first 48 hours than those with anterior circulation aneurysms [9,14]. Individuals with a family history of aneurysmal SAH may also be at risk of a worse outcome. Independent predictors of a good outcome are youth, high GCS and absence of blood on CT.

Conclusions

Although the mortality and morbidity associated with SAH once patients have arrived at hospital is slowly decreasing, the incidence of SAH has changed little. Effective screening and management of patients at risk of aneurysmal SAH require a better understanding of risk factors, the pathogenesis of aneurysms and the natural history of aneurysmal development and rupture. Following rupture, successful outcome in these patients is dependent upon an accurate appreciation of the pathophysiological consequences of aneurysm rupture, close monitoring and prevention of medical complications and secondary cerebral insults. Much of the literature regarding SAH is conflicting and further research is needed to consolidate our knowledge, particularly in identification of "at-risk" groups and clarification of screening protocols, the pathogenesis and management of vasospasm and the role of endovascular treatments in the management of ruptured aneurysms.

Key Points

- *The prevalence of intracranial aneurysms is 0.2–7.9% in the general population, with an annual incidence of SAH of 10–20 per 100,000.*
- *Risks factors for SAH include female gender, family history, connective tissue diseases, smoking, hypertension and sympathomimetic drugs.*
- *Complications specific to SAH include rehemorrhage, vasospasm, hydrocephalus and electrolyte imbalance, particularly hyponatremia.*
- *Early repair of the aneurysm, either surgically or endovascularly, prevents re-bleeding and allows aggressive treatment of vasospasm.*
- *SAH has a high associated mortality and morbidity.*

References

1. Fogelholm R. Subarachnoid hemorrhage in middle-Finland: incidence, early prognosis and indications for neurosurgical treatment. Stroke 1981;12:296–301.
2. Inagawa T, Hirano A. Autopsy study of unruptured incidental intracranial aneurysms. Surg Neurol 1990; 34:361–5.
3. Kojima M, Gagasawa S, Lee Y-E, Takeichi Y, Tsuda E, Mabuchi N. Asymptomatic familial cerebral aneurysms. Neurosurgery 1998;43:776–81.
4. Anonymous. Unruptured intracranial aneurysms: risk of rupture and risks of surgical intervention. New Engl J Med 1998;339:1725–33.
5. Linn FH, Wijdicks EF, van der Graaf Y, Weerdesteyn-van Vliet FA, Bartelds AI, van Gijn J. Prospective study of sentinel headache in aneurysmal subarachnoid haemorrhage. Lancet 1994;344:590–3.
6. Hunt WE, Hess RM. Surgical risk as related to time of intervention in the repair of intracranial aneurysms. J Neurosurg 1968;28:14–20.

7. Drake CG. Report of World Federation of Neurosurgical Societies Committee on universal subarachnoid hemorrhage grading scale. J Neurosurg 1988;38:575–80.
8. Fisher CM, Kistler JP, Davis JM. Relation of cerebral vasospasm to subarachnoid hemorrhage visualized by computerized tomographic scanning. Neurosurgery 1980;6:1–9.
9. Kassell NF, Torner JC, Haley EC Jr, Jane JA, Adams HP, Kongable GL. The International Cooperative Study on the Timing of Aneurysm Surgery. Part 1: Overall management results. J Neurosurg 1990;73:18–36.
10. Huston JD Jr, Nichols DA, Luetmer PH, Goodwin JT, Meyer FB, Wiebers DO et al. Blinded prospective evaluation of sensitivity of MR angiography to known intracranial aneurysms: importance of aneurysm size. AJNR: Am J Neuroradiol 1994;15:1607–14.
11. Newell DW, LeRoux PD, Dacey RG Jr, Stimac GK, Winn HR. CT infusion scanning for the detection of cerebral aneurysms. J Neurosurg 1989;71:175–9.
12. Pickard JD, Murray GD, Illingworth R, Shaw MD, Teasdale GM, Foy PM et al. Effect of oral nimodipine on cerebral infarction and outcome after subarachnoid haemorrhage: British aneurysm nimodipine trial. BMJ 1989;298:636–42.
13. Haley EC Jr, Kassell NF, Torner JC. The International Cooperative Study on the Timing of Aneurysm Surgery: the North American experience. Stroke 1992;23:205–14.
14. Kassell NF, Torner JC, Jane JA, Haley EC Jr, Adams HP. The International Cooperative Study on the Timing of Aneurysm Surgery. Part 2: Surgical results. J Neurosurg 1990;73:37–47.
15. Todd NV, Tocher JL, Jones PA, Miller JD. Outcome following aneurysm wrapping: a 10-year follow-up review of clipped and wrapped aneurysms. J Neurosurg 1989;70:841–6.
16. Solomon RA, Fink ME, Pile-Spellman J. Surgical management of unruptured intracranial aneurysms. J Neurosurg 1994;80:440–6.
17. Guglielmi G, Vinuela F, Dion J, Duckwiler G. Electrothrombosis of saccular aneurysms via endovascular approach. Part 2: Preliminary clinical experience. J Neurosurg 1991;75:8–14.
18. International Subarachnoid Aneurysm Trial (ISAT) Collaborative Group. International Subarachnoid Aneurysm Trial (ISAT) of neurosurgical clipping versus endovascular coiling in 2143 patients with ruptured intracranial aneurysms: a randomised trial. Lancet 2002;360:1267–74.
19. Aaslid R, Markwalder TM, Nornes H. Noninvasive transcranial Doppler ultrasound recording of flow velocity in basal cerebral arteries. J Neurosurg 1982;57:769–74.
20. Kassell NF, Helm G, Simmons N, Phillips CD, Cail WS. Treatment of cerebral vasospasm with intra-arterial papaverine. J Neurosurg 1992;77:848–52.
21. Kassell NF, Torner JC. Aneurysmal rebleeding: a preliminary report from the Cooperative Aneurysm Study. Neurosurgery 1983;13:479–81.
22. Steinke D, Weir B, Disney L. Hydrocephalus following aneurysmal subarachnoid haemorrhage. Neurol Res 1987;9:3–9.
23. Schievink WI. Genetics and aneurysm formation. Neurosurg Clin N Am 1998;9:485–95.
24. Ingall TJ, Whisnant JP, Wiebers DO, O'Fallon WM. Has there been a decline in subarachnoid hemorrhage mortality? Stroke 1989;20:718–24.
25. Le Roux PD, Elliott JP, Downey L, Newell DW, Grady MS, Mayberg MR et al. Improved outcome after rupture of anterior circulation aneurysms: a retrospective 10-year review of 224 good-grade patients. J Neurosurg 1995;83:394–402.

19

Interventional Neuroradiology

Andrew G. Clifton

Summary

Endovascular neuroradiological techniques may be used to treat a wide range of vascular diseases, either in isolation, or as an adjunct to surgery or stereotactic radiosurgery. Techniques include balloon occlusion, embolization using Guglielmi detachable coils, liquid agents or particles, angioplasty and stenting. Rapid technological advancement in the field constantly expands the indications for endovascular treatment. Such treatment should only be undertaken in a neuroscience center, as part of a multidisciplinary team approach. Guidelines for treatment of the acutely ruptured aneurysm vary widely, but coil embolization is increasingly used as an alternative to surgical clipping to prevent early rebleeding. The long term efficacy is as yet unproven, and close follow up is advised. Carotid angioplasty, with or without stenting, is a promising alternative to carotid endarterectomy, but further trials are needed. The value of stents in the treatment of vertebral artery stenosis is uncertain.

Introduction

The indications and techniques for endovascular treatment of diseases of the CNS and head and neck continue to grow. This is in part due to the experience, skill and ingenuity of the interventionalists but also because of the rapid advancement and development of new catheters, wires, coils, balloons and embolic agents, as well as of the X-ray hardware. Biplane and 3-D low-dose digital fluoroscopy and angiography are now commonplace. Because of rapid changes in catheters and embolic agents, this chapter will be a mere snapshot in the evolving story of interventional neuroradiology. As will be described below, endovascular neuroradiological techniques can be used to treat the whole gamut of vascular diseases, either as a sole treatment or cure or as an adjunct to conventional neurosurgery. The techniques should only be carried out by a physician with specific training in interventional neurovascular procedures [1]. When treating neurovascular disease, a multi-disciplinary team approach is the ideal, with the involvement of neurointerventionalist, neurosurgeon, neurologist and neurointensivist.

Principles and Techniques (Tools)

All neurointerventional procedures should be performed in a neuroscience center where there is full surgical (neurosurgical, vascular, and otolaryngology) and neurointensive care back-up. The angiography suite should be digital, ideally biplane. The digital package should include live digital fluoroscopy, as well as road mapping. There should be the facility to perform general anesthesia. Many procedures, such as balloon occlusion, are performed with the patient awake. However, many, such as GDC coiling of aneurysms, are performed under general anesthesia. Ideally, an anesthesiologist should be present for all procedures (even when the patient is awake) but at a minimum should be readily available should the patient not be able to co-operate fully and the procedure need to be converted to general anesthesia.

Consenting

The majority of neurointerventional procedures carry risks of significant morbidity and mortality. The procedure, its risks, its benefits, the goals of treatments (i.e. cure, as an adjunct to surgery) should be fully explained to the patient and, ideally, to the relatives, as they are the ones who "pick up the pieces" should a complication arise. If possible, particularly if a non-acute procedure such as embolization of an AVM or angioplasty of the carotid is to be performed, the patient should be seen as an outpatient and be given time for the information to be taken in and its implications realized. It is not acceptable to obtain consent from a patient on the angio table or in the corridor outside.

Technique

Vascular access is usually gained via the femoral route, although, in certain circumstances, a direct carotid or brachial puncture can be used to facilitate access where vessels are very tortuous. After femoral puncture using the Seldinger technique, a femoral sheath of appropriate size for the guiding catheter is inserted. For most procedures, the patient is then fully heparinized with 5,000iu or 70iu per kg. Ideally, an activated clotting time (ACT) monitor should be in situ in the angiographic suite and the ACT ratio maintained at two to three times normal, depending on the procedure. Full angiography is carried out as appropriate for planning the procedure. The vessel needed to access the lesion (for example, the left internal carotid artery for a left middle cerebral artery aneurysm) is selected and a guiding catheter exchanged into this vessel.

Hemostasis

Once the procedure has finished, it is very important to obtain adequate hemostasis. If the anticoagulation has been adequately reversed, usually with the appropriate dosage of protamine and reference to the ACT ratios, manual pressure may be adequate. However, with the use of larger sheaths, 8 and 9 French, and with continued heparinization, the incidence of hematoma and post-procedure bleeding increases. Rarely, this can lead to emergency open surgical closure of the puncture site and/or marked hypotension, hypovolemia or even death. Devices such as the Fem-stop (Radi-Medical Systems), which is a mechanical pressure device kept at just below arterial pressure, and the Angio-Seal (Sherwood, Davis and Geck, Gosport, Hampshire) have much improved the management of hemostasis post-procedure. The Angio-Seal is easily deployable and consists of a delivery kit and three completely bioresorbable components. Deployment of the device allows mobilization of the patient, if clinically appropriate, after 1–2 hours and obviates the need for prolonged observation of the groin puncture site.

Endovascular Treatment of Intracranial Aneurysms

Occlusion of Aneurysms Using Detachable Balloons

Indications

This technique is performed by sacrifice of the parent artery [2]. To reduce the risk of stroke from the procedure, prior test occlusion of the artery is carried out. The main indications for this form of treatment are symptomatic cavernous carotid aneurysms (treatment is not usually indicated for those picked up coincidentally on MRI or at angiography) or giant aneurysms below the bifurcation of the internal carotid artery not amenable to conventional neurosurgical treatment or unsuitable for treatment with a GDC coil. Other indications for parent artery sacrifice include treatment of carotid cavernous fistula and occlusion of segments of the carotid artery prior to major head and neck surgery. Giant vertebral or basilar artery aneurysms may also be treated by parent artery sacrifice, with consequent reversal of flow through the circle of Willis and thrombosis of the aneurysm.

Test Occlusion

Prior to permanent balloon occlusion, a test occlusion must be performed. Many methods are advocated to assess the efficacy of the intracranial collateral circulation following test occlusion. These include transcranial Doppler ultrasound, Xenon CT, ^{133}Xenon SPECT, ^{99M}Technetium hexamethyl-propyleneamine oxide (HMPAO) SPECT, PET, EEG monitoring, somatosensory evoked potential monitoring, retinal artery pressure measurement and hypotensive challenge. Many of these techniques are, however, complex and time-consuming and cannot be used without transferring the patient from the angio suite [3,4].

The method described here is practiced by the author and is similar to the technique widely practiced in the UK. The patient should be awake and only sedated by a mild intravenous neuroleptic anesthetic agent, such as 5–10 mg diazemuls. Intravenous access with a wide-bore cannula is mandatory. After insertion of bilateral femoral sheaths, the patient is anticoagulated by using intravenous heparin. After anticoagulation, its adequacy is assessed by estimation of the ACT, which should be 2–3 times baseline.

A 7 or 8 French guide catheter is placed in the internal carotid artery supplying the aneurysm or lesion and a non-detachable balloon (e.g. NDSB 1505 Boston Scientific) is inflated as near as possible to the site of permanent occlusion, i.e. near the aneurysm neck, and inflated under road mapping to occlude the artery. Careful clinical assessment is then carried out for up to 30 minutes (ideally by a neurologist or physician, independently from the operator). If neurological symptoms develop, the balloon is immediately deflated. If the patient is asymptomatic, an injection is made into the contralateral internal carotid artery (or vertebral) to assess angiographic collateral flow (Fig. 19.1). There should be a delay of no more than 1 s in venous phase appearance when comparing the occluded side with the opposite injected side. Transcranial Doppler monitoring of middle cerebral artery flow may also be used. As long as decrease in flow does not exceed 30% and the patient passes the other two tests, it is safe to occlude the artery [5].

Permanent Occlusion

Provided the patient passes all three tests, we proceed to permanent occlusion. The temporary balloon is deflated and removed and replaced by a detachable balloon. This is placed in the same position as the non-detachable balloon, i.e. as near to the neck of the aneurysm as possible. The second balloon is then placed proximal to the first balloon. The patient is then transferred to an ICU or HDU for post-procedure care.

Post-operative Care

Post-operative care, particularly during the first 48 hours, is as important as the test occlusion in preventing complications. Hypotension must be prevented and blood pressure therefore continuously monitored. The patient is kept on flat bed rest for 24 hours and kept well hydrated. If symptoms develop, the blood pressure is elevated using inotropes. The patient's blood volume is expanded. If the patient remains asymptomatic, the bed head is elevated and the patient gradually mobilized over the next 5 days. Equally important is the prevention of embolic ischemia. Heparin is continued IV for 48 hours and aspirin commenced.

Complications

Complication rates, including permanent neurological deficit, should be less than 5% if the above regimen is carried out. For example, tying off a carotid artery without test occlusion can cause stroke in the region of 26% of patients [6], whereas figures of 0–5% are reported after test occlusion [3,6,7].

Failure of Test Occlusion

If a patient does fail the temporary occlusion test, extracranial/intracranial (EC/IC) bypass can be performed. I have found this to work only if the patient has barely failed any of the three tests, i.e. failed the clinical test at 20 minutes, or with slight delay in venous return, or passing the clinical test with minor decrease in transcranial Doppler flow by significantly

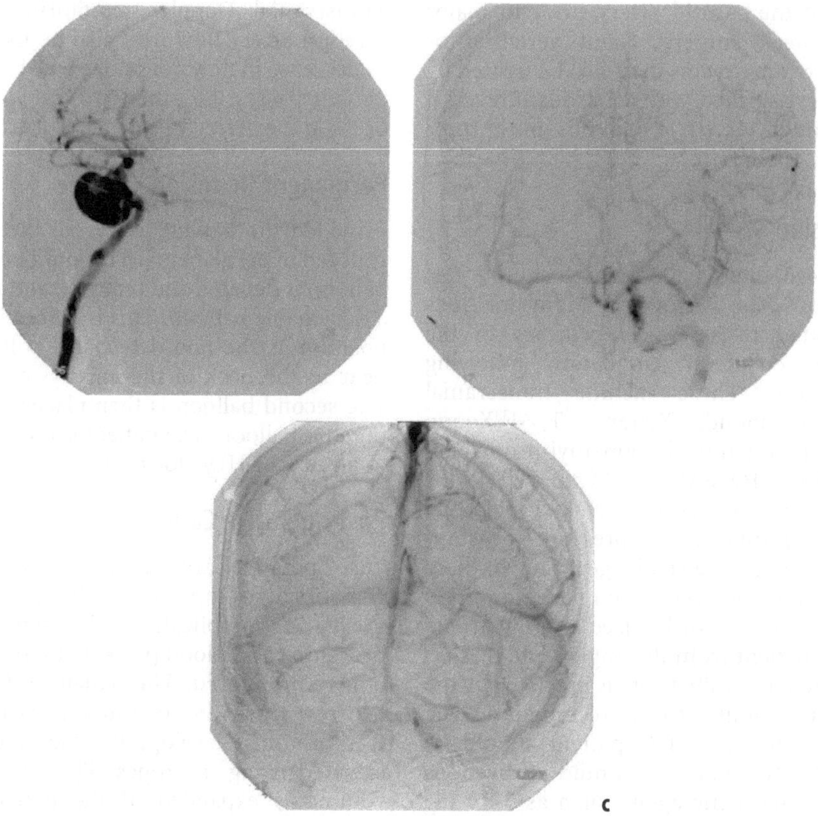

Fig. 19.1. a Right carotid angiogram, showing a large right cavernous aneurysm. **b** Contralateral left carotid angiogram with balloon inflated in the right internal carotid artery, showing excellent crossflow across the anterior communicating artery from the left to fill the right middle cerebral artery. **c** Venous phase of the same angiogram showing symmetrical venous filling.

greater than 50%. If there is an instant failure on occlusion, EC/IC bypass in my experience does not work. There may be a case for direct high-flow bypass here.

Embolization of Aneurysms Using the Guglielmi Detachable Coil

Packing of an aneurysm sac with embolic material to isolate it from the parent vessel whilst preserving the adjacent cerebral circulation is the ideal goal. The occlusion should be permanent, with no recurrence. In the past, embolization of the sac has been performed with balloons, free coils and occasionally liquid agents, but with poor results. Currently, detachable coils, either electrolytic or mechanical, are used. There are many coils on the market but most widely used is the Guglielmi detachable coil. There is vast clinical experience with this and the discussion below shall be confined to this coil [8–11].

It should be noted that endovascular treatment is in continuing evolution and devices such as aneurysm liners, neck bridges, stents and liquid agents are all in experimental use and are now being evaluated on patients in clinical trials. They will certainly find a role in aneurysm treatment in the next decade.

Indications for Treatment

Guidelines for treatment of the acutely ruptured aneurysm vary from center to center and country to country. In some centers, virtually all coilable aneurysms are treated endovascularly and in others all surgically. It is best to employ a multidisciplinary approach with each individual patient, the aneurysm in question being discussed by the neurosurgeon and interventional neuroradiologist. In general, however, GDC is favored in the following circumstances:

Posterior Circulation Aneurysms

Surgical morbidity/mortality for posterior circulation aneurysms is higher than that for anterior circulation aneurysms and may require invasive approaches through the skull base. Morbidity for GDC treatment is similar for both anterior and posterior circulation aneurysms.

Frail or Very Elderly Patients

In frail or very elderly patients at high risk from craniotomy or patients of poor grade: endovascular packing can prevent re-bleeding and allow more aggressive treatment of vasospasm; treatment options at other sites are more controversial. The GDC was initially used to treat aneurysms not suitable for surgery (those thought to be of high surgical risk). It was soon found, however, that coiling small aneurysms that were suitable for surgery had the lowest morbidity and best results.

Anterior Communicating Artery Aneurysms

Opinions amongst neuroradiologists and neurosurgeons vary widely, even in individual centers. There is controversy as to whether neurosurgical treatment of anterior communicating artery aneurysms causes more neuropsychological damage than coiling, or whether damage is due to the hematoma from rupture of the aneurysm itself. Wiebers, in his recent publication on the natural history and treatment of unruptured aneurysms [12], showed significant neuropsychological deficit in patients undergoing elective clipping. There is also controversy as to whether patients undergoing coiling experience less vasospasm than those undergoing surgery [13]. Many centers thus choose coiling for suitable anterior communicating artery aneurysms.

Middle Cerebral Artery Aneurysms

Middle cerebral artery aneurysms have complex anatomy and it is often difficult, because of this anatomy, to adequately image and preserve normal branches during coiling. The consequences of a large MCA stroke are also dire, with 40–50% mortality. Many centers, including ours, do not coil MCA aneurysms unless the patient is elderly or of poor grade.

Posterior Communicating Artery Aneurysms

Posterior communicating artery aneurysms are technically straightforward to clip and usually to coil. Despite the fact that the GDC was first used in 1990 and over 20,000 patients worldwide have been treated, only case series have been presented and published. Case series are unreliable and can be biased, particularly if the operator (surgeon and neuroradiologist) reports the case series [14].

The best way to determine the difference between two treatment modalities is to conduct a prospective randomised control trial. The International Subarachnoid Aneurysm Trial was the first multi-centre prospective randomised clinical trial comparing neurosurgical clipping and endovascular coil treatment for patients with a ruptured cerebral aneurysm causing acute subarachnoid haemorrhage. This was funded primarily by the Medical Research Council, UK. The pilot phase commenced in 1994 and ISAT actively commenced centre recruitment in January 1997, with the aim of enrolling up to 3,000 patients. The ISAT steering committee halted recruitment in May 2002 at 2,143 patients after an interim analysis by the independent data monitoring committee showed a clear advantage to the coiling technique. Follow-up data was available on 1,594 patients overall. 27.2% were dead or dependent, with 30.6% in the neurosurgery arm and 23.7% in the endovascular arm, representing a 22.6% relative risk reduction and a 6.9% absolute risk reduction in the endovascular arm. The overall mortality rate was similar between the two groups, with a 10.1% of the neurosurgical group having died and 8.1% of the endovascular group. What this means for patients in the future is that potentially out of 100 patients treated, around 7 could expect to be better off one year on if they receive endovascular treatment rather than surgery. For many patients, this could be the difference between a return to normal life or substantial disability. Although there has been substantial debate about this trial, particularly about the durability of coiling and the small re-bleed rate, this trial has already impacted on clinical practice in the UK, Europe and the United States. Many centres now choose coiling as the preferred method of treatment of ruptured aneurysms but the debate continues [14a].

Technique

Guglielmi detachable coils consist of a soft platinum coil attached by solder to a stainless steel delivery wire. This allows an individual coil to be repositioned or removed from an aneurysm under fluoroscopic control should its position or size not be correct or optimal. Various coils are available. They vary in the size of the helical diameter (2–20 mm) and length. The diameter of the core wire and primary coil also comes in two sizes: the GDC 10 and the GDC 18. More flexible or soft coils have been developed. A 2-D coil is also available, designed to prevent the first loop of the coil herniating out of the aneurysm into the parent artery. With this coil, the first one-and-a-half loops' helical diameter is smaller than the rest of the coil. A 3-D coil is also available, with a complex shape designed to better pack larger wider-necked aneurysms so that wide-necked aneurysms can be treated.

During the procedure, which is performed under general anesthetic, we aim to maintain heparinization at two to three times baseline. Heparinization prevents intra-arterial thrombosis, which can occur in up to 8% of procedures if unheparinized [15]. Should perioperative rupture occur, heparin can immediately be reversed with protamine sulphate IV [16].

Once the guide catheter is in situ, a microcatheter over a wire is navigated into the aneurysm. The aneurysm is sized, usually using a UK penny or US dime placed on the patient's head. This allows for magnification to a certain degree. The first coil selected should have a helical diameter near the diameter of the aneurysmal sac and be as long as feasible. A

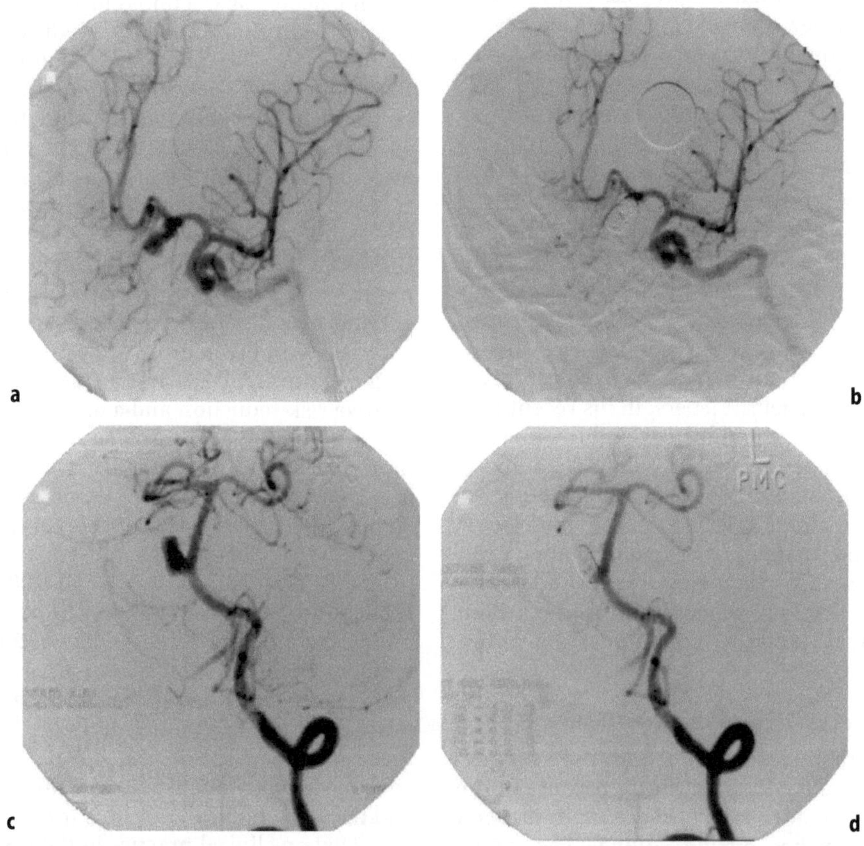

Fig. 19.2. **a** Left internal carotid angiogram, showing large lobular right anterior communicating artery aneurysm. **b** Angiogram showing total occlusion of the aneurysm post-coiling with 5 GDC coils. **c** Left vertebral angiogram, showing a lobular aneurysm arising from the basilar trunk at the origin of the anterior inferior cerebellar artery (AICA). **d** Appearance post-coiling, with preservation of the AICA.

dense packing of the aneurysm is achieved by using additional coils of reduced diameter and length (Fig. 19.2). Some operators advocate that the last coil should be one that is thrown away, i.e. the packing is so dense that the last coil will not fit in the aneurysm.

Post-operative Care

Post-procedure, there is no consensus on heparinization. Some centers continue IV heparin for 48 hours and prescribe aspirin orally. At our center, we do not reverse the heparin but allow it to wear off. We do not continue heparin post-procedure unless coil is seen to protrude into the parent vessel.

Post-operatively, patients should be nursed in an ICU or HDU for at least 48 hours, and longer, obviously, if their clinical grade warrants.

Results

In the initial series of 735 aneurysms treated with GDCs presented for FDA evaluation, the procedure was successful in 75% of cases, with a greater than 90% occlusion of the lumen. Seventy-three percent of the treated patients had good outcomes. The overall morbidity/mortality was 14%. This series was, however, influenced by patient selection. The patients were required to be poor surgical candidates [17].

More recent series [10,18–20] show that ruptured aneurysms may be treated, with better or similar outcomes to surgical series.

According to Cognard et al. [10], 208 patients with 236 intracranial aneurysms underwent endovascular coil embolization. One hundred and fifty patients had SAH at the time of presentation. Follow-up in 152 aneurysms demonstrated total occlusion in 123, subtotal occlusion in 26 and incomplete occlusion in 3. Technique-related morbidity was 4% (seven patients with permanent neurological deficits due to clotting) and mortality 2% (peri-operative rupture in two, hematoma due to urokinase perfusion in one, re-bleeding of the initial hematoma after excessive uncontrolled anticoagulation in one). Re-bleeding occurred in one patient after incomplete occlusion.

A prospective randomized study from Finland [19] included 109 patients with acute (less than 72 hours) SAH caused by ruptured aneurysm. All were suitable candidates for both endovascular and surgical treatment and were randomly assigned to undergo coil embolization. Significantly better primary angiographic results were obtained after surgery in patients with anterior cerebral aneurysms, and after endovascular treatment in those with posterior circulation aneurysms, with no significant difference seen in patients with middle cerebral artery aneurysms. Early re-bleeding occurred after incomplete coil embolization. The technique-related mortality was 4% in the surgical group and 2% in the endovascular group. Clinical outcome (Glasgow outcome score) at 3 months was not significantly different between treatment groups in terms of intended treatment modality.

Recurrence

There are many unresolved questions in relation to endovascular therapy. Whilst GDC coiling, even partial, undoubtedly prevents re-bleeding in the short term, in the long term, efficacy is not yet known, particularly the long-term re-bleeding rate. At best, the late recurrence is converted into an unruptured aneurysm. There is further controversy as recent papers [12,21] suggest that the rupture rate of an unruptured aneurysm is low and treatment unjustified.

Complete obliteration is observed in 50–80% of aneurysms with endovascular treatment. After surgery, complete occlusion is observed in 94% of aneurysms [22]. The risk of hemorrhage from incompletely occluded, surgically treated aneurysms is thought to be less than 1% per year.

The mechanisms of occlusion of an aneurysm by clipping and by coiling are obviously different. In a clipped aneurysm rest, the walls are closely apposed and the remaining aneurysm is completely excluded from the circulation [22]. In contrast, using the endovascular technique, the walls are kept apart by the coils, allowing blood to flow into the sac. In the long term, remnants lead to recurrence. Malesh [15] followed up 100 patients who underwent embolization of 104 aneurysms. Mid-term outcome was obtained for 94 patients (2–6 years, average 3.5 years). Twenty patients required further non-GDC procedures (clipping in 9, parent artery sacrifice in 11).

Follow-up

Our policy is to follow patients with angiography at 6 months and, if the aneurysm is stable and occluded, a further follow up at 2 years.

A paper by Byrne et al. [23] records their 5-year experience using coil embolization for ruptured intracranial aneurysms and looks at outcomes and the incidence of late re-bleeding. In their study during the 5-year period, 317 patients presenting with aneurysmal subarachnoid hemorrhage were successfully treated by coil embolization within 30 days of hemorrhage. The authors followed patients to assess the stability of aneurysm occlusion and its longer-term efficacy in protecting patients against re-bleeding. They showed stable angiographic filling in 86.4% of small and 85.2% of large aneurysms, with recurrent filling in 38 (14.7% of 259 aneurysms). Re-bleeding was caused by aneurysmal recurrence in four patients and by rupture of a coincidental untreated aneurysm in one patient. Annual re-bleeding rates were 0.8% in the first year, 0.6% in the second year and 2.4% in the third year after aneurysm embolization, with no re-bleeding in subsequent years. Re-bleeding occurred in 3 (7.9%) of 38 recurrent aneurysms and in 1 (0.4%) of 220 aneurysms that appeared stable on angiography.

They also state in a discussion of their paper that coil compaction and aneurysm recurrence take time, usually greater than 6 months, to develop. We and others have also observed the fact that coiled aneurysms may appear stable at 6 months and even at the 2-year angiogram, but may re-grow at a later date. Thus, close follow up is strongly advisable.

Embolization of Arteriovenous Malformations

Intracranial arteriovenous malformations remain some of the most challenging lesions to treat by endovascular therapy. They may present with any number of symptoms, including seizures, headache, progressive neurological deficit or intracranial hemorrhage. They are increasingly being detected, particularly on MRI, as an incidental finding when the patient is being scanned for some unrelated reason.

Treatment of AVMs should always be multidisciplinary, with input from the neuroradiologist, neurosurgeon and the radiotherapist. Treatment can consist of embolization, surgery or stereotactic radiosurgery, or a combination of embolization followed by surgery or radiotherapy [24]. The goal of treatment is complete cure. Each patient is different. Factors to take into consideration include age, site (is the AVM in an eloquent area?), size, number of feeding arteries and presenting symptoms. It must never be forgotten that conservative treatment is always an option, particularly for elderly patients and for some large AVMs in eloquent areas.

Technique

AVM embolization can be performed under local or general anesthesia. This is dependent upon the co-operation of the patient and preference of the neuroradiologist. If the patient is co-operative, I perform AVM embolization with the patient awake. With flow-guided catheters, minor neuroleptic analgesia, such as diazemuls IV, is often adequate. With over-the-wire catheters, agents with a short half-life, such as propofol, are administered. These stronger agents are given under the supervision of an anesthesiologist, with standard monitoring of pulse, blood pressure and pulse oximetry.

Provocative Testing

The use of provocative testing is controversial, with many, particularly European, authorities believing it to be unnecessary. However, other, particularly American, authorities consider it useful. I personally perform provocative testing when embolizing AVMs in eloquent areas such as primary motor cortex, language cortex and occipital cortex [25].

With the catheter in a satisfactory position for potential embolization, 40–50 mg of sodium amytal is injected. If a temporary deficit occurs, embolization is not performed. A positive test indicates normal cortex has been perfused. The test remains controversial and many find the anatomical information as good as the physiological from provocative testing.

Embolic Agents

The most commonly used liquid embolic agent is glue. It is a liquid that, when in contact with blood (hydroxyl ions), rapidly polymerizes. The most commonly used glue is N-butyl cyanoacrylate. Glue is injected with lipiodol, an oily contrast medium that not only opacifies the mixture (it is highly radio-opaque) but also slows polymerization. A ratio of 80% glue:20% oil polymerizes very rapidly and such a concentration would only be used in high-flow fistulas. Common concentrations used are 30–60% glue. Flow-guided catheters or over-the-wire catheters can be used. The goal is to occlude the nidus without obstructing venous outflow, which can cause hemorrhage or refluxing into normal vessels.

Once the glue has been injected, the catheter is rapidly pulled or removed to prevent it being glued in place. The catheter is flushed with 5% dextrose to prevent polymerization of glue in the catheter prior to glue injection. Glue embolization is thought to be permanent (Fig. 19.3).

Onyx is a liquid agent increasingly used instead of glue. It consists of ethylene vinyl alcohol copolymer dissolved in the solvent DMSO. It has the advantage of solidifying slowly, allowing better penetration of the nidus. Other agents, such as polyvinyl alcohol particles, silk sutures or micro-coils, are very effective but are strictly for use pre-surgery, as AVMs recanalize after use of these agents.

Complications

Various complication rates are reported in the literature. A very honest appraisal of complications is given in a paper by Wikholm et al. [26]. They present their consecutive series of 150 endovascularly treated arteriovenous

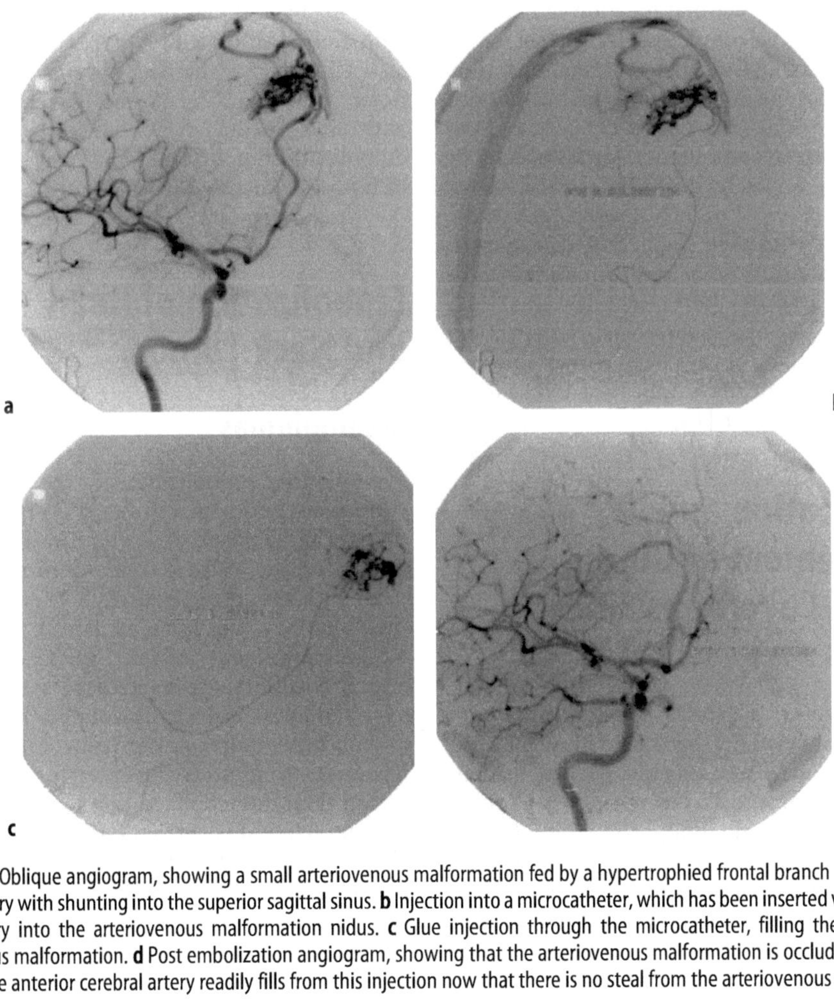

Fig. 19.3. a Oblique angiogram, showing a small arteriovenous malformation fed by a hypertrophied frontal branch of the anterior cerebral artery with shunting into the superior sagittal sinus. **b** Injection into a microcatheter, which has been inserted via the internal carotid artery into the arteriovenous malformation nidus. **c** Glue injection through the microcatheter, filling the nidus of the arteriovenous malformation. **d** Post embolization angiogram, showing that the arteriovenous malformation is occluded by the glue injection. The anterior cerebral artery readily fills from this injection now that there is no steal from the arteriovenous malformation.

malformation patients, most embolizations being performed with glue. A variety of catheters were used. Their mortality rate was 1.3%, and their overall complication rate was nearly 40% (severe 6.6%, moderate 15.3%, slight 17.3%). All the complications occurred in less than 4 days and those were directly related to the procedure. Hemorrhage was found in 14 patients, dissection in 4 patients, vasospasm in 2 patients, untoward embolization of normal brain feeders in 7 patients and thromboembolic complications on the arterial side in 5 patients. No venous occlusion occurred.

No predictors for complications were found, with no difference in rates of complications in relation to the size, location or number of treatment sessions, though they found lower complication rates for arteriovenous malformations of less than 30 mm in diameter. Of particular importance is the fact that location in eloquent areas was not accompanied by an increased incidence of complications after embolization. They occluded the arteriovenous malformations totally in 13.3%, 75% of patients were completely treated in combination with stereotactic radiosurgery and a further 10% were operated on.

With respect to their high complication rate, first, the arteriovenous malformations were large and, second, their complications were assessed strictly by a neurologist, independent assessment having always been shown to give a more "honest" rate of complication than assessment by the operator [14].

Embolization and Management of Dural Carotid Cavernous Sinus Fistulas

Carotid cavernous fistulas are abnormal connections between the carotid artery and the cavernous sinus. They may be bilateral. Presentation is with proptosis, chemosis, retro-orbital pain, bruit and ophthalmoplegia. These lesions may have cranial nerve palsies as their most prominent or sole clinical manifestation [27].

Fistulas may be direct or indirect. Direct fistulas are usually secondary to trauma, often with a single, direct communication between the ICA and cavernous sinus. Indirect fistulas are usually supplied by dural branches of the external carotid artery (ECA) but dural ICA branches may contribute.

Treatment

For direct fistulas, transarterial balloon occlusion is the best option. Detachable balloons can be flow-directed through the fistula with the balloon lodged in the sinus. It is inflated to a larger volume than the fistulous hole, sealing it and preventing prolapse of the balloon back onto the parent vessel. If this fails, transvenous occlusion of the fistula with coils may be attempted. If this fails, occlusion of the ICA may be necessary: this is carried out after test occlusion [28].

With indirect fistulas, if the supply is solely from the ECA, it may be possible to achieve cure with embolization with PVA particles. If there is also ICA supply, the best approach is transvenous embolization of the cavernous sinus with coils [29]. Fig. 19.4 illustrates successful embolization of a dural fistula fed by branches of both external and internal carotid arteries.

Embolization of Head and Neck Tumors

Meningiomas

Pre-operative embolization of meningiomas is commonly performed in the USA, but rarely in the UK and Europe. It is not always necessary, as the feeding arteries to many tumors can be dealt with at surgical approach. Most convexity meningiomas are vascular, whilst many skull base meningiomas are relatively avascular.

Embolization in selected cases is undoubtedly very beneficial, reducing pre-operative bleeding and allowing better tumor control. Devascularized cases usually have less need for blood transfusion than unembolized cases [30].

Embolization is carried out using PVA particles to the tumor bed, using progressively larger particles of 50–150 μ followed by 150–250 μ. Care should be taken to look for hidden anastomoses. The main distal feeding vessel can then be occluded by coils.

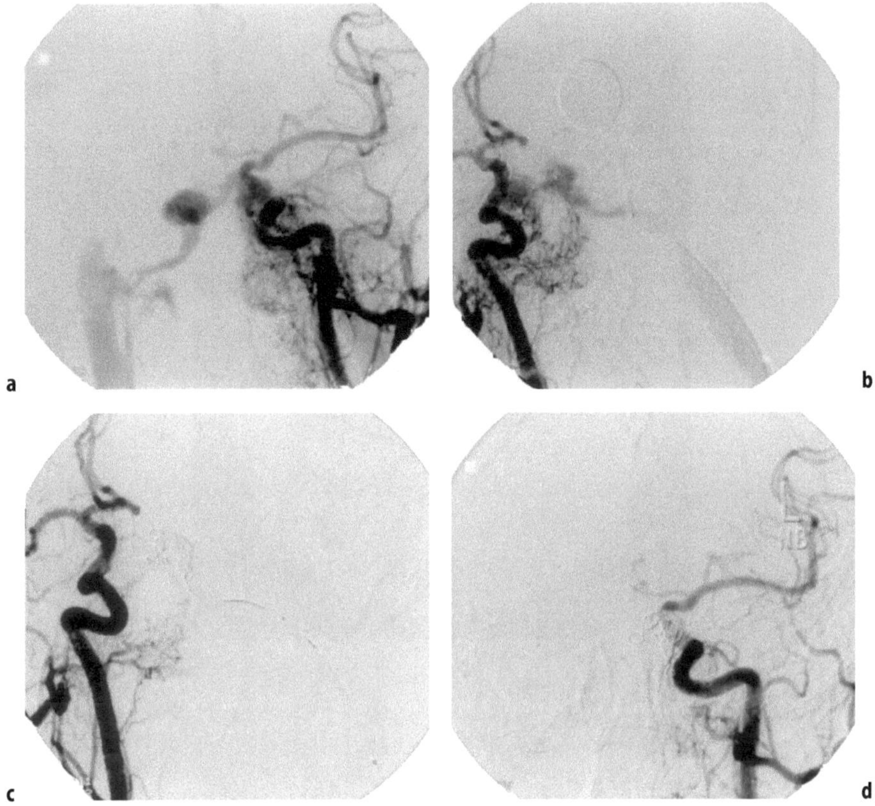

Fig. 19.4. a Left common carotid angiogram, showing a dural fistula which was fed by branches of the external and internal carotid arteries, with shunting into the left cavernous sinus but filling of both cavernous sinuses, with the drainage into both internal jugular veins via the inferior petrosal sinuses. **b** A guiding catheter in the left internal jugular vein and a microcatheter with two tips inserted via the inferior petrosal sinus into the left cavernous sinus. An intra-arterial injection has been made into the right ICA to show the fistula. **c** Insertion of platinum coils into the left cavernous sinus. **d** Post-insertion of micro coils, left carotid injection showing occlusion of the fistula.

Pre-operative embolization is also useful for treatment of juvenile nasopharyngeal angiofibromas, paragangliomas and vertebral body tumors, particularly metastases from the kidney and thyroid.

Fig. 19.5 illustrates embolization of a vascular meningioma.

Carotid and Vertebral Angioplasty and Stenting

Carotid and vertebral angioplasty plus or minus stenting is a relatively new technique and its use remains controversial. Stroke is the third most common cause of death in the UK and atherosclerotic stenosis of the carotid artery close to the carotid bifurcation in the neck causes about 10% of all strokes and transient ischemic attacks. In patients who have had recurrent symptoms associated with severe carotid stenosis, the risk of recurrent stroke over the next 2 years is 20% or more if treated medically and is thought to be greater in patients with very severe stenosis. It may be as high as 28%.

The benefits of secondary prevention in symptomatic patients have recently been convincingly established by the European Carotid Surgery Trial (ECST) [31] and the North American Symptomatic Carotid Endarterectomy Trial (NASCET) [32], showing that the

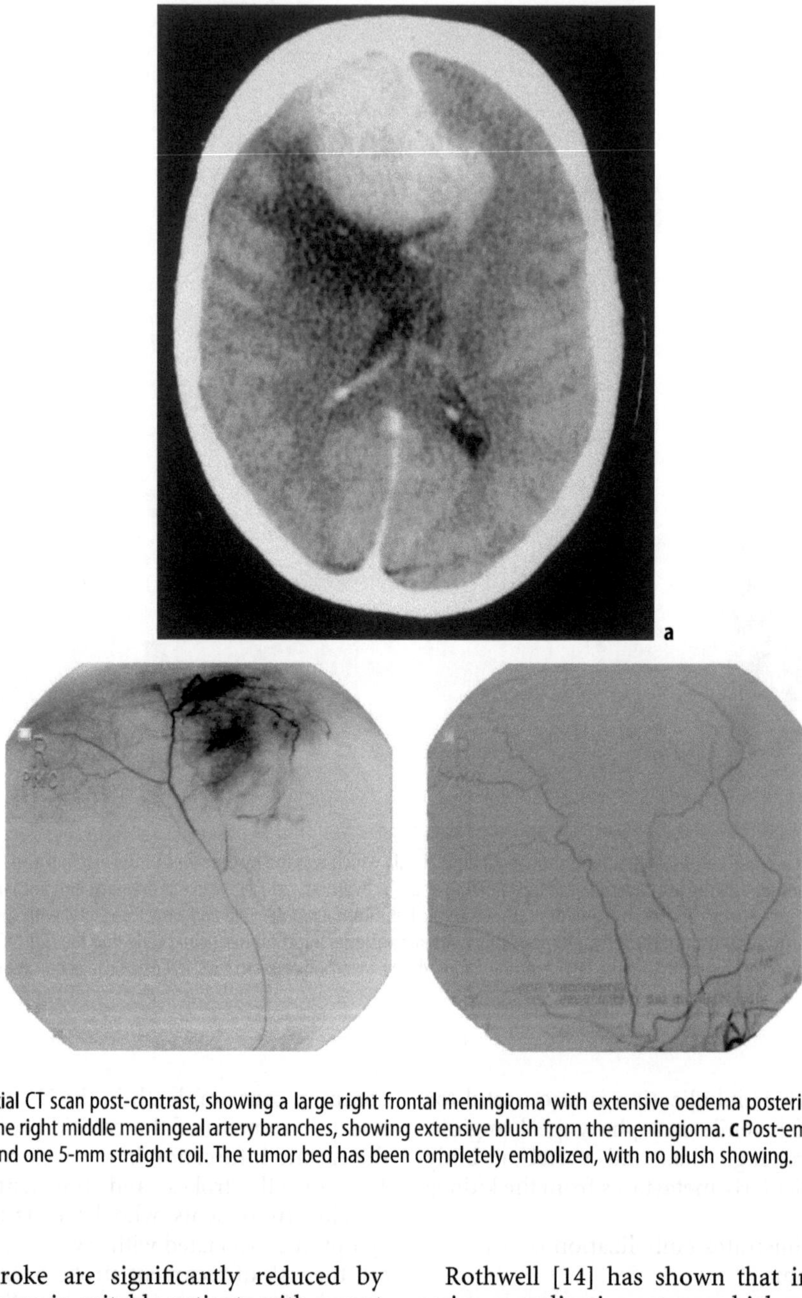

Fig. 19.5. **a** Axial CT scan post-contrast, showing a large right frontal meningioma with extensive oedema posteriorly. **b** Selective injection into the right middle meningeal artery branches, showing extensive blush from the meningioma. **c** Post-embolization with PVA particles and one 5-mm straight coil. The tumor bed has been completely embolized, with no blush showing.

risks of stroke are significantly reduced by carotid surgery in suitable patients with recent symptoms and severe carotid stenosis greater than 70%. These trials establish carotid endarterectomy as a standard treatment for severe symptomatic carotid artery stenosis but not without risk. NASCET had a perioperative stroke and death rate of 5.8% and ECST 7.5%. The risks of surgery are even higher in other reported series (see chapter on ischemic stroke).

Rothwell [14] has shown that in published series, complication rates are highest where they have been assessed by an independent observer, with lower rates from single-author surgeons reporting their own series. Randomized prospective trials probably give the most accurate assessment of risk and benefit.

For asymptomatic stenosis, the risks and benefits are finely balanced. Surgery reduces the risk of stroke by around 30%, with a wide confidence interval from 10 to 50%. Although this relative reduction in stroke risk seems impressive, the absolute benefit is small because the risk of stroke without surgery for asymptomatic stenosis is so low. It is necessary to operate on 50 patients to prevent one stroke, implying a perioperative complication rate of 2%. This is not always achievable, even in the best hands. Charles Warlow, in a *BMJ* editorial in 1998 [33], concludes that for most patients receiving average treatment, the argument is against surgery for asymptomatic carotid stenosis. This argument is easily extrapolated to carotid angioplasty plus or minus stenting.

There are many disadvantages to conventional surgery apart from the perioperative stroke risk. Risks include myocardial infarction, pulmonary embolism, pneumonia, deep vein thrombosis, the side effects of anesthesia and the discomfort of intubation. Cranial nerve palsy also carries risks of significant morbidity, particularly involving the hypoglossal nerve. One of these complications affects at least 10% of patients after carotid endarterectomy.

Whether percutaneous transluminal angioplasty (PTA) plus or minus stenting of the carotid has a place in the routine management of carotid atherosclerosis is still very controversial. There is need for further, ideally randomized, trials between surgery and endovascular treatments. Primary stenting is favored over angioplasty. PTA plus or minus stenting for carotid stenosis has the great advantage of being performed under local anesthesia, avoiding the perils of general anesthesia and the discomfort of an incision in the neck. Carotid angioplasty and stenting can be performed under minimal neuroleptic analgesia and, apart from occasional transient pain on inflation of the balloon, the discomfort of a successful angioplasty is no more than that associated with routine angiography. The patient can be discharged after 24 hours or, in some centers, if the patient is fit, the procedure can be performed as a day case.

The only randomized clinical trial to investigate the risks and benefits of PTA for carotid stenosis in comparison with conventional surgery, the Carotid and Vertebral Artery Transluminal Angioplasty Study (CAVATAS), finished in 1997 [33a]. The trial randomized over 500 patients between surgery and angioplasty between 1992 and 1997. There was no significant difference in the risk of stroke or death related to the procedure between surgery and angioplasty. The rate of any stroke lasting more than 7 days or death within 30 days of first treatment was approximately 10% in both the surgery and endovascular groups. Preliminary analysis of long-term survival showed no difference in the rate of ipsilateral stroke or any disabling stroke in patients up to 3 years after randomization. In CAVATAS, the rates of stroke and death within 30 days in both groups are higher than those reported in the literature but not significantly different from ECST (rate of 7.5%). Long-term follow up is not yet available. Hopefully, centers will continue to follow up CAVATAS-enrolled patients. Long-term 5-year outcome data for angioplasty are scant in the literature. Only when we know how good endovascular treatment is at preventing stroke and death will we be truly able to recommend it.

New randomised trials comparing carotid stenting with carotid endarterectomy are currently ongoing during 2004: the Carotid Revascularisation Endarterectomy versus Stent Trial (CREST) in North America; the Endarterectomy versus Angioplasty in Patients with Severe Symptomatic Carotid Stenosis (EVA-3S) in France; the Stent Protected Percutaneous Angioplasty versus Carotid Endarterectomy (SPACE) in Germany and Austria; the follow-up to the CAVATAS trial, the International Carotid Stenting Study (ICSS) (CAVATAS2 International). It is hoped when these series are analysed that we will be able to have more information as to whether stenting is both as efficacious and durable as carotid endarterectomy. With respect to published series, complication rates from angioplasty and stenting vary from 0–70%. However, data from several series of over 500 patients give a similar risk of stroke and death during carotid PTA as that found as a result of carotid endarterectomy in NASCET and ECST. The mean stroke rate at the time of procedure for these series was 1.5% for minor or non-disabling stroke and 2.1% for major stroke or death, resulting in an overall stroke rate of 3.6%.

Technique

The technique for carotid angioplasty and stenting is variable. My technique has evolved continuously since 1992, both due to increasing experience and to the continued improvement and ingenuity of the available equipment. Manufacturers are now seeing a market for "tools" for carotid angioplasty and stenting and devices are being specifically made for this. I now use a 7 French sheath (Cook's Flexor 7 French Tuohy–Borst sidearm introducer), specifically designed for carotid angioplasty. This sheath provides a firm platform in the common carotid artery (CCA) for negotiation of tortuous vessels and is very stable.

After single femoral access, a standard catheter for selective angiogram is placed in the appropriate common carotid artery. A compass wire plus lock extension is passed into the ECA and the guiding sheath passed into the CCA. If primary stenting is to be performed, which is currently my usual technique, the occlusion is crossed with an 014 wire or with a cerebral protection device. If the stenosis is very tight, pre-dilatation is performed with a profile coronary balloon such as a Savvy (Cordis) with 3mm diameter. The stent is then inserted and post dilated up to the normal diameter of the vessel and the cerebral protection device then removed.

Monitoring During the Procedure

It goes without saying that an anesthesiologist should be present for the procedure with neuroleptic analgesia and to monitor the patient. Heparin is given after femoral access. Atropine is given prior to dilatation. There is monitoring of ECG and blood pressure, as well as transcranial Doppler monitoring of the middle cerebral artery velocity. Heparin is given 24 hours post-procedure. Aspirin is given pre-procedure and for life. There may also be a role for the new anti-platelet agents, such as Clopidogrel.

Both self-expanding and balloon-expanding stents have advantages and the ideal stent is yet to be designed. My personal preference is to use a self-expandable stent. Use of cerebral protection has strongly been advocated and Theron reports excellent results [34]. The main complication of angioplasty and stenting is ipsilateral stroke, thought to be mainly due to embolization of plaque material during the procedure. A balloon occlusion device (Percusurge) and a filter are commercially available and are increasingly used during these procedures.

With respect to PTA or stenting, there are several rationales for primary stenting. Primary stenting has the advantage that the adverse consequences of any dissection or plaque rupture initiated by balloon angioplasty are minimized because the stent maintains a laminar flow across the stenosis and seals the site of dissection, preventing a free intimal flap. In addition, the mesh size may limit the size of any thrombus or debris which may be dislodged.

With respect to re-stenoses, there is little long-term data available for stents. However, a re-stenosis rate of 6% has been shown with a Strecker stent, and our own experience and that of the CAVATAS operators is that, although there is a better immediate result after stenting at 1 month, the re-stenosis rate at 1 and 2 years is similar in the stent and no-stent groups. Re-stenosis is also unlikely to have any correlation with symptoms (Clifton AG (1999) Re-stenosis after carotid angioplasty, stenting and endarterectomy, and its relations to symptomatology. Personal communication/presentation to the Working Group on Interventional Neuroradiology, Val d'Isere, on behalf of the CAVATAS collaborators).

Conclusion

Carotid angioplasty plus or minus stenting is a promising, viable alternative to carotid endarterectomy. Case series and a recent randomized trial suggest the procedure may be as safe as carotid endarterectomy. The results of further ongoing trials are needed before the procedure can be unequivocally recommended.

Fig. 19.6 shows carotid artery stenosis pre- and post-stent insertion.

Vertebral Angioplasty and Stenting

The value of stents in the treatment of vertebral artery stenosis is uncertain [35]. Surgery is rarely carried out because surgical access is poor. Little is known about the natural history of vertebrobasilar disease. Stenoses frequently occur at the vertebral artery origin, which is easily accessible to endovascular technique. Series including 82 vertebral arteries treated with PTA show a procedure-related complication rate of 3.7% for major stroke, with no

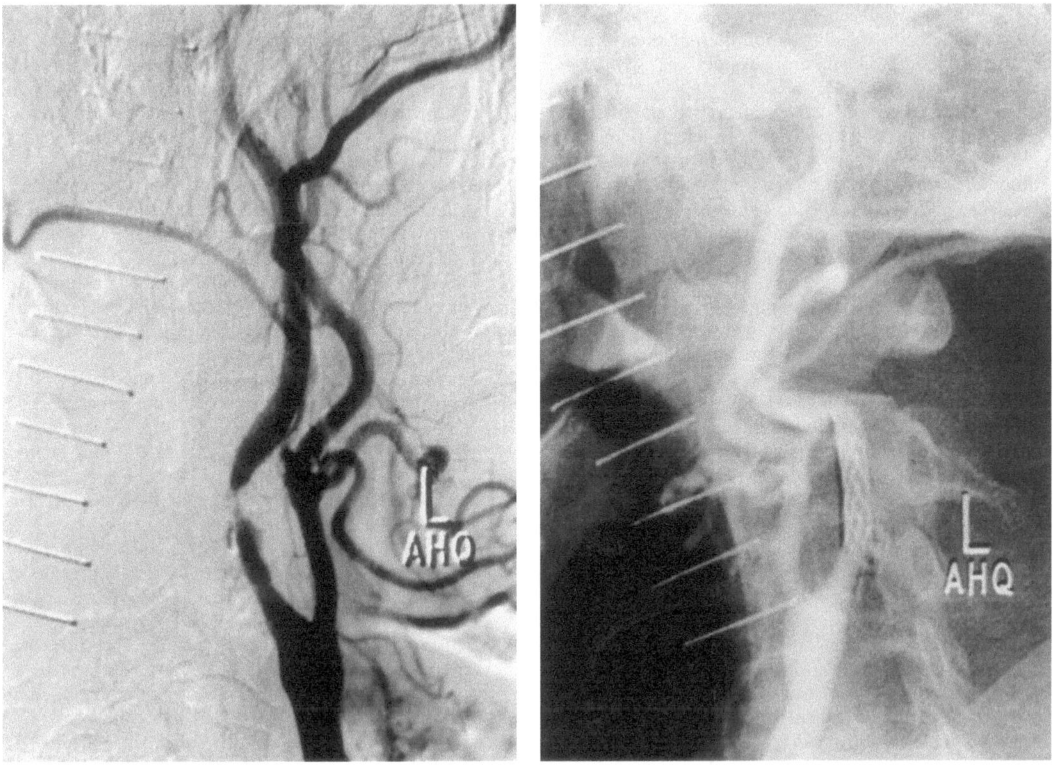

a b

Fig. 19.6. a Left carotid DSA, showing tight stenosis of the proximal internal carotid artery. **b** Excellent appearances post-insertion of stent.

reported minor strokes. There have been reports of a high re-stenosis rate at this site, which has encouraged the use of stents.

Questions

- ☐ What are the indications for balloon occlusion of the internal carotid artery?
- ☐ What methods are available to decide whether a patient can tolerate occlusion of the carotid artery?
- ☐ What are the benefits and the drawbacks of coil embolization of aneurysms?
- ☐ Is there any scientific evidence for stenting a stenotic asymptomatic carotid artery?
- ☐ What is the role of embolization in the treatment of AVMs?

References

1. Lasjaunias P. Education of Interventional Neuroradiologists. Interventional Neuroradiology 1995;1:13–17.
2. Niimi Y, Berenstein A, Setton A, Kupersmith MJ. Occlusion of the internal carotid artery based on a simple tolerance test. Interventional Neuroradiology 1996;2:289–96.
3. Anon VV, Aymard A, Gobin YP et al. Balloon occlusion of the internal carotid artery in 40 cases of giant intracavernous aneurysm: technical aspects, cerebral monitoring and results. Neuroradiology 1992;34:244–51.
4. Mathis JM, Barr JD, Jungreis CA et al. Temporary balloon test occlusion of the internal carotid artery: experience in 500 cases. AJNR 1995;16:749–54.
5. Schneweis S, Urbach H, Solymosie L et al. Pre-operative risk assessment for carotid occlusion by transcranial Doppler ultrasound. JNNP 1997;62:485–9.
6. Linskey ME, Jungreis CA, Yonas H et al. Stroke risk after abrupt internal carotid artery sacrifice: accuracy of preoperative assessment with balloon test occlusion and stable Xenon-enhanced CT. AJNR 1994;15:829–43.

7. Higashida RT, Halbach VV, Dowd C et al. Endovascular detachable balloon embolization therapy of cavernous carotid artery aneurysms: results in 87 cases. J Neurosurg 1990;72:857–63.
8. Byrne JV, Guglielmi G. Treatment by endovascular packing with the Guglielmi detachable coil. In: Endovascular treatment of intracranial aneurysms. Berlin: Springer, 1998; chapter 5, 133–66.
9. Guglielmi G, Vinuela F, Dion J et al. Electrothrombosis of saccular aneurysms via endovascular approach. Part 2. Preliminary clinical experience. J Neurosurg 1991; 75:8–14.
10. Cognard C, Weill A, Castaings L, Rey A, Moret J. Intracranial berry aneurysms: angiographic and clinical results after endovascular treatment. Radiology 1998; 206:499–510.
11. Murayama Y, Vinuela F, Duckwiler G, Gobin P, Guglielmi G. Embolization of incidental aneurysms by using the Guglielmi detachable coil system. J Neurosurg 1999;90:207–14.
12. The International Study of Unruptured Intracranial Aneurysms Investigators. Unruptured intracranial aneurysms: risks of rupture and risks of surgical intervention. N Eng J Med 1998;339:1725–33.
13. Murayama Y, Malisch T, Guglielmi G et al. Incidence of cerebral vasospasm after endovascular treatment of acutely ruptured aneurysm: report on 69 cases. J Neurosurg 1997;87:830–5.
14. Rothwell P, Slattery J, Warlow C. A systematic review of the risks of stroke and death due to endarterectomy for symptomatic carotid stenoses. Stroke 1996;27:260–5.
14a. Molyneux A, Kerr R, Stratton I et al; International Subarachnoid Aneurysm Trial (ISAT) Collaborative Group. International Subarachnoid Aneurysm Trial (ISAT) of neurosurgical clipping versus endovascular coiling in 2143 patients with ruptured intracranial aneurysm: a randomised trial. *Lancet* 2002;360(9342): 1267–74.
15. Malesh T, Guglielmi G, Vinuela F et al. Intracranial aneurysms treated with the Guglielmi detachable coil: mid term clinical results in 100 consecutive patients. J Neurosurg 1997;87:176–83.
16. McDougall CG, Van Halbach V, Dowd CF, Higashida RT, Larsen DW, Hieshima GB. Causes and management of aneurysmal haemorrhage occurring during embolization with Guglielmi detachable coils. J Neurosurg 1998;89:87–92.
17. Vinuela F, Duckwiler G, Mawad M. Guglielmi detachable coil embolization of acute intracranial aneurysm: pre-operative anatomical and clinical outcome in 403 patients. J Neurosurg 1997;86:475–82.
18. Bryan R, Rigamonti D, Mathis JM. The treatment of acutely ruptured cerebral aneurysms: endovascular therapy versus surgery. AJNR 1997;18:1826–30.
19. Vanninen R, Kolvisto T, Saari T et al. Ruptured intracranial aneurysms: acute endovascular treatment with electolytically detachable coils – a prospective randomised study. Radiology 1999;211:322–38.
20. Latchaw R. Acutely ruptured intracranial aneurysm: should we treat with endovascular coils or with surgical clipping. Radiology 1999;211:306–8.
21. Crawley F, Clifton A, Brown MM. Should we screen for familial intracranial aneurysms? Stroke 1999;30:312–16.
22. LeRoux PD, Winn RH. Management of cerebral aneurysms: how can current management be improved. In: Current management of cerebral aneurysms. Part 1. Evaluation and peri-operative care. Neurosurgery Clinics of North America 1998;9(3):421–33.
23. Byrne JV, Sohn M-J, Molyneux AJ. Five year experience in using coil embolization for ruptured intracranial aneurysm: outcomes and incidence of late re-bleeding. J Neurosurg 1999;90:656–63.
24. Flickinejer J, Kondziolka D, Pollock B, Lunsford LD. Radiological management of intracranial vascular malformations. Neuroimaging Clinics of North America 1998;8(2):483–93.
25. Rauch R, Vinuela F, Dion J et al. Pre-embolization functional evaluation in brain AVMs: the superselective Amytal test. AJNR 1992;13:303–8.
26. Wikholm G, Lundquist C, Svendsen P. Embolization of cerebral arteriovenous malformations: Part 1. Technique, morphology and complications. Neurosurgery 1996;39:448–59.
27. Lewis AI, Tomsick TA, Tew JM Jr. Management of 100 consecutive direct carotid cavernous fistulas: results of treatment with detachable balloons. Neurosurgery 1995;36:239–45.
28. Debrun GB, Lacour P, Fox AJ. Traumatic carotid cavernous fistulas: etiology, clinical presentation, diagnoses, treatment, results. Semin Intervent Radiol 1987;4:242–8.
29. Halbach VV, Higashida RT, Hieshima GB, Hardin CW, Pribram H. Transvenous embolization of dural fistulas involving the cavernous sinus. AJNR 1989;10:377–84.
30. Sato H, Hyodo A, Matsumararu Y, Anno I, Kato T, Nose T et al. The evaulation of pre-operative embolization of meningioma. International Neuroradiology 1997;3 (Suppl. 2).
31. European Carotid Surgery Trialists Collaboration Group, MRC European Carotid Surgery Trial. Interim result for symptomatic patients with severe (70–79%) or with mild (0–29%) carotid stenosis. Lancet 1991;337: 1235–43.
32. North American Symptomatic Carotid Endarterectomy Trial collaborators. Beneficial effects of carotid endarterectomy in somptomatic patients with high grade carotid stenosis. N Eng J Med 1991;325:445–53.
33. Warlow C. Carotid endarterectomy for asymptomatic carotid stenosis [editorial]. BMJ 1998;317:1468.
33a. CAVATAS investigators. Endovasccular versus surgical treatment in patients with carotid stenosis in the Carotid and Vertebral Artery Transluminal Angioplasty Study (CAVATAS): a randomised trial. *Lancet* 2001; 357(9270):1729–37.
34. Theron PG, Payelle GG, Coskun O et al. carotid artery stenosis: treatment with protected balloon angioplasty and stent placement. Radiology 1996;201:627–36.
35. Crawley F, Brown MM, Clifton AG. Angioplasty and stenting in the carotid and vertebral arteries. Postgrad Med J 1998;74:7–10.

20

Arteriovenous Malformations

Stephen M. Russell and Peter D. Le Roux

Summary

Cerebral arteriovenous malformations (AVMs), cavernous malformations (cavernomas), developmental venous anomalies (DVAs) and capillary telangiectasias are developmental vascular anomalies of the central nervous system. In particular, AVMs cause significant morbidity and mortality if untreated. These lesions are best treated in specialized neurovascular centers by a multidisciplinary team of neurosurgeons, interventional neuroradiologists and radiation therapists. Treatment needs to be tailored to the individual patient based on the expected natural history and morphology of the lesion.

Introduction

Cerebral arteriovenous malformations (CAVMs) are developmental anomalies of the neurovascular system. There are four main types of CAVMs: arteriovenous malformations (AVMs), cavernous malformations (cavernomas), developmental venous anomalies (DVAs) and capillary telangiectasias. Additionally, there are several rare developmental vascular anomalies such as dural arteriovenous fistulae, pial arteriovenous fistulae and congenital arteriovenous fistulae or vein of Galen malformations.

Each type of vascular malformation has a unique natural history, thus requiring a separate treatment approach. Developmental venous anomalies and capillary telangiectasias are benign lesions, which are discovered incidentally and generally do not require treatment. By contrast, AVMs and cavernous malformations may cause intracranial hemorrhage, seizures, headache or neurologic deficit, and have a poor prognosis if left untreated. A variety of treatment options including microsurgery, interventional neuroradiology, stereotactic radiosurgery or a combination of these modalities are available to treat these lesions. Treatment is optimized by using a multidisciplinary team, including neurosurgeons, interventional neuroradiologists and radiation therapists. In this chapter, we will briefly review the etiology, epidemiology, pathology, and neuroradiographic diagnosis of the four major types of CAVMs. The latter half of the chapter will concentrate on the clinical presentation, natural history and treatment of AVMs.

Etiology and Hereditary Syndromes

Cerebral arteriovenous malformations are thought to arise during fetal development of the neurovascular system. The primitive vascular network first appears adjacent to the developing brain during the third week of gestation. Vascular penetration into neural tissue, however, does not begin until the seventh gestational week. During this vascular penetration, the primitive cerebral vessels elongate, branch, anastomose and regress to create a mature capillary network that irrigates the brain. This vascular penetration and subsequent differentiation continue until the end of the first trimester, during which time CAVMs are thought to develop. Once formed, extrinsic factors such as arterial shunting, growth factors or intracranial hemorrhage may alter a CAVM's morphology.

There are a small number of rare congenital syndromes such as Sturge–Weber, Rendu-Osler–Weber, ataxia telangiectasia and Wyburn–Mason that are associated with CAVMs. Sturge–Weber syndrome, or encephalotrigeminal angiomatosis, has two key pathological components: a cutaneous, facial angioma in the distribution of the trigeminal nerve, and an ipsilateral, parietal-occipital vascular malformation. In Sturge–Weber syndrome, the intracranial vascular malformation is pial based and rarely causes intracranial hemorrhage. However, it may cause intractable epilepsy, mental retardation and progressive encephalomalacia. Rendu–Osler–Weber syndrome, or hereditary hemorrhagic telangiectasia, is an autosomal-dominant syndrome of multiple visceral, mucosal and cerebral vascular malformations. Patients with Rendu–Osler–Weber syndrome usually present with recurrent epistaxis or cerebral infarcts from pulmonary AVM emboli. Ataxia telangiectasia and Wyburn–Mason syndrome may have cerebellar or diencephalic vascular malformations, respectively.

Epidemiology

Autopsy series suggest that the overall prevalence of intracranial vascular malformations is between 1 and 5% [4,9]. Developmental venous anomalies are the most prevalent lesion type and represent nearly two-thirds of all cerebral vascular malformations, whereas capillary telangiectasias, AVMs and cavernous malformations are estimated to occur in 0.9, 0.5 and 0.3% of the population, respectively [9]. Arteriovenous malformations are the most common vascular malformation to become symptomatic and require medical treatment. The incidence of intracranial hemorrhage from AVMs in the general population is estimated to be between 1 and 3 per 100,000 people [12]. Among children, the incidence of AVM-related hemorrhage is lower and is estimated to be 1 per 100,000 children [16].

Neuropathology

The neuropathological features of the various CAVMs are listed in Table 20.1. Several features, including size, location, gross angioarchitecture, vessel wall microscopic appearance, presence and quality of intervening neural parenchyma, evidence of recent hemorrhage, hemosiderin deposition and vessel thrombosis need to be considered when making a neuropathological diagnosis of a suspected CAVM.

Arteriovenous Malformations

Arteriovenous malformations are high-flow cerebrovascular lesions that may occur in any intracranial location and range in size from microscopic to more than 10 cm in diameter. There are three distinct patho-anatomical components to each AVM: (1) arterial feeders, (2) a central nidus, and (3) draining veins [9].

Table 20.1. Neuropathology of cerebral arteriovenous malformations

Characteristic	Arteriovenous Malformation	Cavernous Malformation	Developmental Venous Anomaly	Capillary Telangiectasia
Size	microscopic to >9 cm	1 to 5 cm	1 to 5 cm	1 to 5 mm
Shape	globular or conical, apex towards ventricle	spherical, mulberry	mushroom, umbrella	irregular, patchy
Location	all	all	cerebrum, cerebellum	usually pons
Vessels	thin-walled dysplastic vessels arterialized draining veins	hyalinized sinusoids	normal veins	enlarged capillaries
Parenchyma	gliosis, dysplastic parenchyma	no intervening parenchyma	normal	normal
Hemosiderin	common	always	none	none

Yasargil M: Microneurosurgery, IIIA. Stuttgart: Thieme, 1987

The AVM nidus is a compact tangle of dysplastic, thin-walled vessels of varied length connecting feeding arteries to draining veins. An AVM nidus can either be globular or conical in shape. Within the AVM nidus, arterial blood is shunted directly into draining veins without passage through a normal, high-resistance arteriolar–capillary network. The amount of arteriovenous shunting varies among AVMs and is determined by nidal vessel impedance. There is usually little brain parenchyma within an AVM nidus. However, functional parenchyma may occasionally be found among the vessels of a diffuse nidus. Most intra-nidal parenchyma is densely sclerotic and stained with hemosiderin [9]. Fusiform or pseudo-aneurysms may be present on intra-nidal vessels. Although the weak, dysplastic nidal vessels are usually the source of AVM hemorrhage, concomitant aneurysms represent an independent risk factor for AVM hemorrhage [1].

Each AVM has a variable number of feeding arteries. Each arterial feeder may drain directly into a vein (an arteriovenous fistula), or connect through a mass of dysplastic vessels within the AVM nidus before draining into a vein. Vessels feeding an AVM are frequently histologically normal. However, chronically elevated blood flow may cause accelerated atherosclerosis [11] or flow-related aneurysm formation [1]. These flow-related aneurysms occur on the proximal intracranial vessels and are pathologically similar to saccular aneurysms. Veins draining an AVM are often large and dilated. In addition, direct arterial blood flow into draining veins may promote intimal hyperplasia and subsequently cause venous wall thickening and stenosis. Venous drainage can be directed into deep subependymal or superficial cortical venous systems.

Cavernous Malformations

Cavernous malformations are the second most common CAVM that come to clinical attention. These lesions occur throughout the CNS and are usually between 1 and 5 cm in diameter. Morphologically, cavernous malformations are well circumscribed, round or mulberry-shaped nests of thickly hyalinized sinusoidal vessels [9]. Within a cavernous malformation, there is no intervening neural parenchyma. Extensive areas of micro-hemorrhage and hemosiderin deposition are present.

Developmental Venous Anomalies

Developmental venous anomalies are benign developmental anomalies of the cerebral venous system that rarely hemorrhage [9]. They comprise numerous small veins that drain in a centripetal pattern into a large venous trunk, analogous to the spokes of a bicycle wheel. The venous trunk subsequently drains into a superficial vein that connects to a dural sinus. These lesions are thought to be primitive venous elements that fail to regress during fetal development and so function like normal subcortical veins. Consequently, surgical resection is not indicated. Histologically, DVAs comprise normal, thin-walled venous structures. Vessel wall hyalinization may occur; this, however, is not associated with a worse prognosis. Developmental venous anomalies may be associated with cavernous malformations.

Capillary Telangiectasias

Capillary telangiectasias are benign clusters of dilated capillaries with normal intervening neural parenchyma [9]. Capillary telangiectasias are incidental lesions found at autopsy or during neuroradiographic evaluation of other CNS disorders. Capillary telangiectasias are 1–3 mm in diameter and may occur throughout the CNS. However, the vast majority are found in the posterior fossa, particularly the pons. The capillary walls are histologically normal and hemosiderin staining of the adjacent parenchyma is not present. These lesions do not hemorrhage.

Neuroradiology

Each of the different cerebral arteriovenous malformations has distinct radiographic features. They may be diagnosed non-invasively using CT, MRI or MRA. However, cerebral angiography is necessary for treatment planning when an AVM is diagnosed. Trans-femoral catheter angiography is a safe procedure. The risk of stroke, arterial dissection, lower-extremity ischemia or renal dysfunction is less than 1%. The risk, however, is increased two or threefold for patients with atherosclerotic disease. Other studies, such as fMRI, magnetoencephalography (MEG) or PET scanning, may be useful in selected cases to determine the AVM's relationship to eloquent cerebral cortex.

Arteriovenous Malformations

Arteriovenous malformations commonly present with intracerebral hemorrhage that may be intraparenchymal, intraventricular, subarachnoid or subdural. Consequently, a head CT scan is often the initial radiographic investigation for an AVM and, generally, is the best study to delineate the presence and location of acute intracerebral blood (Fig. 20.2a). In the absence of hemorrhage, an AVM nidus appears slightly hyperdense, sparsely calcified and wedge-shaped on a non-contrast head CT. The apex of a wedge-shaped AVM is directed towards the ventricular system. The arterial feeders, nidal vessels and dilated draining veins are seen on head CT scans after administration of intravenous contrast. MRI is useful in defining the exact anatomic location and size of an AVM. On MRI, the AVM nidus appears as a prominent nest of flow voids within the brain parenchyma (Figs 20.1a, b, c and 20.2b). The large, dilated draining veins adjacent to the nidus are generally well seen. Hemosiderin deposition occurs after AVM hemorrhage; this hemosiderin deposition causes low signal changes on T2-weighted and gradient-echo MRI images and is diagnostic of old hemorrhage. Hemosiderin is not seen on CT scans. Cerebral angiography is necessary for treatment planning. An angiogram fully defines the AVM's angioarchitecture, including its location and size, the number and origin of its arterial feeders, nidal anatomy, direction of venous outflow and the presence of AVM-associated aneurysms (Figs 20.1d–g, 20.2c, d and 20.3a, b). We have not found MRA studies to be useful in treatment planning for AVMs.

Cavernous Malformations

Cavernous malformations are angiographically occult lesions that are best evaluated with MRI (Fig. 20.4a). On T1- and T2-weighted images, cavernous malformations are distinct, popcorn-shaped, heterogeneous masses (Fig. 20.4b, c). The characteristic low-signal ring around cavernous malformations visible on gradient echo MRI sequences is caused by hemosiderin deposition from recurrent micro-hemorrhage. Cerebral angiography is rarely required in the evaluation of cavernous malformations.

Developmental Venous Anomalies

Developmental venous anomalies appear similar on MRI and cerebral angiography. These studies demonstrate a cluster of small veins arranged like the spokes of a wheel, draining into a common venous trunk (Fig. 20.5). This venous trunk points towards the surface of the brain and subsequently drains into a superficial cortical vein.

Capillary Telangiectasias

Capillary telangiectasias generally are too small to be seen on cerebral angiography, CT or MRI scans. Occasionally, they may be observed on MRI scans in the pons as very small high-signal blushes after intravenous gadolinium administration.

Clinical Presentation

The clinical presentation of patients with CAVMs depends in large part on pathology and location of the lesion. Venous malformations are most commonly found incidentally. Rarely, a cerebellar venous malformation may cause intracranial hemorrhage. Capillary telangiectasias are usually found at autopsy. Cavernous malformations often present with seizures and, less frequently, with hemorrhage.

AVMs are the most common vascular malformation to become symptomatic. Most AVMs become symptomatic between 20 and 50 years of age. Less frequently, AVMs first become symptomatic during childhood or in adults greater than 60 years of age. Common presenting features include: hemorrhage (50%), seizures (25%), headache (12%) or progressive neurological deficit (12%) [5,24,25]. The clinical presentation may be predicted by the anatomic location of the AVM [6,24,25]. For example, AVMs located in the basal ganglia, corpus callosum, brain stem and cerebellum present with hemorrhage in greater than 70% of patients. In contrast, AVMs involving the medial temporal lobe and hippocampus generally present with seizures. Furthermore, parietal and occipital lobe AVMs and AVMs with external carotid artery feeders frequently present with headaches in the absence of cerebral hemorrhage.

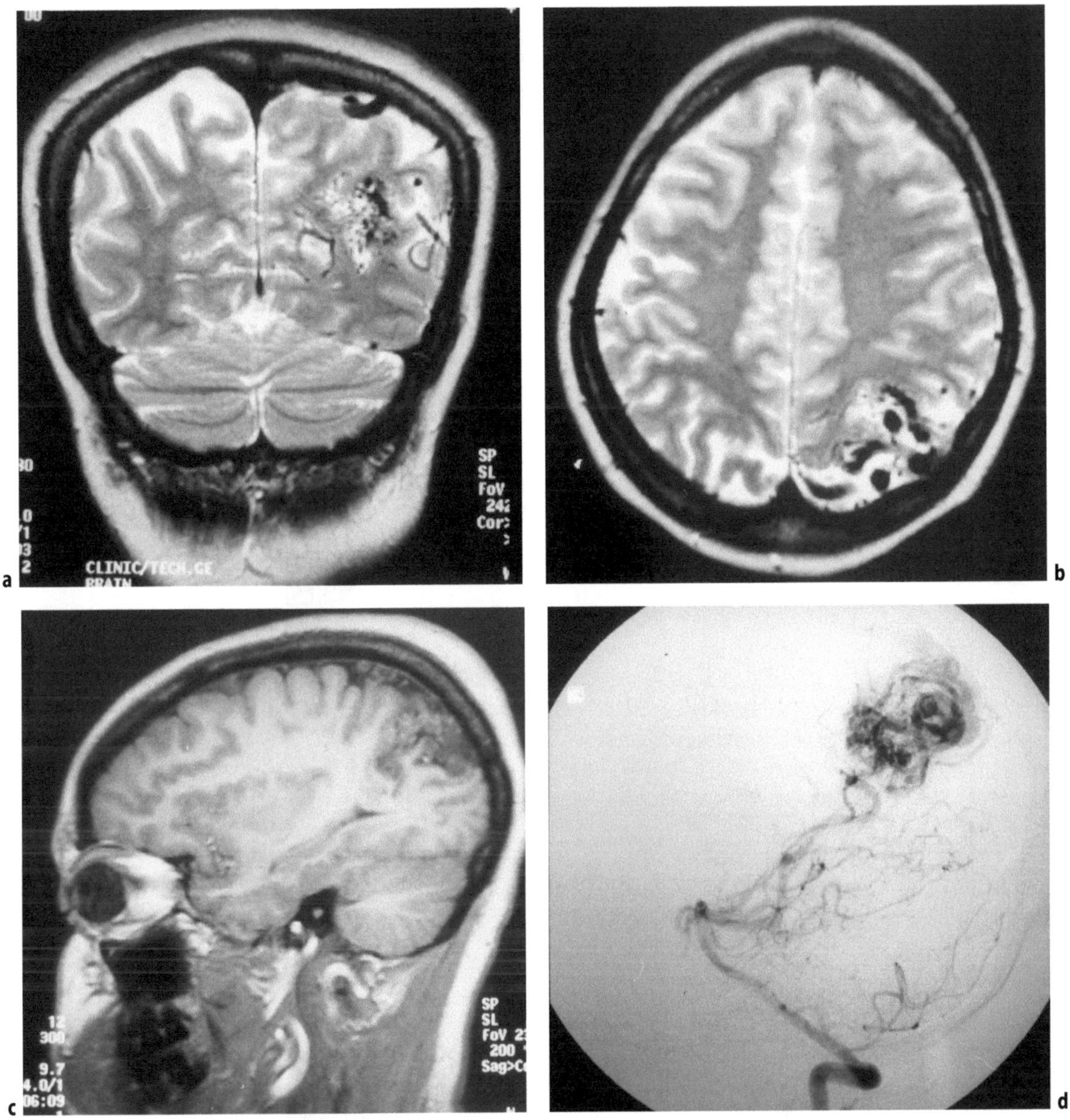

Fig. 20.1. Case 1: A 37-year-old woman presented with a generalized seizure. **a** A T2-weighted coronal MRI was obtained through the posterior cerebral cortex and cerebellar hemispheres. A cluster of flow voids characteristic of an AVM nidus and its draining veins was located in the left parietal-occipital lobe. **b** An axial T2-weighted MRI through the cerebral convexity demonstrated a cluster of large, dilated draining veins in the left posterior parietal lobe. **c** A left parasagittal T1-weighted MRI with contrast administration showed a classic wedge-shaped nidus with the apex pointing towards the lateral ventricle. There was patchy contrast enhancement within the nidus. The nidus was approximately 3–4 cm in diameter. Catheter angiography was performed for treatment planning. **d** A lateral, mid-arterial phase right vertebral artery cerebral angiogram revealed the dysplastic nidal vessels being fed by branches of the left parieto-occipital artery. Early venous opacification was noted superficial to the AVM.

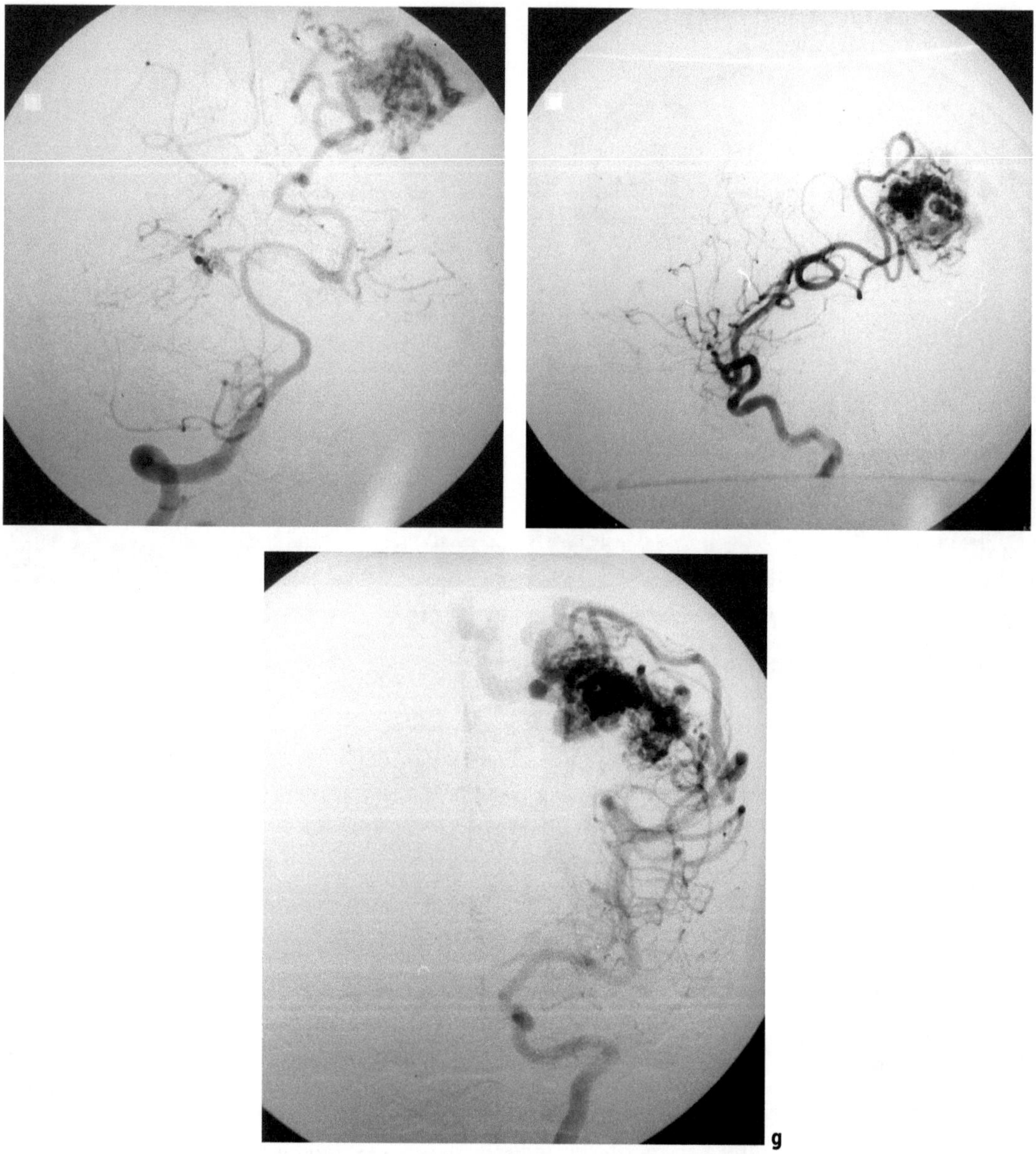

e f g

Fig. 20.1. (*continued*) **e** An anterior–posterior (AP) mid-arterial phase right vertebral artery cerebral angiogram displayed the patchy AVM nidus fed by the left parieto-occipital artery and its branches. **f** The lateral left internal carotid mid-arterial phase cerebral angiogram revealed additional feeding vessels from the middle cerebral artery, most notably large angular and posterior parietal branches. Many of the feeders appeared to be en passant, possibly feeding normal cerebral cortex. **g** An AP left internal carotid artery mid-arterial phase cerebral angiogram defined the arterial feeders from the middle cerebral artery. There was no deep venous drainage or deep arterial feeders present. This AVM was classified as a Spetzler–Martin Grade 3 (2 for size, 1 for eloquence (optic radiations) and 0 for deep venous drainage). This patient received preoperative NBCA embolization, followed by microsurgical excision.

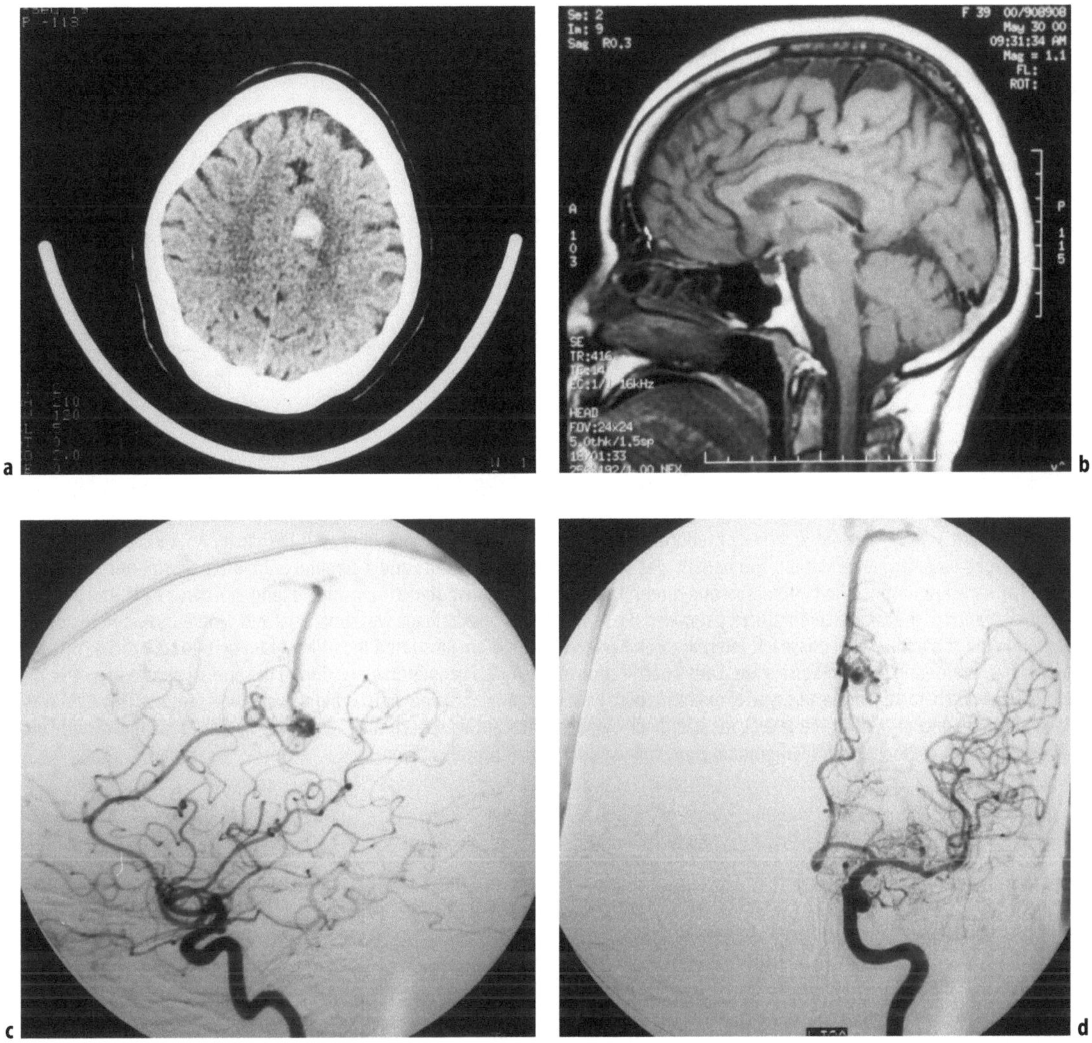

Fig. 20.2. Case 2: A 39-year-old female presented with sudden right-sided hemiparesis and headache. **a** An axial non-contrast CT scan revealed an acute intracerebral hemorrhage in the left medial centrum semiovale. A cerebral angiogram revealed a left-sided 1-cm paracentral lobule AVM. The patient had significant recovery of her hemiparesis from intensive rehabilitation. A MRI and repeat cerebral angiogram was performed 4 weeks after her ictus for treatment planning. **b** A mid-sagittal T1-weighted non-contrast MRI displayed evidence of the AVM. Although small, a collection of vessels was noted at the distal callosomarginal artery territory in the cingulate sulcus anterior–inferior to the paracentral lobule. A prominent linear draining vein was noted in the paracentral sulcus subsequently entering the superior sagittal sinus. The paracentral lobule was markedly atrophic, presumably from her previous hemorrhage. **c** A lateral left internal carotid mid-arterial phase cerebral angiogram revealed a 1-cm AVM, being fed by the callosomarginal artery. Perpendicular to the feeding artery, early opacification of the malformation's draining vein was noted. **d** An AP left internal carotid mid-arterial phase cerebral angiogram further defined the midline AVM. There were no aneurysms or deep venous drainage present. This AVM was classified as a Spetzler–Martin Grade 2 (1 for size, 1 for eloquence (motor cortex) and 0 for deep venous drainage). This patient opted for surgical removal. Frameless stereotaxis was used during the operative procedure to define the nidal margins.

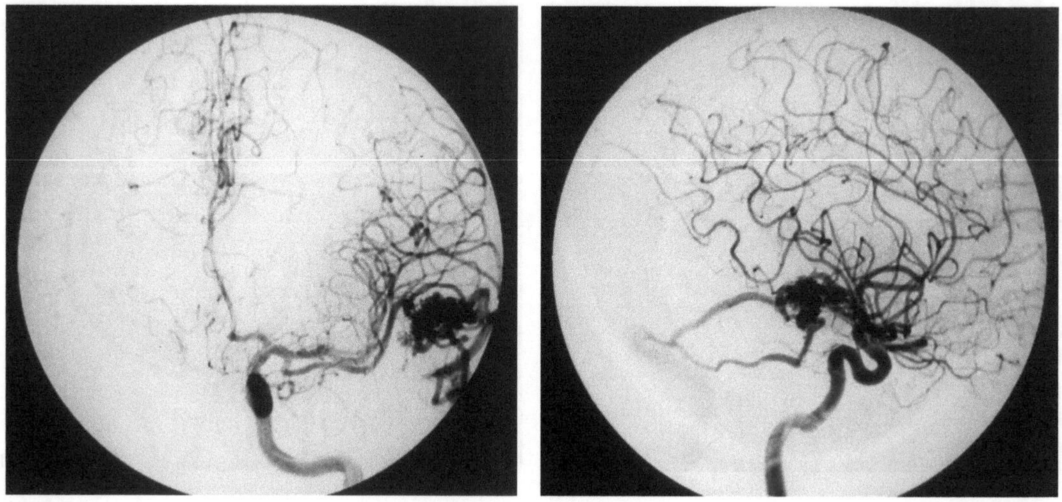

Fig. 20.3. Case 3: A 42-year-old Broadway producer began to experience paroxysms of speech hesitancy. An MRI revealed a left temporal lobe vascular malformation. The patient was started on anticonvulsants and a cerebral angiogram was performed. **a** AP view of an early arterial phase left internal carotid cerebral angiogram demonstrated a 2-cm middle temporal gyrus AVM. The inferior temporal branch of the middle cerebral artery supplied the AVM. The venous drainage was superficial and no aneurysms were noted. **b** Lateral view of a mid-arterial phase left internal carotid cerebral angiogram illustrated the AVM nidus and two superficial cortical-draining veins entering the transverse sinus. Early opacification of the AVM's venous drainage during the arterial phases of a cerebral angiogram was characteristic for this type of malformation. Venous ectasia of the proximal draining veins was present. This AVM was classified as a Spetzler–Martin Grade 2 (1 for size, 1 for eloquence (receptive speech area) and 0 for deep venous drainage). This patient opted for pre-operative NBCA embolization, followed by microsurgical excision.

Hemorrhage

The most common clinical manifestation of an AVM is intracranial hemorrhage. Among young patients who are normotensive and have normal coagulation, AVMs are a common cause of ICH. Most supratentorial AVM hemorrhages are lobar in location, but may also occur in the basal ganglia or thalamus. In the posterior fossa, AVMs cause most cerebellar hemorrhages in normotensive patients less than 40 years old. Brainstem AVMs causing hemorrhage often may be angiographically occult immediately post-hemorrhage. These patients require delayed angiography once the hematoma has resolved in order to define the malformation. Patients with AVMs near the ventricular surface may present with recurrent intraventricular hemorrhage and subsequent hydrocephalus from obstruction of proximal or distal cerebrospinal fluid pathways. Intraventricular hemorrhage from AVMs is often small in volume, with mild clinical manifestations. Pial-based AVMs may cause subarachnoid hemorrhage. In most instances, however, subarachnoid hemorrhage results from the rupture of a primary intraparenchymal bleed through the pial surface. In contrast to aneurysms, basal subarachnoid hemorrhage from AVM rupture is rarely associated with vasospasm [12]. Furthermore, recurrent hemorrhage within the first 2 weeks after AVM rupture is rare and complicates only 1% of patients [12]. The overall mortality rate after each AVM rupture is approximately 10% [10].

Seizures

Seizures are the second most common clinical presentation of a cerebral AVM [24,25]. Nearly three-quarters of patients with AVMs will experience a seizure at some point during their life. AVM-related seizures may be caused by overt intracranial hemorrhage, from hemosiderin deposition following recurrent micro-hemorrhages or secondary to venous hypertension. Seizure type is associated, in part, with AVM location. For example, AVMs located deep in

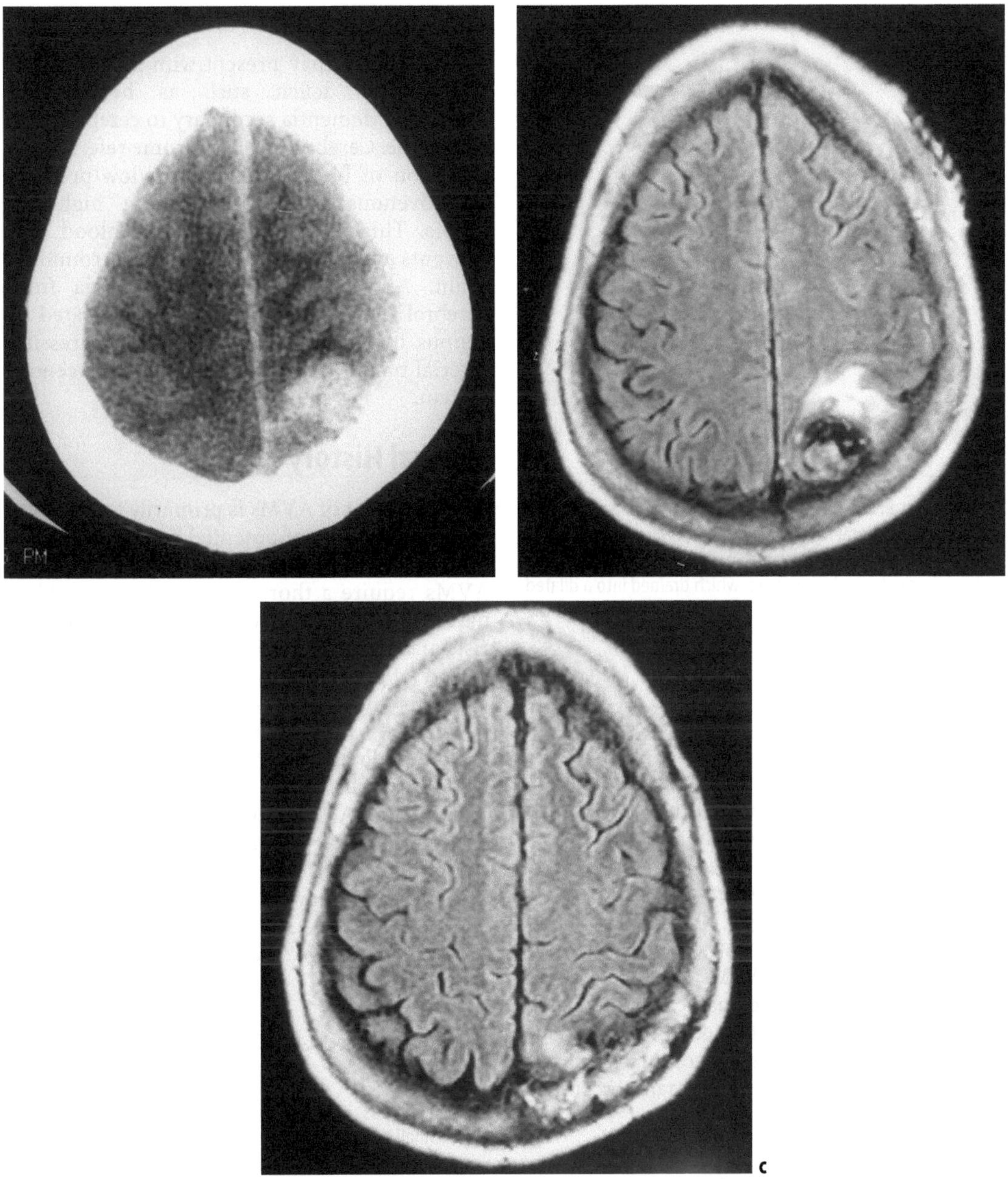

a b c

Fig. 20.4. Case 4: A 65-year-old female presented with sudden headache, confusion and trace right-sided weakness. **a** An urgent axial head CT scan revealed a left-sided parietal hyperdensity. **b** An axial T1-weighted non-contrast MRI through the area of abnormality revealed a 2-cm cavernous malformation with areas of hemorrhage of various chronicity. An acute intraparenchymal bleed was noted anterior to the lesion. The woman was brought to the operating room and the lesion was removed. **c** A post-operative axial T1-weighted non-contrast MRI confirmed the successful resection of her cavernous malformation. With a brief period of rehabilitation, the patient returned to her usual state of good health.

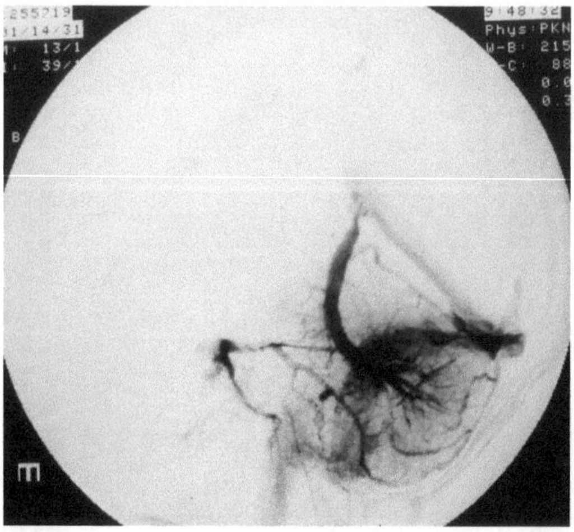

Fig. 20.5. Case 5: A 69-year-old woman with new-onset headaches received an MRI, revealing a cerebellar vascular malformation. Lateral view of a venous phase left vertebral artery cerebral angiogram revealed a centripetal venous cluster in the right cerebellar hemisphere, which drained into a dilated pre-central cerebellar vein that subsequently emptied into the straight sinus. These angiographic features are typical of a DVA. The patient's headaches were medically managed.

the brain or in the posterior fossa infrequently cause seizures, whereas frontal-lobe AVMs may cause generalized seizures, motor strip AVMs may cause Jacksonian seizures and medial temporal lobe AVMs are often associated with complex partial seizures [6]. Most AVM-related seizures respond well to anti-epileptic medication. However, some AVMs, particularly in the medial temporal lobe, may cause medically refractory epilepsy. AVM resection may reduce the frequency of seizures, or completely eliminate the seizure disorder in a small percentage of patients [6].

Headaches

Arteriovenous malformations may also present with headache. Migraine-like headaches commonly are associated with occipital lobe AVMs fed by the posterior cerebral artery, whereas large, superficial AVMs with meningeal supply frequently present with severe ipsilateral headaches [8]. Surgical resection of occipital-lobe AVMs or selective embolization of meningeal feeders is frequently associated with complete relief of the headaches [8].

Neurologic Deficit

Some patients may present with a progressive neurological deficit such as hemiparesis, aphasia or dementia secondary to cerebral steal syndrome. Cerebral steal syndrome refers to the diversion of blood flow through low-pressure arteriovenous connections within high-flow AVMs. This diversion of cerebral blood flow prevents adequate perfusion of the surrounding brain. Additionally, cerebral ischemia from cerebral steal syndrome may be aggravated by venous hypertension caused by high-pressure arterial blood prematurely entering the venous system.

Natural History

The treatment of AVMs is primarily intended to eradicate the risk of potential hemorrhage. The indications and method of invasive treatment of AVMs require a thorough knowledge of AVM natural history and treatment risk. Treatment risk, particularly surgical risk, is defined by a variety of grading systems, the most popular of which is the Spetzler–Martin grading system (Table 20.2) [18]. A predictive grading system for the endovascular management of AVMs is not yet established.

Untreated AVMs have a poor prognosis. For example, Ondra et al. prospectively followed 166 symptomatic but untreated AVM patients [10]. The average follow-up was more than 20 years. During this time, 23% of the patients died from AVM hemorrhage and the combined annual

Table 20.2. Spetzler-Martin AVM grading system

Variable	Score
Size of nidus	
Small (<3 cm)	1
Medium (3–6 cm)	2
Large (>6 cm)	3
Cortical Eloquence	
Yes	1
No	0
Deep vascular component	
Yes	1
No	0

AVM grade = sum (size + eloquence + deep component)
Spetzier R, Martin N: A proposed grading system for arteriovenous malformations of the brainstem. Journal of Neurosurgery 65:476, 1986

morbidity and mortality was 2.7%. In addition, these investigators found that the life expectancy of patients harboring AVMs was significantly reduced. Among AVM patients, the mean age of death from all causes was 51 years compared to 73 years in the general population.

Following rupture of an AVM, the risk of early re-bleeding is significantly lower than that observed after aneurysm rupture. Consequently, AVM treatment can often be delayed for 1 or 2 months after AVM rupture, to allow the patient to recover and undergo treatment under optimal circumstances. However, some authors have observed a two to fourfold increase in the risk of re-bleeding during the first year after AVM rupture than in subsequent years [5]. AVM rupture during pregnancy may have a more malignant natural history, having a high rate of recurrent hemorrhage during the same pregnancy [14]. Consequently, when a ruptured AVM in a pregnant woman is surgically accessible, it should be removed as soon as possible to prevent devastating re-hemorrhage. Embolization and radiosurgery are not options during pregnancy because of potential radiation toxicity to the fetus.

The long-term risk of AVM bleeding for patients with symptomatic AVMs is estimated to be 2–3% per year [10]. This risk may be higher among patients who have had more than one hemorrhage and also in children. Among patients with symptomatic, unruptured AVMs, the risk of hemorrhage is similar to that observed in AVMs that have previously ruptured [10]. The presence of neurologic symptoms does not increase the risk of hemorrhage among patients who have not experienced AVM rupture. Mortality after each AVM rupture is approximately 10% [12]. Long-term, the overall annual mortality rate per year from an AVM hemorrhage is estimated to be 1% for adults and 2% for children [10]. The reasons for an apparently more malignant natural history of symptomatic childhood AVMs have not been defined.

Several anatomic and angiographic characteristics are thought to be associated with a greater risk of AVM hemorrhage. These factors include: (1) smaller AVM size, (2) deep hemispheric location, (3) intranidal aneurysms, (4) deep venous drainage and (5) draining vein stenosis. In contrast, angiomatous change, or angiographically identified vascular hyperplasia of pial vessels being recruited to feed a high-flow AVM, may be associated with a decreased risk of hemorrhage. It is postulated that high-flow AVMs, identified by these angiomatous changes, have low intra-nidal pressures, thus decreasing the risk of AVM rupture.

Between 3 and 14% of AVMs are associated with aneurysms, potentially altering AVM management. High blood flow and subsequent hemodynamic stress may promote aneurysm formation. Aneurysms associated with AVMs may be subdivided as follows: (1) dysplastic, remote aneurysms located at some distance from the AVM that appear anatomically unrelated to major AVM inflow vessels, (2) proximal aneurysms that arise from the circle of Willis or on the proximal portion of major AVM feeding vessels, (3) pedicular aneurysms located on the middle portion of a major feeding pedicle or (4) intra-nidal aneurysms within the AVM. The natural history of these combined lesions is not well understood; however, several studies suggest that the combination of an AVM and cerebral aneurysm is associated with a greater risk of intracranial hemorrhage [1]. For example, Brown et al. observed an annual hemorrhage rate of 2% for AVMs, but 7% among AVMs associated with aneurysms [3]. In general, when these lesions come to attention in the absence of hemorrhage, the aneurysm should be treated first because of the higher morbidity associated with aneurysm rupture. For patients who present with hemorrhage, the symptomatic lesion should be treated first.

A variety of anatomic and physiologic factors, such as AVM size and location, number and distribution of arterial feeders, pattern of venous drainage and flow through the AVM nidus, influence the technical difficulty and consequent risk of surgical, endovascular or radiosurgical treatment of an AVM. These factors have been incorporated into a variety of grading systems that are used primarily in treatment planning to predict surgical risk. Among these various grading systems, the Spetzler–Martin grading system is now most frequently used to predict surgical risk and compare results of clinical series using different treatment modalities (Tables 20.2 and 20.3). The Spetzler–Martin grading system uses three radiographic variables: size of the AVM nidus, pattern of venous drainage and location of the AVM in relation to eloquent cortex. A numerical score is assigned to each variable and one derives the AVM grade,

Table 20.3. Surgical results according to Spetzler-Martin grade

Grade	No. Cases	No deficit	Minor deficit	Major deficit	Mortality
I	23	100%	0%	0%	0%
II	21	95%	5%	0%	0%
III	25	84%	12%	4%	0%
IV	15	73%	20%	7%	0%
V	16	69%	19%	12%	0%
Total	100	86%	10%	4%	0%

Spetzler R, Martin N: A proposed grading system for arteriovenous malformations. Journal of Neurosurgery 65:476, 1986

I through V, by adding the scores. Large AVMs that are intimately associated with eloquent cortex or that are located in the hypothalamus or brainstem may be classified as inoperable Grade VI lesions. Increasing grade is significantly associated with minor and major neurologic deficits post-operatively. Numerous studies have confirmed the reliability of this grading system in predicting surgical outcome. Unfortunately, this grading system is not directly applicable to the endovascular treatment of AVMs, contributing to the difficulty in comparing treatment results of these two modalities.

Treatment

There are several treatment modalities used to manage AVMs: (1) microsurgical excision, (2) endovascular embolization, (3) stereotactic radiosurgery or (4) a combination of these various modalities. The management of a patient with an AVM is best accomplished at specialized neurovascular referral centers where there is a multidisciplinary team, including neurosurgeons, interventional neuroradiologists, radiation therapists, neuroanesthesiologists and neurointensivists. For example, the preoperative use of endovascular embolization may improve the probability and safety of complete microsurgical resection or make an AVM amenable to stereotactic radiosurgical cure. This combined multimodality approach may significantly reduce the risk of AVM treatment and improve outcome.

Several factors influence whether or how an AVM should be treated: (1) patient age and clinical condition, (2) presentation, (3) AVM location, size, morphology and complexity and (4) expected natural history and treatment risks. Management needs to be individualized to each patient and requires careful study of all radiologic images, including CT, MRI and detailed cerebral angiography. Some patients may also require functional imaging studies such as fMRI, MEG or PET scanning to localize eloquent cortex, because several studies have demonstrated that anatomical landmarks to localize eloquent cortex may be imprecise and that these areas may be subject to variability among patients. Alternatively, hemispheric dominance for speech or language can be established by intracarotid sodium amobarbital (Amytal) injection (WADA test). In addition, superselective angiography with amytal injection can establish whether an area of brain supplied by a particular artery is eloquent and so should be preserved. This information may influence whether surgery is selected and influence the use of intraoperative mapping techniques.

Microsurgery

Microsurgical AVM excision is the most effective treatment currently available. However, not every AVM is amenable to or best treated with surgery. Grading systems, such as the Spetzler–Martin grading system, are intended to predict the risk of neurologic deficit after surgery (Table 20.3) [18]. These surgical risks need to be weighed against the patient's age, clinical condition, vocation, psychological factors and expected natural history. For example, small superficial AVMs in silent cortical locations such as the non-dominant anterior frontal lobe are easily resected with little risk, whereas deep AVMs located in the basal ganglia, ventricular system, medial cortical surfaces or brain stem pose a significantly higher risk of neurologic injury during surgery. Similarly, a Grade III AVM in a 25-year-old patient with seizures would be managed differently from a similar lesion in a 75-year-old patient with seizures. In patients where surgical risk exceeds expected natural history, alternative treatments such as stereotactic radiosurgery should be considered, if appropriate. Alternatively, staged embolization may reduce AVM size and complexity, creating an amenable lesion for surgical excision.

There are several general principles and techniques that are useful during AVM surgery. The techniques used to resect AVMs in specific locations, such as perisylvian, parasagittal, medial temporal and parahippocampal, trigonal, intraventricular, basal ganglia or posterior fossa, are beyond the scope of this chapter but are reviewed in detail by other authors. Surgical AVM excision should be an elective procedure, even in patients with ruptured AVMs. In these patients, waiting at least 3 or 4 weeks allows the patient to recover and the hematoma to liquefy, which can greatly facilitate surgery. We routinely administer steroids, anticonvulsants and prophylactic antibiotics before and during AVM resection, particularly for supratentorial AVMs. The use of lumbar CSF drainage or mannitol for brain relaxation is individualized after careful study of all imaging studies. Frameless stereotaxy or intraoperative ultrasound is useful to help localize deep AVMs, whereas electrophysiologic monitoring, such as motor mapping, may be useful when the lesion is located near or within eloquent cortex.

The location of the AVM nidus dictates the operative approach. The relative location of the AVM nidus can be predicted from the preoperative cerebral angiogram. In general, the patient should be positioned with the AVM uppermost and avoiding any vascular obstruction in the neck from head positioning. The craniotomy and dural opening should be wide enough to identify completely the AVM's vascular anatomy. In particular, the surgeon should have enough room to gain access to and differentiate feeding vessels, draining veins, terminal vessels and "en passant" vessels. In addition, the surgical approach should be planned so that the angle of approach is as perpendicular to the major feeding arteries or the dominant nidal plane as possible. A wide opening, however, also allows modification of the angle of view, which is particularly useful when using the microscope or when hemorrhage occurs beyond the immediate surgical site.

The excision of an AVM requires several basic steps. First, the AVM needs to be identified. This is relatively straightforward when the AVM nidus is superficial. When the nidus is below the surface, an arterialized draining vein can be followed to the AVM. Also, a deep AVM nidus may be localized by careful comparison of operative and angiographic vascular anatomy, ultrasound or frameless stereotaxy. Any superficial feeders to the AVM should be secured with bipolar cautery or small clips and divided as close to the nidus as possible. Each vessel, however, must be carefully followed to ensure that it does not supply normal brain.

Second, a circumferential incision is made around the nidus, sparing the normal, adjacent cortex. This dissection is facilitated by use of cisternal and sulcal anatomy to reduce injury to normal brain. During this dissection, it is important to preserve the draining veins until the entire AVM and its feeders is defined because occlusion of venous outflow may increase intra-nidal pressure, causing sudden intraoperative hemorrhage. When there is both superficial and deep venous drainage, it may be possible to eliminate the superficial vein, provided there is adequate deep venous drainage.

Third, any deep feeders should be secured and divided. These vessels lack a muscular coating and tend to retract and continue to bleed into the brain; careful use of the suction and bipolar generally allow these vessels to be identified and secured with micro-clips, when needed. Once all the AVM feeders have been divided, the AVM should collapse and the draining vein should no longer appear "red" and arterialized. The last remaining vascular pedicle (i.e. the draining vein) can then be secured and divided. The resection cavity requires careful inspection to ensure there are no AVM remnants or leaking vessels. The surgical cavity is then lined with a hemostatic agent, such as Surgicel, and a brief period of normotension or a Valsalva maneuver is performed to check hemostasis before closure. Complete AVM excision should be documented by post-operative angiography. In some patients with complex AVMs, intraoperative angiography may be useful. However, intraoperative angiography does not replace the need for post-operative angiography.

Post-operatively, any factors that may increase intracranial, venous or arterial pressure should be avoided. In some patients, particularly those undergoing resection of large and complex AVMs, relative hypotension (90–110 mmHg systolic) during the first 24–48 hours post-operatively may be useful. Similarly, patients at significant risk for normal perfusion pressure breakthrough may benefit from sedation or barbiturate coma. Normal perfusion pressure breakthrough is a rare complication that is postulated to result from impaired autoregulation after excision of a high-flow AVM, which then leads to severe brain edema and hemorrhage, without evidence of residual AVM [19]. Patients at risk for normal perfusion pressure breakthrough generally present with progressive neurologic deficits, suggesting a steal syndrome, have an AVM nidus greater than 4 cm in diameter, have long and large-caliber arterial feeders and lack filling of adjacent normal vasculature on angiography secondary to shunting. The risk of normal perfusion pressure breakthrough may be reduced in these patients, particularly those with large AVMs, by staged embolization prior to surgical resection.

There are several other complications that can occur after AVM surgery. Patients are at high risk for seizures, in part because cortical venous drainage may have been altered by surgery. Generalized seizures can increase the risk of post-operative intracranial hemorrhage; therapeutic levels of anti-seizure medication should therefore be ensured in the immediate perioperative period. The risk of long-term seizures, however, is less than 10%. Prophylactic anticonvulsants can therefore be stopped several weeks after surgery. Post-operative hematomas complicate a small number of patients, usually during the first 48 hours after AVM resection. These hematomas usually result from residual AVM nidus, poor hemostasis or from hemorrhagic conversion of retraction injury. Consequently, when residual AVM is identified on the post-operative angiogram, the residual lesion should be treated without delay. Retrograde venous or arterial thrombosis may occur in rare instances. This complication can be avoided by dividing vessels as close to the AVM nidus as possible and maintaining euvolemia after surgery.

Endovascular Embolization

Endovascular embolization of AVMs is a rapidly evolving technique. This treatment modality is used primarily as an adjunct to surgery or radiosurgery to reduce blood flow and eliminate surgically inaccessible arterial feeders pre-operatively or to incrementally reduce the size of a large AVM nidus, making it amenable to surgical or radiosurgical treatment. The optimal time between embolization and surgery is not defined. Most surgeons, however, operate within 5–7 days after the last embolization to prevent recruitment of new vessels. In some patients, endovascular embolization may be used as a palliative measure to treat headaches or reverse neurologic deficit, whereas, in a small number of select patients, AVM embolization may be curative (Table 20.4). The long-term

Table 20.4. Results of AVM embolization in the contemporary literature

Author	Year	Material	No. Cases	Obliteration rate	Minor deficit	Major deficit	Mortality
Berenstein	1990	IBCA	500	17%	5%	1%	1%
Wilkholm	1996	NBCA/PVA	150	13%	32%	7%	1%
Gobin	1996	NBCA	125	11%	6%	2%	0%
Debrun	1997	NBCA	54	5%	4%	2%	4%
Paulsen	1999	NBCA/PVA	38	3%	6%	6%	0%
Song	2000	silk	230	–	9%	4%	1%

Berenstein A: Cerebral arteriovenous malformations. Am J Neuroradiol 11:220, 1990

Wilkholm G, Lundqvist, Svendsen P: Embolization of cerebral arteriovenous malformations. Part I, technique, morphology, and complications. Neurosurgery 39:448, 1996

Gobin Y, Laurent A, Merienne L: Treatment of brain arteriovenous malformations and radiosurgery. Journal of Neurosurgery 65:476, 1986

Debrun G, Aletich V, Ausman J, Charbel F, Dujovny: Embolization of the nidus of brain arteriovenous malformations with n-butyl cyanoacrylate. Neurosurgery 40:112, 1997

Paulsen R, Steinberg G, Norbash A, Marcellus M, Markss M: Embolization of basal ganglia and thalamic arteriovenous malformations. Neurosurgery 44:991. 1999

Song JK, Eskridge JM, Chung EC, et al: Preoperative embolization of cerebral arteriovenous malformations with silk sutures: analysis and clinical correlation of complications revealed on computerized tomography scanning. J Neurosurg 92:955–960, 2000 results of complete AVM obliteration using endovascular techniques, however, are not known, since there is some suggestion that recanalization may occur [22].

Endovascular embolization usually requires general or neuroleptic anesthesia to keep the patient motionless during the procedure. It also may require several staged procedures. First, a 5–7 French sheath is placed in the femoral artery and a diagnostic cerebral angiogram is performed using standard catheter angiography technique. The AVM characteristics are defined using conventional high-resolution angiography and a micro-catheter is co-axially advanced and placed into the intracranial circulation proximal to the AVM using a flow-directed micro-catheter or guidewire assistance. The AVM can then be further studied using micro-injections to define nidal compartmentalization, presence of aneurysms, location of intra-nidal fistulae and the pattern of venous drainage. Once the AVM anatomy and flow characteristics are understood, arterial feeders to be embolized are micro-catheterized and the embolic material is prepared. Embolization usually is accomplished with cyanoacrylate or, in some instances, silk. Attaching various chemical modulators to its basic structure to change the polymerization rate may modify cyanoacrylate; N-butyl cyanoacrylate (NBCA) is the present agent of choice. Vessel angioarchitecture determines the injection rate, volume and concentration of NBCA during AVM embolization.

The results and morbidity of AVM embolization have been described in several large clinical series [2,17,23]. Overall, between 2 and 18% of AVMs can be completely occluded using endovascular techniques. Procedural risk, however, is high - between 2 and 17% of patients suffer major or minor morbidity and mortality is between 1 and 4%. The overall risk of an ischemic complication per procedure is estimated to be 9.4%. These potential risks need to be considered and included in any decision making when embolization is used as an adjunct to surgery or radiosurgery. Inadvertent glue deposition in normal cerebral vessels, causing infarction, and catastrophic AVM rupture are the two most significant complications encountered during AVM embolization. AVM rupture may result from inadvertent NBCA placement into a draining vein, causing a sudden rise in nidal pressures and consequent hemorrhage. Alternatively, the NBCA bolus itself may rupture the nidus or cause partial nidal occlusion, diverting blood flow and pressure to other nidal segments, leading to rupture. The use of hypotension (60–80 mmHg systolic) for a short period during embolic injections and post-procedure hypotension (90–110 mmHg systolic) for 24–48 hours may help prevent AVM rupture. Thromboembolic complications during AVM embolization may be prevented by the administration of heparin, to achieve ACTs between 250 and 300 s during the procedure.

Stereotactic Radiosurgery

Stereotactic radiosurgery, in particular LINAC or Gamma Knife radiosurgery, can be used in select patients to provide a single, high dose of stereotactically localized radiation to the AVM nidus. This radiation dose causes endothelial damage, smooth muscle cell proliferation, progressive sclerosis and subsequent thrombosis of nidal channels over time. The success of stereotactic radiosurgery depends on AVM size and the radiation dose delivered. Several clinical studies have demonstrated that AVM obliteration can be expected between 1 and 2 years after radiosurgery, provided the AVM nidus is less than 2–3 cm in diameter or has a volume of less than 10 cc (Table 20.5) [7,13,15,20,21]. Long-term angiographic follow-up between 5 and 24 years after radiosurgery suggests that a small number of obliterated AVMs may recur, especially in pediatric patients. Larger AVMs or lesions with a diffuse nidus are generally not amenable to stereotactic radiosurgery. However, the use of specialized collimators, staged radiosurgery, embolization and microsurgery or repetitive radiosurgery may facilitate the treatment of some larger lesions. For example, large AVMs can be incrementally reduced in size with multiple endovascular embolizations until the nidus is smaller than 3 cm in diameter and thus amenable to radiosurgical treatment.

The selection of patients for stereotactic radiosurgery varies among institutions. In general, stereotactic radiosurgery should be considered when (1) surgical AVM excision is associated with an unacceptably high risk, (2) anesthetic risk is high because of the patient's medical condition, (3) surgery with or without

Table 20.5. Results of AVM radiosurgery with gamma knife in the contemporary literature

Author	Year	No. Cases	Obliteration rate	Morbidity	Hemorrhage rate	Mortality
Steiner	1992	239	81%	4%	4%/yr	5%
Freidman	1996	201	–	–	6%/yr	1%
Flickinger	1996	197	72%	–	–	–
Flickinger	1997	307	–	11%	–	–
Karlsson	1997	945	87%	–	–	–
Sasaki	1998	66	86%	7%	5%/yr	1%
Pollack	1999	97	74%	5%	5%/yr	4%

Steiner L, Lindquist C, Adler J, Torner J, Alves W, Steiner M: Clinical outcome of radiosurgery for cerebral arteriovenous malformations. Journal of Neurosurgery 77:1. 1992

Freidman W, Blatt D, Bova F, Buatti J, Mendenhall W, Kubilis P: The risk of hemorrhage after radiosurgery for arteriovenous malformations. Journal of Neurosurgery 84:912. 1996

Flickinger J, Pollack B, Knodziolka D, Lunsford L: A dose-response analysis of arteriovenous malformation obliteration after radiosurgery. Int J radiation Oncology Biol Phys 36:873. 1996

Flickinger J, Pollack B, Knodziolka D, Maitz A, Lunsford L: Complications from arteriovenous malformation radiosurgery: Multivariate analysis and risk modeling. Int J radiation Oncology Biol Phys 38:485. 1997

Karlsson B, Lindquist C, Steiner L: Prediction of obliteration after gamma knife surgery for cerebral arteriovenous malformations. Neurosurgery 40:425. 1997

Sasaki T, Kurita H, Saito I, et al: Arteriovenous malformations in the basal ganglia and thalamus: management and results in 101 cases. Journal of Neurosurgery 88:285, 1998

Pollack B: Stereotactic radiosurgery for arteriovenous malformations. Neurosurgery Clinics of North America 10:281, 1999

embolization was unsuccessful or (4) residual deep AVM remains after surgery. Stereotactic radiosurgery can be particularly useful for patients with deep AVMs, such as those in the basal ganglia or brain stem, or AVMs in critical lobar areas, such as sensorimotor cortex. Radiosurgery becomes the preferred treatment when surgical mortality and morbidity exceed 4 and 12%, respectively. Pregnant patients are not candidates for radiosurgery.

The procedure is relatively straightforward. First, a stereotactic head-frame is placed using local anesthesia and mild sedation. The patient then undergoes an MRI scan and a stereotactic cerebral angiogram. Using these images, the neurosurgeon, radiation physicist and radiation therapist can then plan treatment. The selected target dose depends on the exact configuration of the AVM. In general, a radiation dose of about 20 Gy is administered to the margin of the AVM nidus [21]. Obliteration rates of 70, 80 or 90% have been observed when the radiation dose to the AVM margin is 16, 18 or 20 Gy, respectively. The prescription isodose (radiation dosage)-to-treatment-volume ratio should preferably be less than 2; however, this may be difficult to achieve with irregular contours. After treatment, patients are observed overnight in the hospital. We administer peri-procedural anticonvulsants and steroids to our patients. AVMs are followed after radiosurgery with MRI, until there is no evidence of nidal flow. Once this occurs, follow-up catheter angiography is performed to document AVM obliteration.

Stereotactic radiosurgery is relatively safe and is not associated with the conventional risks of surgery, such as bleeding or infection. Acute, transient radiation risks causing neurologic deficits are uncommon and generally respond to steroids. Instead, the major risks of radiosurgery are delayed. These risks include primary AVM hemorrhage during the latency period before obliteration and the risk of delayed radiation injury. Subtotal AVM obliteration by stereotactic radiosurgery is of no benefit in preventing hemorrhage. This is confirmed by several clinical series demonstrating that the risk of hemorrhage between AVM treatment and obliteration is unchanged from the expected natural history of AVM hemorrhage. It remains between 2 and 4% per year. Successful obliteration can take up to 2–3 years after radiosurgery. Delayed radiation injury, such as radiation necrosis of cortical tissue or cranial nerves surrounding the AVM nidus, is related to the radiation dose, volume treated, patient age and AVM flow characteristics [13]. Radiation-induced tumors are very rare and generally occur many years after treatment. Radiation-related complications are correlated with the volume of brain that receives greater than 12 Gy. In addition, patients with deep AVMs in the basal ganglia or thalamus are more likely to develop radiation-induced complications.

Key Points

- *Each type of vascular malformation has a unique natural history, thus requiring a separate treatment approach.*
- *The clinical presentation of patients with CAVMs depends in large part on pathology and location of the lesion.*
- *The treatment of AVMs is primarily intended to eradicate the risk of potential hemorrhage.*
- *The treatment modalities used to manage AVMs include microsurgical excision, endovascular embolization, stereotactic surgery or a combination of the three.*
- *Treatment needs to be tailored to the individual patient based on the expected natural history and morphology of the lesion.*

References

1. Batjer H, Devous M, Seibert G. Intracranial arteriovenous malformations associated with aneurysms. Neurosurgery 1990;26:570.
2. Berenstein A. Cerebral arteriovenous malformations. Am J Neuroradiol 1990;11:220.
3. Brown R, Wiebers D, Forbes G. Unruptured intracranial aneurysms and arteriovenous malformations: frequency of intracranial hemorrhage and relationship of lesions. Journal of Neurosurgery 1990;73:859.
4. Courville C. Pathology of the central nervous system. Mountainview: Pacific Press, 1945.
5. Fults D, Kelly D. Natural history of arteriovenous malformations of the brain: a clinical study. Neurosurgery 1984;15:658.
6. Heros R, Karosue K, Diebold P. Surgical excision of cerebral arteriovenous malformations: late results. Neurosurgery 1990;26:570.
7. Kjellberg R, Hanamura T, Davis K et al. Bragg-peak proton beam therapy for arteriovenous malformations of the brain. N Engl J Med 1983;309:269.
8. Luessenhop A, Mujica P. Embolization of segments of the circle of willis and adjacent arteries for management of certain inoperable cerebral arteriovenous malformations. Journal of Neurosurgery 1981;54:573.
9. McCormick W. Pathology of vascular malformations of the brain. Baltimore: Williams & Wilkins, 1984.
10. Ondra S, Troupp H, George E. The natural history of symptomatic arteriovenous malformations of the brain: a 24 year follow-up assessment. Journal of Neurosurgery 1990;73:387.
11. Paillas J, Berard M, Sedan R. The relative importance of atheroma in the clinical course of arteriovenous angioma of the brain. Prog Brain Res 1968;30:419.
12. Perret G, Nishioka H. Report on the cooperative study of intracranial aneurysms and subarachnoid hemorrhage: arteriovenous malformations. An analysis of 545 cases of craniocerebral arteriovenous malformations and fistulae reported to the cooperative study. Journal of Neurosurgery 1966;25:467.
13. Pollack B. Stereotactic radiosurgery for arteriovenous malformations. Neurosurgery Clinics of North America 1999;10:281.
14. Robinson J, Hall C, Sedzimir C. Arteriovenous malformations, aneurysms, and pregnancy. Journal of Neurosurgery 1974;41:63.
15. Sasaki T, Kurita H, Saito I et al. Arteriovenous malformations in the basal ganglia and thalamus: management and results in 101 cases. Journal of Neurosurgery 1998;88:285.
16. Schoenberg B, Mellinger J, Schoenberg D. Cerebrovascular disease in infants and children: a study of incidence, clinical features, and survival. Neurology 1978;28:763.
17. Song JK, Eskridge JM, Chung EC et al. Preoperative embolization of cerebral arteriovenous malformations with silk sutures: analysis and clinical correlation of complications revealed on computerized tomography scanning. J Neurosurg 2000;92:955–60.
18. Spetzler R, Martin N. A proposed grading system for arteriovenous malformations of the brainstem. Journal of Neurosurgery 1986;65:476.
19. Spetzler R, Wilson C, Weinstein P et al. Normal perfusion pressure breakthrough theory. Clinical Neurosurgery 1978;25:651.
20. Steinberg G, Fabrikant J, Marks M. Stereotactic heavy charged-particle bragg-peak radiation for intracranial malformations. N Engl J Med 1990;323:96.
21. Steiner L. Treatment of arteriovenous malformations by radiosurgery. In: Wilson C, Stein B, editors. Intracranial arteriovenous malformations. Baltimore: Williams & Wilkins, 1984; 295.
22. Vinters HV, Lundie MJ, Kaufmann JC. Long-term pathological follow-up of cerebral arteriovenous malformations treated by embolization with bucrylate. N Engl J Med 1986;314:477–83.
23. Wilkholm G, Lundqvist, Svendsen P. Embolization of cerebral arteriovenous malformations. Part I: Technique, morphology, and complications. Neurosurgery 1996;39:448.
24. Yasargil M. Microneurosurgery, IIIA. Stuttgart: Thieme, 1987.
25. Yasargil M. Microneurosurgery, IIIB. Stuttgart: Thieme, 1988.

VI
Trauma

21

Management of Severe Head Injury

Bizhan Aarabi, Rajesh Mehta and Howard M. Eisenberg

Summary

The objectives embedded in the management of traumatic brain injury (TBI) include limiting the primary damage and controlling secondary insults, which are thrust upon the brain immediately after an accident. Applying the recommendations of evidence-based guidelines approved by the American Association of Neurological Surgeons attains these objectives. At the scene of accident, airway support, ventilation and oxygenation are strongly recommended in trying to keep the systolic blood pressure (SBP) of the patient at around 100 mmHg [1]. Upon stabilization of the hemodynamic and pulmonary function, the victim is transferred rapidly by surface or air into the closest trauma center. In the emergency department (ED), one must maintain an SBP of at least 90 mmHg with adequate SPO2 before any other diagnostic procedure is performed, including CT of the head. When faced with multiple trauma, surgical prioritization depends on stability of vital signs, clinical evidence of herniation, findings on CT and intracranial pressure. A rapidly deteriorating patient should have infusion of mannitol and short-term hyperventilation en route to the CT suite. To prevent secondary brain insults, especially ischemia and brain swelling, the victim of TBI needs 3–4 weeks of vigilant supportive care in the intensive care unit (ICU), including ICP control and perfusion pressure management, adequate ventilation, infection control, nutritional support, physical and occupational therapy. Physical, mental and occupational rehabilitation in a well equipped center prepares the patient for ultimate social integration.

Epidemiology

Each year, close to 52,000 Americans die from head injury (20/100,000 population). The incidence of severe head trauma (GCS less than or equal to 8) is 100/100,000 population and the prevalence is 2.5–5.6 million (Table 21.1) [2].

Pathogenesis

Translation of kinetic energy into passive parenchymal damage and secondary brain insults is considered TBI. Compressive, tensile and shearing strains heavily contribute to tissue damage in the form of contusion, laceration or diffuse axonal injury. While passive damage is instantaneous, secondary brain insults occur from hours to several days after TBI and significantly alter the prognosis [2]. Transient mechanical microporation, cell rupture, activation of voltage and ligand gated NMDA channels and ischemia result in entry of Ca^{++} and Na^{+} inside cells and egress of potassium ions from cells and altered state of consciousness.

Table 21.1. Epidemiology.

Useful statistics	
Number of patients surviving TBI in USA per year	1.3 million
Number of patients hospitalized with TBI in USA per year	230,000
Firearm-related TBI deaths in the USA during 1995	21,093
Economic burden during 1985	$37.5 billion

Even in concussive states without significant parenchymal damage, the concentration of extracellular K+ is increased fiftyfold. There is a direct relationship between extracellular potassium and mortality. Excess potassium in extracellular fluid (ECF) is sequestered by the glial cells, leading to swelling of the astrocytic footplates, cytotoxic edema, increased ICP and secondary ischemia. Disturbance of calcium homeostasis through inward movement of Ca++ results in metabolic cascades, with dire consequences. Elevated levels of calcium in cytosol results in multimeric transformation of proteins in mitochondrial outer membrane and formation of mitochondrial permeability transition pore (MPTP). MPTP allows abnormal concentrations of calcium in the mitochondrial matrix, disturbance of electron transport, formation of reactive oxygen species and activation of lipases, proteases and endonucleases, hence enhanced cell necrosis. Release of apoptogenic protein from mitochondria, along with intrinsic pathways, signal activation of apoptotic processes which result in programmed cell death [3]. Abnormal concentrations of Ca++ into the axons activates calpain-mediated cytoskeletal damage and axonal transport. The long-term effect of cytoskeletal damage is axotomy and Wallerian degeneration.

Pathology

Mechanical loading of the brain will result in a variety of pathologies, including:

Diffuse axonal injury (DAI).

Transmission of inertial energy in the form of angular acceleration or deceleration results in axonal disruption and immediate coma. CT is such cases is usually without significant intracranial injury but pathological injury indicates retraction balls. DAI is the most frequent finding in patients who die from severe head injury. DAI is seen in younger people, and is usually unassociated with high intracranial pressure [4]. Penetration of axolemma by Ca++ may activate the calpain cascade and disrupt the cytoskeleton, causing chemical axotomy. Microdialysis studies have shown that the concentration of extracellular fluid glutamate in patients with DAI is lower than that encountered in sub-dural hematoma and cortical contusion [5].

Tissue tear hemorrhages (TTH).

Focal contusions.

Focal contusions are usually in the form of high-density lesions. Focal contusions do not occupy much space in the beginning but may blossom within days and cause significant intracranial hypertension. The extracellular concentration of glutamate is higher in patients with focal cortical damage than in patients with diffuse axonal injury.

Intracerebral hematomas.

Intracerebral hematomas are usually in the form of parenchymal contusions. Delayed intracerebral hematomas could have traumatic aneurysms as the main source of bleeding.

Subdural hematomas.

Up to 35–40% of patients with severe TBI have subdural hematomas (SDH). Translational shifts of the hemispheres inside the cranium will result in rupture of cortical veins or arteries and bleeding in the sub-dural space. SDH could be considered as epiphenomena of underlying cortical injuries.

Epidural hematomas.

Depending on the type of the patient population studied, between 1 and 10% of patients with head injury will have epidural hematoma (EDH). EDH is an abnormal collection of blood between the dura and the cranium, usually from a torn middle meningeal artery, but it may be due to torn venous sinuses or bleeding from fracture lines.

Cerebral ischemia, blood flow and metabolism after TBI.

Cerebral ischemia is at the center of the secondary injuries to the brain. Ischemia could have peripheral causes (such as anemia, shock or low SaO2) or central pathogenetic mechanisms (such as low microcirculatory flow, high ICP, diffusion difficulties or problems with electron transfer at the mitochondrial level). More than 90% of the patients who die from head trauma have evidence of hypoxic brain damage at autopsy and up to 36% of patients in the ICU at one point during their hospitalization will have global desaturation, as evidenced by sjvO2 or brain tissue oxygen monitoring [6]. During the first 24 hours after TBI, cerebral blood flow is down, especially during the first 6 hours. After the first day, for the next 3–5 days, CBF will increase and then decrease again within the next 2 weeks. Cerebral metabolism is generally down during the post-injury course of the TBI. Hyperglycolysis and increased CBF immediately after TBI could be part of the restorative mechanisms of membrane instability and could have a relationship with good outcome [7].

Cerebral swelling.

During the first 24 hours after head trauma, cerebral swelling is usually cytotoxic, due to membrane dysfunction and excess extracellular potassium. Astrocytic footplate swelling, evident following oxidative distress, is thought generally to worsen cerebral ischemia.

Clinical Exam

Glasgow Coma Scale (GCS) Score

Following a quick primary and secondary survey and appropriate resuscitation, we must determine the numerical value of the GCS score (Table 21.2) [8]:

Mild head injury: GCS score 13–15.
Moderate head injury: GCS score 9–12.
Severe head injury: GCS score 4–8.
Very severe head injury: GCS score 3.

Pupillary Response to Light

Uncal or central herniation and pressure on the midbrain are usually associated with change in pupillary size and response to light. In uncal herniation, at first, the pupil becomes smaller and then larger, with sluggish reaction to light. Midbrain pupils are irregular and larger and with no or sluggish reaction to light.

Focal Deficit

With focal deficit, one can localize the pathology. It is important to pay attention to any new focal deficit associated with change in GCS score and pupillary change, which may mean uncal or central herniation.

Trauma Scores

Abbreviated Injury Scale (AIS)

AIS is an anatomical scoring system and provides a reasonable way of ranking the severity of injury. Injuries are ranked on a scale of 1 to 6, with 1 being minor and 6 unsurvivable (Table 21.3) [9].

Table 21.2. GCS score.

Points	Best eye	Best verbal	Best motor
6	–	–	Obeys
5	–	Oriented	Localizes pain
4	Spontaneous	Confused	Withdraws from pain
3	To speech	Inappropriate	Flexor (decorticate)
2	To pain	Incomprehensible	Extensor
1	None	None	None

Table 21.3. AIS.

AIS score	Injury
1	Minor
2	Moderate
3	Serious
4	Severe
5	Critical
6	Unsurvivable

Maximum Head AIS (MAIS)

MAIS is the maximum point value that you can give the injury sustained by the brain.

Injury Severity Score (ISS)

For multiple injuries, ISS provides us with the overall injury score [10]. Each injury is assigned an AIS and is allocated to one of six body regions (head, face, chest, abdomen, extremities, spine). Only the highest AIS score in each body region is used. The three most severely injured body regions have their scores squared and added together to produce the ISS score. ISS has values from 0 to 75. If an AIS is 6, the ISS is automatically 75 (Table 21.4).

Revised Trauma Score (RTS)

A physiological indication of injury is expressed as RTS, with a high degree of reliability of prediction of outcome. RTS takes into consideration respiratory rate (RR), blood pressure (SBP) and the GCS score (Table 5):

RTS score = 0.9368 (coded GCS) + 0.7326 (coded SBP) + 0.2908 (coded RR).

The RTS value ranges between 0 and 7.8408 and is heavily weighted towards the GCS score.

Table 21.5. RTS.

GCS	SBP	RR	Coded value
13–15	>89	10–29	4
9–12	76–89	>29	3
6–8	50–75	6–9	2
4–5	1–49	1–5	1
3	0	0	0

RTS = 0.9368GCS + 0.7326SBP + 0.2908RR.

Patients with an RTS of less than 4 should be transferred to a trauma center [11].

TRISS Probability of Survival

Prospective studies indicate that one would be able to calculate the probability of survival if the following variables are available: ISS, RTS, age and the mechanism of injury. The probability of survival (Ps) is expressed by the following formula:

Ps = 1/(1 + e–b), where b = b0 + b1(RTS) + b2(ISS) + b3(AgeIndex).

The coefficients b0–b3 are derived from multiple regression analysis of the Major Trauma Outcome Study (MTOS) databases. AgeIndex is 0 if the patient is under 54 years of age or 1 if 55 years and over. Coefficients b0 and b3 are different for blunt and penetrating trauma. If the patient is under 15 years, the blunt coefficients are used, regardless of mechanism [12].

Studies

CT

CT is the main stay in evaluation of severe head injury. CT of the head is vital in indicating

Table 21.4. ISS.

Region	Injury	AIS	Square top three
Head and neck	Cerebral contusion	3	9
Face	No injury	0	–
Chest	Flail chest	4	16
Abdomen	Ruptured spleen	5	25
Extremity	Fractured femur	3	–
External	No injury	0	–
ISS			50

intracranial bleeds, necessity of surgical exploration and the injury profile. Findings in CT are of significance when it comes to predicting the prognosis. Marshal, in 1991, classified CT findings, taking into consideration basal cisterns, midline shift and the hematoma size (Table 21.6). Obliteration of the basal cisterns is directly related to mortality (Table 21.7).

MRI

MRI may be specifically used to unravel the presence of cortical hypoxia and brain stem finding, both of which are important prognosticating factors. Diffusion-weighted images tell us about the possibility of ischemic injury to the brain.

Cerebral Blood Flow (CBF) Studies

Cerebral blood flow may be of value regionally or globally in verifying the extent of ischemic damage. CBF could be either by Xenon CT or isotope scan. Confirmation of brain death is also possible using CBF studies [7].

Cerebral Oxymetry

Early in the first 6 hours of severe head injury, there is severe brain ischemia, which may be regional or global. Parenchymal sensors may be helpful in diagnosing and alleviating brain ischemia. This is possible by either Licox or Codman cerebral oxymetry. Values lower than 8–10 mmHg of PbrO2 are considered to be confirmation of ischemia and, therefore, indication for corrective measures, such as improvement of FIO2, CPP or lowering of ICP [13].

Cerebral Microdialysis

Evaluation of the microenvironment of neural elements in TBI, although not clinically common practice at the present time, may in the future be of value in management of the TBI. Reversal of the lactate/pyruvate ratio, accumulation of glutamate in the extracellular fluid and significant peaks of potassium have been repeatedly reported in cases of TBI [5].

Table 21.6. Classification of diffuse head injury based on CT.

Category	Initial CT findings
Diffuse injury I	No visible pathology (Fig. 21.2)
Diffuse injury II	Cisterns are present; midline shift <5 mm and/or lesion densities present, no high- or mixed-density lesion >25 ml, may include bone fragments and foreign bodies
Diffuse injury III (swelling)	Cisterns are compressed or absent; midline shift is 0–5 mm; no high- or mixed-density lesion >25 ml (Fig 21.3)
Diffuse injury IV (shift)	Midline shift >5 mm, no high- or mixed-density lesion >25 ml
Evacuated mass	Any lesion surgically evacuated
Non-evacuated mass	High- or mixed-density lesion >25 ml, not surgically evacuated (Fig 21.4)

Marshall et al. [19].

Table 21.7. Correlation of GOS* with basal cisterns.

Basal cisterns	Outcome* Mortality	Vegetative	Severe disability	Moderate disability	Good
	(GOS 1)%	(GOS 2)%	(GOS 3)%	(GOS 4)%	(GOS 5)%
Normal	22	6	16	21	35
Compressed	39	7	18	17	19
Absent	77	2	6	4	11
Not visualized	68	0	11	9	12

*GOS, Glasgow Outcome Scale.

Management

Victims of severe head injury are especially vulnerable to brain hypoxia and ischemia. Traumatic Coma Data Bank studies clearly indicate that even one single recorded SBP of 90 mmHg during pre-hospital rescue or in the emergency department can significantly worsen the neurological outcome after TBI. This was clearly shown in a 1991 reported article by Chesnut et al. [14].

Pre-hospital

One of the basic strategies in treating patients with severe head injury is efficient and timely resuscitation of the victim of TBI. Treatment starts at the scene of the accident by intubation (rapid sequence), oxygenation and support of the airway. The evidence-based guidelines for pre-hospital management of patients with TBI have simplified our approach to these patients [1].

ED

In the ED, primary and secondary surveys will reveal associated injuries and the need for prioritized management. When stable, the following flowchart 21.1 is recommended to be applied for patients with severe head injury [1].

ICP Monitoring

Patients with severe head injury, a GCS score of less than 9 and abnormal CT scan of the head are candidates for ICP monitoring and perfusion pressure management. ICP monitoring is indicated with a normal CT if blood pressure is less than 90 mmHg, the patient is posturing and if the age of the patient is over 40 years [1]. ICP monitoring could be performed by extracerebral, parenchymal or ventricular sensors. Generally speaking, extracerebral and parenchymal sensors have fewer infectious complications but are less accurate than intraventricular sensors. One major advantage of intraventricular cannula (IVC) is the ability to have external ventricular drainage (EVD). Therapy intensity level is roughly related to the CT class of the patient with TBI. As the basal cisterns become less visible on the CT, there is less chance of normal CSF circulation.

Intensive Care Management of a Patient with Severe Head Injury

When hemodynamically secure, with protected airways, optimum oxygenation and no need for urgent decompression, the patient is transferred to the ICU, with an ICP monitoring device in place. In the ICU, based on the level of GCS, CT profile and intracranial pressure, the therapy intensity level (TIL) varies. The victim will be subjected to intense conservative management in order to keep the ICP down and assure adequate cerebral perfusion pressure (CPP). Depending on the need for hemodynamic monitoring, a severe head injury patient may need a triple lumen or Swan–Ganz catheter to ensure adequate hydration and intravascular volume. The type of crystalloids selected should be tailored in such a way as to avoid excessive hemodilution. We try to keep the hematocrit of the patient at between 30 and 33 in order to maintain blood viscosity within the physiological range [15]. Metabolic depression by propofol and morphine is vital to keep the patient calm and lower the intracranial pressure and hamper cough reflex. We titrate propofol from 10–75 (g/kg/hour, based on the degree of restlessness and the intracranial pressure of the patient. Since propofol has a short half-life, it gives us the opportunity to evaluate the patient's level of consciousness frequently [16]. To ensure adequate CPP, we may need to use pressors to keep the mean arterial pressure (MAP) up (Table 21.8). Flowchart 21.2 is a pathway for management of a patient with possible increased intracranial pressure.

Example of TIL

E.H. was a 21-year-old male who was involved in a motor vehicle accident and was transferred to the Shock Trauma Center with a GCS of 7 and a motor score of 5. There was abnormal pupillary response to light. The patient had CT of the head, which was compatible with a diffuse injury 3 (Fig. 21.1). He had already been intubated during his pre-hospital resuscitation. His vital signs were stable. In the trauma resuscitation unit (TRU), he had insertion of a parenchymal ICP monitoring device (Camino, Integra Neurosciences). The patient was sedated and, to further control his ICPs, he needed IVC for external ventricular drainage. Adjustment of his

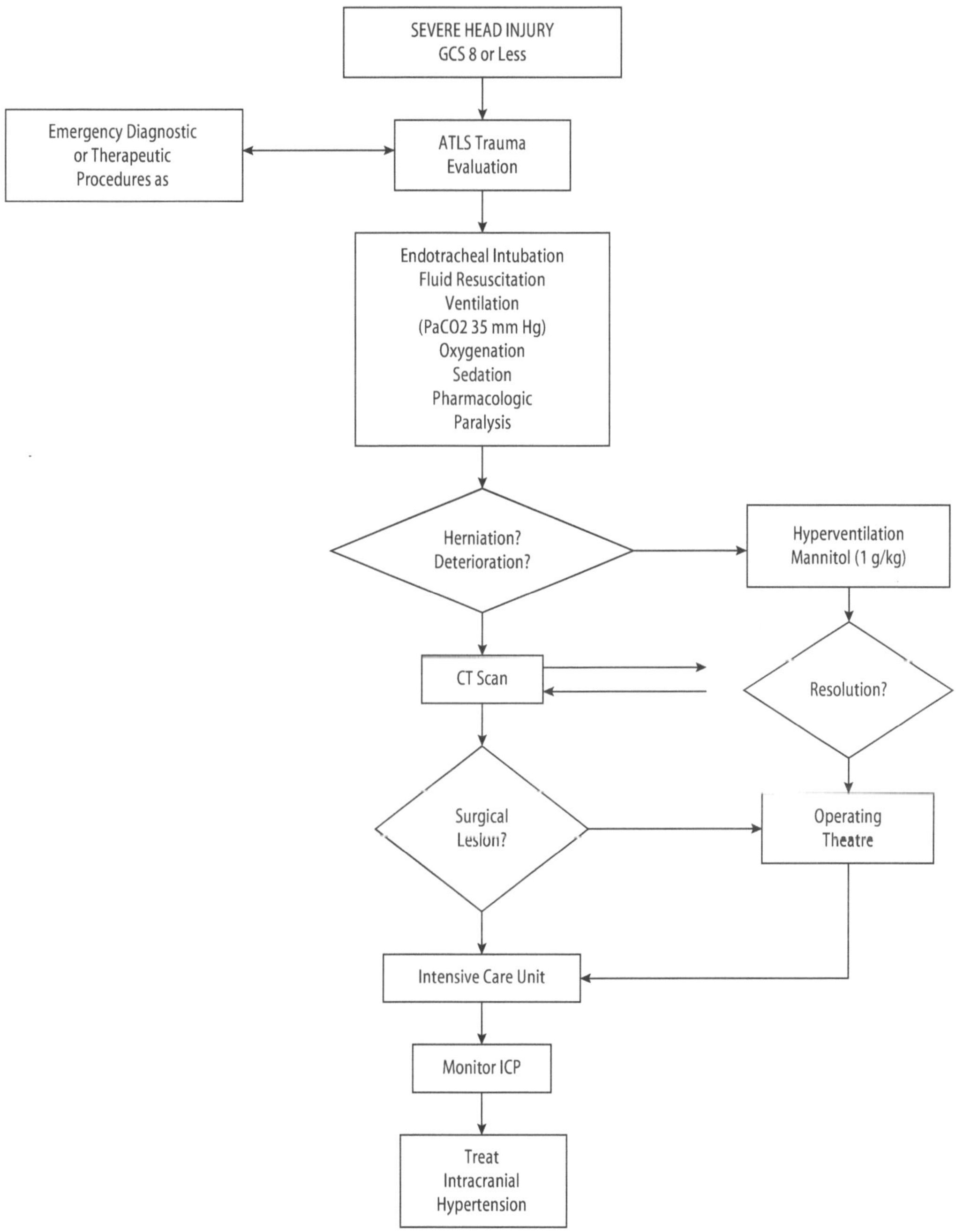

Flowchart 21.1. Initial management of a patient with severe head injury. (Reproduced from Guidelines for Management and Prognosis of Severe Head Injury, with permission.)

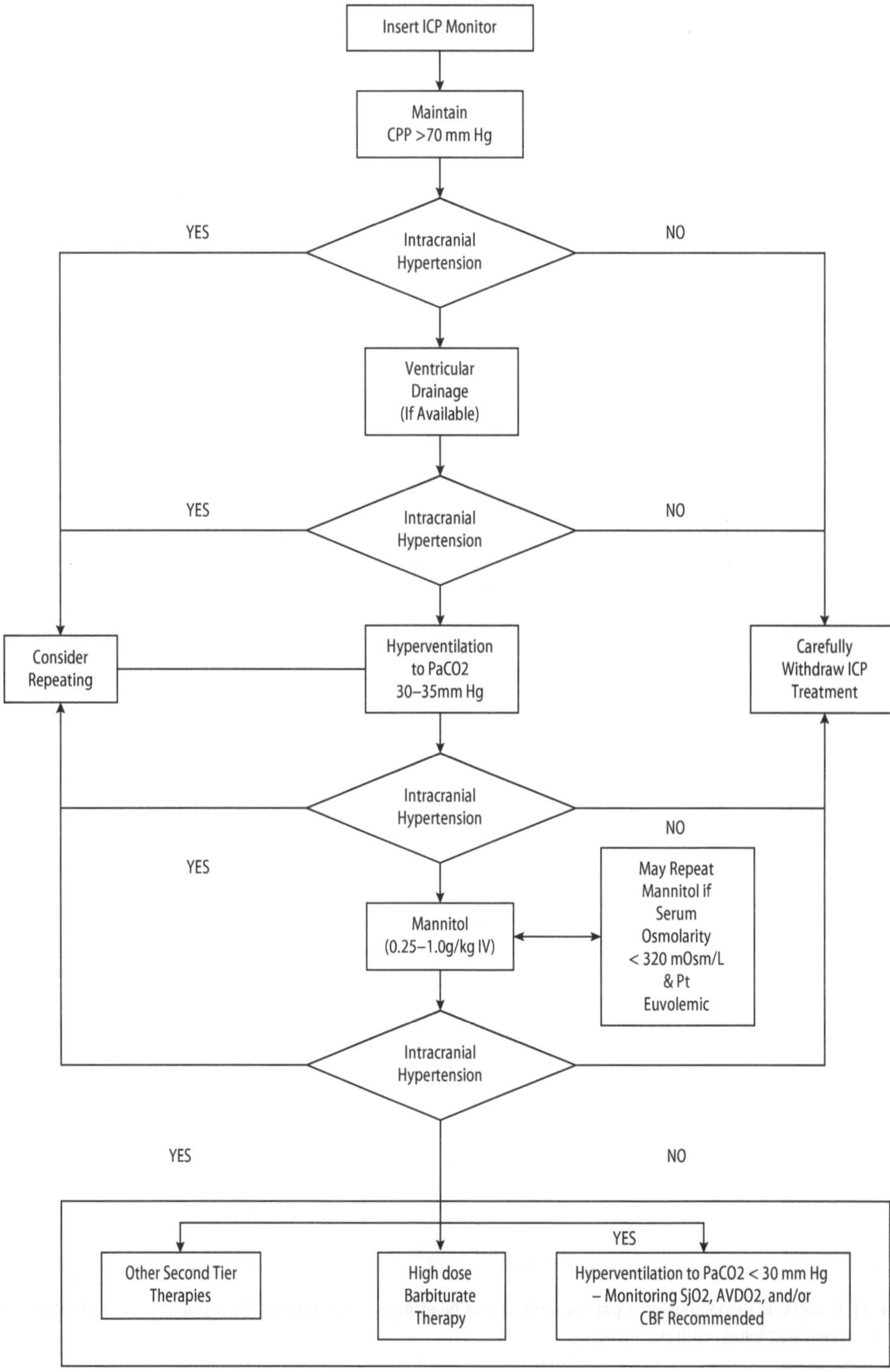

Flowchart 21.2. Steps needed to be taken for ICP control and perfusion pressure management. (Reproduced from Guidelines for Management and Prognosis of Severe Head Injury, with permission.)

Table 21.8. Management of severe head injury in the ICU.

Stepwise progression of therapy intensity level in management of patients with severe head trauma
ATLS protocol, intubation, ventilation, oxygenation and hemodynamic resuscitation.
Sedate the patient with (morphine, propofol); avoid long-term muscle relaxants.
Keep the patients head up 35°.
Maintain normothermia.
Ventilate to a PCO2 of 30–33 mmHg.
Insert ICP monitoring device; keep the ICP at <20 mmHg.
Keep the perfusion pressure at 60–70 mmHg [20].
If needed, administer mannitol or hypertonic saline to maintain an osmolality at 310–320.
Load the patient with phenytoin and continue this medication for about 1 week.
Start nutrition within 72 hours.

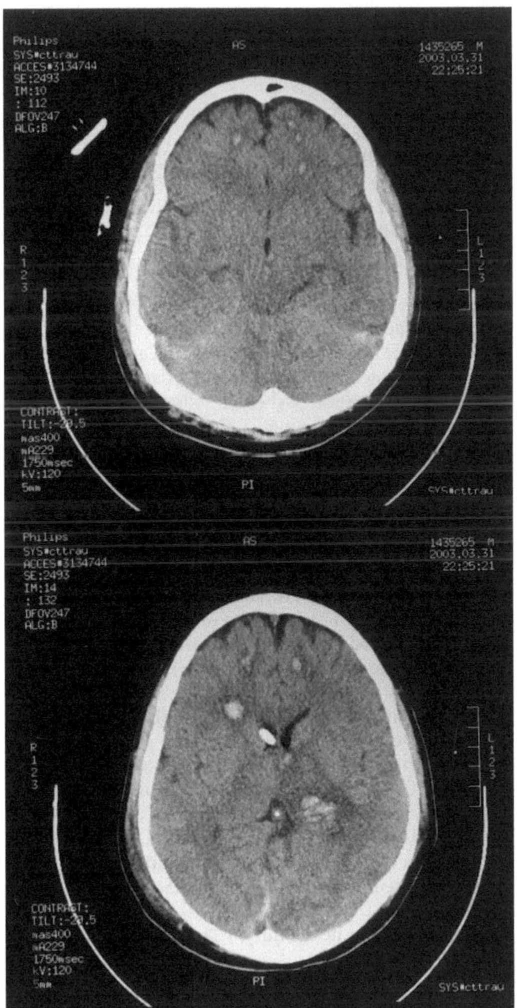

Fig. 21.1. CT scan of head from Case 1, indicating widespread small contusions and compressed basal cisterns.

vent settings kept his PCO2 at around 30–33 mmHg, in addition to osmotherapy with mannitol. His EVD was continued for 12 days until the ICPs were stable and then the IVC was removed. The graph in Fig. 21.2 indicates his therapy intensity level within the first 25 hours of admission.

Prognosis, Rehabilitation and Social Integration

Until the time is right for a pluripotential drug to alleviate the ill effects of secondary brain insults, management of TBI remains primarily supportive and conservative. Mortality still hovers at around 30%. Close to 20% of patients remain in a vegetative state [2].

Key Points

- *Patients with severe head injury should be treated at a trauma center as soon as possible [17].*
- *Pre-hospital resuscitation should assure a SBP of 90 mmHg or above [6,14].*
- *Surgical prioritization must be considered after the multiple trauma patient has stable cardiopulmonary status.*
- *Patients with abnormal CT scan of the head and a GCS of less than 9 should have ICP monitoring [1].*
- *The threshold for intervention is an ICP of 20–25 mmHg and a CPP of 60 mmHg [18].*

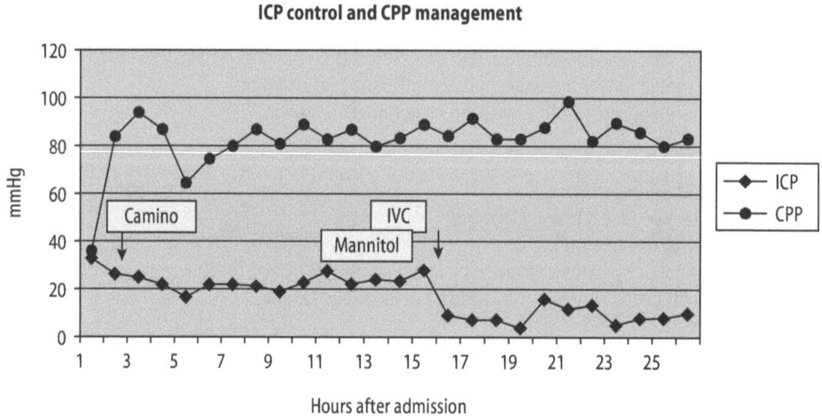

Fig. 21.2. TIL, indicating the need for head elevation, sedation, ventilation, osmotherapy and external ventricular drainage.

References

1. Bullock R, Chesnut RM, Clifton G et al. Guidelines for the Management of Severe Head Injury. J Neurotrauma 1996;13:639.
2. Marshall LF. Head injury: recent past, present, and future. Neurosurgery 2000;47:546–61.
3. Bullock R, Zauner A, Woodward JJ et al. Factors affecting excitatory amino acid release following severe human head injury. J Neurosurg 1998;89:507–18.
4. Adams JH, Graham DI, Murray LS, Scott G. Diffuse axonal injury due to nonmissile head injury in humans: an analysis of 45 cases. Ann Neurol 1982;12: 557–63.
5. Zauner A, Doppenberg EMR, Woodward JJ. Continuous monitoring of cerebral substrate delivery and clearance: initial experience in 24 patients with severe acute brain injuries. Neurosurgery 1999;41:1082–93.
6. Chesnut RM, Marshall LF, Klauber MR. The role of secondary brain injury in determining outcome from severe head injury. J Trauma 1993;34:216–22.
7. Robertson CS, Contant CF, Narayan RK, Grossman RG. Cerebral blood flow, AVDO2, and neurologic outcome in head-injured patients. J Neurotrauma 1992;9 (Suppl 1):S349-S358.
8. Teasdale G, Jennett B. Assessment of coma and impaired consciousness: a practical scale. Lancet 1974; 2(7872):81–4.
9. Association for the Advancement of Automotive Medicine. The Abbreviated Injury Scale, 1990 Revision. Des Plaines, IL: Association for the Advancement of Automotive Medicine, 1990; 1–66.
10. Baker SP, O'Neill B, Haddon W et al. The injury severity score: a method for describing patients with multiple injuries and evaluating emergency care. J Trauma 1979;14:187–96.
11. Champion HR, Sacco WJ, Copes WS. A revision of the trauma score. J Trauma 1989;29:623–9.
12. Boyd CR, Tolson MA, Copes WS. Evaluating trauma care: the TRISS method. J Trauma 1987;27:370–8.
13. Kiening KL, Hartl R, Unterberg AW, Schneider GH, Bardt T, Lanksch WR. Brain tissue PO2-monitoring in comatose patients: implications for therapy. Neurological Research 1997;19:233–40.
14. Chesnut RM, Marshall SB, Piek J et al. Early and late systemic hypotension as a frequent and fundamental source of cerebral ischemia following severe brain injury in the Traumatic Coma Data Bank. Acta Neurochir (Wien) 1993;59 (Suppl):121.
15. Muizelaar JP, Marmarou A, Ward JD, Kontos HA, Choi SC, Becker DP et al. Adverse effects of prolonged hyperventilation in patients with severe head injury: a randomized clinical trial. J Neurosurg 1991;75:731–9.
16. Kelly DF, Goodale DB, Williams J, Herr DL, Chappell ET, Rosner MJ et al. Propofol in the treatment of moderate and severe head injury: a randomized, prospective double-blinded pilot trial. J Neurosurg 1999;90:1042–52.
17. Carrel M, Moeschler O, Ravussin P, Favre JB, Boulard G. Prehospital air ambulance and systemic secondary cerebral damage in severe craniocerebral injuries. Ann Fr Anesth Reanim 1994;13:326–35.
18. Changaris DG, McGraw CP, Richardson JD et al. Correlation of cerebral perfusion pressure and Glasgow Coma Scale to outcome. J Trauma 1987;27:1007–13.
19. Marshall LF, Marshall SB, Klauber MR et al. A new classification of head injury based on computerized tomography. J Neurosurg 1991;75 (Suppl):S14–20.
20. Rosner MJ, Daughton S. Cerebral perfusion pressure management in head injury. J Trauma 1990;30:933–41.

22

Spine Injuries

Dennis A. Velez and David W. Newell

Summary

Spine injuries include injuries to the spinal column and also injuries to the neural structures including the spinal cord and nerve roots. The incidence of spinal cord injury is estimated at 30 to 40 per 1,000,000 persons. Spinal injuries are classified according to location and pattern of disruption of the ligaments and bony elements. Spinal cord injuries are classified according to the level and degree of function using the Frankel or ASIA score. Treatment of spine and spinal cord injuries includes the principles of realignment of the spine and protection of the spinal cord and nerve roots from injury or further injury. A combination of reduction, immobilization and often operative fixation are required to treat the gamut of injuries to the spine. It is important for physicians treating these patients to be familiar with the common and classic patterns of spinal column and spinal cord injuries and the treatment options for each. Pediatric patients represent a group at risk for certain types of injuries, due to unique biomechanical differences between the adult and the pediatric spine.

Introduction

Injury to the vertebral column has the potential for irreversibly damaging the spinal cord. Given the significant morbidity and mortality associated with injuries to the spine and spinal cord, along with the economic, social and psychological consequences, it is of utmost importance that these injuries are recognized, classified and managed expeditiously.

The incidence of spinal cord injury is estimated at 30–40 per 1,000,000 persons, with about 10,000 new cases per year in the USA. The prevalence is approximately 900–950 per 1,000,000. The mortality rate has been estimated at approximately 48%, with about 80% of victims dying at the scene of the accident and an additional 4–15% dying upon admission to the hospital. It is estimated that approximately 250,000 patients with spinal cord injuries are alive now in the USA [1].

Approximately 55% of spinal injuries occur in the cervical region [2]. The most common levels are the middle and low cervical levels, with C-5, followed by C-4 and C-6 as the segments usually injured, due to their mobility and flexibility. Injuries to the thoracic, thoracolumbar and lumbosacral area are equally distributed in terms of incidence. If an injury is located at one level of the spine, it is of utmost importance that the whole spine be evaluated, both clinically and radiographically, since 10–15% of patients will have an injury at another level.

Epidemiology

Trauma to the spine affects both young and older individuals, with a bimodal distribution.

The peak occurs in the 16–24 years of age group. Motor vehicle accidents account for 48% of all injuries in this group, followed by falls (21%) and athletic accidents, diving being the most common, accounting for about 14%. Penetrating injuries and industrial accidents comprise the remaining etiological factor. In individuals older than 55 years, falls, often at home, account for the majority of spine injuries.

These injuries occur most commonly in males during the summer months and at weekends. Regional differences also exist, with most penetrating injuries such as gunshot wounds and stabbing occurring in large cities and diving accidents occurring in more rural areas.

Acute Evaluation and Management in the Emergency Department

As with any trauma patient, a comprehensive and systematic approach, with the primary goals of resuscitation, should be undertaken. In the USA, specialized trauma centers institute the ABCDEs (airway, breathing, circulation, disability, exposure) of the Advanced Trauma Life Support, as dictated by the American College of Surgeon's Committee on Trauma. An emergency airway can be obtained by either oral or nasotracheal intubation. This is performed with the head and neck in a neutral position, with the help of an assistant. This technique of manual in-line traction helps avoid hyperextension of the neck, which, in the case of a cervical spine injury, will prevent worsening of canal stenosis as well as exacerbating motion of fractured segments or dislocations. Trauma to the head, chest, abdomen and musculoskeletal system occurs frequently in patients with spinal injuries. Because of this, some of these patients may present with signs and symptoms of shock. An assessment of pulse rate, skin, mental status and urine output helps to differentiate hemorrhagic from neurogenic shock, both of which present commonly with hypotension. Placement of an arterial line and a Swan Ganz catheter for proper hemodynamic assessment and subsequent management cannot be overemphasized. This helps to guide judicious use of intravenous fluids, which, if excessively administered, can lead to pulmonary edema and acute heart failure, especially in patients with pre-existing heart disease. The use of intravenous vasopressors, such as dopamine and neosynephrine, whether in a bolus or continuous infusion, is useful in reversing the effects of neurogenic shock. This type of shock is usually the result of loss of sympathetic tone in patients presenting with bradycardia and hypotension.

Neurological Assessment

Strict spine precautions, including immobilization, should be maintained until full clinical and radiographic evaluations have been completed. A detailed neurological examination should be done as early as possible during the initial evaluation, with time and date recorded. It is important that, in the awake patient, both motor and sensory function of all extremities be assessed. Grading of muscle strength and sensation to pinprick and light touch need to be recorded using the American Spine Injury Association (ASIA) system. Patients who are unconscious should have their muscle tone, muscle stretch reflexes, long tract signs and priapism in the male patient documented initially. A rectal examination to test sphincter tone, quality of contraction, presence or absence of the bulbocavernous reflex and the anal wink, as well as perineal sensation also, should be part of the initial evaluation.

Placement of a nasogastric tube, as well as a Foley catheter, should also take place in the emergent phase of treatment. This is done since it is common for these patients to develop a paralytic ileus, which places them at risk of aspiration of gastric contents. Not only is the Foley catheter helpful for recording urinary output, but also to prevent bladder distention that frequently accompanies the urinary retention experienced by these patients.

Radiographic Assessment

The radiographic assessment of patients with spinal injuries starts with a lateral cervical spine film. This projection is accurate in identifying significant abnormalities approximately 70–83% of the time. This view should be evaluated for alignment, bone and disc space abnormalities, and soft tissue injuries. Normally, the prevertebral soft tissues are no more than 4 mm in thickness at the C3 level. Attention to pre-vertebral soft tissue swelling is as important as attention to bony anatomy. In some cases, it may be the only radiological sign in 30–40% of patients presenting with an acute central cord syndrome [3]. All seven cervical vertebrae, as well as the C7–T1 junction, need to be visualized [4]. Caudal traction of the arms or a "swimmer's view" might be necessary to visualize this junction. Contraindications to this maneuver include atlanto-occipital, atlanto-axial or other pathologies identified in the initial view. An AP view, as well as an open mouth or odontoid view, are usually all that are needed to adequately visualize the cervical spine. Limitations of plain radiographs include difficulty in identifying injuries to the ligaments, over and underexposure, as well as decreased visualization of the occipitocervical, cervicothoracic and thoracolumbar transitional areas.

Areas not adequately visualized or fractures identified by plain films should be further explored with CT scanning. The advent of spiral CT scanning has made image acquisition more feasible, especially in specialized trauma centers. In our institution, patients who complain of neck pain, in the absence of visible fractures on plain films, have fallen from heights greater than 10 feet, have been involved in high-speed motor vehicle accidents, are unconscious or have an associated head injury, automatically undergo a specialized imaging protocol of the spine, which examines the occiput to T4 with 3-mm cuts and sagittal and coronal reformations through the area [3]. CT scanning is more sensitive for fractures of the posterior elements and bone displacement is also better appreciated with CT scanning [5]. Limitations of this technology include missing fractures that lie parallel to the plane of imaging. The use of reformations has made this less of an issue of concern.

MRI has limited sensitivity for fractures, but it is the study of choice to image the neural elements. It is indicated in the patient with unexplained neurological injury, worsening neurological status and incongruent skeletal and neurological examination. It is also indicated after fracture-dislocations are reduced in the emergent setting. MRI is helpful in showing spinal cord compression, intramedullary edema and hemorrhage, disc disruption, ligamentous injury and vascular occlusion. Chronic responses to injury, such as myelomalacia and syrinx formation, are also better visualized with MRI. Sagittal T2-weighted images are useful in assessing most of the above. MRA has also found a role in the patient suspected of having a vertebral artery injury. This should always be suspected in patients with altered mental status and fractures that involve the transverse processes [6].

Emergency myelography is reserved for situations in which an MRI cannot be obtained or there is a contraindication to MRI, such as a pacemaker.

Emergency Pharmacological Treatment

Pharmacological treatment of the spinal cord injured patient is, at this time, limited to the use of steroids. The NASCIS II and III trials have established a definite benefit in outcome at 6 weeks, 6 months and 1 year in patients with both complete and incomplete injuries [7,8]. Intravenous infusion of methylprednisolone (MPSS) at 30 mg/kg over 1 hour as a loading dose, followed by a continuous infusion of 5.4 mg/kg/hour over 23 hours if this regimen is started within 3 hours of the injury or continued for 48 hours if it is started within 3 and 8 hours of the injury, is the recommended standard of care [9]. Of importance is the fact that steroids are contraindicated for patients whose loading dose would be administered 8 hours after the injury, since the NASCIS II study found worsening in outcome in both motor and sensory scores in this subgroup of patients [8]. Also, no evidence has been found that steroids benefit patients with spinal cord injuries due to penetrating trauma or nerve root injuries.

Although the neuroprotective effects of glucocorticoids like MPSS remain uncertain, their theoretical beneficial effects, such as suppression of vasogenic edema [10], enhancement of spinal cord blood flow, attenuation of the inflammatory response [8], stabilization of lysosomal membranes, inhibition of pituitary endorphin release and alteration of electrolyte concentrations in injured tissue, make them attractive as potential modulators of secondary injury. This is because it is believed that the antioxidant function which these agents seem to convey scavenges lipid peroxidation products from the cell membrane and attenuates the damage done by the production of oxygen, derived free radicals. Their iatrogenic complications, such as gastrointestinal hemorrhage and a higher incidence of wound infections, have prompted the search for compounds which minimize the glucocorticoid and mineralocorticoid effects while preserving their ability to inhibit lipid peroxidation. Tirilizad mesylate, the best known and most extensively studied agent, is a 21-aminosteroid, which, in numerous animal models, has been shown to enhance recovery of motor function. In the NASCIS III study, a 48-hour infusion of tirilizad resulted in improved function similar to that obtained with an MPSS infusion. Since patients that received tirilizad also received a bolus of MPSS, conclusions cannot be reached about its use in acute spinal cord injury [9].

Types of Injuries

General Types of Injuries

In order to appreciate the different kinds of injuries with their associated syndromes, investigators have tried to classify these injuries based on clinical findings. The Frankel grading method is widely accepted because of its ease of use and elimination of subjectivity. Patients are graded as (A) complete, (B) sensory only, (C) motor useless, (D) motor useful and (E) recovery. By this classification, a complete injury has no preservation of motor and/or sensory function in three or more segments below the level of the injury. According to the guidelines published in 1992 by the American Spinal Injury Association, in order for an injury to be incomplete, motor or sensory function or both needed to be present in the sacral segments of S4–S5 [11]. Otherwise, the patient was considered to have a complete injury.

The importance of these definitions lies in the fact that, in terms of prognosis, patients with incomplete injuries have a greater probability of experiencing some functional recovery, whereas those for complete injuries are very modest at best. In reports of large populations of patients with spinal cord injuries, more than half of these patients were classified as having incomplete injuries.

Specific Types of Injuries

Stretching, crushing, compression and vascular compromise account for most of the injury mechanisms to the spinal cord. A subset of spinal cord injured patients would then have findings on initial neurological examination consistent with a specific syndrome that provides more predictive prognostic accuracy.

Hemisection of the spinal cord, usually as a result of some penetrating injury or a stab wound, leads to the Brown–Sequard syndrome. Clinically, patients present ipsilateral motor and proprioceptive loss below the level of the lesion and contralaterally dissociated sensory loss, i.e. loss of pain and temperature sensation, caudal to the lesion. Preservation of light touch is due to the redundancy of the fibers from the anterior spinothalamic tract. Out of all the incomplete syndromes, this one has the better prognosis, with over 90% of patients regaining the ability to ambulate independently.

The most common cervical cord syndrome is usually seen in males, middle-aged or older. It is known as the central cord syndrome, which is usually seen after a hyperextension injury in patients with cervical stenosis, consisting clinically of motor weakness that is greater in the upper extremities than the lower extremities. It involves the distal muscle groups more than it does the proximal groups and the degree of sensory disturbance varies below the level of the lesion. About 50% of patients recover enough function in the lower extremities to ambulate [12]. Upper extremity function, with the ability to exercise fine motor control, is also uniformly poor. Bowel and bladder function, if involved initially, usually recovers. Correlation of MRI findings with both ante-mortem and post-mortem analysis has shown that it is the buckling of the hypertrophied ligamentum flavum which occurs as a result of the hyperextension, which creates a shear type of injury pattern to the spinal cord.

In patients who have suffered a vertical compression or hyperflexion type of injury, cord ischemia in the territory supplied by the anterior spinal artery leads to the anterior cord syndrome. Clinically, the patients have motor and sensory loss below the level of the lesion, but with intact posterior column function. This syndrome has the poorest prognosis for recovery, as only 10–20% of patients recover functional motor control and even fewer recover the ability to ambulate. CT myelography or MRI usually demonstrate anterior canal compromise and cord compression.

The conus medullaris and cauda equina syndromes are usually associated with thoracolumbar spinal cord injuries. These injuries present with a combination of upper and lower motor neuron involvement, since there is injury to the cord as well as the nerve root. Patients with the conus syndrome usually have injuries in the T11–L1 region, whereas in patients with the cauda equina syndrome, the injury is from L1 down through the sacral levels. Patients with conus injuries have the same prognosis as patients with spinal cord injuries, depending on whether the injury is complete or incomplete, with incomplete lesions doing better. In patients with cauda equina, the prognosis is as favorable as those of patients having peripheral nerve injuries. Adequate decompression increases the chances for functional recovery of motor function to an ambulatory status, although chronic intractable pain might be an undesirable outcome for some of these patients.

Injury to the Cervical Spine

The majority of spine injuries occur at the level of the cervical spine, the most mobile portion of the vertebral column. Motor vehicle accidents account for most of these injuries. Fractures and fracture-dislocations are the most common injury patterns, although subluxations and injuries without radiographic abnormalities (SCIWORA), although altogether uncommon, occur more frequently in younger patients [13]. About 60% of patients who have sustained cervical spine trauma have suffered an injury to another organ system which can exacerbate the effects of secondary injury to the spinal cord, such as hypoxia or hypotension.

It is estimated that 15% of patients with trauma to the spine sustain a neurological injury. With the cervical spine being the most commonly affected segment, it is estimated that 40–60% of all trauma to the cervical spine will result in some kind of neurological morbidity and/or mortality. As an example, studies have shown that the mortality, in the field, for patients with occiput–C3 lesions is approximately 25–40%. This is probably due to respiratory compromise secondary to high spinal cord injury.

After clinical and radiographic assessment has been completed, unstable or displaced injuries should be promptly treated with cervical traction by applying Gardner–Wells (GW) skull tongs. The ready availability of MRI-compatible tongs of different sizes in emergency departments and ICUs cannot be overemphasized.

Application of these tongs requires a local anesthetic and skin preparation. The pins are applied 1 cm cephalad to the pinna in line with the external auditory meatus, after careful cleansing of the skin in the area and infiltration of a local anesthetic. The pins are tightened until the spring-loaded pin protrudes 1 mm. This indicates a 30-lb compressive force against the skull. The pins are rechecked and, if necessary, re-tightened only once more, at 24 hours.

Closed reduction can then continue with the patient supine on a stretcher, with caudal traction on both upper extremities. This can be accomplished with a combination of straps and/or surgical tape attached to the shoulders. The use of intravenous analgesics, muscle relaxants and oxygen by nasal cannula is invaluable in accomplishing reduction in responsive patients. The use of portable monitors to assess heart rate, blood pressure and oxygen saturation is helpful when titrating sedatives and muscle relaxants to the desired effect. It is important to keep the patient comfortable but awake enough to co-operate with serial neurological evaluations.

The amount of weight applied at first is always small, to avoid overdistraction. Depending on the level of the injury and the amount of suspected ligamentous damage, to start with 5 lb per vertebral level above the injury is the standard in our institution. Five-pound increments are added until approximately two-thirds of the patient's body weight or about 100 lbs are reached. If these attempts are unsuccessful, open reduction can be indicated.

Cervical traction is associated with complications, such as pin dislodgement, site infections and skull penetration. Contraindications to this procedure include purely distractive injuries, skull fractures and unstable upper cervical spine injuries. In patients with distractive injuries, gentle compression after positioning of a halo ring or the placement of sandbags to secure the head and placing the patient in the Trendelenburg position might provide temporary relief.

Closed reduction with cervical traction should always be done by or with experienced personnel. In our institution, live fluoroscopy is used when the reduction is being performed. Serial plain films after manipulation or when increasing the weight on the traction devices need to be used so as to prevent the potential complications of overdistraction.

Once the reduction is complete, the weight on the traction is reduced so as to maintain the reduction and, after transfer to a Rotobed, the patient undergoes a post-reduction MRI.

Injuries to the Occipital Cervical Articulation

Early and aggressive trauma care, as well as the ready availability of quality imaging, allow for earlier recognition of injuries to this region. Compression, distraction and lateral rotation constitute the primary forces. Falls from a height usually account for the axial compression forces. Rapid deceleration usually accounts for the distractive force, which creates tension in the tectorial membrane and the alar ligaments. Forced lateral bending or axial rotation, failure of the contralateral alar ligament or of the bony attachment to the ligament may occur. These injuries range from a mild ligamentous sprain to a completely unstable fracture pattern with ligamentous disruption, which can compromise adjacent structures such as the brain stem, the vertebral arteries, cranial nerves and the spinal cord. Occipital condyle fractures and atlanto-occipital dislocation are now reviewed.

Occipital Condyle Fractures

First described by Bell in 1817, these are extremely uncommon [14]. The conscious patient may complain of occipito-cervical or neck pain, or may have lower cranial nerve palsies. These injuries are difficult to identify with plain radiographs and require a high index of suspicion. A retropharyngeal hematoma could be the only sign of serious injury. CT with reconstructions provides the definitive diagnosis.

The classification of Anderson and Montesano is the most widely used and divides these fractures into three types (Fig. 22.1) [15]. A type I fracture consists of comminution of the occipital condyle, with minimal to no involvement of the foramen magnum. Axial loading into the atlas is the responsible mechanism. Although the ipsilateral alar ligament may be torn, these are stable fractures due to the integrity of the tectorial membrane and the contralateral alar ligament. An occipital condyle fracture associated with a basilar skull fracture is called a type II injury. Axial CT scanning shows a fracture line involving the skull base and the condyle. As with type I fractures, the mechanism and stability are the same. The type III fractures are avulsion fractures of the condyle by the alar ligament. Usually unstable because of disruption of the tectorial membrane and the contralateral alar ligament, they are the result of excessive rotation and/or lateral bending.

Stable type I and II fractures can be treated in a hard cervical collar or cervicothoracic brace for 6–8 weeks. When in type II fractures the condyle is separated from the occiput, treatment with a halo vest for 12 weeks is indicated. In the case of stable type III injuries, a hard cervical collar or a halo vest provides adequate treatment. Injuries that involve total ligamentous disruption are best managed with a posterior occipital to C2 arthrodesis. The Bohlman wire technique and the posterior occipital cervical fusion with atlanto-occipital (AO) reconstruction plates can be done [16].

The Bohlman wire technique involves careful sub-periosteal dissection of the occiput down to C2. Two parallel troughs, 2–3cm from the foramen magnum, separated by about 5 mm of bone, are drilled. A tunnel is created and a 20-gauge wire is looped around the bone; additional wire is looped around the lamina of C1 and through the spinous process of C2. After harvesting bone of 5 cm long and 1 cm thick and decorticating the occiput, the lamina of C1 and C2, wires are passed through the drill holes placed in the grafts. The wires are then tightened. Post-operatively, the patient wears a halo vest for 12 weeks.

The postero-occipital cervical fusion is done by exposing the medial edge of the pedicle of C2, which is then drilled to a depth of 20–22 mm. Screws are inserted 3–5 mm above the center of C2–C3 facet articulation, with the direction being 20–30° cranial and 15–20° medial. C1 can be fixated using sub-laminar wires. After the length and contour of the plate to be used are determined, it is fixed to C2 with a 3.5-mm screw, 20–24 mm in length. The occiput is then drilled and the usual length of the screw

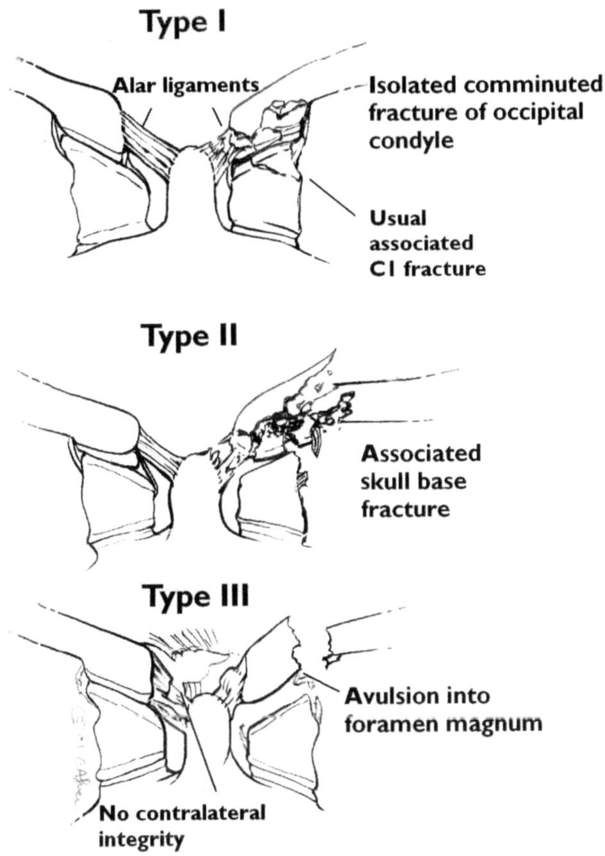

Fig. 22.1. Illustration of the types of occipital condyle fractures according to the classification of Anderson and Montesano, which is the most widely used and divides these fractures into three types.

is 10–12 mm. The holes made are then tapped with a 3.5-mm cortical tap and two screws on each side are placed. The bone grafts harvested are wired to the occiput and C2, as previously described. Post-operatively, patients wear a hard cervical collar for 12 weeks.

Atlanto-occipital Dislocation (AOD)

Until recently, it was uncommon to treat this kind of injury, since patients usually would die at the scene of the accident or promptly upon arrival to the hospital, due to fatal brain stem injury. Aggressive resuscitative efforts at the scene have converted AOD into a potentially survivable injury. The associated morbidity and mortality with missed AOD are quite high, and a high index of clinical suspicion must always be considered. This injury is highly unstable, with the potential for neurological worsening.

A pedestrian struck by a car is a common clinical scenario. Distraction forces are thought to be responsible for the injury to the ligaments that provide stability to this region. Clinically, patients can present with complete tetraplegia and respiratory distress or may be neurologically normal. Sometimes, complaints of occipital pain can be voiced by the conscious patient and lower cranial nerve palsies can be detected. The Brown–Sequard, central cord or Bell's crutiate paralysis syndromes have been described with this injury.

Plain lateral radiographs will show an increased distance between the clivus and the tip of the dens. Displacement of the skull relative to the spine either anteriorly (type I AOD) or posteriorly (type III AOD) can also be seen. Type II AOD consists of a longitudinal distraction separating the occiput from the atlas

(Fig. 22.2). Cervical traction is contraindicated in this type of injury pattern.

The Powers ratio, which is obtained by measuring the distance between the tip of the clivus (basion) and the posterior arch of the atlas and then dividing this measure by the distance between the posterior margin of the foramen magnum to the anterior arch of the atlas, yields a number which is normally 0.7+/− 0.09 in the majority of the population. A value greater than 1 suggests AOD.

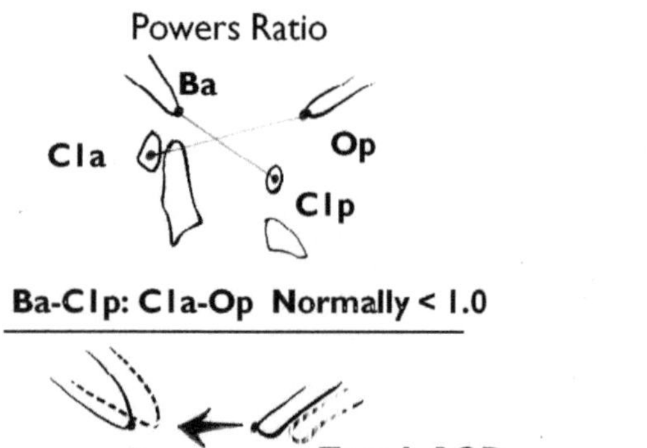

Fig. 22.2. AOD can be detected by using the Powers ratio. This ratio is obtained by measuring the distance between the tip of the clivus (basion) (Ba) and the posterior arch of the atlas (C1p) This measure is divided by the distance between the posterior margin of the foramen magnum or opisthion (Op) to the anterior arch of the atlas (C1a), and yields a number which is normally 0.7+/− 0.09 in the majority of the population. A value greater than 1 suggests AOD. Plain lateral radiographs will also show an increased distance between the clivus and the tip of the dens. Displacement of the skull relative to the spine either anteriorly (type I AOD) or posteriorly (type III AOD) can also be seen. Type II AOD consists of a longitudinal distraction separating the occiput from the atlas.

MRI is not only a valuable tool in assessing alignment, but also in detecting ligamentous disruption. Increased signal intensity in and around the ligaments supports the possibility of ligament damage.

Type I and III AOD injuries might benefit from the use of cervical traction to realign the bony structures and to relieve compression of the spinal canal, especially in cases in which there is a neurological deficit, as reversal of these deficits has been documented with 5 lb or less of traction. Once realignment has occurred, patients can then be placed in a halo vest while they await surgical stabilization using internal fixation.

Atlas Fractures

These fractures account for 5–10% of all cervical spine injuries and 2% of all spine injuries. These are frequently seen in younger age groups and commonly result from motor vehicle accidents. In multiple trauma patients, they are usually associated with head injuries. They usually occur in combination with occipital condylar fractures or fractures of C2, such as dens fractures. A classification involving four types of fracture patterns has been described. These fractures involve the posterior arch, the lateral masses, Jefferson fractures and the horizontal fracture of the anterior arch (Fig. 22.3).

The posterior arch fractures are the most common. They are thought to occur due to a combination of hyperextension forces associated with axial loading. They can be seen in association with anterior teardrop hyperextension injuries of C2. An isolated fracture of this type can be treated safely in a cervical orthotic device for 8–12 weeks, since there is no disruption of the ligamentous structures. The union rates for this kind of injury are very high.

Axial loading associated with lateral bending results in a lateral mass fracture of C1. Usually identified in the open-mouth view, an asymmetry of the lateral masses of the atlas prompts further imaging by way of CT scanning. C2 and condylar fractures can also be better appreciated with CT. Lateral displacement of less than 2 mm usually indicates a stable injury, which can be safely treated with cervical orthosis.

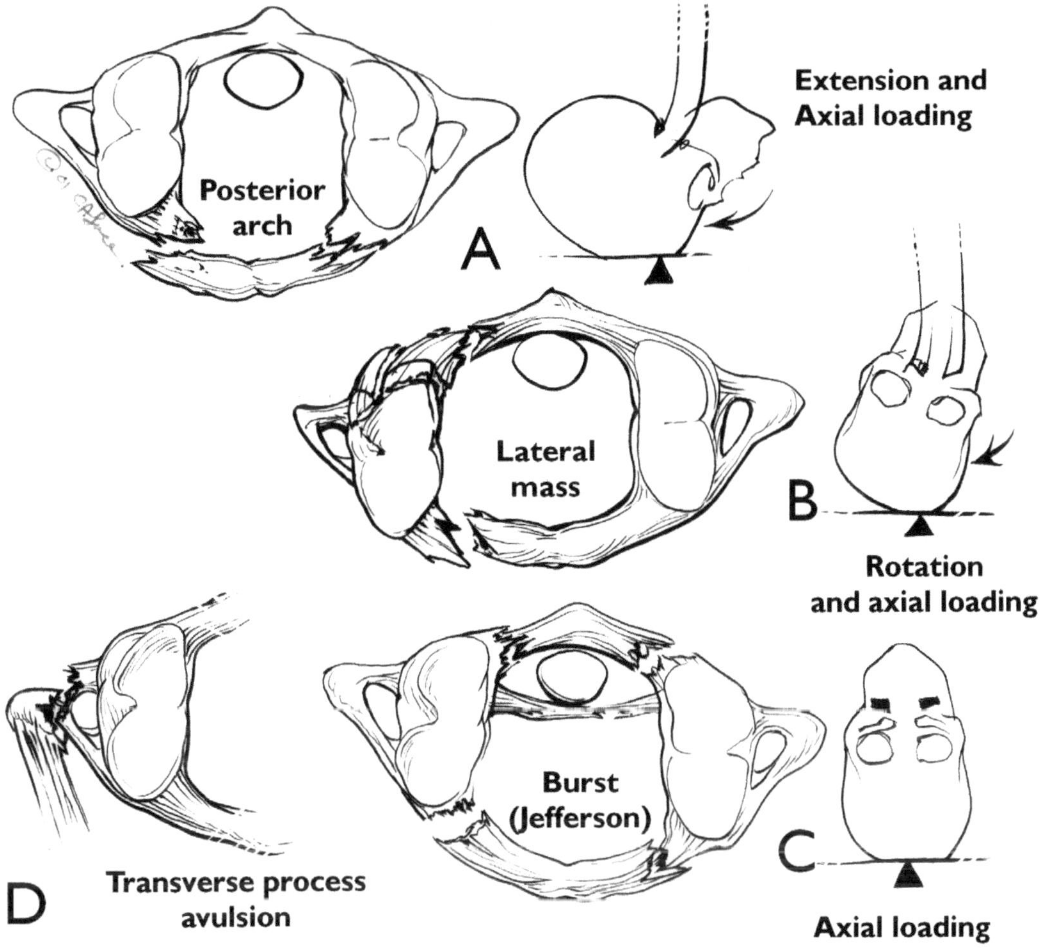

Fig. 22.3. Illustration of the common types of fractures of the atlas, or C1. A classification involving four types of fracture patterns has been described, involving (A) the posterior arch, (B) the lateral masses, (C) Jefferson fractures and (D) the horizontal transverse process fracture of the anterior arch. Extension and axial loading are associated with posterior arch fractures. Extension associated with lateral bending results in a lateral mass fracture of C1. A burst fracture of C1, first described by Geoffrey Jefferson in 1920, is the result of an axial compression, generally with a direct blow on the head, as seen in diving accidents or when an object falls on the head. In this type of injury, there is bilateral spreading of the lateral masses, with both anterior and posterior arches failing. The transverse fracture of the atlas occurs as a result of hyperextension, which results in an avulsion fracture.

A burst fracture of C1, first described by Geoffrey Jefferson in 1920, is the result of an axial compression, generally with a direct blow to the head as seen in diving accidents or when an object falls on the head. An additional fracture of C2, such as a dens fracture, occurs in 41% of Jefferson fractures. In this type of injury, there is bilateral spreading of the lateral masses, with both anterior and posterior arches failing. Clinically, it is rare for patients to have an associated neurological deficit, although this is considered an unstable injury. When lateral displacement of the lateral masses totals a distance of greater than 7 mm, it is presumed that transverse ligamentous disruption has occurred, as described by Spence and associates [17]. CT and MRI can confirm whether there has been an avulsion of the bony attachment of the ligament and integrity of the ligament, respectively. Halo vest placement is advocated for this type of injury. In the cases of severe lateral mass displacement, traction has been recommended to better maintain reduction. If, once the reduction has taken place, there is no further displacement, then placement of the halo is once again indicated.

The transverse fracture of the atlas occurs as a result of hyperextension, which results in an avulsion fracture. The superior oblique portion of the longus colli muscle inserts on the inferior portion of the anterior tubercle of the atlas. In this kind of hyperextension injury, there is an avulsion by the superior oblique portion of the longus colli and the anterior longitudinal ligament. As an isolated injury, this is stable and expected to heal with collar immobilization. Due to the small incidence of these fractures, long-term follow-up and results are currently not available.

Axis Fractures

The anatomy of the C2 vertebra lends itself to a series of unique fracture patterns. These can be divided into fractures of the odontoid process, fractures of the lateral masses, traumatic spondylolisthesis or a combination of these.

Odontoid Fractures

These account for 7–14% of all cervical spine fractures and 18% of odontoid fractures present with other cervical spine injuries. They are usually the result of motor vehicle accidents in young adults. The mechanism of injury in elderly patients is usually falls at home. It is not uncommon for the diagnosis to be delayed because of altered mental status. In younger patients, scalp lacerations, facial trauma or history of concussion should alert the clinician to the possibility of an odontoid fracture. Patients rarely present with neurological deficits, but usually complain of occipital or high cervical pain. Numbness and paresthesia in the distribution of the greater occipital nerve and posterior cervical muscle spasms should lead to further investigation. Lateral plain radiographs may miss these fractures, so careful evaluation of the open-mouth view is critical. The pre-vertebral soft tissues should be examined, although pre-vertebral swelling may not be a common finding in isolated odontoid fractures. The pre-dens space or atlanto-dens interval (ADI) should be less than 3 mm in the adult and less than 4 mm in the child. In the case of CT scanning, the fracture line may be missed on the axial cuts because of its being in the plane of the image. Sagittal and coronal reconstructions are then necessary for further evaluation. Odontoid fractures are commonly classified according to the scheme of Anderson and D'Alonzo (Fig. 22.4) [18].

Type I fractures are characterized by an avulsion of the distal tip of the odontoid. The mechanism of injury is thought to be severe rotational and lateral bending forces, which cause avulsion of bone through the alar and apical ligaments. These are usually uncommon injuries and are not associated with instability. Once an associated distraction injury is ruled out, these patients can be treated safely in a cervical collar. Even when union does not occur, patients are usually asymptomatic and the clinical results are satisfactory.

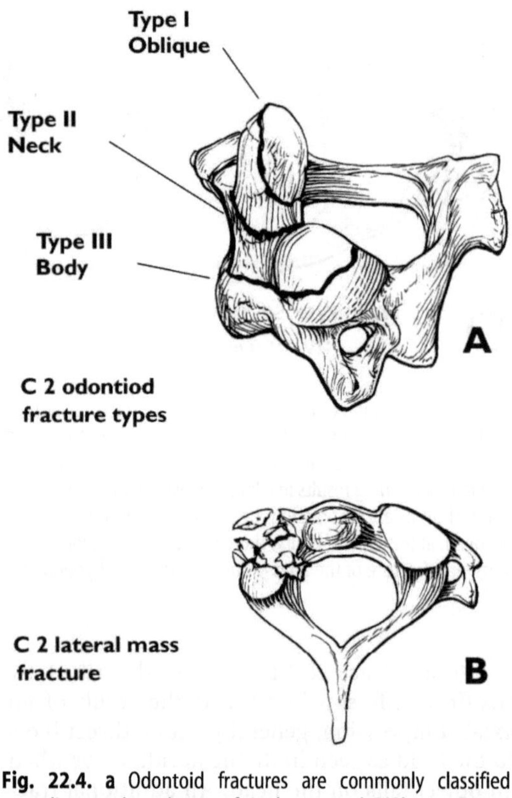

Fig. 22.4. **a** Odontoid fractures are commonly classified according to the scheme of Anderson and D'Alonzo. Type I fractures are characterized by an avulsion of the distal tip of the odontoid. Type II fractures occur through the base of the odontoid, above the body of C2. Type III fractures involve the fracture line passing into the body of C2. **b** The lateral mass fracture of C2, usually produced by an axial loading force, similar to the one producing fractures of C1.

Type II fractures occur through the base of the odontoid, above the body of C2. This is the most common pattern, accounting for approximately 60–90% of odontoid fractures. This type of injury is also associated with the highest rate of non-union. Patients with this kind of fracture are immobilized in a halo for at least 12 weeks. The rates of non-union with this type of treatment range from 11 to 63% [19]. Risk factors identified which promote non-union, besides the poor vascular supply to the distal odontoid, include age greater than 65 years, displacement of greater than 6 mm and, especially, posterior displacement, severe comminution of the fracture site and delay in diagnosis [19].

Surgical options currently used include posterior C1–C2 fusion using either atlantoaxial wiring or transarticular C1–C2 screw fixation. An anterior screw fixation by means of transodontoid lag screw placement can also be done if there is documentation of an intact transverse ligament.

In type III fractures, the fracture line passes into the body of C2. Anterior displacement is commonly seen with this type of fracture. Flexion-type forces have been proposed as the mechanism for this type of injury. These injuries have consistently shown a good overall prognosis when treated with halo immobilization for 12 weeks, with non-union rates of 0–15% in patients treated with other cervical orthoses instead of a halo [20].

Lateral Mass Fractures

An axial loading force, similar to the one producing fractures of the lateral masses of C1, accounts for the mechanism for this type of injury. These injuries are usually treated with a hard cervical collar. The presence of significant comminution or deformity may require cervical traction for reduction and subsequent placement of a halo vest.

Traumatic Spondylolisthesis of the Axis

Also known as hangman's fracture, traumatic spondylolisthesis of the axis consists of a bilateral fracture pattern through the pars interarticularis or pedicles. The fracture line may involve the superior articular surface or the body of C2. It is also frequently seen as a result of motor vehicle accidents. Clinically, patients rarely have an associated neurological deficit. When a deficit is present, it usually occurs as a result of an associated head injury. Instability can be seen with subluxation of C2 on C3 and associated ligamentous attachment. Four types of injury patterns have been identified (Fig. 22.5) [21].

Type I injuries are those fracture patterns in which there is no angulation of C2 on C3 and less than 3 mm of anterior translation. Type II injuries demonstrate greater than 11° of angulation and greater than 3.5 mm of anterior translation. Type IIa injuries, although not associated

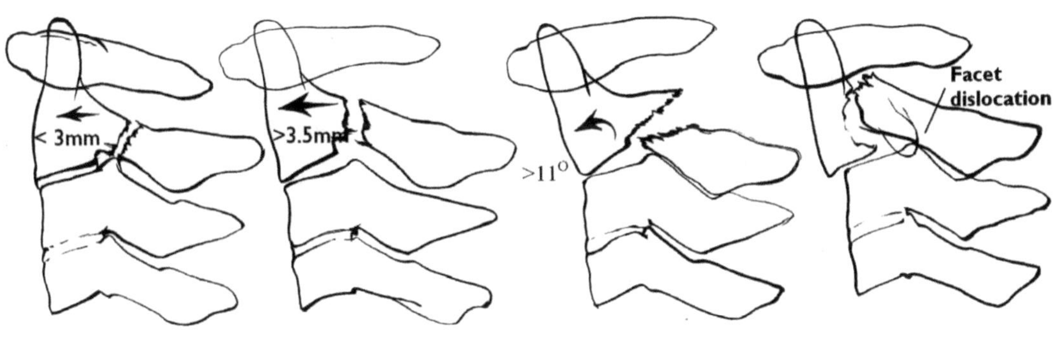

Fig. 22.5. Classification of hangman's fractures, also known as traumatic spondylolisthesis of the axis. Type I injuries are those fracture patterns in which there is no angulation of C2 on C3 and less than 3 mm of anterior translation. Type II injuries demonstrate greater than 11° of angulation and greater than 3.5 mm of anterior translation. Type IIa injuries, although not associated with significant translation, are associated with a high degree of angulation. Type III injuries, although rare, are associated with not only angulation and displacement, but also with facet dislocations of C2–C3. These could be unilateral or bilateral.

with significant translation, are associated with a high degree of angulation. Type III injuries, although rare, are associated with not only angulation and displacement, but also with facet dislocations of C2–C3. These could be unilateral or bilateral.

Type I injuries can be treated in a cervical collar. Types II, IIa, III fractures, if reduced appropriately, can be treated with a halo vest. An anterior fusion between C2 and C3 with plate fixation is the recommended surgical treatment for those injuries not reducible or those that failed conservative treatment with a halo.

Subaxial Fractures and Dislocations

Injuries below C2 are considered together due to the similarity of the vertebrae anatomically and, hence, the injury patterns.

Compression Fractures

These are common injuries, which occur as a result of a mechanism of mild flexion and axial loading. There is failure of the anterior column with sparing of the middle and posterior column, making it a stable injury. These are fractures which are associated with osteoporosis and other degenerative spine diseases and, hence, loss of the cervical lordosis of the spine. Immobilization with a cervical collar is usually the standard treatment.

Burst Fractures

Burst fractures of the cervical spine usually occur as a result of axial loading with the spine in a neutral position. A flexion force may be involved as well. Failure of the anterior and middle columns with retropulsion of bone fragments into the spinal canal is frequently seen, making it an unstable type of injury. Patients who present with an incomplete type of neurological examination might benefit from prompt surgical intervention. For patients who present with a neurologically complete injury, operative fixation using either an anterior or posterior approach or halo immobilization are treatment options.

Teardrop Fractures

These are primarily hyperflexion injuries in which a small piece of bone is avulsed off of the anterior inferior portion of the vertebral body. These are readily recognized using plain radiography. Patients usually present with a neurological deficit. This is an unstable type of injury, since not only the anterior column but also the posterior ligamentous structures are affected. Treatment with a halo vest is a reasonable option; however, an anterior decompression and plating, along with a posterior procedure, might be necessary to provide optimal stabilization.

Unilateral Facet Dislocation

This usually occurs in flexion accompanied by rotation injuries. The facet joint at one level is dislocated so that the inferior articular process of the upper vertebra lies anterior to the superior process of the lower vertebra. Lateral plain radiographs show anterolisthesis of the upper vertebra of less than 25%. Misalignment of the spinous processes is seen on antero-posterior views and facet dislocation is readily seen in oblique projections. These injuries may or may not be associated with a spinal cord injury.

Initial management of this injury is achieved by attempting closed reduction with cervical traction, which, if successful, can then be treated with halo vest immobilization or operative fixation through an anterior or posterior approach. Otherwise, an open reduction followed by fixation is indicated. In this case, the facets are drilled until realignment can be carried out by visual inspection. There is a concern that an acute traumatic disc might occur concurrently with this injury. This is of concern, since the patient can then worsen with closed reduction. This argument has prompted the recommendation than an MRI should be performed prior to attempts at reduction with cervical traction. If a traumatic disc is recognized, surgical removal needs to be carried out before attempts at reduction are made. The reduction can then be performed in the operating room.

Bilateral Facet Dislocation

These injuries are due to a hyperflexion type of mechanism. They are associated with a neurological deficit on clinical presentation. In this case, damage to the posterior ligaments is severe enough to cause both facet complexes to dislocate. Lateral plain films demonstrate a subluxation of greater than 50%, often with a significant angular deformity. These are considered unstable injuries and cervical traction needs to be promptly instituted to reduce the dislocation. If closed reduction is successful, then patients with these injuries can then be either treated with halo immobilization or operative fusion from an anterior or posterior approach. Open reduction with stabilization is necessary when normal alignment cannot be restored with traction.

Hyperextension Injuries

Hyperextension injuries include dislocations, fracture-dislocations and laminar fractures. These are commonly seen in younger patients as a result of motor vehicle accidents and in elderly patients with cervical spondylosis. They usually result from a backward force to the cervical spine as a result of an impact transmitted after an injury to the mandible, face or forehead. This then throws the head and cervical spine into hyperextension. Clinically, patients may not present with any neurological deficits or, in the case of the elderly patient with cervical stenosis that falls forward, they may present with the central cord syndrome.

Due to the fact that the cervical spine might return to its normal alignment after posterior dislocation, the radiological diagnosis might be difficult to obtain. Posterior laminar fractures with avulsion of the anterior longitudinal ligament and retrolisthesis of the vertebral body can be observed. Other signs include pre-vertebral soft tissue swelling, widening or asymmetry of the disrupted intervertebral disc with a small vacuum sign, fractures of the vertebral end plates or small avulsion fractures of the anterior inferior margin of the vertebral body.

In the case of hyperextension dislocation and hyperextension fracture-dislocation, both anterior and posterior longitudinal ligaments may be disrupted. Disruption of the intervertebral disc and displacement of the vertebra above the disc posteriorly may also be appreciated. This can cause compression of the spinal cord against the posterior arch of the spine. Patients can present with focal neurological deficits or complete quadriplegia. Sometimes, abrasions or soft tissue injury to the face and forehead, clinical findings consistent with the central cord syndrome and pre-vertebral soft tissue swelling associated with a normally aligned cervical spine on lateral radiographs are the clues to these types of injury. These are unstable injuries that need surgical stabilization, usually with an anterior approach procedure.

Clay Shoveler's Fracture

The classic fracture consists of an avulsion fracture of the spinous process of C7. However, a fracture of any of the other cervical spinous processes without any other fracture can have this name ascribed. The usual mechanism is a direct blow to the posterior elements, although an avulsion associated with a severe flexion mechanism is recognized as another possibility. Patients usually complain of neck pain, but these are stable fractures that can be safely treated in a cervical collar.

Penetrating Injuries

These usually account for about 10–12% of all spinal injuries, although its incidence might be higher in certain urban areas. Gunshot injuries and stab wounds, usually seen in young men, accounts for these injuries, with 50% of patients with gunshot injuries having a functional cord transection. These injuries, for the most part, do not always compromise the stability of the spine. Operative treatment is indicated in cases of dural tears or when it is necessary to remove an infected foreign body.

Spinal Cord Injury Without Radiographic Abnormality

This entity is defined as clinical evidence of spinal cord dysfunction as a consequence of a traumatic injury, without radiographic evidence of fractures, dislocations or ligamentous injuries.

This type of clinical presentation is seen in adults and children, both of which have different clinical presentations as well as prognoses. In adults, the most likely injury mechanism is hyperextension superimposed on cervical spondylosis, which usually presents clinically with an acute central cord syndrome. Cadaver studies performed by Taylor and associates have demonstrated that the ligamenta flava bulges forward into the canal in hyperextension [22]. This leads to narrowing of the canal diameter and cord injury. Elastic recoil of the paraspinous muscles allows for spontaneous reduction of the associated retrolisthesis, which can occur with anterior longitudinal ligament rupture, yielding to the normal radiographic findings. This type of injury is usually associated with good prognosis for recovery.

In pediatric patients, the mechanisms of injury noted included hyperextension, flexion, repetitive flexion–extension, longitudinal distraction and crush injury [23]. More horizontally oriented articulating facet surfaces, forward wedging of the anterior portion of the vertebral body and increased elasticity and redundancy of the interspinous ligaments, posterior joint capsules and cartilaginous endplates account for the increased susceptibility of the pediatric spinal cord to sustain this type of injury. Usually, these patients present with evidence of complete cord transection or anterior cord syndrome. These syndromes are uniformly associated with a poorer prognosis. Cervical immobilization is the standard treatment.

Injuries to the Thoracic, Thoracolumbar and Lumbar Spine

The thoracic (T2–T10), thoracolumbar (T11–L2) and lumbar (L3–L5) are treated as distinct entities because of their anatomy, biomechanical function and neurological function are different. Although the fracture patterns that occur at each of these segments are similar, the clinical presentation and, hence, the treatment and prognosis varies according to the level of the injury.

Thoracic Spine Injuries

Injuries to the thoracic spine account for 15% of all spinal cord injuries [24]. Although it is difficult to injure the thoracic spine, the contained segment of the spinal cord is very susceptible to injury and has the poorest prognosis for functional recovery. Only 10% of thoracic vertebral body injuries are associated with a spinal cord injury. This is in contradistinction of 39% seen in the cervical spine. Poor collateral circulation and a small spinal-canal-to-spinal-cord ratio account for the severity of the neurological deficits frequently associated with injuries to this region.

In this region, the spinal cord is protected by the ribs, the chest cage and chest wall musculature, the sternum, the back and the costovertebral ligaments. This also adds stability to the thoracic region in the sense that it reduces the amount of physiological movement allowed. For example, the rib cage restricts motion in extension approximately 70% [25]. The rib cage also adds stiffness to the spine as evidenced by data, which demonstrates a fourfold increase in compression tolerance of the vertebral column with an intact rib cage [26]. The ribs also limit the flexion and extension of the upper thoracic area, while the posterior elements mainly resist extension. A physiological kyphosis also occurs due to the greater height of the posterior vertebral wall compared to the anterior vertebral wall. The axis of rotation at a given segment is located in the anterior portion of the vertebral body. Flexion and axial loading account for the majority of osseous injuries to this region, due to a combination of these factors.

Spinal Instability

As defined by White and Panjabi, clinical instability "is the loss of the ability of the spine under physiological loads to maintain its pattern of displacement so that there is no initial or additional neurological deficit, no major deformity, and no incapacitating pain" [26]. For clinical purposes, this definition has rather limited utility. The work of Holdsworth, in which fracture patterns were radiographically identified and stability definition was attempted, based on a two-column stability pattern, was the first attempt at classifying stability in such a way that was accessible to clinicians to determine appropriate treatments [27]. Denis modified this model to include a third column and this is the pattern currently used by many physicians (Fig. 22.6) [28]. As defined, the anterior column is made up of the anterior half of the vertebral body, anterior half of the annulus fibrosus and the anterior longitudinal ligament. The middle column consists of the posterior half of the vertebral body, the posterior half of the annulus fibrosus and the posterior longitudinal ligament. The posterior column comprises the supra- and infraspinous ligaments, the ligamentum flavum, articular processes and joint capsules, the laminae and the spinous processes. This three-column model states that instability results when an injury affects two or more columns.

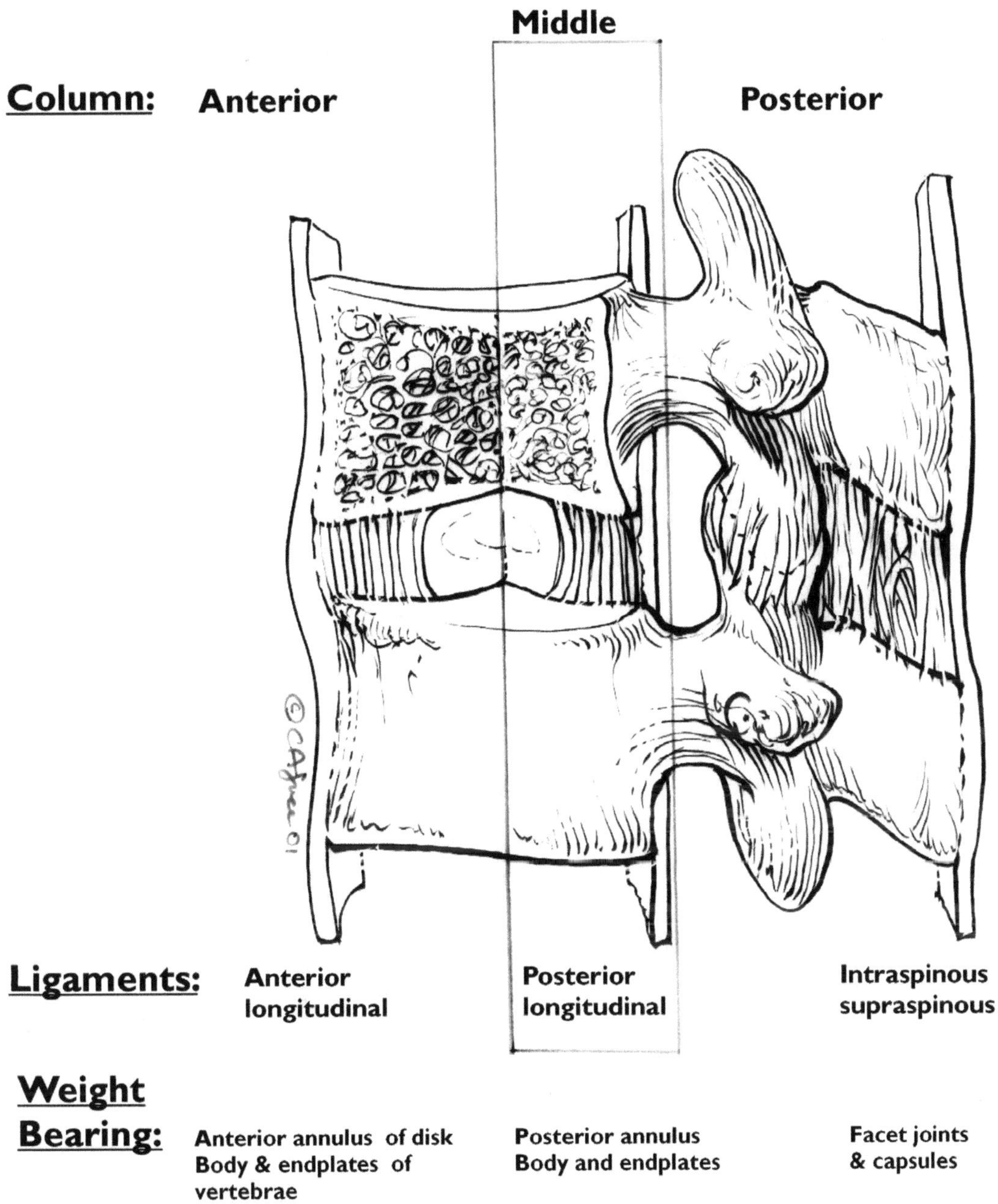

Fig. 22.6. Illustration of the three-column model of Denis, which describes the structural integrity of the thoracic spine. As defined, the anterior column is made up of the anterior half of the vertebral body, anterior half of the annulus fibrosus and the anterior longitudinal ligament. The middle column consists of the posterior half of the vertebral body, the posterior half of the annulus fibrosus and the posterior longitudinal ligament. The posterior column comprises the supra- and infraspinous ligaments, the ligamentum flavum, articular processes and joint capsules, the laminae and the spinous processes. This three-column model states that instability results when an injury affects two or more columns.

Classification of Thoracic Fractures

Four major categories of thoracic fractures have been identified: compression fractures, burst fractures, seatbelt-type injuries and fracture dislocations. Denis advocated that the differences in how the middle column was affected determined what type of fracture would be produced [28].

Compression Fractures

These are the most frequently seen fractures in the thoracic spine and they usually occur as a result of an axial compression load. No pattern of spinal cord injury has been documented with this type of fracture. Radiographically, a reduction in height of the anterior portion of the vertebral body with no involvement of the posterior vertebral body is noticed. Kyphotic angulation and widening of the interspinous processes may be seen (Fig. 22.7). This is generally a stable type of injury, since there is no involvement of the middle column. If, however, the anterior body fracture reduces the height by at least 50%, there is the possibility of posterior column failure [29]. In this case, the middle column acts as a hinge, which results in a tension force on the posterior ligamentous structures. A long-term increase in deformity can be seen when there is associated kyphosis of greater than 30° or the patient has undergone a prior laminectomy. This places the spinal cord and roots at risk and, hence, many surgeons recommend a stabilization procedure to prevent progressive kyphosis. A universal segmental fixation system or the Harrington distraction rod system can correct the deformity and resist the failure associated with the axial loading.

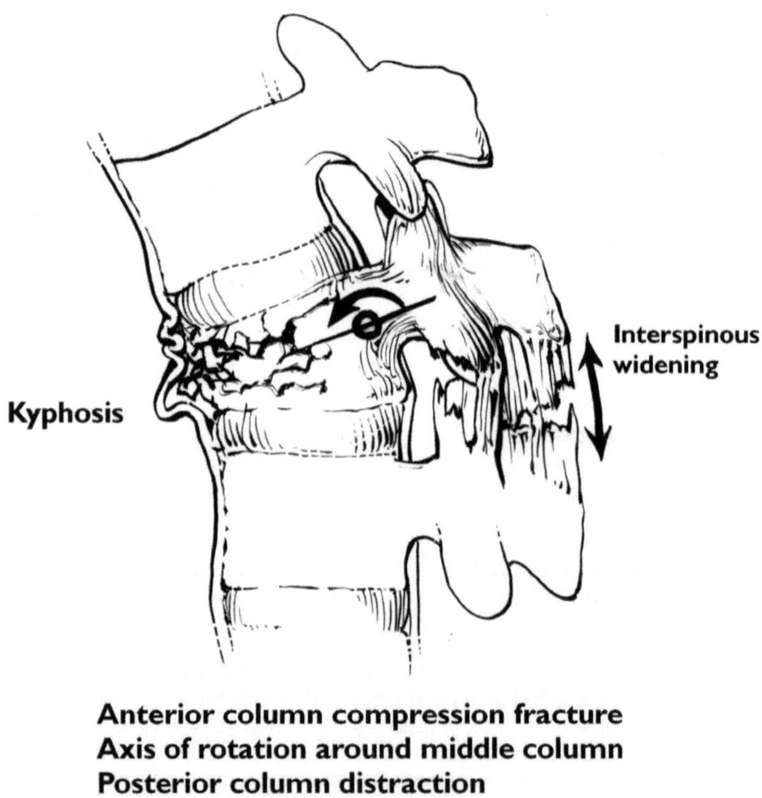

Fig. 22.7. Illustration of anterior column compression fracture showing a reduction in height of the anterior portion of the vertebral body with no involvement of the posterior vertebral body. Kyphotic angulation occurs and widening of the interspinous processes may be seen. In these fractures, the middle column acts as a hinge, which results in a tension force on the posterior ligamentous structures.

In patients with less than 30° of kyphosis and less than 50% loss of vertebral body height, the injury can be treated non-operatively with the use of a thoracolumbar orthosis. Patients can then be mobilized in this brace, which should be used for at least 3 months. Lateral flexion and extension films should then be obtained with the patient out of the brace. In the absence of excessive motion and no progression of the angular deformity, the patient can then be weaned off the orthotic device and physical therapy instituted, to strengthen the atrophied musculature. Progression of the deformity and/or incapacitating pain are indications for surgical stabilization.

Burst Fractures

This type comprises 15–20% of all major vertebral body fractures in most series. It results from failure of the vertebral body under an axial load, with associated flexion. The anterior and middle columns are affected, making it an unstable type of injury. Radiographic features include comminution of the vertebral body, increase of the interpediculate distance, vertical fracture of the laminae, loss of posterior vertebral body height and retropulsion of bone fragment into the canal can be appreciated. This injury has been sub-divided into five different subgroups, according to Denis (Fig. 22.8) [28].

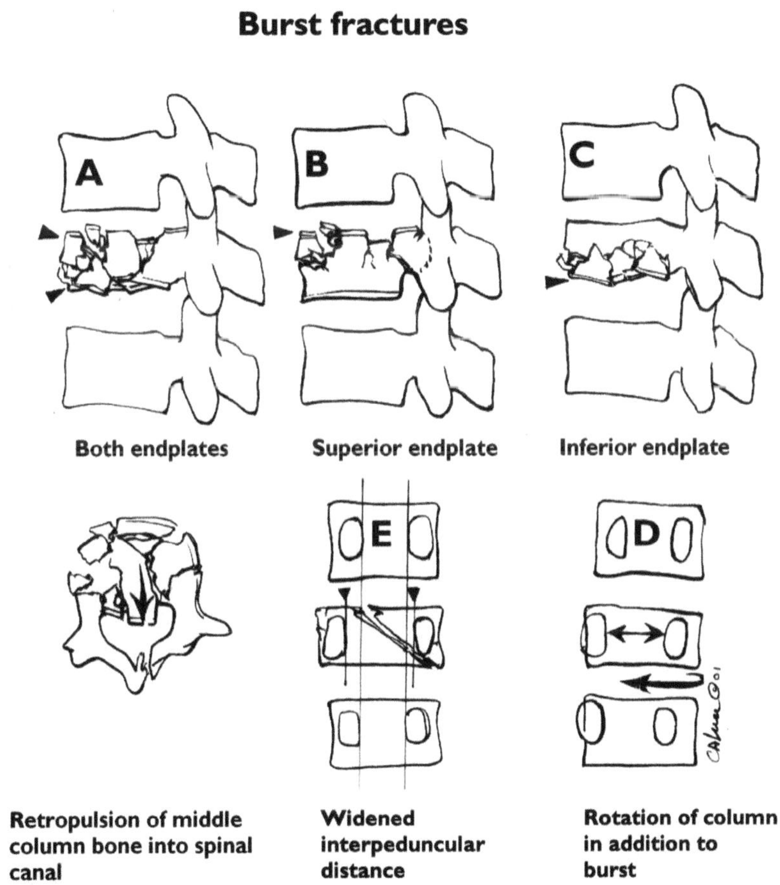

Fig. 22.8. Illustration of the common fracture patterns seen with burst fractures. Burst fractures have been sub-divided into five different subgroups according to Denis. The type A fracture is characterized by fractures of both the superior and inferior end plates, usually as a result of an axial load. The types B and C burst fractures involve the superior and inferior end plates, respectively. These result from an axial load coupled with a flexion load. An axial and a rotational load give rise to a type D burst fracture. The type E fracture is characterized by widened pedicles with a burst and lateral flexion injury.

The type A fracture is characterized by fractures of both the superior and inferior end plates, usually as a result of an axial load. The types B and C burst fractures involve the superior and inferior end plates, respectively. These result from an axial load coupled with a flexion load. An axial and a rotational load give rise to a type D burst fracture. The type A and D fractures appear similar on lateral-plain radiographs, but the AP view shows the differentiating rotational displacement. The incidence of neurological deficits has been reported as high as 47% in patients with this type of injury [28]. These injuries may be unstable and may need surgical stabilization, especially when there is associated injury to the posterior ligaments, the facets, the pars interarticularis or in the presence of paralysis.

There is lack of consensus for the selection of non-surgical or surgical treatment of burst fractures. However, important factors to consider before instituting treatment include the patient's neurological condition, the amount of canal compromise and the degree of angulation. Less than 40% canal compromise in a neurologically intact patient with less than 25° of kyphosis might be reasonably treated in a thoracolumbar orthotic device and allow the patient to freely ambulate. This is used for approximately 3 months, with interval lateral plain radiographs to document any progression of deformity.

In the case of greater than 40% canal compromise, greater than 25° of kyphosis and/or a neurological deficit, surgical therapy is the preferred treatment in most centers. Neurological deficits include lower extremity motor and sensory abnormalities, decreased perineal sensation and bowel and bladder dysfunction.

Any system that helps distract the injured spine segment can be used to treat burst fractures. Harrington distraction rods or the universal fixation system can be used. The Harrington distraction rods usually provide good deformity reduction, as well as long-term maintenance of the reduction. Common complications associated with their use, which has been documented to be as high as 15.5%, include dislodgement of the superior hook from the lamina and failure at the rod–hook interface [30]. Anterior decompression and fusion can be done to treat a burst fracture of a thoracic vertebral body. This can be done if the patient has an incomplete lesion, significant canal compromise, in the absence of, or minimal, kyphosis or significant comminution of the vertebral body associated with disc displacement. However, the presence of posterior column disruption may limit the effectiveness of an anterior decompression as the sole stabilization procedure.

Laminectomies are done in the setting of burst fractures for purposes of decompressing a laminar fracture or to expose a dural tear followed by posterior stabilization. As a sole procedure, a laminectomy would lead to an increase spinal instability and, potentially, worsen a pre-existing neurological deficit.

Seatbelt-type Injuries

These injuries are the result of flexion force vector acting around an anteriorly placed axis of rotation. This is seen when patients, while wearing seatbelts, as a result of the lower spine being fixed against the seat and the upper spine pivoting around an axis anterior to the spine, undergo a distraction injury to the middle and posterior spine elements. When only the osseous elements fail at a single vertebral body, this is classified as a type A injury, or commonly called a Chance fracture (Fig. 22.9) [31]. Involvement of the ligaments at the intervertebral space is called a type B injury. In a type C injury, there is failure of the two bodies and it includes the bony middle column. In the type D injury, there is also failure of the two bodies but it includes the ligament structures.

On plain radiographs, the fracture through the middle and posterior columns is usually evident. These fractures are usually unstable in flexion, although the preservation of the anterior column does not pose an emergent threat to the neural structures.

Treatment of these injuries depends on whether they are primarily osseous or ligamentous in nature. Osseous injuries are commonly managed with bracing devices, whereas those that are primarily ligamentous due to their unpredictability are best treated with a posterior fusion and compressive instrumentation. Decompression is rarely an issue, given that most patients do not present with neurological deficits.

Fracture Dislocation

These fractures are characterized by failure of all three columns as a result of compression,

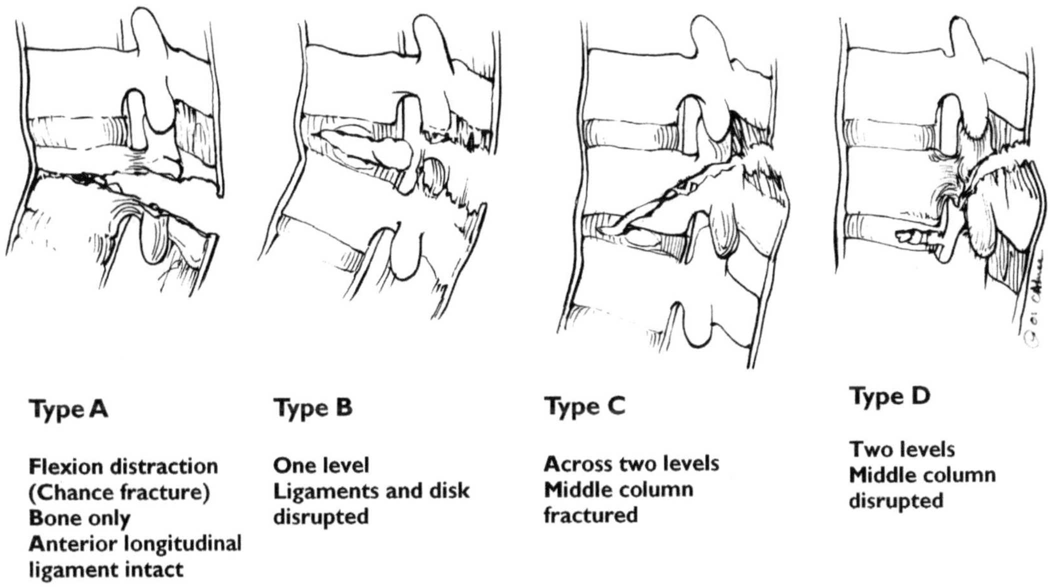

Fig. 22.9. Ilustration of the common types of flexion distraction injuries. These injuries are the result of flexion force vector acting around an anteriorly placed axis of rotation. This is seen when patients, while wearing seatbelts, as a result of the lower spine being fixed against the seat and the upper spine pivoting around an axis anterior to the spine, undergo a distraction injury to the middle and posterior spine elements. When only the osseous elements fail at a single vertebral body, this is classified as a type A injury, or commonly called a Chance fracture. Involvement of the ligaments at the intervertebral space is called a type B injury. In a type C injury, there is failure of the two bodies and it includes the bony middle column. In the type D injury, there is also failure of the two bodies but it includes the ligament structures.

rotation, and extension, shear forces or tension, with a resulting displacement of one vertebral body with respect to the other (Fig. 22.10) [31]. These account for approximately 20% of all spinal injuries and are also associated with the highest incidence of spinal cord injury. Neurological deficits are seen in over 75% of fracture dislocations and approximately 50% of these are complete lesions [32].

The type A fracture-dislocation is due to a flexion–rotation injury and is seen usually the result of a fall or a motor vehicle accident. In CT with reconstructions, rotation of the superior and inferior vertebral bodies can be appreciated on the axial views. Also, disruption of the facets as well as narrowing of the canal can be seen.

The type B injury, which occurs as a result of shear vectors directed from the posterior to the anterior portion of the spine, results in anterolisthesis of the superior body and retrolisthesis of the inferior body, although the opposite can also occur. These are unstable injuries, since they affect all three columns and spinal cord injury is frequently seen.

A third type of injury pattern, characterized by bilateral facet dislocation, is known as the type C injury. The flexion–distraction force injures the anterior column, disrupting the anterior annulus and stripping the anterior longitudinal ligament.

Fracture dislocations are uniformly unstable. This is the reason why most of these injuries necessitate surgical intervention. The surgical procedures performed for these injuries depend on the clinical status of the patient as well as the nature of the injury. Most of these injuries are treated with posterior fixation and fusion, as well as decompression, if needed. Some studies support non-surgical management, with the patient in bed rest for 6–10 weeks [33]. However, patients treated surgically can be mobilized more quickly and have a shorter hospital stay. The purpose of the operation is to realign the spine, repair dural tears if present and to decompress the spinal canal.

Complications, such as overdistraction, overcompression, inadvertent canal compromise due to instrumentation and loss of reduction,

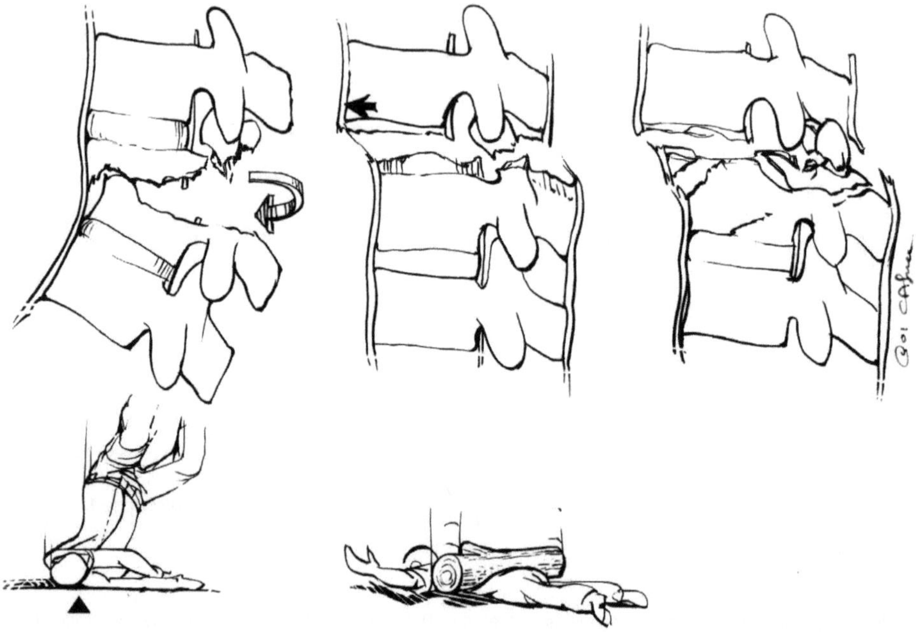

Fig. 22.10. Illustration of three types of fracture dislocation. These fractures are characterized by failure of all three columns as a result of compression, rotation and extension; shear forces or tension with a resulting displacement of one vertebral body with respect to the other. The type A fracture-dislocation is due to a flexion-rotation injury and is seen usually the result of a fall or a motor vehicle accident. The type B injury, which occurs as a result of shear vectors directed from the posterior to the anterior portion of the spine, results in anterolisthesis of the superior body and retrolisthesis of the inferior body, although the opposite can also occur. These are unstable injuries, since they affect all three columns and spinal cord injury is frequently seen. A third type of injury pattern, characterized by bilateral facet dislocation, is known as the type C injury. The flexion-distraction force injures the anterior column disrupting the anterior annulus and stripping the anterior longitudinal ligament.

can be seen with the use of spinal instrumentation in an attempt to effectively treat these injuries.

Other Types of Injuries

Soft tissue injuries, traumatic disc herniations and gunshot wounds to the thoracic spine comprise a small, but significant, subset of injuries to this region.

Only after excluding bony and ligamentous injury can soft tissue injury to the thoracic spine can be diagnosed. A short course of bed rest and non-steroidal anti-inflammatory agents should precede mobilization with physical therapy. Prolonged pain and discomfort can be evaluated with lateral flexion–extension films to exclude a subluxation which could be masked as a result of muscular spasms.

Symptoms such as pain, paresthesias and neurological deficits such as signs of myelopathy or a Brown–Sequard syndrome may be present in patients with thoracic disc herniations. Although these are rare lesions, they are associated with a high morbidity, including paralysis. MRI followed by CT scanning is needed to evaluate the lesion and for preoperative planning. Transthoracic and transpedicular approaches are associated with improvement in neurological condition in 80–90% of patients, while a laminectomy alone has been associated with neurological deterioration as a result of the spinal cord manipulation necessary to remove the disc.

Treatment of patients with gunshot wounds to the thoracic spine should be limited to those in which neurological deterioration is occurring as a result of spinal cord compression. Instability is rarely an issue with these types of injuries and other authors have documented an increase in instability from 0–6%, as well as an increase in the incidence of CSF leaks and infection rates in patients treated with a laminectomy primarily for this type of injury.

Thoracolumbar and Lumbar Spine Injuries

The thoracolumbar junction is situated between the rigid thoracic spine and the more mobile lumbar spine. This predisposes this region to axial compression, flexion and rotational injuries. The latter ones are rare and most osseous injuries are due to axial loading and flexion forces. For example, during axial loading, the thoracic spine deforms in kyphosis while the lumbar spine deforms in lordosis. Hence, the thoracolumbar region is exposed to compressive forces.

In the lumbar region, the vertebral bodies are larger and there is more musculature providing support. This makes lumbar fractures distinctly uncommon, accounting for less than 4% of all spine fractures.

General Management Principles

Injury to this segment of the spine, as in other segments, involves maximization of neurological recovery, stabilization to minimize pain and subsequent deformity and early mobilization for potential rehabilitation. These goals are accomplished along a spectrum of therapies, which range from conservative treatment with bed rest to early mobilization with a brace or after surgical intervention. As discussed previously, initial management goals include maintenance of spinal alignment, treatment and stabilization of concurrent injuries and prevention of complications such as deep vein thrombosis, urinary tract infections, pneumonia and skin breakdown. These complications can be avoided by the use of bladder catheterization, frequent patient repositioning and aggressive pulmonary toiletry.

The decision to institute surgical treatment depends on many factors. Among them, the patient's neurological condition, evidence of instability, clinical and radiographic findings of cord compression and the overall condition of the patient, including age and associated co-morbidities. It has been shown in numerous studies that instrumentation reduces the incidence of pseudoarthrosis, prevents progression of spinal deformity such as kyphosis and allows patients to be mobilized earlier, decreasing hospital time and minimizing post-operative complications such as atelectasis and thrombosis.

Injury to the Lower Spinal Cord, the Cauda Equina and the Role of Surgical Decompression

Patients who present with injuries to the lower spinal cord and the cauda equina may present with complete or incomplete injuries. Generally, decompressive surgery in patients with complete injuries for more than 48 hours does not yield favorable results. Improvement in neurological function has been described in both early and late decompression, making the issue of timing also an unclear subject.

Injury to the T11–L1 Segment

Neural compression is usually anterior. The techniques to decompress this segment of the spine are anterior, postero-lateral and posterior.

Anterior approaches to T11 involve a thoracotomy incision, whereas exposure of T12 and L1 requires a thoracoabdominal approach. This approach may be utilized in incomplete cord lesions or cauda equina lesions with anterior compression. The patient is placed in the lateral decubitus position and the lung is retracted to expose the vertebral column. The pedicle at the fracture site is identified and decompression is accomplished when a vertebrectomy with bone grafting is performed. This procedure is contraindicated when there is evidence of posterior neural compression.

The postero-lateral approaches include the extracavitary and costotransversectomy procedures. Both require the patient to be in the prone position and can be used for cases in which the patient presents with incomplete cord or cauda equina injury with anterior and antero-lateral compression. These techniques also require the removal of at least one rib and transverse processes to gain exposure to the lateral vertebral body. Posterior instrumentation can be accomplished with both techniques, although the extracavitary approach allows for visualization of the level opposite to the pedicle base. Decompression and vertebrectomy with bone grafting follows.

Posterior approaches include laminectomy and transpedicular techniques. With the patient in the prone position, a midline incision is made and a high-speed drill is used to remove portions of the facets and pedicles. Dissection of bone fragments off the cord or the reimpaction of bone fragments anteriorly into the vertebral body can then be accomplished. Large midline bone fragments are difficult to remove with this approach. Intraoperative ultrasound to assess neural decompression is helpful when visualization is compromised. These approaches are associated with the risk of incomplete decompression due to the exposure, as well as increasing the risk of deformity without anterior bone grafting.

Regarding posterior instrumentation and fusion, pedicle screws provide the most rigidity, followed by hooks and sub-laminar wires. At the thoracolumbar junction, rod and pedicle screw placement is preferred because of the larger diameter of the pedicles in this region. At least two levels above and one below the injury site are engaged by pedicle screw fixation. The need for anterior neural decompression leads to the use of anterior instrumentation. In the past, a posterior procedure was always done after an anterior approach because of the low fusion rates and the difficulty associated with maintaining correction of the non-instrumented anterior segment. The use of anterior instrumentation with anterior fixation devices has decreased the need for a staged second procedure. The efficacy of these devices is comparable to that of posterior instrumentation systems. Among the existing systems rods, plates and interbody devices are the most commonly used. They should not be used with fracture dislocations unless supplemented by posterior instrumentation.

Injury to the L2–L4 Segment

These injuries result in cauda equina injuries and, hence, the recovery of function is different. In the presence of neural compression, a laminectomy with transpedicular decompression might provide adequate exposure. A retroperitoneal approach, with an S-shaped incision from the tip of the 12th rib into the lower abdomen, allows for reflection of the peritoneum and the abdominal cavity contents. The psoas muscle is then mobilized and the lumbar segmental vessels are ligated to allow access to the anterolateral aspect of the lumbar spine from L2 caudally. A vertebrectomy with grafting is then performed followed by instrumentation.

The goal of instrumentation in this region is not only to provide stability but also to maintain the physiological lordosis, which, if lost, leads to postural imbalances and a flat back. Rods are contoured to maintain the physiological lordosis and two to three motion segments are then fused, usually two levels above and one below the injury.

Injury to the L5 Segment

At L5, neural decompression is best achieved posteriorly via a laminectomy with a transpedicular approach. In the case of severe neural compression, an anterior decompression can be performed through a paramedian abdominal incision. The lower lumbar spine can then be exposed via a transperitoneal or retroperitoneal approach. The transperitoneal approach provides more extensive exposure but it also entails mobilization of the great vessels and the hypogastric nerve plexus. Mobilization of the latter structure is associated with an increased risk of impotence.

Sacral fixation is needed for L5 fractures. The use of posterior instrumentation with placement of pedicle screws placed at 45° laterally into the ala of the sacrum or medially into the first pedicle provides excellent fixation [34]. Sacral sublaminar wiring is sometimes used to reinforce the construct. Post-operatively, patients are placed in a lumbosacral orthotic device.

Complications Associated with Surgical Management

Neurological deterioration can occur as a result of inadvertent traction on the neural structures, compression, damage to the vascular supply to the spine, graft dislodgement, hemorrhage and hardware displacement. Posterior instrumentation carries a risk of neurological injury of 1–3%, with pedicle screws having a 3% risk of nerve injury.

Injury to the lung, major vessels and abdominal viscera can also occur during exposure. Dural tears can also occur during neural decompression. If the dural tear does not seal on its own by conservative management, an additional procedure might be required to stop the cerebrospinal fluid leak.

Pseudarthrosis can also occur and may lead to progressive deformity, pain and compromise of the neural elements. Dislodgement and breakage of the hardware is usually associated with pseudarthrosis and is expected to occur in 20% of cases in the first 10 post-operative years.

Management of Pediatric Spinal Cord Injury Patients

Incidence

Spinal cord injury in the pediatric age group is rare. The reported incidence of pediatric spinal cord injury ranges from 0.65–10% of all spinal cord injuries [35]. Two age peaks are commonly seen: those younger than 5 years of age and those older than 10 years. The incidence of osseous injury to the spine is greater between the ages of 6 and 15. Under the age of 12, the incidence of spinal injuries has an equal sex distribution, but a significant and dramatic increase in male incidence occurs after the age of 12.

Most of the pediatric spinal cord injuries occur in the summer months. Children of 0–9 years of age usually incur in vehicular versus pedestrian accidents and falls and these account for the majority of the causes in this age group [36]. In the older age group, motor vehicle accidents, including motorcycle accidents, and sport-related injuries are a more common cause. The younger age group of children is also more likely to present with a neurological injury; in fact, younger children are more likely to sustain complete spinal cord injuries than are older children. In this age group, the craniovertebral and upper cervical portions of the spine are more likely to be injured due to the hypermobility of the joints in this age group, especially until the age of 3.

The cervical region is the site most commonly affected, with a higher incidence of spinal cord injury without radiographic abnormality (SCIWORA) in as many as 76% of patients. Multiple non-contiguous spinal injuries have been found in up to 16% of cases, emphasizing the need for complete radiographic evaluation of the vertebral column [2].

Biomechanics of the Pediatric Spine

The pediatric spine is inherently more malleable than its adult counterpart. This in turn allows for considerable movement between vertebral elements without incurring fractures or ligamentous disruption. This, however, occurs at the expense of providing adequate protection to the spinal cord.

In the pediatric spinal cord, several factors account for this physiological hypermobility. The increased elasticity of the ligaments and joint capsules allows for stretching without tearing. The high water content of the annulus and disc also allows for longitudinal traction to occur by as much as 2" without rupture. Translation and flexion and extension occur more easily because the facet joints are both shallower and more horizontally oriented than in the adult. Anterior wedging of the vertebral bodies accounts for the increase in slippage between adjacent segments and lateral and rotational movements are more likely to occur before the age of 10 because of the absence of the uncinate processes in the immature vertebra. The growth zone in the vertebral bodies is found in the end plates. Disruption of this zone can easily occur, even with moderate shearing forces. The large size of the infant's head as well as the delicate nuchal musculature in the absence of full motion control expose the neck to continuous sudden flexion and extension forces. Anthropomorphic data collected on children of different age groups demonstrate that these physiological differences are significant until the pediatric spine undergoes an adult transformation at the age of 8 or 9.

Ligamentous Injuries

Diagnostic criteria for instability in the pediatric spine is not as clearly defined as in the adult patient; however, useful parameters based on clinical and radiographic findings are considered to determine whether ligamentous disruption has occurred.

An atlanto-dens interval of greater than 4 mm is the upper limit of normal for children younger than 8 years of age. In adults, if this interval is greater than 3 mm, instability is likely as a result of rupture of the transverse ligament and a C1–C2 fusion is indicated. Damage to the alar ligaments is likely if the interval is between 5 and 10 mm and an interval greater than 10 mm suggests total ligamentous disruption.

The angle between adjacent vertebrae in adults is usually less than 11°; in pediatric patients, an angle of less than 7° associated with neck pain mandates placement of a rigid collar for 5 days, after which time, in the case of a neurologically normal patient, flexion and extension films need to be undertaken to assess whether there is an accentuation of the angulation. If there is no change, the patient can be kept in a Philadelphia collar for 12 weeks; if there is an increase in the angulation, especially if the angulation is greater than 11°, treatment with halo placement or surgical fusion might be indicated. Pediatric patients who present with greater than 11° of angulation should undergo surgical fusion [37].

Horizontal Translational Displacement

The pediatric spine exhibits more horizontal displacement than its adult counterpart, with subluxation of up to 4 mm considered normal, whereas, in the adult, the upper limit of normal is 3.5 mm [38]. This is most usually seen at the C2–C3 level and, to a lesser extent, between C3 and C4. This is primarily due to the profound elasticity of the surrounding soft tissue and the horizontal orientation of the facets [39]. It is therefore important to remember than in children older than 8 years of age a horizontal displacement of greater than 3.5 mm is a sign of instability. In children younger than 8 years, 4.5 mm is considered unstable. Children less than 8 years of age who present with pain, muscle spasms or neurological deficits and with 3.5 mm of displacement are also considered to be unstable.

AOD

Traumatic AOD in children is associated with 20–35% mortality [40]. It usually occurs as a result of pedestrian versus vehicular trauma. It occurs twice as commonly in children as it does in adults and it is also associated with a good prognosis in those who survive the initial injury, even when presenting with neurological deficits.

The occipito-atlanto-axial junction is relatively unstable in children due to the presence of small occipital condyles, the large surface area of the atlanto-occipital joint and the horizontal orientation of the facet joints. The tectorial membrane, the alar ligaments and the cervical musculature provide the stability for this junction.

Children usually present with signs and symptoms of brainstem and spinal cord injury. Apnea and cardiorespiratory instability can usually be noted at the scene of the accident. Pupillary abnormalities, nystagmus, ocular bobbing, decerebrate posturing, quadriparesis or hemiparesis and cranial nerve palsies have all been described. Injury to the vertebral artery resulting in dissection and thrombosis can also occur, leading to permanent neurological deficits.

Although radiographically gross separation between the occiput and the atlas can be clearly identified, a high index of suspicion needs to be maintained in order for this condition to be identified. Commonly, these patients present with a concomitant head injury which clouds the clinical presentation; hence, aggressive radiographic work-up can lead to early recognition and, potentially, a higher survival rate and eventual functional recovery.

Plain radiography is helpful as an initial screening study, since findings such as a dens–basion interval greater than 14 mm and a Powers ratio greater than 1 are indicative of AOD. A fine-cut CT scan from occiput to C2 with sagittal and coronal reconstruction is helpful, not only in confirming the diagnosis, but also in evaluating the extent of the atlanto-occipital separation.

The preferred treatment is an occiput to C2 fusion. Intraoperative care must be taken to avoid damage to the vertebral artery, which is found 1 cm lateral to the midline. Steinmann pins or Luque rectangles have been advocated to provide immediate internal stability. Postoperatively, a halo is used for at least 12 weeks or until fusion can be confirmed on follow-up radiographs.

Atlantoaxial Rotatory Fixation

This condition has been described in all pediatric age groups. It has been associated with upper respiratory tract infection and with minor trauma. Children usually present with neck pain and torticollis. The position of the head, commonly referred to as the "cock-robin deformity", consists of tilting to one side but rotation towards the other. In this condition, the muscular spasm is on the side to which the chin points. Spasmodic muscular torticollis is the primary differential consideration. In atlantoaxial rotatory fixation, the muscles are attempting to correct the deformity, whereas in torticollis the muscles are causing the deformity.

Although the pathophysiology of this condition is not completely understood, the inflammatory response which occurs as a result of an infection or an effusion from trauma has been theorized to cause an infolding and even a disruption of the synovial folds in the atlantoaxial joints.

Plain radiographs and CT scanning constitute the imaging modalities of choice. AP views show deviation of the spinous process of the axis towards the side of the chin tilt, accompanied by counter-rotation of the subaxial spine. This radiologic finding is known as the "Sudeck's sign". This occurs as the patient makes a conscious effort to realign the deformity. Fine-cut CT scanning from the occiput through C3 help clarify the plain film findings.

Halter traction with incremental weights until the head resumes a midline position constitutes the initial treatment; a post-reduction CT scan is done before the patient is placed in a Guilford brace for 3 months. Recurrence, although unusual, is usually treated with another trial of traction and halo immobilization. Failure of reduction or a second recurrence mandates treatment with a C1–C2 fusion.

Subaxial Cervical Spine Injuries

These tend to occur in adolescent patients as a result of a motor vehicle accident or some sport-related injury. It is important in this age group that, if a cervical fusion is undertaken, single level arthrodesis be attempted to avoid the development of cervical stiffness and reduced range of motion. Also, the exposure of only those posterior vertebral elements needed for stabilization is essential in order to avoid fusion of unwanted segments.

Post-traumatic Spinal Deformity

Children with traumatic spinal injuries are more likely to develop skeletal deformities. The age of the patient and the level of the injury determine the incidence of late deformity. Scoliosis is the most frequent deformity, followed by kyphosis and then by lordosis. Factors such as injury to the osteochondral growth plate, disruption of the posterior ligaments, as well as spinal cord necrosis and syringomyelia, have all been associated with post-traumatic deformity. Pain, progressive neurological deficits and pulmonary complications have been seen in these patients – so close follow-up is essential.

Conclusion

Injuries to the spine have the potential to be neurologically devastating. Immediate recognition in the setting of multiple trauma is essential to prevent neurological worsening. The initial assessment includes airway protection and hemodynamic stabilization, as well as a thorough history and physical examination, including a complete neurological examination. Radiographic identification of life-threatening injuries begins in the emergency department. A high index of suspicion should be maintained at all times to recognize and treat certain injuries, such as atlanto-occipital dislocation.

The cervical spine is the most commonly injured segment of the spinal cord. Recognition and treatment of the injury to this area is imperative, given the high morbidity and mortality associated with injuries to this segment. Closed reduction can be attempted for selected types of injuries which, if successful can be then managed non-operatively.

Other segments of the spine can be injured and can produce a variety of neurological deficits. Injury at one segment should prompt a relentless search for an injury at another segment. Full spine precautions should be maintained during the initial clinical and radiographic evaluation. Pharmacological therapy in the way of steroids is indicated in patients who arrive to the hospital within 8 hours of their injury.

Pediatric patients represent a group at risk for certain types of injuries, which need immediate identification. This is because of the biomechanical differences between the adult and pediatric spines. As in the adult patient, prompt attention to correcting hemodynamic instability, as well as taking into account the anatomical differences, allow for a better outcome on this group of patients.

Key Points

- *Approximately 55% of spinal injuries occur in the cervical region, with the most common levels at the middle and low cervical levels, with C5 followed by C4 and C6 as the segments usually injured. Injuries to the thoracic, thoraco-lumbar and lumbo-sacral areas are equally distributed in terms of incidence.*
- *For spinal cord injury, intravenous infusion of MPSS at 30 mg/kg over 1 hour as a loading dose, followed by a continuous infusion of 5.4 mg/kg/hour over 23 hours if this regimen is started within 3 hours of the injury or continued for 48 hours if it is started within 3 and 8 hours of the injury, is the recommended standard of care. The NASCIS II and III trials have established a benefit in outcome at 6 weeks, 6 months and 1 year in patients with both complete and incomplete injuries.*
- *After clinical and radiographic assessment has been completed, unstable or displaced cervical injuries should be promptly treated with cervical traction by applying GW skull tongs. The pins are applied 1 cm cephalad to the pinna in line with the external auditory meatus after careful cleansing of the skin in the area and infiltration of a local anesthetic. Closed reduction can then continue until definitive treatment with either operative fixation or treatment with external orthosis.*
- *The thoracic, thoracolumbar and lumbar fractures are treated as distinct entities because of their anatomy: biomechanical function and neurological function are different from the cervical spine. Although the fracture patterns that occur at each of these segments are similar, the clinical presentation, treatment and prognosis vary according to the level of the injury.*

References

1. Harrison CL, Dijkers M. Spinal cord injury surveillance in the United States: an overview. Paraplegia 1991;29:233.
2. Young JS, Burns PE, Bowen AM, McCutchen R. Spinal cord injury statistics. Phoenix, AZ: Good Samaritan Medical Center, 1982.
3. Harris, JH. Radiographic evaluation of spinal trauma. Orthop Clin North Am 1986;17:75–86.
4. Nichols CG, Young DH, Schiller WR. Evaluation of cervicothoracic junction injury. Ann Emerg Med 1987;16:640–2.
5. Blackmore CC, Emerson SS, Mann FA, Koepsell TD. Cervical spine imaging in patients with trauma: determination of fracture risk to optimize use. Radiology 1999;211:759–65.
6. Golueke P, Sclafani S, Phillips T et al. Vertebral artery injury: diagnosis and management. J Trauma 1987; 27:856–65.
7. Bracken MB, Shepard MJ, Collins WF et al. Methylprednisolone or naloxone treatment after acute spinal cord injury: one-year follow-up data. Results of the Second National Acute Spinal Cord Injury Study. J Neurosurg 1992;76:23–31.
8. Bracken MB, Shepard MJ, Collins WF et al. A randomized, controlled trial of methylprednisolone or naloxone in the treatment of acute spinal cord injury: results of the Second National Acute Spinal Cord Injury Study. N Engl J Med 1990;322:1405–11.
9. Bracken MB, Shepard MJ, Holford TR et al. Administration of methylprednisolone for 24 or 48 hours or tirilazad mesylate for 48 hours in the treatment of acute spinal cord injury: results of the Third National Acute Spinal Cord Injury Randomized, Controlled Trial. National Acute Spinal Cord Injury Study. JAMA 1997;277:1597–604.
10. Tator CH, Fehlings MG. Review of the secondary injury theory of acute spinal cord trauma with emphasis on vascular mechanisms. J Neurosurg 1991;75:15–26.
11. American Spinal Injury Association. Standards for Neurological and Functional Classification of Spinal Cord Injury, Revised. Chicago: American Spinal Injury Association, 1992.
12. Schneider RC, Cherry G, Pantek H. The syndrome of acute central cervical spinal cord injury. J Neurosurg 1954;11:546–77.
13. Hamilton MG, Myles ST. Pediatric spinal injury: review of 174 hospital admissions. J Neurosurg 1992;77:700–4.
14. Bell C. Surgical observations. Middlesex Hospital Journal 1817;4:469.
15. Anderson PA, Montesano PX. Morphology and treatment of occipital condyle fractures. Spine 1988;13:731–6.
16. Wertheim SB, Bohlman HH. Occipitocervical fusion: indications, technique and long-term results in thirteen patients. J Bone Joint Surg [Am] 1987;69:833–6.
17. Spence K, Decker S, Sell K. Bursting atlantal fracture associated with rupture of the transverse ligament. J Bone Joint Surg [Am] 1970;52:543–9.
18. Anderson LD, D'Alonzo RT. Fractures of the odontoid process of the axis. J Bone Joint Surg [Am] 1974;56: 1663–74.
19. Dunn ME, Seljeskog EL. Experience in the management of odontoid process injuries: an analysis of 128 cases. Neurosurgery 1986;18:306–10.
20. Eichler ME, Vollmer DG. Cervical spine trauma. In: Youmans J, editor. Neurological surgery, Volume 3, 4th Edition. Philadelphia: WB Saunders, 1996; 1962.
21. Cornish BL. Traumatic spondylolisthesis of the axis. J Bone Joint Surg [Br] 1968;50:31–43.
22. Taylor AR. The mechanism of injury to the spinal cord in the neck without damage to the vertebral column. J Bone Joint Surg [Br] 1951;33:543–7.
23. Burke DC. Spinal cord trauma in children. Paraplegia 1971;9:1–14.
24. Tator CH. Epidemiology and general characteristics of the spinal cord injured patient. In: Benzel EC, Tator CH,

editors. Contemporary management of spinal cord injury. Park Ridge, IL: American Association of Neurological Surgeons, 1994.
25. White AA, Panjabi MM. The basic kinematics of the human spine: a review of past and current knowledge. Spine 1979;3:12.
26. White AA, Panjabi MM. Clinical biomechanics of the spine. 2nd Edition. Philadelphia: JB Lippincott, 1990.
27. Holdsworth FW. Fractures, dislocations and fracture-dislocations of the spine. J Bone Joint Surg [Br] 1963;45:6.
28. Denis F. The three-column spine and its significance in the classification of acute thoracolumbar spinal injuries. Spine 1983;8:817.
29. Maiman DJ, Pintar FA. Anatomy and clinical biomechanics of the thoracic spine. Clin Neurosurg 1990; 38:296.
30. Chozick BS, Toselli R. Complications of spinal instrumentation. In: Benzel EC, editor. Spinal instrumentation. Park Ridge, IL: American Association of Neurological Surgeons, 1994; 257–74.
31. Chance CQ. Note on a type of flexion fracture of the spine. Br J Radiol 1948;21:452.
32. Gertzbein SD. Neurological deterioration in patients with thoracic and lumbar fractures after admission to the hospital. Spine 1994;19:1723.
33. Jacobs RR, Asher MA, Snider RK. Thoracolumbar spinal injuries: a comparative study of recumbent and operative treatment in 100 patients. Spine 1980;5:463.
34. Zindrick MR, Wiltse LL, Widell EH et al. A biomechanical study of intrapeduncular screw fixation in the lumbosacral spine. Clin Orthop 1986;203:99–111.
35. Anderson MJ, Schutt AH. Spinal injury in children: a review of 156 cases seen from 1950 through 1978. Mayo Clin Proc 1980;55:499–504.
36. Hadley MN, Zabramski JM, Browner CM et al. Pediatric spinal trauma: review of 122 cases of spinal cord and vertebral column injuries. J Neurosurg 1988;68:18–24.
37. Pang D, Sahrakar K, Sun PP. Pediatric spinal cord and vertebral column injuries. In: Youmans J, editor. Neurological surgery. Volume 3. 4th Edition. Philadelphia: WB Saunders, 1996; 2006.
38. Sullivan CR, Bruwer AJ, Harris E. Hypermobility of the cervical spine in children: a pitfall in the diagnosis of cervical dislocation. Am J Surg 1958;95:636–40.
39. Pang D, Wilberger JE. Traumatic atlantooccipital dislocation with survival: case report and review. Neurosurgery 1980;7:503–8.
40. Alker GJ, Oh YS, Leslie EV. High cervical spine and craniofacial junction injuries in fatal traffic accidents: a radiographic study. Orthop Clin North Am 1978;9: 1003–10.
41. Centers for Disease Control. "Trends in Traumatic Spinal Cord Injury - New York, 1982-1988." MMWR 40 (1991): 535.
42. Feller, BA. "Prevalence of Selected Impairments: United States - 1977." Vital and Health Statistics. DHSS Publication, Feb: Series 10. No 134. (1981): 81-1562.
43. Harvey, C., BB Rothschild, AJ Asmann, T Stripling. "New Estimates of Traumatic SCI Prevalence: A Survey-based Approach." Paraplegia 28 (1990): 537.

23

Rehabilitation of Neurologically Injured Patients

W. S. Lal Gunasekera and June Bendall

Summary

Rehabilitation is an integral component in the management of patients following neurological injury. A brief review of the pathophysiology and process of recovery of damaged neural tissue helps to understand the scientific basis of rehabilitation. The success of a rehabilitation program depends on appropriate timing, patient selection, choice of rehabilitation program, continued medical management and appropriate discharge planning. This is achieved in a multidisciplinary setting in a planned, appropriately equipped rehabilitation department, where medical, nursing, physical therapy, occupational therapy, speech and language therapy, clinical psychology and social work personnel work towards a common goal in a planned and co-ordinated fashion. Several devices, such as the Barthel ADL index, are available to measure the progress and outcomes of the rehabilitation programs.

Introduction

Rehabilitation is a dynamic process of planned adaptive change in lifestyle in response to unplanned change imposed on the individual by disease or traumatic incident. The focus is not on cure but on living with as much freedom and autonomy as possible.

The concept of rehabilitation is not new and dates back from before the birth of Christ. Artificial limbs, one of the first aids to rehabilitation displayed at the Science Museum, London, have been found dating back to about 100 years BC. Most early rehabilitative measures were aimed at getting people back to work, i.e. "Restoring to working order" was an early definition of rehabilitation. Rehabilitation of patients with head injuries, however, was a difficult problem. Until fairly recently, most head injury management meant little more than "containment of the problem". Finding institutional care was the only management available. The psychological problems of patients with head injury were mostly overlooked or unknown. Many patients with behavioral, cognitive and emotional problems were dismissed as unmotivated and irresponsible and ended up in psychiatric institutions. It was after the First World War, when neurosurgery became a separate specialty, that patients with head injury began to be rehabilitated. Currently, the number of patients requiring rehabilitation following traumatic brain injury has increased through modern life style. This, together with improved early care, mean that more people are surviving the initial injury and there is good evidence of "improved" survival following head injury compared with outcomes 10–20 years ago [1].

Although returning to work is still considered an important part of the rehabilitation process, more emphasis is now put on improving the quality of life for patients following head and/or spinal injury. In this context, the terms "impairment", "disability" and "handicap" have to be understood. The United Nations and the Americans with Disabilities Act and the World Health Organization, in its 1980 manual of classification relating to the consequences of disease, made the following distinctions:

> Impairment is any loss or abnormality of psychological, physiological or anatomical structure or function.
>
> Disability is any restriction or lack (resulting from an impairment) of ability to perform an activity in the manner or range considered normal for a human being.
>
> Handicap is a disadvantage for a given individual, resulting from an impairment or disability, that limits or prevents the fulfillment of a role that is normal, depending on age, sex, social and cultural factors, for that individual.

Consequently, The World Health Organization defined "rehabilitation" as a problem-solving and educational process, aimed at reducing the disability and handicap experienced by someone as a result of insult, always within the limitations imposed by available resources and by underlying insult.

Scientific Basis of Neuro-rehabilitation

The understanding of the scientific basis of neuro-rehabilitation would be facilitated by a brief review of the mechanisms of injury to nervous tissue, the pathological sequel and the process of recovery of neural tissue. The pathophysiology of the process of recovery differs in brain, spinal cord and peripheral nerves.

Recovery Following Injury to the Brain

Patients with head injuries form a spectrum. At one end are those with mild head injuries with no neurological or cognitive impairment. At other end are those with severe brain damage, loss of consciousness, often with ventilator support, and sometimes death. Those who survive tend to go through phases over a period of time: off ventilator; slowly improving level of consciousness; improving mobility and possibly back to society with or without any residual deficits. The mechanisms of this process of recovery could be broadly considered as those concerned with the process of resolution and recovery of damaged nervous tissue and those concerned with compensation [2]. As an example, in a patient with dysphasia following damage to the speech area, speech could improve with recovery and resolution of the neural damage. On the other hand, the patient could compensate using alternative methods of communication. Similarly, a right-handed patient with inability to write after a right hemiparesis could improve his writing when the damaged hemisphere recovers. Alternatively, he could compensate by learning to write with his left hand. Rehabilitation harnesses the potential of both of these mechanisms and serves to potentate functional independence. Rehabilitation activities are designed to promote the process of tissue recovery, as well as identify alternative compensatory strategies appropriate for the individual in order to return to the pre-morbid state.

Pathophysiological Process

In head injuries, brain damage is often a product of several associated factors that include the mechanical impact, anoxia , ischemia due to major vessel occlusion in the course of brain displacement or to direct vascular injury and biological agents, due to complicating infection [2]. Mechanical injury may be focal brain damage with relatively small volumes of tissue damage, e.g. penetrating injuries and depressed fractures, or diffuse axonal injury following acceleration deceleration forces, often with more extensive volumes of damaged tissue and more drastic consequences.

Effects of Injury

Pathological changes resulting from such injuries are evident in neurons, axons, glial cells, blood vessels and extra cellular fluid (ECF).

Neuronal Injury

The spectrum of damage to neurons consists of functional impairment with no visible structural alteration at one end and, with greater magnitude of injury, there follows swelling of cells, chromatolysis, disruption of dendritic connections and, finally, death of cells at the other extreme [3].

Axonal Injury

The degree of axonal damage is classified into the following stages [3].

Stage I – Nodal membrane injury at the node of Ranvier, which is the weakest point in the axon, where stretching causes injury with ionic fluxes, influx of Na, Ca and Cl and efflux of K, resulting in conduction block. This may be restored in minutes, with immediate recovery.

Stage II – Reversible cytoskeletal damage follows a greater magnitude of injury. Fluid fluxes to maintain osmolarity, resulting in swelling of axons and impairment of axoplasmic transport but, as swelling subsides, axons recover, restoring function.

Stage III – Secondary axotomy occurs, with even greater injury. Ca and other neurochemicals accumulate and destroy the axoplasm, so that recovery cannot take place.

Stage IV – Primary axotomy with very severe injuries results in immediate disruption of axons.

The ultimate extent of functional recovery depends on the type of mixture in the area of tissue damage. Where the majority of axons have sustained stage I or II damage, structural, and hence functional, recovery could be expected to be satisfactory, as opposed to a situation where the bulk of the axons have sustained stage III or IV damage, where no functional recovery may be expected.

Glial Injury

Unlike neurons and axons, glial cells have the ability to regenerate and form scar tissue. Scar tissue has the potential to act as an epileptic focus.

Extracellular Fluid Changes

Changes in extracellular fluid with injury to neural tissue consists of accumulation of toxic neurochemicals that break down the blood–brain barrier and may contribute to cerebral edema, resulting in raised intracranial pressure, poor cerebral perfusion and further damage to neural tissue [4].

Apart from the above mechanisms, recent investigations have uncovered a process called diaschisis, where depression of brain function takes place in an area remote from the site of primary injury [5]. The mechanism of this phenomenon is not understood but changes have been seen with PET scanning, where functional alterations have been noted in the contralateral hemisphere and cerebellum [6]. Such a situation would magnify the functional disability resulting from the initial injury. However, as the changes are mainly functional, the potential for ultimate recovery could be more favorable.

Sometimes, damaged neurons exhibit denervation super-sensitivity, with exaggerated response to neurotransmitters resulting in altered function [7]. In the brain, such altered function may manifest as central pain syndromes or spontaneous spasms or dystonia with abnormal posturing and impaired mobility.

Thus, the total damage resulting from an injury could be summarized as:

Initial damage, which may be focal or diffuse axonal injury.

Delayed consequences with free radical formation, receptor-mediated responses, Ca flux and inflammatory response.

Secondary damage from hypoxia, hypotension, ischemia resulting from vessel occlusion either due to brain shift or direct vascular injury, raised intracranial pressure following intracranial haematomas, cerebral edema or hydrocephalus, infection, metabolic disorders, dehydration, electrolyte imbalance, hypoglycaemia and possibly the consequences of uncontrolled seizures.

Diaschisis and denervation super-sensitivity.

Effect on target organs, such as contractures, bedsores and disuse atrophy.

Process of Recovery

Structural recovery following injury consists of resolution of the above pathological sequelae, with recovery of damaged neurons, axons, glial tissue and resolution of cerebral edema.

Neuronal Recovery

Restoration of impaired function follows structural recovery, as well as other mechanisms that have been described in recovering neural tissue. Among them are adaptive responses, also called neuronal plasticity, that incorporate the following processes:

Rapid responses, where uninjured neurons assume the function of damaged neurons. This process of unmasking has been demonstrated in PET scans, showing increased cerebral blood flow and metabolism in uninjured areas of brain [8].

Re-learning or long-term potentiation (LTP), which takes place by activity-dependent changes in synaptic efficacy. This influences information storage mediated by neurotransmitters such as NMDA, which facilitates LTP, and GABA, which inhibits LTP. Such phenomena have been seen in the hippocampus and visual cortex [9].

Slow adaptive responses, which consist of rearrangements where several hypothetical models have been proposed [10]:

- Regeneration after axonal damage, with possible regrowth of axons that innervate the target organs [11].
- Pruning, seen in neurons with many axons. When one axon is damaged, other collateral axons innervate the target organs. The evidence for this is more definite in human brains than in hamster brain [12].
- Collateral sprouting, which is the most evident change, consists of outgrowth of axons from undamaged adjacent cells to innervate target organs, forming functioning units [10].
- In-growth, where uninjured neurons from remote areas innervate a target organ. This is commonly observed with injury to sympathetic nerves with the possible consequence of abnormal function [13].

The capacity of neurons to regenerate is very limited and lost neurons are not replaced, resulting in loss of brain volume (atrophy) and replacement with a glial scar, often acting as a focus for epilepsy [14].

Factors Influencing Recovery

Extent of tissue damage [15].

Severity of the initial neurological deficit [16].

Lesion type and size, where focal lesions have better prospects of recovery [4,19].

Location of lesion. Cortical lesions have a better tendency to recover as opposed to subcortical lesions. Lesions of the dominant hemisphere herald a poorer prognosis than non-dominant hemisphere lesions, as do lesions of sensitive areas in medulla and mid-brain [18].

Complications such as raised intracranial pressure, metabolic problems, inter-current infection and uncontrolled epilepsy [19].

Co-existing diseases [20].

Pre-existing mood disorders and psychiatric illness [20].

Age [20].

Racial factors have been suggested following a country-wide survey of stroke patients in the USA. Comparable strokes in blacks were more severe and less likely to recover than in white populations [21].

Genetic factors have been incriminated in relation to different alleles of apolipoprotein E in genes E2, E3 and E4, linked to amyloid deposition in cortex which heralds a tenfold increase in mortality as compared to those who are non-predisposed [22].

Nutritional status [2].

Alcoholism and substance misuse [2].

Pharmaceutical preparations. Experimental evidence suggests that clonidine, haloperidol, prazosin, GABA, diazepam, phenytoin and phenobarbitone have an adverse influence on the process of recovery [23]. Preparations that may promote recovery are still experimental and the likely preparations are norepinephrine, amphetamine and nerve growth factors [24]. Investigations in human subjects where amphetamine was used for treatment following head injury or stroke are of small scale, with variable results [25], but a beneficial effect has been suggested in double-blind studies [26]. Bromocriptine was found to enhance fluency in aphasics [27] but GM1 ganglioside studied in humans revealed no convincing evidence of benefit [28].

Pre-injury education and intelligence. Those with higher pre-morbid IQ and higher levels of education have better prospects of improvement [17].

Appropriate attention by carers and partners and other social factors such as support by friends and family [29].

Forced use of target organs such as limbs and speech is known to promote recovery [30] and emphasizes the place of physiotherapy and rehabilitation.

These factors are important in selecting patients for rehabilitation and planning programs to suit each individual. Elderly patients, those with overwhelming general medical problems, poor nutritional state, poor pre-morbid intelligence and pre-existing psychiatric disorders herald a poor prognosis and such patients may need to be excluded from a general rehabilitation program or managed in special placements.

Recovery Following Injury to the Spinal Cord

The mechanisms of injury and the processes of recovery following spinal cord injury are somewhat different from those of the brain [31]. The causes of injury, however, are similar to brain.

Primary damage from initial injury involves the white matter tracts and gray matter horns. Secondary damage takes place as the result of vascular changes, with loss of auto-regulation and micro-hemorrhages into the white matter tracts and gray matter [31]. Impaired blood–spinal cord barrier function results in the formation of vasogenic and cytotoxic spinal cord edema that would cause spinal cord compression within the confined space of the spinal canal, leading to poor perfusion. Axonal changes consist of membrane alterations, activation of calcium-dependent proteases and arrested or impaired axonal transport. The damaged tissue elicits an inflammatory response, with migration of inflammatory cells and cytokines. In addition, there are biochemical changes, with impaired energy metabolism, excitotoxic mechanisms, arachidonic acid release, free radical production, lipid peroxidation, electrolyte shifts, increased intracellular Ca, increased intracellular K and increased intracellular Na [31].

The process of recovery is similar to that of the brain in broad principles. Often, the added problem of spinal cord compression sets in motion the sequelae outlined above and release of compression favors recovery [32]. Permanent damage results in permanent loss of function. Attempts at reorganization of function may facilitate functional recovery but often result in complications such as paraplegic pain and altered autonomic functions such as autonomic dysreflexia [33].

Recovery of Injured Peripheral Nerves

Peripheral nerves have a greater tendency to recover when compared to the brain and spinal cord. They consist of myelinated axons, which are often mixed: subserving motor, sensory and autonomic functions. The causes of injury are similar to those leading to spinal cord or brain injury, except that peripheral nerves are more robust and withstand injury and ischemia to a much greater extent than brain or spinal cord. Damage to peripheral nerves results in loss of function of target organs innervated by that nerve. The pathological changes following injury lead to the process of Wallerian degeneration, which involves changes in the relevant neuron, the axon distal to the site of damage and the axon proximal to the site of damage, up to the first node of Ranvier.

In the process of regeneration, there follows a reversal of changes to neurons induced by injury. Regrowth of axons occurs along the empty tubes left after the degenerated axoplasm has been removed and an attempt at reinnervation of target organs if growing axons manage to negotiate the site of damage and enter the distal tubes accurately. Axons grow about 1 mm per day. For effective functional recovery, end organs should be kept in prime condition, without atrophy or contractures.

Adverse Effects of "Recovery"

The process of "recovery" of neural tissue sometimes results in several undesirable consequences. In the brain, epilepsy may follow scar formation. Central pain syndromes such as post-stroke pain, dystonia and abnormal posturing – possibly a sequel to abnormal neural connections – can be difficult to treat. Injury to the spinal cord may result in paraplegic pain and autonomic dysreflexia, which may also be from abnormal neural connections. Flexor spasms may follow hyperexcitability of damaged neurons. Phantom limb pain may result from abnormal central organization and reflex sympathetic dystrophy and causalgia may follow abnormal neural connections. In peripheral nerves, neuroma formation may result in neuropathic pain.

The above mechanisms of injury and recovery have widespread implications on several aspects of rehabilitation.

Rehabilitation

Successful outcome from rehabilitation depends on optimum timing, proper patient selection, appropriate choice of the rehabilitation program and its activities in a multidisciplinary setting, proper discharge planning and continued medical supervision after discharge.

Timing of Rehabilitation

The optimum time for rehabilitation to commence would be when mechanisms of recovery are in place, free of complicating factors such as secondary damage from hypoxia, hypotension, ischemia, raised intracranial pressure, uncontrolled epilepsy, etc. The initial pathological processes such as edema, and inflammatory response should be resolving. In the case of spinal injury, possible compressive lesions that may influence recovery are best treated and the spine stabilized, where appropriate [32]. Rehabilitation should not be delayed too long in case other late complicating factors involving target organs such as contractures, bed sores and disuse atrophy set in.

Patient Selection

Appropriate selection of patients is important for the success of a rehabilitation program. Advanced age poses problems of physical fitness and capacity to recover and could hinder the running of a group program. This is important, as most programs are conducted in groups and inability to conform to the group could influence the recovery of the entire group. Similarly, patients with overwhelming complicating factors such as advanced cardiac and respiratory diseases and untreatable malignancies would not be appropriate [20]. Patients are also selected for admission depending on the facilities available in terms of personnel, their expertise in different disciplines and special areas of interest of the center concerned. Most units are inclined towards general neuro-rehabilitation but some units sub-specialize in areas such as cognitive and behavior therapy, spinal injury and appliance technology.

Choice of Rehabilitation Program

Most rehabilitation programs are individually tailored to suit the needs of the individual patient. Those with focal brain injury are likely to have less neurological impairment, with little or no cognitive involvement [4,19], and be able to follow instructions and carry out specific rehabilitation tasks without difficulty. Those with impaired communication skills such as speech and language disorders need a program tailored in such a way as to help overcome these difficulties. On the other hand, cognitive impairment, which tends to follow diffuse axonal damage, poses difficulties with faculties such as memory, where instructions are quickly forgotten. Such patients need intensive cognitive behavioural therapy concurrent with appropriate general rehabilitation. These patients would also have difficulty using ancillary aids such as electronic devices and orthoses and attention should be focused on their safety as well as the safety of others in the rehabilitation unit and in the community. In this context, patients with spinal injury with no cognitive impairment benefit most from use of ancillary devices to improve mobility and environmental control.

Illustrative Case 1

A 53-year-old male who was employed as builder visited a Far-Eastern country on holiday. He failed to return after the holiday and, 3 months later, his friends arranged a search. He was discovered in a poor state of nutrition and in an altered state of consciousness following multiple substance abuse. He had no recollection of his personal identity and was disorientated in place, time and person. He had weakness of both lower limbs and was unable to walk. His friends arranged for repatriation and further investigations revealed that he had a peripheral neuropathy consequent upon substance abuse. His mobility improved with treatment and he was admitted for rehabilitation.

On admission to the rehabilitation unit, he still had difficulty with weight bearing and balance and was unable to walk without assistance. His cognitive functions were grossly impaired, with a very short attention span and loss of short-term as well as remote memory. He was still disorientated in time, place and person.

Initially, he was treated with intensive physiotherapy; his mobility rapidly improved and he was able to walk unaided. However, due to his impaired cognitive functions, he frequently wandered out of the ward and, on several occasions, out of the hospital, requiring police assistance to trace him. As a general neuro-rehabilitiation unit, there were no facilities to ensure security of such high-risk and cognitively impaired patients and his disability imposed great strain on the staff in the unit. He was unable to take part in the rehabilitation program due to the extensive cognitive deficits and had to be transferred to a unit specializing in cognitive behavioral therapy where rehabilitation could be carried out in secure surroundings.

Activities in the Program

There is evidence that repetitive and forced use of target organs and relearning favor recovery [30]. Programs may be tailored to address these issues in relation to daily living activities as well as tasks concerned with employment. Activities are planned in such a way as to facilitate the neural mechanisms of recovery as well as teaching compensatory strategies to overcome the disability.

Continued Medical Management

Medical management focuses on the treatment of intercurrent illnesses such as diabetes, cardiovascular and respiratory diseases, psychiatric disorders and on any factors that may impair recovery. Choice of medications will be important in view of the several pharmaceutical preparations that have been incriminated in delayed recovery [23]. Medical personnel need to be alert to late complications of head injury such as hydrocephalus and chronic pain syndromes, sympathetic dys-synergia following spinal cord injury and reflex sympathetic dystrophy following peripheral nerve damage and seek expert advice where necessary.

Illustrative Case 2

A 24-year-old male sustained extensive head injuries in a road traffic accident. He had diffuse brain injury with traumatic subarachnoid hemorrhage. He recovered gradually and was admitted for rehabilitation.

On admission to the rehabilitation unit, he still had difficulty with communication due to cognitive impairment. He was able to stand with the assistance of two people but his balance was grossly impaired. He required assistance with all activities of daily living but was continent and able to request a bottle for emptying his bladder.

His progress in the rehabilitation program was less than optimal and he failed to reach simple goals. His mobility began to deteriorate and he was unable to stand, even with assistance. On a few occasions, he had been incontinent and was also unaware of bladder emptying. He was then re-investigated and a CT scan showed hydrocephalus with periventricular low-density and effacement of the cortical gyri. He was treated with a ventriculo-peritoneal shunt, following which he improved rapidly. At the conclusion of the rehabilitation program, he was walking unaided and fully independent in his personal care. His cognitive functions had also improved markedly.

Discharge Planning

Planning discharge is an important and sometimes difficult aspect of a rehabilitation program. As the ultimate goal is to return the individual as close as possible to the pre-morbid state, their integration into the community requires special attention. Again, those with diffuse neuronal injury and cognitive impairment pose difficulties in terms of safety. Unless carers at home are prepared to accept responsibility or appropriate community care is available, such patients require long-term placements in appropriate institutions.

Illustrative Case 3

A 45-year-old insulin-dependent diabetic patient suffered a hypoglycemic episode and was admitted as an emergency. Following treatment of the acute episode, he was found to have sustained hypoglycemic brain injury, resulting in spasticity of all four limbs and cognitive impairment, and was admitted for rehabilitation.

On admission to the rehabilitation unit, he was found to be grossly obese, weighing 152 kg. Due to the extent of limb spasticity, he was unable to stand or walk without considerable assistance, which was further complicated by the extreme obesity. The available wheelchairs were unsuitable due to his weight and the first priority was a concentrated effort towards weight reduction. With appropriate dietary management, his weight was reduced to 110 kg, enabling rehabilitation to commence. A suitable wheelchair was also procured, as there was no prospect of achieving independent mobility otherwise.

As part of discharge, a home visit by the rehabilitation team was planned and arranged. His brother, who was also obese, was identified as the long-term carer. Their accommodation was a second-floor, single-roomed flat, shared between the two. Neither he nor his brother was ever employed and both lived on benefits. Basic hygiene had been neglected. There was no wheelchair access to the flat and no space within to ensure wheelchair mobility. There was no possibility of discharge back to the previous accommodation. Alternative accommodation that was suitable for the brother and the patient had to be arranged prior to discharge.

Concept of Multidisciplinary Approach to Modern Neurological Rehabilitation

The success of a rehabilitation program depends on the input of different specialists in related areas in a multidisciplinary setting [34]. The activities of different personnel are tailored to the individual needs of the patient and co-ordinated so as to achieve the maximum benefit in recovery of function and gaining of functional independence.

The multidisciplinary team (MDT) consists of medical personnel, nurses, physiotherapists, occupational therapists, speech and language therapists, clinical psychologists and social workers. In addition, regular services are often required from dietitians, pharmacists, appliance technicians, art therapists and teachers, where appropriate.

Medical Personnel

Medical personnel involved are the rehabilitation specialists and trainees. The services of other specialists are often required, such as neurosurgeons in the event of structural complications like hydrocephalus, and neurologists in the control of epilepsy. Neuro-psychiatrists assist in the management of those with pre-existing depressive and other psychiatric disorders and behavioral problems, as well as with behavior disorders following the brain injury. Plastic surgeons help in cases of difficult pressure sores, orthopedic surgeons in correction of fixed deformities, urologists in cases of genito-urinary complications and general surgeons and physicians in the event of general medical disorders.

In addition to providing medical care during the period of rehabilitation, medical personnel are involved in patient selection, monitoring of general medical progress, with a view to early detection of complications, and appropriate consultation with specialists in relevant areas. The rehabilitation consultant is also responsible for co-ordinating the program activities among the different departments within the multidisciplinary group and also some of the administrative duties in the department.

The Rehabilitation Nurse

Nurses working in a rehabilitation setting have to move away from the traditional role of "caring for the patient" to a major role of working with the patients to enable them to be involved and to share in the rehabilitation process. Working with other members of the MDT is the most effective way to plan, implement and evaluate the rehabilitation process. The nurse must be a good communicator to ensure that the skills learned during therapy sessions are carried over at all times. The relatives need to be involved so that the process continues after discharge.

Physiotherapy (PT)

Physiotherapists play a central role in the MDT. Their activities concentrate mainly on the design of exercises favoring the forced use of target organs. The exercises are also tailored to improve mobility of limbs to maintain a full range of joint movements and to improve balance. The activities are designed in such a way as to be relevant to activities of daily living such as washing, shaving, dressing, toilet, self care, eating and occupation and are closely coordinated with the occupational therapists. In addition, leisure activities in a group setting help the patients to improve confidence and achieve mobility and functional independence.

Physiotherapists also contribute, with hands-on measures to improve spasticity and control of balance. They are involved in the management of chronic pain situations and work towards improvement in overall general fitness. They also recommend the use of devices such as orthoses to assist in mobility and weight bearing and overcoming limb deformities due to abnormal posturing. In this regard, they liaise closely with the technicians who make such devices.

Occupational Therapy (OT)

Occupational therapists are concerned with helping patients to carry out day-to-day activities that are important to them despite their impairments. They work closely with physiotherapists, psychologists and nurses, with due consideration of each individual's impairment and attempt to increase their capacity for self care, productivity and leisure in the context of occupations which are meaningful to each. Activities are carefully graded to gradually increase the demands on the patient's physical and cognitive abilities. Compensatory strategies may be employed to overcome physical and cognitive deficiencies. For example, the simple task of making a cup of tea involves several functions. The patient has to remember where the ingredients are kept and be able to reach them. He has to have sufficient power and co-ordination of limbs to assemble the ingredients on a work surface. The act of boiling and pouring water tests the patient's capacity for safety. The whole process requires sequential thinking and the ability to remember the sequence. Where difficulties exist with physical or cognitive impairment, OT is designed to introduce strategies to compensate for the disability, with appropriate modifications to the environmental setting and the use of appliances. In the above example, modifications to the height of the working table for a wheelchair-bound patient, anti-slip surfaces for those working with one hand and remote-controlled switches to activate different home appliances may be necessary.

To achieve the above objectives, occupational therapists require a clear knowledge of the home setting and workplace in order to plan the goals and tailor activities to achieve these goals. This is facilitated by visits to the patient's home and workplace, where they would be in a position to advise suitable modifications to the environment or the patient's role to compensate for the disability. Home visits also incorporate the carers who would be responsible for the patient in the long term. Occupational therapists, with other members of the MDT, co-ordinate short-term home leave for the patient. This gives the patient, his carers and the MDT an opportunity to assess the ability of the patient to cope within the home environment and to gauge the impact of the patient's disability and rehabilitation strategies on the carers. Where modifications to the home or workplace are required, for instance for wheelchair access, occupational therapists liaise with relevant authorities regarding funding.

Occupational therapists also give advice regarding many of the safety issues in daily living. This involves safety on public transport, driving, crossing roads and the ability to handle money. The safety of the patient in the community has to be assured before arrangements for discharge may be made. Occupational therapists also arrange formal driving assessments, following which appropriate modifications to the car to ensure patient capability and safety may be suggested.

Speech and Language Therapy (SLT)

Many patients with brain injury have difficulties with communication which SLT aims to improve. For this purpose, the speech and language therapists work closely with the clinical psychologists, as communication skills are closely related to cognitive functions. Difficulties in communication have an impact on other issues such as safety in the home, in travelling, marketing and handling money. Improvement of communication following a brain injury parallels structural recovery, as well as the development of compensatory mechanisms and alternative means of communication. Therapy sessions reinforce functional recovery, with improvement in verbal and non-verbal communication. Where improvement fails to occur, alternative means such as visual cues in pictures and word boards have to be considered. Development of electronic technology has greatly improved communications strategies and computer software designed to meet individual needs is now in general use. However, where there is added cognitive impairment, some of these alternative strategies may not be appropriate.

Speech and language therapists work closely with occupational therapists, as some of the activities of daily living (ADL) require sufficient verbal and writing skills and the ability to follow instructions. These factors are taken into consideration during goal planning and review and in planning appropriate discharge.

Severe brain injury may result in swallowing difficulties and the speech and language therapists also assess safety of food intake. They liaise with the nursing staff and dieticians regarding the nature of food that can be consumed and the method of feeding.

Clinical Psychologists

Cognitive impairment is a serious handicap in patients with severe brain injury. Those with diffuse injuries are more likely to suffer loss of cognitive function than those with focal brain damage [17]. A frequently encountered impairment is loss of short-term memory. This results in inability to carry out serial tasks, as the patient forgets what he has done previously. Cognitive impairment has serious implications for safety in ADL as well as taking medication. Patients tend to wander away and be prone to accidents, as well as being a threat to the safety of others. They may lack insight and initiative, show little interest in the rehabilitation program and also exhibit unsociable behavior. They may have poor concentration and difficulty in coping with compensatory strategies and managing devices such as orthoses and electronic equipment.

Psychologists assess patients with suspected cognitive or behavioral difficulties and advise on strategies that are incorporated into goal planning and activities in OT and SLT. In addition, they assist in the management of stress-related disorders and behavioral therapy. Psychological assessment involves a battery of tests to assess memory, anxiety levels, depression, etc. These tests are also used to assess progress and outcome, safety on discharge and may be useful to the neuropsychiatrists who often assist in the management of difficult patients.

Social Workers

Social workers form a key link between hospital services and community services. They liaise with funding organizations and are helpful in identifying care packages to take effect once the patient is discharged into the community. They advise on the choice of placement, taking into account the physical and cognitive disability and the home circumstances. Many patients who are treated in rehabilitation centers are ill for long periods of time and may have financial problems. Social workers assist in these matters and liaise with the appropriate institutions to address such issues.

Dietitians

Patients with neurological injury may have nutritional problems such as under-nutrition or obesity. Under-nutrition may impair the recovery process and delay the process of rehabilitation [2]. It may be due to pre-morbid illness or difficulty in swallowing. In such instances, alternative means of ingestion such as percutaneous endoscopic gastrostomy (PEG) or nasogastric feeding may be necessary. Similarly, excessive weight may hamper the rehabilitation process and may require appropriate dietary advice for weight control. Furthermore, patients with general medical problems such as diabetes may require special diets.

Facilities Required for a Rehabilitation Unit

Many rehabilitation services have been set up in the community and specialized centers have outreach facilities. Careful discharge planning from the specialized unit can help to integrate the disabled person back into a familiar community setting. However, for the early months following severe and moderate injuries, treatment in specialized units is necessary. Such centers are also important for education, training and research.

Purpose-built rehabilitation centers are planned to suit the housing of disabled patients in terms of mobility and safety, with few stairs to negotiate and easily operated lifts, where necessary. Access and doorways must be sufficiently wide for wheelchairs. Special toilets with hoist and bath facilities are required for inpatients who need assistance with transfers. As most patients are likely to be hospitalized for long periods of time, adequate recreational facilities are required for entertainment, as well as indoor games, leisure activities and meeting visitors. There should be sufficient security to ensure that cognitively impaired patients do not wander away into a hostile environment.

Most centers have a gymnasium for physical training, a hydrotherapy pool, OT workshops with facilities for washing, ironing, cleaning and computing, a house-keeping area with a kitchen, and purpose-built gardens for outdoor activity. A garden laid out with elevated flower beds and suitably wide paths to provide wheelchair access would facilitate recreation, as well as improve mobility and co-ordination. An elevated flower bed suits those who are unable to bend due to spinal problems.

An assessment flat gives the opportunity to assess the patient's independence in daily living under supervision. The flat would duplicate equipment and appliances in an ordinary household and the patient's ability to use these facilities and their safety in doing so could be monitored during a short stay. A car may be useful for driving assessment.

The Process of Rehabilitation

The rehabilitation process is structured into sequential stages.

Patient Selection

Those referred for rehabilitation are generally assessed by the entire MDT. This may be done in a single sitting with the relevant team members or in several sittings with individual team members. Medical input is in the nature of advice to the rest of the team regarding the medical problem, prognosis and potential complications consequent upon the medical condition. The suitability of the patient is a decision of the entire team.

Levels of Disability and Grading

Those selected as suitable candidates for rehabilitation are assessed as to their level of disability and need. The need level is assessed using different instruments, e.g. the Northwick Park Dependency Score (NPDS) [35]. For example, a patient with cognitive impairment following a diffuse axonal type of head injury without any focal neurological deficit would have little in the way of physical training needs but a high need for OT, psychology and SLT, whereas those with mainly physical impairments have high physical training and OT needs. Different rehabilitation institutions have their own guidelines for setting levels of disability and need.

Rehabilitation Programs

Most centers have programs in pre-planned packages, such as general for those with head injuries, post-operative neurological deficits and strokes, spinal for those with spinal injuries, cognitive and behavior therapy for those with predominantly cognitive impairment and communications therapy for those with predominantly language and communication impairment. The appropriate package is identified depending on the individual patient's need level.

Goal Planning

Most rehabilitation programs commence with setting of goals appropriate for that patient.

This is done in a multidisciplinary setting, so that each team co-ordinates the goals to be reached by the patient in a specified time frame. This provides the patient with an incentive to work towards the goal and also the satisfaction of achieving it and moving towards a higher target. Goal setting is carried out in discussion with the patient and members of the MDT and tailored to meet the demands of the individual patient. Goal-planning meetings are held at pre-determined periods of time. Such meetings also serve to monitor progress of the patient in the different disciplines of the MDT and adjust the goals according to progress, in consultation with the patient and team members. Goal setting also incorporates discharge planning, as the goals should be appropriate for the discharge destination. For example, a patient who is to be discharged home where access consists of steps leading to the front door and stairs within, will need to have goals set with the objective of managing stairs with safety after a specified period.

The patient is then introduced to the rehabilitation program and provided with a timetable setting out the activities for the week. Some centers appoint a member of the team, to act as a key worker for that patient, who will co-ordinate the activities of the program for that individual. The key worker will also identify other carers, including those who will be involved after discharge.

Assessment of Progress and Outcome Measures

The success of the rehabilitation program is evaluated by frequent monitoring of progress, with regular discussions among the members of the MDT and the patient. Progress and outcome may be monitored using different outcome measures, such as the Barthel ADL index (Table 23.1), Rivermead index, Hodkinson mini mental test scores for cognitive assessment (Table 23.2), Weschler adult score for psychological assessment, Functional Independence Measure (FIM) and Functional Assessment Measure (FAM) [36]. These measures are designed to evaluate the degree of independence in ADL and provide a scaled impression of progress in different activities.

Ancillary Aids, Prosthetics and Orthotics

Some patients with physical disability may be helped with ancillary aids. Technical support for this is usually available from workshops that construct individually suited appliances. Such appliances may be simple splints that overcome lack of tone or deformity or sophisticated electronic devices for environmental control, used to operate household appliances such as the television, telephone and opening and closing curtains and doors. Computers, including voice-activated systems, may assist in alternative means of communication.

Integration with Community Services

The final aim of rehabilitation is to enable the patient to return to the community as closely as possible to the pre-morbid state. This frequently involves the identification of funds for continuing care as well as care packages provided by the community. Modifications often have to be made to home or place of work to suit the needs of the individual patient. The house may require widening of doorways and provision of ramps to improve access. Fixtures such as stair lifts and toilet accessories may be necessary to overcome impaired mobility.

During the rehabilitation process, visitors are encouraged and arrangements are made for short-term home leave. This gives an opportunity to assess the abilities of the patient as well as the carers to cope with the home situation so that necessary adjustments may be made to the relevant goals and the rehabilitation program to suit the individual patient.

Discharge of Patient

Having identified the discharge destination, the rehabilitation goals may have to be modified to meet the requirements for that destination. Personnel must be identified for long-term care. They may be close relatives who live with the patient or care personnel or community workers. Discharge cannot take place until these requirements are met. Return to a hospital environment after rehabilitation would be a retrograde step that should be avoided at all costs, unless medical complications occur that demand separate hospital treatment.

Table 23.1. Illustrates grading of ADL, which can be assessed and recorded at intervals.

BARTHEL ADL INDEX		DATE	HOSPITAL NUMBER			
BOWELS	0 = Incontinent 1 = Occasional accident (one per week) 2 = Continent					
BLADDER	0 = Incontinent or catheterized and unable to manage 1 = Occasional accident (maximum of one per 24 hours) 2 = Continent for over 7 days					
GROOMING	0 = Needs help 1 = Independent, face, hair, teeth, shaving					
TOILET USE	0 = Dependent 1 = Needs some help but can do something 2 = Independent (on and off, dressing, wiping)					
FEEDING	0 = Unable 1 = Needs help cutting, spreading butter, etc. 2 = Independent					
TRANSFER	0 = Unable 1 = Major help (one to two people, physical) 2 = Minor help (verbal, physical) 3 = Independent					
MOBILITY	0 = Immobile 1 = Wheelchair-independent, including corners, etc. 2 = Walks with help of one person (verbal, physical) 3 – Independent (but may use any aid, e.g. stick)					
DRESSING	0 = Dependent 1 = Needs help but can do half unaided 2 = Independent					
STAIRS	0 = Unable 1 = Needs help (verbal, physical, carrying aid) 3 = Independent up and down					
BATHING	0 = Dependent 1 = Independent					
		TOTAL				

Follow-up

As optimum recovery may take several years, it is appropriate to review the patient periodically. This allows monitoring of progress and modification of the services in the community, when required. Depending on progress, consideration of rehabilitation of a different form may become appropriate at different stages. When a patient with a certain level of disability improves with time, a further course of rehabilitation may become appropriate at a different level.

Continued professional support also helps the patients and their families as they adjust to the psychosocial consequences of residual disability.

Table 23.2. Illustrates simple mental tasks which may be evaluated and recorded at intervals.

HODKINSON MENTAL TEST	HOSPITAL NUMBER				
SCORE ONE POINT FOR EACH CORRECT ANSWER	DATE				
Age					
Time (to nearest hour)					
Address (for recall) 42 West Street or 92 Columbia Road	*	*	*	*	*
Name of hospital/area of town					
Year					
Patient's date of birth					
*Month					
Year of First/Second World War					
Name of Monarch/ President					
Count backwards 20 to 1 No errors but can correct self					
Recall address above					
*THIS QUESTION REPLACES "RECOGNIZE 2 PERSONS E.G. DOCTOR AND NURSE"					
	TOTAL				

Questions

- ☐ What do you understand by the terms "impairment", "disability" and "handicap"?
- ☐ What are the pathophysiological factors that determine the severity of brain injury?
- ☐ What pathophysiological processes are involved in recovery of function following injury to brain tissue?
- ☐ Discuss the factors that influence recovery of damaged neural tissue.
- ☐ What influence does the pathophysiology of neural injury have on the process of rehabilitation of patients with neural injury?
- ☐ What factors influence the success of a rehabilitation program?
- ☐ Which type of patients are deemed unsuitable for a rehabilitation program?
- ☐ What is a multidisciplinary team?
- ☐ Who are primary personnel that constitute a rehabilitation team?
- ☐ Discuss the role of three primary members of a rehabilitation team.
- ☐ Of what importance is continued medical care to a rehabilitation program?
- ☐ What facilities are required for a general neuro-rehabilitation unit?
- ☐ What is need level?
- ☐ What is goal planning?
- ☐ What is discharge planning?
- ☐ How would you assess progress of a patient in a rehabilitation program?

References

1. Reilly P, Burlock R. Pathophysiology and management of severe head injury. In: Head injury. London: Chapman Hall, 1997.
2. Finger S, Stein DG. Brain damage and recovery: research and clinical perspectives. New York: Academic Press, 1982; 303–17.
3. Gennarelli TA. The spectrum of traumatic axonal injury. Neuropathology and Applied Neurobiology 1996;22:509–13.
4. Lim R, De La Torre T, Mullan S. Protein and enzyme alteration in experimental brain injury. Archives of Neurology 1972;27:314–17.
5. Feeney DM, Baron JC. Diaschisis. Stroke 1986;17: 817–30.
6. Fiorelli M, Blin J, Bakchine S et al. PET studies of cortical diaschisis in patients with motor hemineglect. J Neurol Sci 1991;104:135–42.
7. Creese I, Burt DR, Snyder SH. Dopamine receptor binding enhancement accompanies lesion induced behavioural supersensitivity. Science 1977;197:596–8.
8. Weiller C, Chollet F, Friston KJ et al Functional reorganisation of the brain in recovery from striatocapsular infarction in man. Neurol 1992;31:463–72.

9. Douglas RM, Goddard GV, Rives M. Inhibitory modulation of long-term potentiation: evidence for a post synaptic locus of control. Brain Res 1982;240:259–72.
10. Cotman CW, Nieto-Sampedro M, Harris EW. Synapse replacement in the nervous system in adult vertebrates. Physiol Rev 1981;61:684–784.
11. Foerster AP. Spontaneous regeneration of cut axons in adult rat brain. J Comp Neurol 1982;210:335–56.
12. Schneider GE, Jhaveri SR. Neuroanatomical correlation of spared or altered function after brain lesion in the new-born hamster. In: Stein DG, Rosen JJ, Butters N, editors. Plasticity and recovery of function in the central nervous system. New York: Academic Press, 1974; 65–109.
13. Crutcher KA. Sympathetic sprouting in the central nervous system: a model for studies of axonal growth in the mature mammalian brain. Brain Res 1987; 434:203–33.
14. Castejon OJ. Electron microscopic study of central axons degeneration in traumatic human brain oedema. Journal of Submicroscopy and Cytology 1985;17:703–18.
15. Graham DI, Generelli TA. Trauma. In: Graham DI, Lantos PL, editors. Greenfild's Neuropathology. London: Arnold, 1996.
16. Lincoln NB, Blackburn M, Ellis S et al. An investigation of factors affecting progress of patients on a stroke unit. J Neurol Neurosurg Psychiatry 1989;52:493–6.
17. Graham J,\Salazar A, Weingartner H et al. The relationship of brain tissue loss volume and lesion location to cognitive deficit. J Neurosci 1986;6:301–7.
18. Lundgren J, Flodstrom K, Sjogren K. Site of brain lesions and functional capacity in recovered hemiplegics. Scand J Rehabil Med 1982;14:141–3.
19. Rose J, Valtonen S, Jannet B. Avoidable factors contributing to death after head injury. BMJ 1977;2:615–18.
20. Kotila M, Waltimo O, Niemi MI et al. The profile of recovery from stroke and the factors influencing outcome. Stroke 1984;15:1039–44.
21. Horner RD, Matchar DB, Divine GW, Feussner JR. Racial variations in ischaemic stroke-related physical and functional impairments. Stroke 1991;22:1497–501.
22. Nicoll JAR. Genetics and head injury. Neuropathology and Applied Neurobiology 1996;22:515–17.
23. Goldstein LB. Pharmacologic modulation of recovery after stroke: clinical data. J Neurol Rehabil 1991;5: 129–40.
24. Feeney DM, Hovda DA. Reinstatement of binocular depth perception by amphetamine and visual experience after visual cortex ablation. Brain Res 1985; 342:352–6.
25. Evans RW, Gualtieri CT, Patterson D. Treatment of closed head injury with psychostimulant drugs: a controlled case study and appropriate evaluation procedure. J Nerv Ment Dis 1987;175:106–10.
26. Crisostomo EA, Duncan PW, Propst M et al. Evidence that amphetamine with physical therapy promotes recovery of motor function in stroke patients. Ann Neurol 1988;23:94–7.
27. Bachman DL, Morgan A. The role of pharmacotherapy in the treatment of aphasia: preliminary results. Aphasiology 1988;3:225–8.
28. Hofbrand BI, Bingley PJ, Oppenheimer SM et al. Trial of GM1 in acute stroke. J Neurol Neurosurg Psychiatry 1988;51:1213–15.
29. Shah S, Vanclay F, Coper B. Prediciting discharge status at commencement of stroke rehabilitation. Stroke 1989;20:766–9.
30. Wolf SL, Lecraw DE, Barton LA et al. Forced use of hemiparetic upper extremities to reverse the effect of learned non use in chronic stroke and head-injured patients. Exp Neurol 1989;10:130–2.
31. Olsson Y, Ahlgren S, Farooque M, Holtz A, Li GL, Yu WR. Pathophysiology of spinal cord trauma: observation on vasogenic oedema and axonal injuries in human and experimental material. Neuropathology and Applied Neurobilogy 1996;22:518 20.
32. Burke DC, Murray DD. The management of thoacic and thoraco-lumbar injury of the spine with neurological involvement. J Bone Joint Surg 1976;58B:72–8.
33. Tator CH. Update on the pathophysiology and the pathology of acute spinal cord injury. Brain Pathol 1995;5:407–13.
34. Semiyen JK, Summers SJ, Barnes MP. Traumatic brain jury: efficacy of multidisciplinary rehabilitation. Archives of Physical Medicine and Rehabilitation 1998;79:678–83.
35. Turner-Stokes L, Tonge P, Nyein K et al. The Northwick Park dependency score (NPDS): a measure of nursing dependency in rehabilitation. Clinical Rahabilitation 1998;12:304–18.
36. Harmon RL, Sheehy LM, Davis DM. The utility of external performance measurement tools in program evaluation. Rehabilitation Nursing 1998;23:8–11.

VII
Hydrocephalus

24

Hydrocephalus and Shunts

Dominic Thompson

Summary

Hydrocephalus occurs as a result of impaired circulation or absorption of cerebrospinal fluid. Hydrocephalus is not a single disease entity but rather the end result of a wide range of congenital or acquired pathological processes. It is important that this etiological heterogeneity is appreciated when evaluating and treating hydrocephalus. The clinical presentation, the rate of evolution and the long-term prognosis of hydrocephalus will vary according to the age of onset and the nature of the underlying cause. It is important that these issues be borne in mind so that the most appropriate management plan can be formulated. This chapter aims to provide an overview of hydrocephalus, its various causes and the use and complications of the shunt devices to treat it. The role of endoscopy in the treatment of hydrocephalus is discussed elsewhere.

Introduction

Numerous definitions of hydrocephalus have been advanced; common to these is an underlying imbalance between the production of CSF and its absorption. Although overproduction of CSF resulting in hydrocephalus is well recognized in association with choroid plexus papillomas, these are rare tumors and, in practice, hydrocephalus is most commonly the result of some impairment of the circulation or absorption of CSF.

The accumulation of fluid in various intracranial compartments was recognized by Hippocrates (BC 460–377) and Claudius Galen (130–200 AD); however, the first morphological description of hydrocephalus, recognizing the ventricular enlargement and brain destruction is attributed to Andreus Vesalius (1514–64). More complete descriptions subsequently appeared in the works of Jean Louis Petit (1664–1750), in Robert Whytt's "Observations on dropsy of the brain" and in the writings of Giovanni Morgani (1682–1771), who described the clinical features of bulging fontanelle and sutural widening in childhood hydrocephalus. The anatomy of the ventricular system and the CSF pathways began to be understood during this period, facilitated in particular by the studies of Thomas Willis (1621–75). It was he who first proposed the choroid plexus as the site of CSF production and who introduced the concept of absorption into the venous system via what he termed the meningeal "glandules", presumed to be the arachnoid granulations. Franciscus Sylvius (1614–72), Alexander Monro (1733–1817) and Francois Magendie (1783–1855) also made important anatomical contributions but it was not until the more physiological investigations of Key and Retzius (1876) that the modern concept of CSF circulation was established.

During this period, crude attempts at treatment of hydrocephalus by means of repeated cerebral puncture were employed but at the cost of great morbidity and mortality. Dandy and Blackfan further contributed, developing experimental models of hydrocephalus, and established a means of classification of hydrocephalus, differentiating between the non-communicating (obstructive) and communicating forms and proposing possible treatment strategies. The treatment options they advanced included extirpation of the choroid plexus, removing obstructive pathologies if these could be identified or the creation of conduits to drain the CSF from the intracranial compartment, either internally by the sub-frontal and sub-temporal routes or extracranially. Early means of CSF diversion included nephrectomy followed by the plumbing of the ureter into the spinal theca, thus draining CSF to the bladder. Other surgical approaches devised at this time included Torkildsen's procedure of draining the lateral ventricle into the cisterna magna, ventriculocisternostomy in cases of aqueductal obstruction and the first descriptions of endoscopic third ventriculostomy by Mixter – a procedure that has recently undergone a renaissance. Morbidity and failure rates, however, remained high. Removing choroid plexus failed to account for the extra-choroidal production of CSF and early artificial conduits were prone to mechanical malfunction. In the 1950s, synthetic, biologically tolerated polymers, in particular silicone elastomer, became available and thus heralded the onset of the shunt era of hydrocephalus management.

Cerebrospinal Fluid Production and Absorption

Although a small proportion of CSF may be produced from the ependyma and brain parenchyma, the predominant site of CSF production is the choroid plexus, contributing 70–80% of the daily volume. Production occurs by a combination of filtration across the capillary endothelium and active secretion of sodium by the choroidal epithelium [1]. Cerebrospinal fluid production does appear to be reduced in the presence of elevated intracranial pressure and reduced cerebral perfusion pressure; however, the effect is small and production is largely independent of pressure under physiological conditions. By contrast, CSF absorption shows a linear relationship to ICP.

The mechanisms of absorption of CSF have been extensively investigated. Direct absorption by the brain parenchyma, the choroid plexus itself and by lymphatic channels in the region of the cribiform plate have been postulated. It is, however, via the arachnoid villi and granulations that most absorption is presumed to take place. Arachnoid villi are herniations of arachnoidal tissue into the dural venous sinuses. For a long time, two models of CSF absorption were debated. The "closed" concept held that the villi were blind diverticulae and absorption of CSF occurred by a process of seepage across their endothelial covering. The alternative "open" model inferred the presence of channels across the villus, opening and closing in a valve-like manner, permitting the unidirectional flow of CSF. Tripathi and Tripathi [2] attempted to reconcile these opposing views and proposed a transmembrane transport mechanism consisting of vacuoles ferrying CSF across the covering endothelial layer. Interestingly, recent work has focused on the role of the CNS microcirculation in the absorption of CSF – a concept that would have major implications for our understanding of the pathogenesis of hydrocephalus [3]. Whilst the precise mechanism of CSF absorption and the relative contributions of the various absorptive pathways currently remain unclear, our classification and management of hydrocephalus is based on traditional concepts of CSF circulation.

Cerebrospinal Fluid Volume and Composition

Cerebrospinal fluid is produced at a rate of approximately 500 ml per day (0.35 ml/min). The total volume of the CSF varies with age and in the adult is 100–150 ml, of which 15–25 ml is contained within the ventricular system.

Etiology and Pathophysiology of Hydrocephalus

An obstruction at any point along the CSF pathway may result in hydrocephalus. It is usual to distinguish between etiologies that lie within the ventricular system or at the fourth ventricular outflow – obstructive hydrocephalus (non-communicating) – and those that impair circulation through the subarachnoid spaces or absorption into the venous system – communicating hydrocephalus. Where the etiology is known, it is possible to further divide hydrocephalus into congenital and acquired forms. Examples of the various types of hydrocephalus are shown in Table 24.1, which includes both adult and pediatric hydrocephalus.

Estimating the true incidence of hydrocephalus is complicated by the etiological heterogeneity, the lack of a precise definition of hydrocephalus and also by institutional factors, such as referral patterns and treatment protocols.

Post-hemorrhagic Hydrocephalus

During cerebral development, the germinal matrix is the site of intense cellular proliferation and the source of both the neuronal and glial elements of the cerebral hemispheres. Situated in the periventricular region, between the thalamus and caudate nucleus, the germinal matrix is a large structure in the early developing brain. From the end of the second trimester, it begins to involute – a process that is almost complete by about 34 weeks; therefore, germinal matrix hemorrhage is unusual after this time. The blood vessels of the germinal matrix are irregular structures that have an immature connective tissue architecture; they also lack the auto-regulatory capacity observed in mature cerebral vasculature. Both these factors are thought to contribute to the propensity for vessel rupture in the premature infant.

The incidence of germinal matrix hemorrhage shows an inverse relationship with gestational age. Hemorrhage is detected in 40–45% of premature infants with birth weight less than 1500 g. In neonatal and pediatric practice, approximately 20% of infants who suffer an intraventricular hemorrhage will go on to require a shunt. Clearly, in a number of cases, the condition resolves following conservative management. The population presenting to the neurosurgeon is selection biased and hence the neurosurgical literature quotes greater rates of shunt placement. The risk of progressive hydrocephalus developing is proportional to the grade of hemorrhage.

The majority of intraventricular hemorrhages occur within the first few days after birth. In addition to prematurity, vigorous resuscitation, respiratory distress syndrome, pneumothoraces and seizures are among the factors associated with an increased risk of development of hemorrhage, with pronounced fluctuations in cerebral blood flow being the possible final pathway. Although hemorrhages may occur in the absence of clinical signs, the more extensive lesions may be associated with seizures, bradycardias and apnoeic spells.

Germinal matrix hemorrhage is readily detected on cerebral ultrasound examination and is graded according to the site of the hematoma and the effect upon the ventricular size [4].

Once germinal matrix hemorrhage has been diagnosed, follow-up by serial ultrasound examinations is required, particularly in the

Table 24.1. Types of hydrocephalus.

Obstructive hydrocephalus	Communicating hydrocephalus
Congenital	**Congenital**
Aqueduct stenosis	Arnold Chiari malformation (type II, less commonly type I)
Dandy Walker cyst	Encephaloceles
Benign intracranial cysts (e.g. arachnoid cysts)	Skull base deformity
Vascular malformations (e.g. vein of Galen aneurysms)	
Acquired	**Acquired**
Tumours (e.g. third ventricle, pineal region, posterior fossa)	Infection (intrauterine, e.g. CMV, toxoplasma, post-bacterial meningitis)
Other mass lesions (e.g. giant aneurysms, abscesses)	Haemorrhage (IVH of infancy, sub-arachnoid haemorrhage)
Ventricular scarring	Venous hypertension (e.g. venous sinus thrombosis, arterio–venous shunts)
	Meningeal carcinomatosis
	Oversecretion of CSF (choroid plexus papillomas)

presence of intraventricular extension or ventricular enlargement. The presence of blood and its breakdown products within the CSF may lead to an ependymal reaction, with blockage at the narrower points of the CSF circulation, such as the aqueduct or the outlet foramina of the fourth ventricle with the subsequent development of an obstructive (non-communicating) hydrocephalus. More commonly, the blood products cause an obstruction at the level of the subarachnoid space and arachnoid villi, leading to a communicating hydrocephalus.

Increasing head circumference and progressive ventricular enlargement indicate the need for intervention. A number of therapeutic options are available. The presence of heavy blood staining or excessive amounts of proteinaceous materials and cellular debris in the CSF precludes the early insertion of a shunt. Moreover, in the premature, low-birth-weight infant, the high risk of shunt infection is an additional concern (see above). Temporizing measures may include serial lumbar punctures or ventricular taps via the fontanelle. If repeated ventricular taps are necessary, there is a risk of causing damage to the cerebral mantle, producing areas of porencephaly. This risk can possibly be minimized by the placement of a ventricular catheter and subcutaneous reservoir. CSF can then be aspirated from the reservoir, thus avoiding repeated cerebral puncture. Recent review of the literature has not found evidence to support the use of repeated lumbar puncture or ventricular taps as a means of either reducing death or disability or the need for shunt placement [4a].

Medical measures to control the ventricular dilation are also employed. Acetazolamide, alone or in combination with furosemide, has been used and some have even suggested that such a regime may avoid the need for subsequent shunt placement. Recent evidence, however, has questioned the clinical efficacy of such regimes [5].

Lately, it has been suggested that intraventricular fibrinolytic therapy, instituted soon after the hemorrhage is diagnosed, may prevent the chemical arachnoiditis that develops in response to intraventricular hemorrhage and thus reduce the number of these infants requiring shunt insertion.

Whatever method of treatment employed, it is important that progress is monitored by means of regular clinical evaluation, head circumference measurements and ultrasonography. If progressive hydrocephalus is present, then once the CSF is clear of blood products, a shunt procedure can be performed.

Hydrocephalus and Myelomeningocele

Hydrocephalus complicates open spina bifida in 85–90% of patients. The key to understanding its etiology in this context is the Chiari (type II) malformation. In the fetus with open spina bifida, the meningocele sac acts as a CSF sump. The constant venting of CSF from the developing brain and spinal cord, beyond the time when the caudal neuropore should have closed, removes the distending force that is normally present within the cranial neurocele. This results in a constellation of features, termed the Chiari II malformation [6]. These include disorganization of brainstem topography, a small posterior fossa and, as cerebellar growth exceeds the confines of the small posterior fossa, herniation of the cerebellum through the foramen magnum and up through the incisura. As a consequence, the normal CSF pathways may be compromised at a number of sites, including the cerebral aqueduct, the fourth ventricular outlet and at the perimesencephalic region, resulting in hydrocephalus.

Hydrocephalus may only become apparent following closure of the myelomeningocele. In addition to the usual presenting features of infantile hydrocephalus, features unique to the myelomeningocele patient are bulging of the back wound, occasionally with CSF leakage and signs of brainstem compression due to the Chiari malformation. These latter signs can include stridor, lower cranial nerve palsies and upper-limb weakness and should prompt the search for progressive hydrocephalus. As well as being presenting signs of hydrocephalus in these infants, these signs may similarly herald a shunt malfunction in the older child. It is important to be aware of these atypical modes of presentation of raised intracranial pressure in the myelomeningocele population.

It is doubtful whether any child with myelomeningocele and shunted hydrocephalus can ever be considered to be truly shunt independent. Even in instances where it appears that the shunt is not being used, there are reports of sudden cardio-respiratory arrest attributable to the combination of raised ICP and the Chiari malformation.

Aqueduct Stenosis

As a result of growth of the tectum and tegmentum, the lumen of the neural tube in the region of the mesencephalon becomes narrowed to form the aqueduct of Sylvius. Because of its small caliber, this area of the CSF pathway is vulnerable to obstruction by a number of congenital and acquired pathologies.

Aqueductal stenosis is responsible for approximately 10% of cases of hydrocephalus in childhood. Presentation may, however, occur at any time from birth to adulthood. In congenital forms of aqueduct "stenosis", the aqueduct, rather than being stenosed, is branched or forked into two or more channels. In some instances, the tectum is also deformed and it has been postulated that, here, the primary pathology is a communicating hydrocephalus in which external pressure on the mesencephalic structures has led to obliteration of the aqueduct secondarily.

Scarring or gliosis in the aqueduct following infection or hemorrhage may lead to an acquired aqueduct stenosis. Tumors arising in adjacent structures, such as the tectal plate, the rostral fourth ventricle, posterior thalamus or pineal region, may not be evident on CT but can similarly result in a picture of aqueduct stenosis. MRI is necessary in such cases.

Imaging reveals a tri-ventricular hydrocephalus, with a small or normal-sized fourth ventricle. In addition, MRI will often reveal a trumpeting of the proximal aqueduct and, moreover, will readily identify associated neoplastic lesions that may not be seen on CT scanning. It is for this reason that MRI scanning should be performed routinely in cases of aqueduct stenosis.

Dandy Walker Syndrome

This syndrome comprises agenesis of the cerebellar vermis with cystic dilatation of the fourth ventricle, enlargement of the posterior fossa and hydrocephalus. The hydrocephalus is often absent at the time of birth but is present in 75% of cases by the age of 3 months. Additional brain malformations are present in over half of the cases. Neurodevelopmental delay is reported in up to 70% of cases.

Some controversy exists among neurosurgeons as to the best surgical treatment of this condition. The principal issue is regarding the placement of the proximal catheter: whether this should be placed in the lateral ventricle, the posterior fossa cyst or indeed whether both compartments should be shunted simultaneously. A further option is to shunt the infratentorial compartment in the first instance and then to treat the supratentorial hydrocephalus endoscopically if the ventricles fail to decompress.

Obstructive Hydrocephalus Due to Tumors

Midline tumors – particularly those of the pineal gland and posterior fossa – commonly result in obstructive hydrocephalus and, indeed, this is one of the principal ways in which these conditions present, especially in children. Although preliminary shunting of the hydrocephalus has been advocated, in the majority of cases, the hydrocephalus will resolve following removal of the obstructive pathology. In their series of posterior fossa tumors with hydrocephalus, Kumar et al. reported that a shunt was required in 18.9% of cases [7]. Young age at presentation, incomplete tumor removal and malignant midline tumors were factors increasing the likelihood of shunt requirement.

In situations where more urgent control of the hydrocephalus is required, insertion of an external ventricular drain, a subcutaneous reservoir or an endoscopic third ventriculostomy can be performed, pending definitive surgical treatment of the tumor.

Post-meningitic Hydrocephalus

Hydrocephalus may occur as the result of a range of infectious or inflammatory processes. The effects of chronic inflammation – organization of the inflammatory exudate with scarring or gliosis – can produce obstruction to CSF flow, both within the ventricular system and in the basal cisterns and cortical subarachnoid spaces. Bacterial, parasitic and granulomatous infections are much more likely to lead to hydrocephalus than viral infections. Ventricular enlargement rather than hydrocephalus may occur due to an ex-vacuo phenomenon. This is a result of the severe white matter damage or encephalomalacia that is commonly seen in the aftermath of bacterial meningitis. The risk of hydrocephalus is greater when treatment has been delayed or is sub-therapeutic.

Purulent infections not uncommonly result in compartmentalization or trapping of parts of the ventricular system (Fig. 24.1). This can make the surgical management of these cases particularly problematic, with the need for multiple ventricular catheters. In some circumstances, neuroendoscopic techniques can be used to fenestrate gliotic septae in an attempt to unify the compartments and thus simplify the shunt configuration.

Hydrocephalus and Venous Hypertension

The role of raised venous pressure as an etiological factor in the development of hydrocephalus has been highlighted in a number of clinical conditions [8], Achondroplasia and syndromic craniosynostosis (e.g. Crouzon and Cloverleaf skull) being the most commonly referred to. The mechanism is thought to be deformity at the skull base, resulting in narrowing of the jugular foramina and impairment of intracranial venous drainage [9]. The raised pressure within the cranial venous sinuses reduces the pressure gradient across the arachnoid villi and granulations impairing the absorption of CSF. In the infant with open sutures and immature myelination, progressive dilatation of the ventricles occurs in these circumstances. By contrast, once the sutures have fused and the cranium is less distensible, a picture more akin to pseudotumor cerebri results.

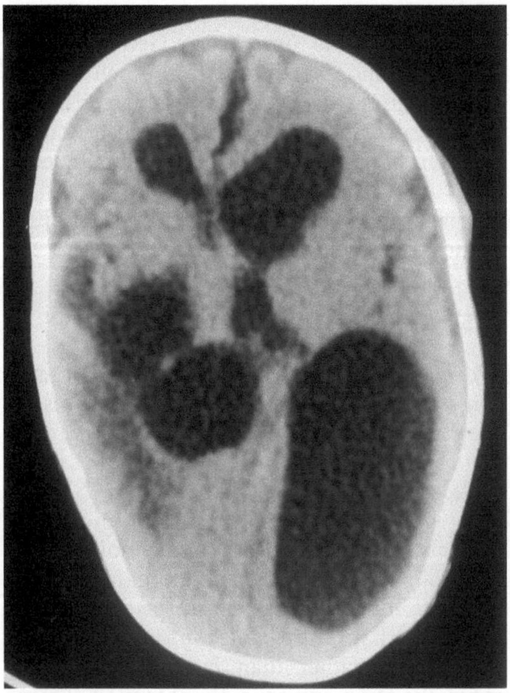

Fig. 24.1. Loculation of the lateral ventricles following bacterial meningitis.

Hydrocephalus commonly accompanies vein of Galen aneurysms. Again, the mechanism is in part the result raised of venous pressure due to arteriovenous shunting. In this instance, shunting the ventricles may be both harmful and unnecessary, since once the primary anomaly has been treated, the hydrocephalus may come under control.

Hydrocephalus Following Subarachnoid Hemorrhage

Hydrocephalus is seen in 10–15% of patients suffering aneurysmal subarachnoid hemorrhage. The incidence is increased where there is intraventricular hemorrhage in addition. Hydrocephalus may appear soon after the initial ictus but must also be considered as a cause of delayed recovery or neurological deterioration later in the illness. Symptomatic hydrocephalus requires intervention, which, in the first instance, will most commonly be by means of external ventricular drainage. There is some concern that the early re-bleeding rate is higher in those patients requiring drainage.

Normal Pressure Hydrocephalus

This condition, most commonly seen in adulthood, is characterized by a clinical picture of gait deterioration, dementia and urinary incontinence in the context of enlarged ventricles on neuroimaging, but relatively normal intracranial pressures. Although in some cases there is a history of subarachnoid hemorrhage, intracranial infection or head trauma, in approximately 60% of cases the etiology remains unknown. The differential diagnosis is wide and the identification of patients that will benefit from shunting is known to be difficult. A number of investigations have been advocated to aid in the selection of patients suitable for shunt treatment. These include isotope cisternography to assess abnormalities of the CSF pathways, infusion tests to detect increased resistance of CSF outflow and ICP monitoring looking at the frequency of Lundberg B waves which seem to be increased in this condition. Clinical features such as short history, predominance of gait disturbance as a presenting feature and a known etiology are though to portend a favorable response to treatment.

Idiopathic Intracranial Hypertension

This condition has previously been termed benign intracranial hypertension (BIH) or pseudotumor cerebri. The intracranial pressure is raised; however, there are no localising signs, no alteration in level of consciousness, the cerebrospinal fluid composition is normal and there is no evidence of hydrocephalus or other cause of raised ICP on neuroimaging. It is thus a diagnosis of exclusion. Chronic meningitis, venous sinus thrombosis and indeed spinal cord tumors may produce a similar clinical picture. An association with various drugs, metabolic and endocrinological disorders is recognized and this needs to be considered during the clinical evaluation of these patients.

Headache and visual disturbance are the usual clinical features. Papilloedema, optic atrophy and reduced visual fields are often present and permanent visual impairment can result. Close ophthalmological surveillance of these patients is mandatory.

Preservation of vision is the main aim of treatment. Treatment options include medical therapies such as acetazolamide. Drainage of CSF, either intermittently with serial lumbar punctures or continuously by placement of a lumbo-peritoneal shunt (or ventriculo-peritoneal shunt if ventricular size permits), may be required where medical therapy fails. Optic nerve fenestration may lead to visual improvement and may be a useful adjunct in the treatment of this condition. The long-term prognosis is generally good, with spontaneous resolution in a number of cases, though the visual loss may persist.

Arrested Hydrocephalus

Occasionally, hydrocephalus may evolve into a chronic state in which ventricular enlargement persists, yet CSF pressure returns to normal. This situation might be more accurately termed "compensated hydrocephalus". In children who have truly compensated, insertion of a shunt may be detrimental, leading to symptoms of low pressure or chronic subdural formation in addition to the usual complications of shunt devices. On the other hand, it is important not to miss the child whose neurodevelopmental progress is being hindered by the presence of hydrocephalus. If a decision is made not to embark upon surgical treatment, close monitoring is required in order to be sure that there is no disproportionate increase in head growth or progression of ventricular size and to ensure that development proceeds at a satisfactory pace.

Hydrocephalus Versus Ventriculomegaly

The term "hydrocephalus" should be used as a clinical term to imply an active process in which either the circulation or absorption of CSF is impaired (or, more rarely, the production of CSF is excessive), leading to an elevation of intracranial pressure. Increased size of the cerebral ventricles on imaging is more appropriately termed "ventriculomegaly" and does not necessarily equate to hydrocephalus requiring treatment. It is important to emphasize that whilst ventriculomegaly can be readily diagnosed by various imaging modalities, such findings must be interpreted in the context of the clinical symptoms and signs in order to permit a firm diagnosis of active hydrocephalus. In some cases, it is necessary to proceed to invasive measurement of intracranial pressure in order to make this distinction [10].

There are other explanations for ventricular enlargement, for example the ex-vacuo effect of cerebral atrophy associated with aging, head trauma or severe infection. In the child, ventricular enlargement may result from hypoxic ischemic insults. Moreover, in the aftermath of various therapeutic interventions such as steroid therapy, radiation therapy and chemotherapy, ventricular enlargement may also be seen. In such cases of white matter loss, there is usually concomitant enlargement of the cortical sub-arachnoid spaces and basal cisterns. The periventricular lucency seen in ventricles under pressure is not usually a feature in these circumstances.

A number of structural abnormalities of the brain, such as colpocephaly, holoprosencephaly and agenesis of the corpus callosum, may also be associated with ventricular enlargement and yet do not necessarily require intervention. Again, correlation with the clinical picture is essential.

Clinical Presentation of Hydrocephalus

The presentation of hydrocephalus differs in the case of the neonate and infant compared with the older child or adult.

Prior to closure of the cranial sutures and obliteration of the fontanelles, hydrocephalus results in disproportionate head growth. Thus, over the first 2–3 years of life, measurement of the occipito-frontal circumference and plotting this on a centile chart provides a simple and sensitive test. Wherever possible, sequential measurements (corrected for gestational age) should be obtained in order that the trend of head growth in relation to the centile lines can be demonstrated. Clinical symptoms are often subtle and include general irritability, poor feeding and slow attainment of milestones. In addition to head size, clinical signs include bulging of the fontanelle, separation of the cranial sutures, prominence of scalp veins and sun-setting of the eyes. This latter clinical sign is attributed to pressure on the mid-brain tectum by CSF in the supra-pineal recess. Papilloedema can be difficult to diagnose in the infant and indeed is not uncommonly absent in infantile hydrocephalus and so is an unreliable sign in this context.

In older children and adults, the classical symptom complex of raised intracranial pressure, headache, vomiting and drowsiness is more likely to herald an underlying diagnosis of hydrocephalus. Where hydrocephalus has developed insidiously, cognitive impairment, poor concentration and behavioural changes occur. Visual obscurations and papilloedema are more common than in the younger age group.

In both groups of patients, the presence of bradycardia, hypertension and irregularities in breathing pattern imply critical elevation of intracranial pressure and should be treated promptly.

Investigation of Hydrocephalus

Cranial Ultrasound Scanning (see Chapter 2)

In the neonate, the supratentorial ventricular system can be reliably evaluated using ultrasound. This is the imaging modality of choice in the investigation and monitoring of the infant with an open fontanelle. Hematomas or other ventricular masses responsible for hydrocephalus can also be identified. Ultrasound provides a non-invasive and readily available tool for both diagnostic purposes and, by means of sequential studies, a way of charting changes in ventricular size.

CT and MRI

In order to more fully evaluate the entire ventricular system and investigate the underlying etiology of hydrocephalus, CT or MRI scanning is required. Clearly, there is a range of normal ventricular size and, indeed, ventricular size changes with age, rendering absolute measurements of ventricular dimensions of little use. No single radiological parameter can be relied upon to distinguish hydrocephalus from the other causes of ventricular enlargement mentioned above. Some features, however, are strongly suggestive, particularly when occurring in combination. Enlargement of the temporal horns of the lateral ventricles and enlargement of the third ventricle, commensurate with the enlargement of the rest of the ventricular system, are findings in favor of hydrocephalus. Obliteration of the basal cisterns and effacement of the cortical sulci further support a diagnosis of hydrocephalus. When the ventricles are under pressure, there may be transependymal flux of CSF into the periventricular parenchyma, particularly at the tips of the frontal occipital and temporal horns. This appears as low density on CT scan or a rim of high signal intensity on the T2-weighted MRI scan (Fig. 24.2).

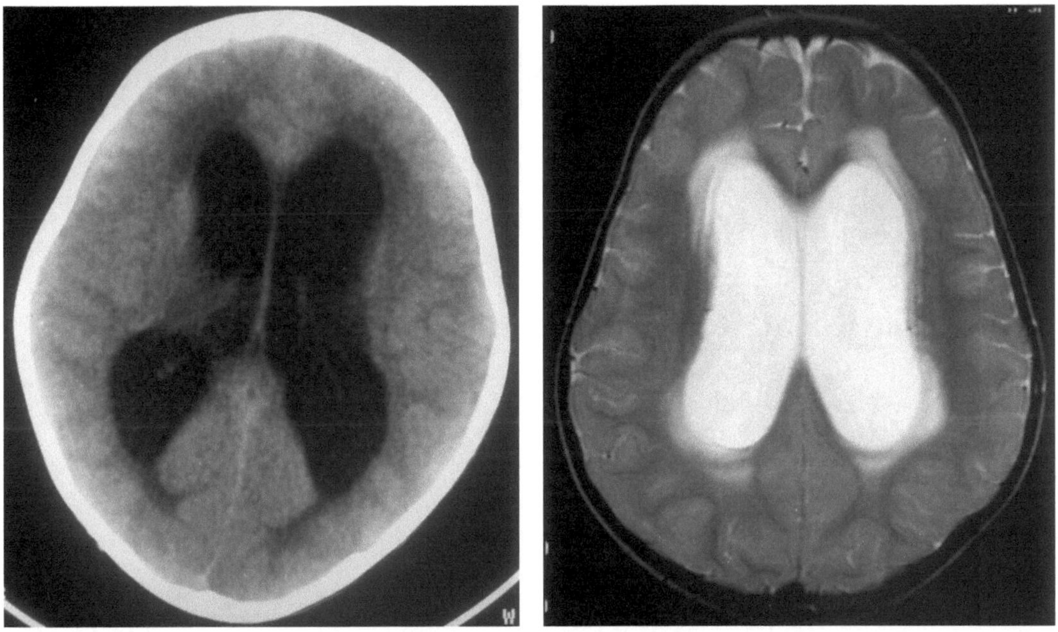

a b

Fig. 24.2. The imaging characteristics of trans-ependymal seepage of CSF in hydrocephalus. On CT, a rim of low density and on MRI, a rim of high-signal intensity on the T2-weighted image.

Treatment of Hydrocephalus

Shunts

Bypassing the site of obstruction to CSF flow or diverting the CSF from the ventricular cavity to a site where it can be more readily absorbed are the basic principles underlying the treatment of hydrocephalus. The ventricular shunt is the mainstay of hydrocephalus treatment and, even in severe hydrocephalus, shunt insertion can have a dramatic effect on the re-expansion of the cortical mantle, particularly in the infant (Fig. 24.3). Neuroendoscopic techniques, in particular third ventriculostomy, also play an important role in the treatment of hydrocephalus and this subject is dealt with in detail elsewhere.

Numerous shunt systems have been devised and marketed, though all have their shortcomings and are prone to similar complications (see below).

The shunt assemblage comprises a proximal catheter, located in the cerebral ventricle, and a distal catheter draining to some alternative site of CSF absorption, most commonly the peritoneal cavity, but drainage to the pleural cavity or right atrium is occasionally employed. Usually, a valve and reservoir are incorporated into the shunt, although the precise configuration is variable.

Proximal Catheter

The most commonly used ventricular catheter comprises a blind-ended silastic tube with a number of side holes adjacent to the catheter tip. Modifications of this basic design will occasionally be encountered, for example flanged catheters. These were designed to protect the side holes from occlusion by tissue at the time of introduction; however, no such advantage has been demonstrated.

A number of devices are available to permit placement of the catheter within the ventricle. A stylet passed down the lumen of the catheter or clipped to its outside is the most simple and widely used. Endoscopes are now available which fit inside specially designed open-ended catheters; these have the advantage of permitting visualization of the ventricular cavity and so aiding optimal placement. Whilst

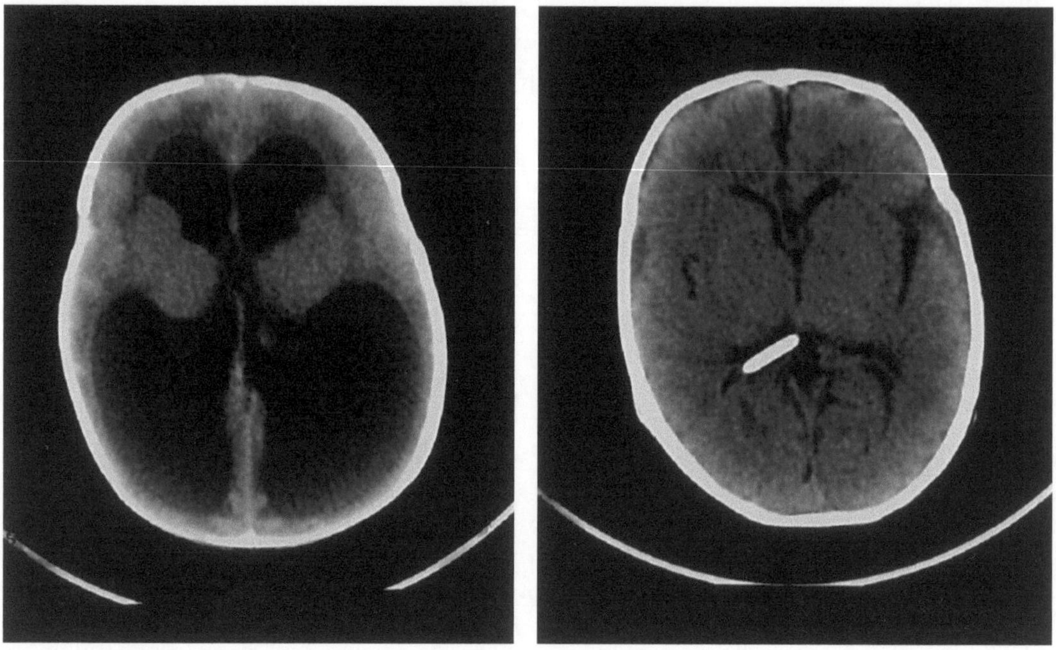

Fig. 24.3. CT scan appearances before (left) and 6 weeks after (right) the insertion of a VP shunt.

this technique may be useful in certain circumstances, it is probably not necessary for routine use.

Valves

A variety of valve designs are currently available (Table 24.2). An array of eponymous names, valve types and manufacturers can lead to great confusion. The table attempts to provide a simple classification of some of the valve designs in common usage but it is by no means exhaustive.

Differential pressure valves are pressure-regulating devices. Pressure regulators maintain a fixed-pressure differential, regardless of flow; this is in contrast to flow regulators that maintain constant flow regardless of pressure. Four types of differential pressure valve are commonly encountered: slit valves, mitre valves, ball and spring and diaphragm valves [11].

For most fixed valves, a low, medium or high-pressure alternative is available. The pressure setting defines the opening or, more commonly, the closing pressure of the valve (the physical characteristics of the valve are the reason for the differences in these two values).

In order to overcome the limitations imposed by fixed-resistance valves, some manufacturers have developed valves whose operating pressure can be varied once the shunt has been implanted. Such devices include the Medos programmable valve (Codman Medos, Le Cocle, Switzerland) and the Sophysa adjustable valve (Sophysa, Orsay, France). An externally applied magnetic field is used to alter the position of an internal rotor and thus vary the pressure setting. The setting is then verified on plain radiograph (Medos) or a compass held over the device (Sophysa).

The pressure gradient across the valve is the difference between the intraventricular pressure and the intra-abdominal pressure in the supine position. In the upright position, the added hydrostatic pressure will increase the differential pressure and so increase the CSF flow through the valve. One of the criticisms of differential pressure valves is that they are subject to this siphoning phenomenon in the upright position.

A number of modifications of shunt design have been devised in order to overcome the problem of siphoning. Anti-siphon or siphon

Table 24.2. Types of CSF shunt valves.

Valve principle	Valve type	Examples
Differential pressure (fixed)	Slit	Codman Holter Codman Denver
	Mitre	Mueller Heyer Schulte in line valve
	Ball and spring	Cordis Hakim valve Codman Medos Hakim valve
	Diaphragm	Mueller Heyer Schulte Pudenz flushing valve PS Medical flow-control valve Codman Accu-flo
	Diaphragm + siphon control device	PS Medical Delta valve
Differential pressure (externally programmable)	Ball and spring mechanism, opening pressure adjusted by externally applied magnetic field.	Codman Medos Programmable Sophysa Adjustable
Flow-control valve	Variable-resistance valve	Cordis Orbis Sigma

control devices (ASDs) can be incorporated in series with the valve. The device, which is placed subcutaneously in series with the valve, houses a mobile membrane that moves in response to a pressure change across it. The outer surface is theoretically at atmospheric pressure. When the pressure within the shunt falls, the membrane moves to occlude the shunt lumen. ASDs are available as separate components to insert below the valve in existing shunts; alternatively they may be incorporated into a valve as in the Delta valve (P.S. Medical Corporation, California, USA) which combines a diaphragm valve and a siphon control device in one.

A different approach to the siphon problem is seen in the Orbis-Sigma valve (Cordis Corporation). By contrast to differential pressure valves, which are pressure regulating, this valve is designed to be a flow-regulating device, permitting a relatively constant flow rate over a wide range of differential pressures.

Unfortunately, at present, there are insufficient data to support many manufacturers' claims of superior function of particular shunt valves. Choice of valve design continues to be, for the most part, a matter of surgical preference, no clear advantages have been consistently demonstrated for any individual model [12].

Distal Catheter

The currently preferred site of drainage is to the peritoneal cavity. Insertion into the peritoneal cavity is either by mini-laparotomy or the use of an abdominal trocar. In childhood, a suitable length of tubing is inserted into the peritoneal cavity in order to compensate for the effects of growth.

Alternative sites include the right atrium, the pleural cavity and the gall bladder. The ventriculoatrial (VA) shunt was the preferred technique prior to the introduction of silastic catheters (previous catheter materials tended to incite a tissue reaction and become occluded); however, the consequences of VA shunt infection, including septicaemia and renal failure, were responsible for significant morbidity and mortality. Furthermore, the positioning of the catheter tip is critical in the atrial shunt (in order to maintain patency) and thus frequent revisions were necessary as the child grew. On occasion, the use of the peritoneal cavity will be precluded, for example following abdominal sepsis or in the presence of extensive post-surgical adhesions, and, in such situations, the atrial site is still used.

Medical Treatment

Medical measures to treat hydrocephalus may be appropriate under certain circumstances. The use of osmotic diuretics such as mannitol is restricted to situations where prompt reduction of intracranial pressure is necessary pending definitive treatment, as in the acute shunt block with neurological deterioration whilst arranging for shunt revision.

Acetazolamide is an inhibitor of the enzyme carbonic anhydrase. The enzyme is present in the choroid plexus epithelium and is necessary for the production of CSF. Acetazolamide is frequently used to reduce CSF production in cases of benign intracranial hypertension (pseudotumor cerebri). It is occasionally used in the management of neonatal post-hemorrhagic hydrocephalus as a temporising measure whilst the child gains weight and the CSF clears of blood products.

Complications of Shunts

The extensive range of shunt models available and the constant search for new alternatives is unfortunately a reflection of the shortfalls of all shunt systems to date. A complex combination of factors relating to the patient, the surgeon and the shunt device itself are likely to be responsible for the complications that are well known to all who treat hydrocephalus.

Mechanical failure and infection together account for the vast majority of shunt complications. A list of some of the more commonly recognized shunt complications is shown in Table 24.3, some of which are discussed below.

Shunt Blockage

Shunt obstruction is the commonest indication for shunt revision and, in the majority of cases, the cause is blockage of the ventricular catheter. Choroid plexus, brain tissue and cellular debris are frequently responsible for the occlusion. Obstruction of the shunt may, however, occur at any level in the shunt assembly. The risk of mechanical failure is related to the time from shunt surgery, with most of these complications occurring in the first post-operative year [13].

The clinical presentation is usually dominated by signs of raised ICP – headache, vomiting and drowsiness are most common. In the infant population group, enlarging head circumference, tense fontanelle, CSF tracking along the course of the shunt and, rarely, seizures are additional indicators of underlying shunt malfunction. The time course of symptom onset is, however, extremely variable; in some, the onset may be insidious over days or weeks whilst in the more shunt-dependent individuals, rapidly progressive symptoms may develop in the space of a few hours.

It has been postulated that the site of insertion of the ventricular catheter has some bearing on the propensity for obstructive complications. The frontal site is preferred by some surgeons, who argue that placement in the frontal horn beyond the foramen of Monro reduces the likelihood of blockage by choroid plexus. This practice does suppose that accurate placement can be attained during blind shunt insertion and that choroid plexus is a major etiological factor in shunt obstructions. Malposition of the ventricular catheter is, however, well recognized and, furthermore, Sekhar has demonstrated that tissues other than choroid plexus, including glial tissue, leptomeninges, chronic inflammatory debris fibrin and thrombus may be responsible for catheter obstruction. In a prospective randomized trial, Bierbrauer et al. [14] failed to show any advantage of frontal placement over the occipital route.

Table 24.3. Commonly encountered complications of shunts.

Complication
Infection
Shunt blockage (proximal, valve, distal)
Fracture or disconnection
Migration
Overdrainage
Isolation (trapping) of ventricles
Malposition
Intracranial haemorrhage
Viscus perforation

CSF Overdrainage

Despite modifications of valve design including on/off control, anti-siphon devices and, more recently, externally programmable valves, shunts cannot reproduce the balance between CSF production and absorption characteristic of normal physiology. Excessive CSF drainage may result in symptoms of headache, nausea and vomiting, diplopia and a generalized lethargy, sometimes with impairment of school performance. These symptoms can be difficult to distinguish from raised ICP. Resolution of symptoms on lying down is an occasional indicator favoring intracranial hypotension.

The consequences of overdrainage include subdural hematoma formation. This may vary from mild extra-axial collections that are often managed conservatively, to larger symptomatic subdural hematomas that may necessitate intervention. Treatment strategies may include burr hole drainage with or without shunt removal, upgrading the valve to a higher pressure or, on occasion, it is necessary to insert an additional (unvalved) sub-dural shunt; this is sometimes plumbed into the existing shunt below the valve.

In the infant, the lowered intracranial tension following shunt insertion may lead to premature closure of the cranial sutures, producing a secondary craniosynostosis with cranial deformity.

Asymmetrical drainage of the ventricles may also be seen to cause trapping or isolation of part of the ventricular system. It may be difficult to distinguish whether this is a true consequence of the shunt or related to compartmentalization of the ventricles as a result of the original pathology, for example post-meningitic hydrocephalus. Trapping of the fourth ventricle is an example of this process and can be seen after apparently successful treatment of hydrocephalus with a shunt. Isolation of the fourth ventricle may be discovered incidentally or may result in symptoms of raised intracranial pressure or cerebellar disturbance. In symptomatic cases, the fourth ventricle can be drained either by inserting an additional shunt system or by placing a catheter into the fourth ventricle and plumbing this into the existing supratentorial shunt via a T or Y connector. It is important that the connection is made above the valve to ensure that the ventricles are drained at the same pressure.

The Slit Ventricle Syndrome

It is important to distinguish between the radiological "label" of slit ventricles, a not uncommonly seen appearance on post-shunt CT scans where the ventricles are barely recognisable but the patient is free of symptoms, and the less frequently encountered clinical symptom complex that may accompany slit-like ventricles. It has been estimated that only 11% of patients with radiologically confirmed slit ventricles demonstrated the clinical syndrome. The clinical syndrome is usually one of episodic headache, which may be positional, vomiting, occasionally with vague gastrointestinal symptoms and the reservoir, if present, may be slow to refill. The symptoms will frequently have a cyclical pattern, episodes lasting from between a few hours to 2 or 3 days, the individual being quite well in between "attacks".

It is postulated that the condition results from a loss of ventricular wall compliance. The small-volume ventricles intermittently collapse around the catheter, temporarily blocking it. Intracranial pressure has to build up in order to distend the non-compliant ventricles; during this period symptoms will be present. Once the ventricle begins to expand, the catheter can again begin to function and symptoms subside.

The syndrome may be accompanied by either low or high intracranial pressure and differentiating these is frequently difficult on clinical grounds alone. A period of ICP monitoring may be a useful aid in the diagnosis and may guide subsequent treatment [10].

If ICP is low then the therapeutic options include upgrading the valve or insertion of an anti-siphon device. Such maneuvres may be associated with re-expansion of the previously collapsed ventricle.

In the presence of raised ICP, clearly it is essential to establish that the shunt is patent. If this is so and symptoms persist, then subtemporal decompression may afford relief. The removal of bone, usually ipsilateral, to the shunt removes some of the constraint upon ventricular dilation, improving compliance and permitting focal expansion of the ventricular cavity. This has been reported to improve symptoms and reduce the number of subsequent shunt-related problems [15].

Abdominal Complications

Numerous complications have been described in relation to the distal shunt catheter. Viscus perforation can occur either as a complication of the initial insertion or may develop as a result of chronic erosion of the catheter tip through the viscus wall. Perforation of the stomach, the large and small bowel, gall bladder and vagina are all described. The presentation may be obvious, with signs of peritoneal sepsis or occasionally with extrusion of the catheter tip at the anus, umbilicus or vagina. Catheters that have become disconnected and lost in the peritoneal cavity can lead to symptoms and will make it difficult to eradicate infection. Retained catheters should be avoided wherever possible.

Intra-abdominal Fluid Collections

It is rare for ascites to develop as a result of the peritoneal cavity failing to cope with the CSF load, except where there is additional abdominal pathology such as adhesions from previous sepsis, surgery or ongoing infection. Hydroceles and an increased incidence of inguinal hernia are recognized complications of ventriculoperitoneal shunts in infants.

More common is the formation of localized CSF collections within the peritoneal cavity. Abdominal pain and distension are common symptoms in the presence of such CSF pseudocysts; these can be readily diagnosed on ultrasound examination. The presence of a CSF pseudocyst should always raise the possibility of underlying infection, which has been reported to occur in two-thirds or more of cases [16].

In such cases, management should be aimed at eradication of the infection, with either removal or externalization of the infected shunt. Although some neurosurgeons have recommended conversion to a VA shunt, a history of pseudocyst formation does not necessarily preclude the continued use of the peritoneal cavity as the distal site.

Shunt Infection

Shunt infection is one of the most common complications encountered and one that carries significant morbidity and even mortality. Shunt infections result in prolonged hospitalization, they increase the risk of subsequent shunt malfunction and can lead to physical disability and impaired intellectual development. Reported shunt infection rates in some instances exceed 20%, although a range of 5–15% would be a more realistic figure, examining larger series of pediatric patients. Rates as low as 1% have been achieved in some centers [17].

The subject of shunt infection is a complex one, and beyond the differences between individual neurosurgical units, there are important variations relating to the heterogeneity of the hydrocephalic population. Whilst shunt infection may afflict adults as well as children, it is in the pediatric population that shunt infection rates tend to be greater and the majority of studies have been performed in this group.

Although there are many factors that appear to contribute to shunt infection, it is generally assumed that contamination of the shunt system occurs at or around the time of shunt surgery. Poor surgical technique, excessive handling of the shunt hardware and inadequate operative environment are among some of the general risk factors frequently cited. Specific factors that appear to have particularly strong correlations with shunt infection are postoperative wound infection and CSF leakage; strenuous measures should be taken to avoid these complications.

Within the pediatric age group, patient age also appears to play a significant role. Pople et al. [18] report an incidence of infection of 15.7% in children less than 6 months of age in contrast to a rate of 5.6% in those older than 6 months. Immunological immaturity, different microbiological flora and physical properties of the skin are among the possible factors increasing the risk of shunt infection in the neonate.

The Presentation of Shunt Infection

Ventriculoperitoneal shunt infection most commonly manifests itself soon after an operative procedure – either shunt insertion or revision. Approximately 70% of shunt infections will have presented within 2 months and 80% by 6 months of the surgical procedure [19]. Rarely, shunt infections present later than this, for example following late perforation of a viscus by the distal shunt, incidental abdominal sepsis (e.g. appendicitis) or in association with wound breakdown or erosion of the shunt through the skin.

A high index of suspicion should be maintained in the weeks following surgery. The mode of presentation is a variable constellation of pyrexia and meningism and general irritability in children.

In the case of ventriculoatrial shunts, infection may manifest early on with an acute, overtly septic illness. A more chronic presentation is also well recognized, characterized by prolonged periods of generalized lassitude, sometimes with a low-grade pyrexia or mild anemia. Vague low-back pain, hematuria and hypertension may herald the onset of "shunt nephritis" – an immune complex-mediated nephritis that can result in renal failure.

In suspected shunt infections, CSF examination is needed to confirm the diagnosis and may be obtained by aspiration from the shunt reservoir – a shunt tap. CSF Gram stain and culture are often diagnostic and will aid in selection of appropriate anti-microbial therapy. It is important to appreciate that if the peritoneal end of the shunt is the source of the infection, a negative CSF result may be obtained in the early stages. Abdominal ultrasound examination, looking for encysted collections of CSF, may be useful in such cases (see above).

Blood cultures are frequently unhelpful in diagnosing VP shunt infection; however, measurement of C-reactive protein (CRP) can be a useful guide, both as part of the initial investigation and as a means of monitoring the effectiveness of treatment.

Organisms Responsible for Shunt Infection

The commensal skin flora is the usual source of pathogens that give rise to shunt infections with the coagulase-negative staphylococci, particularly *S. epidermidis*, the most commonly isolated. *S. aureus* is also well recognized, especially in the context of wound infection or skin breakdown. Enterococci, micrococci and coryneforms account for a significant proportion of the remainder of infecting organisms (Table 24.4).

One of the principal factors which enables coagulase-negative staphylocci to colonize shunt systems is their ability to produce an extracellular slime, which aids adherence of the organisms to the surface of the silicone catheter [20]. This is also one of the main factors responsible for the resilience of these infections to treatment with the shunt in situ.

Treatment of Shunt Infection

Once diagnosed, shunt infection requires prompt and comprehensive treatment with appropriate anti-microbial therapy. Controversy exists, however, as to whether treatment necessitates complete removal of the shunt system or whether the infection can be managed with the shunt in situ. Those who favor treating the infection with the shunt in situ cite the risks of shunt removal, including hemorrhage, from adherent ventricular catheters and the risk of super-added infection associated with temporary external ventricular drainage in support of their policy. The success rates associated with this line of management, however, are poor [21] and the overall morbidity associated with surgical treatment (shunt removal and antibiotic therapy) is lower than with medical therapy alone.

The most common strategy is removal of the shunt and replacement with an external drain for the duration of antibiotic treatment. This permits intrathecal administration of antibiotics if required and serial sampling of the CSF for Gram stain, culture and monitoring of the white cell response. A new shunt is inserted once the CSF is sterilized.

Table 24.4. Organisms responsible for shunt infection.

Organism	Number of cases
Staphylococcus epidermidis	24
Staphylococcus aureus	12
Methicillin-resistant *Staphylococcus aureus*	3
Enterococcus faecalis	2
Escherichia coli	1
Aerococcus viridans	1
Beta-haemolytic Streptococcus group A	1
Pseudomonas putida	1

Data from Great Ormond Street Hospital 1994–97. Courtesy of Dr H. Holzel, Dept of Microbiology (unpublished).

The Role of Antibiotic Prophylaxis in Shunt Surgery

The temporal relationship between time of operation and the occurrence of shunt infection, together with the observation that the commensal skin flora is the commonest source of pathogens, might suggest that antibiotics given at the time of surgery would reduce the incidence of infectious complications. Although there have been numerous studies attempting to demonstrate this, most have failed to reach statistically significant conclusions. One of the principal problems has been enrolling sufficient patients into randomized trials to demonstrate an effect. Two reports have sought to circumvent this problem of type II error using the techniques of metanalysis [22,23]. Both of these reports came out in favor of prophylaxis. Haines and Walters, however, caution that any demonstrable benefit is related to the baseline infection rate; no beneficial effect could be demonstrated when this was less than 5%.

Additional controversy then surrounds the issue of the choice of antibiotic, its route of administration and the duration of prophylaxis. Many antibiotics, including vancomycin, cephalosporins and aminoglycosides, when administered via the intravenous route, fail to achieve significant levels in the CSF, particularly in the absence of inflammation and are thus inappropriate in this respect. Some workers have suggested intraventricular administration or soaking the shunt components in antibiotic solution prior to insertion.

A more recent technique of antibiotic delivery has been to incorporate antibiotics into the silicone tubing. The antibiotic gradually leaches out from the tubing, providing protection in the early post-operative period. In-vitro studies have demonstrated that shunt colonization was delayed for up to 56 days [24]. Shunts containing antibiotic-impregnated silicone tubing using rifampicin and clindamycin are now available for use; however, the results of clinical trials of such devices are awaited.

Miscellaneous Shunt Complications

Seizures

Since the ventricular catheter must, of necessity, traverse the cerebral cortex, there has been concern as to whether this increases the risk of epilepsy for hydrocephalic patients. Whilst a number of studies have attempted to address this question, drawing meaningful conclusions is compromised by the heterogeneity of cases included and variable definitions of epilepsy. Dan and Wade [25] reported that 9.4% of 180 cases of hydrocephalus of variable etiology developed epilepsy after shunting. These authors cite multiple revisions and use of the frontal route of insertion as particular risk factors. Their methodology and conclusions have, however, attracted criticism. Many authors report the incidence of epilepsy in shunted patients to be much greater than this. In an actuarial analysis of 464 patients, Piatt and Carlson [26] found an incidence of epilepsy (defined by the use of anticonvulsant medication) of 12% at the time of diagnosis rising to 33% at 10 years post-shunting. They emphasize that the underlying cause of the hydrocephalus, in particular post-hemorrhage and post-infection, was a far more important predictor of the risk of epilepsy than any surgical factors, including shunt position, number of revisions or history of shunt infection, none of which reached statistical significance. Reporting cases of congenital hydrocephalus only, Noetzel and Blake also favor patient factors, specifically mental retardation and cerebral malformations, as best indicators of long-term epilepsy in shunted patients [27].

Metastases

Extraneural metastasis of primary CNS tumors is an unusual but well recognized phenomenon. Medulloblastoma is the most common of the neural malignancies reported to spread in this way, although germinoma and astrocytoma are also well described. Lymphatic and hematogenous pathways are the most likely routes of spread; however, whether or not shunt systems provide a potential conduit for tumor spread has given cause for concern. Indeed, the incorporation of filters into shunt systems has been advocated to diminish the risk of this. In an analysis of 160 published cases of extraneural spread of medulloblastoma, Jamjoom et al. [28] suggested that the shunt could be implicated in no more than 11 patients. In a further eight cases of extraneural spread in a series of 415 intracranial tumors, Berger et al. [29] failed to identify any increased risk attributable to the presence of a shunt device.

Hemorrhage Related to Ventricular Catheters

Both at the time of initial insertion and particularly during ventricular catheter removal, hemorrhage may occur. Choroid plexus frequently becomes entwined in the catheter and is easily avulsed, leading to intraventricular hemorrhage. It has been suggested that some degree of intraventricular hemorrhage occurs in almost one-third of ventricular catheter revisions. This complication should always be considered when removing catheters, particularly if they have been in situ for a prolonged period of time. Careful evaluation of the pre-operative CT scan may in fact reveal choroid plexus adjacent to the ventricular catheter, highlighting the possible risk of this complication. When an adherent catheter is encountered, it may be necessary to leave it in situ and pass a new one rather than risk choroid plexus avulsion. Passing a stylet along the lumen of the catheter and cauterizing with diathermy prior to withdrawal may help prevent this complication and aid removal of the catheter. Where bleeding does occur, the catheter should be left to drain until the CSF clears; gentle irrigation to prevent occlusion of the catheter with blood clot can be performed. If the blood fails to clear, an external ventricular drain should be left; the patient needs to be closely monitored and scanned post-operatively to assess the extent of the hemorrhage.

Silicone Allergy

Allergic reactions to silicone in ventriculoperitoneal shunts have been reported [30], although is it a rare phenomenon. The presentation may comprise fever and malaise, sometimes mimicking shunt infection. Erythema along the path of the shunt or wound breakdown sometimes occurs. The pathological basis of this condition is a foreign-body giant cell reaction with granuloma formation. Treatment necessitates removal of the shunt and replacement with a silicone-free alternative.

The Prognosis of Shunted Hydrocephalus

Numerous variables influence the long-term neurological and cognitive outcome of shunted hydrocephalus. Whilst a number of studies have attempted to elucidate the relative importance of some of these factors, they need to be interpreted with caution. Donders et al. [31] cite sample bias, variable means of assessment of intellectual outcome, inadequate statistical analysis and the failure to account for coexistent medical problems as the main methodological inadequacies of many of these previous studies. Regression analysis of their own series of patients (in whom they attempted to overcome these design shortcomings) highlighted neonatal problems, including anoxia, respiratory distress, CNS infection and early seizures, and also ocular defects (gaze, movement and refraction) as particularly poor prognostic factors for long-term intellectual outcome.

The timing as well as the nature of the cerebral insult also appear to be important determinants of long-term outcome. A prenatal or neonatal cause for hydrocephalus has been associated with a worse outcome when compared with cases in which postnatal onset was identified or where the etiology of the hydrocephalus was unknown [32].

Academic placement may serve as more tangible criterion of outcome than IQ. In a cohort of 155 shunted patients after a follow-up of at least 10 years, Casey et al. [33] found that over half of the children were able to attend a normal school. Forty-one percent, however, required special schooling. Children whose hydrocephalus was the consequence of intraventricular hemorrhage or infection were much more likely to require special schooling.

In this study, more than half (55%) required one or more shunt revisions during the 10-year follow-up period. Furthermore, a mortality rate of 11% for non-tumor-related hydrocephalus was revealed in this study. Precipitous deterioration and sudden death following shunt blockage are well recognized. The adage *Once a shunt, always a shunt* should at least be assumed to be true and serves as a reminder that when the shunted patient presents with new or unexplained symptoms, the possibility of shunt malfunction must be borne in mind and investigated promptly.

Key Points

- *Hydrocephalus is not a single disease entity. Treatment should be formulated based on an understanding of the underlying condition.*
- *Ventricular size is not the sole index by which hydrocephalus and the need for treatment should be evaluated; always correlate with the clinical picture before embarking on surgery.*
- *A wide range of shunt products are available for the treatment of hydrocephalus; it is recommended that the clinician becomes familiar with the use of a particular shunt system and reserves the more novel shunt valves for specific problem cases.*
- *The clinical presentation of shunt malfunction is extremely variable; shunt malfunction should always be considered in the presence of new or unexplained symptoms.*
- *When presented with cases of shunt malfunction, consider whether there is an opportunity to simplify complex shunt systems or perform endoscopic third ventriculostomy.*

References

1. Davson H, Welch K, Segal MB. The physiology and pathophysiology of the cerebrospinal fluid. Edinburgh: Churchill Livingstone, 1987.
2. Tripathi BJ, Tripathi RC. Vacuolar transcellular channels as a drainage pathway for cerebrospinal fluid. J Physiol 1974;239:195–206.
3. Greitz D, Greitz T, Hindmarsh T. A new view on the CSF-circulation with the potential for pharmacological

treatment of childhood hydrocephalus. Acta Paediatr 1997;86:125–32.
4. Papile LA, Burstein J, Burstein R, Koffler H. Incidence and evolution of subependymal and intraventricular hemorrhage: a study of infants with birth weights less than 1,500 gm. J Pediatr 1978;92(4):529–34.
4a. Whitelaw A. Repeated lumbar or ventricular punctures in newborns with intraventricular hemorrhage. Cochrane Database Syst Rev. 2001;(1):CD000216.
5. Kennedy CR, Campbell M, Elbourne D, Hope P, Johnson A. International randomised controlled trial of acetazolamide and furosemide in posthaemorrhagic ventricular dilatation in infancy. Lancet 1998;352:433–40.
6. McLone DG, Knepper PA. The cause of Chiari II malformation: a unified theory. Pediatr Neurosurg 1989; 15:1–12.
7. Kumar V, Phipps K, Harkness W, Hayward RD. Ventriculo-peritoneal shunt requirement in children with posterior fossa tumours: an 11-year audit. Br J Neurosurg 1996;10(5):467–70.
8. Portnoy HD, Branch C, Castro ME. The relationship of intracranial venous pressure to hydrocephalus. Child's Nerv Syst 1994;10:29–35.
9. Thompson DNP, Hayward RD, Harkness WJ, Bingham RM, Jones BM. Lessons from a case of Kleeblattschadel: case report. J Neurosurg 1995;82:1071–4.
10. Fouyas IP, Casey AH, Thompson D, Harkness WF, Hayward RD, Rutka JT et al. Use of intracranial pressure monitoring in the management of childhood hydrocephalus and shunt-related problems. Neurosurgery 1996;38(4):726–32.
11. Drake JM, Sainte-Rose C. The shunt book. Cambridge: Blackwell Science, 1995.
12. Drake JM, Kestle JRW, Milner R, Cinalli G, Boop FA, Piatt JJ et al. Randomized trial of cerebrospinal fluid valve design in pediatric hydrocephalus. Neurosurgery 1998;43(2):294–305.
13. Sainte-Rose C, Hoffman HJ, Hirsch JF. Shunt failure. Concepts in Pediatric Neurosurgery 1989;9:7–20.
14. Bierbrauer KS, Storrs BB, McLone DG, Tomita T, Dauser R. A prospective, randomized study of shunt function and infections as a function of shunt placement. Pediatr Neurosurg 1990;16(6):287–91.
15. Holness RO, Hoffman HJ, Hendrick EB. Subtemporal decompression for the slit-ventricle syndrome after shunting in hydrocephalic children. Childs Brain 1979;5:137–44.
16. Ersahin Y, Mutluer S, Tekeli G. Abdominal cerebrospinal fluid pseudocysts. Child's Nerv Syst 1996; 12(12):755–8.
17. Choux M, Genitori L, Lang D, Lena G. Shunt implantation: reducing the incidence of shunt infection. J Neurosurg 1992;77(6):875–80.
18. Pople IK, Bayston R, Hayward RD. Infection of cerebrospinal fluid shunts in infants: a study of etiological factors. J Neurosurg 1992;77(1):29–36.
19. George R, Leibrock L, Epstein M. Long term analysis of cerebrospinal fluid shunt infections. J Neurosurg 1979;51:804–11.
20. Bayston R, Rogers J. Production of extracellular slime by *Staphylococcus epidermidis* in the stationary phase of growth and its association with adherence to implantable devices. J Clin Pathol 1990;43:866–70.
21. James HE, Walsh JW, Wilson HD, Connor JD. The management of cerebrospinal fluid shunt infections: a clinical experience. Acta Neurochir 1981;59(3-4):157–66.
22. Langley JM, LeBlanc JC, Drake J, Milner R. Efficacy of antimicrobial prophylaxis in placement of cerebrospinal fluid shunts: meta-analysis. Clin Infect Dis 1993;17(1):98–103.
23. Haines SJ, Walters BC, McComb JG. Antibiotic prophylaxis for cerebrospinal fluid shunts: a metanalysis. Neurosurgery 1994;34(1):87–93.
24. Bayston R, Lambert E. Duration of protective activity of cerebrospinal fluid shunt catheters impregnated with antimicrobial agents to prevent bacterial catheter-related infection. J Neurosurgery 1997;87(2):247–51.
25. Dan NG, Wade MJ. The incidence of epilepsy after ventricular shunting procedures. J Neurosurgery 1986; 65(1):19–21.
26. Piatt-JH J, Carlson CV, Wyler AB, Engel J, DeGiorgio CM. Hydrocephalus and epilepsy: an actuarial analysis. Neurosurgery 1996;39(4):722–8.
27. Noetzel MJ, Blake JN. Seizures in children with congenital hydrocephalus: long-term outcome. Neurology 1992;42(7):1277–81.
28. Jamjoom ZA, Jamjoom AB, Sulaiman AH, Naim UR, al Rabiaa A. Systemic metastasis of medulloblastoma through ventriculoperitoneal shunt: report of a case and critical analysis of the literature. Surgical Neurology 1993;40(5):403–10.
29. Berger MS, Baumeister B, Geyer JR, Milstein J, Kanev PM, LeRoux PD. The risks of metastases from shunting in children with primary central nervous system tumors. J Neurosurg 1991;74(6):872–7.
30. Jimenez DF, Keating R, Goodrich JT. Silicone allergy in ventriculoperitoneal shunts. Child's Nerv Syst 1994; 10(1):59–63.
31. Donders J, Canady AI, Rourke BP. Psychometric intelligence after infantile hydrocephalus. Child's Nerv Syst 1990;6:148–54.
32. Fernell E, Hagberg G, Hagberg B. Infantile hydrocephalus epidemiology: an indicator of enhanced survival. Arch Dis Child 1994;70(2 Suppl.):F123–8.
33. Casey A, Kimmings EJ, Kleinlugtebeld AD, Taylor WAS, Harkness W, Hayward R. The longterm outlook for hydrocephalus in childhood: a ten year cohort study of 155 patients. Pediatr Neurosurg 1998;27:63–70.

VIII
Pediatrics

25

Craniosynostosis

John A. Jane, Jr, Aaron S. Dumont,
Kant Y.K. Lin and John A. Jane, Sr

Summary

Craniosynostosis results from the premature fusion of one or more cranial sutures. The authors discuss historical aspects and treatment of craniosynostosis. Classic syndromes have been described based on the sutures involved and the resultant deformities. Treatments have evolved over the years and are tailored to the individual patient, with the goal of surgery being to restore a normal skull contour and allow continued growth of the brain to reshape the skull. All of this requires a multidisciplinary effort to achieve the desired results.

Introduction

Craniosynostosis results from the premature fusion of one or more cranial sutures. This untimely fusion produces progressive and characteristic craniofacial abnormalities. The etiology may be either sporadic (of non-syndromic nature) or secondary to a distinct syndrome. Recent advances in molecular biology and genetics provide clues as to the possible causes of this disorder. Craniosynostosis is diagnosed clinically and confirmed with radiographic and other studies. Although predominantly a problem of cosmesis, craniosynostosis may also be complicated by neurological dysfunction. Procedures used to correct it may properly be termed "reconstructive".

The treatment of this disorder is undertaken as a multidisciplinary effort, increasingly in specialized craniofacial centers. Treatment paradigms have evolved over time and are tailored to the individual patient. In general, simple strip craniectomies have been superseded by complex calvarial reconstructions. These are necessary because single-suture closure causes not only the primary impaired growth at the fused suture, but also secondary compensations that affect the entire skull. The goal of surgery is to restore a normal skull contour and allow continued growth of the brain to reshape the skull.

History

Since antiquity, various cultures have focused on individuals with abnormal cranial contour. Allusions to aberrant skull shape have been noted in writings connected with the ancient Chinese gods of good fortune and long life (Fukurokuju and Shou Lao), by Homer in "The Iliad" and by Hippocrates and Galen [1] and others. Nearly 200 years ago, Sommerring reported the first scientific investigation of cranial deformities [2]. He discussed cranial sutures, recognized their primary importance in skull growth and asserted that premature suture fusion produced cranial deformity. In

1830, Otto postulated that premature suture closure gives rise to cranial deformity, with compensatory expansion elsewhere [3]. In an extension of Otto's observations, Virchow published his seminal work on skull deformity that provided the basis for future scientific study of cranial deformity and craniosynostosis [4]. Although not the first to make these observations, Virchow noted that cranial growth occurs along suture lines and premature fusion arrested growth perpendicular to the fusion, producing skull deformity .

Over the next century, understanding of craniosynostosis burgeoned. Reports of craniosynostosis were increasingly disseminated [1] and ophthalmological perspectives were introduced. Authors also described craniosynostosis in association with other anomalies and provided the impetus for future classification of syndromic craniosynostosis. Apert [5] and Crouzon [6], among others, described those syndromes that continue to bear their names. In the late nineteenth century, Lane [7] and Lannelongue [8] reported the first modern surgical corrections of skull deformity resulting from premature suture closure. From these original pioneering experiences, subsequent advances in treatment have continued into contemporary times.

Virchow's hypotheses concerning craniosynostosis remained the standard for nearly a century. However, in the mid-twentieth century, van der Klaauw and Moss questioned the primacy of the calvarial sutures as the antecedent mediator of skull deformities [9, 10]. Based on his original ideas, subsequent work and the efforts of others, Moss proposed that the primary anomaly in craniosynostosis arose in the cranial base. He hypothesized that the *primary* abnormality arose in the cranial base, and this resulted in the *secondary* fusion of the cranial vault suture(s). His arguments were fourfold [10–12]: (1) on occasion, suture patency was found at surgery, despite pre-operative suspicion of premature suture fusion and characteristic skull configuration [13]; (2) characteristic anomalies of the cranial base were associated with specific calvarial suture closures; (3) experimental removal of normal cranial vault sutures resulted in no significant change in overall skull shape; and (4) cranial base development and maturation precede those of the cranial vault. Additionally, Moss believed that the primary force driving the sutures' deposition of bone (with consequent expansion and modeling of the skull) was growth of the underlying brain. This was termed the "functional matrix theory" [12].

Further work by Persson and others endeavored to clarify the primary locus of craniosynostosis. Persson et al. demonstrated that experimental restriction of a suture's growth produced skull deformities that mimicked craniosynostosis in humans [14]. In addition, cranial base and facial abnormalities appeared to occur in response to the cranial suture restriction [15]. This suggested that craniofacial anomalies were primarily the result of suture fusion – not the cranial base, as Moss had proposed. Marsh and Vannier reported that pre-existing cranial base abnormalities resolved after surgery in which only cranial vault alteration was undertaken [16]. Collectively, considerable data have accrued against Moss's stance that suggest, at least in most cases of non-syndromic craniosynostosis, that the cranial vault sutures assume a major inciting role in the pathogenesis of craniosynostosis. In states of syndromic craniosynostosis (e.g. Apert or Crouzon syndromes), however, a more generalized pathologic process involving the cranial vault sutures and cranial base may exist.

Work by Opperman and colleagues emphasized the critical influences of mesenchymal tissues, including the dura mater and periosteum, at the suture site in regulating and maintaining suture patency during development [17–18]. Recognition of this dynamic interaction and the existence of factors, including matrix and cytokine influences (fibroblast growth factors (FGF), fibroblast growth factor receptors (FGFR) and transforming growth factor beta (TGF-β), have been instrumental in the refinement of our contemporary molecular understanding of craniosynostosis [19].

Classification

A multitude of classification schemes for craniosynostosis have been proposed, often reflective of the particular time period and representative specialty of the classifier(s). The reader is referred to an excellent discussion by Cohen [1].

The authors have adopted a practical classification scheme (Table 25.1). Craniosynostosis is first divided into syndromic and non-syndromic types. Over 90 syndromes have been

Table 25.1. Classification of craniosynostosis.

Type	Deformity
Syndromic	
Over 90 identified	Variable
Non-syndromic	
Simple	
Sagittal	Scaphocephaly
Unilateral coronal	Frontal plagiocephaly
Metopic	Trigonocephaly
Unilateral lambdoid	Posterior plagiocephaly
Compound	
Two or more sutures	Variable
Bilateral coronal	Turribrachycephaly
Bilateral lambdoid	Brachycephaly

identified and are beyond the scope of this discussion [20]. Apert and Crouzon syndromes are two more common examples of syndromic craniosynostosis. Non-syndromic craniosynostosis is classified based upon the location and extent of the involved suture(s). Detailed descriptions of the appearances of each category are provided in the ensuing sections.

Epidemiology

The birth prevalence of craniosynostosis is estimated at 343–476 per 1,000,000 live births (i.e. affecting 1 in 2,100 to 1 in 2,900 newborns) [20, 21]. Non-syndromic craniosynostosis represents the most prevalent form. Involvement of the sagittal suture is the most common form and accounts for between 40 and 60% of cases. This is followed by coronal synostosis, which occurs in approximately 20–30% of cases. Unilateral coronal synostosis outnumbers bilateral involvement by a 2:1 margin. Metopic craniosynostosis is estimated to comprise less than 10% of cases and true lambdoid craniosynostosis is much rarer [20]. Two or more sutures may be involved in 4–8% of non-syndromic craniosynostosis.

Syndromic craniosynostosis is much less common, although new syndromes are becoming increasingly recognized. Syndromic craniosynostoses typically involve multiple sutures. There are more than 90 syndromes characterized by craniosynostosis and various associated anomalies [20]. The birth prevalence of the two more common syndromes – Apert and Crouzon – are estimated at 13.7–15.5 per 1,000,000 [22] and 15.5–16.5 per 1,000,000 [22], respectively.

Etiology

Syndromic craniosynostosis arises from a known disorder and is well discussed elsewhere [23]. As is evident in Table 25.2, a myriad of conditions may lead to secondary craniosynostosis. For example, in malformations such as microcephaly, lack of growth stretch is postulated to cause secondary craniosynostosis. In infants with hyperthyroidism, premature osseous fusion is thought to result in premature suture closure.

Study of syndromic craniosynostoses has been invaluable in advancing contemporary insight into the molecular pathophysiology of craniosynostosis. For many of the craniosynostosis syndromes, the underlying genetic defects have already been identified. For example, mutation in a member of the homeobox gene, *MSX2*, has been identified in Boston craniosynostosis and studies in transgenic mice reveal that this mutation also causes craniosynostosis in this model. In addition, mutations in the *TWIST* gene have been discovered in

Table 25.2. Disorders with secondary craniosynostosis.

Hematological disorders
Polycythemia
Sickle cell anemia
Thalassemias
Iatrogenic disorders
Shunted hydrocephalus
Malformations
Encephalocele
Holoprosencephaly
Microcephaly
Metabolic disorders
Hyperthyroidism
Rickets
Mucopolysaccharidoses and related disorders
α-D-mannosidase deficiency
β-glucuronidase deficiency
Hurler syndrome
Morquio syndrome
Mucolipidosis III
Teratogens
Aminopterin
Cyclophosphamide
Diphenylhydantoin
Fluconazole
Retinoids
Valproate

Saethre–Chotzen syndrome. Furthermore, mutations in FGFR 1 and 2 have been demonstrated in Apert, Crouzon, Pfeiffer and Jackson–Weiss syndromes [19].

In turn, an understanding of these mutations has provided impetus for delineating the molecular substrates and basis of suture and cranial development, and has directed our thinking pertaining to the pathogenesis of non-syndromic craniosynostosis. The pathogenesis and etiology are complex and heterogeneous and, in the majority of cases, the cause(s) remain obscure. Although craniosynostosis is mostly sporadic, likely resulting from de-novo autosomal-dominant mutations [20], familial cases are well documented. Continuing studies of molecular genetics may elucidate the genes involved in these non-syndromic cases.

FGFRs are expressed during development in the calvarial sutures and both FGFRs and FGFs are important in osteogenesis and differentiation. FGFs and FGFRs may maintain the integrity of suture formation and patency. The *TWIST* gene probably functions as a transcription factor and is implicated in the embryogenesis and development of the head and limbs [19]. The *MSX2* gene is expressed during embryogenesis and has been specifically localized to the osteogenic front in developing cranial sutures [19]. An increasing body of evidence suggests the existence of a dynamic interaction between *MSX2* and FGRF2 that may regulate suture and cranial development. More recently, *TWIST* has been postulated to interact with FGFR and *MSX2* in a common signaling pathway involved in head mesenchyme formation at distinct steps [19]. Associated mutations in these genes may precede development of craniosynostosis. Other putative molecular mediators of suture morphogenesis, closure and craniosynostosis have been proposed, including TGF-β and bone morphogenetic proteins (BMPs) [19]. Although considerable progress has been made in our understanding of the molecular basis of syndromic and non-syndromic craniosynostosis, further probing into these quintessential mechanisms is warranted.

Much attention has focused on the genetic basis of craniosynostosis. However, this certainly does not preclude the existence of environmental influences on the genesis of this disorder. For example, fetal head restraint has been thought to underlie simple craniosynostosis in some cases, both clinically and experimentally [24].

The pathoetiological basis of craniosynostosis is complex. Although there are many known causes of craniosynostosis, in the majority of cases the underlying factors remain elusive. Advancements in our molecular understanding of syndromic craniosynostosis have facilitated progress in our understanding of basic suture biology and calvarial development and, consequently, in our understanding of primary non-syndromic craniosynostosis.

Diagnosis

The diagnosis of craniosynostosis is made clinically, although adjunctive imaging studies may confirm the diagnosis and aid in the planning of further care. Craniosynostosis must be differentiated from deformational molding, as the latter is much more common than true craniosynostosis and often amenable to conservative management [20, 25, 26]. This is particularly true of lambdoid synostosis. Over the last decade, most cases that were thought to be lambdoid synostosis are now recognized as positional molding. Unless severe, this masquerading plagiocephaly may be treated conservatively.

CT scanning, particularly with three-dimensional reconstruction, readily defines the characteristic head shapes and delineates associated cranial base anatomy effectively. It also permits visualization of changes within and around suture(s). We have also found that CT angiography effectively defines dural sinus anatomy and allows appropriate operative planning and complication avoidance [27]. This is particularly important in the syndromic forms, where jugular foramen atresia and subsequent enlargement of emissary veins may present formidable obstacles. The modified prone position requires significant neck extension, and dynamic cervical spine films are employed to screen for cranio-cervical junction instability. Others have suggested the use of high-resolution tomography, TCD ultrasonography and PET as pre-operative studies. Their clinical utility awaits further confirmation.

Molecular genetic testing is becoming increasingly feasible and some have correlated molecular diagnosis with phenotype, natural history and in their analyses of surgical results. A multidisciplinary team, usually in the context of a craniofacial center, should evaluate patients with craniosynostosis. These teams include specialists from medical photography, medical genetics, neuropsychology, physical therapy, social work, radiology, ophthalmology, otorhinolaryngology, plastic surgery and neurological surgery. Patients are continually followed during their pre- and post-operative periods in this network.

Compensatory Skull Growth

A precise prediction of characteristic craniofacial abnormalities associated with premature closure of a specific suture assists in differentiating true craniosynostoses from deformational molding. The phenotypic appearance of each individual with craniosynostosis is hardly random. Several basic tenets can be used to predict the characteristic craniofacial abnormalities associated with the premature closure of a given suture [28, 29].

Fusion of a single suture does not simply cause arrest of growth perpendicular to the suture. Metopic synostosis does not cause only a narrow forehead, coronal synostosis does not produce just a unilaterally shortened skull and sagittal synostosis does not simply result in a narrow skull. Instead, compensatory growth occurs at neighboring unfused sutures as well [28]. When the adjacent suture is parallel to the fused suture, bone is deposited symmetrically on either side of the suture. If the adjacent suture is more or less perpendicular to the fused suture, most of the growth will occur in the bone that is distal to the fused suture. In the case of anterior fusion of the sagittal suture, the metopic and coronal sutures are the adjacent sutures (Fig. 25.1a). The metopic suture is parallel to the sagittal suture and the compensatory growth tends to symmetrically widen the frontal bone. Because the coronal sutures are perpendicular to the sagittal suture, the majority of the compensatory growth occurs, not in the parietal bone, but distal to the sagittal suture, creating frontal bossing.

Treatment

General Considerations

The primary message emanating from these rules is that single-suture closure affects the entire skull. It follows that surgery cannot then focus only on the fused suture; it must address the compensatory changes primarily. Correction, regardless of the fused suture, should effect a normal contour.

The optimal time for surgical correction is prior to the fusion of the non-pathologic sutures. Early repair benefits from the pliability of infant skull – a quality that diminishes significantly near the end of the first year. The pliable skull may be re-contoured using either radial or barrel-stave osteotomies combined with controlled fractures and the Tessier rib bender. Early correction also takes advantage of the corrective influences of the growing brain. After surgery has restored normal contour, further brain growth tends to re-contour the skull appropriately. During the first 6 months, brain volume doubles, and triples by 2.5 years, at which time the brain has attained approximately 80% of its ultimate size. Early surgery also prevents the compensatory growth from being fully manifested. It is evident from our studies on the natural history of synostoses that, without correction, cranial deformity worsens with time [19]. Our previous recommendations were to perform surgery at 3 months. Currently, primarily to maximize fortitude and to benefit from pliability of the bone, surgery is delayed until 6 months of age.

After normal contour is restored, the expanding brain promotes persistent normal contour. This has been facilitated by the introduction of absorbable plates. These plates maintain the initial correction, but re-sorb prior to restricting the natural correction influenced by the expanding brain. When correction is performed late – after fusion of the sutures and after the majority of brain growth has occurred – the correction is designed to reflect the end result and may be rigidly fixed.

A constant consideration during these procedures is the location and status of the underlying venous sinuses. An unfused, non-pathologic suture remains adherent to the underlying dura. Prior to the craniotomy or bringing the bone

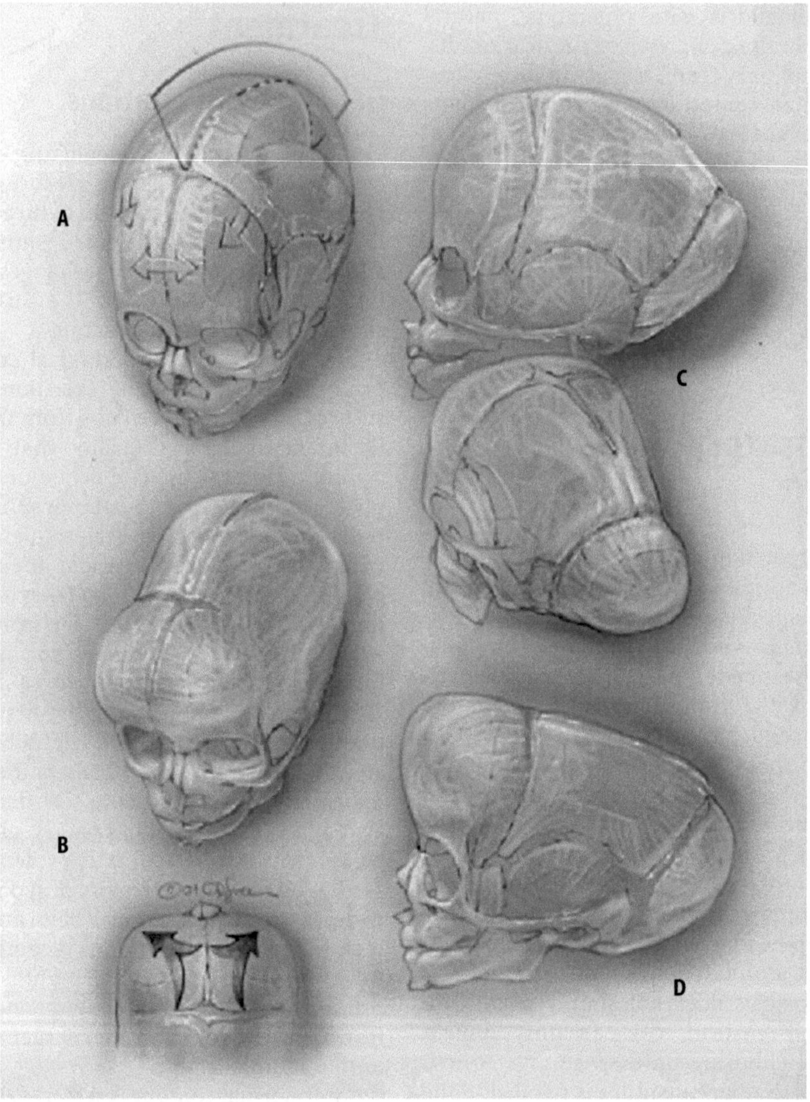

Fig. 25.1. Varieties of sagittal synostosis. **a** Compensatory changes. **b** Anterior sagittal synostosis. **c** Posterior sagittal synostosis. **d** Complete sagittal synostosis.

together, the sagittal, transverse and confluence of sinuses must often be carefully separated from the overlying suture. Otherwise, there is significant risk of entering these sinuses with the craniotome or kinking them when remodeling the skull. CT venography is especially useful in establishing the location of these important venous structures. This technique also changes the relationship between the pathological dura and the overlying skull and may interrupt the signals that would otherwise cause restenosis.

Patients are positioned supine for anterior corrections, prone for posterior corrections and in a modified prone position for simultaneous correction of anterior and posterior abnormalities. In order to shorten operative procedures and the surgical stress upon the patient, there may be a tendency to perform anterior and posterior corrections in stages. This often has sub-optimal results and every effort should be made to effect a normal skull contour with a single operation. The modified prone position is particularly useful for correction of complete sagittal synostosis and bilateral coronal synostosis. The primary limitation is that, in this position, access is limited to the inferior orbital rims.

The following is a summary of the surgical correction of the most common single-suture closures. The techniques discussed herein are offered not as absolutes but as alternatives. Just as the entity of sagittal synostosis is protean, so should be the treatments [30-32]. The goal should be a normal contour of the skull. To that end, strict adherence to rehearsed techniques should be prohibited.

Metopic Synostosis

Premature closure of the metopic suture causes a narrow and flattened frontal bone. There is temporal narrowing, recession of the superior orbital rims and varying degrees of hypotelorism (Fig. 25.2a). Often, there is a prominent metopic ridge. Compensatory growth at the coronal sutures occurs away from the metopic suture, expanding the parietal bones. Compensatory growth also occurs symmetrically at the sagittal suture and further enlarges the parietal bones.

The extent of the surgical correction varies greatly for this disorder. At times, when the compensatory growth and hypotelorism are mild and only a large metopic ridge is evident, the surgery involves only burring down the stenotic ridge. More involved techniques are required when the full range of primary and secondary effects of suture closure are evident (Fig. 25.2). Surgery must restore normal contour to the forehead, bringing the orbital rims forward, widen the skull in the temporal region and attend to the hypotelorism.

Children are placed supine and a bi-coronal incision is fashioned. To minimize blood loss, dissection is carried out in a supra-periosteal plane, to a level approximately 1 cm above the supraorbital ridges. A sub-periosteal plane is then developed in continuity with the periorbita, exposing the supraorbital rims. The temporalis muscle is elevated and the frontal process of the zygoma and the inferior orbital rim are exposed. The hypoplastic frontal bone is generally addressed first. A bi-fronto-parietal craniotomy that includes the coronal suture is fashioned, with an attempt to remove the bone as a single unit (Fig. 25.2b). This flap is refashioned using radial osteotomies, controlled fractures and the Tessier rib bender.

To perform the orbital advancement, the orbital rims are removed in a single unit. Bilateral orbital osteotomies are fashioned through the orbital roof and the lateral-orbital wall below the fronto-zygomatic suture. Bone graft is used to refashion the orbital rims and to correct the hypotelorism (Fig. 25.2c and d). When advancing the orbital rims, it is important to re-attach the temporalis muscle anteriorly to prevent the appearance of temporal wasting post-operatively (Fig. 25.3e). The re-contoured frontal craniotomy is then fixed to the orbital rims. This flap is most often not fixed posteriorly, in order to allow the expanding brain to move the frontal bone and orbital rims as a single unit. If the skull continues to appear narrow, barrel-stave osteotomies may be out-fractured in the temporal bone.

Coronal Synostosis

Unilateral Coronal Synostosis

Fusion of the coronal suture causes flattening of the ipsilateral frontal and parietal bones (Fig. 25.3a). Compensatory growth at the sagittal suture causes contralateral parietal bone overgrowth. Symmetric growth occurs at the contralateral coronal suture, causing unilateral frontal bossing. The ipsilateral squamosal suture causes overgrowth of the temporal bone. To restore normal contour to the frontal region, surgery must advance the ipsilateral orbital rim, expand the ipsilateral fronto-parietal region and contract the contralateral side.

In the supine position, a bi-frontal craniotomy, including the coronal sutures, is fashioned and remodeled using radial osteotomies and controlled fractures (Fig. 25.3b). The ipsilateral greater sphenoid wing, which is often thickened and displaced superiorly, is rongeured or drilled to the level of the superior orbital fissure (Fig. 25.3c). A unilateral orbital rim advancement is performed on the fused side using orbital osteotomies, as described for metopic synostosis (Fig. 25.3d). The temporalis muscle is moved anteriorly and affixed to the advanced lateral orbital rim (Fig. 25.3e). If the ipsilateral temporal region has overgrowth, a temporal craniotomy is performed and the bone is re-contoured using radial osteotomies.

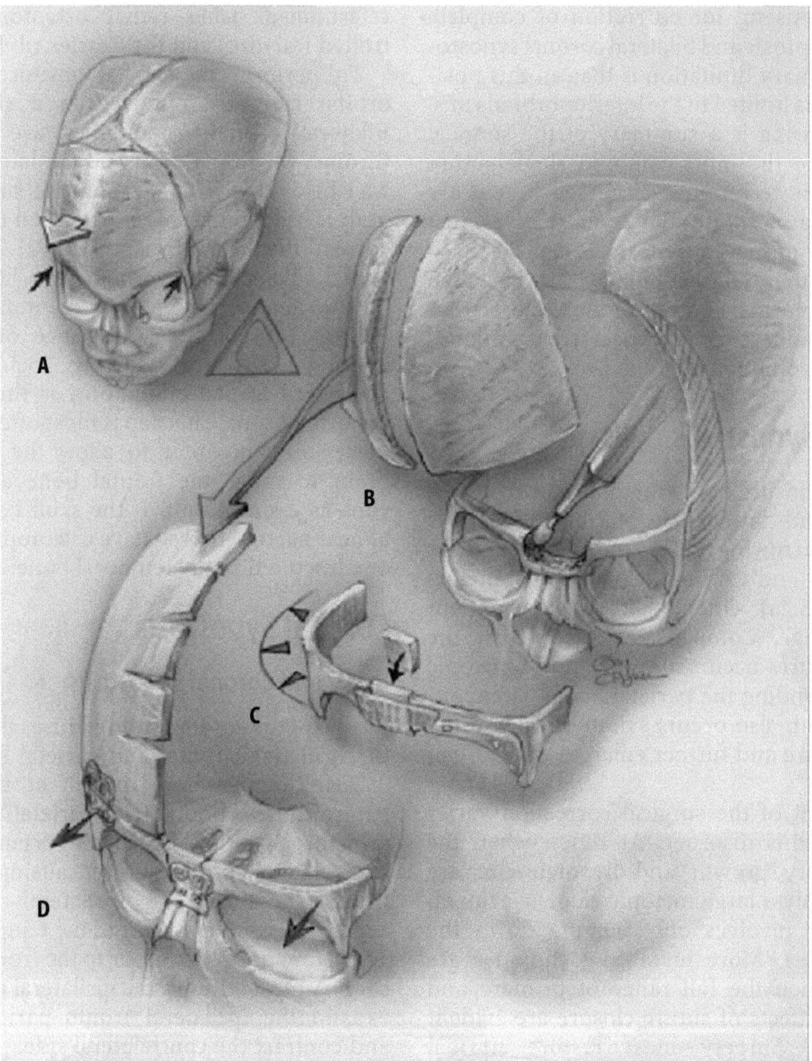

Fig. 25.2. Metopic synostosis. **a** Primary pathology and compensatory changes. **b** Bi-frontal craniotomy. **c** Orbital rim reconstruction. **d** Orbital rim and frontal advancements.

Bilateral Coronal Synostosis

Bilateral coronal synostosis causes restricted antero-posterior growth of the skull. Compensatory growth occurs at the metopic, sagittal and squamosal sutures, which increases the height of the skull and results in turribrachycephaly (Fig. 25.4a). Surgery must shorten the protracted cranial height and expand the restricted orbito-frontal region.

To decrease the skull height and increase its antero-posterior dimension, a near calveriectomy is required (Fig. 25.4b). In the modified prone position, a bi-frontal craniotomy is fashioned, removing the flap as a single unit. A similar bi-parieto-occipital flap is performed, leaving only the sagittal suture and two parietal struts between the anterior and posterior craniotomies. The anterior and posterior craniotomies are refashioned using radial osteotomies and controlled fractures. The remaining occipital bone is out-fractured using barrel-stave osteotomies, expanding the skull posteriorly. Bilateral orbital rim advancements are

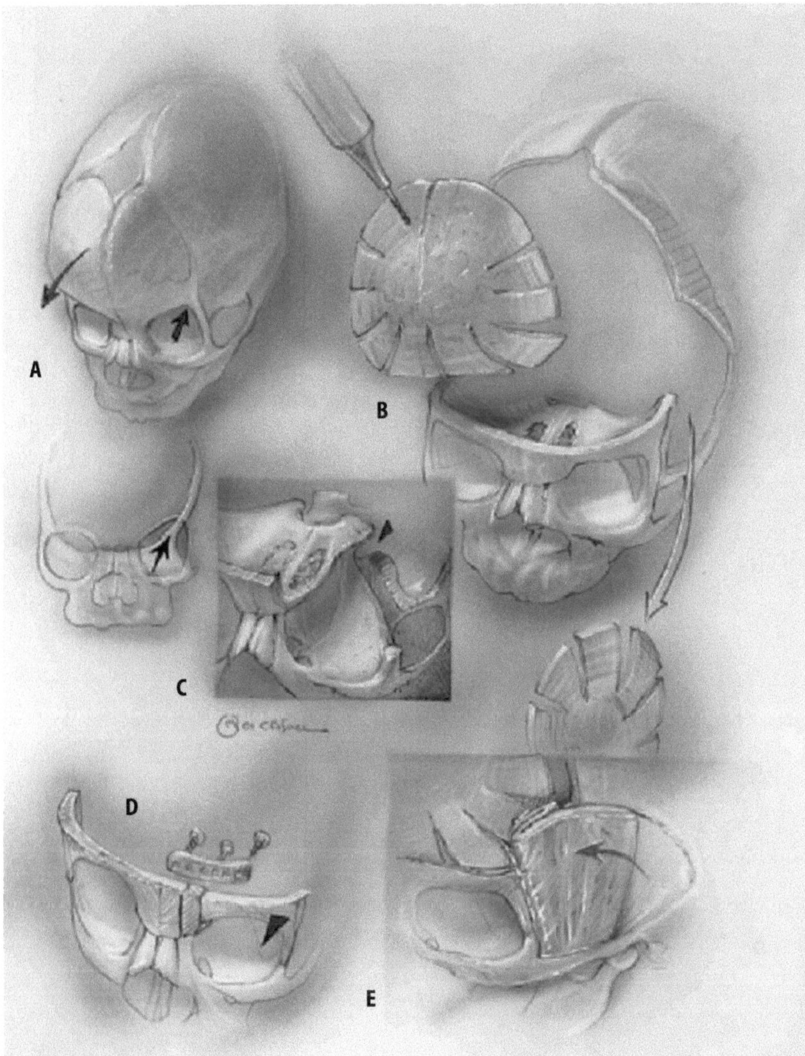

Fig. 25.3. Unilateral coronal synostosis. **a** Primary pathology and compensatory changes. **b** Bi-frontal craniotomy and remodeling. **c** Drilling to superior orbital fissure. **d** Orbital rim advancement. **e** Temporal muscle advancement.

performed, similarly expanding the skull anteriorly (Fig. 25.4c). The skull height is diminished by removal of bone from the two parietal struts and re-affixing the struts to the temporal bone (Fig. 25.4d and e).

Sagittal Synostosis

Common Presentations

Sagittal synostosis has several common presentations, each of which requires an operation that is designed for the individual deformity. The primary abnormality associated with premature fusion of the sagittal suture is the narrow skull. Compensatory growth occurs at the coronal and lambdoid sutures and increases the antero–posterior dimension of the skull, termed "dolichocephaly" or "scaphocephaly". These are not the only changes, however.

Sagittal synostosis has many different forms; the specific phenotype depends on the location along the sagittal suture that fuses prematurely. Fusion may be anterior, posterior or complete

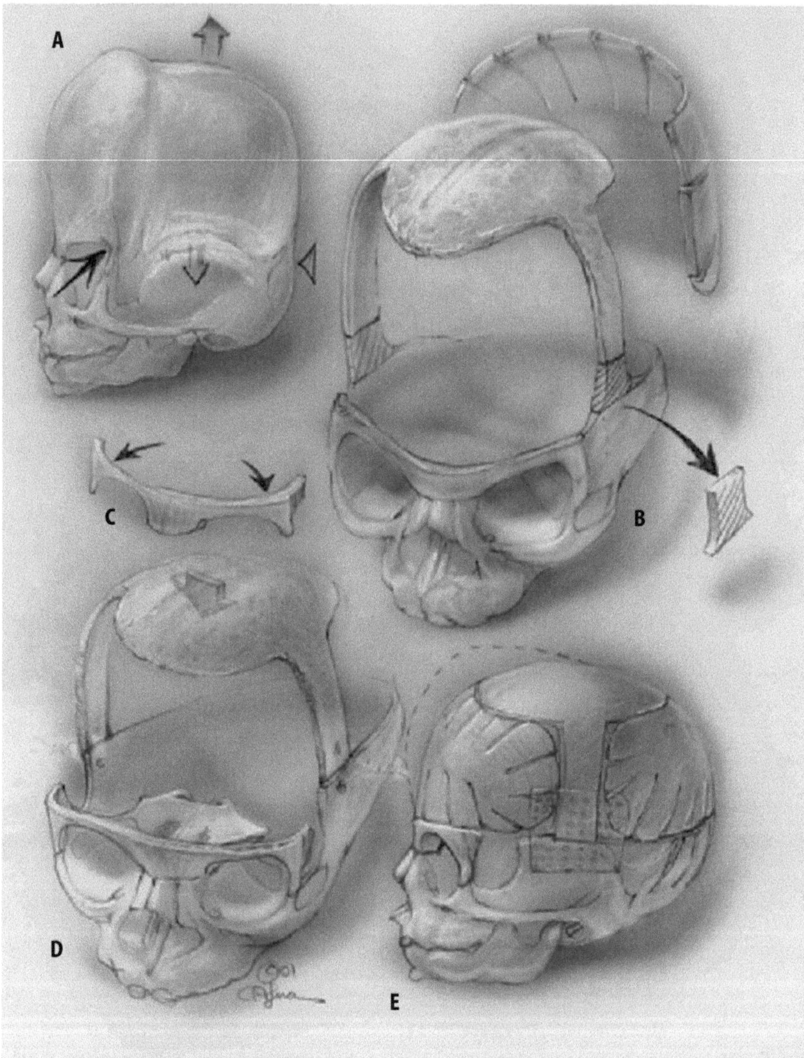

Fig. 25.4. Bilateral coronal synostosis. **a** Primary pathology and compensatory changes. **b** Bi-fronto–parietal and parieto–occipital craniotomies. **c** Orbital rim reconstruction. **d** Vault reconstruction. **e** Reconstruction of vault.

(Fig. 25.1). Anterior fusion causes excessive growth at the coronal and metopic sutures, resulting in varying degrees of frontal bossing.

Likewise, posterior sagittal synostosis causes varying degrees of deformity in the occipital bone. Closure of the posterior portion of the sagittal suture occurs less commonly and requires different surgical approaches. There are several variants, each demanding individual consideration. The most basic deformity is the so-called occipital knob. In such a circumstance, the occipital bone, because it is distal and perpendicular to the fused suture, experiences the compensatory overgrowth. The "golf tee" deformity is more than simply an exaggerated form of the occipital knob. The skull is narrower posteriorly and protrudes more prominently. In addition, the unfused anterior portion of the sagittal suture can widen the parietal bone anteriorly, accentuating the occipital narrowing. Bathrocephaly – another variant of posterior sagittal synostosis – is characterized by the appearance of a podium in the occipital region. The posterior portion of the parietal bone slants inferiorly, while the occipital bone juts superiorly. In its most extreme form, complete closure of the sagittal suture causes deformity fore and aft.

Anterior Closure

When the anterior portion of the sagittal suture closes prematurely, the compensatory growth causes frontal bossing and an extensive craniotomy is required. The craniotomy must expand the narrowed skull, shorten the protracted anterior–posterior distance and attend to the bossing (Fig. 25.5a).

One option is to perform the so-called anterior Π procedure. In the supine position, separate bi-parietal flaps are fashioned, whose anterior and posterior limits are the coronal and lambdoid sutures (Fig. 25.5a). The coronal suture and the bone overlying the temporal fossa are then rongeured, leaving a craniotomy in the shape of a Π (Fig 25.5b). Notably, the pathological sagittal suture is not excised; the operation focuses on the compensations, and not the fused suture. The remaining elements are united, slanting the frontal bone posteriorly, thus correcting the skull length and the frontal bossing. Barrel-stave osteotomies are fashioned in the parietal and temporal bones and are then out-fractured so that when the remaining bony elements are brought together, the width of the skull can expand (Fig. 25.5c and d).

There are a number of variations in this procedure, depending on the degree of frontal bossing. When dramatic, the frontal bone must be removed and reshaped using radial osteotomies and careful infracturing of the frontal bone. At times, other techniques are used. The skull may be foreshortened by removing a narrow bi-parietal flap that contains the sagittal suture. This flap is then shortened and rotated 90° to increase the width of the skull. Skull on either side of the coronal and lambdoid sutures is rongeured and, after the remaining bone edges are united, the skull is shorter and rounder.

Posterior Closure

Occipital Knob

To correct the long and posteriorly narrow skull, a reverse Π procedure may be employed (Fig. 25.6a). Similar to the anterior Π technique but in the prone position, after the bi-parietal flaps are removed, the bone is rongeured across the posterior portion of the sagittal suture and across the lambdoids. The resultant craniotomy appears as a reversed Π. Care must again be taken to release the dura along the remaining unfused portions of suture. Radial osteotomies in the occipital bone may be required to correct the knob. The results can be quite good and the normal contour can be re-established.

Golf Tee

To correct this more dramatic deformity, the skull must not only be shortened, but the occipital region must be widened as well (Fig. 25.6b). An occipital craniotomy is performed and a paramedian bi-parietal flap containing the sagittal suture is fashioned. A laterally oriented vaulted arch accomplishes the widening of the region and radial osteotomies allow the occipital bone to be refashioned.

Bathrocephaly

Surgical correction requires not only a shorter skull, but also one that has a normal contour (Fig. 25.6c). After bi-parietal flaps are established, the sagittal and lambdoid sutures are separated from the underlying dura. A paramedian vault is created that normalizes the relationship between the posterior parietal and occipital bones. Radial cuts across the lambdoid sutures allow the occipital bone to be fractured outward and result in a wider occipital region.

Complete Sagittal Synostosis

In severe cases of anterior and posterior deformity, patients are positioned in a modified prone position. Surgical correction must involve the entire skull, correcting the scaphocephaly, frontal bossing and occipital knob (Fig. 25.7a). This gives access to the entire skull. A near calveriectomy must be fashioned, removing bi-frontal, bi-occipital and two parietal flaps (Fig. 25.7b). The flaps are remodeled using radial osteotomies and replaced, creating a shorter and rounder skull. Barrel-stave osteotomies in the parieto-temporal region can also increase the skull width (Fig. 25.7c).

Other techniques are also available and commonly employed for patients presenting with scaphocephaly. Sagittal synostosis may also be addressed using an "I"-shaped calveriectomy. After the dura is separated from the overlying

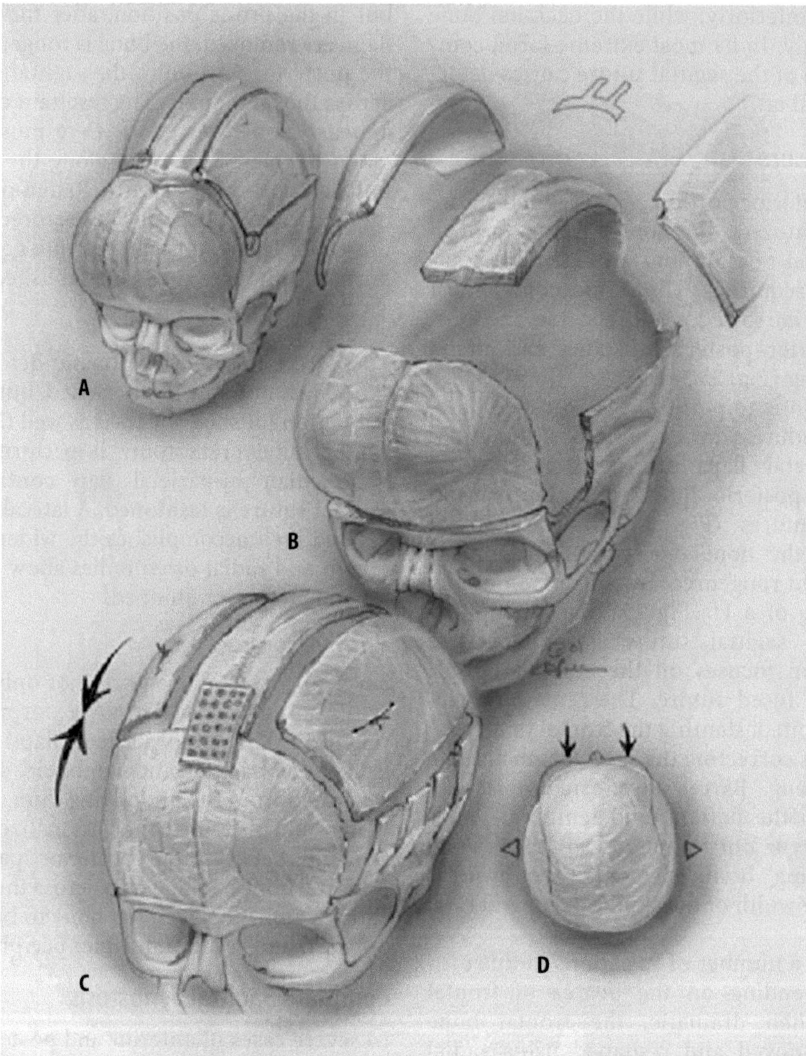

Fig. 25.5. Anterior sagittal synostosis. **a** Primary pathology, compensatory changes and craniotomy. **b** Bone remodeling. **c** Bone fixation. **d** Conceptualization of correction.

sutures, bone is removed across the coronal, sagittal and lambdoidal sutures. The removed bone is interposed in the midline to widen the skull and the remaining frontal, parietal and occipital bones are cinched together. The result is a shorter and wider skull. When frontal bossing or posterior deformities are significant, this procedure may be combined with frontal or parieto-occipital craniectomies for their respective remodeling.

Unilateral Lambdoid Synostosis

In our experience, true lambdoid synostosis is rare. In true lambdoid synostosis, there is flattening of the ipsilateral parietal and occipital bones (Fig. 25.8a). Compensatory growth at the sagittal and contralateral lambdoid suture expands the contralateral parietal bone. Asymmetric growth also occurs at the ipsilateral squamosal suture, causing a temporal bulge and antero-inferior displacement of the pinna.

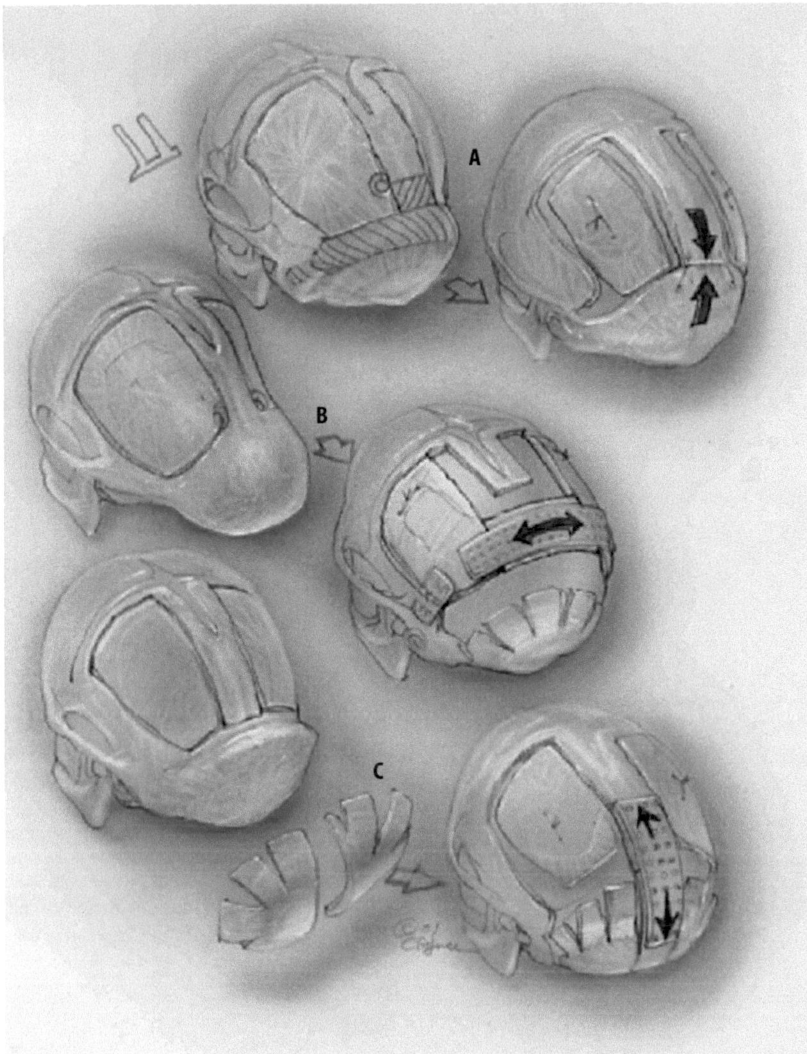

Fig. 25.6. Posterior sagittal synostosis. **a** Occipital knob, pathology (left) and correction (right). **b** Golf tee deformity, pathology (left) and correction (right). **c** Bathrocephaly, pathology (left) and correction (right).

In a prone position, a bi-parieto-occipital craniotomy is performed and remodeled using radial osteotomies and controlled out-fractures (Fig. 25.8b). Bilateral occipital barrel-stave osteotomies are performed. Controlled out-fractures are fashioned ipsilateral, and in-fractures contralateral to the fused lambdoidal suture.

What had once been called lambdoid synostosis is now recognized as positional plagiocephaly. In positional plagiocephaly, the skull affects a parallelogram shape (Fig. 25.8c). The ear and frontal bones are forward, creating an ipsilateral occipital flattening and frontal bossing. Unless severe, this entity does not require surgery. Some patients, however, with severe positional molding have significant ipsilateral frontal bossing and are unlikely to correct with conservative treatment. These patients are placed in a modified prone position. The posterior correction proceeds as with true lambdoid synostosis. The anterior correction is

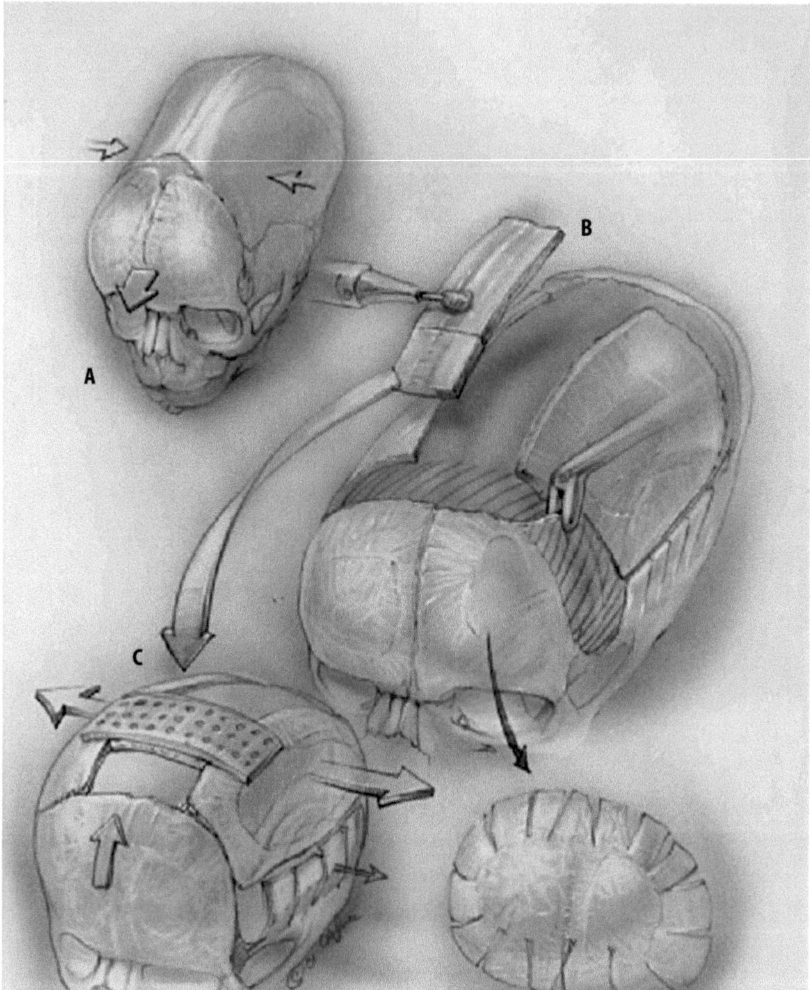

Fig. 25.7. Complete sagittal synostosis. **a** Primary pathology and compensatory changes. **b** Craniotomy and remodeling. **c** Fixation of remodeled bone.

performed using a bi-frontal craniotomy (Fig. 25.8d). The bone is remodeled using radial osteotomies and re-attached to the superior orbital rims.

Conclusion

Abnormal head shape has captured our interest for centuries. Craniosynostosis results from the premature fusion of one or more cranial sutures. The underlying pathoetiology is complex, although considerable progress has been realized in recent years, with the advent of refined techniques of molecular biology. Premature suture closure produces characteristic craniofacial abnormalities that can be precisely predicted. Although each form of synostosis conforms to certain clinical rules of compensatory growth, surgeons are cautioned to avoid using pre-determined surgical procedures. Regardless of the particular technique employed, the goal of surgery should be a normal and pleasing skull contour.

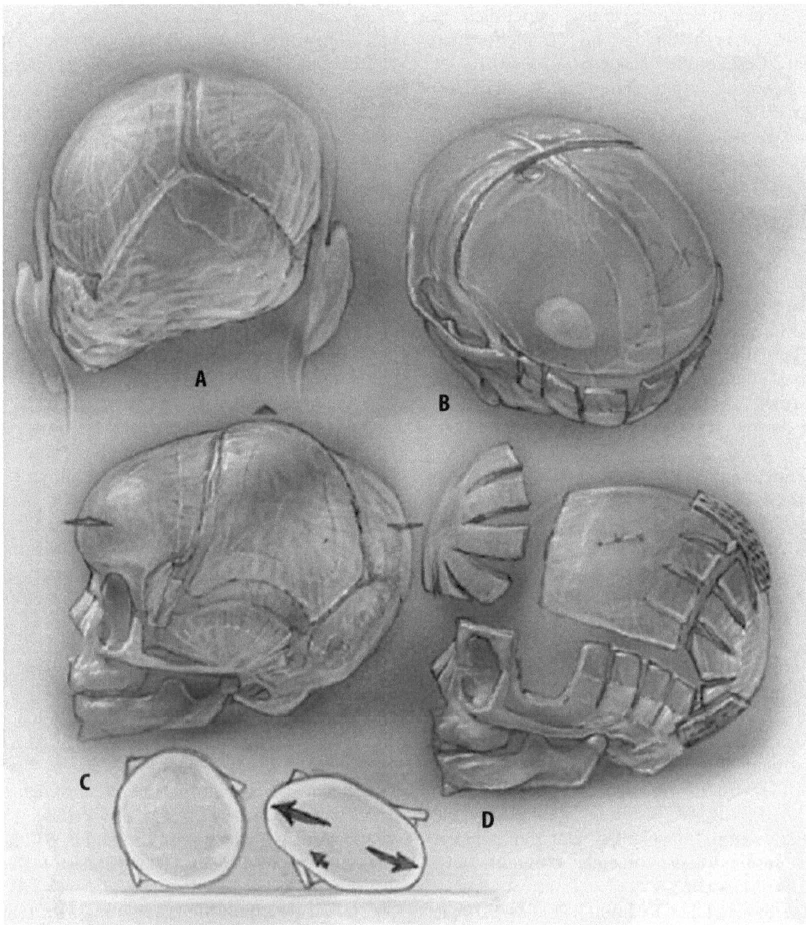

Fig. 25.8. Lambdoid synostosis and positional plagiocephaly. **a** Lambdoid synostosis pathology. **b** Correction of lambdoid synostosis. **c** Positional plagiocephaly pathology. **d** Correction of positional plagiocephaly.

Key Points

- *The goal of surgery is to restore a normal skull contour and allow continued growth of the brain to reshape the skull.*
- *Simple strip craniectomies have been superseded by complex calvarial reconstructions because single-suture closure prevents not only growth at the fused suture, but also causes secondary compensations that affect the entire skull.*
- *The diagnosis is made clinically, although adjunctive imaging studies may confirm the diagnosis and aid in the planning of further care.*
- *Each form of synostosis conforms to certain clinical rules of compensatory growth; surgeons should be cautioned to avoid using predetermined surgical procedures.*

References

1. Cohen MM Jr. History, terminology, and classification of craniosynostosis. In: Cohen MM Jr, MacLean RE, editors. Craniosynostosis: diagnosis, evaluation, and management. 2nd Edition. New York: Oxford Press, 2000; 103–11.
2. Sommerring, ST. Vom Baue des Menschlichen. 2nd ed. Leipzig, Voss, 1839.
3. Otto AW. Lehrbuch der Pathologischen des Menschen und der Thiere. Berlin, Rucker, 1830.

4. Virchow R. Ueber den cretinismus, namentlich in Franken: Und euber pathologische Schadelformen. Verh Phys Med Gesane Wurzburg 1851;2:230–71.
5. Apert E. De l'acrocephalosyndactalie. Bull Soc Med Hop Paris 1906;23:1310.
6. Crouzon O. Dysostose craniofaciale hereditaire. Bull Soc Med Hop Paris 1912;35:545.
7. Lane LC. Pioneer craniectomy for relief of mental imbecility due to premature sutural closure and microcephalus. JAMA 1892;18:49–50.
8. Lannelongue M. De la craniectomie dans la microcephalie. CR Acad Sci 1890 ;110 :1382-1385.
9. van der Klaauw CJ. Cerebral Skull and facial skull. Arch Neerl Zool 1946;7:1–37.
10. Moss ML. The pathogenesis of premature cranial synostosis in man. Acta Anat 1959;37:351-370.
11. Moss ML. Growth of the calvaria in the rat: The determination of osseous morphology. Am J Anat 1954;94: 333–62.
12. Moss ML. Functional anatomy of cranial synostosis. Child's Brain 1975;1:22–33.
13. Bolk L. On the premature obliteration of sutures in the human skull. Am J Anat 1915;17:495–523.
14. Persson KM, Roy WA, Persing JA, Rodeheaver, Winn HR. Craniofacial growth following experimental craniosynostosis and craniectomy in rabbits. J Neurosurg 1979;50:187–97.
15. Persing JA, Morgin EP, Cronin AJ, Wolcott WP. Skull base expansion: Craniofacial effects. Plast Reconstr Surg 1991;87:1028–33.
16. Marsh JL, Vannier MW. Cranial base changes following surgical treatment of craniosynostosis. Cleft Palate J. 1986;23(Suppl 1):9–18.
17. Opperman LA, Persing JA, Sheen R, Ogle RC. In the absence of periosteum, transplanted fetal and neonatal rat coronal sutures resist osseous obliteration. J Craniofacial Surg 1994;5:327–32.
18. Opperman LA, Sweeney TM, Redmon J, Persing JA, Ogle RC. Tissue interactions with underlying dura mater inhibit osseous obliteration of developing cranial sutures. J Dev Dynam 1993;312–22.
19. Alden TD, Lin KY, Jane JA. Mechanisms of premature closure of cranial sutures. Childs Nerv Syst 1999;15: 670–5.
20. Sun PP, Persing JA. Craniosynostosis. In: Albright AL, Pollack IF, Adelson PD, editors. Principles and practice of pediatric neurosurgery. New York: Thieme, 1999; 219–42.
21. Cohen MM Jr. Epidemiology of craniosynostosis. In: Cohen MM Jr, MacLean RE, editors. Craniosynostosis: diagnosis, evaluation, and management. 2nd Edition. New York: Oxford Press, 2000; 112–18.
22. Cohen MM Jr, Kreiborg S. New indirect method for estimating the birth prevalence of the Apert Syndrome. Int J Oral Maxillofac Surg 1992;21:107–9.
23. Cohen MM Jr. Sutural pathology. In: Cohen MM Jr, MacLean RE, editors. Craniosynostosis: diagnosis, evaluation, and management. 2nd Edition. New York: Oxford Press, 2000; 51–68.
24. Koskien-Moffet L, Moffet BC, Graham JM Jr. Sutures and intra-uterine deformation. In: Persing JA, Edgerton MT, Jane JA, editors. Scientific foundations and surgical treatment of craniosynostosis. Baltimore: Williams and Wilkins, 1989:96–106.
25. Persing JA, Jane JA. Craniosynostosis. In : Youmans JR, editor. Neurological Surgery : a comprehensive guide to the diagnosis and management of neurosurgical problems. 4th Edition. Philadelphia: W.B. Saunders, 1996;995–1011.
26. Huang MH, Mouradian WE, Cohen SR, Gruss JS. The differential diagnosis of abnormal head shapes: separating craniosynostosis from positional deformities and normal variants. Cleft Palate Craniofac J 1998;35: 204–11.
27. Simmons NE, Lanzino G, Phillips CD, Jane JA, Lin KY. Use of preoperative computed tomography-angiography in cranial remodeling : technical note. Neuro surgery 1998;43:970–2; discussion 972–3.
28. Jane JA, Persing JA. Neurosurgical treatment of craniosynostosis. In: Cohen MM, editor. Craniosynostosis: diagnosis, evaluation, and management. 1st Edition. New York: Raven Press, 1986;249–320.
29. Delashaw JB, Persing JA, Broaddus WC, Jane JA. Cranial vault growth in craniosynostosis. J Neurosurg 1989; 70:159–65.
30. Jane JA Sr, Jane JA Jr. Treatment of craniosynostosis. Clin Neurosurg 1996;43:139–62.
31. Jane JA, Persing JA. Neurosurgical treatment of craniosynostosis. In: Cohen MM, editor. Craniosynostosis: diagnosis, evaluation, and management. 2nd Edition. New York: Raven Press, 2000; 209–27.
32. Francel PC, Jane JA. Image reconstruction and craniofacial repair. In: Salcman M, editor. Current techniques in neurosurgery. 2nd Edition. Philadelphia: Current Medicine, 1996;30–51.

26

Syndromic Craniosynostosis

Francis R. Johns, John A. Jane Sr and Kant Lin

Summary

The common features in syndromic craniosynostoses are premature coronal suture closure and abnormal cranial base morphology. Over 90 syndromes have been identified. The authors focus on six of these syndromes – Crouzon, Apert, Pfeiffer, Saethre–Chotzen, Carpenter and Kleeblattschadel.

Introduction

Syndromic craniosynostoses consist of a group of synostotic malformations occurring in conjunction with a constellation of facial, skeletal or other organ abnormalities. These craniofacial dysostoses are familial disorders and may present with single or multiple fused cranial vault sutures. Each syndrome may display extreme variability in clinical presentation in terms of its severity and outcome. This is due to complex interactions between genetic factors, cellular events and local forces affecting normal growth and development [1–3].

The common features in syndromic craniosynostoses are premature coronal suture closure and abnormal cranial base morphology. This results in a characteristic brachycephaly and mid-face retrusion. There is controversy, however, over which factor (closed cranial vault suture or cranial base suture) is the initiating process resulting in the characteristic clinical features.

The classification systems for syndromic craniosynostoses are based upon either genetic and etiologic factors or clinical features. Cohen's system categorizes according to gene malformations, chromosomal defects or teratogenic-induced mutations [1]. Mutations in FGFR genes have been demonstrated in several syndromes. These are a family of heparin-binding polypeptides that stimulate mitogenesis, induce differentiation in cells and exhibit angiogenic activity. Presently, specific mutations in FGFR2 have been associated with Apert, Crouzon and Pfeiffer syndromes. Pfeiffer syndrome has also been associated with a mutation in FGFR1 [4]. Other classification systems, on the other hand, categorize by morphologic characteristics. These may be more useful clinically by facilitating surgical planning and decision making.

The various syndromic craniosynostoses often undergo similar reconstructive procedures to improve craniofacial form, proportionality, balance and symmetry. Each patient, however, should be approached with an individualized reconstructive strategy, in order to address the craniofacial dysostosis as well as the particular needs of the patient. Quantitative analysis with CT scans, surface anthropometry or cephalometry can be helpful in treatment planning. One should understand that the reconstruction may in fact correct the presenting deformity, but does not address the underlying growth abnormality. As a result, the goals of any reconstruction should be to address the immediate needs while minimizing the number of future surgical interventions.

Functional Considerations

The primary functional consideration in the treatment of craniofacial dysostosis is normal brain development. Premature sutural fusion can lead to elevated ICP and potential retardation of brain development, with mental dysfunction. Renier et al. have determined that 42% of untreated children with more than one prematurely fused suture and 14% of untreated children with one prematurely fused suture had significantly elevated ICP [5]. Another important functional consideration with elevated ICP is papilledema and subsequent optic atrophy and blindness. As a result, consideration should be given to monitoring all infants who have multiple or syndromic craniosynostosis during the neonatal period, since clinical indicators of elevated ICP (irritability, failure to thrive, papilledema) may occur late. It is often necessary to perform a surgical expansion of the intracranial capacity to decompress the brain in order to prevent these functional problems.

Hydrocephalus is often associated with syndromic craniosynostosis, particularly in Crouzon syndrome, Apert syndrome and Kleeblattschadel anomaly. The etiology is not clear but may be related to a generalized cranial base stenosis, with constriction of all foramina. Close clinical monitoring for signs of elevated ICP in this patient population is imperative. Invasive forms of monitoring include performing a small craniotomy to place an epidural pressure monitor or lumbar puncture monitoring. Others perform CT scanning or ultrasonography of the ventricles in the perioperative period to facilitate the diagnosis and management of hydrocephalus. Early surgical intervention, consisting of a strip craniectomy in those patients with elevated ICP, may allow for more normal brain development.

Visual problems commonly associated with craniofacial dysostosis include proptosis, strabismus, hypertelorism, exposure keratitis and decreased visual acuity related to papilledema. Shallow orbits may lead to proptosis, with risk of exposure and corneal ulceration as well as the risk of trauma to the globe. These can be managed with eye lubricants or tarsorrhaphy, until permanent measures such as orbital advancement can be performed. Severe orbital hypertelorism as well as convergent or divergent strabismus may compromise visual acuity and restrict binocular vision. Pre-operative visual assessment and baseline measurements should be determined for all infants. Also, early surgical correction is important to enable proper afferent input and prevent amblyopia.

Airway obstruction can occur in syndromic craniosynostosis secondary to mid-face hypoplasia (with nasopharyngeal narrowing), choanal stenosis, elongated soft palate, glossoptosis and laryngotracheomalacia. Previous measures for managing these problems included prolonged intubation or tracheostomy. Due to the inherent problems with these measures, they are avoided if possible by conservative means, such as patient positioning, nasal stents and continuous positive airway pressure. Alternative surgical measures for those that are refractory to these therapies include adenotonsillectomy, palatal expansion, uvulopalatopharyngoplasty and mid-face advancement.

Speech and language problems occur commonly in those individuals with craniofacial dysostosis due to peripheral and not CNS factors. These include speech resonance abnormalities and articulation problems secondary to abnormal anatomy, such as maxillomandibular disproportions, a constricted maxilla, dental crowding, a large tongue and a cleft palate with velopharyngeal insufficiency.

Hearing deficits are also commonly associated with syndromic craniosynostoses. Conductive hearing loss secondary to eustacian tube dysfunction and chronic otitis media are the most common causes. Apert syndrome, in particular, may be associated with hearing deficits related to stapedial footplate fixation in addition to middle-ear disease. Audiologic testing should be routinely performed, in order to diagnose these problems early so that appropiate therapy can be undertaken.

Extremity anomalies are also common in syndromic craniosynostoses, which can lead to significant functional deficits. These anomalies include broad thumbs and great toes, complex compound syndactylism of the digits, partial soft tissue syndactylism and pre-axial polysyndactyly of the feet.

Crouzon Syndrome

Crouzon syndrome was first described by a French neurosurgeon in 1912. It is the most frequent form of craniofacial dysostosis, occurring in approximately 1 per 25,000 births. About half of the cases occur as sporadic mutations and the remaining are familial and inherited as an autosomal-dominant trait [6,7]. There is occasional difficulty in differentiating between severe and mild forms of Crouzon syndrome, due to its variable expressivity (Fig. 26.1).

Seizures occur in approximately 12% of those with Crouzon syndrome but actual mental deficiency is found in only 3%. The association of increasing hydrocephalus is rare [1]. Conductive hearing deficits occur in 55% and cervical spine anomalies occur in approximately 30%, along with sacral and rib anomalies [7].

Crouzon syndrome is characterized by craniofacial skeletal anomalies; however, there is no clear characteristic pattern of limb involvement. A small proportion of Crouzon syndrome patients will have elbow abnormalities (ankylosis or radial head sub-luxation) and minor hand abnormalities (short or malaligned fingers). Brachycephaly is the typical cranial form secondary to bilateral coronal synostosis. Other sutures may be involved, such as the lambdoid, sagittal and metopic sutures. There are also abnormal growth centers in the cranial base and facial sutures, leading to orbital, zygomatic and maxillary hypoplasia with normal soft tissue development. Often, there is associated upper-lid ptosis present, with significant exophthalmos, strabismus, exorbitism and hypertelorism. Associated with the mid-face hypoplasia, constricted maxilla, dental crowding and class III malocclusion is a paradoxical retrogenia. Intelligence is usually normal and the incidence of clefting is low. There are some general similarities in the craniofacial features displayed with Apert syndrome but, as a rule, Crouzon syndrome is a much less severe deformity, with a few distinct differences.

The initial surgical procedure for Crouzon syndrome is usually cranio-orbital decompression and reshaping. This is usually performed at 6–12 months, unless signs of elevated ICP

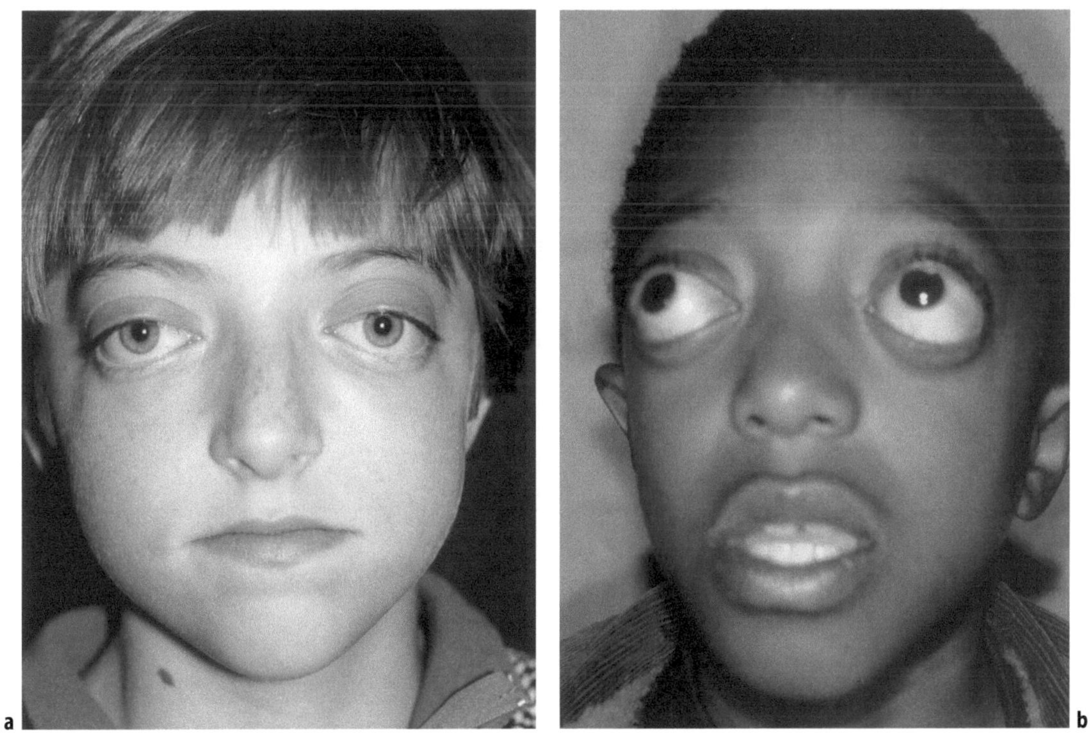

Fig. 26.1. a Mild form of Crouzon syndrome. **b** Moderately severe form of Crouzon syndrome.

are evident earlier, at which point a limited cranial vault expansion may be indicated. The cranio-orbital decompression consists of bicoronal suture release and osteotomies of the anterior cranial vault and orbits, with reshaping and advancement. The purpose is to decompress the brain and increase orbital volume, to decrease globe protrusion. The child is then followed clinically at intervals and further decompression with reshaping is performed if there is evidence of elevated ICP. The site of brain compression is determined and cranial vault expansion is performed in this area, either anterior or posterior. Later in childhood (at 5–7 years of age), correction of the mid-face hypoplasia, along with final cranial vault reshaping, can be performed through a LeFort III, monobloc or facial bipartition. Selection of the procedure depends upon the presenting deformity and should be customized accordingly. More commonly, LeFort III and monobloc procedures are performed for Crouzon syndrome. Final correction of the malocclusion through orthognathic surgery should be reserved until skeletal maturity, to avoid recurrence of the malocclusion and also creation of severe enophthalmos in an attempt to correct the bite at an early age.

Apert Syndrome

Apert syndrome was first described by a French neurologist in 1906. It is also known as acrocephalosyndactyly, referring to its characteristic features of craniosynostosis, mid-facial hypoplasia and symmetric compound complex syndactylism of the hands and feet (Fig. 26.2). The majority of cases occur sporadically, as fresh mutations. Increased paternal age has been associated with sporadic cases [8]. There is also an autosomal-dominant inheritance pattern, with complete penetrance. The incidence of Apert syndrome is about 1 per 100,000 births [9]. This does not account for the high mortality rate in the neonatal period, which equates to an incidence in the general population of 1 per 2 million [10].

The craniofacial features of Apert syndrome include bilateral coronal suture synostosis at birth, resulting in turribrachycephaly, with a high, flat forehead and transverse frontal skin furrow above the supraorbital ridges. There is also a wide midline calvarial defect in the area of the metopic and sagittal suture, present until the third year of life. The cranial base is malformed and asymmetric, with a short clivus and

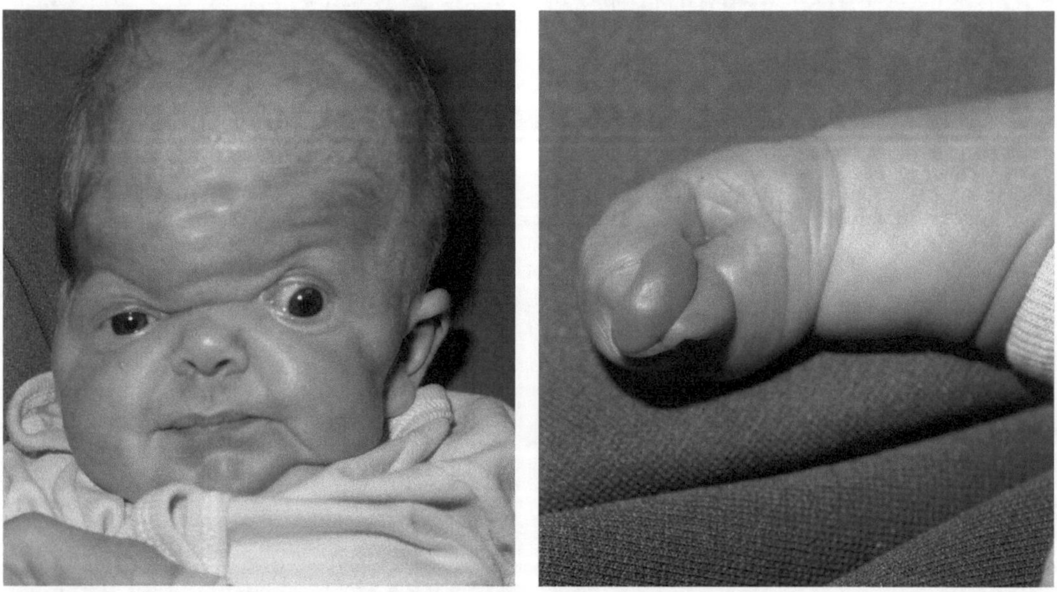

a b

Fig. 26.2. **a** Apert syndrome, with hypertelorism, exorbitism, strabismus, turribrachycephaly and maxillary hypoplasia. **b** Apert syndrome, with severe syndactyly anterior cranial fossa. The sella is enlarged and the greater wings of the sphenoid are protruded. There is an expanded ethmoidal labyrinth, with orbital hypertelorism and shallow orbits, with proptosis. Down-slanting palpebral fissures and strabismus are frequently present. The ocular motility disturbances may be due to mechanical factors or structural alterations of the extraocular muscles.

Mid-face hypoplasia is also characteristic of this syndrome, resulting in a depressed nasal bridge, mandibular prognathism and a class III malocclusion, along with maxillary arch constriction. This results in a V-shaped maxillary dental arch, dental crowding and thickening of the alveolar ridges. Consistent with these deformities, there is often a posterior cross-bite and an anterior open bite. There is often delay of dental eruption and frequent supernumerary teeth. The palate is short, highly arched and often has a median furrow. The incidence of cleft palate is also high, occurring in 30% of those afflicted [11]. This results in eustachian tube dysfunction and frequent otitis media. Congenital stapedial foot plate anomalies, along with frequent middle-ear infections, result in an increased risk of hearing deficits. The soft palate is longer and thicker than in normal subjects. The nasopharynx is also reduced in size, placing these patients at risk of airway obstruction.

Mental retardation occurs in a significant number of those with Apert syndrome. The average IQ in one series was 73, with a range of 52–89 [12]. Structural CNS malformations may be partly responsible for the mental deficiencies, such as absence of the corpus callosum, hypoplasia of the cerebral white matter and abnormalities of the limbic structures and pyramidal tracts [13]. Progressive hydrocephalus is uncommon and is often confused with non-progressive ventriculomegaly, due to an embryonic malformation or abnormal brain shaping by the malformed skull [14].

Other findings in this patient population are four-limb symmetric complex syndactylies of the hands and feet, with brachydactyly and joint stiffness. Malformations of other joints, including the elbows and shoulders, may also be found. At birth, height and weight are increased; however, final height is below average due to deceleration of limb growth. Cardiovascular defects can also occur, as well as other visceral anomalies. Lastly, acne vulgaris, extending to the forearms, chest, back and upper arms, commonly occurs.

The initial surgical procedure for Apert syndrome is cranio-orbital decompression and reshaping. It consists of bi-coronal suture release and osteotomies of the anterior cranial vault and orbits, with reshaping and advancement. The purpose is to decompress the brain and increase orbital volume, to decrease globe protrusion. This is usually performed at 6–12 months, unless signs of elevated ICP are evident, in which case a strip craniectomy, limited cranial vault expansion and/or shunt is placed within the first month of life. The child is then followed clinically at intervals and further decompression with reshaping is performed if there is evidence of elevated ICP. Commonly in Apert syndrome, there is need for posterior cranial vault decompression and reshaping. Correction of the mid-face hypoplasia, along with final cranial vault reshaping, are best performed no sooner than at 5–7 years of age. These can be performed through a LeFort III, monobloc or facial bipartition. The facial bipartition allows for more complete correction of the deformities of the orbits (exorbitism and hypertelorism), forehead and mid-face. These procedures are most often performed through distraction osteogenesis, in order to decrease the incidence of post-operative relapse. Final correction of the malocclusion should be reserved until skeletal maturity, to avoid recurrence of the malocclusion and also creation of severe enophthalmos in an attempt to correct the bite at an early age.

Pfeiffer Syndrome

Pfeiffer syndrome was first described in 1964 and has characteristic features of broad thumbs and great toes, partial soft tissue syndactyly of the hands/feet and also craniosynostosis [15]. Other features include maxillary hypoplasia, with a class III malocclusion, hypertelorism, exorbitism, strabismus, downward-slanting palpebral fissures, depressed nasal bridge, beaked nose and turribrachycephaly due to the bilateral coronal synostosis (Fig. 26.3). Additional findings which have been described include fused cervical and lumbar vertebrae and abnormalities of the humerus, pelvis and radioulnar joint, as well as cleft palate.

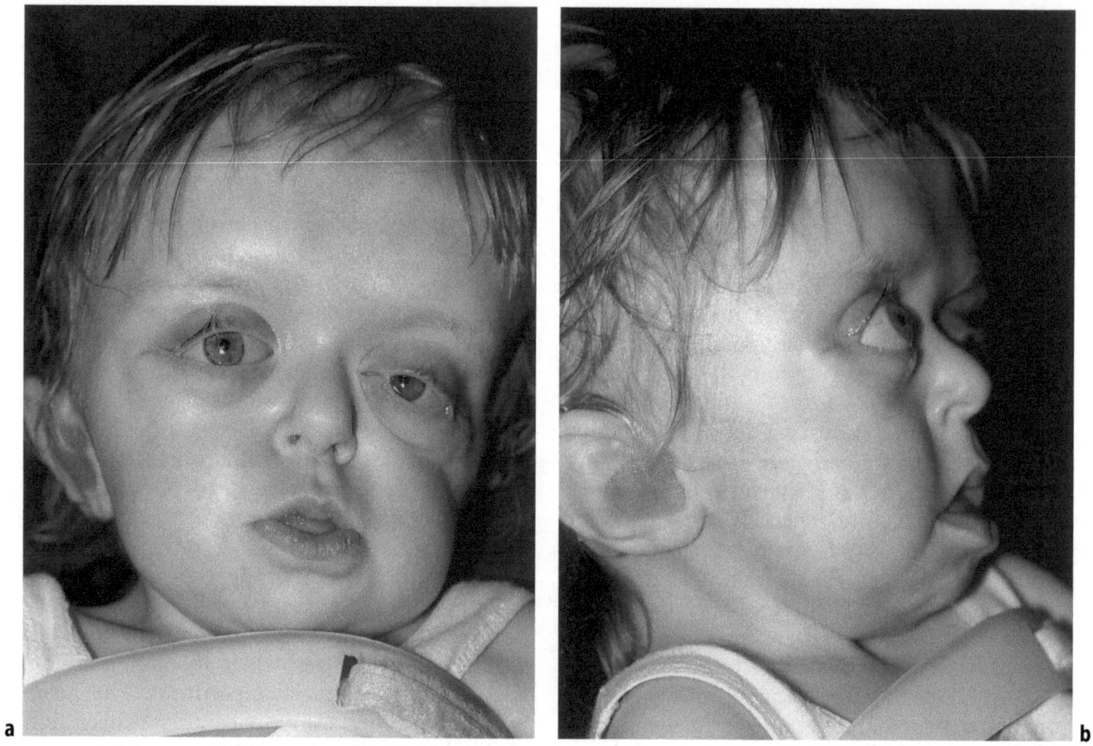

Fig. 26.3. Pfeiffer syndrome, with maxillary hypoplasia, hypertelorism, exorbitism, downward-slanting palpebral fissures, depressed nasal bridge, beaked nose and turribrachycephaly.

The inheritance pattern is most commonly autosomal-dominant, with complete penetrance and variable expressivity. Sporadic cases have also been reported and tend to be more severe in nature [16,17]. The severity of craniofacial deformity in the usual form of Pfeiffer syndrome is lower than that found in Apert syndrome.

The intelligence is usually normal in Pfeiffer syndrome; however, other CNS abnormalities have been reported, such as seizures, hydrocephalus and Arnold–Chiari malformations [18]. Sporadic cases of cloverleaf skull have also been reported in association with Pfeiffer syndrome. These cases often have additional anomalies that are not found in the usual form of Pfeiffer syndrome [1].

Saethre–Chotzen Syndrome

Saethre–Chotzen was first described in 1931 as a syndrome displaying coronal or lambdoidal craniosynostosis and characteristic features, including a low-set frontal hairline, upper-eyelid ptosis, facial asymmetry, deviated nasal septum and partial soft tissue syndactyly of the hands [13,19]. Inheritance is autosomal-dominant, with a high degree of penetrance and variable expressivity [11,20].

Craniofacial features include a brachycephaly or an anterior plagiocephaly due to bilateral or unilateral coronal suture involvement, respectively. Craniosynostosis is, however, not obligatory to the syndrome. Other cranial features that may be present include frontal bossing, parietal bossing, a flattened occiput, enlargement of the sella turcica and large and late-closing fontanelles. Maxillary hypoplasia and a flattened nasofrontal angle, with a beaked, deviated nose, are also common (Fig. 26.4). Oral findings can include a cleft palate, supernumerary teeth and enamel hypoplasia. Orbital findings may include ptosis of the eyelids, strabismus, blepharophimosis, hypertelorism, epicanthal folds, down-slanting palpebral fissures and sparse eyebrows medially.

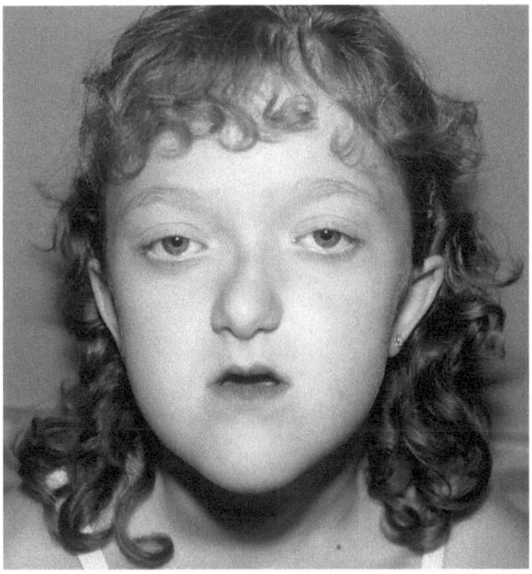

Fig. 26.4. Saethre–Chotzen syndrome with maxillary hypoplasia and a flattened nasofrontal angle, with a beaked, deviated nose.

In most cases, intelligence is normal; however, mild to moderate mental retardation can also occur. Other findings may include defects of the cervical and lumbar spine, dilatation of the lateral ventricles, as well as epilepsy and schizophrenia.

Carpenter Syndrome

This syndrome was first described in 1901; however, it was not recognized as a distinct genetic entity until 1966 [21,22]. Inheritance is different from the other syndromic craniosynostoses in that it is autosomal-recessive. It is characterized by craniosynostosis, polysyndactyly of the feet, brachydactyly of the phalanges, clinodactyly and occasional partial soft tissue syndactyly, cardiac anomalies, low-set ears, short obese neck, short stature, obesity and mental deficiency (Fig. 26.5).

The synostotic pattern most commonly involves the sagittal and lambdoidal sutures, but less commonly the coronal. It often results in significant malformation of the cranium. Unilateral synostosis of the coronal or lambdoidal suture may also occur, causing significant cranial asymmetry. Mental retardation has been associated with many patients with Carpenter syndrome. This may be related to a primary brain abnormality or as the result of elevated intracranial pressure that is untreated. Orbital findings include down-slanting palpebral fissures, epicanthal folds, optic atrophy and corneal opacity. Cardiovascular anomalies are also common, including atrial septal defect, ventricular septal defect (VSD), pulmonic stenosis, patent ductus arteriosus (PDA) and tetrology of Fallot.

Kleeblattschadel Anomaly

The word Kleeblattschadel is German for cloverleaf and describes the most severe form of craniosynostosis. It consists of a trilobular-shaped skull (Fig. 26.6), with synostosis of multiple sutures, which most commonly involves the cranial base, facial and cranial vault sutures, with the sagittal, squamosal and metopic remaining open, leading to compensatory bulging through them. The degree of severity varies with the involvement of the different sutures. There can also be a complete cranial vault synostosis (pansynostosis). The etiology is heterogeneous in that it may present as an isolated anomaly or together with other anomalies, making up various syndromes. Approximately 40% of all cases represent thanatophoric dysplasia and approximately 20% represent Pfeiffer syndrome [23].

Craniofacial features include recessed supraorbital rims, frontal bone hypoplasia, maxillary hypoplasia, severe exorbitism, hypertelorism, down-slanting palpebral fissures and also convexity of the squamous portion of the temporal bones. The ears are displaced downward, the nasal bridge is low and the eyelids often fail to close, leading to corneal ulceration and venous distention of the scleras. Radiographically, the skull is trilobular, with a honeycomb appearance and a thin distorted vault.

Hydrocephalus is common, as well as psychomotor retardation, cerebellar hypoplasia and herniation, along with other brain anomalies [24]. Other malformations may include blindness, obstructed nasolacrimal ducts, facial clefting, cleft lip/palate, absent external auditory canals, PDA and ASD. Early death has been noted in most cases, with few surviving into adolescence, often due to airway abnormalities that may be present at multiple levels.

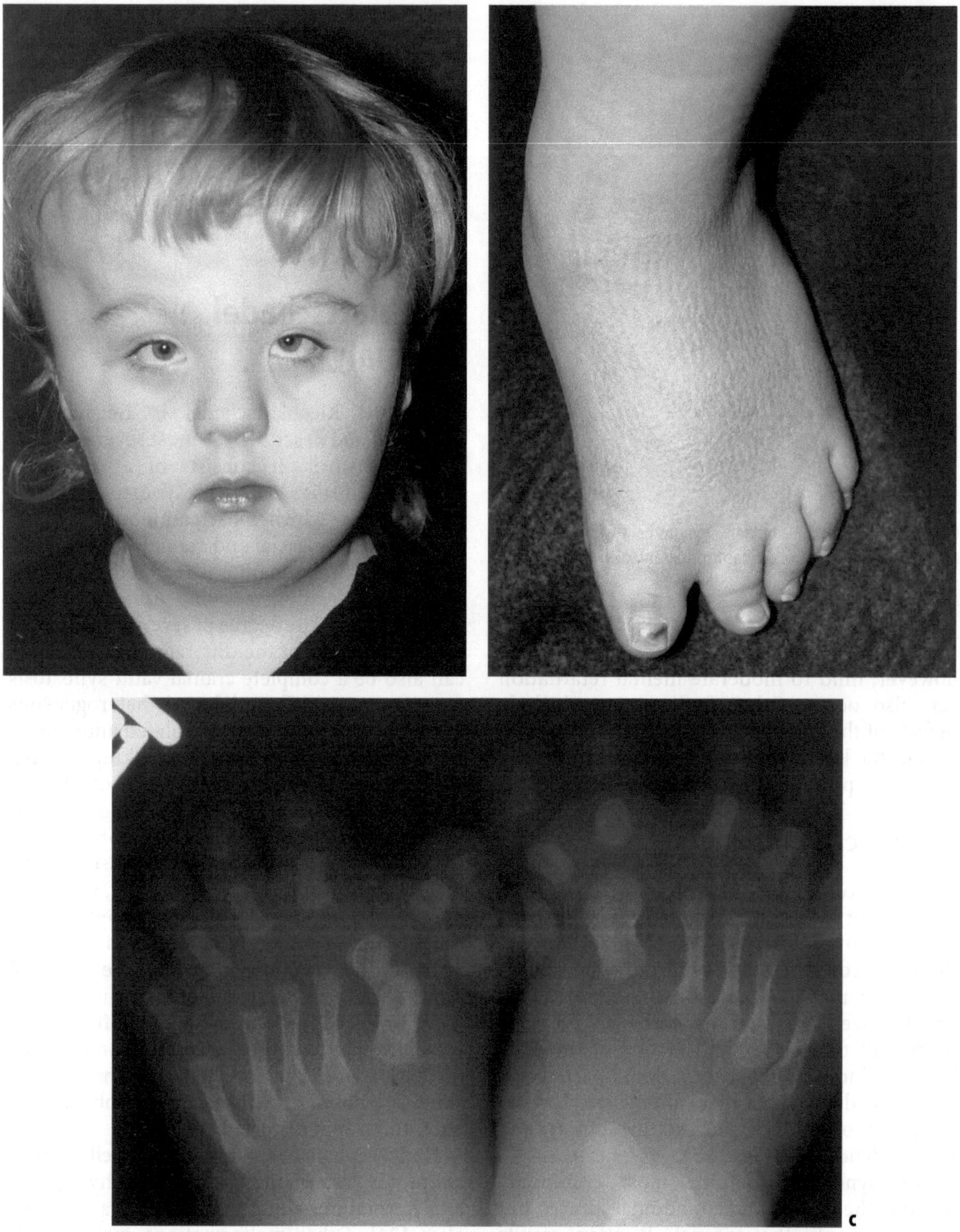

a b c

Fig. 26.5. a Carpenter syndrome with lambdoidal craniosynostosis, low-set ears, short neck, obesity, down-slanting palpebral fissures and epicanthal folds. **b** Carpenter syndrome, with brachydactyly of the phalanges and partial soft tissue syndactyly. **c** Carpenter syndrome, with polysyndactyly of the feet.

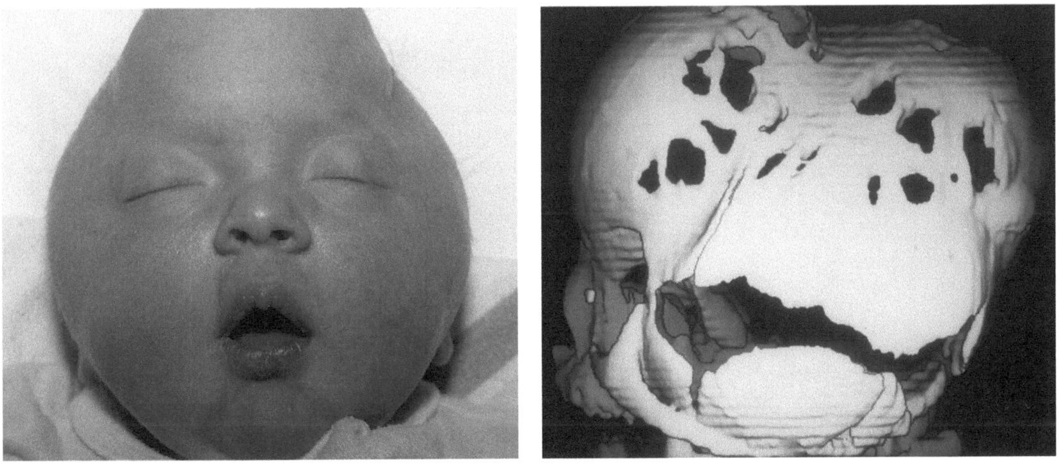

Fig. 26.6. Kleeblattschadel anomaly, with trilobuar skull.

Diagnosis and Clinical Evaluation

The comprehensive care of craniofacial patients requires the efforts of a multidisciplinary craniofacial team, including the pediatric neurosurgeon, craniofacial surgeon, geneticist, speech pathologist, nutritionist, orthodontist, oral surgeon, pediatrician, ophthalmologist and pulmonologist, in order to accurately diagnose, evaluate and treat their challenging problems. A careful history (including family, pregnancy and birth) and systemic evaluation, as well as a functional and aesthetic assessment, are vital to a successful outcome. Key physical-examination findings include height, weight, head circumference, head shape, head positioning, muscle tone, movements, airway noises, globe position, fundoscopic findings, intra-oral findings, facial morphology and extremity morphology. Imaging studies are an invaluable aid in evaluating patients with syndromic craniosynostosis. A skull series can help evaluate cranial sutures for signs of fusion; however, CT is more diagnostic in assessing the cranial vault as well as the brain. Three-dimensional reformatting can provide improved visualization of the deformity. MRI can provide a better view of the brain in assessing for signs of increased intracranial pressure.

Surgical Reconstruction

There are many different techniques and modifications of surgical procedures used to correct the deformities associated with syndromic craniosynostosis. There are also differences in opinion regarding the timing for the surgical corrections of the various anatomic regions. These complex problems require the close cooperation between the craniofacial surgeon, neurosurgeon and pediatric anesthesiologist. We will review the approach at the University of Virginia to the treatment of these deformities by anatomic region.

Early calvarial decompression for syndromic craniosynostosis is primarily directed towards release of the fused suture. In addition to this, frontal bone reshaping/advancement, superior–lateral orbital rim reconstruction with advancement of 10–20 mm and possible cranial vault reshaping, when necessary in cases of severe brachyturricephaly, can be accomplished (Fig. 26.7). Fixation of the osseous segments has evolved to resorbable fixation plates in all cases, in addition to using resorbable suture suspension. Synostotic suture release is indicated before 18 months of age and preferably in early infancy, before the first year of life. There are differences in opinion regarding the optimal time within the first year of life to perform this calvarial reconstruction, however. Some

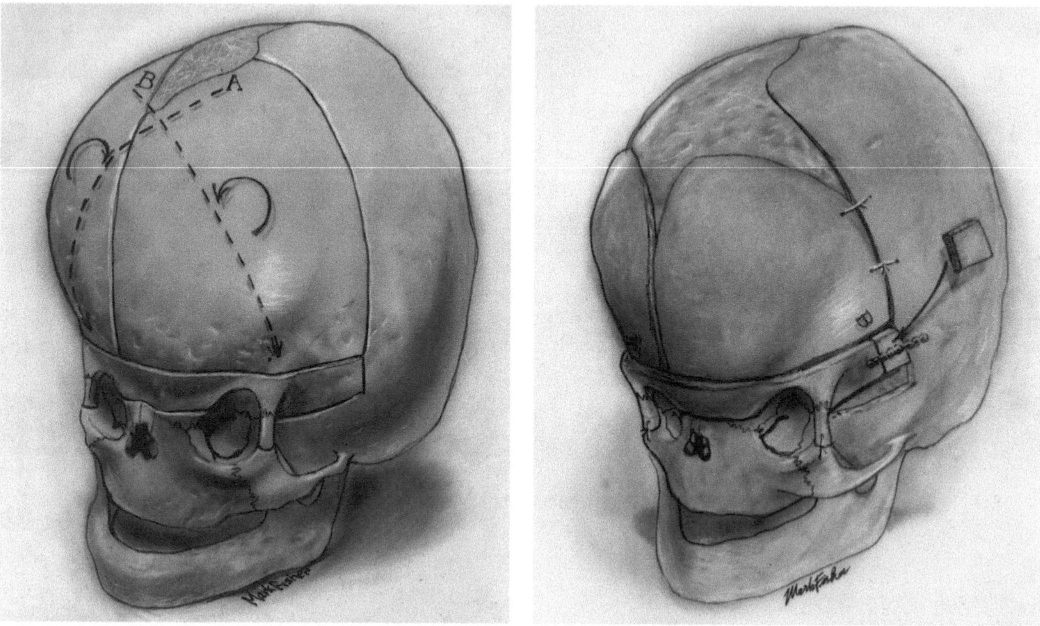

Fig. 26.7. Illustration demonstrating frontal–orbital advancement, with 180° rotation of the frontal bone flaps and fixation of the orbital bar, with resorbable plates in the area of bone graft.

advocate performing it before 6 months of age, in order to avoid compensatory changes in the skull, while others advocate between 6 and 12 months of age, in order to accomplish more effective fixation and avoid high re-operation rates. If, however, there is evidence of increased intracranial pressure or pansynostosis, sutural release is mandated in the neonatal period as soon as possible.

Mid-facial advancement may be performed alone through an extracranial LeFort III osteotomy or simultaneously with a frontal bone advancement as a monobloc unit. The timing of these procedures depends upon the facial morphology that results after primary fronto-orbital advancement. If the exophthalmos is severe or nasal obstruction is present, then a LeFort III advancement can be performed in early childhood (4–6 years of age). In most instances, it is performed in mid-childhood (7–14 years of age). If the supraorbital position is not acceptable with exorbitism or there is hypertelorism, then a monobloc or a staged fronto-orbital advancement performed in the early childhood years (4–6 years of age) followed by a LeFort III osteotomy in the mid-childhood years may be performed.

The fixation of osseous segments in monobloc and LeFort III procedures originally utilized wires and then rigid metallic plate fixation. These methods carried the risk of migration or extrusion of the fixation device as the child grew. Presently, distraction osteogenesis is performed, which utilizes a temporarily placed metallic fixation device that is activated daily (Fig. 26.8). This avoids the need for harvesting bone grafts and improves post-operative stability by slowly expanding the soft tissues, which reduces the potential for relapse. These devices will most likely be completely resorbable in the future, obviating the need to remove the device in a subsequent surgery, following an adequate consolidation phase.

The monobloc fronto-facial advancement can be used to correct severe orbital/mid-facial retrusion (Fig. 26.9). This procedure, however, carries the risks of prolonged surgery and higher infection rates, especially when performed with a midline osteotomy (bipartition) due to an opening between the nasal cavity and cranial vault. As a result, the monobloc is contraindicated in those patients with a shunt or with frontal sinus development. The advantage of a bipartition, which can be performed in a

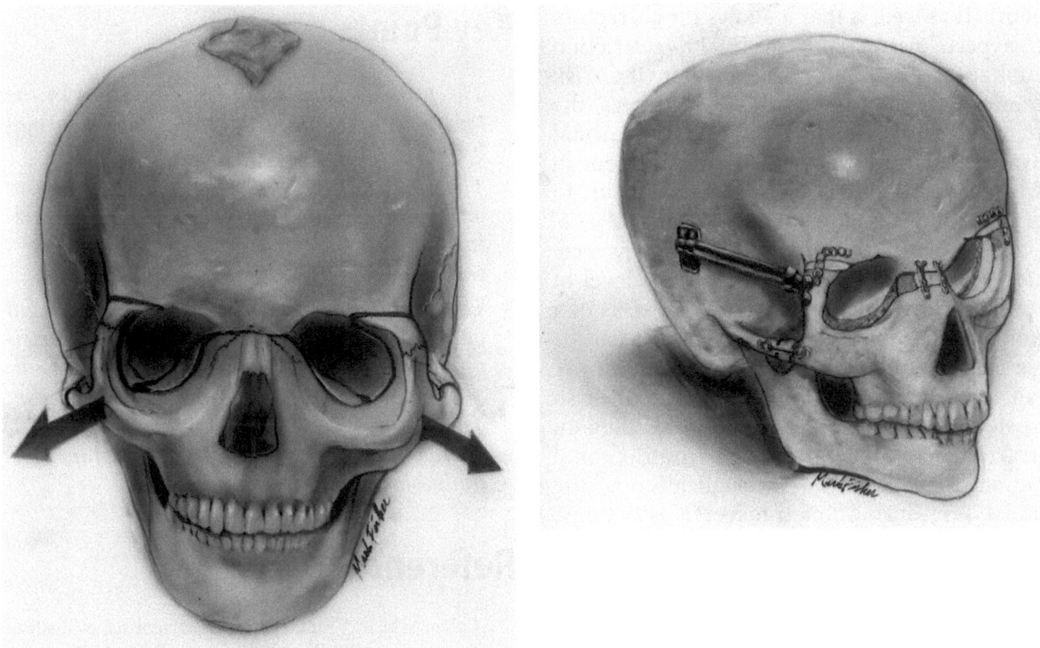

Fig. 26.8. Illustration demonstrating LeFort III advancement of mid-face, which can be fixated with either resorbable plates and bone grafts in advanced position or can be advanced over several weeks, with internal metallic distractor (also demonstrated).

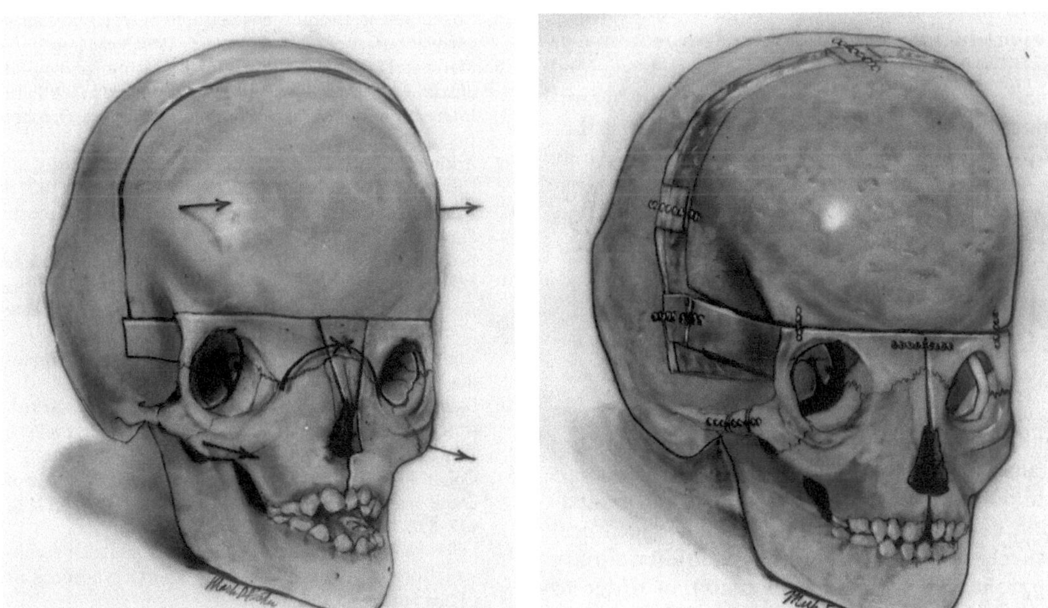

Fig. 26.9. Illustration demonstrating monobloc advancement of mid-face and frontal bone, performed through an intracranial approach.

LeFort III as well, is that it allows for correction of hypertelorism and maxillary restriction simultaneously. Some believe that the risk of infection and its inability to address the occlusion are reasons to stage fronto-orbital advancement and a LeFort III advancement in early and mid-childhood, respectively, or to perform them simultaneously.

The LeFort III procedure utilizes a transverse osteotomy at the nasal root below the level of the cranial base, in order to avoid the risks of a monobloc. The level of the cranial base can be assessed pre-operatively by a coronal-cut CT scan. If the cranial base is low, leading to the risk of osteotomizing into the cranial base, then an intracranial approach through a fronto-orbital craniotomy will allow for visualization of the cranial base during this transverse osteotomy. The intracranial approach also provides access to the lateral and superior orbital walls for osteotomies, if necessary. As mentioned earlier, a bipartition may be performed in a LeFort III procedure as well.

The occlusal relationship cannot be precisely controlled with the monobloc or LeFort III procedures. In addition, the patients are usually in a mixed dentition, with additional growth of the jaws remaining at the time of these procedures. As a result, orthognathic surgery, including a LeFort I and often a mandibular osteotomy, is performed during adolescence after skeletal maturity is complete. This is performed in conjunction with pre-surgical orthopedics/orthodontics for precise occlusal alignment. It may require segmental osteotomies to correct transverse and/or vertical disproportions, as well as residual cleft palate abnormalities, if present.

Conclusion

The treatment of syndromic craniosynostoses and its myriad of malformations and deformations is one of the most challenging areas of craniofacial surgery. The diagnosis and evaluation, as well as the strategy, timing and technical aspects of surgery, require a multidisciplinary approach in a craniofacial center in order to ensure that the individual needs of each patient are considered, to achieve the best outcome.

Key Points

- *The primary functional consideration in the treatment of craniofacial dysostosis is normal brain development.*
- *The goal of any reconstruction should be to address the immediate needs while minimizing the number of future surgical interventions.*
- *The comprehensive care of craniofacial patients requires the efforts of a multidisciplinary craniofacial team, including the pediatric neurosurgeon, craniofacial surgeon, geneticist, speech pathologist, nutritionist, orthodontist, oral surgeon, pediatrician, ophthalmologist and pulmonologist.*

References

1. Cohen MM Jr. Craniosynostosis: diagnosis, evaluation and management. New York: Raven Press, 1986.
2. Slavkin HC, Bonner JJ. Genetic control mechanisms during early oral facial development. In Stewart RE, Prescott GH, editors. Oral facial clefts. St Louis: CV Mosby, 1976; 1.
3. Higginbottom MC, Jones KL, James HE. Intrauterine constraint and craniosynostosis. Neurosurgery 1980; 6:39.
4. Cohen MM Jr. Craniosynostosis: phenotypic/molecular correlations. Amer J Med Genetics 1995;56:334–9.
5. Marchac D, Renier D. Functional and morphological outcome in 62 Apert's syndrome. Presented at the Fifth International congress of Craniofacial Surgery, October 1993, Oaxaca, Mexico.
6. Atkinson FRB. Hereditary craniofacial dysostosis, or Crouzon's disease. Med Press Circular 1937;195:118–24.
7. Kreiborg S. Crouzon syndrome. Scand J Plast Reconstr Surg 1981;(Suppl 18):1–198.
8. Erickson JD, Cohen MM Jr. A study of parental age effects on the occurrence of fresh mutations for the Apert syndrome. Ann Hum Genet (London) 1974;38: 89–96.
9. Tunte W, Lenz W. Zur Haufigkeit und Mutationstrates des Apert-syndroms. Hum Genet 1967;4:104–11.
10. Blank CE. Apert's syndrome: observations on a British series of thirty-nine cases. Ann Hum Genet 1969;24: 151–64.
11. Cohen MM Jr. An etiologic and nosologic overview of craniosynostosis syndromes. Birth Defects 1975;11(2): 137–89.
12. Lefebvre A. A psychiatric profile before and after reconstructive surgery in children with Apert's syndrome. Br J Plast Surg 1986;39:510–13.
13. Gorlin R, Cohen MM Jr, Levin L. Syndromes with craniosynostosis in syndromes of the head and neck. 3rd Edition. New York: Oxford University Press, 1990; 520–1.

14. Fishman MA. The concurrence of hydrocephalus and craniosynostosis. J Neurosurg 1971;34:621–9.
15. Pfeiffer RA. Dominant erbliche Akrocephalosyndaktylie. Z Kinderheilkd 1964;90:301–20.
16. Asnes RS, Morehead CD. Pfeiffer syndrome. Birth Defects 1969;5(3):199–203.
17. Cremers CWRJ. Hearing loss in Pfeiffer's syndrome. Int J Pediatr Otorhinolaryngol 1981;3:343–53.
18. Saldino RM. Familial acrocephalosyndactyly (Pfeiffer syndrome). Am J Roentgenol 1972;116:609–22.
19. Pantke OA, Cohen MM Jr, Witkop CJ Jr, Feingold M. The Saethre–Chotzen syndrome. Birth Defects 1975; 11(2):190–225.
20. Cohen MM Jr. Craniosynostosis and syndromes with craniosynostosis. Birth Defects 1975;15(5b):85–9.
21. Carpenter G. Two sisters showing malformations of the skull and other congenital abnormalities. Rep Soc Study Dis Child (London) 1901;1:110–18.
22. Temtamy SA. Carpenter's syndrome. Acrocephalopolysyndactyly: an autosomal recessive syndrome. J Pediatr 1966;69:111–20.
23. Hodach RJ. Studies of malformation syndromes in man. XXXVI. The Pfeiffer syndrome: association with Kleeblattschadel and multiple visceral anomalies. Z Kinderheilkd 1975;119:87–103.
24. Angle CR. Cloverleaf skull: Kleeblattschadel-deformity syndrome. Am J Dis Child 1967;114:198–202.

27

Spinal Dysraphism

Simon Stapleton

Summary

Spina bifida represents a spectrum of conditions of disordered development of the spine and spinal cord. In its most severe form - open myelomeningocele - the neurological deficits can be profound, with implications for repeated and lifelong management, although, with the concerted effort of a multidisciplinary team, the outlook for quality of life may be good. The incidence of this condition is declining and may be reduced further with the introduction of periconceptual folic acid supplements.

Less obvious forms of spina bifida occur and may not be immediately apparent at birth - occult spinal dysraphism - although there may be cutaneous manifestations of the underlying condition. The concept of "tethering" of the spinal cord by a dysraphic condition has proved useful in the understanding of the generation of symptoms and in the rationale for treatment of these disorders.

Introduction

The term "spinal dysraphism" covers a range of developmental conditions of the spinal cord and its surrounding structures. Often also referred to as either spina bifida or neural tube defects, spinal dysraphism is sufficiently all-encompassing to allow for the scope and complexity of these conditions, which the other two terms fail to convey. Spinal dysraphism includes both conditions obvious at birth or before, such as myelomeningocele (spina bifida aperta), and conditions of the spine which may or may not be apparent on closer inspection. This latter group includes so-called occult dysraphism (spina bifida occulta), when the only hint of an underlying spinal abnormality may be a cutaneous lesion or the development of orthopedic or urological symptoms.

Substantial progress has been made in the understanding and management of these conditions in recent years. Effective treatment of hydrocephalus and the multidisciplinary approach to the needs of children with myelomeningocele have led to improvement in the outlook for those affected. The realization of the importance of tethering as a mechanism for deterioration in dysraphic states has meant an improvement in the management of these conditions, directed at the underlying neurological problem, rather than the acceptance of inevitable deterioration. A fall in the incidence of dysraphic lesions, improvements in diet and the use of preconception folic acid, as well as a better understanding of the genesis of these conditions, will hopefully mean that fewer children are affected in the future.

Epidemiology

Estimates of the true incidence of neural tube defects occurring in pregnancy are difficult to ascertain, since a proportion of severely affected fetuses are undoubtedly aborted spontaneously, early in pregnancy. Nevertheless, worldwide, the prevalence of neural tube defects occurring at birth appears to be falling. This can be partly attributed to screening programmes and possibly to improvements in nutrition, but the rate also seems to be declining for unexplained reasons. In the UK, the prevalence throughout the country is falling from an overall level of approximately 4 per 1,000 live births in the 1970s to in the region of 0.3 per 1,000 live births now. There remains a significant geographical variation in the prevalence of cases in this country, with the highest rates occurring in the west of the country, namely in western Scotland, Wales and Northern Ireland, where the incidence may be more than twice as high as elsewhere, but the incidence in these areas is also falling. Elsewhere in the world, the prevalence rates are generally lower, ranging down to about 1 in 10,000 in sub-Saharan Africa.

There is a significant genetic component to the development of neural tube defects, since, if either parent has had an affected child or if either parent is affected by the condition, there is an approximately 10% risk of further offspring having a neural tube defect. If two affected pregnancies occur, the risk to a further pregnancy is increased about 20-fold. Secondary prevention of further affected pregnancies requires screening techniques, including alphafetoprotein sampling and ultrasound, with selective termination of affected pregnancies. Primary prevention, however, requires the prevention of neural tube defects occurring in the embryo in the first place, even in pregnancies not at higher risk of such an occurrence. Since the 1960s, it has been recognized that women with an affected pregnancy had significantly lower red cell folate levels than those with unaffected pregnancies. The Medical Research Council Vitamin Study of 1991 [1], in which women who had had a previous pregnancy affected with a neural tube defect were randomized to receive folic acid (4 mg daily) or placebo, with or without other multivitamin supplements, demonstrated that the rate of affected subsequent pregnancy was significantly reduced in the folic acid group (relative risk 0.29). It is now, therefore, recommended that in order to prevent a recurrence of a neural tube defect in subsequent pregnancies, 5 mg daily of folic acid should be supplemented to the diet prior to conception. In order to prevent a first occurrence of a neural tube defect, all women should be advised to take 400 mg of folic acid daily prior to conception, as well as increasing their dietary intake of foods rich in folic acid, continued until the 12th week of pregnancy (food high in folate includes green vegetables, yeast, beef extract and breakfast cereals fortified with folic acid) [2].

Etiology

There is clearly a familial tendency to the development of neural tube defects, although this is probably a polygenic mechanism. Siblings of an affected individual have an approximately ten times greater chance of also being affected (2.5% vs approximately 0.2% risk in the general population – see above). The children of healthy siblings of an affected child are known also to be at increased risk.

Nutritional factors are thought to play a role and may explain partly the social class differences in incidence. The use of preconception folic acid stems from the concept that low maternal folate intake is implicated in the etiology of neural tube defects (see above). Numerous teratogens have been identified in animal models, including anticonvulsants such as valproate and phenytoin, other folate antagonists such as aminopterin, hypervitaminosis A, alcohol and mitomycin C. The extent to which these factors operate in humans remains uncertain.

Recently, abnormalities in homeobox genes have been implicated in the genesis of neural tube defects in mice. In particular, the human analogue of the mouse Pax3 gene has been identified. It is unknown, however, whether this is a sine qua non in humans [3].

Embryology

Under normal circumstances, development of the neural tube proceeds as follows. The supposed relevant deviations from this related to specific forms of dysraphism are described in the appropriate section.

The primitive streak develops at the caudal end of the bilayered embryonic disc by developmental day 14. From the primitive streak, cells migrate between the layers of ectoderm and endoderm to form the embryonic mesoderm. Hensen's node is located at the cranial end of the primitive streak and, from here, the notochordal process develops in a cranial direction between the two embryonic layers by day 17. The solid notochord becomes a hollow cylindrical structure, which transiently fuses with the underlying layer of endoderm. There exists, therefore, a communication between the amniotic cavity dorsally and the yolk sac ventrally via the primitive pit, known as the neurenteric canal. This communication closes as the notochord again separates from the endoderm by day 20. At this time, Hensen's node and the primitive streak regress with growth of the embryonic disc, in a caudal direction, ultimately to lie in the low sacral or coccygeal region.

The notochord induces the overlying ectoderm to thicken and cells heap up to form the neural plate. The neural groove develops in the neural plate, producing lateral folds which ultimately meet in the midline as the neural groove deepens, to form the neural tube. This is the process of primary neurulation. Closure of the neural tube begins in the mid-thoracic region and extends both cranially and caudally. At the cranial end of the neural tube (the future lamina terminalis), closure of the anterior neuropore occurs by day 24, while closure of the caudal or posterior neuropore occurs by day 28. The location of the posterior neuropore is a matter of some debate but probably lies in the region of L1 or L2. Caudal to this level, development of the spinal cord does not occur by primary neurulation. In this region, Hensen's node and the primitive streak give rise to an undifferentiated clump of cells known as the caudal cell mass, destined to form the conus medullaris and the filum terminale. This occurs by a rather poorly defined process – secondary neurulation – of vacuolation, condensation and subsequent fusion to the spinal cord formed by primary neurulation. The significance of this process in the human remains rather uncertain.

As the process of primary neurulation occurs, the ectoderm lateral to the developing neural plate fuses in the midline to cover the neural tube, while embryonic mesoderm from the sclerotome at each level of the embryo migrates towards the midline to surround the notochord and the neural tube to give rise ultimately to the vertebral bodies and neural arches, as well as the dural sheath. The process of secondary neurulation (vacuolation, condensation and fusion of the caudal cell mass) occurs after the overlying ectoderm has fused to form the skin.

Myelomeningocele

This is the single most common form of spinal dysraphism and is synonymous with spina bifida aperta or an open neural tube defect. It is the most severe form of spinal dysraphism and presumably represents a failure of closure of the neural tube at approximately day 21 of development (primary neurulation).

Clinical Presentation and Assessment

Unless detected antenatally by ultrasound or maternal screening, open myelomeningocele is immediately apparent at birth (Fig. 27.1). This manifests usually as a defect on the back, with evidence of a neural placode representing the open spinal cord, often with normal- and

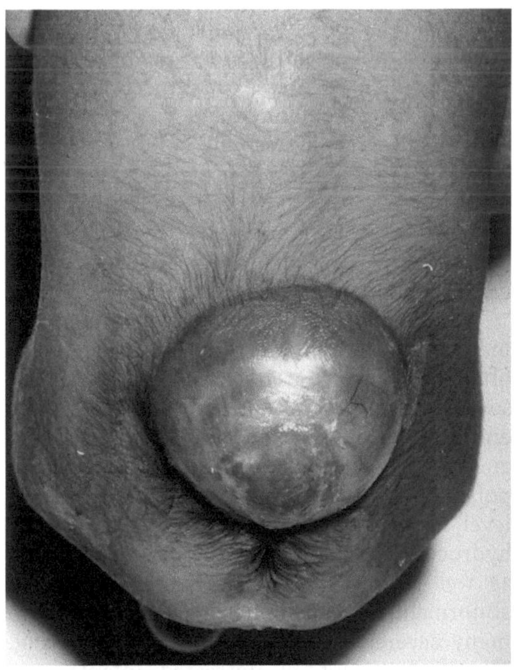

Fig. 27.1. Myelomeningocele in the lumbar region of a neonate. Note the cystic appearances, with fragile blood vessels visible.

abnormal-appearing nerve roots coursing from it ventrally and surrounded by arachnoid adhesions, an incomplete dura and associated paravertebral soft tissues. The central canal of the spinal cord may be visible at the rostral end of the placode; the defect may be covered by a thin epithelial or arachnoid layer, but this may have ruptured and CSF will be seen to leak from the defect.

There may be associated developmental anomalies, usually of the nervous system. Most infants will develop hydrocephalus and a Chiari II malformation is very common. Abnormalities of cerebral gyration, of the posterior fossa contents and agenesis of the corpus callosum, as well as associated vertebral anomalies, may also occur. Unsuspected, more rostral "occult" forms of dysraphism may coexist.

Delivery of an infant with a suspected open myelomeningocele should be by Cesarean section, in order to avoid the risk of infection during passage along the birth canal; the child should be nursed on its front or side, with a sterile moist dressing covering the defect, and kept warm. Having examined the defect itself, clinical assessment aims at determining the neurological deficit, both sensory and motor. Much of this can be done by observation and gentle stimulation of the limbs to ascertain sensation and movement. Bladder and bowel function are difficult to assess with any certainty but a good urine stream may suggest an incomplete deficit, although almost all children will go on to have some degree of bladder and bowel disturbance. Further examination is directed towards possible associated congenital anomalies and hydrocephalus, as well as general cardiopulmonary status.

Without closure of the myelomeningocele, meningitis is likely to develop within a few days, often with fatal consequences. In view of the severe, often devastating neurological deficits and the poor outlook for a fulfilling, self-caring and dignified existence, Lorber [4] proposed a policy of selective non-treatment, based on the level of the lesion, the severity of associated hydrocephalus and degree of spinal deformity, as well as the presence of other congenital abnormalities. This policy has clearly led to many severely affected infants not surviving. Nevertheless, not all untreated infants succumb, with the effect that they may go on to survive, with more severe disabilities than had they been treated initially. McLone [5–7] has presented evidence that, with a concerted multidisciplinary team approach whereby all open myelomeningoceles are closed at birth, the overall outcome with respect to mortality, intellect and mobility is not improved by selective non-treatment.

Surgery for open myelomeningocele is aimed at protecting the existing neural structures and preventing infection. Surgery will not restore neurological function; nevertheless, it is essential to preserve any functioning nervous tissue that does exist. Because of the risk of infection, closure of the defect should be carried out within 48 hours of birth. Closure of the defect involves defining the neural placode and freeing this from arachnoid adhesions. Some surgeons reconstitute the neural tube by folding over and suturing the neural placode in an attempt to prevent future cord tethering; however, this procedure is not essential and may unnecessarily damage the delicate existing nervous tissue if the sutures are inappropriately placed. It should be ensured that there are no skin appendages attached to the placode. The extradural space is identified, the dura is mobilized and this plane developed around the defect to allow closure of the dura in a watertight fashion. If necessary, a dural graft may be required to close the dura, without compromising the neural structures and maintaining the closure free from tension The muscle and fascia on either side of the defect are mobilized; this may require lateral releasing incisions if the defect is large, and then approximated. The skin is then closed in a watertight manner. For very large defects, plastic surgical procedures with myofascial or cutaneous flaps may be required to achieve adequate closure. At all stages of the closure, it is essential that the tissue layers are not approximated under tension, otherwise wound breakdown and CSF leakage will occur.

Approximately 80% of children with myelomeningocele will require a shunt at some stage. For those with obviously severe hydrocephalus, this may need to be carried out within several days of closure of the spinal defect. For those children less severely affected, observation, with head circumference measurements and assessment of signs of raised intracranial pressure, will dictate the need for and the timing of shunt insertion. The majority of children who will need a shunt will do so by the age of 5 months [8].

Long-term Care and Outcome in Open Myelomeningocele

The long-term care and follow-up of children with myelomeningocele requires the input of many disciplines, preferably in a combined multidisciplinary clinic devoted to the management of children with spina bifida and its complications. This will include assessment of all aspects of physical, as well as cognitive, development.

Overall survival with myelomeningocele after the first 4 years appears to stabilize at approximately 85% [6], although there continues to be a significant mortality. This can be related to many of the associated problems faced by these children, including hind-brain disturbance, causing respiratory distress, apneic spells and gastro–esophageal reflux with tracheal aspiration, shunt malfunction and infection, and bladder and renal problems.

Myelomeningocele itself does not appear to have a significant impact on intelligence. Although the average IQ of affected children is below the mean, the majority fall within the normal range, with only 9% having an IQ score below 70 in McLone's series, followed up for over 15 years. Factors which do seem to affect intelligence include initially severe hydrocephalus, neonatal ventriculitis and shunt infections, as well as the level of the lesion. Hydrocephalus and Chiari malformations presumably also account for the consistently found deficits in fine motor function in the upper limbs and in visuo–spatial processing, as well as changes in age-related language ability. Two-thirds of children, with appropriate support, can be kept in mainstream education. Ultimate employment opportunity seems to be related more to intellectual ability than to physical disability [9].

Numerous factors contribute to mobility. The ability to walk will depend not only upon the level of motor and proprioceptive deficit, but also on factors such as spasticity, deformity, ataxia and obesity, as well as intelligence, support and motivation. In McLone's series, 75% of surviving children by school age were mobile without a wheelchair; nevertheless this figure declines with age [10], largely due to increasing difficulty and effort required to maintain posture, especially with weight increasing proportionately faster than strength.

Again, bladder and bowel continence depends chiefly upon the level of the neurological lesion. Most children manage the bladder with clean intermittent catheterization and many are able to perform this for themselves. Management of the bowel depends upon a combination of bulk laxatives and enemas, avoidance of constipation and the use of a Shandling catheter [11].

The long-term care and assessment of children with myelomeningocele requires attention to many details of their development, with particular scrutiny for the possible complications which may arise in time. From a neurological perspective, aside from the ever present risk of shunt malfunction and Chiari malformation and syringomyelia-induced problems, this will include the possibility of cord re-tethering.

Re-tethering of the spinal cord (see below) following closure of a myelomeningocele or after any other "untethering" operation, such as after surgery for lipomeningocele, should be considered in any child with a clinical deterioration. Re-tethering may manifest as a deterioration in motor power or gait, pain, altered sensation or deformity in the legs, or with changes in bladder function. Increasing scoliosis has also been considered to result from re-tethering.

Most neural placodes or lipomas probably adhere to the dura soon after the initial operation; however, it is only with continued traction on the cord that symptoms are likely. Re-tethering remains a clinical diagnosis, since static MRI will only show the location of the conus, rather than its mobility.

Re-operation to release the cord should be considered in any child with a significant clinical deterioration. There are often dense adhesions and thick scar, making surgery difficult, and consideration to expanding the dura with a patch should be given. The results of surgery are reported to be gratifying in that most children can be stabilized and pain is often improved [12].

"Occult" Spinal Dysraphism

The term "occult dysraphism" implies that the presence of the dysraphic condition is not immediately apparent, as it is in "open" myelomeningocele. This may or may not be so at birth, but most dysraphic conditions of the spine become apparent in one way or another in childhood or adolescence. The diagnosis may be suspected at birth by the presence of a lumbosacral lipoma or cutaneous lesion with abnormal pigmentation in the midline. Commonly, infants are referred with a sacral dimple with a question as to the presence of a dysraphic condition. Shallow dimples, tethered inferiorly, in the natal cleft are generally innocent. Any midline dimple above the natal cleft should be treated with suspicion, particularly if there is any history of discharge. Cutaneous lesions often have abnormal pigmentation and may have an associated hairy patch.

Other manifestations of "occult" dysraphism include orthopedic problems such as scoliosis, pes cavus or inequality of calf girth or foot size. Neurological abnormalities such as leg weakness or numbness are common presentations, usually with variable loss of lower-limb reflexes. In older children, adolescents and adults, sensory abnormality in the feet may lead to trophic changes, with smooth, shiny skin and occasionally with ulcers which are slow to heal. The child may be referred as being generally clumsy on his or her feet. Disturbances of bladder or bowel function are also seen frequently. Constipation requiring regular laxatives and delay in toilet training may be apparent after the age of 5 years, when the child may still not be dry by day as well as by night. There may be evidence of a poor urinary stream and frequent urinary tract infections. Pain as a feature of spinal dysraphism is uncommon in children but is a frequent occurrence in adults either with a known dysraphism or who may present for the first time in adulthood (see below).

Occult dysraphism may be suspected at birth by the presence of a visible abnormality but frequently presents during subsequent periods of rapid spinal growth, at approximately age 6 years and in adolescence. Occasionally, presentation may occur acutely at times of excessive spinal motion, such as in sporting activities, after being placed in the lithotomy position, after childbirth and as an unsuspected underlying condition following surgical correction of scoliosis. Such modes of presentation support the idea that symptoms and signs in dysraphic conditions are the result of "tethering" of the spinal cord by the underlying abnormality, preventing the normal ascent of the spinal cord and conus relative to the bony spine during postnatal growth and development. Coupled with the repeated stretching of an already "taut" cord during everyday activity, this leads to neurological dysfunction and the development of the associated orthopedic and urological features.

Spinal Cord Tethering

Central to an understanding of the development of symptoms in occult dysraphism is the concept of spinal cord tethering. This is a dynamic problem with the spinal cord and cannot therefore be identified per se on static imaging such as MR or CT. Nevertheless, that tethering may exist can be inferred by the presence of an abnormality such as a lipoma, bony spur or thickened filum terminale, producing an abnormally long spinal cord with a low-lying conus. The implication is that the cord has been held in its original position and prevented from ascending within its thecal sac during growth of the individual. There are a number of possible explanations of why this should lead to neurological dysfunction:

- sustained traction on the cord with growth of the bony spine leads to stretching of the cord itself and disruption of neuronal function;
- ischemia of the cord leads to abnormalities of oxidative metabolism [13];
- repeated hyperflexion (e.g. during sporting activities) of the spine causes acute injury to neuronal processes at the level of the tethering lesion.

Attempts have been made to "visualize" tethering clinically using MR CSF pulsatility studies [14] or to demonstrate motion of the conus using CT myelography in both prone and supine positions, but the diagnosis remains a clinical one, based on the presence of a presumed tethering lesion and evidence of neurological dysfunction.

If tethering is the underlying cause of neurological deterioration in many dysraphic conditions, the principle of surgical treatment is to untether the spinal cord and to prevent it retethering. This is generally achieved by removing the tissue responsible for the tethering or detaching the spinal cord from it, as described in the specific sections below.

Tight Filum Terminale

The simplest and perhaps the most easily imagined form of spinal cord tethering is that produced by a thickened, fatty, filum terminale. This may present with asymmetric neurological or orthopedic abnormalities in the lower limbs and is well seen on sagittal and axial T1-weighted MRI as high signal within the filum associated with a low-lying conus. Treatment simply involves division of the filum, ensuring that no nerve roots are attached to it. On occasion, at operation, the proximal end of the filum may spring out of view superiorly, providing convincing evidence of the tethering process.

Lipomeningocele

Lipomeningocele is an abnormality of the spine characterized by a low-lying conus medullaris, infiltrated with fatty tissue, which extends through a bony dysraphic defect and into the subcutaneous tissues. It is thought to occur as a result of an abnormality of secondary neurulation of the caudal cell mass, whereby pluripotential mesenchymal cells fail to regress and may lead to lipomas, hamartomas and teratomas in the lumbosacral region. The lipoma is invariably covered by skin but may have pigmentation, hair or cutaneous dimples on it. They often lie asymmetrically across the midline in the lumbosacral region and can reach a very large size. Intradurally, the lipoma may be attached to the dorsal surface of the cord or it may be inserted into the terminal end of the conus. The lipoma may enlarge in infancy or may be associated with obesity. Although uncommon, lipomeningoceles may be associated with other developmental anomalies, including syringomyelia, Chiari malformation and anal and genitourinary malformations. The lesion is considered to lead to tethering of the spinal cord, thereby producing symptoms.

The cutaneous abnormality is frequently obvious at birth but, in the past, has not always been recognized for what it is. Progressive, often asymmetrical neurological deterioration in the legs is a common mode of presentation, as well as discrepancies in foot size and leg length in older children. Bladder and bowel dysfunctions are also frequent complaints. As with other forms of dysraphism, pain tends to be a feature in adulthood. Similarly, acute neurological deterioration has been described.

The approach to treatment of lipomeningocele depends largely upon the perceived natural history of the condition. Arguments in favor of prophylactic untethering include the fact that many infants appear to be neurologically normal, whereas most adolescents and adults present with some neurological deficits. In one study [15], all children were symptomatic by the age of 4 years. The condition therefore appears to carry a high risk of progressive deterioration, while the risks of surgery remain relatively low. Once neurological deficits or orthopedic deformity have occurred, they tend not to be reversible, even with surgery, and there is a background risk of acute deterioration and paraplegia without surgery. For these reasons, many neurosurgeons consider untethering the cord before the age of 6 months or do so as soon as the lesion is recognized thereafter [16,17]. Counter to this argument is the fact that not all children with lipomeningoceles do deteriorate as demonstrated by the occasional unsuspected adult presentation; that surgery does carry some risk of neurological damage; and that acute paraplegia in the absence of any preceding symptoms is rare. Added to this is the frequent problem of re-tethering after surgery. There has therefore been a reappraisal of the need for early prophylactic untethering and consideration of surgery only at the onset of the development of symptoms. This requires close and regular assessment of all patients with lipomeningoceles, to detect any neurological change [18,19]. There is little argument over the place of surgery in preventing further deterioration in those presenting with progressive neurological deficits. Recently, Chumas [20] has summarized these arguments and emphasized the need for long-term follow-up of all these patients if a consensus is to be achieved.

Pre-operative assessment requires careful neurological examination of the legs and urodynamic assessment. MRI in the sagittal plane clearly demonstrates the lesion (Fig. 27.2a) and will also show an associated hydromyelia. Axial images reveal the relationship of the lipoma to the cord itself (Fig. 27.2b).

Surgery is aimed at untethering the spinal cord, reducing the bulk of the lipoma and reconstituting the dura to enable the conus to lie freely. This may require a dural patch to try to

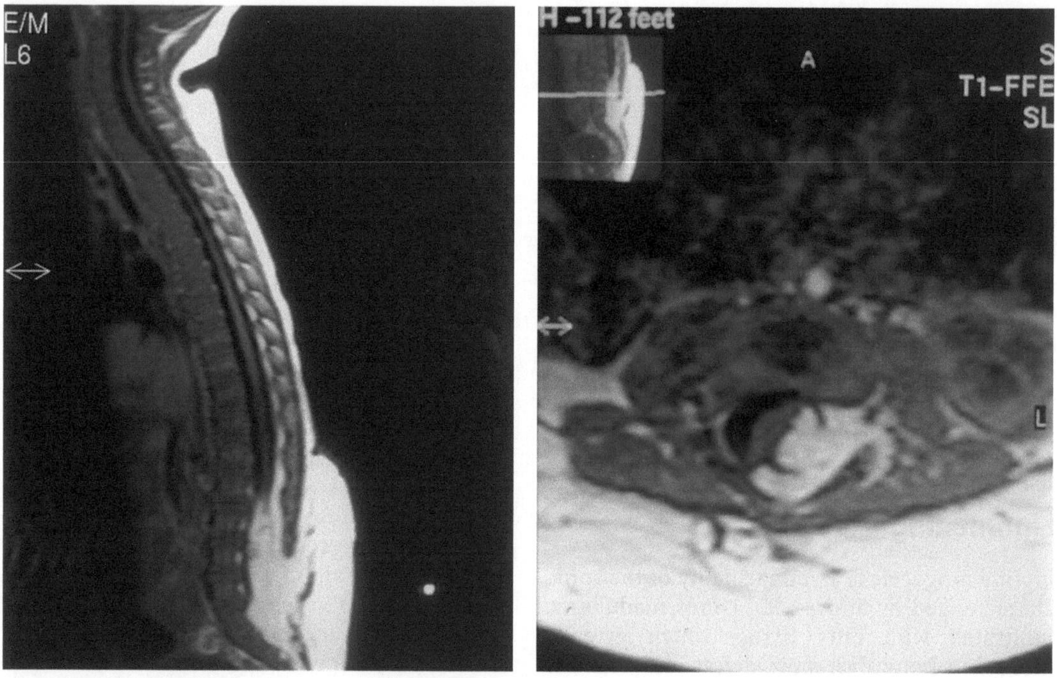

a b

Fig. 27.2. **a** Lumbar lipomeningocele. Sagittal T1-weighted MR scan, demonstrating a low-lying conus associated with a lipomeningocele. The spinal cord ends in a lipoma, which itself is continuous with the subcutaneous tissues and is coupled with a defect in the lumbar laminae. **b** Lumbar lipomeningocele. Axial T1-weighted MR image, revealing the relationship between the conus and the lipoma itself.

prevent re-tethering by local scar tissue. Surgery is generally carried out through a midline incision, although plastic surgical considerations may need to be taken into account in large lesions. The first normal lamina above the lesion is identified and the dura here exposed. The dura is then opened to expose the attachment of the lipoma to the cord and the opening continued around the exiting fatty defect. The line of fusion of the lipoma with the cord can then be identified and, with the exiting nerve roots anterior to this line, the lipoma can be detached. The bulk of the lipoma can then be removed and the dura closed, ensuring that the mobility of the conus is not compromised by the closure. The frequent difficulty in obtaining a satisfactory dural closure leads to the two chief complications of the procedure: CSF leakage and re-tethering. The former is generally manageable with CSF drainage and re-suturing, if need be. The latter may become apparent within months or many years of the initial surgery and is characterized by the onset of neurological deterioration or pain. Since the conus, following even successful surgery, may not change position on MRI studies, re-tethering can be difficult to prove radiologically and re-exploration may be necessary on clinical grounds alone (see above).

Surgery carries a low risk for neurological deterioration (less than 5%) and appears to prevent the subsequent development of neurological deficits. In those with clinical signs of tethering, surgery appears to be effective at preventing further deterioration and, for early intervention, may reverse some of the neurological dysfunction. For long established deficits with orthopedic deformity, surgery will not lead to improvement but can effectively prevent a worsening deficit.

Split Cord Malformations

"Split cord malformation" is a term used to describe a number of congenital abnormalities of the development of the spinal cord and its coverings, characterized by a division of the cord into two, not always equal, parts. The general term "split cord malformation" is preferable to the potentially confusing terms used to describe the conditions often referred to as diastematomyelia and diplomyelia. The abnormality may take the form either of a division of the spinal cord within a single dural sac (diplomyelia, type II split cord malformation) or of splitting of two hemicords, each with its own dural covering, by a septum, usually made up of a bony spur and/or fibrocartilagenous band (type I split cord malformation).

The embryological origin of split cord malformations remains unclear. The presence of two hemicords within a single dural tube has been considered to occur as a result of a doubling of the neural tube without fibrous tissue dividing the cords and therefore without the potential for causing tethering. On the other hand, two hemicords, each with its own dural sheath and surrounding bony structures, have been thought to be due to splitting of the notochord by an interposed adhesion between the primitive endodermal and ectodermal layers or of incomplete persistence of an accessory cranial neurenteric canal. This leads to a septum splitting the cord and, with growth, tethering as the bony spine lengthens relative to the cord itself. However, Pang has considered that all split cord malformations represent a spectrum of a single abnormal embryological process [21,22]. This is characterized by the formation and persistence to a variable degree of an abnormal connection between the endodermal and ectodermal layers of the embryo, resulting in an endomesenchymal tract. The endomesenchymal tract results in the independent development of two heminotochords and two hemineural tubes. The degree to which the invading mesoderm (future meninges) is associated with the endomesenchymal tract between the two developing neural tubes affects the extent to which the two future hemicords are split. If both hemicords are each surrounded by invading mesoderm, then two separate dural tubes result, with associated bony and fibrocartilaginous tissue producing the dividing spur. Pang has termed this the "split cord malformation type I". If the mesoderm of the future meninges is not associated with the endomesenchymal tract dividing the hemicords, then a single dural sac is created, with only thin sagittal fibrous bands, representing the remains of the endomesenchymal tract, attaching the hemicords to the dural sleeve. This Pang terms the "split cord malformation type II". The implication here is that both types of split cord malformation represent tethering lesions and therefore both require surgical exploration in order to prevent subsequent neurological deterioration.

Split cord malformations are characteristically associated with a midline hairy patch or "horse's tail". This is much more commonly found in split cord malformations than with other forms of "occult" dysraphism (Fig. 27.3). There may occasionally be an associated dermal sinus or pigmented skin lesion. The spur is generally found in the lumbar or lower thoracic region. Clinically, this may produce one leg with muscle wasting or sensory loss, with or without orthopedic manifestations, such as pes cavus. One or both ankle jerks are often absent. There may be involvement of the bladder and bowels, particularly in those children presenting in early adolescence. Scoliosis may also occur, as may other vertebral anomalies. The anatomy of the defect is demonstrated on MRI scans; particularly well seen on axial imaging are the two hemicords. Once the level has been established,

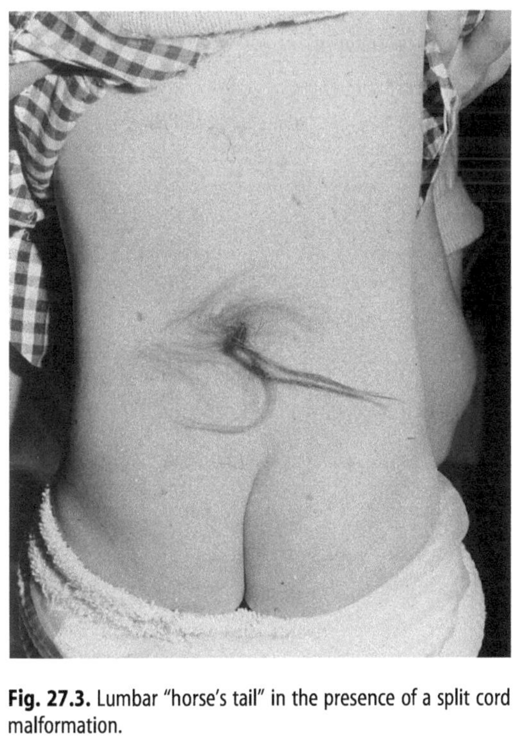

Fig. 27.3. Lumbar "horse's tail" in the presence of a split cord malformation.

and this may not be the level of the cutaneous stigma (an important point preoperatively), CT scanning with intrathecal contrast may demonstrate a bony spur. Nevertheless, with modern MRI, CT myelography is generally no longer necessary.

Neurological deterioration in split cord malformations is generally considered to be a result of tethering, although associated lesions such as hydromyelia may contribute. The aim of surgery, therefore, is to remove the bony or fibrocartilaginous spur and to excise the dural sleeve surrounding it. In cases with separate dural tubes, each containing a hemicord (type I split cord malformations), the tethering spur is found at the caudal end of the divided dural tube (Fig. 27.4a). The cutaneous mark may not necessarily lie over the bony abnormality but there is usually an abnormal lamina present. Surgery involves identifying the lowermost normal lamina and then carrying out a laminectomy of the abnormal lamina below, it usually being necessary to include the lowermost normal lamina. The spur is then isolated and removed down between the two dural tubes. The stalk and surrounding epidural veins can bleed briskly and this should be anticipated. Once the stalk has been removed, the dura is opened around the cleft, revealing the hemicords, which usually unite just below the location of the spur. Pang emphasizes the importance of dividing any fibrous bands and median nerve roots, which are non-functioning, coursing dorsally to tether the hemicords. These bands may continue to the subcutaneous tissues, forming the entity known as a meningocele manqué [23]. The dural sleeve around the spur should be excised to ensure that the union of the hemicords is free to “ride up”. It is not necessary to close the ventral dura but the

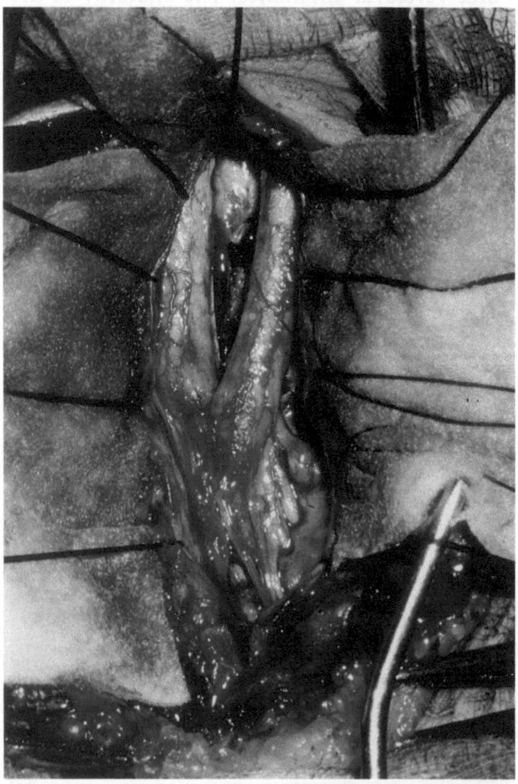
a

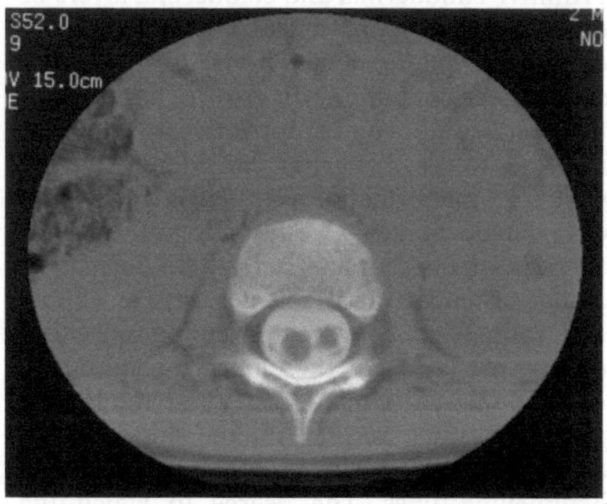

b

Fig. 27.4. a Type I split cord malformation at operation. The two dural tubes containing the hemicords unite just below the dividing spur, with associated nerve roots visible. **b** Type II split cord malformation. Two hemicords visible within a single dural tube on CT myelography. The lateral nerve roots are well seen.

dorsal dura may need a patch to obtain satisfactory closure without constriction of the intradural contents. Since the hemicords usually unite below the spur, a single, thickened filum terminale may be present. This should be sought and divided through a separate incision inferiorly, if necessary.

Two hemicords within a single dural tube (type II split cord malformations) generally do not require surgical exploration unless there is evidence of a thickened filum or of dorsal intradural fibrous bands (Fig. 27.4b). Pang, however, argues that all these malformations should be explored since, in all 18 of his reported cases, intradural tethering bands were found, even in their apparent absence on preoperative investigations. This is clearly an area which awaits further clarification.

Congenital Dermal Sinus

Infants are frequently referred to the pediatric neurosurgeon with a midline spinal dimple, occasionally with discharge from the tract. This may be the initial presentation of many congenital dermal sinuses but a significant number present with meningitis due to skin or gut organisms. Multiple episodes of meningitis may even occur before the diagnosis is made, since the cutaneous opening of the tract may be minute. Nevertheless, meningitis due to organisms such as Staphylococcus aureus or Escherichia coli in an infant rather than a neonate should arouse suspicion and, particularly after recurrent episodes, a concerted effort to identify a sinus tract should be made. The opening may be anywhere along the midline of the spine and may even occur in the occiput.

Many infants are referred with a dimple in the natal cleft, fixed inferiorly. These are generally innocent and should not be explored surgically because of their benign nature and, if surgery is carried out, they almost always become infected.

The congenital dermal sinus is an epithelial-lined tract that may end in the soft tissues or may extend deeper, to be attached to or penetrate the dura; may end in the subarachnoid space; or, more commonly, be attached to the filum terminale and end at the conus medullaris. There may be inclusion dermoid material, forming a mass anywhere along the tract.

There is rarely any neurological deficit, unless a dermoid cyst has compressed local nerve roots or meningitis has caused a deficit. MRI scanning reveals the extent of the tract and any associated dysraphic abnormality (Fig. 27.5). Contrast media or probes should not be inserted along the tract.

Surgical excision of the tract is indicated both because this may be a tethering lesion and because of the risk of meningitis. This should be carried out without undue delay. If meningitis occurs, this should be treated as appropriate first, and only when the inflammation has resolved should surgery be undertaken. Once meningitis has occurred, the tract and subarachnoid spaces may be scarred, making the operation technically more difficult.

The object of surgery is to excise the tract in its entirety. This involves excising its cutaneous orifice and following this to its termination. This may require opening the dura and excision of the attachment to the filum terminale. Any associated dermoid cyst, either intradural or extradural, should also be excised.

Complete excision achieves a cure and neurological outcome is generally very good, with few, if any, long-term problems [24].

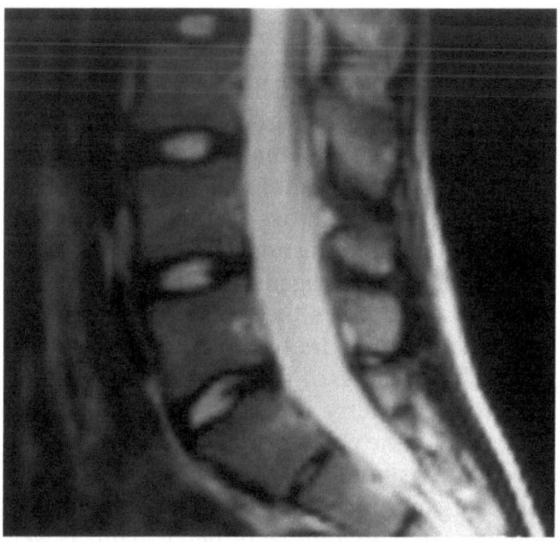

Fig. 27.5. Sagittal T1-weighted MR image of a 14-year-old boy with a congenital dermal sinus entering the theca at the L4 level. He had had two episodes of staphylococcal meningitis prior to referral.

Neurenteric Cyst

Neurenteric cysts are epithelial-lined cysts derived from the neurenteric canal, which transiently connects the embryonic yolk sac with the amniotic cavity during the third week of embryonic development (see "Embryology" section). Due to the endodermal origin of the cyst lining, gastrointestinal or respiratory epithelium may be found and associated abnormalities of the gut, respiratory tract and vertebrae may occur. Such cysts (also called, for this reason, enterogenous cysts) tend to present as intradural extramedullary lesions situated ventrally in the cervical region. They may also be found in the thoracic region, where a dorsal intradural location is more often seen. Clinically, these lesions generally present in adolescence or early adulthood with neck pain and spinal cord compression, causing a cervical myelopathy. MRI scanning reveals the cyst and its location, allowing surgical excision, which can usually be achieved from a posterior approach. Even if a complete excision cannot be achieved safely, due to dense attachments to the cord or nerve roots, partial excision and cyst drainage provide lasting benefit, since re-accumulation is extremely slow. The prognosis for improvement in neurological function is generally very good.

Anterior Sacral Meningocele

An out-pouching of dura containing CSF may occur through a defect in the body of the sacrum (anterior spina bifida). This may be an isolated defect or may be in association with a more severe developmental abnormality of the whole caudal region of the embryo, as in caudal agenesis, where abnormalities of the genitourinary tract, rectum and anus may also occur in association with sacral agenesis. Presumably, the defect in the bone is the primary abnormality and, with the pressure of CSF, the meningocele gradually enlarges. The meningocele may contain sacral nerve roots. As the meningocele enlarges into the pelvis or retroperitoneal space, it produces symptoms of compression of the pelvic organs, including constipation, urinary frequency and abdominal or pelvic pain, as well as low back pain. Anterior sacral meningoceles are more common in females and may present as an incidental mass identified on pelvic examination or ultrasound. The diagnosis is established by CT myelography, which will confirm the connection with the spinal theca and reveal the bony anatomy well. MRI scanning will demonstrate the presence of the mass and its relationship with the pelvic organs, but may not identify the neck of the sac. It is important to distinguish these masses from other pelvic masses such as an ovarian cyst or other tumor, and, similarly, no attempt should be made to aspirate the cyst through a potentially infected area.

Symptomatic cysts are best treated by sacral laminectomy, aspiration and ligation of the cyst neck. If access is not possible posteriorly, an abdominal approach may be indicated, but it is not necessary to excise the meningocele wall. Asymptomatic cysts may require no treatment, although progressive enlargement with time may be expected.

Spinal Dysraphism in Adults

Adult patients with spinal dysraphism include those with new symptomatic onset of a previously unsuspected occult dysraphic condition and those with a known dysraphic lesion in childhood but with symptom onset only in adulthood. In both groups, unlike in childhood, pain is the most frequent presenting symptom. This may be poorly localized and bilateral, and coupled with weakness in the legs as well as sensory disturbance. Problems with bladder control, as well as erectile dysfunction, also occur frequently. Not infrequently, the problem only comes to light as a result of excessive stretching of the conus, as may occur in childbirth or trauma [25]. In those with a known dysraphic lesion, presentation in adulthood may be with a progressive scoliosis or foot deformity, although these features are generally not seen in an adult with a previously unsuspected dysraphism.

There is often no cutaneous clue to an underlying dysraphic lesion, which may take the form of a thickened or tight filum, or an intradural lipoma, as well as containing dermoid material.

As for childhood dysraphism, surgical untethering is recommended for symptomatic adults. This usually involves division of the filum or release of adhesion and debulking of a lipoma.

Pang and Wilberger [25] have reported very satisfying improvements in pain following surgery in adults, with reasonably good results for motor and sensory improvement but, as in childhood, bladder and bowel dysfunction tends not to improve significantly with surgery. Surgery for fixed orthopedic deformities does not improve, although it may prevent progressive deterioration

Key Points

- *The incidence of open myelomeningocele is in decline.*
- *Periconceptual folic acid supplements reduce the risks of neural tube defects.*
- *A combined multidisciplinary team approach can lead to a good long-term outlook for patients with open myelomeningocele.*
- *Midline cutaneous lesions should raise the suspicion of an underlying occult spinal dysraphism.*
- *"Tethering" of the spinal cord is considered to be the underlying mechanism for the development of clinical problems in most occult dysraphism and the surgical approach to treatment, therefore, has been aimed at "untethering" the spinal cord.*

References

1. The MRC Vitamin Study Group. Prevention of neural tube defects: results of the Medical Research Council Vitamin Study. Lancet 1991;238:131–7.
2. Folic acid and the prevention of neural tube defects. Report from an expert advisory group. Department of Health, 1992.
3. Goulding M, Paquette A. Pax genes and neural tube defects in the mouse. In: Boch G, Marsh J, editors. Neural tube defects. CIBA Foundation Symposium. Number 181. Chichester, UK: John Wiley, 1994; 103–17.
4. Lorber J. Results of treatment of myelomeningocele: an analysis of 524 unselected cases, with special reference to possible selection for treatment. Dev Med Child Neurol 1971;18:279–303.
5. McLone DG, Dias L, Kaplan WE, Sommers MW. Concepts in the management of spina bifida. In: Humphreys RP, editor. Concepts. Pediatr Neurosurg 1985;5:97–106.
6. McLone DG. Continuing concepts in the management of spina bifida. Pediatr Neurosurg 1992;18:254–6.
7. McLone DG. Treatment of myelomeningocele and arguments against selection. Clin Neurosurg 1986;33: 359–70.
8. Rekate HL. To shunt or not to shunt? Hydrocephalus and dysraphism. Clin Neurosurg 1984;32:593–607.
9. McAndrew I. Adolescent and young people with spina bifida. Dev Med Chld Neurol 1979;21:619–29.
10. McLone DG. Disorders of the pediatric spine. Pang D, editor. New York: Raven Press Ltd, 1995; Chapter 9, 137–57.
11. Shandling B, Gilmour RF. The enema continence catheter in spina bifida: successful bowel management. J Pediatr Surg 1987;22:271–3.
12. Herman JM, McLone DG, Storrs BB, Dauser RC. Analysis of 153 patients with myelomeningocele or spinal lipoma reoperated upon for a tethered cord. Pediatr Neurosurg 1993;19:243–9.
13. Yamada S, Iacono RP, Andrade T, Mandybur G, Yamada BS. Pathophysiology of tethered cord syndrome. Neurosurgery Clin North America 1995;6(2):311–23.
14. McCullough D, Levy L, DiChiro G et al. Toward the prediction of neurological injury from tethered spinal cord: investigation of cord motion with magnetic resonance. Pediatr Neurosurg 1990;16:3–7.
15. Hoffman HJ, Taecholarn C, Hendrick EB, Humphreys RP. Management of lipomyelomeningoceles. J Neurosurgery 1985;62:1–8.
16. LaMarca F, Grant JA, Tomita T, McLone D. Spinal lipomas in children: outcome of 270 procedures. Pediatr Neurosurgery 1997;26:8–16.
17. McLone D. Occult dysraphism and the tethered spinal cord. In: Pediatric Neurosurgery, 1999; 61–78.
18. Zerah M, Pierre-Kahn A, Catala M. Lumbosacral lipomas. In: Pediatric Neurosurgery, 1999; 79–100.
19. Pierre-Kahn A, Zerah M, Renier D et al. Congenital lumbosacral lipomas. Childs Nerv Syst 1997;13:298–335.
20. Chumas PD. The role of surgery in asymptomatic lumbosacral spinal lipomas. Brit J Neurosurg 2000;14:301–4.
21. Pang D, Dias MS, Ahab-Barmada M. Split cord malformation: Part I: A unified theory of embryogenesis for double spinal cord malformations. Neurosurgery. 1992 Sep;31(3):451–80.
22. Pang D. Split cord malformation. Part II: clinical syndrome. Neurosurgery 1992;31:481–500.
23. James CCM, Lassman LP. Spinal dysraphism: spina bifida occulta. London: Butterworths, 1972.
24. Kanev PM, Park TS. Dermoids and dermal sinus tracts of the spine. Neurosurg Clin N America 1995;6(2): 359–66.
25. Pang D, Wilberger JE Jr. Tethered cord syndrome in adults. J Neurosurg 1982;57:32–47.

28

Pediatric Neuro-oncology

Kevin L. Stevenson, J. Russell Geyer and
Richard G. Ellenbogen

Summary

Tumors of the CNS are, as a group, the second most frequent malignancy of childhood and the most common solid tumor in this age group. In this chapter, the epidemiology, clinical presentation, surgical considerations, chemotherapy and radiation therapy options regarding pediatric brain tumors will be reviewed. In addition, we will specifically focus on several of the major categories of pediatric CNS malignancy and the late effects resulting from current treatment regimens.

Introduction

Tumors of the CNS are, as a group, the second most frequent malignancy of childhood and the most common solid tumor in this age group. In general, children with brain tumors have not shared in the remarkable improvement in prognosis that has characterized other childhood malignancies. In this chapter, the epidemiology, clinical presentation, surgical considerations, chemotherapy and radiation therapy options regarding pediatric brain tumors will be reviewed. In addition, we will specifically focus on several of the major categories of pediatric CNS malignancy and the late effects resulting from current treatment regimens. In conclusion, the future directions in pediatric brain tumor management will be discussed.

Epidemiology

CNS tumors represent approximately 17% of all malignancies in the pediatric age range, including adolescents. Approximately 2,000 children younger than 20 years of age are diagnosed annually with tumors of the CNS [1]. Brain tumors in childhood are a heterogeneous group. Astrocytomas are the most frequent, accounting for approximately 52%, while primitive neural epidermal tumors account for approximately 21%, ependymomas 9% and other tumor types represent the remaining 15%. While in older children and adults the most frequent site of malignant brain tumors is supratentorial, young children have a relatively high occurrence of tumors in the cerebellum and brain stem. The incidence of CNS tumors is greater in those children younger than 8 years of age - approximately 35 cases per million children - than it is in children from 8 to 17 years of age - approximately 20 per million [1].

Over the last two decades, CNS cancer incidence in children appears to have increased. While this has provoked concern that there may be changes in environmental exposures responsible for this increasing incidence, epidemiologic evidence to support this hypothesis is lacking. Alternatively, the increase in incidence could be related to improving diagnostic technology. There are several known risk factors predisposing to the development of CNS tumors in childhood. Therapeutic doses of radiation utilized in the treatment of leukemia or previous brain tumors are clearly implicated as a risk factor. Patients with several inherited genetic conditions have greatly increased risk of brain tumors, specifically neurofibromatosis, tuberous sclerosis and the Li–Fraumeni syndrome. Taken as a whole, these known risk factors account for a small percentage of pediatric brain tumors; for the great majority of brain tumors in childhood, there is no specific risk factor known to be related to their incidence.

Medulloblastoma/Primitive Neuroectodermal Tumor

PNETs of the CNS are a group of embryonal tumors that histologically comprise poorly differentiated neural epithelial cells. These tumors occur predominantly, though not exclusively, in childhood and constitute approximately 20–30% of all childhood brain tumors [1]. This group of tumors shares the biologic propensity of dissemination throughout the subarachnoid space, in addition to recurrence or progression at the primary site.

Tumors of this histology are most common in the posterior fossa and, in this location, are commonly called medulloblastomas (Fig. 28.1a). However, tumors that histologically appear identical to those found in the posterior fossa can occur in other locations throughout the CNS, where they are referred to as supratentorial PNETs, pineoblastomas in the pineal region and retinoblastomas in the eye [2]. While PNETs of the posterior fossa and of other sites share a common histologic appearance and a similar propensity for a pattern of metastases, the issue of whether these tumors share a common origin in biology remains quite controversial [2]. Recent studies examining the

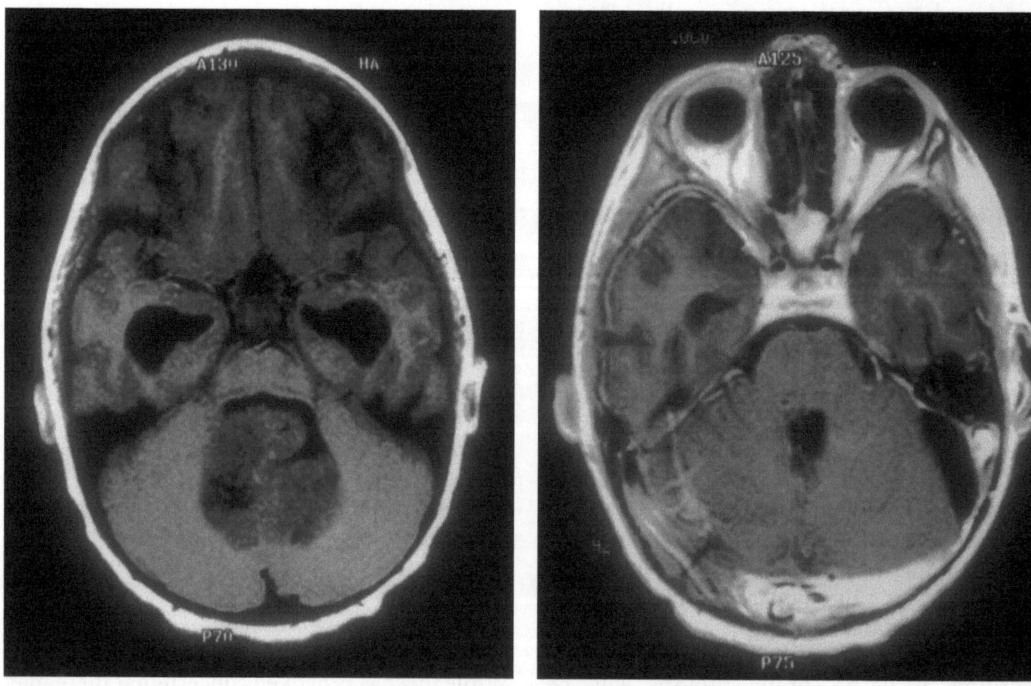

a b

Fig. 28.1. **a** Axial MRI (T1), showing moderately sized medulloblastoma. Typical of medulloblastomas, this tumor involves the roof of the fourth ventricle, without invading the floor. Also note the markedly enlarged temporal horns of the lateral ventricles. **b** Post-operative axial gadolinium-enhanced MRI (T1), showing resection of the fourth ventricular tumor, as well as resolution of hydrocephalus.

molecular biology of these tumors suggest that there may be differences, in spite of the common histologic appearance. Nonetheless, treatment strategies over the last decade have combined supratentorial PNETs and medulloblastomas.

Clinical Presentation

The vast majority of children with medulloblastomas present with signs and symptoms of hydrocephalus: headache, nausea, vomiting and lethargy. It should be kept in mind that this symptom triad is not unique to medulloblastomas; any posterior fossa tumor can produce this symptom complex. Headaches tend to be worst in the morning upon awakening, and are often accompanied by nausea. Vomiting will often temporarily decrease or eliminate the headache, perhaps due to hyperventilation-induced hypocarbia. It is not uncommon for children to have several months of headache, nausea and/or vomiting prior to diagnosis. During this time, more common etiologies of these symptoms are often investigated, including migraines, primary gastrointestinal disorders, and even psychiatric disorders. In addition to hydrocephalus, etiologies of lethargy in medulloblastoma include dehydration and direct brainstem compression/invasion by the primary lesion. Other common signs and symptoms of medulloblastomas include papilledema, ataxia, dysmetria and diplopia. As 15–20% of children with medulloblastomas will have spinal disease ("drop metastases") at the time of diagnosis [3], back pain may uncommonly be the initial complaint.

Surgery

Despite advances in the non-surgical management of medulloblastomas, surgical resection remains the primary initial treatment of these tumors. In addition to providing histologic diagnosis and relief of tumor burden, surgical resection of medulloblastomas can provide immediate relief of neurologic signs and symptoms due to hydrocephalus and direct brainstem compression. Because 90% of children present with hydrocephalus, and up to 30% will require chronic CSF diversion [4], an EVD is inserted prior to tumor resection, regardless of the degree of hydrocephalus present on imaging. More recently, endoscopic third ventriculostomy may be another appropriate approach to relieving the block of CSF flow at the level of the aqueduct of Sylvius. Typically arising from the roof of the fourth ventricle, medulloblastomas invade the floor of the ventricle in up to 36% of cases [5]. Unlike ependymomas (discussed later), tumor residual in the brainstem does not adversely affect outcome [6] and most pediatric neurosurgeons will resect the tumor flush with the floor of the fourth ventricle, without entering the brainstem (Fig. 28.1b). Adjuvant technology, such as the operating microscope, intraoperative cranial nerve/SSEP monitoring and post-resection intraoperative ultrasound are essential in our institution for achieving the goal of radical resection of these tumors. For staging purposes, a lumbar puncture can be performed with the child still anesthetized. In these authors' experiences, immediate lumbar puncture after tumor resection does not lead to false-positive results.

Radiation Therapy and Chemotherapy

Recognition that metastatic failure throughout the sub-arachnoid space was second only to local recurrence as a site of failure in children with medulloblastoma led to the use of cranio-spinal radiation as adjuvant treatment by the mid-1950s. Several clinical studies demonstrated a dose–response relationship in regard to the dose of radiation required to control disease at the primary site, with doses of less than approximately 5,000 cGy resulting in higher rates of failure [7]. Until recently, however, the cranio-spinal dose–response relationship was unclear, but, by convention, most children received doses from 3,000 to 3,600 cGy. Following surgical resection and cranio-spinal radiation at these doses, durable survival was reported in approximately 30–50% of children by the mid-1970s.

Two large co-operative trials treating children with medulloblastoma were conducted in the late 1970s: one by the Children Cancer Group (CCG), in the USA, and one by the Society of International Pediatric Oncology (SIOP), conducted in Europe [8,9]. In both studies, patients were randomly assigned to receive irradiation alone or irradiation plus adjuvant chemotherapy, which, in both studies, consisted of vincristine and lomustine. More than 500 patients were accrued between the two studies and the 5-year-of-entry survivals of approximately 50% in both studies were very similar. Overall, neither study demonstrated survival advantages of the use of adjuvant chemotherapy. However, chemotherapy did show a benefit in subgroups of patients in both the CCG and SIOP studies. Those with partial resection brainstem involvement and large tumors and the other patients with extensive disease, i.e. large tumors and sub-arachnoid metastases, had superior survival when treated with adjuvant chemotherapy in addition to irradiation. These studies delineated a group of patients at higher risk for disease progression, i.e. those with larger partially resected tumors and those with metastatic disease at diagnosis, and confirmed the value of adjuvant chemotherapy for this high-risk group. As a result of these studies, post-surgical staging of the subarachnoid space, initially with myelogram and more recently with gadolinium-enhanced MRI has become standard, as has the use of adjuvant chemotherapy in the patients at high risk.

The issue of appropriate dose of neuraxis irradiation was addressed in a prospective study conducted by the Pediatric Oncology Group (POG) and the CCG in the mid-1980s [10]. In this study, children with medulloblastoma without high-risk features were randomly assigned to receive either standard-dose irradiation to the neuraxis (3,600 cGy) or reduced-dose irradiation (2,300 cGy). All children received a total dose of posterior fossa irradiation of 5,400 cGy. In the final analysis, eligible patients receiving standard-dose neuraxis irradiation had a 67% event-free survival at 5 years, while those patients receiving reduced neuraxis had only a 52% event-free survival at 5 years. Thus, at least when used as the only adjuvant treatment modality, the dose of cranio–spinal irradiation has been defined as 3,600 cGy. Unfortunately, this same study demonstrated that, at least for those children younger than 8 years, treatment with the higher dose of neuraxis radiation resulted in greater intellectual morbidity than those treated with the lower dose. Efforts to develop treatment approaches that allow a lower dose of radiation to be administered to the neuraxis continue to be investigated.

As noted above, the first randomized studies demonstrated that the addition of adjuvant chemotherapy to neuraxis radiation was of benefit for those patients at higher risk of tumor progression, i.e. those with significant residual post-operative tumor and those with metastatic disease. A number of single-arm studies, as well as randomized studies, have been conducted in an effort to optimize adjuvant chemotherapy. In a single-institutional study, children with medulloblastoma and high-risk features were treated with standard-dose cranio–spinal irradiation, as well as with CCNU, vincristine and cisplatin. The 5-year progression-free survival was greater than 70% [11]. A randomized trial in the CCG compared adjuvant therapy with CCNU, vincristine and prednisone with a multiple-drug regimen, which included vincristine, CCNU and cisplatin. Overall, the study demonstrated a 5-year progression-free survival in patients with non-metastatic disease of greater than 70% but those children with metastatic disease had an approximately 40% event-free survival at 5 years [12]. In addition, in this study, the complex regimen was clearly inferior to the two-drug regimen. In an attempt to improve survival outcome for children with average-risk medulloblastoma, as well as to effectively utilize reduced-dose neuraxis irradiation, a study treated children with average-risk disease with reduced-dose radiotherapy (2,300 cGy), as well as vincristine, cisplatin and CCNU.

The 5-year event-free survival from this study was approximately 80%, suggesting that reduced-dose neuraxis radiation can be safely employed if combined with adjuvant chemotherapy [13]. An ongoing, randomized trial in the Childrens Oncology Group (COG) is comparing two regimens of chemotherapy, both in the context of reduced-dose neuraxis radiation for those children with average-risk medulloblastoma.

The survival outcome of children with high-risk medulloblastoma, particularly those with metastatic disease, remains poor. Ongoing trials are investigating the role of high-dose chemotherapy with stem cell rescue in combination with standard irradiation. Another trial is investigating the concomitant addition of carboplatin with the radiation in an attempt to radiosensitize the tumor.

Successful treatment of children with recurrent medulloblastoma remains problematic, with the 2-year survival rate following initial relapse being less than 10% in most studies [12]. High-dose chemotherapy with stem cell rescue has shown promise in limited studies as a salvage regimen for those children with local recurrence; this appears to be of limited benefit in those with sub-arachnoid metastatic recurrence.

Astrocytomas

Astrocytomas account for approximately 50% of CNS tumors in childhood. Of these, approximately 10–20% are high-grade astrocytomas and thus the majority are low-grade astrocytomas.

High-grade Astrocytomas

High-grade astrocytomas represent a rare group of primary brain tumors in children. While the majority of pediatric astrocytomas occur in the posterior fossa, the minority are high-grade, representing 4–8% of all cerebellar astrocytomas [14,15]. Supratentorial astrocytomas, while less common than those in the infratentorial space, are more likely to be pathologically high-grade, with 20% of all hemispheric tumors being high-grade gliomas [16]. Anaplastic (WHO Grade III) gliomas histologically show marked nuclear pleomorphism, anaplasia and hyperchromasia, with variable degrees of mitoses and endothelial proliferation, while glioblastoma multiforme (WHO Grade IV) displays similar characteristics, with areas of necrosis.

Low-grade Astrocytomas

The low-grade astrocytomas of childhood can be further sub-divided into pilocytic astrocytomas, which account for approximately 75% of the group of low-grade astrocytomas, and other histologies, including fibrillary, protoplasmic and gemistocytic tumors, make up the remaining 25%. Pilocytic astrocytomas are histologically composed of fusiform astrocytes, loosely interwoven in a fine fibrillary background. These tumors frequently have a microcystic component, Rosenthal fibers and large macrocysts. While the most common location of pilocytic astrocytomas is in the cerebellum (Fig. 28.2), they can be found in other locations within the CNS, notably the visual pathway and optic chiasm, the brain stem and the cerebral cortex. The biologic behavior of these pilocytic tumors can be quite indolent and, in fact, spontaneous cessation of growth, as well as regression without treatment, has been observed. More commonly, however, these tumors progress slowly and present with symptoms

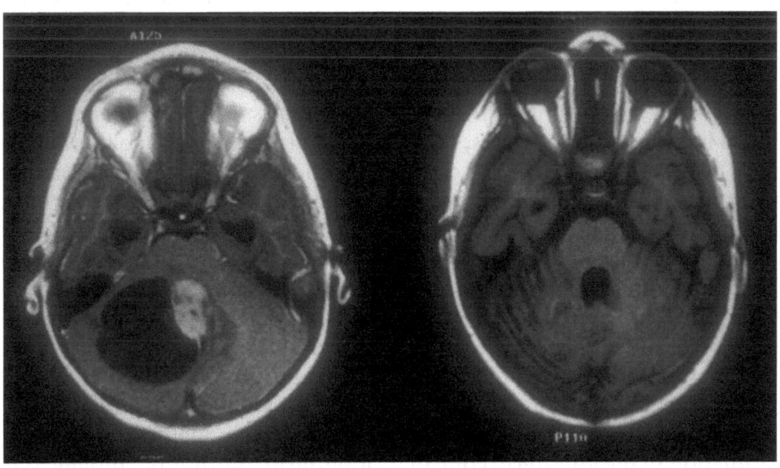

Fig. 28.2. (Left) Axial gadolinium-enhanced MRI (T1), showing a vermian juvenile pilocytic astrocytoma. Typical of pilocytic astrocytomas, the majority of the mass effect is due to the large cyst, while the enhancing solid portion contributes much less. (Right) Post-operative axial MRI (T1) after gross total resection of the solid portion of the astrocytoma. As the cyst wall is not composed of tumor cells, it is unnecessary, and potentially morbid, to resect the cyst wall.

characteristic of their site of origin, i.e. hydrocephalus and ataxia for those of the posterior fossa and visual abnormalities associated with those tumors of the visual pathway, including the optic chiasm.

Management

In general, complete resection of pilocytic astrocytomas results in long-term disease control in the great majority of patients. For example, resection of cerebellar pilocytic astrocytomas has resulted in more than 95% of the patients being free of disease 5 years from the time of surgical intervention in most series. Therefore, adjuvant therapy following gross total resection of these tumors is not indicated. The natural history of pilocytic astrocytomas was the subject of a recent large co-operative group trial. In this study, patients with low-grade astrocytomas, principally pilocytic astrocytomas, who underwent a complete surgical resection were observed. The progression-free survival at 5 years was 85%. Those patients who were unable to undergo a complete resection were observed and did not, in most instances, receive either adjuvant radiation or chemotherapy. The 5-year progression-free survival for this group of patients was 60%. Thus, while progression following a subtotal resection, or no resection, of pilocytic astrocytomas occurs much more frequently than is observed following gross total resection, it is by no means inevitable. Therefore, achieving a gross total resection at the expense of significant morbidity is not indicated in the management of these tumors. Furthermore, given that a substantial proportion of patients do not inevitably progress, even following limited or no resection, it is not clear that adjuvant radiation or chemotherapy is required for these patients. In the asymptomatic patient, serial observations, including neuroimaging, is often employed, withholding adjuvant therapy for clear evidence of either neurologic or radiographic progression. Should progression of subtotally resected or unresectable pilocytic astrocytomas occur, a number of studies have demonstrated the value of involved field radiation in the long-term control of these tumors [17]. In one study, 5-year progression-free survival was greater than 90%, as was 10-year progression-free survival. Thus, involved field radiation therapy remains important adjuvant therapy for the treatment of progressive pilocytic astrocytomas.

Inasmuch as these tumors often occur at a very young age, particularly those tumors originating in the visual pathway and chiasm, concern over the late effects of radiation therapy has led to investigation of alternative modalities of treatment, when required. Initial trials of chemotherapy with vincristine and dactinomycin were modeled on treatment protocols utilized for non-CNS low-grade tumors and demonstrated tumor stabilization and, in some cases, initial tumor regression in patients with tumor recurrence after radiation therapy and subsequently in newly diagnosed patients with progressive disease prior to radiation therapy. Subsequent protocols have utilized other alternative chemotherapeutic regimens. The largest data set exists for the use of carboplatin and vincristine. In a prospective study of these agents in children with progressive low-grade astrocytomas (primarily of the visual pathway), the 3-year progression-free survival was over 50% [18]. Subsequent resumption of tumor growth after several years is not uncommon and radiation can be then employed, but it is hoped that delaying radiation therapy for even several years in a very young child might ameliorate late toxicities. Currently, a randomized trial comparing carboplatin and vincristine to a multi-drug regimen consisting of vincristine, procarbazine, thioguanine and CCNU is being evaluated within the COG. While the utility of delaying radiation therapy in the younger child is reasonably clear, the benefits of such an approach in adolescents are less obvious. Nonetheless, utilization of chemotherapy either as front-line or salvage therapy in the instance of progression of low-grade astrocytoma in the adolescent should be considered. Children with low-grade astrocytomas, particularly those with pilocytic histology, can have a chronic course, requiring multiple interventions. A principle guiding therapeutic intervention should be that of minimizing morbidity. Therefore, avoiding adjuvant therapy in the asymptomatic patient without demonstrated progression, utilizing the modality of treatment with the least long-term morbidity initially (i.e. chemotherapy) and avoiding rapid institution of a therapy change based on minimal changes in imaging studies are important strategies. The long-term outcome in terms of survival for these tumors is good but the potential for significant morbidity, both as a result of progressive disease, i.e. visual loss in the case of those patients with visual pathway tumors, or morbidity related to therapy, is considerable and requires ongoing management by an experienced neuro-oncology team. Non-pilocytic low-grade astrocytomas, such as those with fibrillary histology, are less frequent in childhood and outcome is somewhat less predictable. A similar approach to that described above for pilocytic astrocytomas is reasonable.

Ependymoma

Approximately 10% of childhood brain tumors are ependymomas [1]. This tumor is most frequent in young children, with approximately half of the cases occurring before age 5 years. This tumor type appears to be approximately twice as common in males as in females, with an incidence rate of approximately 3.5 per million amongst males and 1.8 per million amongst females. Histologically, ependymomas are composed predominantly of neoplastic ependymal cells, where there is great variability of morphologic appearance. The WHO grading system recognizes four tumor types: subependymoma and myxopapillary ependymoma (Grade I tumor), low-grade ependymoma (Grade II tumor) and anaplastic ependymoma (Grade III tumor) [19]. However, there is great variability in the classification of ependymomas within these grades and the recognition of the malignant variant is not easily reproducible. Reports in the literature in terms of frequency of the anaplastic variant show wide variation. Several reports using the WHO classification had failed to link poor histologic grade with poor outcome. Thus, the prognostic significance of histology in ependymoma remains unclear.

Management

The pattern of recurrence of ependymoma is primarily local, with less than 10% of relapses occuring distant from the primary site. Furthermore, most recent series have demonstrated complete resection to be the most important favorable prognostic sign [20,21]. Therefore, aggressive surgery is the primary modality in the treatment of ependymomas (Fig. 28.3). So important is total tumor resection that serious consideration should be given to

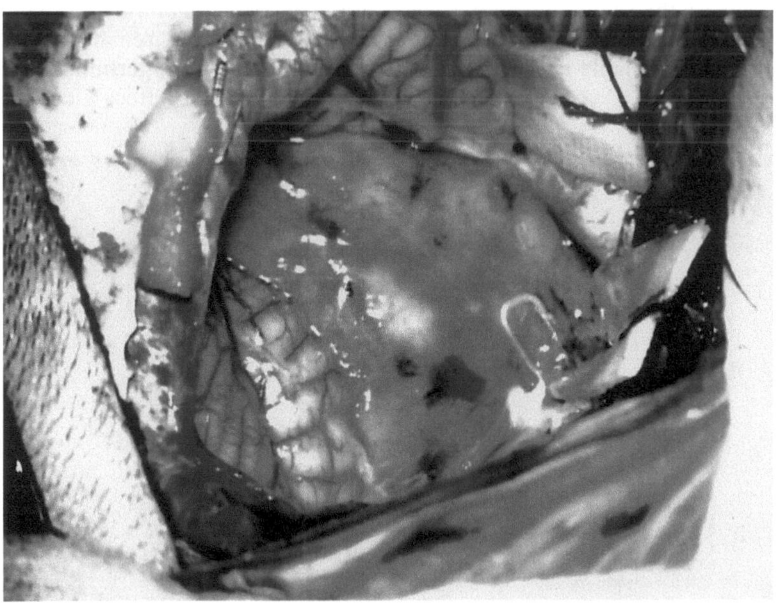

Fig. 28.3. Intraoperative photograph of an ependymoma. This tumor originated in the fourth ventricle and grew dorsally into the cisterna magna, as well as laterally to encase cranial nerves IX, X and XI on the right.

radical resection, including the tumor infiltrating the brainstem. While this approach offers a significantly greater chance of long-term survival, it also significantly increases the risks of serious and permanent neurologic disability; the risks of such an aggressive approach must be thoroughly discussed with the family.

Although several small series have suggested that some patients with ependymoma treated only by gross tumor resection are long-term survivors [22], most clinicians have followed surgical resection with radiation therapy. Several single-institution studies have shown durable progression-free survival in greater than 50% of patients receiving focal radiotherapy following gross total resection, while children with significant post-surgery residual tumor have considerably worse survival, even with radiotherapy [23].

While several chemotherapeutic agents have demonstrated activity in ependymoma, no randomized trials have shown that the addition of chemotherapy to post-operative radiotherapy improves prognosis. When an aggressive chemotherapeutic protocol was used without radiation therapy in the treatment of infants with ependymoma, the 5-year progression-free survival was 34% [24]. Thus, the role of chemotherapy in the treatment of ependymoma has yet to be defined. A study soon to open in the COG will evaluate the use of chemotherapy in patients with incompletely resected tumors to render these tumors resectable at second-look surgery.

Germ Cell Tumors

Germ cell tumors originate in the primordial germ cells, which may undergo either germinomatous or embryonic differentiation. They are biologically diverse and range from benign teratomas to the malignant germinomas and non-germinomatous germ cell tumors. These tumors are located primarily in the midline, with the majority occurring outside the CNS. Approximately 5% of germ cell tumors in children occur within the CNS, most frequently in the pineal and suprasellar regions [1] (Fig. 28.4). Germinomas account for approximately 60% of these tumors, teratomas 30% and the malignant embryonal carcinoma, choriocarcinomas and endodermal sinus tumors approximately 10%. The non-germinomatous malignant germ cell tumors are often characterized by secretion of either beta HCG, alphafetoprotein or both. Significant elevation of one or both of these tumor markers, in association with a tumor located in the characteristic region, are sufficient to make a diagnosis. However, in the absence of such tumor marker elevation, tumor biopsy is required.

Surgery

Surgical resection of the benign teratomas is the only treatment required in the majority of cases. On the other hand, germinomas require adjuvant treatment to effect a cure. In fact, these

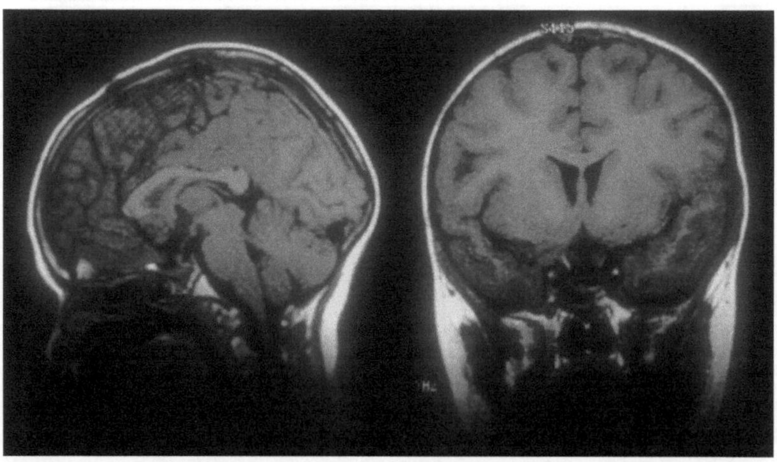

Fig. 28.4. Sagittal (left) and coronal (right) MRI (T1), showing a suprasellar germinoma. Typically located in the midline, the pineal region is also a common location for germinomas.

tumors are highly radiation and chemotherapy sensitive and the surgical approach should be limited to obtaining diagnostic tissue; aggressive resection is contraindicated. In the setting of co-existant hydrocephalus, a combined endoscopic third ventriculostomy (ETV) with tumor biopsy can be attempted if the tumor resides within the third ventricle. Although an attractive approach, this strategy is not uniformly successful due to the difficuty in reaching the tumor from the standard ETV trajectory. We have successfully utilized both flexible endoscopy and a more anterior burr hole for our rigid endoscope to achieve the goal of endoscopic third-ventricle fenestration and biposy. An alternate approach is an image-guided stereotactic approach to biopsy of presumed germinomas, treating the hydrocephalus in a second stage, if needed.

The role of resection in malignant non-germinomatous germ cell tumors is controversial. While most series suggest that obtaining a complete response with the use of combined modality treatment, including surgery, is necessary to achieve long-term disease control, these tumors are often locally invasive and initial complete resection not feasible. While these tumors are less chemo- and radiosensitive than are germinomas, significant and even complete responses have been obtained utilizing chemotherapy; this modality should be employed prior to definitive attempt at resection, in preference to a radical initial approach if there is significant likelihood of morbidity [25].

Radiation Therapy

There is no established role for adjuvant radiation therapy in the management of the resected teratoma. On the other hand, germinomas are highly radiosensitive and radiation therapy is curative in the majority of patients. Subarachnoid dissemination of germinomas is well recognized but, in the absence of dissemination at diagnosis, subarachnoid spread occurs infrequently and the role of cranio–spinal irradiation is controversial.

Malignant non-germinomatous germ cell tumors are much less radiosensitive and the use of radiation therapy as a stand-alone adjuvant modality results in tumor recurrence in the majority of cases. However, combination therapy with radiation and chemotherapy has resulted in long-term disease control in the majority of patients in several recent series [25].

Chemotherapy

As is the case with non-CNS malignant germ cell tumors, tumors in the CNS are quite responsive to chemotherapy, particularly cisplatin-based treatment. Complete responses occur in the majority of patients with germinomas and in a high percentage of patients with non-germinomatous malignant germ cell tumors of the CNS [26]. However, chemotherapy without radiation therapy for both germinomas and non-germinomatous malignant germ cell tumors has resulted in tumor recurrence in the majority of patients [26]. Recognizing the activity of chemotherapy in germinomas, as well as the potential toxicity of radiation therapy, several recent studies have investigated the use of chemotherapy and reduced-volume and dose-of-radiation therapy in the treatment of germinomas, with good results [27]. The definitive role of chemotherapy in the treatment of germinomas of the CNS remains controversial. As noted above, radiation therapy alone is insufficient to effect a cure in the majority of patients with malignant non-germinomatous germ cell tumors of the CNS. Several recent studies combining platinum-based chemotherapy with radiation therapy and, often, second-look surgery have significantly improved the prognosis of patients with these tumors, such that over 50% long-term progression-free survival has been reported [25].

Other CNS Tumors of Childhood

Craniopharyngioma

Despite benign histopathology and their relative rarity (6–9% of all pediatric brain tumors), craniopharyngiomas often prove one of the most difficult pediatric tumors to cure without significant neurologic morbidity. Due to their intimate association with the ventricular system, visual pathways, hypothalamus and pituitary, craniopharyngiomas commonly present with signs and symptoms of hydrocephalus, visual disturbance (occasionally blindness) and/or endocrine dysfunction. While some degree of endocrine dysfunction is noted in up to 90% of newly diagnosed patients, only a minority come to medical attention secondary to their endocrinopathy, most commonly short stature, diabetes insipidus and hypothyroidism. The most common histology seen in pediatric craniopharyngioma is the adamantinomatous type, composed of epithelial cells, keratin, microcalcification and cholesterol clefts. Grossly, and on imaging, craniopharyngiomas can be primarily cystic, primarily solid or, most commonly, a mixture of the two (Fig. 28.5) and it is not uncommon for a rim of calcium to be seen on CT scan.

Surgery

Craniopharyngioma is primarily a surgical disease. Gross total resection is reported in up to 70%, with 90% of this group going on to enjoy a surgical cure [28]. Because of their sellar/parasellar location and the tendency for the tumor to adhere to adjacent structures (optic apparatus, hypothalamus, pituitary stalk), post-operative neurologic morbidity can be as high as 30%, panhypopituitarism develops in up to 90% and overall operative mortality reaches 12% [28]. Operative mortality associated with recurrent craniopharyngioma surgery has been reported to be as high as 42% in the best of hands [29], including late mortality related to chronic endocrinopathy and shunt malfunction. By limiting surgical resection, neurologic morbidity decreases, as does tumor control. In light of the significant morbidity and mortality associated with craniopharyngioma resection, many pediatric neurosurgeons have used minimally invasive techniques to effectively treat these lesions, with far fewer operative complications. Endoscopic endonasal transphenoidal techniques have been successfully employed in a select patient population, with promising results, primarily in patients with sella-based lesions. Increasingly, stereotactic techniques are being used, with excellent results in cystic craniopharyngiomas. Stereotactic intracavitary irradiation with ^{32}P or ^{90}Y has shown complete cyst resolution in 80% of patients, while installation of bleomycin can provide adequate tumor control in approximately 70%. Finally, stereotactic radiosurgery has shown to be effective treatment for the non-cystic craniopharyngiomas, either as initial treatment or for treatment of the solid portion of mixed tumors following intracavitary treatment and cyst involution. Tumor control rates of 90% have been achieved when combined intracavitary and stereotactic irradiation are used as first-line therapy, and tumor control rates of approximately 60% have been shown in recurrent craniopharyngiomas using stereotactic radiosurgery alone. Given the low rate of post-operative complications, these minimally invasive techniques offer new options in the surgical management of this tumor.

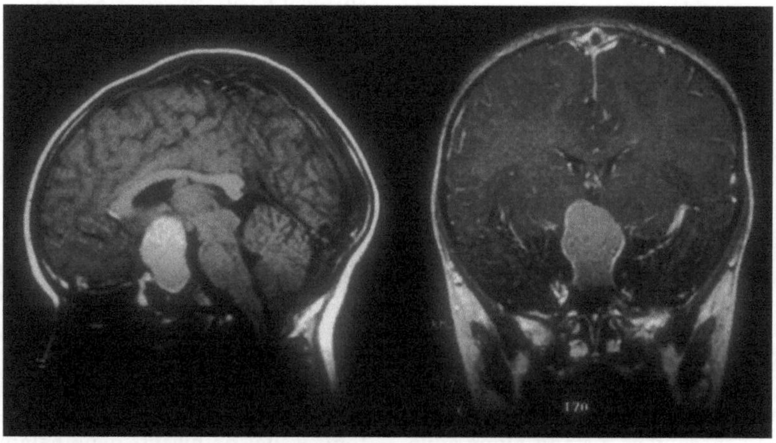

Fig. 28.5. Sagittal (left) and coronal (right) gadolinium-enhanced MRI (T1), showing a craniopharyngioma. This example is entirely cystic in appearance, with pronounced enhancement of the wall.

Radiation Therapy

Subtotal, or planned, limited resections of craniopharyngiomas without post-operative radiation therapy will lead to recurrence and growth of the tumor, residual in the majority of cases. Conventional radiation therapy for residual craniopharyngioma consists of fractionated therapy to 5,500 cGy at 180 cGy/fraction. At doses of more than 5,400 cGy, the recurrence rate after fractionated radiation therapy is 15%, and doses greater than 6,100 cGy are associated with unacceptably high complications, making 5,500 cGy an acceptable dose.

Brainstem Gliomas

Brainstem gliomas account for approximately 10–20% of childhood CNS malignancies. Of these tumors, 64–75% are intrinsic to the brainstem, centered in the pons and histologically low-grade – the so-called "diffuse brainstem glioma". These tumors tend to present after a rapid course of subtle, progressive ataxia and cranial nerve dysfunction, most commonly V, VI, VII, IX and X. Focal tumors of the brainstem are much less common than diffuse brainstem tumors in the pediatric population and tend to be slowly progressive in nature. Signs and symptoms are related to the involved brainstem region, and low-grade lesions far outnumber high-grade malignancies in this group. A subtype of focal brainstem tumor is the tectal glioma. Typically coming to neurosurgical attention due to late-onset hydrocephalus due to acquired "aqueductal stenosis", these children typically have an essentially normal brain on imaging, with the exception of obstructive hydrocephalus. A third category of brainstem tumor is the dorsally exophytic tumor. Arising from the subependyma of the fourth ventricle and growing dorsally, these patients present similarly to patients with medulloblastomas and ependymomas of the posterior fossa: headache, nausea and vomiting due to hydrocephalus. These tumors grow primarily into the fourth ventricle, rather than invading the brainstem, and are most commonly pilocytic astrocytomas on pathological examination (Fig. 28.6). Exophytic tumors that grow laterally and/or ventrally are more likely to be high-grade in nature, and typically present after a shorter course of neurologic symptoms.

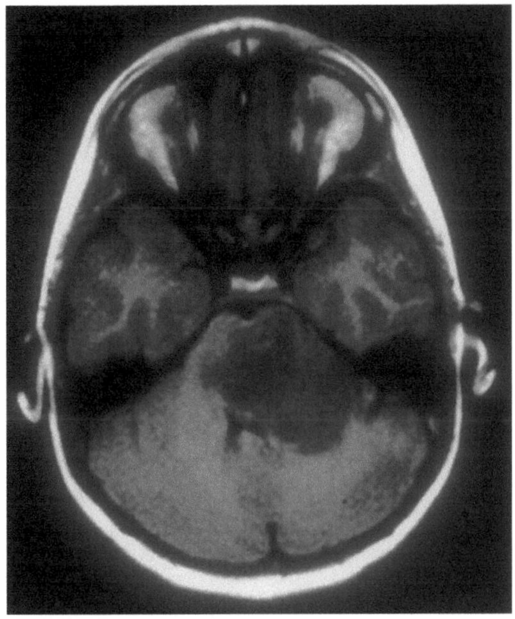

Fig. 28.6. Axial MRI (T1) of an exophytic brainstem glioma. Note the paucity of mass effect, edema and hydrocephalus, typical of these indolent lesions.

Summary

The role of surgery in the intrinsic brainstem glioma is limited to the occasional necessity for permanent CSF diversion. Biopsy has not proven to add important information which will alter therapy and, given the high potential for morbidity, is not recommended. On the other hand, focal lesions of the brainstem can often be approached surgically (Fig. 28.7). In most cases, a subtotal resection is all that can be safely accomplished. Even in the absence of post-operative adjuvant treatment, generous central debulking of focal brainstem tumors can provide significant disease control and surgical success should be based on neurologic outcome from surgery, rather than the amount of tumor resected. Exophytic tumors of the brainstem should be approached like other fourth-ventricular tumors until the fourth ventricle is free of tumor. A decision to enter the brainstem should only be made after confirmation of low-grade histology and then surgery should proceed as described above for focal brainstem tumors.

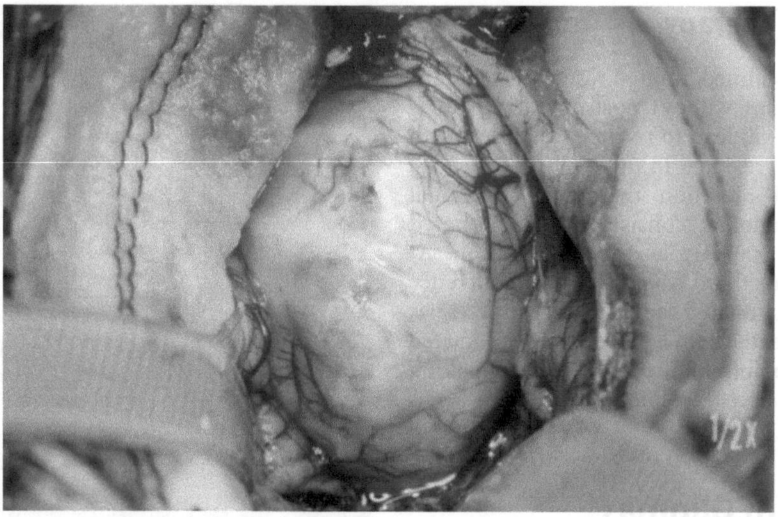

Fig. 28.7. Intraoperative photograph of a focal brainstem glioma arising from the pons and growing into the fourth ventricle.

Radiation Therapy

The only modality that is demonstrated effective for intrinsic brainstem gliomas, albeit transiently, involves field radiation therapy of doses exceeding 50 GY. Use of this modality often results in symptomatic improvement but, in the vast majority of children, progression occurs despite completion of radiation therapy. Radiation therapy for focal brainstem lesions results in a high degree of disease control, which is not surprising given that the majority of these tumors are pilocytic in histology. Radiation therapy can be employed should there be progression after surgical resection or in those instances in which the risk of severe neurologic compromise is sufficiently high from re-operation.

Chemotherapy

Intrinsic brainstem gliomas are quite refractory to chemotherapy. Responses in phase II trials have been infrequent and, in the only randomized trial comparing radiation and chemotherapy with radiation therapy alone, no survival advantage was demonstrated for the use of chemotherapy.

Recent approaches have attempted to improve the activity of radiation therapy by utilizing concomitant chemotherapy but, as yet, these approaches have not resulted in demonstrable improvement in survival.

Choroid Plexus Tumors

Neoplasms of the choroid plexus account for approximately 3% of brain tumors in children and are much more common during the first year of life. The majority of these tumors originate in the lateral ventricles (specifically the trigone), but they can occur in the fourth, and rarely the third, ventricle as well. Choroid plexus papillomas are slow-growing tumors and complete resection, possible in the majority of patients, is generally curative. The choroid plexus carcinoma is an anaplastic choroid plexus neoplasm and constitutes approximately 15% of choroid plexus neoplasms. This histology is much more invasive than the papilloma and has propensity for sub-arachnoid metastasis. Long-term survival following complete resection has been well documented but survival following incomplete resection, in spite of the use of either radiation, chemotherapy or both, is infrequent. The role of chemotherapy as an adjuvant therapy is unclear, although several series have documented the utility of chemotherapy in the incompletely resected choroid plexus carcinoma, in an attempt to improve the resectability at second-look surgery by decreasing vascularity and size of the tumor.

Rhabdoid Tumors

Rhabdoid tumors of the CNS, also called atypical teratoid tumors, are recently described neoplasms characterized by monosome 22. These tumors are likely related to the renal rhabdoid tumor of infancy. The majority of these tumors occur in children of less than 2 years of age and more than half are supratentorial in location. These tumors are locally aggressive and approximately 25% of cases will display sub-arachnoid metastasis. Long-term survival is infrequent, even with the use of aggressive adjuvant chemotherapy and, in the absence of complete resection, extremely unlikely. The role of radiation therapy is unclear and the young age of these children has precluded aggressive radiation therapy approaches.

Late Effects

Survivors of childhood brain tumors are at risk for long-term complications, both from their tumors and their therapies. In fact, significant evolution of therapy over the last two decades has been an attempt to reduce the morbidity of treatment. Of principal concern is the effect of radiation therapy on the developing CNS. It is quite clear that impairment of cognitive function can result from cranial irradiation. Volume (i.e. whole-brain vs focal irradiation), age (i.e. young children vs older children) and total dose of radiation all play roles in predicting a higher likelihood of significant neurocognitive sequelae [30]. This has led to ongoing attempts at reducing radiation doses, at times by substituting chemotherapy, or at decreasing the volume of radiation with new radiotherapy techniques characterized by recent and ongoing investigations. Those children who have received cranial irradiation require careful neurocognitive follow-up and involvement with the educational process. Cranial irradiation can also result in multiple endocrine abnormalities, principally growth hormone and thyroid deficiencies. Fortunately, replacement therapy can ameliorate many of the long-term consequences but it is imperative that these children receive timely evaluation by an endocrinologist experienced in the management of these problems. Second malignant neoplasms are well described, particularly following radiation therapy for both CNS and other malignancies. Such second malignancies are often high-grade astrocytomas and quite refractory to salvage therapy.

Conclusion and Future Directions

Significant improvement in the diagnosis and management of pediatric CNS tumors has occurred over the last several decades and the majority of children with CNS tumors will be long-term survivors. Nonetheless, improvements in prognosis and quality of life for many children with CNS tumors has been less dramatic than that seen for other childhood malignancies. This lack of progress probably has several causes. Although CNS tumors in childhood constitute the most common solid tumor as an aggregate, the multiple histologies involved make any single tumor type relatively infrequent. The need for enrolment of every eligible patient in co-operative group trials if at all possible is imperative, given the relative infrequency of these tumors. The lack of understanding of the basic biology of these tumors has been hampered by inadequacies of tissue availability. As new molecular techniques have become available for further understanding the basic genetic abnormalities of CNS tumors, the necessity for obtaining tumor tissue from as many patients as possible for evaluation in ongoing biologic studies is critical. Care of children with CNS tumors is complex, requiring multimodality treatment, with experts in a range of medical and supportive areas. Improvement in outcome has been demonstrated in studies in which a dedicated pediatric neuro-oncology team is available to provide expertise in diagnosis, management and long-term follow-up care.

References

1. Ries L, Kosary C, Hankey B. SEER cancer statistical review, 1973–1994. National Cancer Institute, SEER Program NIH Publication Number 97-2789, 1997.

2. Rorke LB, Gilles FH, Davis RL, Becker LE. Revision of the World Health Organization classification of brain tumors for childhood brain tumors. Cancer 1985; 56:1869–86.
3. O'Reilly G, Hayward R, Harkness W. Myelography in the assessment of children with medulloblastoma. Br J Neurosurg 1993;7:183–8.
4. Albright A. Medulloblastomas. In: Albright A, Pollack I, Adelson P, editors. Principles and practice of pediatric neurosurgery. New York: Theime, 1999; 591–608.
5. Park T, Hoffman H, Hendrick B, Humphreys R, Becker L. Medulloblastoma. Clinical presentation and management: experience at the Hospital For Sick Children, Toronto, 1950–1980. J Neurosurg 1983;58:543–52
6. Albright AL, Wisoff JH, Zeltzer PM, Boyett JM, Rorke LB, Stanley P. Effects of medulloblastoma resections on outcome in children: a report from the Children's Cancer Group. Neurosurgery 1996;38:265–71.
7. Hughes EN, Shillito J, Sallan SE, Loeffler JS, Cassady JR, Tarbell NJ. Medulloblastoma at the joint center for radiation therapy between 1968 and 1984: the influence of radiation dose on the patterns of failure and survival. Cancer 1988;61:1992–8.
8. Evans AE, Jenkin RD, Sposto R, Ortega JA, Wilson CB, Wara W et al. The treatment of medulloblastoma: results of a prospective randomized trial of radiation therapy with and without CCNU, vincristine, and prednisone. J Neurosurg 1990;72:572–82.
9. Tait DM, Thornton-Jones H, Bloom HJ, Lemerle J, Morris-Jones P. Adjuvant chemotherapy for medulloblastoma: the first multi-centre control trial of the International Society of Paediatric Oncology (SIOP I). Eur J Canc 1990;26:464–9.
10. Thomas PR, Deutsch M, Kepner JL, Boyett JM, Krischer J, Aronin P et al. Low-stage medulloblastoma: final analysis of trial comparing standard-dose with reduced-dose neuraxis irradiation. J Clin Oncol 2000;18:3004–11.
11. Packer RJ, Sutton LN, Elterman R, Lange B, Goldwein J, Nicholson HS et al. Outcome for children with medulloblastoma treated with radiation and cisplatin, CCNU, and vincristine chemotherapy. J Neurosurg 1994;81: 690–8.
12. Zeltzer PM, Boyett JM, Finlay JL, Albright AL, Rorke LB, Milstein JM et al. Metastasis stage, adjuvant treatment, and residual tumor are prognostic factors for medulloblastoma in children: conclusions from the Children's Cancer Group 921 randomized phase III study. J Clin Oncol 1999;17:832–45.
13. Packer RJ, Goldwein J, Nicholson HS, Vezina LG, Allen JC, Ris MD et al. Treatment of children with medulloblastomas with reduced-dose craniospinal radiation therapy and adjuvant chemotherapy: a Children's Cancer Group Study. J Clin Oncol 1999;17:2127–36.
14. Steinbok P, Mutat A. Cerebellar astrocytomas. In: Albright AL, Pollack IF, Adelson PD, editors. Principles and practice of pediatric neurosurgery. New York: Thieme, 1999.
15. Wisoff JH, Boyett JM, Berger MS, Brant C, Li H, Yates AJ et al. Current neurosurgical management and the impact of the extent of resection in the treatment of malignant gliomas of childhood: a report of the Children's Cancer Group trial Number CCG-945. J Neurosurg 1999;90:1147–8.
16. Pollack IF. Brain tumors in children. N Engl J Med 1994;331:1500–7.
17. Shaw EG, Daumas-Duport C, Scheithauer BW, Gilbertson DT, O'Fallon JR, Earle JD et al. Radiation therapy in the management of low-grade supratentorial astrocytomas. J Neurosurg 1989;70:853–61.
18. Packer RJ, Ater J, Allen J, Phillips P, Geyer R, Nicholson HS et al. Carboplatin and vincristine chemotherapy for children with newly diagnosed progressive low-grade gliomas. J Neurosurg 1997;86:747–54.
19. Kleihues P, Burger P, Scheithauer B. Histological typing of tumors of the central nervous system: WHO International Histological Classification of Tumors. 2nd Edition. Berlin: Springer-Verlag, 1993.
20. Duffner PK, Krischer JP, Sanford RA, Horowitz ME, Burger PC, Cohen ME et al. Prognostic factors in infants and very young children with intracranial ependymomas. Pediatr Neurosurg 1998;28:215–22.
21. Healey EA, Barnes PD, Kupsky WJ, Scott RM, Sallan SE, Black PM et al. The prognostic significance of postoperative residual tumor in ependymoma. Neurosurgery 1991;28:666–71.
22. Hukin J, Epstein F, Lefton D, Allen J. Treatment of intracranial ependymoma by surgery alone. Pediat Neurosurg 1998;29:40–5.
23. Perilongo G, Massimino M, Sotti G, Belfontali T, Masiero L, Rigobello L et al. Analyses of prognostic factors in a retrospective review of 92 children with ependymoma: Italian Pediatric Neuro-oncology Group. Med Pediat Oncol 1997;29:79–85.
24. Geyer R: , 2002.
25. Robertson PL, DaRosso RC, Allen JC. Improved prognosis of intracranial non-germinoma germ cell tumors with multimodality therapy. J Neuro-oncol 1997;32: 71–80.
26. Balmaceda C, Heller G, Rosenblum M, Diez B, Villablanca JG, Kellie S et al. Chemotherapy without irradiation. A novel approach for newly diagnosed CNS germ cell tumors: results of an international cooperative trial. The First International Central Nervous System Germ Cell Tumor Study. J Clin Oncol 1996;14:2908–15.
27. Allen JC, Kim JH, Packer RJ. Neoadjuvant chemotherapy for newly diagnosed germ-cell tumors of the central nervous system. J Neurosurg 1987;67:65–70.
28. Hoffman HJ, DeSilva M, Humphreys RP, Drake JM, Smith ML, Blaser SI. Aggressive surgical management of craniopharyngiomas in children. J Neurosurg 1992; 76:47–52.
29. Yasargil MG, Curcic M, Kis M, Siegenthaler G, Teddy PJ, Roth P. Total removal of craniopharyngiomas: approaches and long-term results in 144 patients. J Neurosurg 1990;73:3–11.
30. Duffner PK, Cohen ME. Long-term consequences of CNS treatment for childhood cancer. Part II: clinical consequences. Pediat Neurol 1991;7:237–42.

IX
Spine

29

Management of Spinal Tumors

Karl F. Kothbauer, George I. Jallo and
Fred J. Epstein

Summary

This chapter describes the treatment approach to patients with intradural spinal tumors, with the most common being nerve sheath tumors and meningiomas, representing a combined 55%. The remaining 45% of intradural tumors are intramedullary. Surgical management of these tumors may include the application of the Cavitron ultrasonic aspirator and the laser. Many intramedullary tumors are amenable to gross total resection using an aggressive approach. Techniques for surgical resection and monitoring techniques are discussed.

Introduction

The first successful resection of an intramedullary spinal cord tumor was performed in 1907 in Vienna, by Anton von Eiselsberg [1]. The first publication appeared in 1911 in New York, by Charles Elsberg [2]. He developed a strategy for a two-stage operation: a myelotomy was performed at the first surgery and, by the second surgery (about a week later), the tumor had already partly extruded itself from the cord substance, facilitating further resection. The first intradural extramedullary tumor resections are credited to William Macewen in 1883 and Victor Horsley [3].

After the work of these pioneers, the neurological risk of surgery for intramedullary neoplasms was considered unacceptably high. This led to the development of a conservative treatment concept with biopsy, dural decompression and subsequent radiation therapy, regardless of the histological diagnosis. Intradural–extramedullary tumors were commonly regarded as surgically resectable tumors.

The microscope and microsurgery have revolutionized all neurosurgery and also opened the door to innovation in the treatment of spinal cord tumors. CT and particularly MRI have dramatically improved pre-operative planning and significantly contributed to the development of modern treatment strategies of both intra- and extramedullary spinal cord tumors. In particular, the conservative treatment strategy for intramedullary tumors changed to an aggressive approach. Since the large majority of these tumors are histologically benign, complete or near complete, resection results in long-term progression-free survival, with acceptable neurological morbidity [4–7]. More recently, the application of intraoperative neurophysiological monitoring techniques has made a significant impact on the treatment management of both intra- and extramedullary tumors [8,9].

This chapter describes the treatment approach to patients with intradural spinal tumors.

Epidemiology and Pathology

Intradural spinal cord tumors have a prevalence of 3–10 per 100,000 per year. They predominantly occur in the middle third of life. The most common tumors are nerve sheath tumors, which account for about 30%, and meningiomas, which account for another 25%. The remainder includes sarcomas, epidermoids and dermoids. Intramedullary tumors are rare – approximately 20–35% of all intradural neoplasms, with a higher percentage (55% of all intradural neoplasms) in children [10]. The most common intramedullary tumors are astrocytomas and ependymomas. Hemangioblastomas, cavernomas, epidermoids and lipomas are rare.

Intradural Extramedullary Tumors

Nerve sheath tumors (Fig. 29.1) usually arise from the dorsal roots. They are relatively avascular, globoid and without calcification. The dorsal root of origin is most often intimately adherent to the tumor and can rarely be preserved during surgical resection. In patients with neurofibromatosis, these tumors are multiple and occur at numerous levels of the spinal canal. When located in the area of the intervertebral foramen, they may assume a characteristic dumbbell configuration, with an extra- and an intradural component (Fig. 29.1).

Meningiomas [11] (Fig. 29.2), unlike nerve sheath tumors, arise from arachnoid cluster cells and thus are usually separate from the nerve roots. These tumors tend to have a lateral or ventrolateral location relative to the spinal cord. They may arise in any age group, mostly occurring between the fifth and seventh decades of life, and are seen more frequently in women. They are most often located in the thoracic spine.

Intramedullary Tumors

Astrocytomas (Fig. 29.3) are the most common intramedullary tumors. They can occur at any age but are most frequent in the first three decades. The majority of these neoplasms are benign, being either low-grade fibrillary or pilocytic astrocytomas. They usually are not well demarcated from the surrounding neural tissue and they may contain cystic areas, as well as adjacent, non-neoplastic cysts.

Gangliogliomas (Fig. 29.4) are benign neoplasms, mostly occurring in children and young

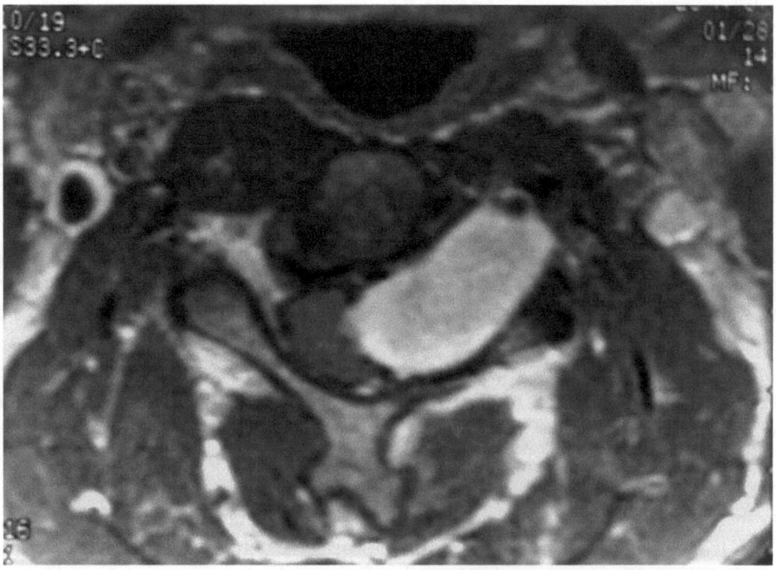

Fig. 29.1. Axial T1-weighted MRI after contrast administration shows a dumbbell-shaped cervical spinal schwannoma.

a 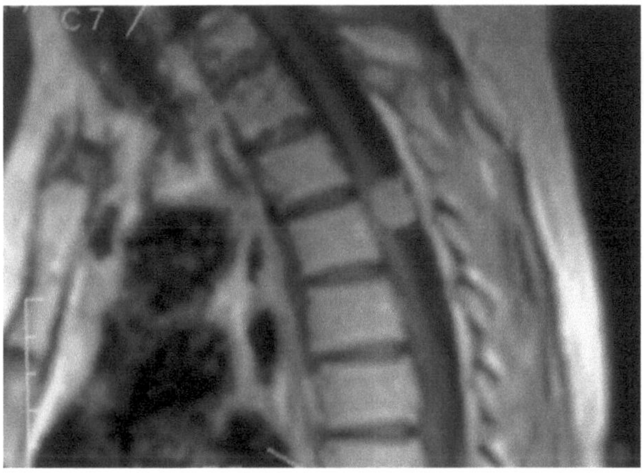

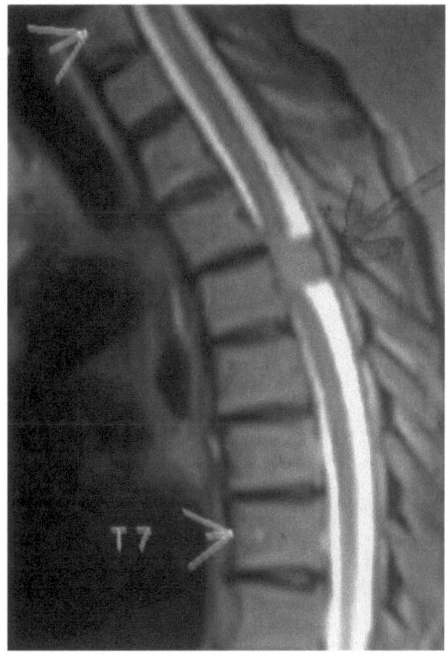

b

Fig. 29.2. **a** Sagittal T1- and **b** T2-weighted images of a typical thoracic spinal meningioma.

a 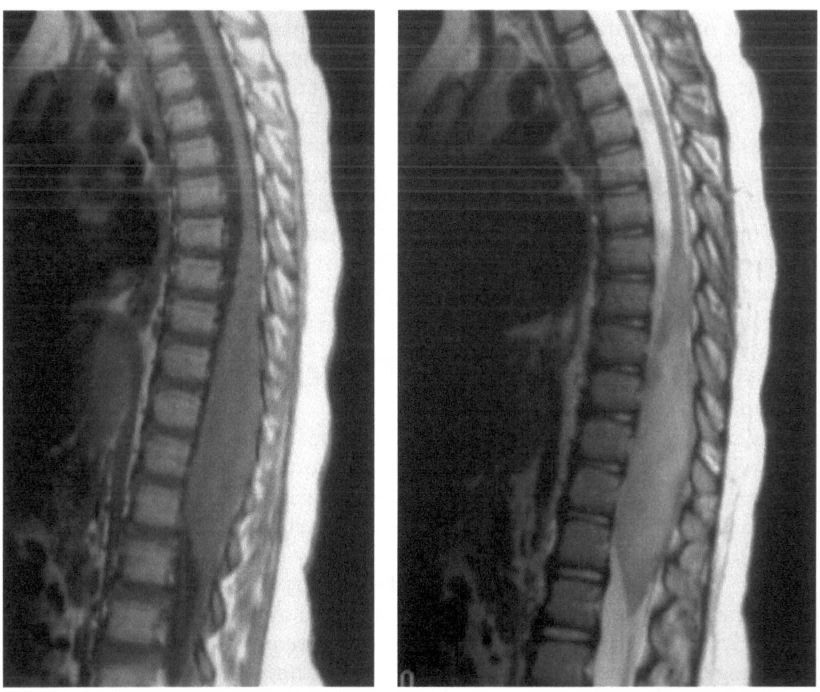 b

Fig. 29.3. Spinal cord low-grade astrocytoma.

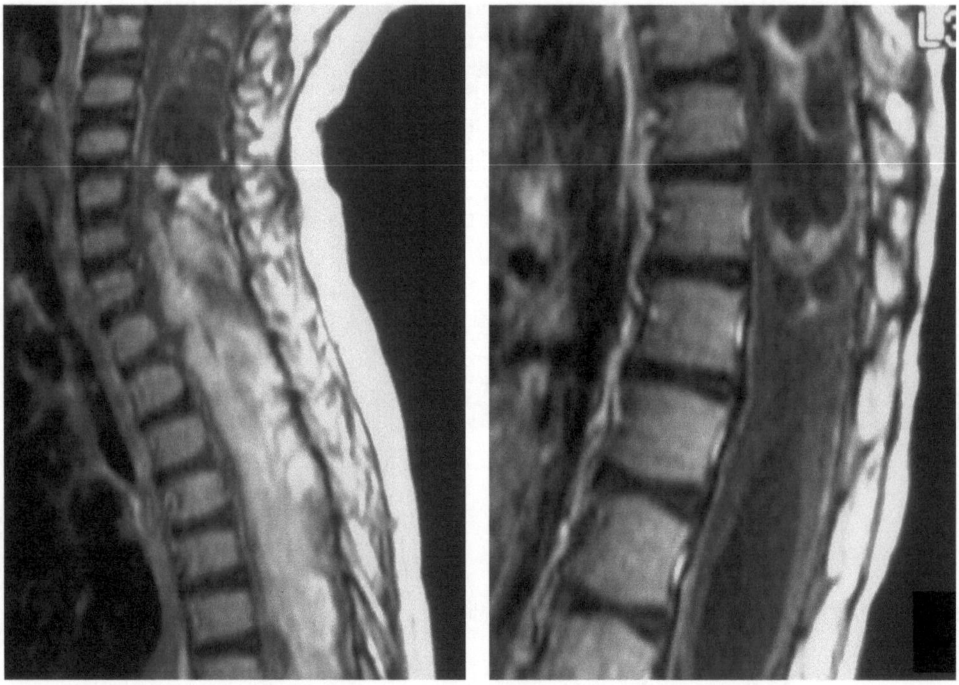

a b

Fig. 29.4. Large spinal cord ganglioglioma involving the entire cord with **a** the solid and **b** the cystic portion.

adults. They consist of well differentiated neoplastic neurons and astrocytes. The neurons have characteristic nuclear and nucleolar features, abundant cytoplasm and argyrophilic neuritic processes. Their expression of neuronal markers like synaptophysin and neurofilament proteins also serves to identify these abnormal neurons. Most gangliogliomas grow slowly and have an indolent course.

Ependymomas (Figs 29.5 and 29.6) are the most common intramedullary neoplasms in adults [12,13], while in children they account for only 12% of all intramedullary tumors. Ependymomas typically have a central location in the cord. They occur throughout the spinal axis. They are well delineated from the surrounding spinal cord and often have rostral and caudal non-neoplastic cysts that cap the tumor poles. Virtually all of them are histologically benign.

Myxopapillary ependymomas (Fig. 29.7) are a subgroup of ependymomas with characteristic microcystic histologic features. Their typical location is the conus-cauda region [14]. Located in the filum, they may grossly enlarge the filum and displace the nerve roots laterally and anteriorly. In spite of their benign histology, a small percentage of them tend to sub-arachnoid dissemination.

Hemangioblastomas account for 3–7% of intramedullary spinal cord tumors. They occur throughout the spinal canal. Spinal cord hemangioblastomas are mostly sporadic, but up to 25% of the patients have von Hippel–Lindau disease.

Clinical Presentation

Intramedullary spinal cord tumors may remain asymptomatic for a long time and may increase to a considerable size before they are detected. The onset of symptoms is often insidious and they may be present for months or even years before the diagnosis is established. Symptoms may also appear at the time of a trivial injury. Not infrequently, exacerbations and remissions occur. A common early symptom is back or neck pain, occurring in up to two-thirds of patients. The pain may be either diffuse, in

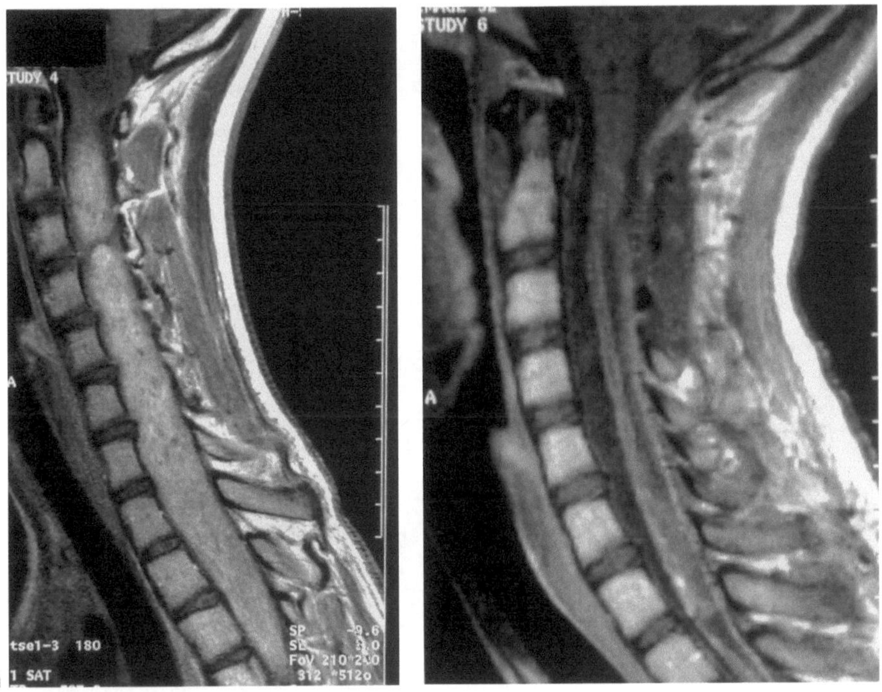

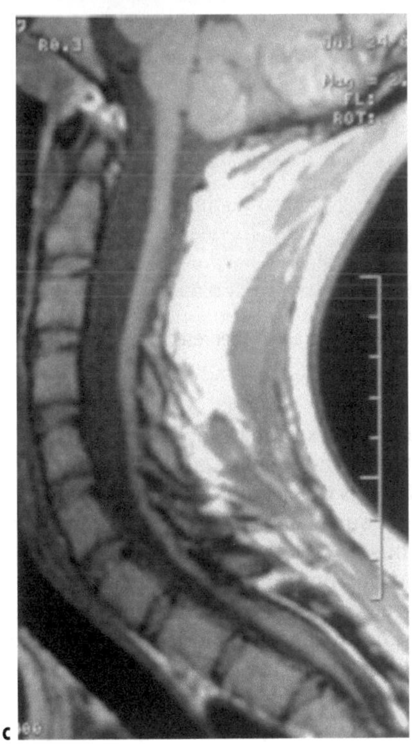

Fig. 29.5. a Pre-operative, **b** immediate post-operative and **c** 3-year follow-up sagittal T1 contrast-enhanced images of a large cervical intramedullary ependymoma.

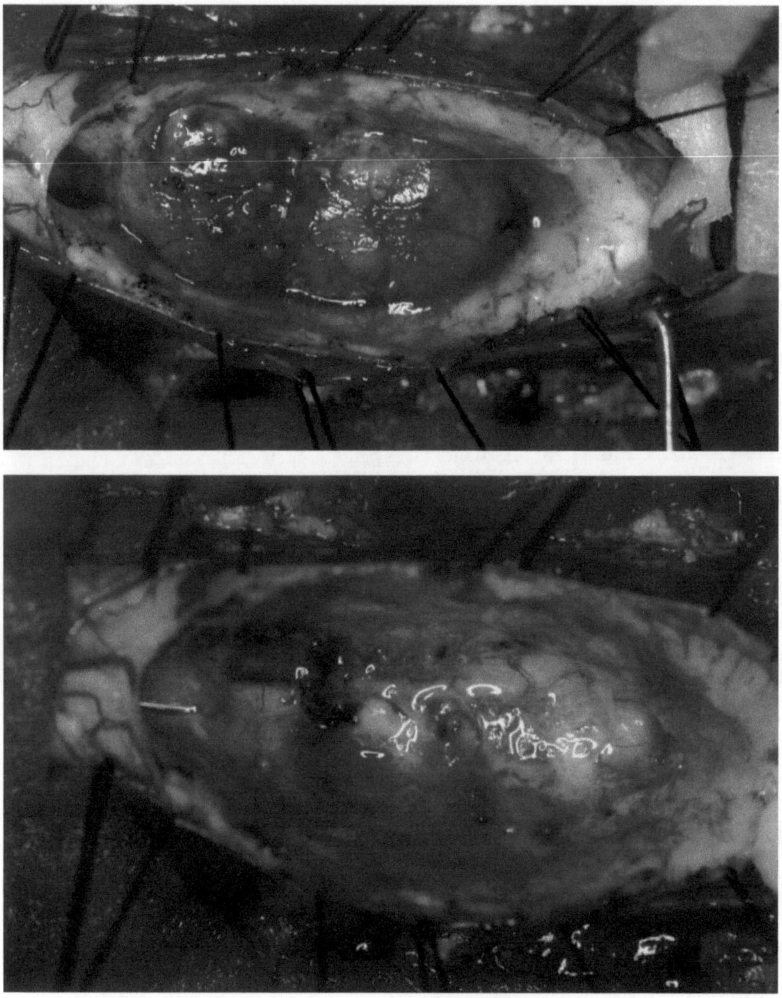

a

b

Fig. 29.6. Intraoperative view of an ependymoma **a** before and **b** after resection.

which case an intramedullary tumor is the more likely cause, or it may have a radicular distribution, which is more common in intradural extramedullary lesions [15]. Young children may even present with abdominal pain as a non-specific symptom that makes finding the correct diagnosis particularly difficult. Pain is characteristically more severe in the horizontal position, thus causing nighttime pain.

Motor function appears to be affected early [5,16] in younger children: this may manifest as motor regression, i.e. refusal to stand or crawl after having learned to walk, or as gait abnormality. Young adults present with lower-extremity weakness, clumsiness or frequent falls. On examination, the majority of these patients show some mild to moderate motor deficit, as well as upper motor neuron-type findings, such as spasticity, hyperreflexia and clonus.

About one-third of the patients have some degree of spinal deformity, most of them with tumors in the thoracic region. Paraspinal pain is common in this group and attributed to the scoliosis. Torticollis was seen in about one-fifth of the pediatric patients.

Sensory symptoms, mostly dysesthesias, described as unpleasant hot or cold sensations, are also found in about 20% of the patients. In glial tumors, as opposed to ependymomas, the

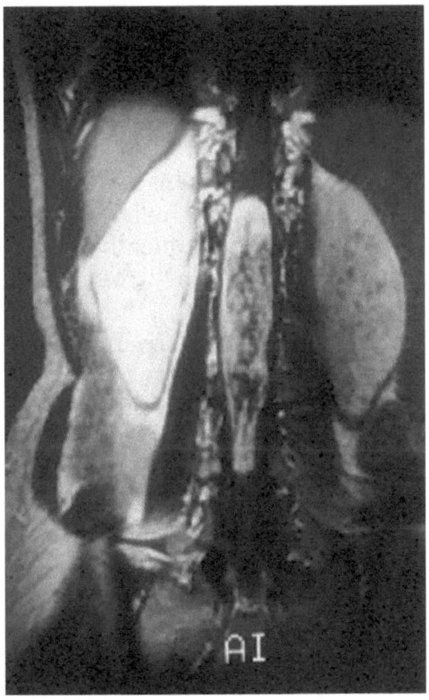

a

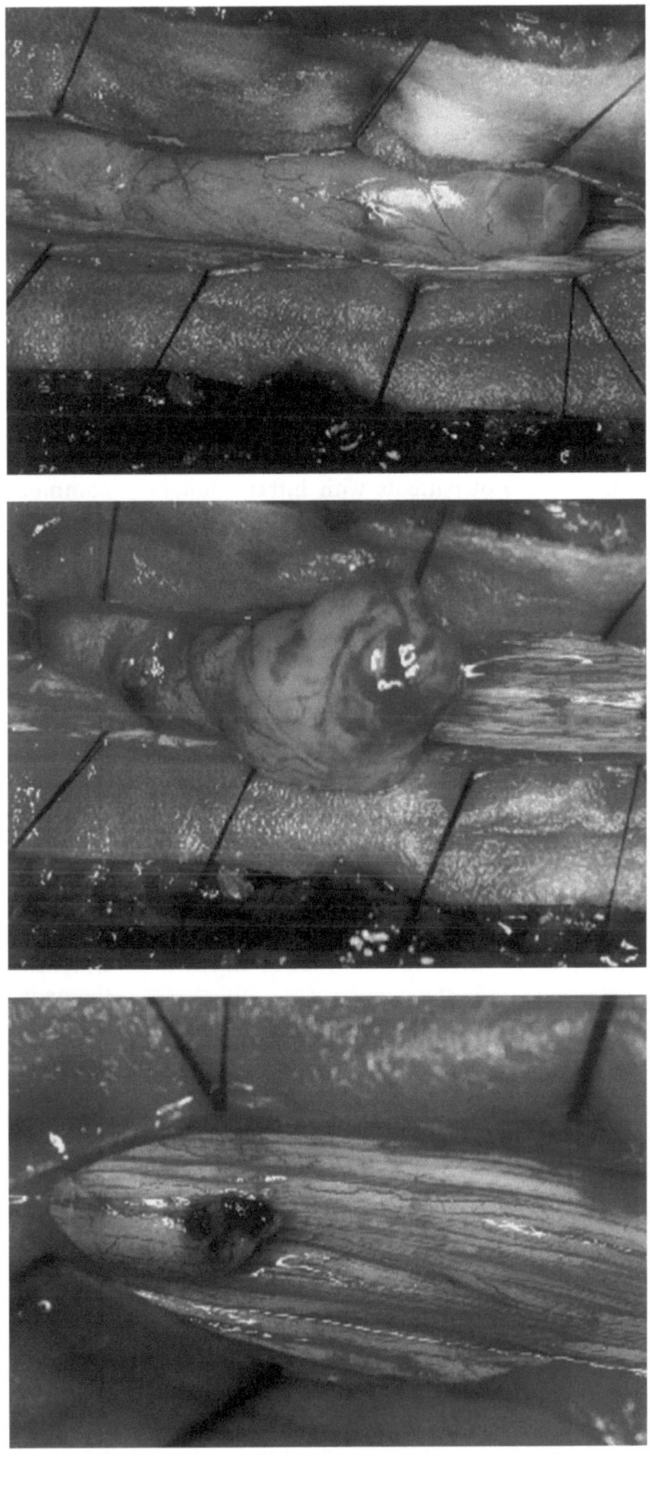

b

c

d

Fig. 29.7. Myxopapillary ependymoma of the filum on **a** MRI and **b** and **c** during resection.

sensory symptoms are frequently asymmetric. Sphincter dysfunction is present late in the clinical course, except for tumors located in the conus medullaris. Malignant intramedullary gliomas are rare [7,16–18]; their symptomatology is similar, but with a significantly shorter history.

Almost all patients with extramedullary tumors have pain, which most commonly has a radicular distribution. The number of patients with mild motor deficits at presentation is high, but only a minority are severely impaired [11].

Hydrocephalus

Hydrocephalus has been reported to occur in as many as 15% of patients with intramedullary tumors. The mechanisms for hydrocephalus include an increased concentration of protein in the cerebrospinal fluid, arachnoidal fibrosis and sub-arachnoid dissemination. The incidence of hydrocephalus is substantially higher in patients with malignant tumors (approximately 35%) than in those with low-grade tumors (approximately 15%). Patients with cervical tumors are more likely to develop hydrocephalus, probably secondary to obstruction of the fourth ventricle outlets.

Diagnostic Studies

MRI

MRI is the study of choice to identify both intra- and extramedullary spinal cord neoplasms [4]. Extramedullary lesions are readily identified as such and their relation to the cord, attachment to dura and displacement of the cord are visualized.

MRI scans should be performed before and after intravenous administration of contrast agents (gadolinium diethylene-triamine-pentacetic acid), with T1-weighted images in multiple planes [19]. These images demonstrate the solid tumor component. T2-weighted images optimally show the cerebrospinal fluid and tumor-associated cysts. While MRI does not allow for a certain histologic diagnosis preoperatively, the more common tumors have typical patterns of imaging appearance.

Ependymomas usually enhance brightly and homogeneously (Fig. 29.5), frequently have rostral and caudal cysts and, not uncommonly, a hemosiderin “cap” at their poles. On axial view, they are usually seen in the center of the cord. Astrocytomas (Fig. 29.3) and gangliogliomas (Fig. 29.4), on the other hand, enhance less frequently and, if enhancement is seen, it is more often heterogeneous. On axial images, these neoplasms are more frequently found to be eccentric in the cord. They may cause asymmetric enlargement of the cord. Hemangioblastomas (Fig. 29.8) characteristically show bright enhancement of a tumor nodule and associated cysts, often with significant cord edema adjacent to it. Meningiomas (Fig. 29.2) and nerve sheath tumors (Fig. 29.1) may have similar appearance on MRI and they commonly enhance brightly. Schwannomas sometimes show large cysts, while meningiomas often can be identified by a broad dural attachment.

Plain Radiographs

Spinal X-rays should be taken, particularly in patients who present with scoliosis. These films serve as a baseline for the future management of the spinal deformity. Intradural extramedullary tumors can thin or cause sclerosis of the pedicles. A tumor that extends through a neural foramen enlarges that foramen, which can be seen on oblique films. Intramedullary neoplasms may show a diffusely widened spinal canal, with associated erosion of the pedicles and scalloping of the vertebrae.

Myelography and CT

Myelography with water-soluble contrast agent combined with CT was used extensively in the evaluation of suspected intraspinal lesions [7]. Today, CT–myelography is reserved for the rare cases where MRI may be impossible to perform (e.g. due to metallic implants) or impossible to interpret due to image distortion from metallic artifacts.

Angiography

Angiographic evaluation of the vascular supply and venous drainage is strongly recommended before the removal of a spinal cord hemangioblastoma (Fig. 29.8) is attempted.

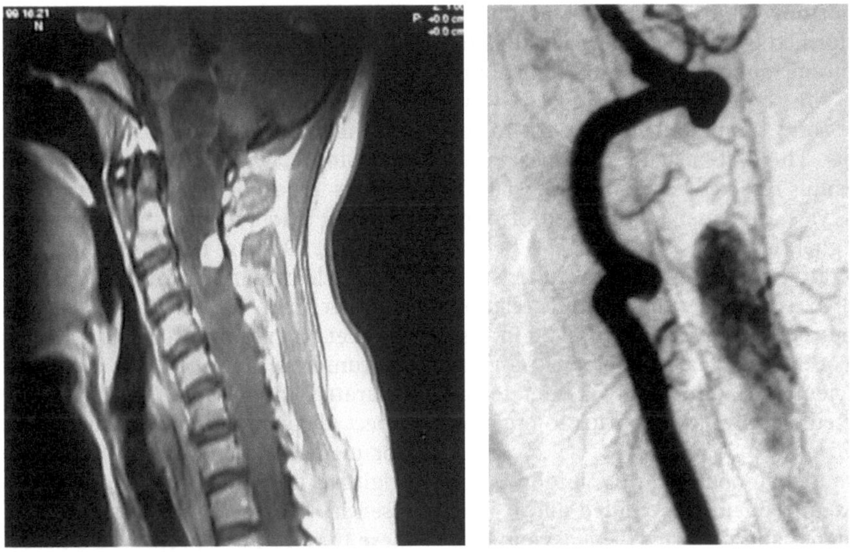

a b

Fig. 29.8. **a** Intramedullary hemangioblastoma with bright enhancing nodule and cyst on the sagittal T1-weighted image. **b** The angiogram depicts the vascular anatomy of the lesion.

Surgical Management of Intradural Tumors

Surgical Instruments

Suction and bipolar cautery are used, together with a set of specialized instruments that aid in minimizing surgical trauma to normal neural tissue. Some of these specialized instruments have become essential for the microsurgical resection of spinal cord tumors.

Ultrasonic Aspirator

The application of the Cavitron ultrasonic aspirator (CUSA) system was a significant advancement in the removal of spinal cord tumors. It uses high-frequency sound waves to fragment the tumor tissue, which is then aspirated by the suction apparatus at the tip of the device. This allows much easier and quicker removal of a bulk of tumor tissue, with less manipulation of the adjacent neural tissue as compared to the suction–cautery technique.

Laser

The laser is an excellent surgical adjunct for spinal cord surgery. We prefer the Nd:YAG Contact Laser^{TM} System (SLT, Montgomeryville, PA) to other available laser technologies. This system has a handpiece and contact probes, and can be used as a microsurgical instrument. The laser is particularly useful as a scalpel to perform the myelotomy, demarcate the glial–tumor interface and remove residual tumor fragments. Firm lesions, such as meningiomas, neurofibromas or rare types of intramedullary tumors, can only be removed with reasonable safety when the laser is available. These lesions cannot be manipulated with the bipolar and scissors because of inevitable manipulation of the adjacent spinal cord tissue, and they are too firm for the CUSA for internal debulking. For the rare spinal cord lipoma, the microsurgical laser is the instrument of choice for vaporization of fat and internal debulking.

Surgical Technique

Surgery is performed with the patient in a prone position. A rigid head-holder (Sugita or Mayfield) is utilized for cervical and cervicothoracic tumors, to secure the head in a neutral position. The horseshoe headrest should be avoided because it does not secure a neutral neck position.

A laminectomy or osteoplastic laminotomy [20] is performed with a high-power drill using the craniotome attachment, round burr and rongeurs. The bone removal must always expose the solid tumor but not the rostral or caudal cysts. The cysts usually disappear after the neoplasm is resected, since the cyst walls of "capping" cysts are usually composed of non-neoplastic glial tissue.

Intraoperative sonography (Fig. 29.9) visualizes the full extent of the tumor and its relation to the bone removal, as well as cysts and displacement of the cord [21]. If the bone removal is not sufficient, the laminectomy is extended to expose the entire solid tumor prior to opening the dura.

The dura is then opened in the midline. The spinal cord is frequently expanded and it may even be rotated and distorted. The asymmetric expansion and rotation of the spinal cord may make identification of the midline raphe difficult. However, it is important to localize this raphe because this is the most frequent approach into the spinal cord. An alternative approach for extremely asymmetrical tumors is to enter the spinal cord through the dorsal root entry zone. This is an approach used sometimes when an asymmetric deficit is present; thus, it is essential to preserve the "good" arm and hand while the other upper extremity is already severely impaired, and deafferentation adds little morbidity.

If the tumor is not visible on the surface, the microsurgical laser is used to perform the myelotomy, with minimal neural injury. The various types of intramedullary tumors have different macroscopic appearances. Ependymomas (Fig. 29.6) are red or dark gray in color and have a clear margin from the spinal cord. This interface can be separated with the plated bayonet or the microsurgical laser. One pole of the tumor is identified and the cleavage plane separated in an axial direction. The ventral aspect of ependymomas is adherent to the anterior median raphe because the feeding vessels originate from the anterior spinal artery. It is essential to preserve this vessel. The majority of these tumors can be removed en bloc [6].

Astrocytomas or gangliogliomas have a gray–yellow glassy appearance. They must be removed from the inside out, until the glial–tumor interface is recognized by the change in color and consistency of the tissue. Rarely, a true plane between tumor and normal spinal cord exists, and futile efforts to define this interface result in hazardous manipulation of normal spinal cord tissue [18]. Their resection is usually started at the midportion rather than at the

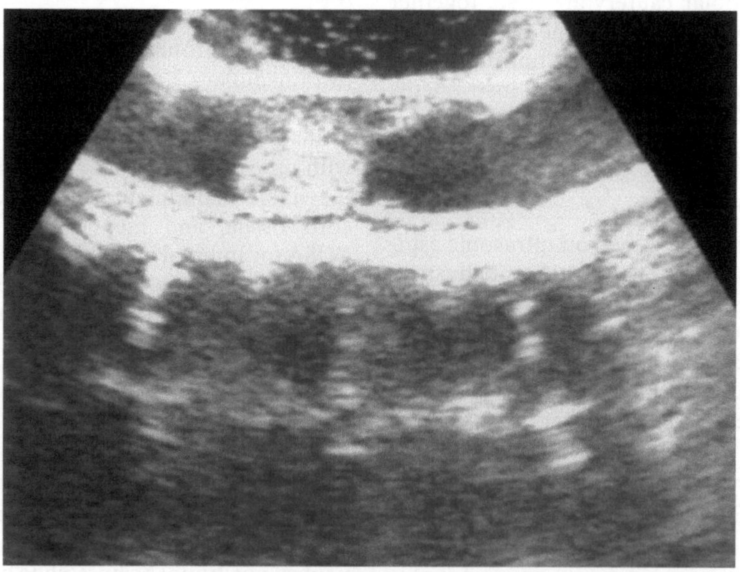

Fig. 29.9. The intraoperative sonographic view of an intramedullary ependymoma allows for identification of the solid and cystic components.

poles. The rostral and caudal poles are the least voluminous and manipulation there may be dangerous to the normal tissue.

Intramedullary lipomas appear well demarcated from the adjacent spinal cord, but they are intimately adherent to the normal tissue. Therefore, total removal is impossible without incurring neurological deficits and should not be attempted. The microsurgical laser is the instrument of choice for debulking a spinal cord lipoma. The laser vaporizes fatty tissue without surgical trauma to the spinal cord. The debulking of the lipoma may result in improvement of pain but rarely in improvement of neurological function. Further growth of a lipoma is unlikely or at least very slow. However, in adolescence, probably due to endocrine factors, lipomas of the cord may increase in size and may, at that time, cause progressive neurological dysfunction.

Following tumor removal, hemostasis is obtained with saline irrigation and local application of microfibrillar collagen (Avitene(r), C. R. Bard, Inc., 730 Central Avenue, Murray Hill, NJ). The dura is closed primarily in a watertight fashion. If an osteoplastic laminotomy was performed, the segments of bone are replaced and secured with a non-absorbable suture on each lamina bilaterally. One tissue layer must be closed in a cerebrospinal fluid (CSF)-tight fashion. The muscle and fascial closure must not be under tension. A subcutaneous drain is placed in large incisions, and particularly in reoperations, or when the patient had undergone prior radiation therapy. The skin is closed with running, locked sutures. Patients who have had previous surgery and received radiation therapy are at higher risk for wound dehiscence and CSF leak.

The resection of extramedullary tumors follows these same lines. The vast majority of them are tackled with a posterior approach. Dorsolateral approaches are rarely needed and anterior approaches are only required in the exceptional case. After laminectomy or laminotomy, adequate bony exposure and location of the lesion are assured with the intraoperative ultrasound. Depending upon their individual locations, schwannomas, meningiomas or myxopapillary ependymomas can be removed in toto. Large tumors, particularly when located ventrally or ventrolaterally, may require piecemeal resection. Firm texture of the tumor, particularly in meningiomas, requires use of the microsurgical laser. We have found the use of this instrument to be by far the safest way to resect firm tumor attached to the cord. Manipulation of a firm mass with forceps, scissors or the CUSA may cause significant injury to the cord. The dural attachment of meningiomas need not be resected [11]; extensive coagulation of the dural layer after excision of the tumor bulk appears to be associated with the same small recurrence rate.

The most important strategy for the resection of completely intradural schwannomas is to sacrifice the nerve root that they are arising from. This greatly facilitates their resection and does not usually result in a significant neurological deficit.

In toto, resection of myxopapillary ependymomas of the filum should be attempted whenever the tumor has not yet spread into the arachnoid space (Fig. 29.7). Only disseminated ependymomas need to be resected in a piecemeal fashion, mostly using bipolar and suction. In this situation, there is invariably some residual tumor tissue left on the pia or the nerve root epineurium.

Intraoperative Neurophysiological Monitoring

Intraoperative monitoring with motor evoked potentials (MEPs) is a direct motor tract monitoring technique which is now the most important monitoring tool for spinal cord surgery [8,9]. Motor potentials are evoked with transcranial electrical stimulation of the motor cortex in two ways: a single-stimulus technique and a multipulse technique (Fig. 29.10). With a single stimulus, a single volley of signals in fast conducting corticospinal axons is generated, which is then recorded with an electrode placed on the spinal cord, usually in the epidural space. This signal is called a D-wave, because it results from *D*irect activation of these fast-conducting axons. The D-wave's amplitude is a relative measure of the number of fast-conducting corticospinal fibers (Fig. 29.11). The multipulse or train stimulus technique [21] evokes a muscle response in target muscles (thenar, anterior

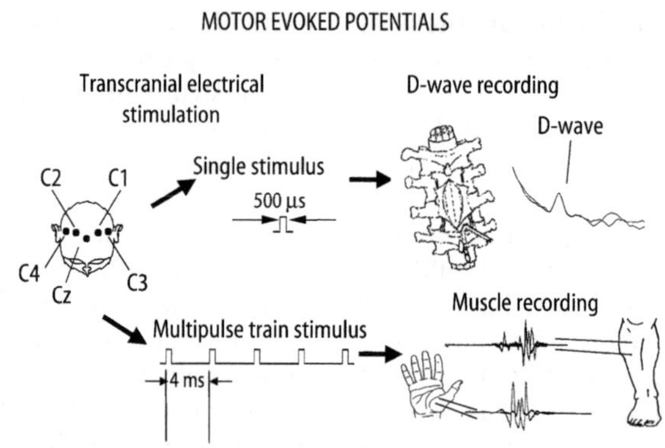

Fig. 29.10. Principles of MEP monitoring. MEPs are elicited with transcranial electrical stimulation (left) using two distinct stimulus techniques. The single-stimulus technique allows recording of D-waves (top), and the multipulse technique allows recording of muscle responses.

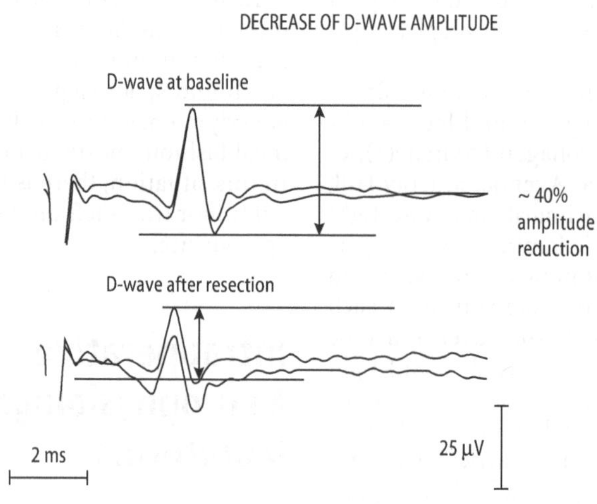

Fig. 29.11. The amplitude of D-waves is a measure of the number of fast-conducting fibers in the corticospinal tract. This amplitude is the primarily monitored parameter for intraoperative assessment of the functional integrity of the motor system in the spinal cord. A decrease of up to 50% from the baseline amplitude is associated with intact motor control in all instances.

tibialis). These muscle MEPs are interpreted in an all-or-none fashion. Their presence indicates intact functional integrity of the voluntary motor system in the spinal cord. Their absence indicates jeopardized functional integrity of the motor pathways, highly associated with an at least temporary disruption of voluntary motor control. The stimulation and recording of D-waves and muscle MEPs can be repeated every second. Therefore, the feedback information is provided in real time. Figure 29.4 summarizes the technique of stimulation and recording.

D-waves and muscle MEPs must be interpreted together. Loss of muscle MEPs during a spinal cord tumor resection indicates at least a temporary disruption of motor function of the spinal cord. The more incremental change of the D-wave amplitude then allows further interpretation of the motor outcome. A loss of muscle MEPs is highly associated with a temporary motor deficit in the lower extremities, even if the D-wave amplitude is unchanged. In the majority of cases, this is even side specific. As long as the D-wave amplitude remains above a cut-off value of about 50% of its baseline value, this motor deficit is temporary, with the patient recovering to pre-operative strength within hours to days, or sometimes weeks. A further decline in D-wave amplitude or its loss is associated with a long-term severe motor deficit [9].

The short-term neurological morbidity of intramedullary tumor surgery is about 30%. The combined use of epidural and muscle MEP recording has been shown to intraoperatively detect all post-operative motor deficits [8]. Most importantly, the combination of epidural and muscle MEPs allows for the neurophysiological identification of a reversible motor deficit. Thus, MEPs are giving information about injury to the motor system *before* this injury results in permanent, irreversible neurological deficit.

In particular, the resection of ventrally located intradural–extramedullary lesions requires some degree of spinal cord retraction. With the use of motor monitoring, this can be done safely, as the degree of retraction that is tolerated "functionally" can be assessed. This allows resection of anteriorly located extramedullary lesions via a simple posterior approach.

Somatosensory evoked potential (SEP) recording is of use to assess the functional integrity of the sensory system. The correlation of SEPs with post-operative motor function, however, is poor and, particularly in intramedullary surgery, SEPs tend to disappear when the midline myelotomy is performed and are then of no further use for the critical assessment of the motor system.

Electromyographic mapping of nerve roots, that is direct electrical stimulation of exposed nerves with a handheld probe and recording from lower extremity and sphincter ani muscles, is useful during resection of tumors in the conus/cauda equina region.

Continuous monitoring of the bulbocavernosus reflex (BCR) provides information on the functional integrity of oligosynaptic reflex arches involved in sphincter control. This has been shown to be feasible during general anesthesia, and there is good correlation of BCR data to post-operative sphincter control.

Surgical Complications

Functional Outcome

The feared complication after intraspinal and, in particular, intramedullary tumor surgery is paralysis. The incidence of this occurrence is related to the pre-operative functional status. Patients who have no or minimal pre-operative motor deficits have less than 3% incidence for this complication. On the other hand, patients who already have a significant motor deficit are more likely to deteriorate post-operatively [9].

While complete resection of extramedullary tumors should be attempted and is possible in almost all cases, the resection radicality in intramedullary surgery is lower. In fact, complete removal, particularly of the last fragments of tumor tissue, has a high risk of resulting in major neurological deficits. In the senior author's experience of intramedullary tumors, a gross total resection was feasible in about 70–80% of cases and a subtotal (80–97%) in the remainder. There was no surgical mortality. The short-term deterioration of motor function is significant. One-third of patients experience a transient motor deficit, which resolves within hours to days [8]. The long-term functional motor outcome is much better and directly related to the pre-operative neurological function [9]. Therefore, it is advisable that patients with intramedullary tumors undergo surgery before the development of significant neurological deficits.

Impaired joint position sense may be a serious functional disability and is more commonly seen after ependymoma rather than astrocytoma resection. Patients who have impaired proprioception may require extensive physical therapy to learn to compensate for this deficit. In addition, patients may experience a variety of pain syndromes, autonomic symptoms and decreased strength for prolonged physical activity.

Post-operative Spinal Deformity

Another potential problem is spinal deformity. Scoliosis and kyphosis may evolve after surgery [22]. This is particularly important for the pediatric patients, of whom about one-third with a significant deformity eventually require a stabilizing orthopedic operation. Several surgeons recommended osteoplastic laminotomy for all children, to reduce the incidence of spinal deformity [20]. In a study of 58 patients younger than 25 years of age who underwent multi-level laminectomy for various conditions, deformity occurred in 46% of patients younger than 15 years, and in 6% of children older than 15 years. In this series, 100% (nine of nine) of children who had a cervical laminectomy developed a post-operative deformity as compared to 36% for thoracic laminectomy, and none of six patients after lumbar laminectomy. It is therefore essential that children be followed particularly closely with plain radiographs and receive orthopedic evaluation. Surgical indications for spinal fusion should be regarded as more urgent in these patients than in those with idiopathic deformity. Furthermore, patients who develop progressive deformity should also undergo a new MRI to rule out tumor recurrence.

A spinal deformity may also be a result of radiation therapy used to treat epidural tumors. Mayfield et al. reported that 32 of 57 children with neuroblastoma treated with radiation therapy and chemotherapy developed significant spinal deformities. A higher rate of deformity was associated with younger age at time of radiation, doses greater than 20 Gy and asymmetrical radiation fields. This emphasizes that radiation therapy cannot be regarded as a "non-invasive" alternative to surgically treatable spinal cord tumors.

Cerebrospinal Fluid Leakage

This complication is very rare in patients who have not previously been operated on or received radiation therapy. However, after radiation therapy and/or previous surgery, there is a significant risk for wound dehiscence and CSF leak. Experiences with wound-healing problems revealed that meningitis resulted in the utilization of plastic surgical techniques with bilateral mobilization of the spinal muscles for wound closure. The fascia must be closed in a watertight fashion, without tension. Relaxing incisions laterally may be necessary to provide a tension-free closure. A sub-fascial or subcutaneous drain must be placed for several days to allow healing of the wound.

Oncological Outcome

It must be emphasized that in intramedullary tumor surgery, despite gross total resections, residual microscopic fragments are left in the resection bed. This residual tissue (in particular for glial neoplasms) may remain dormant or may involute over time. The clinical significance of these small fragments remains to be determined.

Long-term survival is better for low-grade neoplasms when compared to the high-grade group. The 5- and 10-year survival rates were 88 and 82%, respectively, for the low-grade neoplasms in the senior author's series. The cause of death in these patients was progression of disease and systemic complications after chemotherapy. The patients with high-grade neoplasms fared poorly, with an 18% 5-year survival, despite surgery and adjuvant therapy.

Intradural extramedullary tumors generally have a very favorable prognosis, with low recurrence rates (6%) after complete, and even after incomplete (17%), resection [11], unless the patient has neurofibromatosis [23].

Adjuvant Therapy

The deleterious effect of radiation has been mentioned above and no study has convincingly demonstrated a beneficial effect of radiation therapy on survival or neurological function for low-grade tumors. Although some authors still recommend radiotherapy for intramedullary spinal cord tumors, no study has been performed comparing the effects of radiation therapy for intramedullary neoplasms. Thus, these tumors should be recognized as a surgical disease, both at presentation and at time of recurrence. Stein also did not recommend radiotherapy for adult patients with low-grade intramedullary neoplasms, regardless of the extent of removal, and emphasized the deleterious effects of radiation on the spinal cord tissue adjacent to the tumor site. The results are similar to others who have reported myelopathy in children who have received doses of 30 Gy. Thus radiation therapy is reserved for patients with malignant tumors, those with documented post-operative rapid tumor regrowth or for those with substantial residual tumor who are not candidates for further surgery. Intramedullary ependymomas should be resected and radiotherapy is not an option for these patients.

We employ total neuraxis radiation for the malignant tumors. Unfortunately, it has been shown that glioblastomas invariably progress. Despite aggressive radiotherapy and chemotherapy, patients with these neoplasms have a median survival of 12 months.

Adjuvant therapy is usually not used for patients with intradural extramedullary tumors. However, for instance, patients with meningiomas of the rare clear-cell variant should be radiated after resection of a recurrent tumor [24]. Radiotherapy for the recurrent and nonresectable meningioma must also be considered.

Key Points

- *The strategy for intramedullary tumors has changed from a conservative to an aggressive approach with the improvement in preoperative planning.*
- *Intramedullary spinal cord tumors may remain asymptomatic for a long time and may increase to considerable size before they are detected.*
- *MRI is the study of choice to identify both intra- and extramedullary spinal cord neoplasms.*

References

1. Eiselsberg Av, Marburg O. Zur Frage der Operabilität intramedullärer Rückenmarkstumoren. Arch Psychiatr Nervenkr 1917;59:453–61.
2. Elsberg CA, Beer E. The operability of intramedullary tumors of the spinal cord: a report of two operations with remarks upon the extrusion of intraspinal tumors. Am J Med Sci 1911;142:636–47.
3. Gowers WR, Horsley V. A case of tumour of the spinal cord: removal and recovery. Med-Chir Trans 1888;53: 377–428.
4. Brotchi J, Dewitte O, Levivier M, Baleriaux D, Vandesteene A, Raftopoulos C et al. A survey of 65 tumors within the spinal cord: surgical results and the importance of preoperative magnetic resonance imaging. Neurosurgery 1991;29:651–6; discussion 656–7.
5. Epstein FJ, Epstein N. Surgical treatment of spinal cord astrocytomas of childhood. J Neurosurg 1982;57:685–9.
6. Greenwood J. Surgical removal of intramedullary tumors. J Neurosurg 1967;26:276–82.
7. Guidetti B, Mercuri S, Vagnozzi R. Long-term results of the surgical treatment of 129 intramedullary spinal gliomas. J Neurosurg 1981;54:323–30.
8. Kothbauer KF, Deletis V, Epstein FJ. Motor evoked potential monitoring for intramedullary spinal cord tumor surgery: correlation of clinical and neurophysiological data in a series of 100 consecutive procedures. Neurosurg Focus 1998;4:Article 1 (http://www.aans.org/journals/online_j/may98/4-5-1).
9. Morota N, Deletis V, Constantini S, Kofler M, Cohen H, Epstein FJ. The role of motor evoked potentials during surgery for intramedullary spinal cord tumors. Neurosurgery 1997;41:1327–36.
10. Yamamoto Y, Raffel C. Spinal extradural neoplasms and intradural extramedullary neoplasms. In: Albright AL, Pollack IF, Adelson PD, editors. Principles and practice of pediatric neurosurgery. New York: Thieme Medical Publishers, 1999; 685–96.
11. Solero CL, Fornari M, Giombini S, Lasio G, Oliveri G, Cimino C et al. Spinal meningiomas: review of 174 operated cases. Neurosurgery 1989;25:153–60.
12. Fischer G, Mansuy L. Total removal of intramedullary ependymomas: follow-up study of 16 cases. Surg Neurol 1980;14:243–9.
13. McCormick PC, Torres R, Post KD, Stein BM. Intramedullary ependymoma of the spinal cord. J Neurosurg 1990;72:523–32.
14. Schweitzer JS, Batzdorf U. Ependymoma of the cauda equina region: diagnosis, treatment, and outcome in 15 patients. Neurosurgery 1992;30:202–7.
15. Murovic J, Sundaresan N. Pediatric spinal axis tumors. Neurosurg Clin North Am 1992;4:947–58.
16. Constantini S, Miller DC, Allen JC, Rorke LB, Freed D, Epstein FJ. Radical excision of intramedullary spinal cord tumors: surgical morbidity and long-term follow-up evaluation in 164 children and young adults. J Neurosurg (Spine) 2000;93:183–93.
17. Cohen AR, Wisoff JH, Allen JC, Epstein F. Malignant astrocytomas of the spinal cord. J Neurosurg 1989; 70:50–4.
18. Epstein FJ, Farmer J-P, Freed D. Adult intramedullary astrocytomas of the spinal cord. J Neurosurg 1992; 77:355–9.
19. Goy AMC, Pinto RS, Raghavendra BN, Epstein FJ, Kricheff II. Intramedullary spinal cord tumors: MR imaging, with emphasis of associated cysts. Radiology 1986;161:381–6.
20. Raimondi AJ, Gutierrez FA, Di Rocco C. Laminotomy and total reconstruction of the posterior spinal arch for spinal canal surgery in childhood. J Neurosurg 1976;45:555–60.
21. Taniguchi M, Cedzich C, Schramm J. Modification of cortical stimulation for motor evoked potentials under general anesthesia: technical description. Neurosurgery 1993;32:219–26.
22. Yasuoka S, Peterson HA, MacCarty CS. Incidence of spinal column deformity after multilevel laminectomy in children and adults. J Neurosurg 1982;57:441–5.
23. Klekamp J, Samii M. Surgery of spinal nerve sheath tumors with special reference to neurofibromatosis. Neurosurgery 1998;42:279–90.
24. Jallo GI, Kothbauer KF, Silvera VM, Epstein FJ. Intraspinal clear cell meningioma. Diagnosis and management: report of two cases. Neurosurgery 2001;48: 218–22.

30

Management of Extradural Spinal Tumors

David A. Lundin, Charlie Kuntz and Christopher I. Shaffrey

Summary

The pathology and pathophysiology of both primary bony tumors and metastatic lesions that commonly invade the axial skeleton of the spinal canal and involve the spinal column are examined. A detailed description of possible lesions, diagnostic evaluation and treatment paradigms is included.

Introduction

There are a large number of tumors that involve the spinal column, spinal cord or the peripheral nerves near the axial skeleton. Despite the extensive differential diagnosis, there are factors such as age, location, incidence and pathology that provide important clues in correctly diagnosing each specific condition. The ability to effectively treat lesions involving the spinal column or spinal cord has increased dramatically over the past 15 years, if an early and accurate diagnosis is achieved.

For lesions involving the bony spinal column, younger patients tend to present with benign bone tumors more frequently than do those over 30 years of age. Adults, especially the elderly with spinal column lesions, are much more likely to have a malignancy. Malignant lesions involving the spinal column (whether primary tumors or metastases) occur more often in the vertebral body. Benign tumors usually originate in the spinous processes, laminae or the pedicles of the vertebrae. The incidence of skeletal metastases outweighs the incidence of primary malignant bone tumors by a margin of 25–40:1 [1–6].

A variety of parameters can be used to narrow the differential diagnosis for spinal cord and peripheral nerve tumors. Intramedullary tumors are much more common in children and represent approximately half of the intradural tumors. In adults, less than one-third of intradural tumors are in an intramedullary location. Taken as a whole, approximately two-thirds of spinal cord tumors are extramedullary and one-third are intramedullary. Intramedullary tumors are typically of glial origin – predominantly astrocytoma and ependymoma. In children, astrocyomas are more common, but in adults, ependymomas predominate. Extramedullary tumors are then divided into those which are intradural and those which are extradural. Intradural lesions are twice as frequent as extradural lesions, and primarily consist of nerve sheath tumors and meningiomas. Here, we will concentrate on those tumors arising in the extradural space. These consist of primary bone neoplasms and metastatic disease to the spine.

Primary Bony Neoplasms

Primary bony neoplasms of the spine can be either benign or malignant, and optimal management depends upon a precise diagnosis. Unfortunately, many of these lesions are located in poorly accessible places and the approaches for direct or percutaneous biopsy can have substantial risks. When approaching spinal neoplasms, the principles of tumor staging and oncologic resection should be considered. In general, patients presenting with a short duration of symptoms and a rapid progression of neurological findings are more likely to have a malignancy than are those with the slow onset of symptoms. Typically, benign lesions are found in the posterior elements of younger patients, whereas lesions found in the vertebral body in older patients are worrisome for malignancy. One study found that 75% of primary bony tumors involving the vertebral body were malignant, as opposed to 35% when the posterior elements alone were involved. This same study found that 80% of primary tumors were malignant in patients older than 18 years and only 32% were malignant when the patient was younger than 18 years [5].

Benign Tumors of the Spinal Column

Benign tumors of the axial skeleton are most commonly found in children and adolescents. When they occur in adults, they are generally found in individuals between 20 and 30 years of age, in a posterior location. The more common types of benign lesions - osteochondroma, osteoid osteoma and osteoblastoma - have a lower incidence of recurrence if a complete excision can be obtained. Unlike malignant tumors that require resection of a wide margin of normal tissue surrounding the lesion, resection of the benign tumor itself is usually curative. There are other "benign" tumors that can be associated with systemic disease, occur in multiple locations or are locally aggressive, including eosinophilic granulomas, giant cell tumors, aneurysmal bone cysts and hemangiomas, respectively.

Osteochondroma is a cartilage-capped, bony protuberance that is thought to develop from an adjacent physis or a cartilaginous remnant of the physis. Osteochondromas are the most common of the benign bone tumors. Over 50% of symptomatic spinal lesions occur in the cervical region, and they almost always involve the posterior elements. Osteochondromas can be a manifestation of multiple hereditary osteochondromatosis, which is one of the more common skeletal dysplasias. Clinical presentation varies from individuals reporting a dull backache (smaller tumors) to decreased motion or deformity (larger tumors). Neurological compromise is rare; however, when present, the cervical spine, followed by the thoracic spine, are the most common lesion locations, with resultant myelopathic symptoms. Plain radiographs demonstrate a protruding lesion, with well demarcated borders in the posterior elements. Treatment for this condition is usually observation, because the natural history is of very slow progression. On rare occasions, pain, neurological deficit or an accelerated growth pattern may necessitate surgical removal. Prognosis is usually excellent when complete curettage of the affected periosteum and surrounding cartilage is performed. Osteochondromas will occasionally degenerate into malignant chondrosarcomas (usually in patients with multiple lesions) [2–4].

Osteoid osteoma and osteoblastoma share a common pathologic origin but differ in size and incidence of spinal involvement. These tumors are thought to be a chronic inflammatory reaction rather than true neoplasms. Osteoid osteoma accounts for 2.6% of all excised primary bone tumors and up to 18% of axial skeletal primary lesions. By definition, osteoid osteomas are less than 2 cm in size; otherwise, the lesions are classified as osteoblastomas. Approximately 40% of spinal osteoid osteomas occur in the lumbar region, and the majority occur in the posterior elements. Most patients with symptomatic lesions are young and male. Half of all symptomatic lesions present in the second decade of life. On clinical presentation, patients report a dull ache, which is exacerbated at night. This condition is believed to be the result of prostaglandin production by the tumor - thus, the classic pain relief with aspirin. Neurological deficits are rare but osteoid osteoma is the most common lesion of painful scoliosis in adolescents. Radiologically, a radiolucent area with a central nidus and an appropriate degree of surrounding sclerosis characterizes the lesion. The treatment is excision. Instrumentation and fusion may be required if there is severe scoliosis, although minor deformities will resolve with resection alone. Overall, there is an excellent prognosis, with marginal recurrence rates related to inadequate excision of the nidus [1–4,6].

Osteoblastomas differ from osteoid osteomas in their attaining greater size (more than 2 cm). Histologically, the two lesions cannot be differentiated. Less common than osteoid osteomas, osteoblastomas represent less than 2% of primary benign bone tumors, but have a greater propensity for axial skeletal involvement. Approximately 30–40% of osteoblastomas involve the axial skeleton. The lesions are distributed throughout the longitudinal axis of the spine, occur most commonly in the posterior elements and have a propensity to produce spinal deformity (Fig. 30.1). In 90% of cases, osteoblastomas present in patients of 30 years of age or younger; these lesions have a male to female predominance of 2:1. Clinical presentation characteristically involves a higher incidence of neurological deficit, secondary to lesion size. Treatment is en-bloc resection, usually with resolution of scoliotic deformity. Prognosis is favorable with adequate removal. Long-term recurrence rates approach 10% [1–4,6].

Giant cell tumors (GCTs) are benign lesions of unknown cell origin. These aggressive tumors carry some malignant potential and a high incidence of local recurrence. They are responsible for 21% of all primary benign bone tumors and affect the spinal axis in 8–11% of all cases. They most commonly occur in the sacral region, when the spinal column is involved. Unlike the majority of primary bone tumors, GCTs are generally found in individuals in the third and fourth decades of life, with decreasing frequency in later years. Women are affected slightly more commonly than are men. Plain radiographs demonstrate cortical expansion, with little reactive sclerosis or periosteal reaction. MR images reveal homogeneous signals, while CT studies can better delineate the degree of vertebral bone involvement and define surgical margins. Because of the non-distinct histological characteristics of GCTs, a thorough evaluation, including radiographic investigation coupled with histopathology, is important, to differentiate this condition from other primary bone tumors. Treatment is usually an aggressive en-bloc resection, with consideration of adjuvant radiation therapy. There is a relatively poor prognosis because of the high recurrence rates (50%). These tumors have the potential for malignant transformation, especially after local radiation if surgical margins were inadequate [1–4].

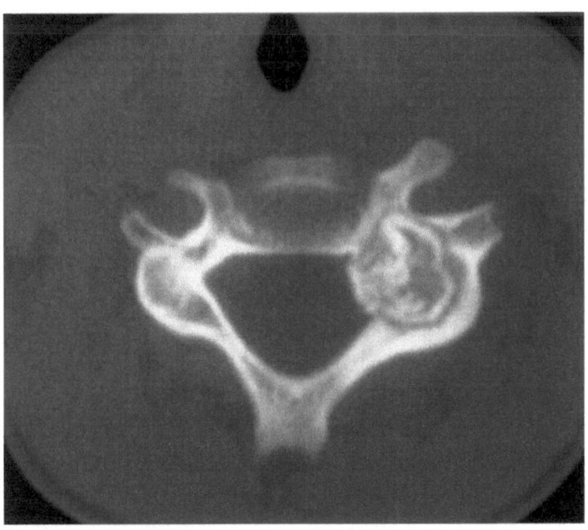

Fig. 30.1. Axial CT scan of an osteoblastoma. The patient is an 11-year-old male with a 6-month history of progressive neck pain.

Aneurysmal bone cysts (ABCs) are benign, non-neoplastic proliferative lesions. Although only responsible for approximately 1–2% of all primary bone tumors, ABCs affect the axial skeleton in 12–25% of all reported cases. The pathogenesis is unclear, but accepted theories include an underlying tumor or traumatic arteriovenous malformation, with subsequent development of a cyst. Histologically, ABCs contain fluid-filled spaces, separated by fibrous septa. The incidence of ABCs is greater in the thoracolumbar region. As in the majority of benign osseous lesions, posterior location predominates, with 60% of spinal aneurysmal bone cysts occurring in the posterior elements. ABCs typically present in young patients who are in their second decade of life, with a slight predominance in women. Radiographic imaging with MRI and CT demonstrates a multiloculated, expansile, highly vascular osteolytic lesion with a thin, well demarcated, eggshell-like cortical rim (Fig. 30.2). Multiple-level vertebral involvement may occur in up to 40% of cases. Treatment involves pre-operative embolization and surgical resection, or embolization alone

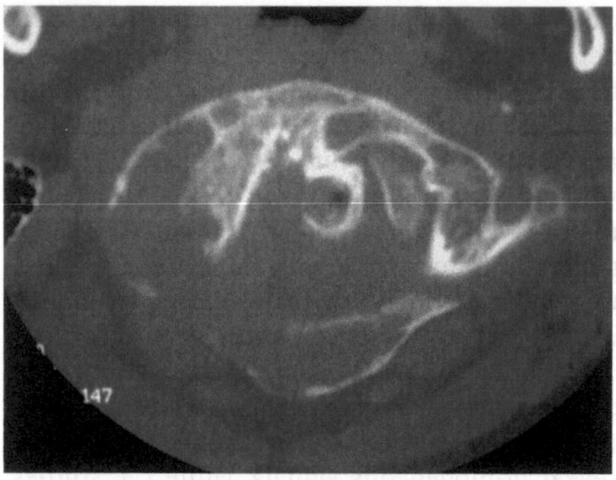

Fig. 30.2. Axial CT scan of an ABC. The patient is a 7-year-old female with a 3-month history of neck pain and torticollis.

for areas of the spine that are difficult to approach surgically. Post-operative radiation may have a role if inadequate margins were obtained during surgical resection. Recurrence rates vary from 6 to 70%, depending on the extent of surgical resection and administration of post-operative radiation [1–4,6,7].

Hemangiomas are benign tumors of vascular origin and are probably the most common benign tumor of the spine. General autopsy studies have found hemangiomas of the axial skeleton in 10–12% of cases. Characterized by slow growth and a female predominance, vertebral hemangiomas occur most commonly in the thoracolumbar spine and have a predilection for the vertebral body. Symptomatic vertebral hemangiomas are exceedingly rare but, when they do present, the most common initial symptom is back pain, with or without radiation into the lower extremities. There is a loose relationship between pregnancy and expansile vertebral hemangiomas that produce a neurological deficit. This is believed to be the result of the physiological volume increase of the circulatory system during pregnancy, which results in expansion of a previously asymptomatic lesion. Diagnosis of symptomatic lesions is best made with MRI, while asymptomatic lesions are discovered incidentally during other radiographic investigations. Treatment for symptomatic lesions involving the spine incorporates a combination of embolization, surgical resection and possibly radiotherapy, and is generally performed in cases of pathological fracture or neural impingement [1–4,6,8].

Eosinophilic granuloma (EG) is the solitary osseous lesion in a continuum of disorders (histiocytosis X, Letterer–Siwe and Hand–Schuller–Christian diseases) characterized by an abnormal proliferation of Langerhans cells. EGs are uncommon lesions of the axial skeleton, occurring most frequently in the vertebral body. Most EGs occur in the pediatric population, with a peak incidence at between 5 and 10 years of age. MRI and CT are the investigative procedures of choice, with ultimate diagnosis relying on biopsy. Treatment is somewhat controversial but commonly includes surgical curettage. Adjuvant radiotherapy or chemotherapy is reserved for disseminated versions of this uncommon disease of the axial skeleton [1–4,6,9].

Malignant Tumors of the Axial Skeleton

Malignant tumors of the axial skeleton can either be primary (arising from the bony skeleton itself) or metastatic. The most common metastatic spinal column tumors are breast, lung and prostate malignancies, while multiple myeloma, chordoma, chondrosarcoma, osteogenic sarcoma and Ewing's sarcoma are the more common primary malignant axial skeletal neoplasms. Metastasis can result from direct extension or hematogenous spread. Primary malignant axial skeletal neoplasms and metastatic tumors most frequently involve the vertebral body. Malignant tumors of the spinal column are 25–40 times more likely to be metastatic than primary [1–4,6].

Chordomas, originally described by Virchow, are tumors originating from the primitive notochord. Being tumors of the axial skeleton and the skull base, chordomas account for 1–2% of all skeletal sarcomas. Chordomas are histologically low-grade, locally invasive tumors; however, metastases may occur in 5–43% of chordoma cases. More than 50% of these lesions are located in the lumbosacral region, 35% in the clival and cervical area, and the remainder are spread throughout the vertebral column. Chordomas are the most common primary neoplasms of the sacrococcygeal region and occur predominantly in the fifth and sixth decades of life. Neurological deficit in the form of bowel and bladder dysfunction may be present at the time of diagnosis. MRI is probably the radiographic modality of choice for total tumor evaluation, because of the ability to evaluate soft-tissue involvement. CT remains the modality of choice for imaging the extent of bony destruction (Fig. 30.3). Diagnosis is based upon CT or fluoroscopic-guided biopsy. Treatment is en-bloc resection, when feasible. Radiation is usually reserved for local recurrence and surgically inaccessible disease. There is considerable debate on pathological subtypes with respect to grade, recurrence and outcome. Age at presentation is probably the best prognostic indicator for disease-free survival following surgery, with younger patients having a better prognosis [1–4,6,10,11].

Chondrosarcomas are rare, malignant, cartilage-forming neoplasms, arising from cartilaginous elements. These tumors primarily affect the adult appendicular skeleton, with rare spinal involvement (6% of cases). Chondrosarcomas arise either primarily or from pre-existing solitary osteochondromas, hereditary multiple exostosis or Paget's disease. There is an even distribution of tumor involvement among cervical, thoracic and lumbosacral locations.

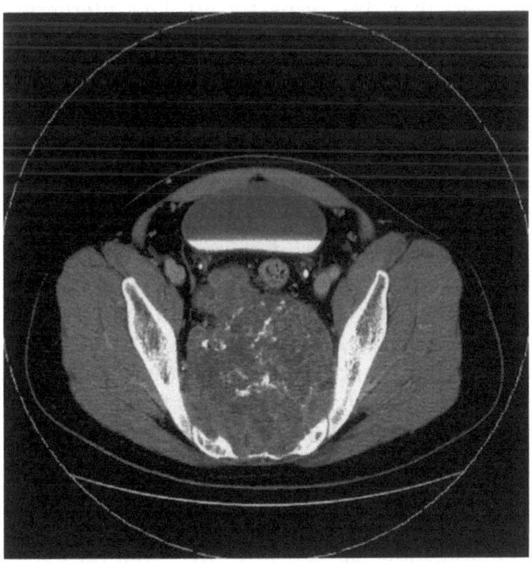

Fig. 30.3. Axial CT scan of a large sacrococcygeal chordoma. The patient is a 43-year-old male who presented with a 2–3-year period of progressive sacral pain. The patient went on to undergo an anterior L5/S1 discectomy, with bilateral sectioning of the sacroiliac ligaments, followed by posterior total sacrectomy, followed by L3 through iliac reconstruction.

Primary and secondary chondrosarcomas usually arise in middle-aged and older patients, and show a predilection for males. Diagnostic characteristics on MRI and CT radiographic imaging include bone destruction, associated soft-tissue mass and characteristic flocculent calcifications in the soft tissue mass. Definitive diagnosis is based upon biopsy of the tumor. Treatment is en-bloc resection, if feasible. Neither radiation therapy nor chemotherapy is of much benefit. Prognosis correlates with tumor extension and grade. Unresectable chondrosarcoma has a 5-year survival rate of only 20% [1–4,6,12].

Osteogenic sarcomas are primary malignant tumors of bone that are exceedingly rare in the axial skeleton. Only 2% of all osteogenic sarcomas arise in the spine. When they do involve the vertebral column, osteogenic sarcomas are more likely to be metastases than primary tumors. Osteogenic sarcomas may arise primarily or secondarily. The vertebral body is involved in over 95% of cases and these lesions are distributed evenly throughout the spine. The majority of cases of primary osteogenic sarcoma present in the first 20 years of life; secondary sarcomas arise in the fifth to sixth decades, as a result of irradiated bone or pre-existing Paget's disease. This neoplastic disease has a slight predilection for males. Radiologically, osteogenic sarcomas typically exhibit combined lytic and sclerotic lesions, with cortical destruction and ossification in the tumor mass. CT or fluoroscopic-guided biopsy will provide a diagnosis and guide pre-operative adjuvant therapy. Pre-operative embolization, chemotherapy and surgical extirpation with adjuvant radiotherapy are the current treatment modalities. Overall prognosis is poor, with a life expectancy of 10 months to 1.5 years, although there are a few long-term survivors [1–4,6].

Ewing's sarcomas are small, blue cell tumors of bone, whose cell of origin remains unclear (Fig. 30.6). Only 3–4% of Ewing's sarcomas arise within the axial skeleton, and Ewing's sarcomas only account for 6% of all primary malignant bone tumors, making these rare primary neoplasms of the spinal column. The incidence of spinal column involvement decreases from caudal to rostral, with more than 50% of Ewing's sarcomas arising within the sacrum. Vertebral body involvement is most common. Ewing's sarcoma is primarily a disease of the pediatric population, with over 85% of cases occurring during the first two decades of life. Males are affected more frequently than females, with a ratio of 2:1. Radiological imaging with MRI and CT will usually reveal a lytic lesion, with possibly a blastic component. Diagnosis is based upon biopsy of the tumor. Treatment involves a multidisciplinary approach that combines surgical extirpation, radiation and chemotherapeutic protocols. Younger patients tend to have a better prognosis. Survival at 5 years for younger patients approaches 75% [1–4,6,13].

Multiple myelomas (MMs) and solitary plasmacytomas are two manifestations on a continuum of B-cell lymphoproliferative diseases. Spinal involvement leading to extradural compression is a common finding in multiple myelomas. MMs are the most common malignant neoplasms of bone in adults and affect the spine in 30–50% of reported cases. The thoracic spine is affected most commonly, followed by the lumbar spine and, rarely, the cervical spine (less than 10%). The vertebral body is usually the site of tumor involvement. MM is primarily a disease of the fifth, sixth and seventh decades of life. There is an equal distribution for MM among males and females; however, approximately 75% of solitary plasmacytomas occur in males. Unlike the classic axial skeletal tumor presentation of pain with recumbency, MM lesions are sometimes relieved by rest and aggravated by mechanical agitation, mimicking other degenerative sources of pain. Diagnosis for MM is based upon characteristic serum protein abnormalities and radiological imaging. Plain radiographs and CT can be almost solely diagnostic because of the characteristic osteolytic picture without sclerotic edges involving the vertebral body and sparing the posterior elements. Treatment and prognosis vary greatly, depending on whether the diagnosis is a solitary plasmacytoma or the systemic MM. Both conditions are exquisitely radiosensitive, but with significantly longer survival rates for solitary plasmacytoma [1–4,6].

Metastatic Spinal Disease

Cancer is a leading cause of death in the USA, claiming nearly half a million deaths each year. The vast majority of these patients will have some evidence of metastatic disease. In fact, spinal metastases occur in virtually all types of systemic carcinomas. Although certain cancers are more likely to spread to the spine, surgical or autopsy studies have found that as high as 90% of patients with systemic carcinomas have spinal metastases. Between 5 and 20% of these patients will have epidural compression secondary to this, leading to neurological compromise [2,14–23].

Overall, metastatic lesions are equally spread throughout the thoracic and lumbosacral spine; however, the number of symptomatic thoracic metastases is greater. Epidural compression leading to neurological compromise is found in the thoracic region in roughly 70% of cases and in the lumbar region 20% of the time. Most series report symptomatic cervical lesions occurring in only 6–8% of patients. The axiom, however, that acute neck or back pain in a patient with a known malignancy is metastatic disease until proven otherwise remains a prudent guideline. The majority of patients have involvement at a single level, although 15–20% of patients have compression at two or more sites [2,14–23].

The vertebral body is involved most commonly (85%), with the posterior elements and epidural space involved less frequently (10–15% and less than 5%, respectively). The intervertebral disk is almost universally spared from metastatic disease, even when the vertebral body is completely destroyed. Two factors have been proposed to explain this distribution. First has been the high concentration of growth factors found in the rich medullary bone of the body to both attract tumor cells and promote their growth. Many of these factors, such as basic fibroblast growth factor (bFGF), hepatocyte growth factor (HGF) and tumor necrosis factor-((TNF-(), are well known to facilitate angiogenesis and subsequent tumor growth. The second mechanism involves the draining of the venous plexus of the thoracic, abdominal and pelvic viscera, as described by Batson [2,14–23].

Most frequently, metastases result from hematogenous spread into the vertebral body. To establish a presence in the medullary bone, tumor cells must bypass the filters of the liver and lungs to reach the capillary system of the bone. This explains the fact that in a significant number of patients with spinal metastasis, additional lesions are found in those organs.

Another potential route is via direct flow from segmental arteries from the lungs or through Batson's para-vertebral venous plexus. A mechanism of retrograde flow though this plexus has been described with Valsalva's maneuvers, such as coughing or straining. This hypothetically allows for direct implantation of tumor cells into the spinal column. The final pathway is via direct extension into the bony column from the cancer's primary site. This is seen in lung cancer that extends into the thoracic spine and occasionally in rectal cancer that spreads into the sacrum [2,14–23].

The most common metastatic spinal column tumors are breast, lung and prostate malignancies. Additional cancers that also frequently metastasize to the spine include renal cell, thyroid cancer and multiple myeloma. Although there has been some argument between authors as to whether the latter lesions represent true metastasis or primary lesions of the medullary bone, we have included it in our section on primary bony malignancies [2,14–23].

A variety of studies have compared the results of radiation therapy and surgical management of metastatic disease. Many of these studies compared laminectomy to radiation therapy. Over the past 10 years, there has been a re-evaluation of the surgical approach to vertebral metastasis. The principal site of neural compression in metastatic spine disease is from an anterior or antero-lateral direction. Laminectomy further destabilizes an already compromised spinal column, resulting in progressive deformity and pathological fracture. Laminectomy also results (at best) in incomplete resection of the metastatic disease. Recent studies using aggressive anterior surgical approaches and current instrumentation techniques have shown very promising results in reducing pain, improving function with a relatively low complication rate [24] (Figs 30.4 and 30.5).

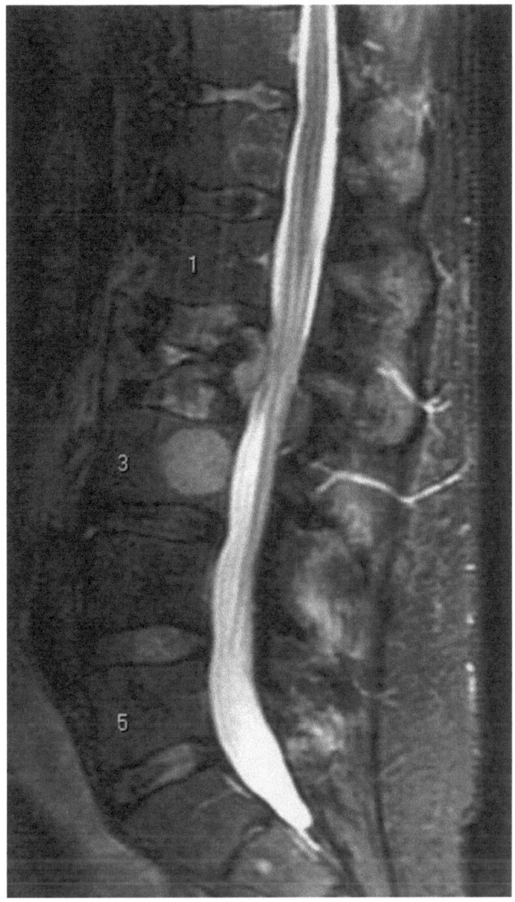

Fig. 30.4. Sagittal T2-wieghted MRI (for patient's details, please see Fig. 30.5).

Breast Carcinoma

By far the most prevalent of all metastatic tumors found in the spine, breast cancer has been cited to spread to the spinal column in 85% of all cases. However, the natural history of these tumors varies considerably. Some patients may present with a prolonged course of minimal symptoms, while others deteriorate rapidly. Local, radicular and referred pain are the most common symptoms seen in patients with metastatic breast cancer. This is reasonably tied to the biologic activity and, potentially, the hormonal sensitivity of the primary lesions. It is therefore useful to know the degree to which estrogen and progesterone receptors are present, as this can have a considerable impact on the modality of treatment that patients are offered. In such patients, hormonal manipulations via medical treatment are often used.

Often leading to osteolytic lesions, breast carcinomas are the primary cause of pathologic fractures due to metastatic disease. In certain series, breast carcinomas have been cited as being responsible for more than 50% of pathologic fractures.

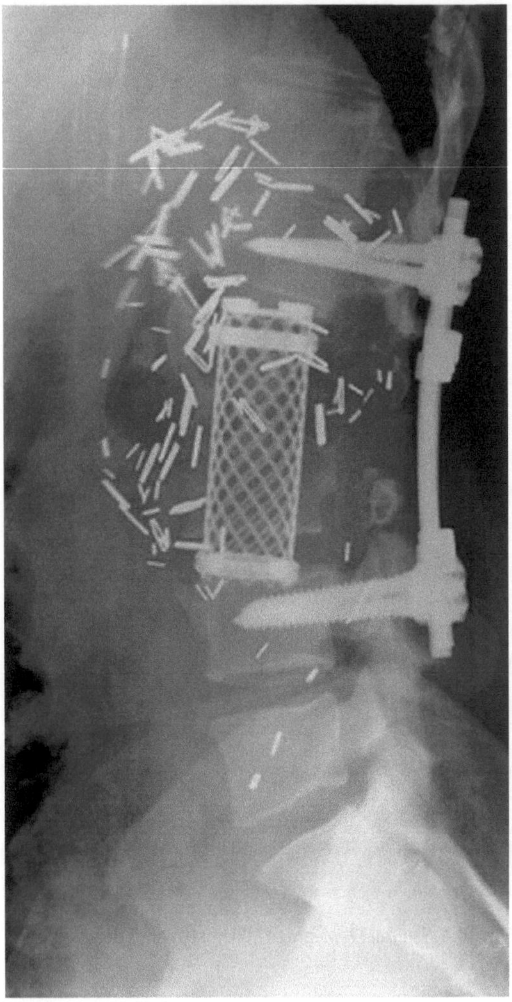

Fig. 30.5. Post-operative lumbar radiograph of a 42-year-old male with a history of metastatic renal cell carcinoma. The patient initially underwent radiation therapy but continued to have severe intractable pain and progressive neurological deficits. The patient went on to undergo a two-stage procedure, including L2 and L3 laminectomies, with L1–L4 posterior segmental instrumentation, followed by a right-sided retroperitoneal approach to the lumbar spine, followed by L2 and L3 corpectomies, with L1–L4 anterior reconstruction using a titanium cage. Prior to surgery, the patient underwent angiography and tumor embolization.

Many patients with previously diagnosed and treated breast cancer have undergone some form of radiotherapy. It is therefore important for the clinician to evaluate the patient's cardio-pulmonary function prior to consideration of further therapy. Pulmonary function often can be significantly impaired in patients with parenchymal pathology, either from radiation to the chest wall or from primary lymphangitic spread of the breast cancer itself.

Most cases of breast carcinoma are fairly radiosensitive; therefore, radiation is the first-line treatment for spinal metastasis. Surgery is reserved for cases in which clear instability or neurological deficit is present, severe pain that is unresponsive to conservative measures, tumors that have not responded to radiation treatment or when previous irradiation fields overlap with areas of new disease, making further irradiation contraindicated [2,14–20].

Prostate Carcinoma

Prostate cancer is second only to lung cancer as the leading cause of cancer-related deaths in men. Histological evidence of prostate cancer is directly related to increasing age. The incidence of occult disease has been shown to be as high as 30% in patients over the age of 50 years and over 70% in patients over the age of 80 years. The presence or absence of metastases primarily determines the prognosis of prostate cancer. The highest incidence of prostate metastases is found in bone, and lesions in the spine are felt to precede those in other areas of the body, such as the lung or liver. Kuban et al. found that spinal cord compression occurs in approximately 7% of all men with prostate cancer. Many argue for a backward venous spread of tumor to the spine. This is felt to account for the gradual decrease in spine involvement from the lumbar to the cervical spine (from 97 to 38%).

New onset of back pain in elderly men should be carefully evaluated for evidence of metastatic prostate cancer. For those patients with a known medical history of prostate cancer, back pain should also lead the clinician to entertain a diagnosis of recurrence, with metastases. In such patients, it is often helpful to routinely check the serum prostate-specific antigen (PSA) level. If the serum PSA level is greater than 100 ng/ml, then the positive predictive value for bony metastasis is 74%. Conversely, a level of less than 10 ng/ml indicates a negative predictive value of 98%. As the PSA level is a relative marker for extent of disease, it is useful to have prior levels and trends to compare current levels with.

Prostate cancer is distinct from other bony metastasis in that it produces mainly osteoblastic lesions. Whereas most cancers typically produce osteolytic lesions, this is true in only 5% of cases of metastatic prostate cancer. The proposed mechanism of this is related to the production of peptide growth factors, such as insulin-like growth factors (IGFs).

Most prostate metastases are fairly radiosensitive; thus, surgical management is generally reserved for those cases that have responded poorly to radiation or where spinal instability or pathological fracture is present. Surgery may also be indicated when a patient's prior prostate radiation fields preclude the use of additional radiation. The latter is not an uncommon event for lesions found in the lumbar spine, due to the close proximity to the prostate. Since most patients present later in life, the overall medical condition and medical co-morbidities which could complicate surgery must be carefully weighed against the patient's expectations from surgery [2,14–19,21].

Lung Carcinoma

Metastasis to bone is the most frequent extrapulmonary site of recurrence in patients with non-small cell lung carcinoma, accounting for as many as 43% of all distant recurrences. Of these, metastases to the spine are the most significant and potentially debilitating. Lung carcinoma may invade the spinal column, through direct extension or via hematogenous routes. Most frequently, metastases produce osteolytic lesions, which result from a variety of acid phosphatases, acid hydrolases and alkaline phosphatases. Lung carcinoma follows the typical pattern of spread, with the thoracic spine being most commonly involved, followed by the lumbar spine and finally the cervical spine.

The ultimate biologic activity of the subtypes of lung carcinoma is directly linked to their presumed cell of origin. Squamous cell carcinoma is thought to arise from the basal cell of the bronchial epithelium; adenocarcinoma from the CLARA cell of the bronchiole; bronchoalveolar carcinoma from the type II pneumocytes; and for small (oat) cell carcinoma, the neuroendocrine cells of the bronchoalveolar system are felt to be responsible. The cell of origin for large cell carcinoma is yet to be clearly defined. Of these, however, the spine surgeon rarely encounters those patients with disease other than non-small cell adenocarcinoma. This is due to the rarity of some lesions, such as large cell carcinoma, and to the exquisite sensitivity to radiation for small cell tumors. Patients with squamous cell disease typically have very aggressive disease that is widely disseminated in the lungs and liver, with overall survival looked at in terms of months.

Overall, the prognosis of patients with vertebral metastasis from lung carcinoma remains poor. With the exception of some patients with small cell carcinoma, in which significant responses or even remissions may be seen after chemotherapy and radiation, for the majority of patients with non-small cell disease, the goal of therapy is palliation and prevention of neurological deficits. Due to the relative radio-insensitivity of non-small cell carcinoma compared to breast or prostate cancer, patients may more frequently require surgical intervention to attain these goals [2,14,15,17–19,22].

Renal Carcinoma

Although renal cell carcinoma (RCC) is relatively rare compared to lung, breast or prostate cancer, it is an aggressive malignancy that frequently metastasizes. The approximately 30,000 cases of renal cell carcinoma account for only 2.5% of all cancer patients. However, as many as 50% of these patients will have evidence of metastatic disease at the time of diagnosis [25]. Although metastatic renal cell carcinoma is found in multiple organs, there is a disproportionately high number of metastases to the spine, making it the fourth most common cancer to affect the spine, and the most common type to present with a neurological deficit as an initial presentation [25].

In contrast with breast and prostate cancer, however, the majority of RCCs are highly resistant to systemic chemotherapy and radiation therapy. In a minority of patients, immunotherapy such as interferon- or interleukin-2 will show a partial response. Therefore, at many institutions, surgery is considered to be the primary treatment option.

Surgery is most often indicated in patients with severe, medically intractable pain, neurological deficit or spinal instability. Classically, RCC is richly vascularized in comparison to other metastatic tumors of the spine. Therefore, many patients undergo pre-operative tumor angiography and embolization to minimize the degree of blood loss during surgery. Although the effectiveness of pre-operative embolization has been debated, it is typically performed prior to non-emergent surgery in patients with large tumors.

Due to the absence of effective systemic therapy, the prognosis of metastatic RCC remains poor, with less than 15% survival at 5 years. Surgical resection and stabilization can provide effective pain relief and neurological preservation or improvement, and the goal of therapy is palliation and prevention of neurological deficits, rather than increase in length of survival [2,14,15,17–19,25].

Diagnosis

The first symptom of bony metastasis is often back pain. In fact, pain is the most common presenting symptom for tumors involving the axial skeleton and spinal cord. The hallmark of neoplastic lesions of the axial skeleton is localized spinal pain, associated with recumbency and night pain. Pain in the axial skeleton occurs in up to 85% of patients in the larger series of vertebral column tumors and usually begins well prior to any radicular pain or neurological deficit. However, ultimate diagnosis relies on a combination of laboratory investigation, radiographic studies and, potentially, tumor biopsy.

Diagnostic imaging is a cornerstone in the diagnosis of metastatic lesions of the spine. Typically, patients with known carcinoma are staged using multiple modalities of imaging, although, frequently, the spinal axis is not routinely screened unless symptoms are present.

The initial work-up for all patients should include plain radiographs of the spine. Anterior–posterior and lateral X-rays of the region in question can often give important information in the diagnosis of malignancy and can typically be done in an expedited fashion, with little cost to the medical system or patient. Pathologic compression fractures, the presence of a blastic lesion or destructive process within the vertebral bodies, or the destruction of the pedicle on AP views are often characteristic of spinal metastasis. Further, important information on sagittal alignment, including the presence of a kyphotic or scoliotic deformity, is best seen with plain X-rays. These caveats can be helpful in determining a requirement for stabilization or corrective procedures.

CT scanning of an involved area is also often warranted. The sensitivity of CT scanning is higher than that of plain films, although this modality is used most commonly to further define the degree of bony involvement and/or destruction. The detail of bony anatomy is useful in surgical planning, especially if instrumentation will be used for stabilizing the spine. Finally, in patients in which MRI is not an option, such as those with known metal fragments in their body or incompatible devices such as pacemakers, CT scanning with the administration of intrathecal contrast can help to define the degree of epidural extension

Recently, MRI has become the gold standard for radiological diagnosis of spinal metastasis. The ability of MRI to clearly visualize both the soft tissue, extradural and intradural contents in multiple planes makes this modality unique. Further, pending any contraindications to MRI, it enables the surgeon to evaluate the neural elements, with little or no risk to the patient. As MRI technology advances and as MRI-incompatible devices and hardware become less common, the utility of invasive tests such as myelography is sure to become more limited.

Another screening test that is commonly used in patients thought to have bony metastasis is isotope Tc99m bone scan. Often, bone scans are used as an adjuvant to standard screening examinations for patients with cancer. While these tests are useful in detecting bony lesions in patients with metastatic disease, the specificity of them is poor, as patients with degenerative processes or infectious processes can have lesions that are similarly bright on bone scan [2,14–23].

Treatment

The primary goal in treating all of the above malignancies remains palliation rather than cure. Therefore, relief of pain and preservation of neurological function should be optimized. Treatment options for metastatic disease of the spine include medical therapy, radiation and surgical intervention. Operative intervention is palliative, with pain control and maintenance of function and stability as the goals.

Surgery is usually reserved for neurological compromise, pathological fracture, intractable pain, radiation failure, spinal instability or uncertain diagnosis. The patient's pre-operative functional status and level of activity directly correlate with the post-operative result. When neurological deficit is present, those patients who suffer progressive neurological deficits, occurring within a 24-hour period, have a higher chance of permanent paraplegia, while those with slowly evolving deficits are more likely to regain ambulatory function. Overall prognosis is directly related to neoplastic type, spinal location and extent of systemic involvement [2,14–23].

Key Points

- *Tumors of the axial skeleton arise primarily from the bone or spread to the bone via hematogenous routes.*
- *Primary bone tumors can be benign or malignant; benign lesions are typically found in patients who are younger than 30 years of age and are more commonly found in the posterior elements; malignant lesions are typical in older patients and most commonly found within the vertebral body.*
- *The most frequent metastatic lesions to the spine arise from malignancy of the breast, prostate and lung.*
- *Diagnostic studies include physical examination, plain roentgenography, CT scanning and MRI, with the latter being the gold standard in imaging.*
- *Treatment for metastatic disease is primarily palliative; initial treatment is typically radiation therapy, with surgical treatment reserved for unclear diagnosis, intractable pain, spinal instability or neurological deficit.*

References

1. Dreghorn CR, Newman RJ, Hardy GJ, Dickson RA. Primary tumors of the axial skeleton: experience of the Leeds Regional Bone Tumor Registry. Spine 1990;15: 137–40.
2. Boden SD, Laws ER. Tumors of the spine. In: Boden S, editor. The aging spine: essentials of pathophysiology, diagnosis, and treatment. Philadelphia: WB Saunders, 1991; 221–52.
3. Boriani S, Weinstein JN. Differential diagnosis and surgical treatment of primary benign and malignant neoplasms. In: Frymoyer JW, editor. The adult spine: principles and practice. 2nd Edition. Philadelphia: Lippincott-Raven, 1997; 951–1014.
4. Ebersold MJ, Hitchon PW, Duff JM. Primary bony spinal lesions. In: Benzel EC, editor. Spine surgery: techniques, complication avoidance, and management. New York: Churchill Livingstone, 1999; 663–77.
5. Weinstein JN, McLain RF. Primary tumors of the spine. Spine 1987;12:843–51.
6. Weinstein JN. Tumors of the spine. In: Simeone FA, editor. The spine. 3rd Edition. Philadelphia: WB Saunders, 1992; 1279–319.
7. Gupta VK, Gupta SK, Khosla VK, Vashisth RK, Kak VK. Aneurysmal bone cysts of the spine. Surg Neurol 1994;42:428–32.
8. Faria SL, Schlupp WR, Chiminazzo H Jr. Radiotherapy in the treatment of vertebral hemangiomas. Int J Radiat Oncol Biol Phys 1985;11:387–90.
9. De Schepper AM, Ramon F, Van Marck E. MR imaging of eosinophilic granuloma: report of 11 cases. Skeletal Radiol 1993;22:163–6.
10. Bjornsson J, Wold LE, Ebersold MJ, Laws ER. Chordoma of the mobile spine: a clinicopathologic analysis of 40 patients. Cancer 1993;71:735–40.
11. O'Neill P, Bell BA, Miller JD, Jacobson I, Guthrie W. Fifty years of experience with chordomas in southeast Scotland. Neurosurgery 1985;16:166–70.
12. Slater G, Huckstep RL. Management of chondrosarcoma. Aust N Z J Surg 1993;63:587–9.
13. Sharafuddin MJ, Haddad FS, Hitchon PW, Haddad SF, el-Khoury GY. Treatment options in primary Ewing's sarcoma of the spine: report of seven cases and review of the literature. Neurosurgery 1992;30:610–18; discussion 618–19.
14. Gerszten PC, Welch WC. Current surgical management of metastatic spinal disease. Oncology (Huntingt) 2000;14:1013–24; discussion 1024, 1029–30.
15. Welch WC, Jacobs GB. Surgery for metastatic spinal disease. J Neurooncol 1995;23:163–70.
16. Benjamin R. Neurologic complications of prostate cancer. Am Fam Physician 2002;65:1834–40.
17. Healey JH, Brown HK. Complications of bone metastases: surgical management. Cancer 2000;88(Suppl.12): 2940–51.
18. Ratanatharathorn V, Powers WE. Epidural spinal cord compression from metastatic tumor: diagnosis and guidelines for management. Cancer Treat Rev 1991;18: 55–71.
19. Byrne TN. Spinal cord compression from epidural metastases. N Engl J Med 1992;327:614–19.
20. Landreneau FE, Landreneau RJ, Keenan RJ, Ferson PF. Diagnosis and management of spinal metastases from breast cancer. J Neurooncol 1995;23:121–34.
21. Osborn JL, Getzenberg RH, Trump DL. Spinal cord compression in prostate cancer. J Neurooncol 1995; 23:135–47.
22. Greenberger JS. The pathophysiology and management of spine metastasis from lung cancer. J Neurooncol 1995;23:109–20.

23. Jahroudi N, Greenberger JS. The role of endothelial cells in tumor invasion and metastasis. J Neurooncol 1995;23:99–108.
24. Gokaslan ZL, York JE, Walsh GL, McCutcheon IE, Lang FF, Putnam JB Jr et al. Transthoracic vertebrectomy for metastatic spinal tumors. J Neurosurg 1998;89: 599–609.
25. Jackson RJ, Loh SC, Gokaslan ZL. Metastatic renal cell carcinoma of the spine: surgical treatment and results. J Neurosurg 2001;94(Suppl.1):18–24.

31

Degenerative Disease of the Cervical Spine

Paul J. Marcotte and Mark G. Burnett

Summary

This chapter will focus on cervical spondylosis and the resulting symptomatology, including pain, nerve root and spinal cord compression. The pathophysiology, imaging diagnostics and treatments for cervical spine degeneration are discussed. A variety of operative and non-operative treatment modalities are available, including rest, anti-inflammatories, decompressive surgery and fusion surgery, with the goal of treatment being to diminish pain, restore neurological function and re-establish spinal stability.

Degeneration of the cervical motion segments is an inevitable consequence of aging. The configuration and extent of the degenerative process vary from patient to patient, as do the clinical manifestations. Recent advances in the understanding of cervical spondylosis, biomechanics, imaging techniques and surgical procedures have led to more effective management of symptomatic patients. This chapter will discuss the current concepts of cervical spondylosis, management strategies and some of the consequences associated with surgical treatment of spondylosis.

Pathophysiology and Biomechanics

The cervical region is a highly mobile segment of the spine. At rest, in a neutral position, the normal cervical spine has a gentle lordotic configuration, due to increased disc height anteriorly. In this neutral position, the balance point between flexion and extension of the spine runs through the center of the vertebral body of C2 and the odontoid process at the occipital–cervical junction, and extends down to the cervical–thoracic junction. In this neutral position, there is a balance between flexion and extension forces across the cervical spine segment, so that minimal muscle contraction is required to maintain neck position. When the neck becomes more forward-flexed and kyphotic, more tonic paraspinal muscle contraction is required to maintain the head in the upright position.

The subaxial cervical spine facet orientation enables movements in all three primary planes. The joint spaces are flattened and horizontal, with a posterior and an inferior inclination. This configuration of the cervical facet joints enables a wide range of motion in all primary directions, including flexion/extension, lateral bending and rotation. Some of these movements can be purely in one direction and others are compound movements in which there is spinal movement in more than one plane simultaneously. From a functional point of view, the cervical spine can be divided into two segments, based upon the different anatomic characteristics of each component. The atlantoaxial complex is unique in that its major articulation involves the odontoid process and transverse ligament complex. Although a minimal amount of flexion and lateral bending can occur across the atlantoaxial complex, the dominant movement is rotation. Fifty percent of cervical rotation takes place across C1 and C2.

Stability of the cervical spine motion segments is primarily dependent upon the ligamentous structures and paraspinal musculatures. The facet joint capsules, anterior and posterior longitudinal ligaments and annulus limit the physiological range of motion of the cervical spine. The paraspinal musculature also contributes to stability, in addition to its obvious function of inducing spinal movement.

Degeneration of the cervical spine motion segments results from an accumulation of repeated movement, stress and strain on the osseoligamentous structures. Genetic and developmental factors may have an influence on the vulnerability of the cervical spine to degenerative change. Although all the mobile components of the cervical spine are susceptible to degenerative change, the subaxial cervical spine is most often (and severely) affected compared to the atlantoaxial complex. In particular, the lower cervical motion segments at C5–C6, C6–C7 and, to a lesser extent, C4–C5 typically incur maximal degenerative change. These segments are most vulnerable because they incur the widest degree of range of motion and the maximal amount of axial stress of the cervical spine motion segments. The precise pathogenesis of cervical spondylosis is not clearly understood. Current concepts suggest that changes in the disk initiate the cascade of changes in cervical spondylosis. Degeneration of the facets and ligaments and reactive bony changes follow the primary diskogenic pathology.

Initial changes in the disk include loss of water content and changes in the relationship of the glucose aminoglycans and other polymers within the disk (Fig. 31.1). The volume of the disk is diminished and the biomechanical characteristics are altered. In a normal disk, the central component of the disk bears and transmits most of the weight across the motion segment. As the disk degenerates, the nature of the weight-bearing function of the disk changes and becomes more diffuse throughout the cross-sectional surface area of the disk. These changes put more stress and strain on the underlying peripheral endplates of the adjacent vertebrae. Loss of volume of the disk reduces tension on the annulus. The laxity of the annulus and the longitudinal ligaments and alterations of the disk change the character of movement across the interspace. Instead of pivoting across a stationary focal instantaneous axis of rotation, the axis of rotation becomes more widespread and its location varies, depending on the configuration of the motion segment.

The altered dynamics of motion across the disk are transmitted through the pedicles, to affect the relationship of the facet articulations posteriorly. The apposition of the facet joint surfaces is altered by the anterior changes and abnormal asymmetric stresses are placed upon the joint surfaces, which causes deterioration of the cartilaginous surfaces of the joints and promotes synovial tissue and bony reactive changes.

In response to the disk and facet changes, the ligaments and capsules which bridge the adjacent vertebrae are placed under abnormal stress and strain, and change in consistency and compliance. Traction spurs can result at the site of insertion of the ligaments, as another form of reaction to the biomechanical stress. Bony changes also result from the disk and facet joint changes. This takes the form of sclerosing of these bones and the accumulation of osteophytes and bone spurs.

In addition to the typical forms of spondylosis discussed above, two other unique forms of cervical degeneration have been observed: ossification of the posterior longitudinal ligament (OPLL) and diffuse idiopathic skeletal hypertrophy (DISH). Both of these disorders are considered forms of spondylosis, which take specific patterns. The reason for the characteristic manifestations of each is uncertain. Patients with OPLL have a preferential accumulation of calcium in the posterior longitudinal ligament (Fig. 31.2). The accumulation of calcium is not confined to the disk space, but can extend vertically for a variable distance along the posterior longitudinal ligament. The volume of calcification observed in this a 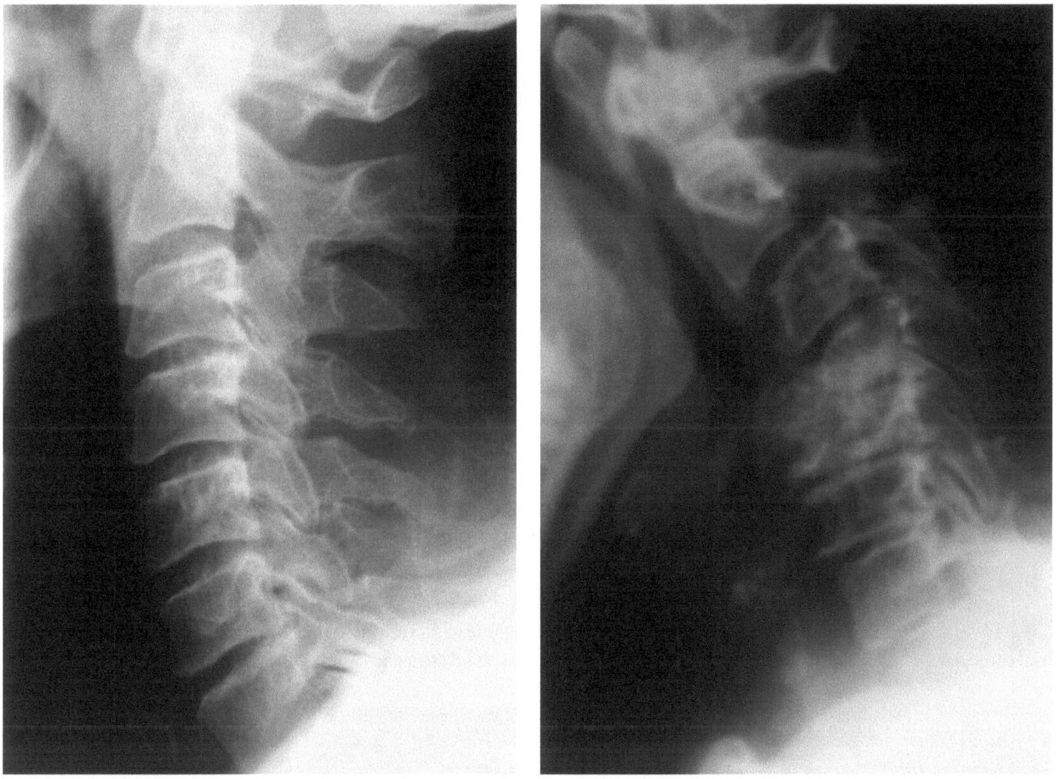 b

Fig. 31.1. Lateral X-rays of a normal (**a**) and degenerate (**b**) cervical spine. The normal cervical spine has a gentle lordotic curvature, with a neutral axis located along the posterior aspects of the vertebral bodies. Advanced degenerative changes **b** are seen in the mid-cervical spine. The cervical lordosis is lost and there is a kyphotic deformity from C3 to C5. There are advanced degenerative changes affecting disks, with significant loss of disk space height and sclerotic changes involving the vertebral bodies. Osteophytes are present both anteriorly and posteriorly at C4–C5 and C5–C6.

condition is quite variable and can be extreme. A patient with DISH has an exuberant accumulation of anterior osteophytes and calcification along the vertebral bodies (Fig. 31.3). In addition to the distinct changes of each of these conditions, the patients have advanced degenerative changes involving the disk spaces. OPLL is more commonly seen in the Asian population. No specific cause has been determined. DISH is somewhat more common in African-American males.

Clinical Manifestations and Differential Diagnosis

The consequences of the spondylitic process include diminished range of motion of the neck, pain or neurological deficits. The diminished range of motion of the neck results from the diminished volume of the disk, accumulation of osteophyte and change in consistency of the ligamentous and capsular structures. Crepitus can also be appreciated in some patients. This also results from accumulation of osteophyte and changes in the consistence of ligamentous structures and joint surfaces.

Pain is the most common manifestation of spondylosis. The character, severity and distribution of the pain are variable. In some people, the degenerative changes are painless. Pain can result from inflammation and reaction to the osseoligamentous changes or from irritation or compression of nerve roots or dural structures. Depending on the origin of the pain, it can be axial and/or appendicular in distribution. Ascertaining the origin of the pain can be problematic.

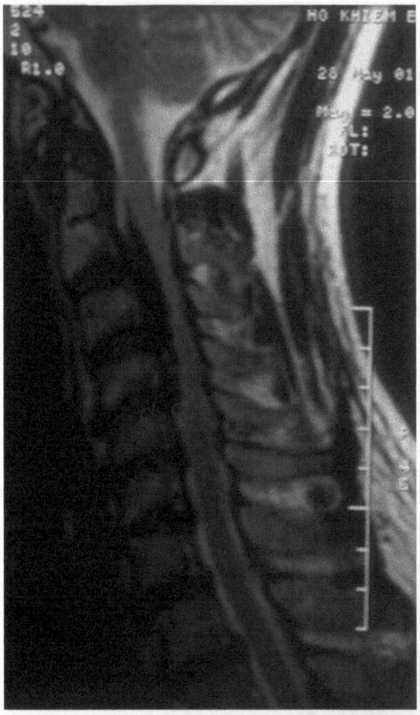

a

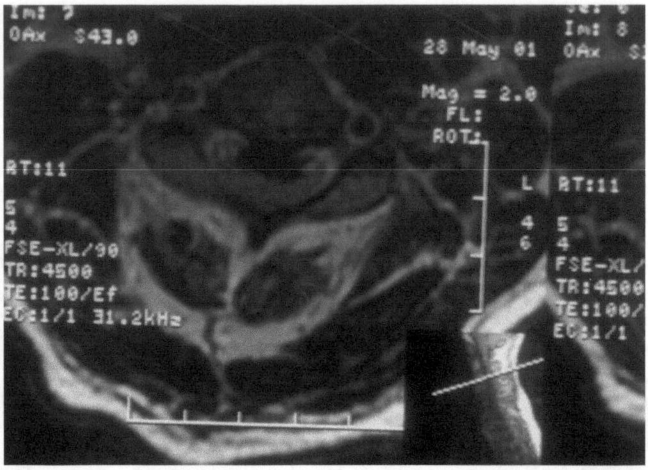

b

Fig. 31.2. OPLL. Sagittal **a** and axial **b** MRI images of the cervical spine. There is significant thickening and calcification of the posterior longitudinal ligament from C2 to C5, with severe stenosis and spinal cord compression.

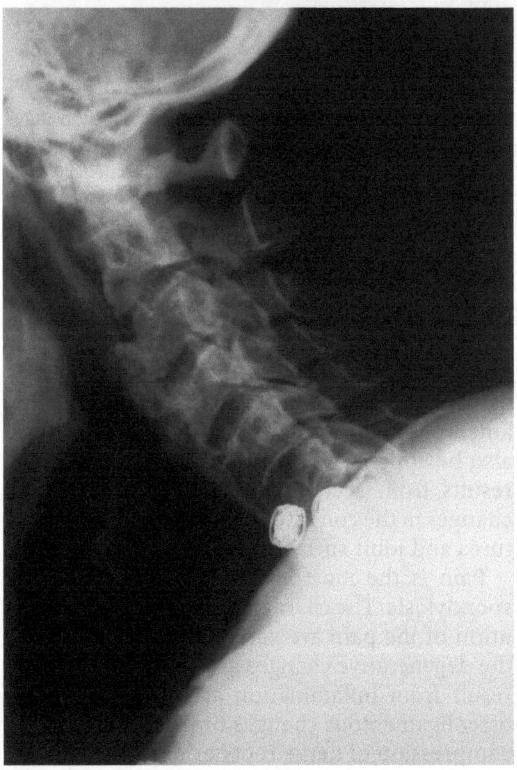
a

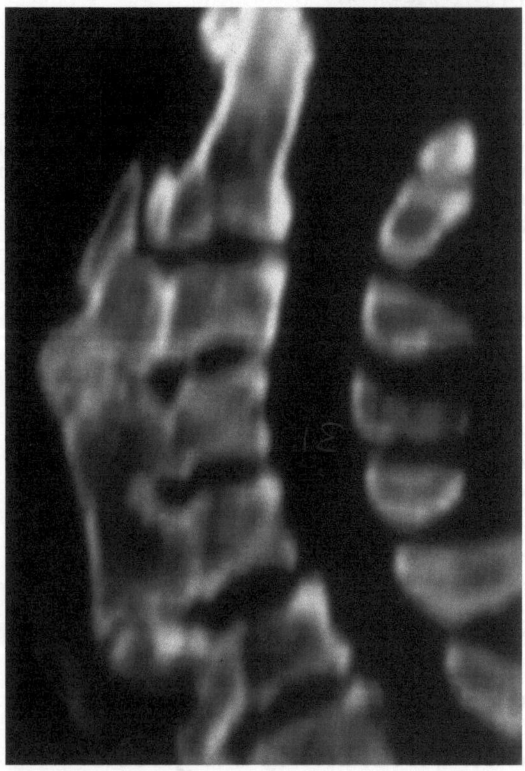
b

Fig. 31.3. DISH. Lateral X-ray **a** and CT scan reconstruction **b** of the cervical spine, demonstrating thick ossification anterior to the vertebral bodies from C2 to C6. The process involves the anterior aspect of the vertebral bodies only, without encroaching upon the spinal canal. This patient presented with dysphagia.

Pain radiating to the distal aspects of the arm is highly suggestive of ongoing cervical nerve root compression. This typically results from encroachment upon the exiting nerve root in the lateral aspect of the spinal canal or the intervertebral foramen. Compression can result from a disk herniation, uncovertebral joint hypertrophy or foraminal stenosis from facet hypertrophy. If the pain clearly conforms to the distribution of an isolated nerve root, or if it is associated with neurological deficit in an appropriate distribution, the origin of the pain can be attributed to nerve root compression. Pain involving the proximal aspects of the arm is less specific with respect to origin. It may result from cervical nerve root compression, or it may represent a referred phenomenon from the osseoligamentous changes of degeneration.

Axial and proximal, non-radicular arm pain can be the consequence of the degenerative changes described above. The pain results from a number of sources. Biomechanical strain of the osseoligamentous structures, inflammation and muscle fatigue can all contribute to this form of pain. The pain is probably manifested through pain fibers of the posterior rami of the cervical nerve roots. The posterior ramus innervates the vertebral bodies, annulus, facet joints and the bridging ligamentous structures of the cervical motion segments. The distribution of the pain is variable and can be widespread. There can be a radiating and/or referred component to the pain. A clear-cut cutaneous pattern to the referred phenomenon usually is not observed. Axial pain is typically in the posterior cervical region, but can extend cephalad to the sub-occipital and occipital–parietal regions. Pain can also radiate caudad into the interscapular and scapular regions. Lateralization of the pain can involve the suprascapular and trapezius areas, the proximal arm and also the anterior chest region. Headaches are also a possible manifestation of spondylosis, but there is no consistent or typical character to the headaches. Continuous pain, unaltered by position, may be more typical of pain of an inflammatory origin, whereas activity-related and/or positional pain would be more typical of a mechanical phenomenon.

The neurological manifestations of spondylosis include radiculopathy or myelopathy, or a combination of the two. As discussed above, nerve root compression can occur at the level of the lateral aspect of the canal or the intervertebral foramen from osteophyte or disc material. Sensory symptoms (pain and/or numbness) or motor deficits can result.

Cervical cord compression can result from static or dynamic factors (Fig. 31.4). The typical cause of cord compression is an accumulation of osteophyte or a disk herniation causing an AP narrowing of the spinal canal. Typically, if the AP diameter is less than 12 mm, the patient can have signs and symptoms of myelopathy. Also, the presence of anterior encroachment upon the spinal cord without absolute AP diameter stenosis can cause symptomatic myelopathy. The cord is most vulnerable to anterior compressive pathology in the presence of a kyphotic cervical configuration [1]. Under such circumstances, the spinal cord is draped over the anterior compressing pathology. A dynamic cord compression can also result from overt instability or micro-instability of a motion segment. Secondary changes to the ligamentous structures which bridge the bony elements of the motion segment can render them lax and no longer able to perform their function of limiting physiological spinal movement. Under such circumstances, repeated mechanical force can be applied to the spinal cord, resulting in dysfunction.

The differential diagnosis of spondylosis is extensive and includes peripheral nerve entrapment syndromes, neurodegenerative disorders and infectious processes. Patients manifesting with distal arm numbness and/or weakness and pain may have peripheral entrapment neuropathy, involving median and/or ulnar nerves. The distribution and character of the symptoms and the findings on examination can assist in the differential diagnosis. Carpal tunnel syndrome typically presents with pain and/or numbness and occasionally weakness, predominantly involving the hand. Pain from carpal tunnel syndrome can radiate proximally to involve the forearm. It is atypical but possible for carpal tunnel pain to extend up to the shoulder. In the latter instance, proximal nerve or nerve root involvement must be considered. Another typical feature of carpal tunnel syndrome is an exacerbation of the numbness and pain at night. Bilateral hand symptomatology could be a manifestation of bilateral carpal tunnel syndrome. However, cervical cord compression could also manifest with bilateral hand symptomatology in its early stages.

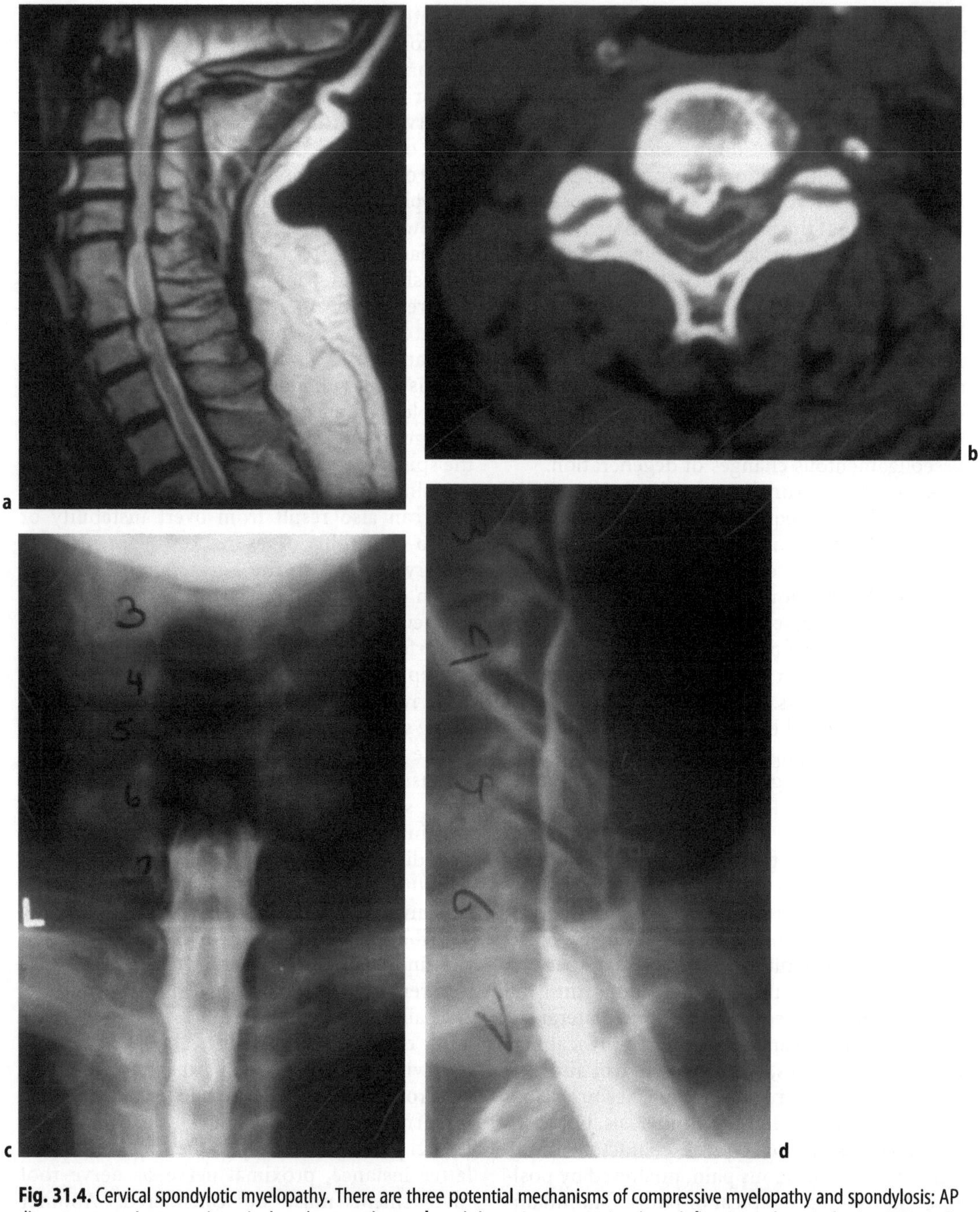

Fig. 31.4. Cervical spondylotic myelopathy. There are three potential mechanisms of compressive myelopathy and spondylosis: AP diameter stenosis **a**, anterior spinal cord encroachment **b** and dynamic compression (**c** and **d**). **a** Lateral cervical spine MRI study demonstrating narrowing of the spinal canal from C3 to C5, due to congenital narrowing of the canal compounded by bulging disk and osteophytes at the interspaces. **b** Post-myelogram CT scan axial view, demonstrating an anterior osteophyte indenting and deforming the anterior aspect of the spinal cord. (**c** and **d**) An AP X-ray demonstrates a complete block at the C6–C7 level **c**. With the head flexed, the dye passes across the level of the obstruction to the upper cervical spine, and there is no focus of compression seen in this image **d**.

Ulnar neuropathy can manifest with numbness and/or pain along the medial aspect of the forearm and hand, and, in more severe cases, as hand intrinsic weakness. A C8 radiculopathy can also produce similar symptoms. Proximal arm involvement would favor C8 radiculopathy, whereas provocative testing over the ulnar groove is more typical of an ulnar neuropathy. Electrophysiological testing should be able to distinguish between these two clinical entities. The presence of numbness alone along the medial forearm and hands, in the authors' experience, is relatively non-specific in the absence of neurological deficits. This is a typical site of referred pain or paresthesias in patients with spondylosis involving the lower cervical motion segments.

Left-upper-chest and arm pain can be seen in a C7 radiculopathy, but may also be a manifestation of cardiac ischemia. An appropriate cardiac evaluation can help to identify the latter. A lung apex tumor can also present with upper-chest pain radiating into the arm, mimicking cervical radiculopathy. The presence of supraclavicular lymphadenopathy and focal pain in the superior chest region supports this diagnosis and imaging studies (chest X-ray and CT scan) are needed for confirmation. Thoracic outlet syndrome is a difficult diagnosis to confirm, but should be considered in patients with radiating arm pain and numbness along the medial aspect of the forearm, extending to the hand. Associated electromyogram (EMG) and nerve conduction studies showing weakness and brachial plexus (lower-trunk) deficits support the diagnosis.

A number of neural degenerative disorders can mimic the manifestations of cervical spondylosis. In particular, multiple sclerosis and amyotrophic lateral sclerosis can involve the arms. Guillain–Barre syndrome and transverse myelitis can also affect cervical spinal cord function. The clinical manifestations of each disorder, supplemented by electrophysiological and imaging studies, can also distinguish spondylosis from these other entities. Coexistence of these entities has been reported.

Multiple sclerosis can be used to explain any focal or non-focal neurological deficit. Although an inflammatory plaque could symmetrically involve the cervical spinal cord at one level and manifest with a relatively symmetric deficit, this would be a less typical manifestation of multiple sclerosis. One would expect asymmetries and more patchy involvement from this disorder. Also, multiple foci of involvement and multiple flare-ups of acute symptoms would be required to confirm a diagnosis of multiple sclerosis. A lumbar puncture to look for oligoclonal banding would support a diagnosis of multiple sclerosis. MRI studies of the brain and spinal cord should also enable one to distinguish between the two disorders. The absence of significant cord compression and signal change in the cord or the white matter of the brain parenchyma would indicate a demyelinating disorder.

Amyotrophic lateral sclerosis (motor neuron disease) presents with motor deficits in the absence of a sensory phenomenon or pain. The process can affect both upper and lower motor neurons. Hence, the clinical manifestations can vary from patient to patient. One can get asymmetric limb involvement. On examination, the patients typically have no sensory deficit. They may have significant wasting of muscle groups and fasciculations. In particular, involvement of multiple muscle groups with fasciculations, especially if the legs are also involved, would be typical of motor neuron disease with a preferential involvement of the lower motor neurons. In spondylosis, it is not common to have diffuse fasciculations. In isolated radiculopathy, fasciculations can be seen in a radicular distribution. Involvement of bulbar musculature would confirm the diagnosis of motor neuron disease and exclude spondylitic myelopathy.

The other possible causes for upper limb symptoms or gait disturbances include thoracic spinal cord compression, peripheral neuropathy, joint osteoarthritis and connective tissue disorders, particularly rheumatoid arthritis.

Imaging and Investigations

A variety of imaging techniques are available to study the anatomy and pathology of the cervical spine for spondylosis and other spinal disorders. Although the primary objective of the imaging studies is still to identify the foci of compression of the spinal cord and nerve roots and determine the stability of the spine, other manifestations of the spondylotic process can be investigated in an attempt to identify focal pain generators. The advent of computer-assisted imaging studies has significantly improved the ability to delineate the extent of spondylosis involving the motion segments of the cervical spine.

Plain films are typically used as the initial study in a patient with symptomatic spondylosis. The alignment and stability of the cervical spine can be outlined on the lateral X-ray in dynamic and static views. Bony changes associated with spondylosis, including sclerosing of the endplates and accumulation of osteophyte, can be seen directly. Encroachment upon the intervertebral foramina, and sometimes the central spinal canal, can be seen on the plain films. Some of the degenerative changes of the disk can be indirectly identified on the plain X-rays.

A spinal canal study is required to determine the patency of the central spinal canal and the intervertebral foramina. An MRI or myelogram, followed by a post-myelogram CT scan, provide visualization of these areas. The quality of the MRI studies obtained on the high-resolution machines has significantly improved since the advent of MRI scanning. The ability to obtain multiplanar imaging of the spine and the ability to directly visualize the spinal cord and its relation to surrounding osseoligamentous tissues has made this a very sensitive and specific means of visualizing the cervical spinal canal for evidence of cord and/or nerve root compression. This non-invasive technique has eliminated the need for myelography in a number of cases. Some perform myelogram/CT scanning for delineating the extent of nerve root and spinal cord compression. The AP post-myelogram X-ray can enable visualization of the nerve roots as they exit the spinal canal through the proximal aspect of the foramen and outline the foci of compression. Flexion/extension views in a lateral projection can identify dynamic foci of compression of the spinal cord in the central canal.

Detailed study of the osseoligamentous structures of the spine can be obtained using MRI and CT scanning. These two forms of computer-assisted imaging provide complimentary information. The extent of disk desiccation, the presence of reactive changes in the endplates and the accumulation of fluid in the facet joints can be clearly seen on the MRI study. Sclerosing of the vertebral body endplates and accumulation of osteophyte at the disk space or associated with the facet joints can be seen on the CT scan.

The presence of degenerative change in the cervical spine does not always correlate with the presence of symptoms and often does not specify the location of the pain generator in a situation where the patient has more than one level of degenerative change. The challenge to the physician is to correlate the patient's symptomatology with the imaging findings. In the presence of a neurologic deficit from spinal cord compression or isolated nerve root compression, a focus of spinal cord or nerve root compression which conforms to the distribution of the neurological deficit is usually sufficient to establish a correlation between the clinical and imaging findings. In other cases, ancillary testing and diagnostic procedures may be required to obtain a clinical pathological correlate. Electrophysiological testing and diagnostic nerve root and facet blocks and diskography may be helpful in assessing the origin of a patient's pain.

Electrophysiological testing can be effective in identifying the origin of arm pain. A peripheral entrapment neuropathy, brachial plexus abnormality or a radiculopathy should be distinguishable on an EMG/nerve conduction study. The EMG/nerve conduction study can assist in identifying the precise nerve root involved in a patient with radicular pain and deficit, although this should be apparent by the clinical assessment. Also, the EMG/nerve conduction study can be helpful in identifying the origin of proximal arm pain, which could either be radicular or a referred phenomenon from the cervical spondylosis [2].

The percutaneous injection of steroids and/or local anesthetics can be of diagnostic and, in some cases, therapeutic benefit [3]. Selective injections blocking conductivity through nerve roots or the facet joint can determine if the specific structure injected is contributing to axial and/or appendicular pain. The techniques should be performed under fluoroscopy to optimize the specificity of the procedure. Despite safeguards and meticulous technique, the procedure is not completely specific and sensitive.

Diskography is a controversial diagnostic technique to evaluate the presence of pain of diskogenic origin. The concept of diskogenic pain is also controversial. Innervation of the annulus and the endplates provides a substrate for transmission of painful impulses from the anterior complex structures. The indication for diskography is the presence of pain, thought to be emanating from spondylotic changes of the cervical disk in the absence of a neural compressive cause for the pain. The distribution of the pain could either be axial or appendicular. The anatomy of the disk can be outlined on a diskogram. This information in some cases supplements information from the MRI studies [4]. The most important component of the diskogram test is the provocative phase of the study. The provocation of pain while injecting dye under pressure into the interspace is the endpoint in determining a correlation between the patient's pain and the degenerative changes. However, some point to confounding factors, such as psychological influences, in determining the validity of the test [5].

Treatment

The potential clinical manifestations of cervical spondylosis are quite variable with respect to the degree of pain and neurological disability. A variety of operative and non-operative treatment modalities are available to treat clinically symptomatic and significant spondylosis.

The goals of treating patients with symptomatic cervical spondylitic disease include diminishing pain, restoring neurological function and re-establishing spinal stability. Many people have degenerative changes in the cervical spine on imaging studies without symptoms. Treatment is not required for the radiograph findings, but should only be considered for disabling symptoms [6]. It is unclear whether exercise can diminish the progression of cervical spondylosis or if it acts to prevent the development of symptoms. Augmenting paraspinal muscle tone and conditioning will improve the stability of the cervical spine and its resistance to abnormal movement. However, exercise would not alleviate the forces upon the disks and joints of the cervical motion segment complex. In fact, repeated activity and strain, theoretically, could promote degeneration of the joint complexes.

Rarely is there a need for prophylactic surgery to prevent neurological dysfunction in the presence of spondylosis. A clear indication for considering prophylactic surgery would be the presence of instability. Based on the trauma criteria for stability, if the patient has greater than 3.5 mm of translational movement between adjacent vertebrae, then instability exists and should be treated surgically. The need to decompress the intervertebral foramina or the central spinal canal in an asymptomatic patient is not clear. The nerve roots are quite tolerant of compression, as many patients have significant radiographic foraminal stenosis without associated symptoms. It is possible that compensation by the nerve roots takes place during the slow progressive compression. Incidental central spinal canal stenosis is more controversial. This entity is becoming a more frequent finding with the widespread use of MRI studies. A percentage of physicians recommend decompression to prevent an acute spinal cord injury from head or neck trauma, but there are no studies substantiating the merits of prophylactic surgery in these cases. In all likelihood, a patient with focal stenosis from spondylosis has a higher risk of incurring a spinal cord injury from trauma than the general population, but the magnitude of this risk is difficult to define. Given the ubiquity of cervical spondylosis, the increased risk is probably minimal and probably in the same range as the risk of incurring a spinal cord injury during a surgical procedure. Therefore, patient factors should be considered carefully when determining the need to decompress a patient with asymptomatic stenosis. An active patient who participates in high-impact sports and activity may be a suitable candidate for prophylactic decompression [7].

Pain and neurological deficit are the typical manifestations of symptomatic cervical spondylosis, as discussed above. The presence of a significant neurological deficit in the form of motor or sensory impairment or signs of cord compression require primary surgical treatment, without consideration of a course of non-operative treatment to optimize the chance of neurological recovery. Except in extreme cases, those patients presenting with pain should first be considered for non-surgical treatment.

Non-operative Treatment

The various non-operative treatment modalities available for cervical spondylosis include physical treatments, oral and percutaneous pharmaceutical administration and other alternative techniques [8]. A wide spectrum of opinions regarding the optimal non-operative treatment techniques for symptomatic spondylosis exists. The approach utilized is determined by the nature of the symptoms, patient factors and the preference of the treating physician.

The nature and chronicity of the symptoms determine the etiology of the pain and the sequence of treatment. Radicular pain can present either as an acute event or with chronic pain. The distribution of the pain suggests irritation of the cervical nerve root. Anti-inflammatory and analgesic use would represent the mainstay of preliminary treatment. A decrease in the severity of the patient's pain will optimize function and enable the patient to sleep and perform activities of daily living. Presumably, a component of inflammation exists, especially in the acute setting of radiculopathy, and the anti-inflammatory effect could be beneficial. Physical treatments may also be of assistance. Immobilization of the neck and limiting activity and movement would be a logical treatment modality in the presence of an acutely inflamed nerve root. Cervical traction in some cases is beneficial, as it could enlarge the intervertebral foramen and alleviate some tension on the nerve root. However, this effect is probably only temporary, during the application of traction. Active strengthening and range of motion exercises of the neck or the affected limb is an illogical approach in the acute setting. Movement of acutely inflamed tissue would likely exacerbate the pain and does not alleviate the tension on the nerve root. Therefore, these authors would not advocate active exercises in the presence of an acute radiculitis.

Neck and axial pain may also present acutely or chronically. The origin of such pain is less certain. Such symptoms may emanate from the paraspinal musculature, soft tissue structures of the motion segment unit (tendons and ligaments), the facet joint, disks or other osseous structures of the vertebrae. Compression of the major cervical nerve roots within or as they exit the cervical spine may also contribute to axial pain, although verifying such a mechanism is difficult. The probable mediator of axial pain in spondylosis is the posterior ramus of the cervical nerve roots. Again, in an acute setting, the use of immobilization, anti-inflammatories and analgesics represents the primary treatment modality. In the presence of true muscle spasms, which are episodic, intense, cramp-like pains, muscle relaxants can be of value. For chronic, continuous pain, the theoretical benefit of a muscle relaxant is less clear. Spasm is typically not a component of such pain. The medication frequently has a sedating effect, which can be beneficial for rest but can impair one's ability to function throughout the day. An exercise program should be considered for patients with chronic axial pain to optimize paraspinal muscle conditioning and range of motion. Muscle fatigue manifests as chronic burning pain, provoked by prolonged activity and upright posture. Improving the paraspinal muscle conditioning can diminish this component of the pain. Loss of range of motion can be a consequence of spondylosis, as the patient splints his neck because of the pain. Loss of range of motion can have a functional consequence and also can contribute to the pain. Therefore, undertaking a range of motion exercises can counteract these adverse effects of limited movement and improve comfort.

Anti-inflammatories and analgesics can be of benefit as preliminary modalities of treatment for the manifestations of cervical spondylosis. Also, the judicious use of physical measures can be of benefit in selected cases. The use of injectable steroids has become widespread as a treatment modality for spondylosis. These techniques are typically considered when the preliminary treatment for spondylosis has failed. Injectable techniques vary with respect to the location of the steroid placement. The options include epidural, trigger-point or selected nerve root and/or facet injections. The role of steroid injections is controversial. They function to counteract the inflammatory component of the pain. Theoretically, the specificity of the injection should optimize the effect of the injection and also be of some diagnostic value. Epidural injections involve installation of the steroid into the epidural space. Presumably, the medication diffuses throughout the epidural space and can gain access to the nerve roots and the outer surfaces of the joints and other soft tissue structures of the spine. Trigger-point injections involve placement of the needle into a focal site of pain. The pain point may be in the axial spine or over the scapular or shoulder regions. A direct effect on the pain generator may be achieved by injecting into the cervical spine.

The peripheral trigger-point injection could be expected to treat a non-cervical cause of appendicular pain. If the peripheral trigger point is a point of referred pain from the cervical spine, one would not expect the trigger-point injection to be beneficial. Selected injections involving the nerve roots and/or facet joints can be both of diagnostic and therapeutic value. The use of such injections is logical in cases where the patient has localized neck pain or referred pain in a nerve root distribution.

The subjective nature of pain, the diversity of the manifestations of cervical spondylosis and the variable natural history have made the objective study of the results of steroid injections difficult and inconclusive. Theoretically, the steroids can act as potent anti-inflammatories for a finite period of time at a site of inflammation. The injections are not treating the cause of the inflammation directly and do not act to decompress the neural elements when this mechanism is contributing to the pain. When the steroid has been absorbed and metabolized and is no longer present at the injection site, if the process which produces the pain remains active, the pain should recur. In those instances where the patient has alleviation of the symptoms, it is possible that the underlying cause has become inactive or has been resolved by intrinsic mechanisms. Therefore, steroids probably do not alter the natural history of symptomatic spondylosis, but can temporarily moderate symptoms which are the result of inflammation.

A wide variety of alternative treatments have also been utilized for treatment of symptomatic spondylosis. Often, these treatments are invoked if preliminary conventional methods have failed or if the patient wants to avoid surgery. Acupuncture, deep muscle stimulation, chiropractic manipulation, biofeedback and other such methods remain alternatives. The rationale and results of such techniques are beyond the scope of this chapter. In the authors' experience, some patients appear to obtain some improvement of their pain symptoms from such techniques. It is unclear, however, if this represents the natural history of the disease since, again, as for steroid injections, the techniques involved do not appear to directly alter the underlying pathophysiology of the pain.

In summary, non-operative treatments represent the first line of treatment for patients with pain from cervical spondylosis in the absence of a significant neurological deficit. A variety of non-operative treatment modalities have been used. Objective data regarding the merits of each modality are limited, due to the subjective nature of pain and its associated disability and the various pain generators underlying the symptoms. Immobilization, anti-inflammatories and the judicious use of analgesics are a logical first line of treatment for acute and chronic pain syndromes. Active physical therapy and exercise can be effective in selected cases of chronic axial pain, for reactivation after an acute episode of pain or prophylactically to diminish the likelihood of recurrent pain after an acute episode. Steroid injections can help reduce a focus of acute inflammation. The treatment does not directly treat the underlying cause of the pain and the effect is probably temporary. Its use and that of alternative therapies must be studied more closely to determine their usefulness in the treatment of spondylosis.

Surgical Treatment

Surgical treatment is considered for those patients with spinal instability or neurologic deficit from spondylosis, or in those patients who present with pain and have failed non-operative treatment. A variety of surgical techniques have been developed for the treatment of symptomatic cervical spondylosis. Many factors and considerations have to be taken into account to determine the type and extent of surgery required in a given case. Regardless of the specific factors, however, the principles of surgery for spondylosis are similar to those for the treatment of cervical trauma and other spinal disorders. These principles include neural decompression, reduction and stabilization. Utilizing these guidelines, surgical treatment alternatives can be planned for symptomatic spondylosis.

Neurological deficit for spondylosis results from compression of the nerve roots and/or spinal cord. The compression can be either static or dynamic. Neurological deficit constitutes a clear indication for surgery. Decompression is accomplished by removing the compressive pathology, expanding the channel through which the neural element is passing or by reduction of a deformity which is causing encroachment upon the spinal cord or nerve roots.

As described earlier, the sources of pain from spondylosis include nerve root compression or stress injury, or inflammation of the osseoligamentous component of the motion segment. The character and distribution of the pain often define the source of the pain. Neural compressive pain is usually quite well defined and, if the distribution of symptoms correlates with compressive pathology on the imaging studies, an affirmative outcome can be expected if an adequate decompression is achieved at surgery. The origin of non-radicular distribution arm pain or axial pain is much more difficult to determine. Non-radicular distribution pain may represent a referred phenomenon from the cervical spine. In isolated cases, in patients who have a combination of axial pain and radicular pain, focal neural decompression can sometimes alleviate or reduce axial pain. However, in many cases, the axial pain is not due to neural compression and does not respond to decompressive surgery. In selected cases, some believe that segmental fusion can be of benefit in the treatment of axial pain [9]. These concepts are quite controversial and do not constitute clear indications for surgery in the neurosurgical literature. The treatment of axial pain with fusion surgery has been promoted by some and has been a concept considered more commonly by orthopedic surgeons.

After a determination of the extent of the degenerative disease has been made, the type of surgery required to achieve the objectives of surgery has to be formulated. A variety of factors influence the nature of the operative procedure, including the nature, location and extent of the pathology and patient factors. The surgeon must determine where the degenerative pathology is located in relation to the neural elements and how this is most directly and safely accessed. The patient's age, bone quality, spinal curvature and general health can influence the approach and extent of surgery required.

Decompressive surgery is typically a component of an operative procedure for cervical degenerative disease. Decompression of the spinal cord and/or nerve roots may be required in a given case. Access for decompression of either of these elements can be achieved by an anterior or a posterior approach. The initial techniques available for spinal cord and nerve root decompression involved a posterior approach by complete or partial laminectomy. These techniques involved a midline incision and retraction of the paraspinal musculature off the laminae and spinous processes. The laminae would be removed to expand the AP diameter of the cervical canal to decompress the spinal cord. If the nerve root requires decompression, a foraminotomy could be performed by extending the laminectomy lateral over the medial aspect of the given facet joint, which would overlie the intervertebral foramen. The foraminotomy could be performed alone or in combination with a midline laminectomy.

Long-term analysis and follow-up of patients who have undergone cervical laminectomies for stenosis and myelopathy have demonstrated that this technique is not universally applicable for all patients with stenosis. Some patients fail to improve, despite the intervention, or could experience a delayed deterioration following the intervention [10]. The cause of myelopathy from stenosis is not only determined by the degree of the AP canal diameter narrowing. In some cases, anterior compression, especially in the presence of a straightened or kyphotic cervical spine or the presence of micro-motion, can contribute to myelopathy. These two factors are not directly addressed by a laminectomy (Fig. 31.5). The soft tissue dissection required to access the laminae and the subsequent bony resection can increase the degree of instability of the spine resulting from a laminectomy. The patient may experience further micro-trauma to the cord from the instability or develop a kyphotic deformity of the cervical spine, which can contribute to anterior compression of the spinal cord or predispose to a cervical pain syndrome [11]. Based on these potential limitations of the laminectomy, supplementing the posterior decompression with fusion or effecting decompression by an anterior approach has been considered in certain cases [12].

Posterior cervical foraminotomy was the initial technique developed for cervical nerve root decompression. The posterior aspect of the intervertebral foramen is unroofed. Enlargement of the foramen by this technique, in some cases, is all that is required to effect decompression of the nerve root. Typically, the compressing pathology in foraminal stenosis is located anterior to the nerve root. In the case of a herniated disk, a soft fragment of disk can be

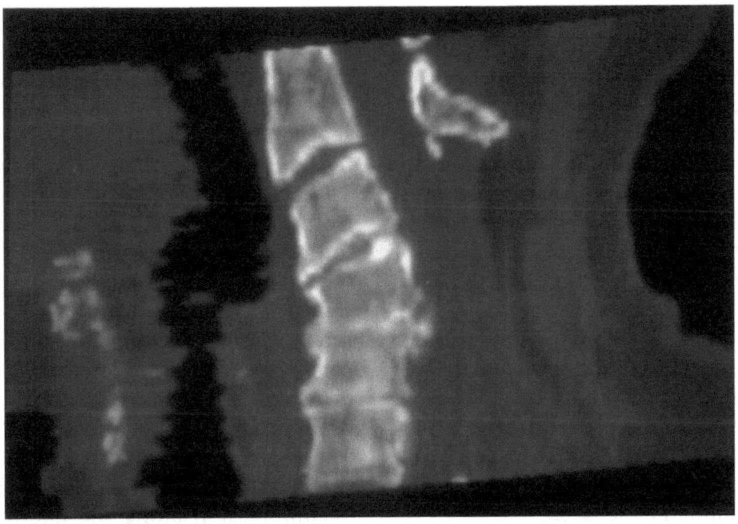

Fig. 31.5. A sagittal CT scan reconstruction of the mid-cervical spine. The patient underwent a previous laminectomy and had transient improvement of his symptomatology, followed by progressive myelopathy. The kyphotic configuration of the spine and the anterior osteophyte have prevented adequate decompression of the spinal cord by the laminectomy.

retrieved by retracting the nerve root and incising the posterior ligament, which typically contains the herniated fragment. Osteophyte usually cannot be removed by the posterior approach.

The genesis of anterior decompressive procedures has contributed significantly to the ability to directly decompress the neural elements in the cervical spine. Most degenerative pathology originates anterior to the thecal sac or the cervical nerve roots. In particular, the degenerative process typically begins in the disk space. Spinal cord and/or nerve root compression can result from the accumulation of osteophytes or from protruding disk material. Facet hypertrophy can also contribute to foraminal compression, although this is much less common in cervical spondylosis as opposed to its frequency in lumbar spondylosis. Compressive pathology can also be located posterior to the vertebral body, contributing to canal stenosis. Disk material can herniate vertically and be positioned behind the vertebral bodies. Osteophyte can proliferate from the interspace and extend behind the vertebral body, as can ossification of the posterior longitudinal ligament. Since compressive pathology typically originates anterior to the spine, the anterior decompressive techniques are a logical option to directly decompress the neural elements.

If the compressive pathology is confined to the level of the interspace, either in the central canal or the intervertebral foramen, a diskectomy and osteophytectomy confined to the interspace can be utilized to effect spinal cord and/or nerve root compression, respectively. The original anterior decompression technique was devised by Cloward, where a large burr-type hole was made over the mid portion of the disk, extending into the adjacent vertebral bodies and extending posteriorly to the annulus [13]. From this midline channel, lateral decompression could be carried out to decompress the lateral aspects of the spinal canal and perform foraminal decompressions. Following the decompression, a bone dowel was harvested from the iliac crest and placed into the hole to effect fusion. A modification of the Cloward procedure has since been devised and is called the Smith–Robinson technique [14,15]. Instead of a cylindrical hole, disk material and the endplate are removed in a rectangular shape. The decompression can be extended laterally to perform foraminotomies. Following the decompression, bone graft can be inserted into the interspace to maintain the disk space height and produce a fusion. Some authors perform decompression without fusion. Apparently, a majority of patients who do not have fusion bone inserted following the decompression will go on to a spontaneous fusion [16]. It is not uncommon to develop collapse across the interspace following a decompression without fusion. This can result in a cervical kyphosis or foraminal stenosis [17].

In an attempt to eliminate the extent of disk removal for radiculopathy, a technique for lateral diskectomy and foraminal decompression has been developed [18,19]. The technique involved a lateral exposure to the anterior aspect of the spine and resection of the lateral aspect of the disk and uncovertebral joint to access the intervertebral foramen. The rationale for this procedure is to avoid a complete diskectomy and maintain the mobility of the motion segment. The risks of the procedure are injury to the vertebral artery and nerve root, and probably a higher risk of incomplete decompression because of the limited exposure.

Re-establishment of normal spinal alignment, or reduction of spinal deformity, has been a principle of spinal reconstructive surgery for trauma. In the setting of trauma, spinal realignment frequently achieves neural decompression. Besides decompressing the spinal cord and nerve roots, reduction of spinal deformity and re-establishment of a normal cervical lordosis appear to have other benefits in patients with cervical spondylosis. Cervical kyphosis, as discussed above, can contribute to anterior compression of the spinal cord, contributing to myelopathy. In addition, kyphosis probably also contributes to the likelihood of axial pain from spondylosis. In a kyphotic configuration, the paraspinal musculature, positioned posterior to the spine, is at a mechanical disadvantage and requires continuous contraction to maintain the head in a neutral position. This increased paraspinal muscle activity can contribute to axial neck pain. A posterior decompression, with removal of the posterior bony elements and detachment and manipulation of the posterior musculature, can also diminish the effectiveness of the extensor musculature and contribute to a progressive cervical kyphosis. Based on these biomechanical factors, a laminectomy in the presence of cervical kyphosis can predispose to delayed complications.

The presence of kyphosis also adds to the amount of translational force applied to the individual motion segments. This can accelerate the deformity, as discussed above, but also impair the ability to achieve fixation and fusion of the cervical spine. The translational biomechanics of the cervical fixation device are somewhat limited; hence, fixation failure is more likely to occur in the presence of kyphosis.

In order to achieve reduction and attempt to re-establish cervical lordosis, the involved motion segments of the spine have to be mobile. The relative mobility of the deformity varies from patient to patient. Some are fixed deformities and others are mobile. Mobilization must be effected prior to correction of the deformity. Typically, the deformity occurs across the interspaces. Achieving mobility between adjacent vertebrae by diskectomies, facetectomies or osteotomies is carried out in order to effect mobilization. Application of axial force re-establishes a normal spinal alignment. The presence of osteophyte that is inaccessible to decompression along the lateral aspect of the vertebral bodies and the facet joints may sometimes limit reduction. The loss of anterior vertebral body height can also contribute to kyphosis. Resection of the trapezoidal-shaped vertebrae and reconstruction with a rectangular bone graft can treat this component of the deformity.

The need to perform a fusion in the setting of cervical spondylosis depends upon the nature of the spondylotic disease, patient factors and the extent and type of surgery required for decompression. The general indications for fusion surgery for spondylosis include deformity correction, treatment of instability or the presence of axial or mechanical neck pain. The presence of instability or neurological deficit caused by abnormal spinal movement is a clear indication to proceed with fusion surgery. Criteria to determine whether or not axial or mechanical pain should be treated by fusion surgery are much less clear and are controversial. The ability to localize the site of the pain generator and the severity of the pain and the associated disability are factors which determine the need and feasibility of segmental fusion for pain. Since the outcome of such surgery is somewhat unpredictable, this form of therapy should be considered only if the patient fails non-operative treatment and is quite limited by the pain. Also, segmental fusion likely predisposes to premature degeneration of the adjacent motion segments, which could result in a pain syndrome or neurological deficits in the future. Therefore, the decision to operate for axial pain must be made carefully.

The principles of fusion include adequate preparation and decortication of the host site, a source of bone graft (which, if possible, should be placed under compression) and immobilization of the osseous elements involving the fusion. Typically, the ability to effect fusion in the cervical spine is good, as compared to fusion success rates in the lumbar spine [20].

Fusion can be achieved by an anterior or posterior approach. The induction of fusion implies bony bridging between adjacent vertebrae. Bone graft provides a scaffolding upon which osteoblasts migrate between the two adjacent vertebrae. Immobilization of the involved segment is critical to allow for proper bony fusion. A rigid cervical collar or a halo brace are the external fixators most commonly utilized. Internal fixation is now frequently used as an adjunct to promote fusion.

The instrumentation devices available for the cervical spine are strictly internal fixation devices, with no reduction capability. Therefore, cervical manipulation, either by external or internal force application, and placement of the bone graft produce reduction and spinal re-alignment. The fixation device contributes to immediate stabilization of the segment intended to be fused. Long-term stabilization depends upon maturation of the fusion.

As for the previously described decompressive procedures, cervical fusion procedures were initially performed by a posterior approach. The placement of on-laid bone graft supplemented with a halo represents one of the earliest techniques for effecting fusion. Fixation by wiring the posterior elements in various configurations represented some of the early internal fixation techniques [21] (Fig. 31.6). The effectiveness of these procedures is limited and loss of reduction and fixation can occur. An interspinous wire would recreate the extensor tension band posteriorly and limit motion in flexion and extension. In cases of ligamentous injury in trauma, this confers some stabilization to the involved motion segments. Sub-laminar wiring would also have a similar effect, with a high risk of spinal cord injury during the sub-laminar pass. The translational biomechanics of these techniques are limited and dependent upon the integrity of the facets. The Bowman

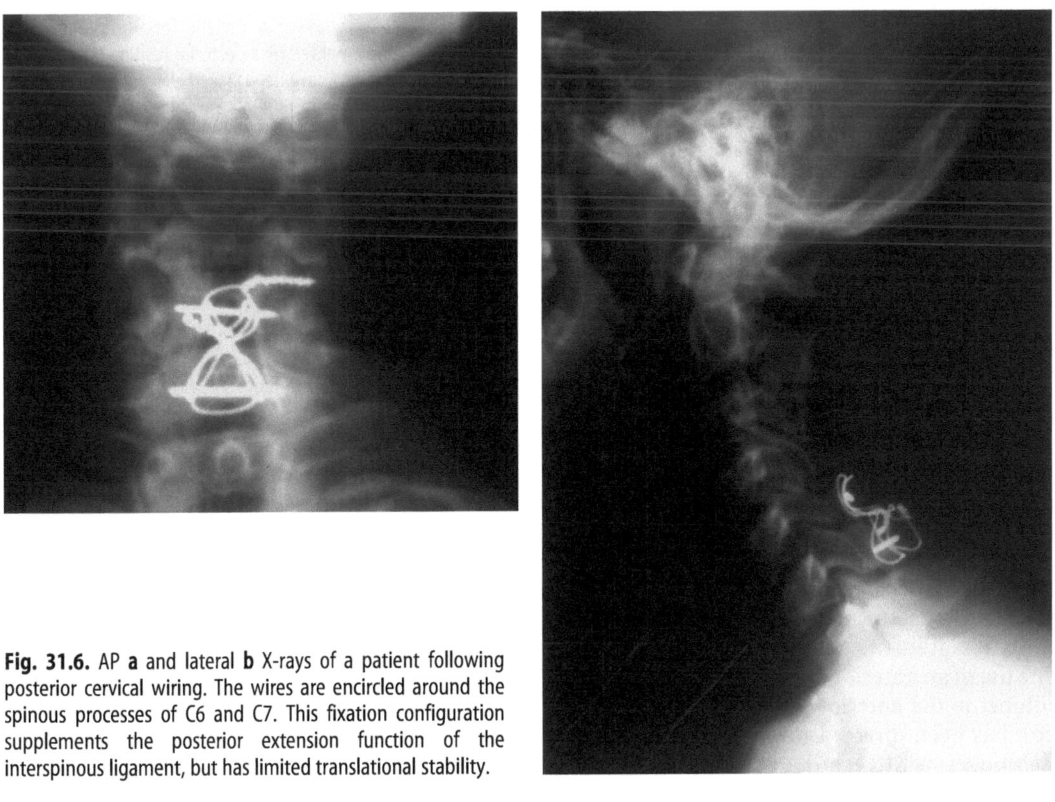

a

b

Fig. 31.6. AP **a** and lateral **b** X-rays of a patient following posterior cervical wiring. The wires are encircled around the spinous processes of C6 and C7. This fixation configuration supplements the posterior extension function of the interspinous ligament, but has limited translational stability.

triple-wire technique, where struts of bone are wired to the spinous processes over the motion segments, improves translational stability [22]. Besides the biomechanical problems with posterior element wiring, the frequent need to undertake decompression at the time of fixation/fusion requires removal of the spinous processes and laminae, making them unavailable for such wiring techniques. Based upon the limitations of midline wiring, lateral mass fixation procedures emerged.

Facet wiring, although somewhat technically demanding, if it can be accomplished, is the most stable wiring technique available. It is not dependent upon the integrity of the laminae or the spinous processes. The technique involves making holes through the inferior aspect of the lateral mass and facet of the adjacent vertebrae and passing wires through these holes and up through the facet joint space [23].

Lateral mass plating techniques were developed approximately 25 years ago. The procedure involves placement of a screw through the lateral mass of the vertebrae. The entry point of the screw is in the anatomical center of the lateral mass. The screw direction is oriented superior and lateral in the lateral mass to avoid the nerve root and vertebral artery, respectively. With the plates secured to the posterior aspect of the lateral masses by the lateral mass screws, both extensor tension band and translational stability across the motion segment are enhanced. The initial lateral mass-plating techniques involved semi-rigid devices, where the screw head was not rigidly fixed to the plate (Fig. 31.7). The newer-generation devices have connecting links which secure the screw heads to rods in a rigid manner. This increases the stability of the fixation.

Anterior fusion techniques involve the use of bone graft which is at least partially composed of cortical bone, to allow for structural stability of the fused segment in compression. The size of the graft is dependent upon the extent of disk and/or bone removal required for the decompression. An interbody graft is used following diskectomy and a more lengthy cortical cancellous strut graft is used for vertebral body replacement following vertebrectomies. The use of an anterior cervical plate is a frequent adjunct to the anterior bone graft. Much attention has been directed towards anterior fusion techniques with regard to factors influencing

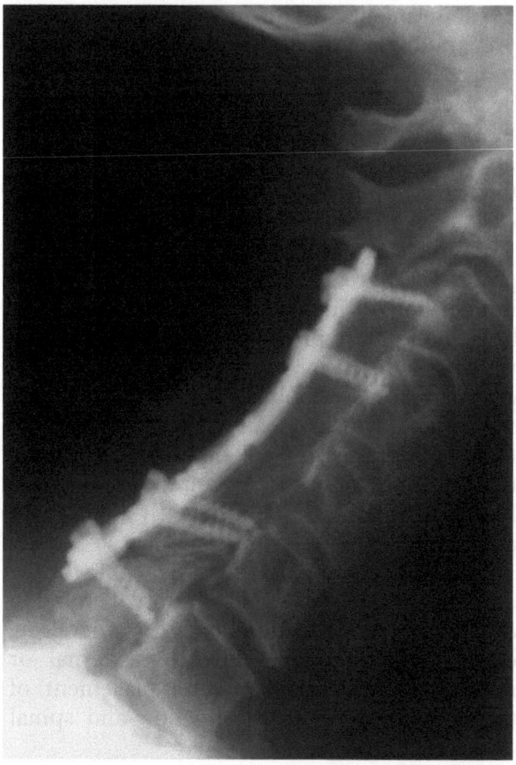

Fig. 31.7. Lateral X-ray of a patient following a cervical laminectomy supplemented by a posterior fusion with fixation. The lateral mass screws have been placed into the lateral masses of C3, C4, C6 and C7. The facet joints are obliterated from C3–C4 to C5–C6, but remain patent at C6–C7, suggesting a non-union at the latter.

graft migration and fixation failure [24]. Evaluation of the results of anterior fusion have indicated that there is an incidence of collapse across the grafted segment, referred to as subsidence, and an incidence of graft extrusions. Obviously, the extrusion of a graft can result in a non-union and esophageal obstruction. Subsidence can produce a kyphotic cervical deformity, which predisposes to axial pain and, in more extreme circumstances, neurological complications. Many factors are involved in the likelihood of graft subsidence and/or extrusion, including the type of graft, its length and cross-sectional size and its positioning. Patient factors, including the configuration of the spine, the segment of spine involved in the fusion and the bone quality, also can influence the likelihood of subsidence. The use of a plate and the characteristics of the given plate utilized can also have some bearing on the likelihood of subsidence or graft extrusion [25].

The modulus of elasticity of the grafting material can influence the likelihood of its compressing into the adjacent vertebral endplates. Cortical bone, as seen in the fibular strut graft, is relatively rigid compared to the endplates and underlying cancellous bone in the vertebral bodies. Theoretically, this substrate is more likely to subside than cortical cancellous allograft. The cross-sectional diameter of the bone graft is also relevant: the smaller the cross-sectional diameter, the greater the pressure per square unit of volume exerted by the bone graft on the endplates. Therefore, the larger the graft, the less likely it is to sink into the endplate. Ideally, a graft of at least two-thirds of the cross-sectional diameter of the disk space should be used. The positioning of the bone graft within the decompression channel may also have some bearing on its tendency to subside. Placement of the cortical portion of the graft anteriorly, in alignment with the anterior aspect of the vertebral bodies, probably reduces the likelihood of subsidence. When the graft is placed in this fashion, the vertical force exerted on it through the superior vertebrae is transmitted through the cortical portion of the graft, which is in continuity with the cortex of the adjacent vertebrae. This configuration allows for a relatively non-compressible cortex/cortex construct.

The complication rate of insertion of a lengthy bone graft, involving three or more motion segments, is higher than that for shorter bone grafts. This is especially true when the bone graft extends down to the cervical thoracic junction, where the spine curvature is in transition from the cervical lordosis to kyphosis. The translational force across the inferior aspect of the bone graft at the cervical thoracic junction predisposes to anterior extrusion of the inferior aspect of the graft.

Anterior cervical plating technology has evolved significantly over the past 15 years. The Caspar plate (Aesculap Incorporated, Center Valley, Pennsylvania, USA) was the first type of anterior cervical plate to be used for a broad range of cervical problems (Fig. 31.8). The coupling between the screws which fixed the device to the vertebral bodies was semi-rigidly attached to the plate. In order to augment the stability characteristics of the fixation,

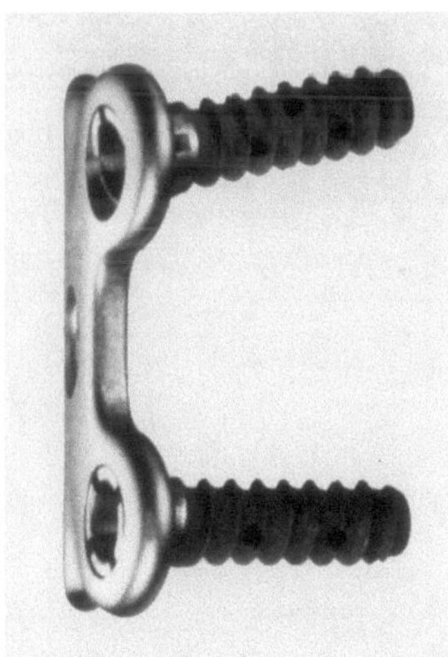

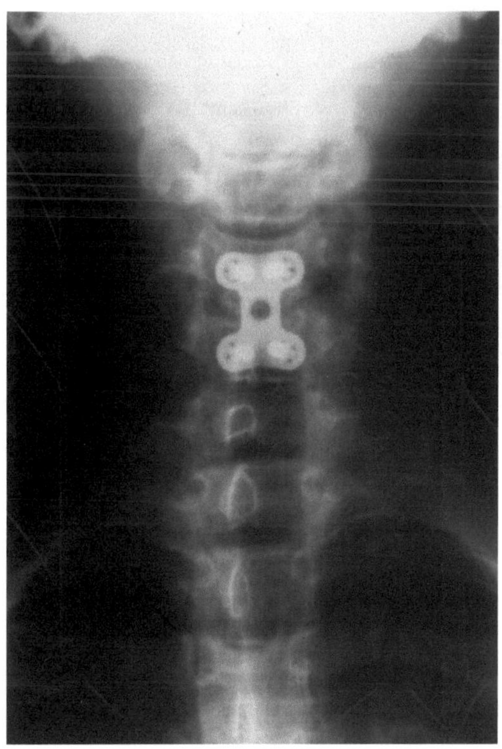

Fig. 31.8. Caspar cervical plate (Aesculap Incorporated, Center Valley, Pennsylvania, USA). A first-generation anterior cervical plate. The screws are not rigidly linked to the cervical plate and require bi-cortical purchase in order to optimize the fixation.

bi-cortical screw purchase was required. Obtaining bi-cortical screw purchase, incorporating the posterior cortex of the vertebrae, increased the risk of spinal cord injury, with encroachment upon the spinal canal by the screw. Despite the bi-cortical screw purchase, there remained a percentage of failure with these plates, especially in cases where the bone quality was poor or a long plate was required for a lengthy anterior fusion.

Based on limitations of the Caspar plate, newer generations of plates have been devised (Fig. 31.9). Although the conventional plates carry similar biomechanical characteristics, most of the plates, except for the DOC plate (Johnson and Johnson/DePuy AcroMed Corp., Cleveland, Ohio, USA), incorporate a rigid coupling of the screw to the plate. Various devices to achieve this locking of the screw to the plate have been devised, including internal screws to expand the head and/or shaft of the screw, cam-locking mechanisms and interference-type screws. Rigid coupling has decreased the failure rate of plates and reduced the likelihood of subsidence; however, complications from plating have not been eliminated. Screw back-out is very uncommon in the newer-generation plates. Screw fracture or interosseous migration can result if the forces promoting subsidence overcome the resistance provided by the graft and the fixation device (Fig. 31.10). Newer-generation dynamic plates (e.g. DOC Plate) have been designed to allow for some degree of settling of the graft, without putting direct stress upon the bone/metal interface of the screws (Fig. 31.11).

The decision to proceed with an anterior/posterior (a combined fusion) procedure is determined by a number of factors, including the

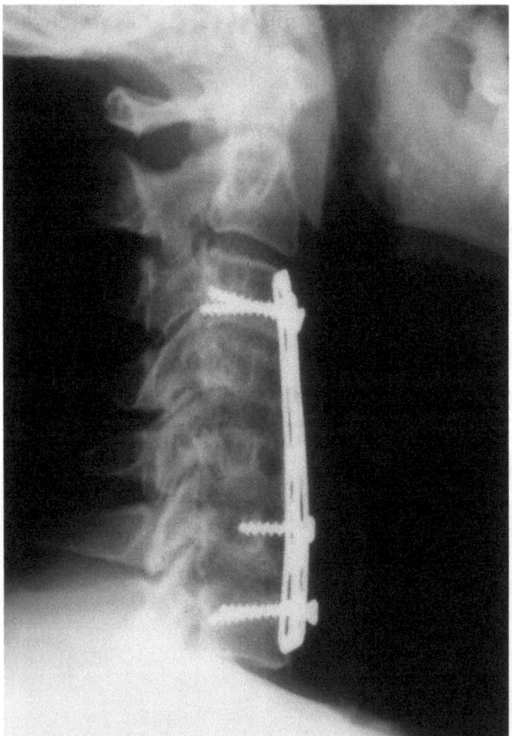

Fig. 31.9. CLSP plate (Synthes Incorporated, Paoli, Pennsylvania, USA). Lateral view of a CLSP plate (a). The heads of the screws are locked to the plate with an expanding screw, placed co-axially into the inner perforation of the bone screws. An AP X-ray (b) of the cervical spine following an interbody fusion supplemented with an anterior cervical plate.

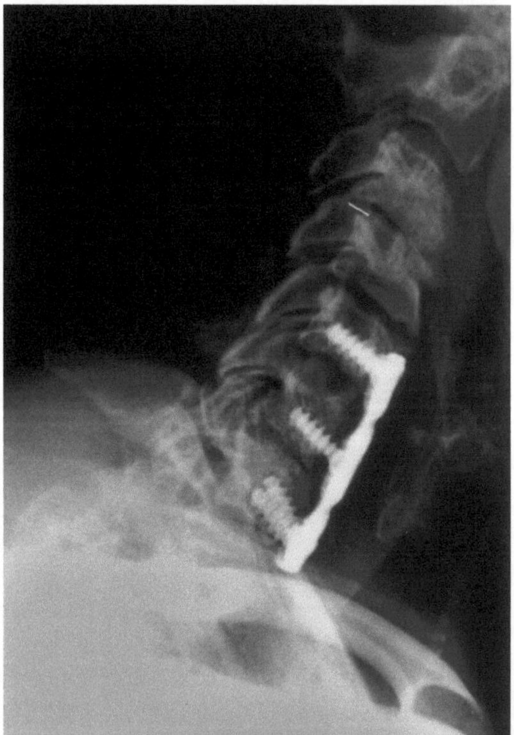

Fig. 31.10. A post-operative lateral cervical spine X-ray approximately 1 year following a two-level diskectomy and interbody fusion at C5–C6 and C6–C7. There is clear lucency across the interspace at C6–C7. The inferior screws and the plate have toggled as the disk space of C6–C7 settled, with resorption of the graft.

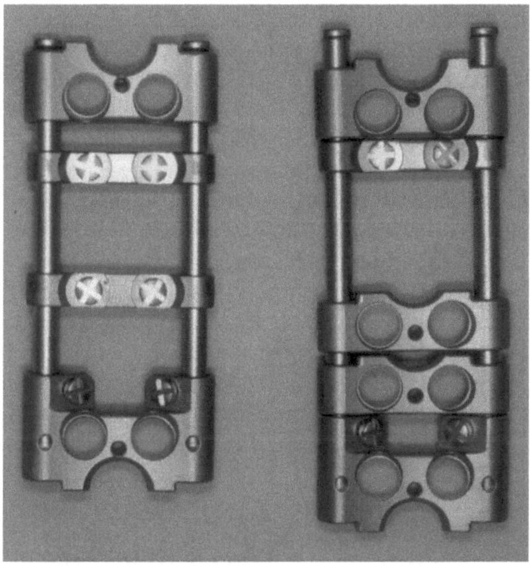

Fig. 31.11. The DOC plate (Johnson and Johnson/Depuy-Acromed Incorporated, Cleveland, Ohio, USA). Anterior views of two DOC plates. The DOC plate is a dynamic device which compensates for subsidence across the fusion segment. The plate on the left demonstrates the upper crosslink device, which attaches to the vertebral bodies in the upright position. On the right, the upper crosslink has migrated inferiorly to the limiting crosslink, which is the amount of the subsidence allowed by this plate. The inferior crosslink is attached to the inferior vertebral body along the segment of fixation and the middle two crosslinks, seen on the right-hand side of the plate, are used to attach intervening vertebral bodies or the bone graft.

extent of fusion required, the presence or absence of a deformity and the extent of its correction and patient factors. In the presence of a cervical kyphosis, attempt at reduction of the kyphosis is optimal. As discussed earlier, correction of the kyphosis would reduce the likelihood of mechanical pain and reduce the amount of translational and compressive force on the fixation device. Both anterior and posterior fixation devices have a limited capacity to resist translational movement. In the setting of cervical spondylitic disease, spinal deformity typically takes the form of kyphosis, due to loss of disk space or vertebral body height. It is very difficult to correct and maintain correction of kyphosis by a posterior approach. Therefore, a component of the fixation/fusion for kyphosis usually involves anterior surgery, utilizing either interbody grafts or a vertebrectomy strut. Adequate immobilization is required following implantation of the interbody grafts. Many would consider an anterior plating procedure to supplement the interbody graft. The plate stabilizes the involved motion segment and the bone graft. It also acts as a load-sharing structure, where some of the axial force placed upon the fused segment is transmitted through the screws and the vertical member of the fixation device, and not solely through the bone graft. This reduces the likelihood of graft subsidence and subsequently the loss of kyphosis correction.

Posterior fixation and fusion for degenerative disease is considered to prevent subsequent kyphosis following laminectomy or to correct and stabilize an unstable motion segment. Utilization of a posterior fixation/fusion technique alone for the correction of a mobile kyphosis has a significant likelihood of fixation failure. Anterior instrumentation can be used to supplement the posterior fixation and fusion to augment the stabilization and likelihood of achieving fusion in such a circumstance.

Laminoplasty is another technique utilized to effect spinal stenosis decompression. The technique involves mobilizing the posterior elements without completely detaching the lamina from the lateral masses. Complete transsection of the lateral aspect of the lamina, combined with a partial scoring of the lamina of the contralateral side, will enable the lamina to be cracked back across the partially transected lamina to expand the canal size. Another technique involves splitting the posterior elements in half down the spinous process. The two halves of the spinous process or the laminae are then spread apart. In both techniques, a bone graft is interposed between the cracked fragments of bone to maintain the patency of the canal following the decompression.

The advantages of laminoplasty are in diminishing the accumulation of epidural scar tissue and maintaining some of the extensive compartment function, by enabling the paraspinal musculature to reinsert upon the posterior elements. Some preliminary studies indicate that the likelihood of inducing kyphosis is lower with a laminoplasty when compared to laminectomy alone or laminectomy combined with segmental fusion. Also, patients who have undergone laminoplasty remain mobile and unfused, which is a more physiological state. Biomechanical studies have not clearly determined if the hypothetical goals of laminoplasty are realized.

Ossification of the posterior longitudinal ligament is a variation of degenerative disease in the neck, involving significant hypertrophy and calcification of the posterior longitudinal ligament. It typically manifests with symptoms and/or signs of myelopathy. It is more frequently seen and reported in the Japanese literature. There also appears to be some predisposition in the African–American population. Spinal canal decompression is a primary goal in the treatment of such patients. Ideally, a resection of the ossified ligament which is encroaching upon the canal is the goal of surgery. However, the site and the vertical extent of the calcified ligament can make it difficult to adequately decompress the canal without significant morbidity. It is not uncommon to see that the calcified posterior ligament is fused to the dura, which can result in a dural perforation during the decompression, which increases the likelihood of spinal cord injury. In more severe cases, which extend over multiple motion segments, laminectomy with or without fusion can be utilized as a less optimal form of treatment.

Summary

The degenerative process can affect the cervical spine morphologically and clinically in a variety of ways. The cervical disc is probably the first element involved in this process and its degeneration predisposes the remainder of the motion segment to spondylotic changes. The accumulation of osteophytes, alteration of spinal curvature and instability can all produce symptoms. The clinical manifestations of spondylosis are typically pain or neurological symptoms or signs. As part of the work-up for the cause of axial arm pain or neurological deficit, one must consider intrathoracic pathology, appendicular joint osteoarthritis and peripheral entrapment neuropathies in the differential diagnosis. The correlation between symptoms and signs should be made with imaging findings, demonstrating ongoing neural element compression, advanced degenerative change or instability. Except in the presence of significant neurological deficit or myelopathy, non-operative treatment should be considered initially. Rest, anti-inflammatories and analgesics are often effective for treating acute neck and arm pain from spondylosis. These modalities are less efficacious for the treatment of chronic cervical pain.

A variety of surgical options are available for the treatment of symptomatic cervical spondylosis refractory to non-operative measures. Cervicoradicular pain resulting from cervical nerve root compression is usually amenable to decompressive surgery. Anterior and posterior decompressive approaches are available. The procedure selected is dependent upon the location of the compressive pathology and the need to undertake fusion at the time of decompression.

Fusion surgery is required in cases where spinal instability is contributing to symptoms or to reconstruct the segment of the spine that was resected for decompression. The role of spinal fusion for the treatment of axial neck pain is controversial. In a highly selected population, segmental fusion can be effective for treating axial pain if the location of the pain generator is clear. Internal fixation devices are an effective adjunct to achieve immediate stabilization of a segment which is intended to be fused.

Key Points

- *The degenerative process can effect the cervical spine morphologically and clinically in a variety of ways.*
- *The clinical manifestations of spondylosis are typically pain or neurological symptoms or signs.*
- *A variety of surgical options are available for the treatment of symptomatic cervical spondylosis refractory to non-operative measures.*

References

1. Batzdorf U, Batzdorf A. Analysis of cervical spine curvature in patients with cervical spondylosis. Neurosurgery 1988;22:827–36.
2. Bohlman HH, Emery SE. The pathophysiology of cervical spondylosis and myelopathy. Spine 1988;13:843–6.
3. Dooley JF, McBroom RJ, Taguchi T, Macnab I. Nerve root infiltration in the diagnosis of radicular pain. Spine 1988;13:79–83.
4. Grubb S, Kelly C. Cervical discography: clinical implications from 12 years of experience. Spine 2000;25:1382–9.

5. Block AR, Vanharanta H, Ohnmeiss DD, Guyer RD. Discographic pain report: influence of psychological factors. Spine 1996;21:334–8.
6. Kadanka Z, Bednarik J, Vohanka S et al. Conservative treatment versus surgery in spondylotic cervical myelopathy: a prospective randomised study. Eur Spine J 2000;9:538–44.
7. Torg JS, Ramsey-Emrhein JA. Management guidelines for participation in collision activities with congenital, developmental, or post-injury lesions involving the cervical spine. Clin Sports Med 1997;16:501–30.
8. Chapman-Smith D. Nonoperative treatment of neck and arm pain. Spine 1999;15:2746–54.
9. Palit M, Schofferman J, Goldthwaite N et al. Anterior discectomy and fusion for the management of neck pain. Spine 1999;24:2224–8.
10. Fairbank J. Trials and tribulations in cervical spondylosis. Lancet 1998;352:1165–6.
11. Kaptain GJ, Simmons NE, Replogle RE, Pobereskin L. Incidence and outcome of kyphotic deformity following laminectomy for cervical spondylotic myelopathy. J Neurosurg 2000;(Spine 2)93:199–204.
12. Kumar VGR, Rea GL, Mervis LJ, McGregor JM. Cervical spondylotic myelopathy: functional and radiographic long-term outcome after laminectomy and posterior fusion. Neurosurgery 1999;44:771–8.
13. Cloward RB. The anterior approach for removal of ruptured cervical discs. J Neurosurg 1958;15:602–17.
14. Aronson N, Filtzer DL, Bagan M. Anterior cervical fusion by the Smith-Robinson approach. J Neurosurg 1968;29:397–404.
15. Clements DH, O'Leary PF. Anterior cervical discectomy and fusion. Spine 1990;15:1023–5.
16. Benini A, Krayenbuhl H, Bruderl R. Anterior cervical discectomy without fusion: microsurgical technique. Acta Neurochir (Wien) 1982;61:105–10.
17. Bertalanffy H, Eggert HR. Complications of anterior cervical discectomy without fusion in 450 consecutive patients. Acta Neurochir (Wien) 1989;99:41–50.
18. Jho HD. Microsurgical anterior cervical foraminotomy for radiculopathy: a new approach to cervical disc herniation. J Neurosurg 1996;8:155–60.
19. Johnson JP, Filler AG, McBride DQ, Batzdorf U. Anterior cervical foramenotomy for unilateral radicular disease. Spine 2000;25:905–9.
20. Cauthen JC, Kinard R, C., Vogler JB et al. Outcome analysis of noninstrumented anterior cervical discectomy and interbody fusion in 348 patients. Spine 1998;23:188–92.
21. Hadra BE. The classic wiring of the vertebrae as a means of immobilization in fractures and Pott's disease. Clin Orthop 1975;112:4–8.
22. Weiland DJ, McAfee PC. Posterior cervical fusion with triple-wire strut graft technique: one hundred consecutive patients. J Spinal Disord 1991;4:15–21.
23. Roy-Camille R, Saillant G. Chirurgie du rachis cervical. 1. Generalites: luxations pures de articulaires. Nouv Presse Med 1972;1:2330–2.
24. Fernyhough JC, White JI, LaRocca H. Fusion rates in multilevel cervical spondylosis comparing allograft fibula with autograft fibula in 126 patients. Spine 1991;16:S561–4.
25. Aebi M, Zuber K, Marchesi D. Treatment of cervical spine injuries with anterior plating: indications, techniques, and results. Spine 1991;16:S38–45.

X
Peripheral and Cranial Nerves

32

Peripheral and Cranial Nerve Injury

Gavin Wayne Britz, Todd McCall,
Gerald Grant and Michel Kliot

Summary

The peripheral nervous system is an integral component of the neural connection between the CNS and the end organs. Injuries involving this system are often complex and require a thorough understanding of the management strategies of these injuries to help optimize recovery. Recent advances in MRI may lead to its becoming a useful tool in managing peripheral nerve injuries; however, good clinical acumen and the understanding of the anatomy and classification of nerve injuries remain the most important aspects. This chapter will therefore address the anatomy of a peripheral nerve, the classification of nerve injuries and the utility of MRI in diagnoses of peripheral nerve injuries and discuss the evaluation and treatment of injuries to peripheral and cranial nerves.

Anatomy of the Peripheral Nervous System

The peripheral nervous system consists of those structures containing nerve fibers or axons that connect the CNS to motor, sensory, somatic and visceral end organs. This includes the cranial nerves (III–XII), spinal nerves, cervical, brachial and lumbosacral plexus and nerves of the extremity. These nerves are mostly mixed nerves (motor and sensory). In the peripheral nervous system, excluding the cranial nerves, they have their origin as a spinal nerve that is formed by the union of ventral and dorsal roots. The ventral root is largely formed by efferent fibers that innervate somatic musculature, but also contain some pre-ganglionic autonomic fibers that innervate blood vessels, smooth muscle and glandular epithelium. The dorsal root contains most of the afferent fibers from the somatic and visceral system. These spinal nerves then emerge from the neural foramina in the vertebral column and form extensive plexuses in which radical re-grouping of fibers occurs. Each of the peripheral nerves arising from these plexuses contains fibers contributed by two, three, four or even five ventral rami. As a result, the cutaneous areas supplied by the peripheral nerves do not correspond to the cutaneous area supplied by the individual dorsal roots. Similarly, several ventral roots may contribute fibers to a single muscle and conversely several muscles may receive fibers from a single ventral root.

The integral component of the neural connection between the CNS and motor, sensory, somatic and visceral end organs is the axon, which is the "cable" that makes the connection possible (Fig. 32.1). Axons may be surrounded by a myelin sheath (myelinated) or not (un-myelinated) and are surrounded by a fine connective tissue layer called the endoneurium.

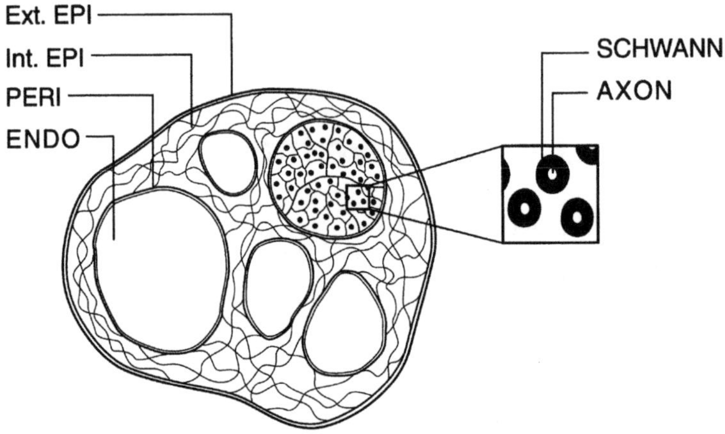

Fig. 32.1. Schematic cross-sectional view of a peripheral nerve. These are the axons, which may be surrounded by a myelin sheath (myelinated – presence of schwann cell) or not (unmyelinated) and are surrounded by a fine connective tissue layer called the endoneurium (ENDO). These are bundled together into fascicles and surrounded by a further layer of connective tissue called the perineurium (PERI). Multiple nerve fascicles are then further bundled together within soft connective tissue called the mesoneurium or internal epineurium (Int. EPI) and covered by a firmer layer of connective tissue called the epineurium (EPI).

These are bundled together into fascicles, which are surrounded by a further layer of connective tissue called the perineurium. Multiple nerve fascicles are then further bundled together within soft connective tissue called the mesoneurium and covered by a firmer layer of connective tissue called the epineurium.

Classification of Peripheral Nerve Injuries

The classification of peripheral nerve injuries was developed as a means of allowing the treating physician to objectively grade the injury, predict clinical outcome and determine the optimal type of treatment. This also allowed for an objective method for following the recovery process. A number of grading schemes have been proposed to fulfill these objectives, of which two have been found to be the most useful. The first is that described by Seddon [1] in 1943, in which he described three types of injury that correlate with damage to specific components of the peripheral nerve; this grading system was also found to be helpful in predicting prognosis of an injury and therefore determining appropriate management of it (Table 32.1).

Table 32.1. Classification of nerve injuries by Seddon.

Injury	Anatomical injury	Electrodiagnostic evaluation	Prognosis
Neurapraxia	Focal loss of myelin, otherwise normal structure	Normal nerve conduction distal to site of injury, but impaired across	Recovery complete within hours to months
Axonotmesis	Disruption of axon and myelin sheath but normal connective tissue structures, with Wallerian degeneration distal to the site of injury	No conduction, either proximal or distal to site of injury	Functional recovery generally occurs over months to years; may not be complete.
Neurotmesis	Complete disruption of connective tissue, axon, myelin, with complete Wallerian degeneration distal to site of injury	No conduction, either proximal or distal to site of injury	Spontaneous regeneration is impossible; functional recovery may occur with surgical aid, but complete recovery very unusual

The least severe grade in Seddon's classification of peripheral nerve injuries is neurapraxia (Fig. 32.2). This level of injury is due to the loss of a functional myelin sheath, while the axon and the surrounding connective tissue remain intact. This leads to the disruption of propagating action potentials across the site of injury. With re-myelination almost always occurring following trauma or removal of the underlying cause, neurapraxic injuries generally have a high level of recovery, which occurs in days to weeks. Possible etiologies of a neurapraxic injury include mechanical compression, metabolic derangements, demyelinating diseases and ischemia.

The intermediate grade in terms of severity is an axonotmetic injury which involves disruption of both the myelin sheath and axon, with Wallerian degeneration occurring distal to the site of injury (Fig. 32.2). Subsequently, there is no conduction of an electrical stimulus distal to the site of injury. Recovery of axonotmetic injuries does occur, as the axon can regenerate along the path of the previous axon. Typically, the rate of recovery is 1–1.5 mm per day, or approximately 1 inch per month. Thus, functional recovery generally takes place over a period of months, with more proximal injuries taking longer to recover from. Clinically, this regenerating axon can be demonstrated by the progression of the point at which a Tinel sign is present.

The functional recovery following an axonotmetic injury may not be complete, as several factors can potentially influence the ability of a regenerating axon to reach the proper target [2]. First, anatomically complex nerves with more branching have a decreased chance of proper re-innervation compared to less complex nerves. Secondly, functionally complex nerves with both motor and sensory components less accurately re-innervate compared to nerves that are only motor or sensory. Thirdly, the need for precise innervation to maintain function varies between nerves. For example, clinical recovery from a distal tibial nerve injury often gives a more gratifying result compared to a distal ulnar nerve injury, because proper hand function is dependent on more precise innervation.

The most severe grade in Seddon's classification is neurotmesis. In this injury, the myelin sheath, axon and connective tissue encompassing the nerve are all disrupted (Fig. 32.2). This connective tissue surrounding the nerve, as described in the anatomy section, can be conceptualized as a "highway" that regenerating axons can follow to reach the appropriate target. Thus, when the connective tissue highway is damaged, peripheral nerves can no longer regenerate along the proper path, resulting in poor or absent functional recovery. This is often complicated by extraneural and/or intraneural fibrosis that further hinders the recovery by blocking axon regeneration [2].

Sir Sydney Sunderland's classification is another scheme that is often utilized and involves his proposed five grades of degree of injury [3] (Table 32.2). The first- and second-grade degrees of injury in Sunderland's scheme correspond to neurapraxic and axonotmetic injuries, respectively. The third-grade degree of injury is characterized by endoneurial damage, in addition to Wallerian degeneration. Recovery occurs at a similar rate to a second-grade-degree injury but is not as complete, because the compromised endoneurium no longer provides a clear conduit that the regenerating axons can follow. A fourth-grade-degree injury involves a nerve with continuity maintained, but with scar tissue disrupting the endoneurium and perineurium. Fascicular disorganization leads to minimal spontaneous functional recovery, because regenerating axons no longer reach their original targets. A fifth-grade-degree injury is complete transection of a nerve. This degree of injury is typically easy to diagnose because it is associated with an open traumatic injury, along with complete loss of motor and sensory function of the injured nerve.

Management of Peripheral Nerve Injuries

The management of peripheral nerve injuries is largely determined by understanding the mechanism, and grade of injury. This involves evaluating an associated laceration and classifying the grade of the injury utilizing one of the schemes described above. The authors personally believe that most traumatic peripheral nerve injuries can be logically managed by utilizing the Seddon three-tier grading scheme, as described earlier [3]. The crux of this evaluation is that it is essential to differentiate between neurapraxic/axonotmetic grades of injury and neurotmetic injuries, as the first can recover

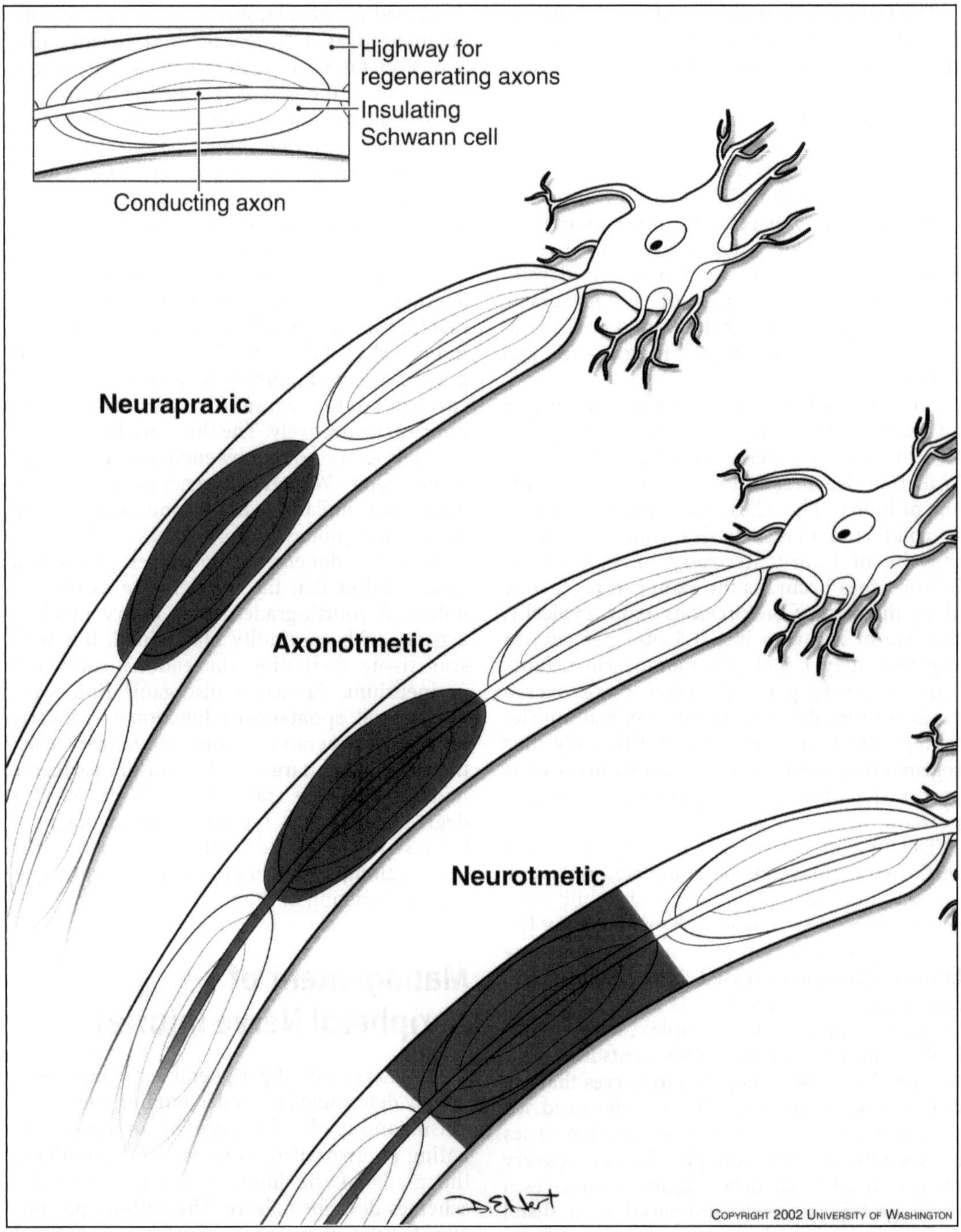

Fig. 32.2. Schematic diagram of the three grades of injury and anatomical elements involved. The neurapraxic injury is due to the loss of a functional myelin sheath, while the axon and the surrounding connective tissue remain intact. The axonotmetic injury involves disruption of both the myelin sheath and the axon. The neurotmetic injury involves the myelin sheath, axon and connective tissue encompassing the nerve.

Table 32.2. Classification of nerve injuries by Sunderland.

Injury	Anatomical injury	Electrodiagnostic evaluation	Prognosis
First degree	Focal loss of myelin, otherwise normal structure	Normal nerve conduction distal to site of injury, but impaired across	Recovery complete in hours to months
Second degree	Disruption of axon and myelin sheath but normal connective tissue structures, with Wallerian degeneration distal to site of injury	No conduction, either proximal or distal to site of injury	Functional recovery generally occurs over months to years; may not be complete
Third degree	Endoneurium disrupted, epineurium and perineurium intact; nerve may not appear seriously damaged on gross inspection	No conduction, either proximal or distal to site of injury	Recovery may range from poor to complete and depends on degree on intrafascicular fibrosis
Fourth degree	Interruption of all neural and supporting elements; epineurium intact; nerve is usually indurated and enlarged	No conduction, either proximal or distal to site of injury	Spontaneous regeneration is nearly impossible. Functional recovery may occur with surgical aid, but complete recovery very unusual
Fifth degree	Complete disruption with loss of continuity of the nerve	No conduction either proximal or distal to site of injury	Spontaneous regeneration is impossible. Functional recovery may occur with surgical aid, but complete recovery very unusual

spontaneously but a neurotmetic injury requires surgical intervention. This differentiation is made with serial neurological and electrodiagnostic evaluations. The initial neurological evaluation often demonstrates a complete neural injury and the differentiation may be made by documenting improvements in neurological function. Early complete recovery signifies a neurapraxic injury, while later recovery, even if incomplete, suggests an axonotmetic rather than a neurotmetic injury. This information is often supplemented by serial electrodiagnostic conduction studies. In a neurapraxic injury, the electrical stimulation of the nerve distal to the site of injury will elicit a response, since the axon remains in continuity, while electrical stimulation proximal to the lesion will not elicit a response (or elicits a reduced response in the case of a partial neurapraxic injury). Neurotmetic and axonotmetic injuries cannot be differentiated using electrodiagnostic studies, as no response is elicited with stimulation proximal or distal to the lesion. In centers with expertise in MRI, as discussed later in the chapter, further information can be obtained to enhance the diagnosis of these types of injury.

In situations where the skin integrity is maintained, the peripheral nerve injuries are often no less acute; due to repetitive stretching and/or compression of the nerve, a lesion in continuity is more common than a transected nerve. The management of closed nerve injuries is still based on properly categorizing the injury as neurapraxic, axonotmetic or neurotmetic. As discussed earlier, a neurapraxic injury is often readily distinguished, based on clinical and electrodiagnostic studies, since this grade of injury has distinct electrodiagnostic findings compared to the other grades of injury. Neurapraxic injuries due to trauma should be managed medically without surgery and excellent recovery can be expected.

Axonotmetic and neurotmetic injuries can be difficult to differentiate because both grades of injury involve disruption of the axon, resulting in similar initial electrodiagnostic findings and muscle denervation. However, it is important to determine whether a peripheral nerve injury is axonotmetic or neurotmetic because the former does not require surgical repair while the latter does, as reconstruction of the "highway" is needed to facilitate axonal regeneration (Figs 32.1 and 32.2). Therefore, patients with these types of nerve injury should be closely followed with serial neurological examinations and electrophysiological studies that will evaluate for the presence of axon regeneration and muscle reinnervation. If there is no evidence of recovery within 3–4 months, then a neurotmetic injury is more probable and a surgical exploration is indicated. This recommendation for surgical exploration in the 3–4 months following injury is not arbitrary but is predicated on the observation that muscles not reinnervated within 2 years following nerve injury have poor recovery of useful motor function [4]. After 2 years, muscles undergo irreversible atrophy and are replaced by adipose tissue. Thus, regenerating nerves must be allowed adequate time to reinnervate to their appropriate target, remembering that regeneration occurs at the rate of approximately 1 inch per month [3].

In nerve injuries associated with skin disruption, clinical evaluation of the wound is important, in addition to identifying the source of injury, as this will largely determine the management of these patients. An open lesion with the nerve in continuity should be managed with surgical repair of the wound and serial neurological, electrodiagnostic and imaging examinations, as this nerve injury most likely represents either a neurapraxic or an axonotmetic injury. In situations where the nerve is clearly disrupted, a neurotmetic injury is evident and, in those lesions, the mechanism of injury determines the timing of surgical management. In a situation where there is a sharp transection of the nerve, such as occurs with lacerations from glass or a knife, immediate surgical repair with an end-to-end suture repair, where possible, without producing tension, is indicated. In situations where blunt trauma is responsible for the transection, as occurs in complex extremity fractures or power saw injuries, then a delayed repair is indicated. This delay should be for at least 2–3 weeks following the injury, as this allows for the maturation of the injury so that the damaged, scarred, non-viable nerve can be readily distinguished from the undamaged, unscarred nerve. The damaged, scarred nerve segment can then be resected and the nerve, with viable proximal and distal ends, can be surgically repaired with or without a nerve graft, depending on the gap length.

Surgical Repair of Peripheral Nerve Lesions

When the decision is made to explore an injured nerve, it is important that the surgeon understands the thought process involved. First, it is paramount that this surgical exploration be performed with the utilization of intraoperative electrophysiological monitoring to aid in the decision making. Usually, the decision to explore the nerve is based on the assumption that a neurotmetic injury exists or, unless this occurs in the case of an open wound, there is clear evidence of neural disruption.

Therefore, once the nerve is exposed both proximally and distally to the injured segment, direct electrical stimulation of the nerve should be performed. In situations where this results in a recordable response across a lesion, this suggests the presence of functioning nerve fibers (at least several thousand) and often, therefore, implies either a neurapraxic or an axonotmetic lesion [5]. Axonotmetic lesions should be managed medically and recovery usually occurs within weeks to months, as remyelination and/or regeneration occur, and the wound should be closed. In neurotmetic lesions, no conduction will be recorded across the lesion and, in this case, surgery is indicated.

The surgical repair of neurotmetic peripheral nerve injuries has evolved in the past three decades, with significant advancements. First, microsurgical techniques have developed, including intraoperative magnification, microinstruments and fine suture material [6]. Secondly, the use of grafts has re-emerged, allowing surgeons to perform tension-free nerve repairs [7]. Thirdly, factors such as timing of surgery and fascicular anatomy are now better appreciated.

A principle tenet of peripheral nerve surgery is that a repair must be tension free. Tension can diminish the intraneural blood supply and compromise the clinical outcome of a peripheral nerve repair [7].

A primary nerve repair is desirable, but use of a nerve graft is indicated if an end-to-end repair cannot be made tension free. Positioning of an extremity should be neutral and not altered to accommodate a tension-free primary nerve repair, because the nerve must be able to remain tension free during flexion and extension of the extremity through a full range of movements.

No consensus exists as to a specific length of nerve gap (the distance between two nerve ends) that requires a nerve graft [6]. This is largely due to the variability between anatomic locations.

For example, a 1-cm gap in a digital nerve cannot be overcome without a nerve graft, while the same gap in the forearm can be overcome with mobilization of the nerve proximally and distally. Anterior transposition of the ulnar nerve can provide up to 5 cm to span a nerve gap. There is also no clear relation between the length of nerve graft and clinical outcome. However, small-caliber grafts do appear to result in better outcome when compared to whole-nerve grafts [7]. The most popular choice for a nerve graft is the sural nerve. Excision of the sural nerve results only in sensory deficits along the lateral foot, which resolve partially with time, and the nerve graft can be long enough to bridge a nerve gap of 30–40 cm. Other nerves frequently harvested for nerve grafts include the lateral antebrachial cutaneous nerve and the anterior division of the medial antebrachial cutaneous nerve in the upper arm.

Another consideration in the repair of peripheral nerves is the determination of whether an epineurial or fascicular repair is more appropriate. Several experimental [8] and clinical [9] studies have addressed the issue of whether epineurial or fascicular repair is more effective, with no conclusive evidence suggesting the superiority of one over the other [2]. Studies examining the specificity of muscle reinnervation of rat sciatic nerve have demonstrated that fascicular repair resulted in more accurate regeneration as compared to epineurial repair [10,11].

However, primate studies comparing fascicular and epineurial repair did not find a significant difference between the two techniques [12]. Clinical studies have failed to demonstrate a significant difference in recovery of function when comparing fascicular to epineurial repair, although no randomized trial with sufficient clinical and electrophysiologic evaluations has been undertaken [2]. Theoretically, fascicular repair should provide more specific paths through which peripheral nerves can regenerate. However, this potential benefit of fascicular repair is probably not realized, due to the difficulty of accurately aligning fascicles.

MacKinnon [2] suggests that aspects of both fascicular and epineurial repair should be employed, depending on the circumstances. Factors to consider include the timing of the repair and the location of injury. Acute injuries can generally be managed with epineurial repair, as anatomic markings visible on the nerve provide guidance for proper alignment. The location of the injury can be important regarding proximal versus distal injury. Proximally, nerves tend to be monofascicular or oligofascicular and, in such circumstances, an epineurial repair is indicated. Distally, nerves are more polyfascicular and often arranged in groups. A surgeon can then match groups of fascicles to minimize the use of sutures and additional trauma. The application of Tisseel™ fibrin glue has allowed surgical repairs to be performed with the placement of fewer sutures.

Brachial Plexus Injury

The brachial plexus classically arises from the fifth to the eighth cervical spinal nerve roots and the first thoracic nerve root, and is responsible for innervation of all muscles of the upper extremity. These spinal nerves roots form three trunks (upper, middle and lower), which then divide to form divisions, cords and, finally, peripheral nerves. These peripheral nerves include the musculocutaneous, radial, median and ulnar nerves. Traumatic lesions of the brachial plexus are often due to excessive traction, resulting in root avulsion. However, any of the aforementioned components of the brachial plexus may be involved with a traumatic injury and in various combinations.

Injury to the upper roots of the brachial plexus results in weakness of the deltoid, biceps, brachialis and brachioradialis muscles. Clinically, injury to the upper trunk of the brachial plexus presents with an adducted shoulder, medially rotated forearm and extended elbow, which, together, are referred to as an Erb–Duchenne palsy. Injury to the lower trunk of the brachial plexus results in a clawhand deformity, due to injury of the short muscles of the hand, which is called Klumpke's palsy. Injury to the proximal lower spinal roots and/or nerves may also result in a Horner's syndrome with ptosis, miosis and anhydrosis. Proximal nerve root injury can also manifest as elevation of the ipsilateral diaphragm (phrenic nerve), scapular winging (long thoracic nerve) and weakness of the rhomboid muscles (dorsal scapular nerve).

Diagnosis of brachial plexus injury is based on clinical, electrophysiological and imaging findings. Neuroradiological studies used for the pre-operative diagnosis of root avulsion include CT–myelography and MRI. The accuracies of CT–myelography and MRI for diagnosing cervical root avulsion have been estimated to be 85 and 52%, respectively [13]. Post-traumatic meningocele may not always accompany a root avulsion, and the presence of a post-traumatic meningocele does not necessarily imply the presence of a root avulsion. Furthermore, supraclavicular exploration is not always reliable, because extradurally intact roots may be avulsed intradurally. Neuroradiologic findings may be supplemented with intraoperative electrodiagnostic studies, including nerve action potentials and somatosensory evoked potentials. Still, intradural surgical inspection remains the gold standard for the diagnosis of avulsed cervical roots.

Complete restoration of arm function is usually unrealistic following significant brachial plexus injury. Therefore, the surgeon must prioritize which functions to attempt to restore in cases involving multiple cervical roots and spinal nerves. Elbow flexion (musculocutaneous nerve) and shoulder abduction (suprascapular and axillary nerves) are generally considered the most beneficial functions for improving patient quality of life [14].

Proximal brachial plexus lesions may be classified as either post-ganglionic or pre-ganglionic and this is an important distinction when choosing the method of surgical repair. With post-ganglionic lesions, the continuity of the spinal–cervical root is maintained. In such cases where there is continuity of the spinal–cervical root with the spinal cord, a nerve graft may be useful. Studies using sural nerve to reconstruct the musculocutaneous nerve have helped to identify factors affecting the outcome of nerve graft surgeries in cases of post-ganglionic brachial plexus injury [13].

The time interval between brachial plexus injury and surgery should be emphasized as an important factor influencing the success of surgical intervention. In a retrospective study involving 54 cases of musculocutaneous nerve reconstructed with sural nerve grafts, reinnervation of the musculocutaneous nerve occurred in 75% of patients undergoing surgery within 6 months after injury, compared to a reinnervation rate of 25% with surgery more than 12 months following injury [15]. Factors that may be detrimental to the success of surgery after a prolonged post-injury interval include degeneration of muscle fibers, fibrosis or scar tissue formation and chronic degeneration of the distal nerve pathway. Length of nerve graft has not been found to be a significant factor in nerve graft repair of the musculocutaneous nerve, although a trend towards better outcomes with shorter grafts has been documented [13,15].

Samii proposed that the length of nerve graft required increases with the severity of injury. Therefore, poor outcomes with longer grafts may be due to the severity of injury, and not caused by the length of graft [15]. Revascularization of nerve grafts occurs from surrounding tissue, such that the increased length of a nerve graft should not be expected to increase ischemia [16].

In cases of pre-ganglionic injury, the avulsed nerve root cannot be used for the reconstruction of a nerve. In these instances, neurotization of the brachial plexus has been used in an attempt to restore function. Options for neurotization of the brachial plexus include the accessory, intercostal, phrenic and hypoglossal nerves [14,17,18].

Use of the accessory nerve is favored by some because, if transected distally, function of the trapezius is not significantly compromised [13]. The accessory nerve may be used either directly with the suprascapular nerve or in conjunction with a free sural nerve graft to reinnervate the musculocutaneous nerve. Use of the phrenic nerve is often discouraged due to possible loss of pulmonary function [13]. As with nerve grafts, outcome following neurotization of the brachial plexus is dependent upon the time interval between injury and surgery [18].

Recently, Carlsted [19] described ten patients who underwent re-implantation of ventral nerve roots into the spinal cord following pre-ganglionic brachial plexus injury. Regeneration and reconnection with muscle were demonstrated in nine of the ten patients, and three of the ten patients recovered some useful function. Co-contraction between antagonistic muscles limited recovery, although there was a decrease in difficulty with co-contractions over time. Again, early surgical intervention within the first month, if possible, was an important prognostic indicator. Direct re-implantation of avulsed roots into the spinal cord is still experimental, but it may become another viable option for surgeons in the repair of severe brachial plexus injuries.

MRI Evaluation of Peripheral Nerve Trauma

The majority of serious peripheral nerve injuries do not lead to actual transection of the nerve, but rather leave the nerve in continuity. As described earlier, initially it may be difficult to distinguish closed nerve injuries that recover on their own (neurapraxic and axonotmetic grades) from those that do not (neurotmetic grade) and therefore require a surgical repair. Serial clinical and electrodiagnostic evaluations, often over a period of months, have traditionally been the mainstay of decision making in the management of closed traumatic peripheral nerve injuries.

MRI has been used to evaluate muscle signal changes in the clinical setting of a variety of peripheral nerve disorders (Fig. 32.11) [20–22]. MRI was shown to detect increased signal in denervated muscle groups that is most prominently seen using short tau inversion recovery (STIR) or T2-weighted pulse sequences [23]. The increased signal intensity correlates with the degree of muscle denervation seen on EMG and weakness found on clinical examination. In general, the threshold for producing an increased STIR signal is weakness graded at 3 or less out of 5 (i.e. at or below antigravity on the Medical Research Council grading scheme) and conspicuous muscle denervation changes of 3+ or more seen on the EMG [20,23]. The MRI muscle signal changes occur as early as 4 days following a traumatic nerve injury, in contrast to the 2–3 weeks required for EMG evidence of denervation to develop in muscle. These signal changes normalize with muscle reinnervation, as assessed both clinically and by electrodiagnostic studies.

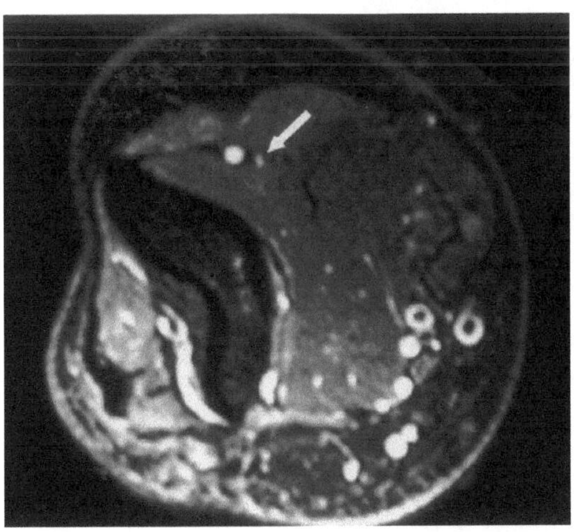

Fig. 32.3. Axial STIR MR image through the proximal forearm of a patient with clinical and electrodiagnostic evidence of a radial neuropathy. Note the increased signal of the radial nerve (white arrow) (from Reference 13).

In the setting of pure neurapraxic injuries (i.e. demyelination without axonal loss) or disuse muscle atrophy, the involved muscles exhibit normal signal characteristics on STIR and T2 pulse sequences. In contrast, in severe axonotmetic and neurotmetic injuries, both of which involve loss of axons, increased STIR and T2 signal appears in the affected muscles as a result of muscle denervation. MRI of muscle, therefore, can be useful in distinguishing neurapraxic from the more severe axonotmetic and neurotmetic grades of injury soon after trauma. In chronically denervated muscles, atrophic changes eventually occur, with the development of fatty infiltration after several months, which is best visualized on T1-weighted images, along with the eventual normalization of signal on T2 and STIR pulse sequences.

We have been attempting to determine whether MRI can be used to localize and determine the grade of a traumatic peripheral nerve injury, and thereby help to determine whether surgery would be of benefit in a more expeditious manner. Soon after traumatic nerve injuries, electrodiagnostic testing can reliably identify neurapraxic injuries by virtue of the ability of such injured nerves to conduct nerve action potentials distal to the site of partial or complete conduction block. Neurapraxic injuries also exhibit no electromyographic or MRI evidence of muscle denervation [23]. In contrast, electrodiagnostic studies cannot distinguish between complete axonotmetic and neurotmetic grades of nerve injury soon after acute trauma.

Using high-resolution MRI techniques, we have found that traumatic injuries produce increased signal in nerves on T2 and STIR pulse sequences that are usually greatest at the site of injury. These MR signal changes have been useful to us in visualizing damaged nerve segments, such as in the setting of traumatic brachial plexus avulsion injuries. We have found that the absence of increased T2 or STIR nerve signal changes, in the clinical setting of severe trauma with complete loss of function, is usually associated with the intraoperative finding of extensive fibrosis, which can make it difficult to distinguish peripheral nerve elements from the surrounding tissues. These severe types of nerve injury are also characterized by the loss of nerve fascicular structure that

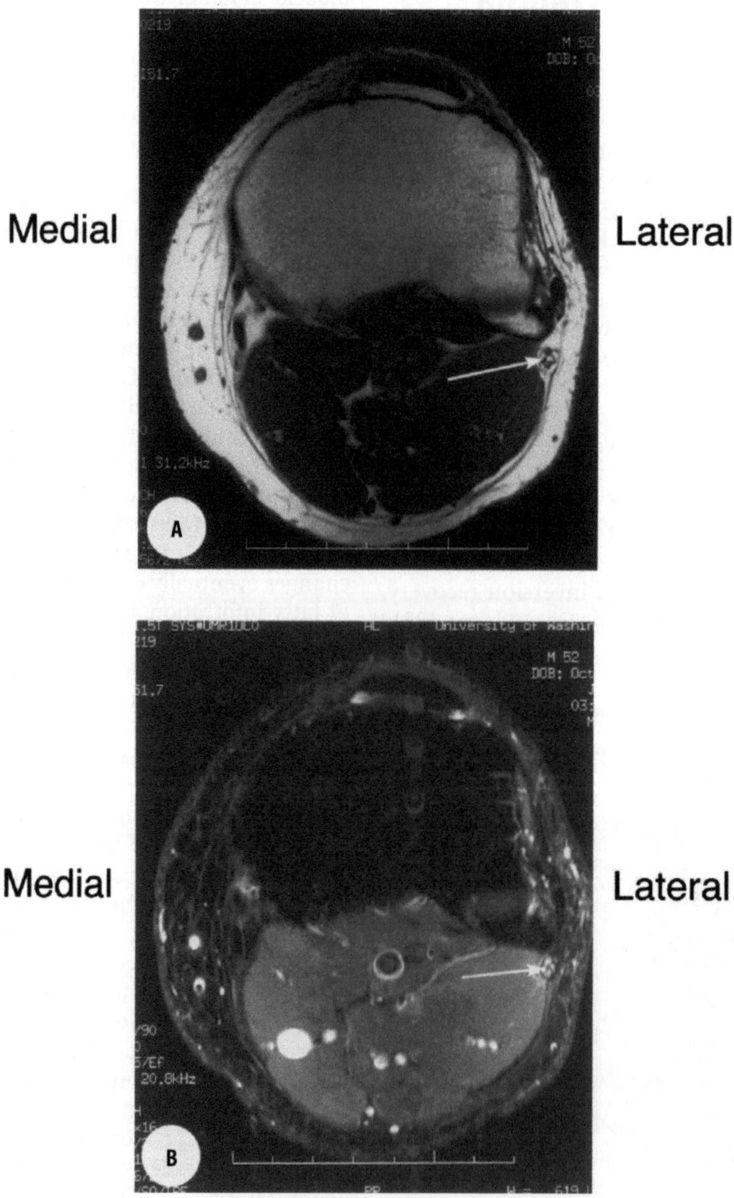

Fig. 32.4. Axial MR images through the lower extremity at the level of the fibular head in a patient with a traumatic peroneal neuropathy. The T1-weighted sequence **a** visualizes the common peroneal nerve, surrounded by fat (white arrow). This nerve was found to display increased signal on the STIR sequence image **b** (from [13]).

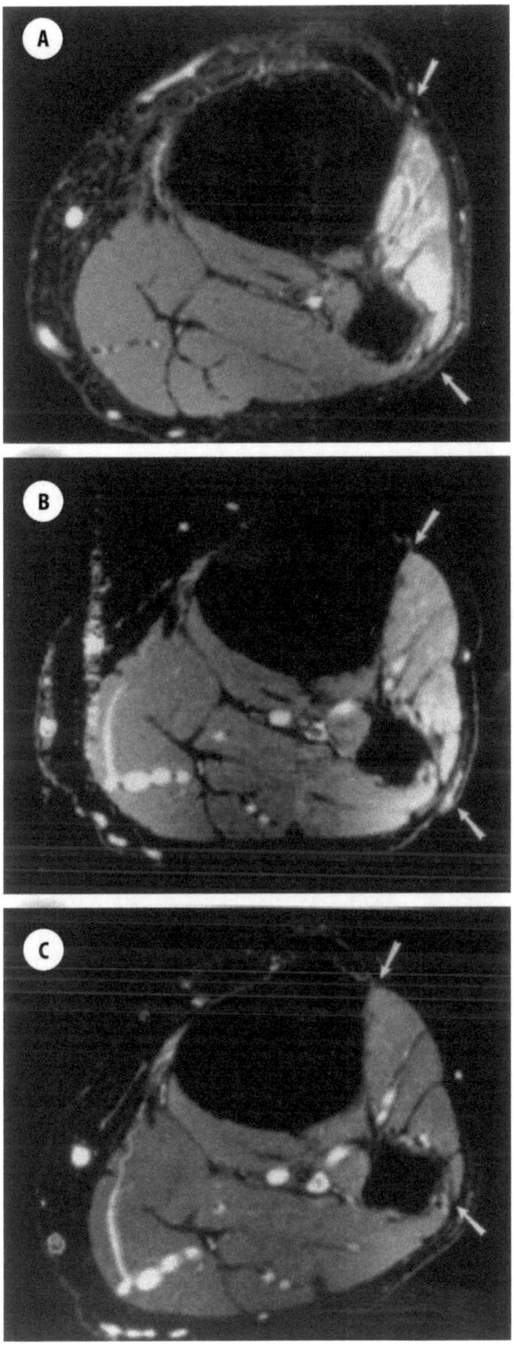

is usually best seen on cross-sectional (i.e. axial) T1 pulse sequence images.

An important question is whether an MRI of a nerve can distinguish between axonotmetic and neurotmetic grades of nerve injury. Both grades of injury are characterized by absent nerve conduction responses and muscle denervation, seen both on EMG and MRI studies [23]. Following traumatic nerve injuries of sufficient magnitude to produce distal loss of axons, increased signal on T2 and STIR pulse sequences occurs in the nerve, at and distal to the site of injury (Fig. 32.12). These nerve signal changes, however, can be transient. For example, increased nerve signal was shown to slowly normalize over a period of many months, as axonal regeneration with concomitant recovery of function, confirmed both clinically and electrodiagnostically, occurred in a patient following a nerve graft repair operation. In chronically and severely damaged nerves, we have seen examples in which peripheral nerves retain increased T2 and STIR signal for several years, such as following a pre-ganglionic brachial plexus avulsion injury or in the nerve graft segments of surgically repaired nerves. However, we have also seen clinical examples of chronically degenerated peripheral nerve where the increased signal eventually normalizes over months, even in the absence of functional recovery.

In summary, MRI can be used to non-invasively evaluate recovery in the peripheral nervous system following axonal injury in a manner that either confirms or supplements information gained from electrodiagnostic studies. MRI signal changes in nerve and muscle correlate with phases of axonal degeneration and regeneration, muscle denervation and reinnervation, and loss and recovery of function following peripheral nerve injury. Our results demonstrate the potential of MRI to non-invasively visualize and distinguish traumatic peripheral nerve injuries that recover through axonal regeneration (i.e. an axonotmetic grade)

Fig. 32.5. Axial STIR MR images through the lower leg of a 40-year-old male patient who spontaneously developed a severe peroneal nerve palsy. **a** STIR image of the right lower leg 2 weeks after the onset of symptoms shows bright signal in peroneal-supplied muscles (between white arrows). Motor strength in these muscles was MRC Grade 2. No denervation changes on EMG were present at this time. **b** At 8 weeks after the onset of symptoms, the STIR signal in the peroneal supplied muscles remained increased but less so than in **a**. Motor strength had improved to Grade 4 in the involved muscles. Denervation potentials were now present on EMG at this time. **c** At 20 weeks after the onset of symptoms, the STIR signal was normal in all muscles. Strength and EMG studies were normal as well [23].

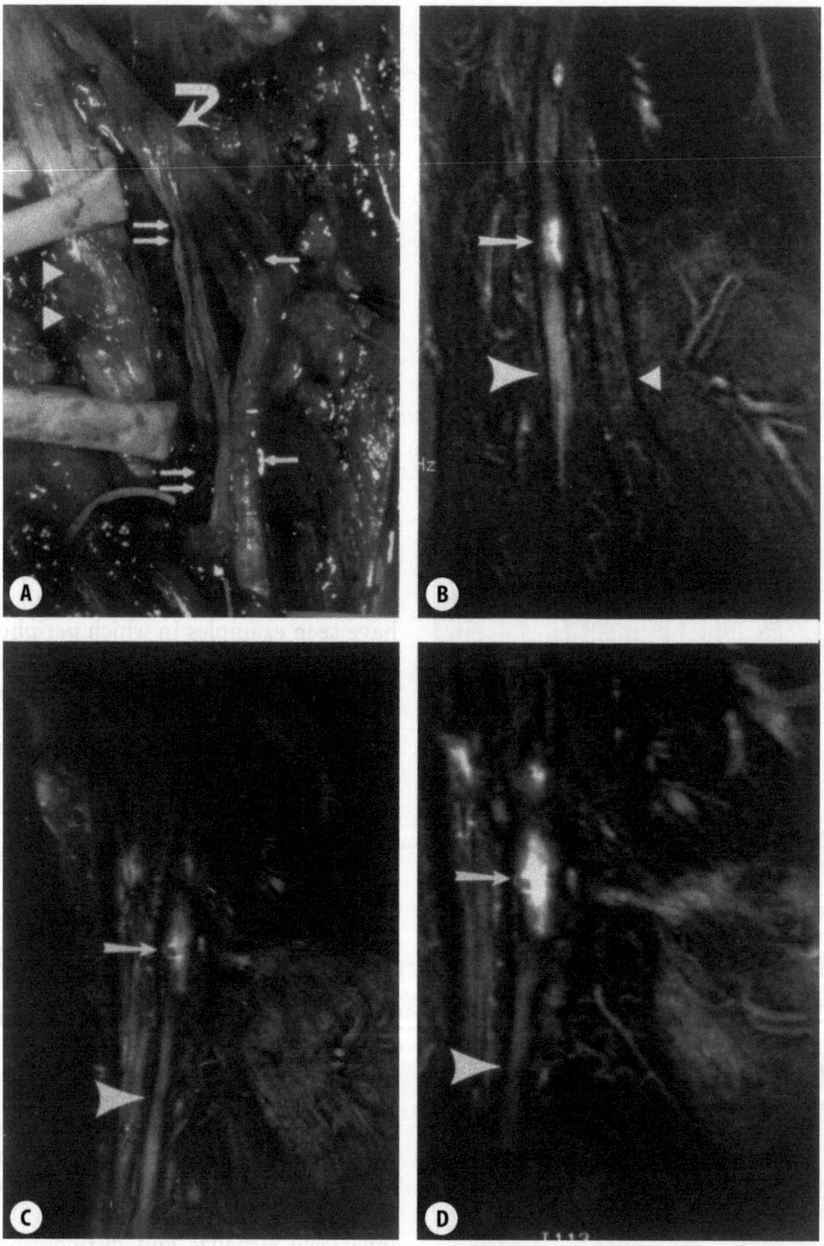

Fig. 32.6. A 29-year-old man suffered a traumatic laceration to his right peroneal nerve, just above the popliteal fossa, resulting in a complete foot drop that had been suture repaired. He failed to recover peroneal nerve function and, 6 months later, a coronal T2-weighted MR image **b** visualized high signal in the nerve at (white arrow) and distal to (white arrowhead) the suture repair site. At the second operation **a**, performed 8 months after the first, no nerve conduction response could be recorded across the scarred suture-repaired segment of the peroneal nerve. This scarred segment was excised and the resultant gap bridged by two sural nerve grafts (**a**, double white arrows), leaving several sensory fascicles intact (**a**, single arrows). Eight months later, the patient began to show clinical and electromyographic evidence of muscle reinnervation and a coronal T2 MR image **c** showed partial return to normal of the bright signal in the distal peroneal nerve (white arrowhead). By 16 months, strength in peroneal-supplied muscles was near normal, the EMG confirmed additional muscle reinnervation and the coronal T2 MR image showed further normalization of signal in the distal peroneal nerve (white arrowhead), while signal remained high at the graft repair site (**c** and **d**, white arrow). (from [13]).

from those that do not and therefore require a surgical repair (i.e. a neurotmetic grade). However, before MRI can do so in a clinically useful manner, we must develop techniques that can more reliably distinguish regenerating nerve from chronically degenerating nerve. New and improved MRI techniques employing diffusion weighting, magnetization transfer and MR spectroscopic pulse sequences, as well as new contrast agents that can label nerves may make such an important goal possible. Such a non-invasive diagnostic modality would significantly improve the treatment of patients with traumatic peripheral nerve injuries by providing earlier and more accurate diagnosis and prognosis, thereby reducing the need for exploratory surgery.

Cranial Nerve Injury

Cranial nerves are similar to peripheral nerves biologically, including the capacity to regenerate following injury. However, surgical repair is often more difficult with cranial nerves due to decreased accessibility. As with peripheral nerves, the ability of surgical intervention to successfully restore function of an injured cranial nerve is largely dependent upon the complexity of the nerve. For example, the trochlear and abducens nerves are each responsible for the innervation of only one muscle. Therefore, regeneration of the proximal nerve stump is more likely to reach the proper target muscle, compared to a more complex nerve such as the trigeminal.

Correctable cranial nerve injury is usually iatrogenic, occurring during surgery. The trochlear nerve has a long course in the lateral wall of the cavernous sinus and therefore may be damaged during surgery in this area. Several cases have been reported in which the trochlear nerve was injured during surgery for an aneurysm or neoplasm and subsequently repaired either end to end [24] or with a peripheral nerve graft.

In general, trochlear nerve repairs have been successful in restoring superior oblique function, both with primary anastamosis and the use of a nerve graft. The abducens nerve is similar to the trochlear nerve in that it only has one target muscle, and therefore a good functional outcome is possible with surgical repair. As with the trochlear nerve, successful repairs of the abducens nerve have been reported using both primary anastamosis and interpositional nerve graft. Fibrin glue is often utilized in both trochlear and abducens repair, since suture may inhibit nerve regeneration.

A common iatrogenic cause of facial nerve injury is vestibular schwannoma resection. Surgical repair of the facial nerve in cases where the proximal nerve is available may be attempted by sural nerve graft, transplantation to the mastoid segment or transplantation to the stylomastoid segment. If the proximal portion of the facial nerve is not available, then neurotization re-animation with the hypoglossal nerve or contralateral facial nerve may be attempted. In a series of 60 patients with facial nerve injury following vestibular schwanoma resection, more than 70% of patients achieved a satisfactory result with intracranial nerve reconstruction or neurotization reanimation [25]. In this case series, Samii emphasizes early reconstruction if the facial nerve is severed and a comprehensive follow-up program.

Key Points

- *In the management of peripheral nerve injuries, understanding the anatomy of a peripheral nerve and classification of the grade of a peripheral nerve injury are crucial.*
- *Serial electrodiagnostic and neurological evaluations are important, to distinguish between neurapraxic injuries that recover spontaneously and axontometic/neurotmentic injuries that may require surgical intervention.*
- *MRI may further aid in distinguishing the grades of nerve injury when making this diagnosis.*
- *Surgical repair should be reserved for those lesions that are documented to be neurotmetic or in those axonometic injuries that have not recovered within the appropriate time.*
- *Surgical repair should entail a tension-free repair that utilizes grafts, if required.*

References

1. Seddon HJ. Three types of nerve injury. Brain 1943;66:237–88.
2. Mackinnon SE, Dellon AL. Nerve repair and nerve grafts. In: Surgery of the peripheral nerve. New York: Thieme, 1988; 89–129.
3. Sunderland S. Nerves and nerve injuries. 2nd Edition. New York: Churchill Livingstone, 1978.
4. Kline DG, Hudson AR. Surgical repair of acute peripheral nerve injuries: timing and technique. In: Morley, editor. Controversies in neurosurgery. Philadelphia: W.B. Saunders Co., 1976; 184–97.
5. Kline DG, Hudson AR. Lower extremity nerve: operative care and technique. In: Nerve injuries. Philadelphia: W.B. Saunders Co., 1995; 117–46.
6. Samii M. Use of microtechniques in peripheral nerve surgery: experience with over 300 cases. In: Handa, editor. Microneurosurgery. Tokyo: Igaku Shoin Ltd., 1975; 85–93.
7. Millesi H. Reappraisal of nerve repair. Surg Clin North Am 1981;61:321–40.
8. Snyder CC. Epineurial repair. Orthop Clin North Am 1981;12:267–76.
9. Bora FW Jr, Pleasure DE, Didizian NA. A study of nerve regeneration and neuroma formation after nerve suture by various techniques. J Hand Surg (Am) 1976;1:138–43.
10. Brushart TM, Henry EW, Mesulam MM. Reorganization of muscle afferent projections accompanies peripheral nerve regeneration. Neuroscience 1981;6:2053–61.
11. Brushart TM, Mesulam MM. Alteration in connections between muscle and anterior horn motoneurons after peripheral nerve repair. Science 1980;208:603–5.
12. Grabb WC, Bement SL, Koepke GH et al. Comparison of methods of peripheral nerve suturing in monkeys. Plast Reconstr Surg 1970;46:31–8.
13. Penkert G, Carvalho GA, Nikkhah G et al. Diagnosis and surgery of brachial plexus injuries. J Reconstr Microsurg 1999;15:3–8.
14. Berger A, Becker MH. Brachial plexus surgery: our concept of the last twelve years. Microsurgery 1994; 15:760–7.
15. Carvalho GA, Nikkhah G, Matthies C et al. Diagnosis of root avulsions in traumatic brachial plexus injuries: value of computerized tomography myelography and magnetic resonance imaging. J Neurosurg 1997;86: 69–76.
16. Seddon HJ. Surgical disorders of the peripheral nerves. London: Churchill Livingstone, 1975.
17. Dolenc VV. Contemporary treatment of peripheral nerve and brachial plexus lesions. Neurosurg Rev 1986;9:149–56.
19. Carlstedt T, Anand P, Hallin R et al. Spinal nerve root repair and reimplantation of avulsed ventral roots into the spinal cord after brachial plexus injury. J Neurosurg 2000;93:237–47.
20. Britz GW, Haynor DR, Kuntz C et al. Carpal tunnel syndrome: correlation of MRI, clinical, electrodiagnostic, and intraoperative findings. Neurosurgery 1995;37: 1097–103.
21. Britz GW, Haynor DR, Kuntz C et al. Ulnar nerve entrapment at the elbow: correlation of magnetic resonance imaging, clinical, electrodiagnostic, and intraoperative findings. Neurosurgery 1996;38:458–65.
22. Shabas D, Gerard G, Rossi D. Magnetic resonance imaging examination of denervated muscle. Comput Radiol 1987;11:9–13.
23. West GA, Haynor DR, Goodkin R et al. Magnetic resonance imaging signal changes in denervated muscles after peripheral nerve injury. Neurosurgery 1994;35: 1077–86.
24. Ferrier R, Padmanabhan V, Hunn A et al. Successful outcome following anastomosis of a severed trochlear nerve in the middle fossa. Aust N Z J Ophthalmol 1992;20:133–6.
25. Samii M, Matthies C. Management of 1000 vestibular schwannomas (acoustic neuromas). The facial nerve: preservation and restitution of function. Neurosurgery 1997;40:684–94.

XI
Functional Neurosurgery

33

Pain

Tom Hollway and Katherine Brosnan

Summary

The management of pain is a complex process. This can be helped by understanding the mechanisms of pain, both neurophysiological and bio-social. When pain occurs in the absence of a diagnosis that would define a specific treatment resulting in cure and relief of the symptoms, then the focus necessarily falls on the pain itself. Management of this may include local treatments, such as nerve blockade, but an equal effort must be directed at the bio-social aspects. This may involve the use of drugs such as anti-depressants, complementary therapies and techniques to improve the sufferer's ability to manage their pain, most clearly demonstrated in the concept of the Pain Management Programme.

Basic Concepts

Definitions and Taxonomy

Pain has been defined by the Subcommittee on Taxonomy of the International Association of the Study of Pain (IASP). The definition is as follows: "An unpleasant sensory and emotional experience associated with actual or potential tissue damage or described in terms of such damage."

Pain is always subjective – a learned experience that, very early on, the individual associates with actual or potential tissue damage. It not only has a pathological component but also a psychological component, the latter becoming more important as the pain becomes more chronic.

Acute pain is relatively short-lived and normally associated with a reversible underlying pathology, for example post-operative pain. Although it may be severe, the likelihood of successful treatment is high, as one is not troubled by the problems of long-term therapy (habituation, attenuation of response, etc.).

Pain becomes chronic when it persists beyond a reasonable length of time after the underlying pathology has healed or recovered. The time quoted varies between different authors, the range being 1–6 months. The pain is unresponsive to common modes of treatment and, as the condition persists, it begins to affect the individual's ability to function, with dramatic effects on family, work and social status. The individuals tend to be withdrawn, suffer from anxiety and depression and, because of fear and reduced mobility, become increasingly dependent on family members and other outside resources, leading to economic as well as psychological stresses in the home and workplace. The patients often no longer have realistic treatment aims and require education, with more emphasis being placed on managing their symptoms and condition in relation to their life than on seeking a cure. The IASP developed a list of pain terms and definitions, which was first published in 1979. These terms arose as a result of agreement between various specialties, including anesthesiology, neurology, neurosurgery, psychiatry and psychology. The following list may prove useful in the further reading of this chapter [1].

Allodynia	is pain due to a stimulus that does not usually provoke pain. Allodynia involves a change in the quality of sensation such that a sensation that is normally non-painful becomes so. The stimulus may be mechanical, e.g. light touch, or thermal.
Analgesia	is the absence of pain in response to stimulation that would normally be painful.
Anesthesia dolorosa	is pain in an area or region that is anesthetic.
Causalgia	is a syndrome of sustained burning pain, allodynia and hyperpathia after a traumatic nerve lesion, often combined with vasomotor and sudomotor dysfunction and later trophic changes.
Central pain	is pain associated with a lesion of the CNS.
Dysesthesia	is an unpleasant abnormal sensation, whether spontaneous or evoked. This definition encompasses allodynia and hyperpathia.
Hyperpathia	is pain characterized by increased reaction to a stimulus, especially a repetitive one.
Hyper/hypoalgesia	is an increased/decreased response to a stimulus that is normally painful.
Neuralgia	is pain in the distribution of a nerve or nerves.
Neuropathy	is a disturbance of function or pathological change in a nerve; in one nerve, mononeuropathy; in several nerves, mononeuropathy multiplex; if diffuse and bilateral, polyneuropathy.
Nociceptor	is a receptor preferentially sensitive to a noxious stimulus or to a stimulus that would become noxious if prolonged.
Paresthesia	is an abnormal sensation, whether spontaneous or evoked. This is different from dysesthesia, as it describes an abnormal sensation that is not unpleasant.

Structure and Function

Pain transmission and perception is not a rigid wiring diagram, as was once thought. It is a system in which peripheral stimulation brings about adaptive changes in neuronal connections and physiology that can be temporary or permanent. Information from the periphery is passed along with other sensory input to make up a whole injury picture. Onward information is affected by inhibiting and facilitating mechanisms before the final situation is perceived and appropriate behavioral responses occur.

Peripheral Pain Perception

When tissue damage occurs in the periphery, then both inflammatory and neuronal responses occur which are intimately linked with the inflammatory process profoundly altering the physical and chemical response of the sensory fibers. Pain is perceived in the periphery by nociceptive nerve endings. Very few nociceptors respond entirely to noxious stimuli, but also respond to other sensory modalities, such as heat. Pain impulses are carried by the slowly conducting unmyelinated C fibers and the relatively faster-conducting, lightly myelinated A-delta fibers; classification of fibers is shown in Table 33.1.

The information about tissue damage, however, is not only conveyed by nerve impulses in sensory fibers, but also by the slow transport of chemicals along axons, e.g. neurotrophins to dorsal root ganglion cells. The unmyelinated C fibers are particularly involved with this type of transmission, responding to chemicals, which then change the metabolism and chemistry of the cell cytoplasm and membrane.

Inflammatory Mediators

The algogenic or pain-producing substances include H+, K+, prostaglandins and leukotrienes in tissues, bradykinin in plasma and substance P in nerve terminals. These chemicals profoundly alter the physical and chemical

Table 33.1. Nerve fiber types and conduction velocities.

Fiber type	Function	Conduction velocity (m/s)	Myelin sheath
Aα	Proprioception, somatic motor	70–120	Yes
Aβ	Touch, pressure	30–70	Yes
Aγ	Motor to muscle spindles	15–30	Yes
Aδ	Pain, cold, touch	12–30	Yes
B	Pre-ganglionic autonomic	3–15	Yes
C dorsal root	Pain, temperature, autonomic reflexes, some mechanoreceptors	0.5–2	No
C sympathetic	Post-ganglionic sympathetic	0.7–2.3	No

stimuli to which sensory fibers normally respond. They cause their effects by changing membrane ion channel function or by receptor-coupled second messenger cascades.

Substance P

Substance P is a polypeptide found in primary neurones and their terminals, as well as in parts of the gastrointestinal tract and CNS. In the periphery, it increases the response of cells activated by noxious cutaneous stimuli, contributing to hyperalgesia. Centrally, it stimulates second-order neurones in the dorsal horn.

Nerve Growth Factor

Nerve growth factor (NGF) is a member of a small family of secretory proteins called neurotrophins and is present in many tissues of the body. NGF is necessary for the survival of sympathetic and small-diameter sensory neurones. NGF concentration is increased by inflammatory conditions and may produce hyperalgesia by both peripheral and central effects. It is also thought that NGF may have a different role in chronic pain resulting from cell death or atrophy, e.g. post-herpetic neuralgia. At an early stage of injury, NGF can form part of an adaptive response. If, however, neurotrophic support to fibers starts to diminish, then the adaptive response is lessened and this may contribute to the development of chronic pain.

Central Pain Modulation

The Dorsal Horn

Sensory neurones enter the spinal cord via the dorsal spinal roots and synapse with cells in the gray matter of the dorsal horn. The gray matter is divided into ten layers, or laminae, some of which are involved in pain transmission. In particular, polymodal C-fibers enter into laminae I, II and V, with A-fibers entering into laminae I, II, V and X. The laminae have direct inputs from the periphery and also connections with other laminae; thus, information is not only received in the dorsal horns, but is also subject to a degree of modulation before onward transmission. Neurotransmitters within the dorsal horn include the excitatory amino acids glutamate and aspartate, acting via N-methyl-d-aspartate (NMDA) channels, substance P and calcitonin gene-related peptide (CGRP). These substances not only stimulate second-order neurones, but also increase the response of cells to noxious peripheral stimuli.

Ascending Pathways

Information is conveyed to the brain by the primary nociceptive pathways, consisting of the spinomesencephalic tract, the spinothalamic tract and the spinoreticular tract.

The lateral system consists of the lateral spinothalamic tract. It consists of long, myelinated axons that are rapidly conducting. There is a discrete somatic organization within these pathways, allowing information on the precise location of the stimulus, as well as intensity and duration of injury. The pathway relays in the thalamic nuclei before projecting onto the sensory cortex.

The medial system consists of the medial spinothalamic tract, the spinoreticular tract and the spinomesencephalic tract. These tracts contain both long and short fibers, are multisynaptic and relatively slow to conduct. The system lacks organization and is thought to be responsible for the diffuse, persistent quality of pain. The system relays in the reticular formation, peri-aqueductal gray matter, hypothalamus, medial and intra-laminar thalamic nuclei, before projecting to the limbic forebrain. Part of the tract originating from the substantia gelatinosa (also known as Lissauer's tract) becomes continuous with the spinal tract of the trigeminal nerve before reaching the thalamic nuclei.

Supraspinal Control

Transmission from the dorsal horn is not only modulated by activity in the same and other segments, but also by descending tracts from the brain and brainstem.

Descending pathways originate in the cortical and diencephalic system, the peri-aqueductal gray matter, raphe nuclei and locus ceruleus and medullary dorsal horn. Descending control of pain involves, among other substances, 5-hydroxytryptamine (5HT), noradrenaline (NA), γ-amino-butyric acid (GABA) and opioids.

5HT pathways arise in the raphe nuclei and other nuclei in the pons and medulla, terminating in laminae I, II, IV and V. Depletion of 5HT from these neurones blocks the action of systemic opiates. Noradrenergic pathways descend from the locus ceruleus and other brainstem sites to laminae I, II, IV, VI and X. Both pathways act by inhibiting nociceptor neurones and interneurones in the dorsal horns.

Naturally occurring opioids (enkephalins, dynorphins and β-endorphins) can be found at both spinal and supraspinal levels, causing modulation of both ascending and descending pathways. The mechanism of action is not clear, but may be by effects on the descending noradrenergic and serotinergic pathways or by inhibiting release of primary afferent neurotransmitters in the spinal cord [2,3].

Chronic Pain Development

As already stated, many physical and chemical changes occur within sensory fibers following tissue injury, e.g. new protein expression for ion channels and enzyme induction. Noxious stimulation is also followed by a rapid change in gene expression within the dorsal horn neurones. *c-fos* is an inducible gene controlling the expression of other genes, the products of which can form the substrate for long-term changes in neuronal excitability. Another factor that is thought to be responsible for the development of chronic neuropathic pain following injury is the NMDA receptor. Repeated C-fiber activity causes NMDA receptor activation, resulting in massive depolarization of the cell, with amplification and prolongation of response. These two things, together with ongoing abnormal peripheral input, may well contribute to the development of chronic pain.

Therapeutic Aspects

In cases of acute or post-operative pain, the site, intensity and character of pain will be clear. Management will involve removing the cause, if possible, e.g. by stabilizing a fracture, and administration of an appropriate analgesic regime. In this situation, the underlying condition is not expected to persist; thus, little consideration need be given to long-term effects, such as habituation, drug dependency, etc. The regime can include conventional oral and parenteral analgesia, as well as targeted regional techniques. It is beyond the scope of this article to identify all drugs and techniques but it is wise to become familiar with a limited number of agents and techniques from each class.

Patients with a longstanding painful condition will show a greater range of problems – physical, psychological and social. All aspects need to be considered, even if it may not be possible or appropriate to answer them all.

Conventional Analgesics

Conventional analgesics play an important role in the management of pain, both acute and chronic, although they may not be the mainstay of treatment. As patients suffering from chronic pain are likely to be taking the prescribed drugs for months or years, some important factors must be considered before selecting the drug and its mode of delivery.

These include the degree of potency required from the analgesic, tendency to drug dependency, patient compliance and side effects. It is sensible to start with the less potent agents and work up the "analgesic ladder", as required. It is a general rule of thumb that side effects increase with increasing potency. Drug dependency can become a problem in patients with longstanding pain and care should be exercised in prescribing potent narcotic analgesics, although they are by no means contra-indicated. The type of analgesia required will determine the first-choice drug, e.g. inflammatory pain may be more likely to respond to a non-steroidal analgesic. Patient compliance can be improved by the use of sustained-release preparations, and knowledge of side effects can help sustain compliance by allowing the patient to evaluate better the gains and losses from any therapeutic regime.

Non-steroidal Anti-inflammatory Drugs (NSAIDs)

There are many drugs within this group. They have an analgesic effect, produced peripherally by reduction in the effect of inflammatory mediators, such as bradykinin, histamine, serotonin and substance P, the mechanism for this being an inhibition of prostaglandin synthesis. Central analgesic effects are present, again mediated by inhibition of prostaglandin (PG) synthesis, PG being capable of enhancing the action of excitatory neurotransmitters, leading to pain perception. However, their efficacy is limited by their side effects, which include gastrointestinal (GI) toxicity, ranging from mild epigastric discomfort to GI hemorrhage, renal toxicity, precipitation of bronchospasm and platelet dysfunction. Recently, new nonsteroidals, e.g. rofecoxib, which selectively inhibit the inducible form of cyclooxygenase COX-2, while avoiding COX-1, which is essential for maintaining gastric mucosal protection and renal blood flow, have been introduced. Their place in therapy has yet to be fully evaluated, with cost being an important factor. Their benefit will be most apparent if used in patients at higher risk of GI side effects, such as the elderly, female group.

NSAIDs are available as sustained-release preparations and may be administered orally, rectally or transdermally. They have been classified on the basis of chemical structure (salicylates - *aspirin*, pyrazoles - *phenylbutazone*, indenes - *indomethacin*, proprionic acids - *ibuprofen*, fenamates - *mefenamic acid*, oxicams - *piroxicam*, acetic acids - *diclofenac*), although this gives little help in drug selection for a particular patient. The individual practitioner should develop a shortlist of those drugs with which he/she is wholly familiar as to dose schedules, side effects and contra-indications and confine prescribing to this list.

Paracetamol has no obvious anti-inflammatory effect, yet appears to have both central and peripheral analgesic effects, the mechanism of action being unclear. It is a useful drug, as its low incidence of side effects gives good compliance. Hepatotoxicity is a rare and potentially fatal result of overdose. Paracetamol is often combined with an opiate to reduce the dose, and thus side effects, of the latter drug [4].

Opioids

The opioids can be classified by potency - strong, e.g. *morphine*, or weak, e.g. *codeine*. They may also be described in terms of their receptor affinity. There are three opioid receptor sites $-\mu$, κ and δ. μ site agonists include *morphine* and *fentanyl*.

Buprenorphine acts at the μ receptor as a partial agonist, i.e. a drug that binds with the receptor but activates it at a level below maximal. *Pentazocine* is a partial agonist at the κ receptor, whilst, at the same time, is a partial antagonist at the μ receptor. This combination is known as a mixed agonist–antagonist. *Naloxone* is an antagonist at all three receptor sites. *Tramadol* binds weakly to the μ receptor, at which it is an agonist; however, at least a part of its analgesic effect is probably modulated through 5HT-mediated pathways.

It is conventional to start with opioids of low potency and work up the analgesic ladder, as needed. Combining opioids with NSAIDs is a useful method of reducing opioid requirements.

Morphine is normally administered orally; it is well absorbed and effective systemic levels can normally be achieved. It is not common to require parenteral routes of administration, unless swallowing is difficult or vomiting is frequent. Where pain is constant, then administration should be regular rather than on a "wait for pain" basis. Morphine is available as a sustained-release preparation, which some patients find useful in reducing the variability of effect that occurs over time with shorter-acting preparations and also overnight. It can be helpful to use additional doses of shorter-acting opiate drugs, e.g. Sevredol, to cover breakthrough pains. These can be prescribed on an as-required basis.

Side effects are common with opiate analgesic drugs. Sedation, inattention, respiratory depression are all loosely dose related, while dysphoric effects are idiosyncratic. Respiratory depression is associated with doses in excess of those required to control pain; it does not occur when ineffective doses are used. Fear of respiratory depression is not a reason to withhold opiate therapy. The degree of effectiveness of analgesia diminishes with time (habituation). Gastrointestinal effects are, largely, secondary to reduced peristalsis and are manifested by gastric fullness, lack of appetite and constipation. These effects can be reduced by the use of appropriate drugs, e.g. metoclopramide, laxatives and stool softeners [5].

Co-analgesics

Many patients with chronic pain do not respond or respond inadequately to conventional analgesia, but do gain relief from the following groups of drugs, either alone or in combination with conventional analgesics.

Anti-depressants

Tricyclics, e.g. *amitriptyline and imipramine.*

Newer anti-depressants, e.g. *fluoxetine.*

Monoamine oxidase inhibitors (MAOIs), e.g. *phenelzine.*

These drugs act by altering the activity of monoamines at a synaptic level. Tricyclics prevent the uptake of NA and serotonin, whereas the MAOIs prevent their breakdown. The newer anti-depressants are selective serotonin uptake inhibitors. Of all the antidepressants, most experience has come from using *amitriptyline*, which has been shown to be of benefit in certain chronic pain syndromes, e.g. post-herpetic neuralgia, and anecdotal evidence supports its more widespread use in this field. Although the newer agents are being used, less is known about their clinical effect. Much smaller doses are used to treat chronic pain than those needed to treat depressive illness. It is common practise to start at the smallest dose, e.g. amitriptyline 10 mg nocte, and increase slowly, by for example 10 mg every 3 days, until a useful effect has been achieved. It is rarely necessary or desirable to exceed 75 mg daily. The whole dose can be given at night, which fits well with many sufferers from chronic pain conditions who frequently have a marked sleep disturbance. Side effects can be a problem, with the most common complaint being that of a dry mouth. Other problems include daytime drowsiness, constipation, worsening prostatism and orthostatic hypotension. Patients should also be advised not to stop taking the drugs abruptly, as withdrawal symptoms can occur [6].

Anticonvulsants

A number of anticonvulsants have been used to treat painful conditions: *phenytoin*, *carbamazepine*, *sodium valproate*, *lamotrigine* and *gabapentin.*

The method of action is unique to each drug, but includes membrane stabilization, interference with ion conduction and enhancement of GABA activity. Anticonvulsants have traditionally been used for pain of a lancinating or stabbing nature, hence their well established use in trigeminal neuralgia. If one drug is unsuccessful or side effects are intolerable, it is worth trying a different anticonvulsant before dismissing this group of drugs. As with the antidepressant drugs, starting dose should be low, with incremental increases. It may be necessary to monitor plasma levels in some cases. Side effects of the drugs vary, but it is prudent to warn patients of the potentially fatal hematological problems that can occur [7].

Major Tranquilizers

This group of drugs includes the phenothiazines (e.g. *chlorpromazine*) and the butyrophenones (e.g. *haloperidol*). Their method of action is by dopaminergic blockade. They are useful in the treatment of painful diabetic neuropathy, but are otherwise used as an adjuvant to other drugs, e.g. anti-depressants. These compounds can cause extrapyramidal reactions and drug-induced parkinsonism, as well as anti-cholinergic side effects.

Others

Increased muscle tone is associated with pain in certain chronic pain syndromes, e.g. prolapsed intervertebral disc. Muscle relaxants such as *baclofen* may prove useful, although objective evidence is lacking.

Anxiolytics, e.g. benzodiazepines, have a role in promoting sleep and alleviating anxiety, but they have limited use in long-term treatment and may lead to dependence in some patients.

Capsaicin is a naturally occurring alkaloid obtained from the chilli pepper. When applied to the skin, it causes excitation of C-fibers, with release of substance P and other neuropeptides, e.g. CRGP. Initially, it causes burning on application to the skin but, after repeated use, nerve endings become reversibly depleted of substance P and this effect lessens. The burning may be reduced by prior application of anesthetic creams (*EMLA cream or Ametop*). Capsaicin is produced as a 0.025 or 0.075% cream, which is applied to the skin 3–4 times daily. It has been reported to be helpful in the pain associated with post-herpetic neuralgia and diabetic neuropathy.

New Drugs

Potential treatment targets for the future include NMDA antagonists such as *ketamine* and derivatives, neurokinin receptor antagonists or α_2-receptor agonists such as *clonidine*.

Transcutaneous Electrical Nerve Stimulation (TENS)

TENS consists of a pulse generator or stimulator attached to the patient via Aβ-fibers to modulate onward pain transmission in the spinal cord. The pulse generator has controls for frequency (2–250 Hz), pulse width and for selecting the type of TENS required.

The main variants of TENS are:

Continuous. This is a continuous high-frequency/low-intensity stimulation. Patients should experience a strong but comfortable sensation, akin to non-painful paresthesiae in the affected area.

Pulsed. This results in stimulation as above, with the stimulus coming in bursts.

Acupuncture-like. This is low-frequency/high-intensity TENS. Patients should experience muscle twitching when utilizing this mode.

Most devices allow modification of the above modes by varying the amplitude and pulse-width. There is no correct setting for TENS. Patients should receive initial instruction on how to use the unit, before experimenting at home with pad position, type and intensity of stimulation. It is important that the machine is worn for at least an hour for benefit to occur and can be worn throughout the day. Side effects are few, allergy to the electrodes being the commonest. The effect tends to wane with time but, if a useful benefit is maintained to 3 months or so, long-term benefit is likely.

TENS should not be given to patients with pacemakers (unless a cardiologist is consulted), pregnant women (unless in labor) or to patients who have difficulty understanding the machine. Patients may experience minor skin irritation from the pads and burns have been reported.

There are no clear indications for this therapy. For every series purporting to show benefit, one can find one showing no effect.

Alternative Therapies

Acupuncture (AP) is a form of traditional Chinese medicine, which uses fine needles to stimulate AP points that lie on specific lines or meridians. Once placed, a small electric current can be used to stimulate the points through the needle or the needle may be twitched or oscillated by hand.

Signals from AP needles probably enter the spinal cord through Aβ-fibers, causing inhibition of onward transmission of painful stimuli at both a spinal and central level, via descending pathways and central endorphin release. Conditions said to respond well to AP include osteoarthritis and headaches [8].

The list of alternative therapies grows each year; osteopathy and chiropractic have long held a place in the management of musculoskeletal disorders. In recent years, homeopathy, reflexology, aromatherapy and others have all claimed their place in the sun in the field of chronic disease.

Pain Management Programs

These programs have been developed to rehabilitate chronic pain sufferers, and are run by a team consisting of physicians, physiotherapists, occupational therapists, specialized nurses and clinical psychologists.

Programs consist of a number of aspects. Physical activity is designed to increase stamina and range of function. Education about the patient's condition will help in the realization of what is possible and help to defer fears about the significance of the pain ("When it hurts am I damaging myself?"). Psychological approaches include help in confidence building, relaxation techniques and coping strategies for pain. Goals are agreed for each aspect with the patient, these goals being set in a co-ordinated way by the therapists running the program.

Careful selection of patients for these programs is important. Before acceptance, the patient will undergo a medical interview, as well as a psychological assessment. Patients also require a level of mobility to match the others in the group. Part of the success of pain programs is the group experience, so careful selection is essential, otherwise a disruptive patient will unsettle the whole group.

Patients who are most likely to benefit from the programs are those who refrain from any other form of treatment while participating in the program. Success is unlikely if the patients lack motivation, have unrealistic aims or are seeking a cure or second opinion.

The programs normally require attendance every day over several weeks, with some being residential. Support days are usually arranged in the months following programs in order to provide ongoing encouragement and reinforce learned techniques. The involvement of the workplace is useful [9,10].

Peripheral Nerve Blockade

Peripheral nerve blocks are used frequently in the management of the chronic pain patient with varying success. Nerve blocks may be used as a diagnostic tool, but can be employed to provide symptomatic relief on a temporary or more permanent basis. Injection of local anesthetic around a nerve can often provide relief in chronic pain patients that is beyond the normal expected duration of the blockade. The blocks may be repeated over the course of weeks or months. If good results are obtained, more destructive methods can be used to provide more lasting results. However, a good result with local anesthetic does not always mean a successful block by more permanent means.

Neurolytic Solutions

Phenol and absolute alcohol are both used to provide more permanent neural blockade. Phenol is available as a 5–6% solution in water, as a hyperbaric solution of 5–10% in glycerol, or of 5–10% in non-ionic X-ray contrast medium. It causes temporary nerve degeneration by coagulating proteins in the nerve sheath. It is used for lumbar sympathectomy, para-vertebral and peripheral nerve blocks and for epidural and intrathecal blocks. Phenol is toxic at high doses, with hepatic and cardiac complications. It can cause painful neuralgias, well described in the ileo-inguinal neuralgia that may follow lumbar sympathetic blockade. Absolute alcohol produces a more lasting block than phenol by causing axonal degeneration. It is associated with a higher incidence of neuralgia. Alcohol is used for celiac plexus blocks (50% alcohol), cranial neural blockade (trigeminal nerve and branches) and intrathecal neurolysis. Absolute alcohol is hypobaric with respect to CSF and thus is useful for intrathecal neurolysis at the thoracic level.

Radio Frequency Lesioning

Radio frequency (RF) lesioning uses heat to destroy nervous tissue. The nerve to be lesioned is identified using appropriate surface markings and radiological guidance. The RF needle is placed at the appropriate site. The RF generator has modes that allow testing of temperature, impedance and response to physiological stimuli to be undertaken. Confirmation of position of the needle tip is done by stimulating at tetanic rates (about 50 Hz) and at low twitch rates (about 2 Hz). The higher rates give good appreciation of the spread of the paresthesiae, which should be in the same distribution of the target nerve, whilst the lower rates give visual evidence of motor nerve involvement. When correct placement is shown, by appropriate paresthesiae at low voltage (e.g. less than 0.5 V for trigeminal lesioning), a radiofrequency current (of 300 kHz) is then passed through the thermocouple probe for 60 seconds at a power to raise the tip temperature, as measured by thermocouple or thermistor, to 60–80°C, depending upon the nerve to be treated. Repeat lesions may be required, depending on the outcome of post-lesion re-testing. Radiofrequency lesioning is used for facet joint denervation, ganglion blockade and blockade of spinal dorsal roots [11].

Cryotherapy

Cryotherapy produces axonal degeneration (Wallerian) that is not permanent. Regeneration usually occurs. The cryoprobe consists of two tubes, one inside the other. CO_2 or N_2O is passed under pressure through the outer tube, which has a tapered end. As the gas emerges from the tapered end, it expands, causing a drop in temperature and an ice ball to form on the end of the probe. This temperature drop (to about -60°C) causes freezing of the immediate surrounding tissues. Nerves to be blocked are again identified using surface markings with the aid of an image intensifier, if appropriate. Stimulation of the nerve can also be used but is not always possible. Each nerve is then subjected to a period of freezing, followed by a defrost period of 1 minute and then another freezing period. These periods vary from 1 to a few minutes, depending upon the vascularity (and thus degree of heat sink) of the area targeted. Cryotherapy is used for facet joint denervation, intercostal, occipital, ileoinguinal, genitofemoral and peripheral trigeminal nerve blockade. The crucial requirement is the ability to place the probe within 1–2 mm of the nerve as the temperature gradient within the ice ball is of the order of 10°C/mm. Temperatures to cause a lesion need to be below -20°C to -30°C.

Spinal Cord Stimulation

This technique involves the placing of one or more electrodes in the epidural space, percutaneously or at open surgery. Stimulation of the electrode(s) with varying electrical current in the frequency range 20–200 Hz produces analgesia in the area where the stimulus is appreciated. The mode of action remains obscure, despite four decades of research.

Indications for this treatment are unclear but current opinion would support its use in the following conditions - deafferentation syndromes, chronic regional pain syndrome (CRPS), arachnoiditis, failed back surgery, radicular pain and vascular disease (peripheral and angina).

There are no randomized controlled trials (RCTs) to support its use, not least because it is impossible to blind patient and operator as to the treatment. The technique is expensive and is therefore used erratically, depending upon the sources of healthcare funding. At various consensus meetings for its use in conditions such as angina pectoris, it has been placed low in the list, often coming to represent a last resort. It is said to be relatively free from major deleterious side effects, but most series report significant incidences of complications, largely related to electrode positioning, movement and breakage. The patients are thus often continuingly dependent on the implanting physician for aftercare.

Patient selection for these treatments has proved difficult, with psychological assessment being said to be important but with little objective evidence for the benefit of this.

The technique involves the placement of a trial electrode percutaneously, such that the electrode tip is at or near the appropriate dermatomal level. Trial stimulation allows manipulation of the electrode to obtain ideal placement. In many centers, the trial electrode is then connected to an external pulse generator to allow prolonged testing (in some series up to 2 weeks) of effect. If benefit by a previously agreed yardstick with the patient is obtained, then permanent implantation is undertaken by fashioning a subcutaneous pocket, usually on the abdominal wall, for the pulse generator. The electrode is connected by tunnelling the catheter from the spine. Firm anchoring of the catheter is important, as movement is a common cause of failure. The electrode can also be placed on and stitched to the dura under general anesthesia and mini-laminectomy, but this is more prone to inaccurate siting of the electrode.

Various electrodes are available that are able to cover differing amounts of the spinal cord. Multi-electrode devices allow for fine tuning post-implant and will, to a certain extent, compensate for some movement post-procedure.

The devices are battery powered and have, therefore, a limited life, depending on usage, power settings, etc. The modern devices allow the patient some freedom to alter stimulation parameters and turn the device on and off [12].

Implantable Drug Delivery Systems

With the improvements in implantable materials and the miniaturization of computing systems, it has become a realistic possibility to implant devices for the continuous or intermittent injection of drugs into the CSF. The technology is ahead of the pharmacology. Implantable drug delivery systems for intrathecal baclofen administration in the field of spasticity management are common, if not quite routine. The technology works, catheter complications are at an acceptable level (approximately 10%) and good studies exist for efficacy, cost benefit and patient satisfaction. The same level of information does not exist for the use of these systems in pain, despite a longer history of use.

Patient selection is not clear; consensus suggests that this is an end-of-the-line treatment, to be used when all else fails. Naturally, the list of underlying conditions for which this has been used is long and covers the full range of patients seen in a chronic pain service.

The patients can be categorized into two groups: pain secondary to malignant disease and the non-malignant pain group.

With pain due to *malignant disease*, relatively simple intraspinal techniques may suffice, as they are unlikely to be required in the long term; epidural infusions of opiate with or without local anesthetic are popular and effective in well chosen patients. The potential problems of long-term intraspinal drug administration need not be addressed.

In the case of *chronic non-malignant pain*, the long-term issues of neurotoxicity, dependence and the ever present possibility of intrathecal infection are real. The numbers of reported patients are not yet large enough for us to pronounce on these with any certainty. Patients need to be aware of the experimental nature of the therapy and it must be doubtful if any treatment on these lines should be undertaken outside of a clinical trial setting. The very minimum assessment should include psychiatric and psychological evaluation. Trials of efficacy of single-dose opiate (or other chosen drug) should be undertaken, possibly even including placebo administration. If all trials are positive, then implantation of continuous drug delivery systems is a simple task; attention to detail is important, especially concerning catheter fixation, as movement or "plumbing" problems dominate the complication list.

There is a tendency for dose requirements of opiates to rise with time and, if other drugs are included in the mixture (e.g. clonidine), then it may require complete emptying of the reservoir to enable dose changes to be made, thus losing some of the elegant advantages of the implantable computerized systems (*Synchromed*) available from Medtronics (Minneapolis/St Paul)[13–15].

Some Conditions of Special Interest to Neurosurgery

Back Pain

It is well known that back pain is one of the largest causes of time absent from work, resulting in loss of revenue from industry, as well as increased work load for general practitioners, hospital doctors, physiotherapists and other supporting staff. Back pain can be classified into acute (of less than 6 weeks' duration), sub-acute (of between 6 and 12 weeks' duration) and chronic (of greater than 12 weeks' duration). Pain practitioners tend not to be involved in the care of acute back pain, which is generally managed by patient education, physical rehabilitation with early return to normal activity, manipulation and simple analgesia. Most referrals to the pain clinic are for the management of mechanical or degenerative problems and are from general practitioners, orthopedic and neurosurgeons and rheumatologists, with the patients having generally been thoroughly examined and investigated. This section will outline the pain clinic management of non-specific mechanical back pain, as well as discuss in slightly greater detail the management of facet joint pain and radicular pain.

Assessment

General evaluation of the patients includes time of onset, precipitating events, type of pain, site and radiation, aggravating and relieving conditions and associated symptoms, e.g. weakness, paresthesiae, etc. It is also important to establish the effect of the pain on the patient's social life and work, treatments already tried, as well as any ongoing litigation. The available special investigations (MRI, CT scan, etc.) should be reviewed. The diagnosis is rarely definite, the imaging results and clinical symptoms and signs may not be in harmony and psychological disorders may be apparent. In this situation, the resort to focused invasive procedures may be ineffective at best, positively harmful at worst. The practitioner must be aware of the pressure from patient and colleagues to "do something, anything must be better than this". Good evidence for benefit is lacking for most invasive procedures in the management of back pain.

This assessment will normally allow the patient to be placed into one of three loose diagnostic categories: back pain with evidence of nerve root induced sciatica, mechanical back pain from posterior spinal structures (e.g. facet joint syndrome) or non-specific back pain not referable to any particular anatomical structure.

Non-specific Back Pain

In many pain relief clinics, this represents a high proportion of referrals. The clinical picture is necessarily varied. The history may be short (months) but, more commonly, the story can be traced back some years. Frequently, an initial injury or working practice is remembered, but the connection with the present state appears weak. The initial injury or degenerative changes have led to a cycle involving limitation of movement, resulting in decreased muscle usage, reduced joint mobility and abnormal posturing.

Patients complain of discomfort across the lower back, usually in an L3–S1 distribution with associated buttock and lateral back pain. The pain may radiate into the legs and be associated with non-specific paresthesiae. The relationship with exercise, rest and posture is varied. Some will complain that any movement is painful and they may, in extreme cases, take to a wheelchair, whilst, at the other end of the spectrum, continual gentle movement is reported as beneficial, leading to a lifetime of fidgeting and moving to "get comfortable". There is usually a long history of analgesic use, partially effective at best. Most patients will have undergone outpatient physiotherapy and many will have attended alternative practitioners (chiropractic, osteopathy, acupuncture, etc.). Treatments will frequently be described as effective, but only in the short term, or becoming less effective over the years.

Physical findings are non-specific, with no demonstrable neurologic deficit or signs of nerve root irritation.

Management

The aim of treatment is to reduce the amount of pain to a level at which function can be improved and a normal lifestyle (social and work) resumed. If the pain is of relatively recent onset, simple analgesics should be prescribed (NSAIDs) and narcotic analgesics avoided. For more persistent symptoms, physical therapy should be included, activity encouraged and bed rest, which may be harmful if prolonged, should be avoided. Early return to work should be advised, if at all possible. The objective evidence for this approach is lacking, save for analgesic/NSAID use; however, it represents a consensus view, with similar guidelines appearing across the Western world.

For the more chronic sufferers, short-term measures are unlikely to produce benefit. Analgesic drugs are often reported to be ineffective. Simple physiotherapy is avoided, as "it makes the pain worse". Where do we go from here? The last two decades have seen the widespread introduction of multidisciplinary pain management programs targeted at this group of patients. There is good evidence for benefit from this approach. It is, or can be, expensive and, at present, is therefore available to a small percentage of the problem patients.

Other treatments – TENS, acupuncture, chiropractic, etc. – may be tried, with benefit in some. There is no known way of predicting success and no objective RCT evidence of benefit. Where there is little danger of inflicting harm, it may be reasonable to try these techniques.

Although many patients will be using analgesic drugs, they probably are of little benefit, apart from in managing acute or chronic exacerbations. Amitriptyline or other tricyclic drugs may have a role at night in patients who are experiencing sleep difficulties because of pain.

Specific interventional treatments – trigger-point injections, sacroiliac injections, nerve-root injections, facet-joint injections, lumbar and caudal epidurals – should be avoided, as there is no sustainable evidence for benefit [9,10].

Mechanical Low Back Pain Related to Facet Joints

Whether there is a true facet joint syndrome is unclear. It does, however, figure as a common diagnostic entity amongst medical practitioners, physiotherapists, osteopaths and chiropractors. Patients complain of low back pain, which may be referred to the thigh. There is usually increased pain with lumbar hyperextension and lateral flexion and there may be tenderness over the joints themselves, with limited straight-leg raising. Pain may be referred to the leg but not usually below the knee. Radiological investigations are not particularly helpful, degenerative change being common in the population as a whole and not necessarily related to pain.

The facet joints protect the intervertebral discs from excessive shear and axial rotation, but, with increasing age, the discs lose height and the facet joints may take on more of the compressive load, thus leading to pain. Facet joints are innervated by the medial and intermediate branch of the dorsal primary ramus at a segmental level and also from the medial branch of the dorsal primary ramus from the level above.

General management of "facet joint pain" is the same as for non-specific back pain. Many practitioners will offer injections or denervation of these joints as well.

Facet Joint Injections

Facet joints may be injected blindly but it is more usual to inject with the help of X-ray imaging. The patient is placed prone on the X-ray table and, using an image intensifier, the patient is rotated, with the side to be blocked uppermost, until the posterior portion of the facet joint is visible. The degree of rotation varies between patients (0–45°) and tends to increase as one descends down the spine. With appropriate local anesthesia and sedation (required in a few patients), a 22-gauge needle can be passed in the line of the X-ray beam into the joint. Placement can be confirmed by injecting small quantities (0.1–0.5 ml) of X-ray contrast medium. The joint can then be filled with local anesthetic, depo-steroid or both; volumes should not normally exceed 1 ml or so. The patient may report pain similar to his/her normal pain on injection; this may be a useful pointer to a facet joint pain syndrome. After the procedure, the patient is re-examined to assess effect, then allowed to go home and report at a later date the efficacy or otherwise of the injection(s). If beneficial, it is worth instituting an exercise regime to try to build on the gains from the procedure. In the event of good-quality but short-term relief being obtained, consideration should be given to a destructive lesion of the nerves supplying the appropriate joints.

In some patients, many months of relief may be obtained from the anesthetic/deposteroid injections themselves; in these cases, it is probably simpler to repeat the injections occasionally, as required.

Facet Denervation

Facet joints may be denervated using cryotherapy or radiofrequency lesioning to destroy the medial branch of the posterior primary ramus. The medial branch of the posterior primary ramus crosses the transverse process in a groove and supplies the joint both at the level of the joint itself and the level below. The nerves are blocked at the superior edge of the transverse (the eye of the Scottie dog) process using X-ray control. Stimulation is used to confirm correct probe placement before lesioning takes place; pain or strong paresthesiae in the correct segmental level can be elicited at 0.5 V with a frequency of 50–100 Hz. Absence of motor response in the leg should then be confirmed by ensuring that no twitching is elicited at a frequency of 2 Hz and a voltage of less than 1 V. There is no difference in success rates between the cryogenic or RF techniques, but neither should be tried until local anesthetic blockade of the facet joints has shown successful pain relief [11,16].

Lumbar Disc Disease

Lumbar disc disease is another frequently encountered problem in the pain clinic. Patients with prolapsed discs often recall a specific event precipitating the onset of the pain. The pain is exacerbated by standing and increases in abdominal pressure, whilst it may be relieved by lying flat. It may radiate into the leg in a dermatomal distribution and, if significant nerve root compression is present, this may well be the dominant complaint. Sensory, motor and reflex changes may also accompany the pain. Straight-leg raising may produce radicular pain when the leg is raised to greater than 40°. Positive crossed straight-leg raising produces pain in the affected side by raising the contralateral side. CT and/or MRI scanning will demonstrate disc prolapse, if present, and the presence or absence of nerve compression. The patients can be divided into two groups – those with symptoms, signs and radiological evidence of nerve compression at one (occasionally more) level, and those in whom the findings are inconsistent, e.g. symptoms referable to a different disc prolapse than seen radiologically; or those with no radiological lesion.

The management of "disc induced" sciatica follows the standard guidelines for back pain but more focused treatments are available for persistent or severe problems. Discectomy is discussed elsewhere. Epidural steroid injections are widely practiced. It is difficult to establish the number of these procedures performed but, in the UK, the figures will be measured in the tens of thousands annually. There is remarkably little useful literature on the subject, given the numbers performed. There have been a number of reviews of the available information and even these fail to reach consensus. It can be said that although epidural steroid injections give modest help to acute sciatica, long-term benefit is not apparent. What, therefore, is their place? It is reasonable to offer patients with short-term sciatica (of, say, less than 1 year) an epidural that can be repeated once or twice if benefit accrues, but does not last. It is also the authors' practice to offer epidurals to all patients on the waiting list for surgery for decompression of nerve roots (discogenic or spondylotic). Long waiting lists are a particular peculiarity of UK healthcare [17,18].

Lumbar Steroid Epidural Injections

Epidural injection techniques vary widely; there is no evidence in favor of any method over another, provided both are properly practiced. The authors use the lumbar rather than the caudal route, trying to place the steroid–anesthetic mixture as close to the affected level as possible. Once the epidural space is located, the chosen mixture of steroid, with or without local anesthetic, is injected. It is the authors' practice to use 5–10 ml (depending on age, infirmity, etc.) of 0.375% plain bupivacaine plus 80 mg Depomedrone (methylprednisolone). The choice of local anesthetic or saline, methylprednisolone or triamcinolone, volume of injectate and route (caudal or lumbar) is operator dependent. There is no helpful scientific evidence. Neither steroid compound has a license for epidural use in the UK.

Despite the widespread use of epidural steroids, controversy still exists as to their mechanism of action and potential beneficial effects. Possible mechanisms of action include inhibition of phospholipase A2 (phospholipase A2 activity increases in the area of disc herniation, causing release of arachidonic acids from cell membranes, from which inflammatory mediators are then manufactured), blockade of C-fiber transmission, mast cell stabilization and changes in capillary permeability. There are a few contraindications to the procedure, including sepsis close to the injection site, allergy to the planned drugs and bleeding diathesis of whatever cause. Problems that may occur when using epidural steroids include arachnoiditis, if accidental sub-arachnoid injection occurs, and systemic effects – worsening diabetes, Cushing's syndrome and later adrenal suppression if large and repeated doses are used. Menstrual irregularity has been reported. Serious side effects are rare and include infection (the incidence of this is unknown) and reports in the literature are sporadic. Accidental dural puncture, which occurs in 1% of cases, is a nuisance rather than a serious event. Management is bed rest and copious fluids by mouth for 24 hours. Rarely, epidural blood patch will be needed to cope with a persistent CSF leak headache [17,18].

Pain in the Cervical Spine

The principles of management of pain arising from the cervical spine are essentially the same as those described above for the lumbar spine. The increased mobility of this part of the spine and the greater use of paraspinal muscles for stabilization, however, place a greater emphasis on functional treatments in the management of chronic cervical spine pain. Although, theoretically, the approach to nerve root compression and irritation is the same as that for the lumbar spine, the use of invasive therapies such as epidural injections is more limited. This is at least partly because the technique of epidural injection in the cervical spine is more difficult and the potential risks (para- or quadri-paresis, secondary to epidural hemorrhage or infection) are more severe. They may be considered for the treatment of cancer-related cervical spine pain and radicular-type pain. The procedure is carried out using an 18-gauge Tuohy needle and a loss-of-resistance technique to locate the epidural space. Local anesthetic and steroid may be injected. Much smaller volumes of local anesthetic (5 ml or less) than in the lumbar region should be used because of the disastrous consequences of uncontrolled spread. Careful patient observation is required following the procedure, to detect any untoward respiratory, cardiovascular or neurological events. The combination deters all but the enthusiast.

Cervical Facet Joint Injections

Injection of the cervical facets can be a useful tool in the management of patients with degenerative disease. Patients complain of pain radiating to the occiput, shoulder, arm or scapula, depending on the site of pathology, with the pain being exacerbated by rotation and hyperextension. Local anesthetic and steroid can be placed into the joint capsule in a similar fashion to lumbar facet joint injection, under X-ray control from C3 to C7. Careful aspiration is required prior to injection, as the epidural space lies immediately medial to the joint, with the vertebral artery lying lateral. Again, as with lumbar facet joint injections, if good pain relief is obtained following joint injections, consideration should be given to facet joint denervation for more permanent relief. The C3–C4 facet joints to C7–T1 are supplied by the medial branch of the posterior cervical rami, both from the corresponding level and the level above. The C2–C3 facet is supplied by the posterior ramus of C2 and the third occipital nerve from C3.

Cervical facet joint injections are more difficult than in the lumbar spine and, frequently, injections are directed at the nerve supply to the joint at the point where the nerve winds backwards around the lateral mass. Results, as in the lumbar spine, are equivocal but the technique is low-risk and worth trying in those patients with a mechanical pain of a non-radicular nature.

As in the lumbar spine, the use of the multidisciplinary approach to chronic cervical pain has become established, although there is little objective evidence for education-based techniques or muscular relaxation in these patients [19,20].

Trigeminal Neuralgia

Trigeminal neuralgia (TN) is the term used to describe pain in the distribution of the trigeminal nerve, affecting 4 in 100,000 of the population per year.

Clinical Features

The pain is described as an electric shock-like sensation, lasting from a few seconds to several minutes. Patients also experience allodynia in the distribution of the nerve root and, occasionally, aching in between episodes. Attacks are precipitated by innocuous stimuli such as touch, cold, the wind, stress, eating and shaving, typical trigger zones being the angle of the mouth and nasolabial folds, which result in a profound aversion to anything touching the face. The pain can also precipitate facial spasm, hence the term "tic douloureux". Attacks do not occur every day and patients may experience spontaneous remission lasting weeks or years. In 97% of cases, the pain is unilateral, the majority of attacks being in the distribution of the second (maxillary) and third (mandibular) divisions of the trigeminal nerve.

Pathogenesis

The majority of TN (80–90%) is caused by compression of the nerve in the root entry zone by a blood vessel (usually the superior cerebellar artery) or by a space-occupying lesion. Because of the possibility of a space-occupying lesion, patients should have an MRI scan as part of their initial assessment. Patients should also be questioned directly about any episodes of visual disturbance, weakness, sensory and bladder disturbance, as a small percentage of patients have a demyelinating condition as the cause of their neuralgia. It is also important to exclude any dental problems that the patient may have, as dental pain may mimic TN.

Treatment

After assessment, patients should at least initially be treated conservatively with oral medication. Depending on the patient's age, fitness and the underlying cause of the neuralgia, information should be given on, and a discussion undertaken about, the more invasive treatments available.

Carbamazepine is the first-line treatment for TN. The patient should be started on a small dose at night, which is then gradually increased until relief occurs. Relief normally occurs quite quickly, typically at doses below 1000 mg/day. Once relief is obtained, the patient is maintained on that dose, although occasional increases may be necessary to treat breakthrough pain. It may be possible in time to reduce the maintenance dose. If carbamazepine treatment fails or the drug is not tolerated due to side effects or drug reaction, other anticonvulsants should be tried. *Phenytoin* is long established as a second-line therapy but the introduction of *gabapentin* has provided alternatives. *Lamotrigine* is also used and there are reports of pain relief with *baclofen*. The drugs may be used in combination, if required.

In the event of failure with conservative therapies, there is a wide range of reported treatments of varying degrees of invasiveness. There has long been use of peripheral cryoblockade of trigeminal branches, commonly infra-orbital, supra-orbital and supra-trochlear nerves. These techniques may keep the condition under control where peripheral trigger points for the pain are suitably sited.

Gasserian Ganglion Lesions

There are three techniques widely used for trigeminal gangliolysis: gangliolysis with anhydrous glycerol, selective retroGasserian RF lesioning and balloon compression of the ganglion. In recent years, stereotactic radiosurgery to the trigeminal ganglion has been developed. The three percutaneous injection techniques share the same anatomical approach as that described by Sweet. An image intensifier is used to identify the foramen ovale in the supine anesthetized patient. A 20-gauge spinal needle (glycerol gangliolysis), RF cannula (RF lesion) or Fogarty catheter (balloon compression) is inserted approximately 3 cm lateral to the corner of the mouth. The needle is advanced in a cephalad direction towards the base of the skull (taking care not to pierce the buccal mucosa), using the medial border of the pupil as an anterior–posterior guide and a point 2.5 cm anterior to the tragus of the ear as a lateral guide. The needle is then "walked off" into the foramen ovale (the position being confirmed by X-ray).

For *glycerol gangliolysis*, free-flowing CSF is obtained, indicating that the needle now lies within the trigeminal cistern in Meckel's cave. The patient (still anesthetized) is then moved with due care from the supine to the sitting position. Radio opaque dye is injected to outline the bucket shape of Meckel's cave, confirming correct needle placement and also to ascertain the volume of Meckel's cave. Glycerol is then injected according to the volume of the cave. As the glycerol is hyperbaric, the sitting position ensures that the solution is placed at the bottom of the cave, around the maxillary and mandibular branches. Following injection, the patient needs to remain sitting with the head flexed for 1–2 hours following the procedure, to ensure that the solution remains in the correct place.

RF lesioning requires the patient to be conscious, with the needle in Meckel's cave for sensory and motor testing to take place to establish precise positioning of the probe tip. When this has been achieved, anesthesia is reinstituted and lesioning at 60°C for 1 minute takes place. Frequently, flushing of the skin over the lesioned area will be seen. Waking the patient confirms the adequacy or otherwise of the procedure. Repeat lesions may be required at higher temperatures.

Balloon compression requires the passage through the foramen ovale of a Fogarty catheter, which can be inflated with X-ray contrast medium such that a pear-shaped shadow is seen lying in Meckel's cave; compression is maintained for 1 minute.

There are minimal differences between these techniques in terms of outcome; the choice is made with regard to operator experience and training. Some patients find the sleep/wake/sleep routine of an RF lesion too distressing and will opt for the greater comfort of full general anesthesia, available with balloon compression or glycerol injection.

Radiosurgery is totally non-invasive and may represent the future as equipment becomes more widely available.

Problems associated with Gasserian gangliolysis include reduced sensation in the distribution of the nerve roots (trauma to the lips may occur due to inadvertent biting; corneal ulceration may follow ophthalmic division anesthesia), anesthesia dolorosa (the pain, which may be worse than the original pain), infection, hemorrhage, Horner's syndrome and activation of herpes zoster. Success with neurolysis is good (approximately two-thirds of patients experience permanent or long-lasting relief). However, pain may recur at any time, requiring further interventions or medication. Subsequent procedures may be more difficult, especially in those requiring free flow of CSF.

In patients who are relatively fit, microvascular decompression (Janetta's procedure) is used with good results. The procedure involves using sponge to elevate the vessel causing compression of the nerve at the root entry zone. If no vessel is found, then some surgeons will "traumatize" the nerve as a treatment for the pain. Of all the treatments for TN, surgery is associated with the lowest rate of recurrence; however, the main disadvantage is that it involves all the complications associated with posterior fossa surgery [21–23].

Conditions Accompanied by Neuropathic Pain

There is a diverse group of conditions in which pain is described as neuropathic. These are central disorders, such as post-stroke pain, spinal cord damage or disease; more peripheral conditions, such as nerve trauma, phantom limb pain, post-herpetic neuralgia; and even conditions with no known neural insult, such as Sudecks atrophy. The principles of management are broadly the same for all.

Some of these disorders have been gathered together under two categories, known as Complex Regional Pain Syndrome I and II (CRPS I, II). Both types show spontaneous pain, hyperalgesia and/or allodynia in the territory of, and frequently spreading beyond the territory of, a single peripheral nerve. They show or give a history of blood flow changes and trophic changes to skin, nails and/or hair. There may be, or have been, edema. CRPS II (causalgia) follows nerve injury; CRPS I (reflex sympathetic dystrophy) follows any noxious event.

There is, however, no agreement on the cause of each syndrome or the best treatment. Both syndromes consist of neuropathic pain. Following an initiating event, it seems that changes take place in both the somatic and sympathetic nervous systems, consisting of structural changes both peripherally and centrally, alteration in the chemical contents of afferent nerve cells and the development of adrenergic sensitivity.

The pain associated with these syndromes is neuropathic in nature and out of proportion to any injury. It is described as burning in nature and has features of dysesthesia, paraesthesia, mechanical allodynia and hyperalgesia to cold stimuli. The clinical course is divided into three stages.

Stage 1 consists of pain, the affected extremity being either warm or cold, along with accelerated nail and hair growth. The symptoms come on at any time, from hours to weeks after the original injury.

Stage 2 (the dystrophic phase) consists of continuing pain in the affected limb, which is cold and cyanotic. Nails become rigid and brittle and osteoporosis develops. Finally, lack of use of the affected limb leads to Stage 3, the atrophic stage. This consists of continuing pain, muscle wasting, development of contractures and demineralization of bone.

The presence of autonomic changes, typically mimicking an overactive sympathetic state (a cold, sweaty, poorly perfused periphery) in these conditions, has been the catalyst to attempts at reversing the process by the use of sympathetic blockade. Intravenous phentolamine has been used in an attempt to show whether a sympathetic component is present; if pain is relieved, then a sympathetic block (temporary or permanent) is performed [24].

Management of Neuropathic Pain

Management of patients with neuropathic pain follows the usual rules of assessment and treatment of any reversible causes, although these are rarely to be found. First-line drug treatment is with tricyclic antidepressants, commonly *amitriptyline*, starting at a low dose of 10 mg, rising in 10-mg steps to 75 mg nocte. Occasionally, higher doses of up to 150 mg/day may be used in younger patients. The onset of analgesia with these drugs is faster than their antidepressant action (a few days, as opposed to a few weeks). If this is not or only partially successful, then the addition of an anticonvulsant is indicated. *Gabapentin*, starting at 300 mg/day and rising in 300-mg steps to 2,400 mg/day, is the first choice for one of the authors, as its side-effect profile is more benign than that of *carbamazepine*, which represents a sensible second-line therapy. If benefit is only partial, then it is possible to increase the dose yet further to 3,600 mg/day. Other anticonvulsants may be tried, but if two have failed, the third rarely succeeds.

Membrane-stabilizing drugs (lignocaine and mexiletine) have been used. Side effects are common with mexiletine and it probably represents a last-chance therapy. *Lignocaine* is used as a trial drug for *mexiletine*, being given as an infusion for a limited period (hours). Benefit with lignocaine can be followed by oral mexiletine therapy.

Capsaicin can be tried, although the early reports of benefit in diabetic neuropathy have not really been borne out in everyday practice.

TENS and acupuncture may be tried, although there is no objective evidence of benefit.

Analgesic use is controversial with regard to opiates. There has been a feeling that opiate analgesics were ineffective in neuropathic pain and that their use would predispose patients to addiction. These fears, while not groundless, have been overstated and there is evidence from RCTs that, at least in the short term, narcotic analgesics have a place in the management of neuropathic pain. It would seem, therefore, reasonable to try narcotic analgesics for patients with neuropathic pain that has not responded to the more conventional approaches outlined above [2,3,6,7].

Invasive Therapies

Interventional techniques have been used – both somatic and autonomic blockade. Permanent somatic block, where feasible, does not normally produce long-lasting relief and has largely fallen out of favor.

Sympathetic blockade may be achieved paravertebrally or by a simpler, less invasive regional approach. This technique can be used in both the upper and lower limbs (although sedation will be needed for lower-limb blockade, as it can be extremely uncomfortable). The limb is exsanguinated and a double cuff applied, inflated to 100 mmHg above the patient's systolic blood pressure. *Guanethidine* (5–10 mg) mixed with prilocaine is then injected intravenously, with the cuff left inflated for 10–15 minutes. Guanethidine depletes the sympathetic nerve endings of noradrenaline, the local anesthetic being added to provide pain relief during the procedure, as it can be very uncomfortable. Other drugs used include *ketanserin* and *bretylium*.

The sympathetic supply to the upper limb can easily be blocked by injection of local anesthetic around the stellate ganglion lying on the transverse process of C6. The sympathetic supply to the lower limbs can be blocked, either by an epidural or by a lumbar sympathetic block. The sympathetic supply to legs and lower gut lies on the lateral aspects of the bodies of L2–L4. Using X-ray control and contrast, needles can be accurately placed in order to inject either local anesthetic or neurolytic solutions (although caution should prevail before injecting neurolytic solutions in younger patients because of the incidence of genitofemoral neuralgia). Sympathetic blockade should be accompanied by active physiotherapy to increase function within the affected limb.

There is no one, single, proven successful treatment of CRPS and, indeed, there is a group of patients in which treatment will never be successful. It is also worth remembering that the longer the condition is left untreated, the more difficult it becomes to treat, as disuse leads to further pain and the development of a more permanent disability. The majority of patients can expect to be incapacitated for 12–18 months before return to normal function occurs.

Key Points

- *Pain is a symptom with both neuro-physiological and bio-social causes.*
- *Never ignore the secondary impact of mood changes.*
- *The characteristics of the pain, e.g. allodynia, may lead to more specific drug use, e.g. anticonvulsants.*

Questions

- ☐ Plan your management of recent-onset trigeminal neuralgia in a 65-year-old patient with long-standing MS.
- ☐ What NSAID would you recommend to an elderly lady with pain from osteoarthritic change in the spine?
- ☐ How would you manage neuropathic pain in the arm following successful treatment of a Colles fracture?
- ☐ Give an outline of your treatment plan for acute sciatica with no neurologic deficit.
- ☐ Do injection techniques have any place in the management of back pain?
- ☐ What other specialties and therapies will you need to add to neurosurgery when establishing a spinal surgery service?
- ☐ What risks are associated with anticonvulsant therapy in chronic pain management?
- ☐ Under what circumstances would you consider implantation of an intrathecal opiate delivery system?

References

1. Turk CT, Okifuji A. Pain terms and taxonomies of pain. In: Loeser JD, editor. Bonica's management of pain. Lippincott Williams & Wilkins, 2001; 17–25.

2. McCormack K. Signal transduction in neuropathic pain, with special emphasis on the analgesic role of opioids. Part I: the basic science of phenotype expression in normal and regenerating nerve. Philadelphia PA: Pain Reviews 1999;6:3–34.
3. McCormack K. Signal transduction in neuropathic pain, with special emphasis on the analgesic role of opioids. Part II: moving basic science to a new pharmacotherapy. Philadelphia PA: Pain Reviews 1999;6:99–133.
4. Moore A, McQuay HJ. Cox-2 round up. In: Bandolier. http://www.jr2.ox.ac.uk/bandolier/band75/b75-2.html.
5. Moore A, McQuay HJ. League table of analgesics. In: Bandolier. http://www.jr2.ox.ac.uk/bandolier/booth/painpag/Acutrev/Analgesics/Leagtab.html.
6. McQuay HJ, Moore RA. Antidepressants in neuropathic pain. http://www.jr2.ox.ac.uk/bandolier/booth/painpag/Chronrev/antidc/CP072.html.
7. Wiffen P, Collins S, McQuay H, Carroll D, Jadad A, Moore A. Anticonvulsant drugs for acute and chronic pain (Cochrane Review). In: The Cochrane Library, Issue 2. Oxford: Update Software, 2001.
8. Linde K, Melchart D, Fischer P, Berman B, White A, Vickers A et al. Acupuncture for idiopathic headache (Cochrane Review). In: The Cochrane Library, Issue 2. Oxford: Update Software, 2001.
9. van Tulder MW, Ostelo RWJG, Vlaeyen JWS, Linton SJ, Morley SJ, Assendelft WJJ. Behavioural treatment for chronic low back pain (Cochrane Review). In: The Cochrane Library, Issue 2. Oxford: Update Software, 2001.
10. Karjalainen K, Malmivaara A, van Tulder M, Roine R, Jauhiainen M, Hurri H et al. Multidisciplinary biopsychosocial rehabilitation for subacute low back pain among working age adults (Cochrane Review). In: The Cochrane Library, Issue 2. Oxford: Update Software, 2001.
11. Kline MT. Radiofrequency techniques in clinical practice. In: Waldman SD, Winnie AP, editors. Interventional pain management. W.B. Saunders, 1996; 185–217.
12. Simpson BA. Spinal cord stimulation. Philadelphia PA: Pain Reviews 1994;1:199–230.
13. Gilmer-Hill HS, Boggan JE, Smith KA, Wagner FC Jr. Intrathecal morphine delivered via subcutaneous pump for intractable cancer pain: a review of the literature. Surg Neurol 1999;51:12–15.
14. Staats PS. Neuraxial infusion for pain control: when, why, and what to do after the implant. Oncology (Huntingt) 1999;13(5 Suppl. 2):58–62.
15. Krames ES. Practical issues when using neuraxial infusion. Oncology (Huntingt) 1999;13(5 Suppl. 2):37–44.
16. Nelemans PJ, Bie RA de, Vet HCW de, Sturmans F. Injection therapy for subacute and chronic benign low back pain (Cochrane Review). In: The Cochrane Library, Issue 2. Oxford: Update Software, 2001.
17. Watts RW, Silagy CA. A meta-analysis on the efficacy of epidural corticosteroids in the treatment of sciatica. Anaesthesia and Intensive Care 1995;23:564–9.
18. McQuay HJ, Moore RA. Epidural steroids for sciatica. Anaesthesia and Intensive Care 1996;24:284–5.
19. Lord SM, Barnsley L, Wallis BJ, McDonald GJ, Bogduk N. Percutaneous radio-frequency neurotomy for chronic cervical zygapophyseal-joint pain. N Engl J Med 1996;335:1721–6.
20. McDonald GJ, Lord SM, Bogduk N. Long-term follow-up of patients treated with cervical radiofrequency neurotomy for chronic neck pain. Neurosurgery 1999;45:61–7; discussion 67–8.
21. Perkin GD. Trigeminal neuralgia. Curr Treat Options Neurol 1999;1:458–65.
22. Maesawa S, Salame C, Flickinger JC, Pirris S, Kondziolka D, Lunsford LD. Clinical outcomes after stereotactic radiosurgery for idiopathic trigeminal neuralgia. J Neurosurg 2001;94:14–20.
23. Brown JA, Gouda JJ. Percutaneous balloon compression of the trigeminal nerve. Neurosurg Clin N Am 1997;8:53–62.
24. Walker SM, Cousins MJ. Complex regional pain syndromes: including “reflex sympathetic dystrophy” and “causalgia”. Anaesth Intens Care 1997;25:113–25.

Recommended Further Reading

Waddell G. The back pain revolution. Churchill Livingstone, 1998. ISBN 0 443 060398

34

Epilepsy Surgery

Christopher L. Chandler and Charles E. Polkey

Summary

Evaluation of patients being considered for epilepsy surgery is based on a multidisciplinary approach, with access to neuroimaging, neurophysiology (both invasive and non-invasive), neuropsychology and functional imaging, in addition to careful clinical assessment. Surgical interventions aim to either resect a structural abnormality or to modify brain function so as to improve the control of the patient's epilepsy. Resective surgery can result in cure of seizures in up to 80% of patients, whilst functional procedures may produce significant seizure control in between 30 and 80% of patients.

Introduction

The surgical treatment of epilepsy has developed from empirical observations and theoretical proposals. Surgical interventions fall into two groups: resective surgery, in which an area of brain is removed, generally because it contains a structural abnormality; or functional surgery, in which brain function is modified so as to improve the control of epilepsy.

Between the first attempts at epilepsy surgery in the late 1800s and the modern era over 150 years later, the surgical treatment of epilepsy has been determined by the available methods of investigation and surgical techniques, against the background of current neuroscience knowledge.

The concept of the pathology underlying focal epilepsy emerged in the 1950s and 1960s. The detailed work by Murray Falconer and neuropathological colleagues revealed the pathological substrates underlying temporal lobe epilepsy. These substrates are an excellent predictor of outcome.

In the mid-1970s, direct brain imaging by CT and MRI scanning permitted direct visualization of brain pathology. Early CT scans could only be relied upon to demonstrate gross brain pathology and so a concept of lesional epilepsy and lesional surgery appeared. Even now, the published literature distinguishes between lesional epilepsy from hamartomas and DNET tumors and non-lesional epilepsy, even when there may be clear pathology, such as mesial temporal sclerosis (MTS). Because MTS is predominantly, but not exclusively, unilateral, its demonstration with direct brain imaging is more complex than other pathologies, with the exception of cortical neuronal migration disorders. However, continued advances in MRI imaging have allowed the better delineation of both these conditions. At present, resective surgery is based upon a multidisciplinary approach, with a heavy emphasis on underlying pathology and direct brain imaging. Stereotactic methodology, both with frame-based and "frameless" stereotaxy, has gained a place in lesion-directed surgery.

Functional operations modify the pathophysiology of epilepsy and they are less frequent and less effective than resective operations, but they offer some relief to a group of patients who would otherwise be untreated. Stereotactic lesioning for epilepsy has been largely unproductive. Cerebellar stimulation has fallen into disuse, having been shown to be ineffective, and vagus nerve stimulation (VNS), first described in 1990, is now a recognized technique. Recently, deep brain stimulation has been described in the thalamus and proposed in the sub-thalamic nucleus. Callosotomy was introduced in 1940 and has proved useful, as has multiple sub-pial transection, introduced by Morrell and his colleagues.

The essence of a successful epilepsy surgery program is first to identify a focus of the seizure disorder and then to establish the safety of resecting the focus. Many different strategies for achieving these aims have been used.

Presurgical Assessment

Despite the great changes in knowledge over the past 20 years, the criteria for admission to a presurgical assessment program have changed little from those proposed by Rasmussen before 1975. These are "when adequate medical treatment in a patient with (focal) epilepsy has failed to give satisfactory control of the attacks, which interfere significantly with the patient's ability to lead a normal or near normal life". The main purpose of surgery is to decrease the seizure tendency rather than to "cure" the epilepsy and the patient and their relatives must have sufficient motivation because the investigation and surgery require the patient's complete and enthusiastic co-operation. In dealing with large numbers of patients with a variety of epilepsies, it is possible to use a structured scheme of management which, at each stage, allows the team to decide whether a patient can be offered surgery, withdrawn from the program or be further investigated. This is illustrated in Table 34.1.

Non-invasive Assessment

Clinical Assessment

The importance of a good clinical assessment cannot be over-emphasized. The interictal component of the history, including past medical history, will indicate the pathology. Falconer

Table 34.1. Structured management of pre-surgical assessment.

	Investigation	Stop	Possible resective operation	Possible functional operation
Phase 1A	Clinical history	Generalized seizures	Lesionectomy Temporal lobectomy Hemispherectomy or hemispherotomy	Anterior callosal section VNS
	Routine and sleep EEG	Generalized EEG		
	Basic neuropsychology			
	Structural MRI	No lesion (including MTS)		
Phase 1B	Amytal test for speech and memory	Inconsistent findings	Temporal lobectomy or selective AH	
	MRI temporal lobe protocol and 3-D rendering	No lesion		
	FDG–PET	No lateralization		
	Ictal SPECT	No localization		
	Scalp or FO telemetry Or sub-dural strips	No localization	Frontal vs temporal resection	
Phase 2	Major invasive recording to test a specific hypothesis	Hypothesis not confirmed	Local resection and/or MST	MST

clearly established that the pathology plays an important part in the outcome of epilepsy surgery [1] and earlier work by Ounsted showed that a careful clinical history could reveal the underlying pathology. By contrast, the ictal history will indicate the origin and spread of the seizure within the brain. The semiology of simple or complex partial seizures arising within the temporal lobe or frontal lobe has been frequently and well described [2]. Outside of the temporal and frontal lobes there are good pointers to seizures arising in the primary sensory or motor areas, in other supplementary areas [3] and in the occipital lobe [4]. Finally, the effect of seizures upon speech and the significance of transient neurological deficit following a seizure, known as a Todd's paresis, are important.

Structural Brain Imaging

MRI scanning must now represent the gold standard because it reveals over 95% of structural abnormalities within the brain. This has also lessened the need for invasive neurophysiological recording. Mesial temporal sclerosis varies in its severity and laterality [5] and the ability to demonstrate this lesion will vary according to the MRI technique available. The subtle changes of mesial temporal sclerosis can now be shown using sophisticated analysis. In addition to sequences in which the change is obvious, when the condition is severe, there are a number of other analyses and sequences, such as volumetric analysis and FLAIR sequences, which are helpful in delineating this condition. Cortical neuronal migration disorder can exist in diverse forms, some of which are amenable to focal resective surgery and others which are not [6]. MRI can also show when pathology is more widespread or multiple, as in cortical neuronal migration disorder or when there may be dual pathology. If the demonstrated lesion in a particular patient does not correspond to the other data, then other modalities of the pre-surgical assessment must be used to resolve the matter.

MR spectroscopy has been shown to be useful in three areas. It can demonstrate bilateral disease, loss of neuronal function both in mesial temporal sclerosis [7] and cortical neuronal migration disorder, and it is often lateralized to the same side as other indicators of the epileptic focus. However, the techniques for determining N-acetylaspartate NAA, creatinine and choline and their ratios are difficult and, essentially, this is likely to remain a research tool.

Neurophysiology

Modern brain imaging has led to a major reappraisal of the place of neurophysiology in pre-surgical assessment, certainly as far as resective procedures are concerned. An interictal record, even using semi-invasive electrodes and drug activation, can often be clearly focal but, if it is not, there can still be a surgically remediable lesion. Invasive neurophysiology is clearly indicated when there is a lack of concordance between investigations or observations in Phase 1 and when there is a discrepancy between the interictal neurophysiological findings and the suspected seizure origin. Seizures originating from the mesial surface of the cerebral cortex may be difficult to detect by simple scalp telemetry and, therefore, a negative result does not necessarily exclude surgery. In certain patients, who may be candidates for functional procedures, the interictal EEG may be an important selection criterion, as with bilateral synchronous spike wave discharges for callosotomy and "electrical status epilepticus of slow sleep" (ESESS) in Landau–Kleffner syndrome. With temporal lobe epilepsy, non-invasive tests make selection for surgery accurate and effective but outside the temporal lobe, invasive neurophysiology plays a more important role, both in recording seizures and in allowing stimulation of the cerebral cortex to determine seizure origin and to locate eloquent areas. Major intracranial neurophysiological investigations are more hazardous and, therefore, these are placed in Phase 2.

Functional Brain Imaging

There are two well validated techniques of functional brain imaging in use: PET and SPECT. Functional techniques using MR and MEG for cerebral localization are still in the development stage.

There are a number of different PET techniques but the most useful in pre-surgical assessment uses fluoro-deoxy-glucose (FDG) as the ligand. In temporal lobe epilepsy, in the interictal state, there may be an area of hypometabolism on the same side as the epileptic focus and this corresponds well with lateralization from other investigations, including depth electrode exploration. Patients with bilateral hypometabolism on FDG–PET have a worse outcome from temporal lobe surgery than those with unilateral hypometabolism. Hypometabolism with flumazenil C11 PET detects mesial temporal sclerosis and is more precise than FDG–PET, although not necessarily more efficient. It has been shown to give additional useful information in certain situations, as described by Ryvthin et al. [8]. In patients with some forms of cortical neuronal migration disorder, FDG–PET abnormalities may be seen when the MRI appears normal. Such a focal PET abnormality was first described in neonates who appeared to have non-focal epilepsy and it has been suggested that it may be useful in hemimegalencephaly. It has also been shown that in patients with tuberose sclerosis, those tubers which are likely to be epileptiform can be identified using C11, labelled tryptophan.

The use of SPECT for imaging in epilepsy patients is more complex. The usual ligand is HMPAO and Bonte first described abnormalities in epilepsy in 1983. Studies indicate that interictal SPECT demonstrating hypometabolic activity is unreliable, except when it correlates well with other tests. Ictal SPECT, obtained after the ligand had been administered during or close to a seizure, demonstrates hypometabolisms more reliably. Further studies showed that if the time course of the changes in relation to the seizure was taken into account, ictal SPECT was very useful in non-invasive assessment of temporal lobe epilepsies. There has been a lot of interest in the use of SPECT in frontal-lobe epilepsy. The necessity to mix chemicals to produce the ligand was a time-limiting factor, but a pre-mixed version is now available. However, the brief duration and rapid spread of frontal-lobe seizures still make capture with SPECT difficult, since some may be of briefer duration than the circulation time of the tracer. However, co-registration of SPECT on MRI has been described as useful in extratemporal epilepsies by O'Brien et al. [9].

Neuropsychology

Basic neuropsychological tests have been used for many years to assess verbal and non-verbal intelligence and memory. These tests may help to evaluate the potential effect of resective surgery on brain function.

Invasive Procedures

The use of invasive techniques has been much reduced by improved understanding of the pathology of epilepsy and the development of modern brain imaging. These invasive procedures fall into three groups: pharmacological activation or inactivation procedures, minor and major invasive intracranial electrodes.

Carotid Amytal Test

The carotid amytal test is used to assess hemispheric speech dominance and also to assess memory reserve and distribution. Although the standard test involves injection of sodium amytal into the internal carotid artery, a number of selective amytal tests have also been described. A good review of the use of the carotid amytal test has been written by Jones-Gottman and colleagues [10].

The intracarotid amytal test can also be used to demonstrate bilateral secondary synchrony, in which an epileptic focus in one hemisphere is thought to be driving activity in the other hemisphere. Some believe that the administration of barbiturates to the point of electrical silence on EEG will reveal the true spike focus. These tests are certainly useful in certain circumstances, such as in working up a patient with Landau–Kleffner syndrome for multiple sub-pial transection, but the large amounts of barbiturates administered require proper supervision and anesthetic assistance.

Intracranial Electrodes

Invasive electrode placements may be used with videotelemetry to clarify the nature and origin of a patient's seizures. The extracranial ones include sphenoidal leads and epidural peg electrodes. Foramen ovale electrodes, placed through the foramen ovale to lie close to the mesial surface of the temporal lobe, can be used to provide lateralization, to distinguish temporal from extratemporal onset of seizures and mesial temporal from lateral temporal onset. Complications are few but include disturbance of facial sensation, usually transient, and, very rarely, hemiparesis, possibly more common after previous operation. Bilateral sub-temporal strip electrodes are also used for the investigation of temporal lobe problems and, in the authors' practice, have been preferred in recent years, since they allow a wider coverage and have fewer complications.

Major invasive electrode placement serves a number of purposes and can be divided into two groups. Stereotactically determined placement of multi-contact wire electrodes may be used primarily to explore an area of brain, surface and depth, in order to delineate the epileptogenic zone, and may include some stimulation protocols for functional localization and to provoke seizures. The placement, either epidurally or, more frequently, sub-durally, of arrays of point contacts embedded in silastic strips or grids delineates an epileptogenic zone and allows detailed mapping of the primary motor and sensory cortex and assessment of speech lateralization and memory function. Technical details of these methods will be found in appropriate reviews [11].

The interpretation of data obtained from intracranial recordings needs a sophisticated technological set-up with video-EEG, including an adequate number of recording channels. Experienced neurophysiologists with a wide knowledge of seizure semiology and of the clinical data relating to the particular patient under investigation are essential.

The use of depth electrodes has decreased with the advent of good MRI and varies considerably between centers, dependent upon their case-mix, other facilities and previous experience. Stimulation through depth electrodes gives valuable information about seizure thresholds, as well as functional information about motor function and, in the temporal lobe, cognitive function.

Conclusion

Adherence to such a scheme of pre-surgical assessment is important if candidates for epilepsy surgery are to receive the best advice. The fate of 210 adults and children going through such an assessment scheme is shown in Table 34.2.

Table 34.2. Fate of 210 patients assessed for epilepsy surgery, 1990–1995.

Action	Phase		
	1A	1B	2
Stop	81	21	4
Operation	32	50	22
To next Phase	97	26	0

Note: Phase 1A: Clinical history, interictal EEG, basic neuropsychology, structural MRI. Phase 1B: Volumetric and spectroscopic MRI, FDG–PET, video-telemetry, including foramen ovale electrodes, intracarotid sodium amytal test. Phase 2: Major invasive recording with sub-dural and depth electrodes or sub-dural grids or mats.

Resective Surgical Procedures

The application of resective techniques varies in extent and site and it is probably best to classify procedures into three groups: temporal resections, extratemporal resections and major resections. The use of local anesthesia to permit localization during epilepsy surgery is used less frequently because the use of the grid electrodes described above has resolved many localization problems. If it is necessary to explore the central area under local anesthesia, whatever the age of the patient, it is often best to perform the craniotomy under general anesthesia on one day and re-open it a few days later under local anesthesia. The range of resective operations carried out at the Maudsley Hospital between 1976 and 1995 is shown in detail in Table 34.3.

Temporal Resections

The mechanism of chronic temporal lobe epilepsy probably differs from focal epilepsy in other parts of the brain and this is important in assessing the value of various procedures. In temporal lobe epilepsy associated with mesial temporal sclerosis, there is good evidence for the "amplifier" mechanism proposed by Wieser and Engel, which hypothesises that a normal parahippocampal gyrus is part of the neurophysiological circuit responsible for the persistence of the epilepsy and will need to be removed to obtain a cure [12].

Table 34.3. Resective operations in adults and children, 1976–1995.

Operation	Total Number	%	Adults (73%) Number	%	Children (27%) Number	%
Temporal resections						
"En bloc"	223	56.6	180	62.3	43	41
Extended	16	4	12	4.2	4	3.8
Selective amygdalo–hippocampectomy	44	11	42	14.5	2	1.9
Total	283	71.6	234	81	49	46.5
Other resections						
Frontal	40	10.1	22	7.6	18	17.2
Parietal	21	5.3	14	4.8	7	6.7
Central	5	1.3	1	0.3	4	4.0
Occipital	4	1	1	0.3	3	2.8
Total	70	17.7	38	13	32	30.7
Major resections						
Multilobar	10	2.5	4	1.4	6	5.7
Hemispherectomy	31	7.9	13	4.5	18	17.1
Total	41	10.4	17	5.9	24	22.8
GRAND TOTAL	394		289		105	

Note: Children are aged less than 16 years at operation.

Most temporal resections involve removal of both superficial and deep structures and it is the extent of that removal which varies. Most temporal lobectomies are two-stage procedures: first, resection of the neocortical structures, followed by removal of the hippocampus and parahippocampal gyrus, and it is only the relative extent of lateral and medial resection which varies. Certain anatomical boundaries are imposed upon the surgeon. In the dominant hemisphere, the majority of the superior temporal gyrus must be preserved. The insular cortex must remain undisturbed if the risk of a manipulation hemiplegia is to be avoided. The posterior extent of the resection is governed by the risk of hemianopia. In adults, the limit is around 6.5 cm; in smaller children, it is convenient to use the height of the temporal lobe at the mid-Sylvian point as the posterior extent of the resection. Spencer has described a technique for gaining access to the posterior mesial temporal structures without undue neocortical destruction [13]. Complete removal of benign tumours, dysembryonic neuroepithelial tumours (DNETs), hamartomas and the like is very desirable but, where they are adherent to important vessels and removal could cause hemiplegia if these vessels were damaged, a small portion may be left without detriment to the outcome. Some surgeons use the microscope and the CUSA for the deep parts of a temporal lobe removal.

The en-bloc temporal lobectomy described by Falconer provides a large specimen, which is suitable for both physiological and pathological analysis. The standard procedure performed in the authors' unit obtains a block specimen using the technique described by Spencer to maximize hippocampal removal. The patient is supine, with a sandbag under the ipsilateral shoulder, with the head turned to the contralateral side to achieve a horizontal. A question-mark incision starts just anterior to the level of the zygoma, curving superiorly and posteriorly behind the ear and extending forwards to just superior to the external angular process of the frontal bone. The surgeon may then elevate either an osteoplastic or a free flap. It is important to position the inferior limit of the bone flap as close to the floor of the middle fossa as possible. The inferior burr-hole should be placed just superior to the zygoma and the anterior burr-hole as close to the base of the sphenoid wing as possible.

The craniotome can then be used to cut a bone flap based along the sphenoid wing which extends several centimetres behind the ear. Further bone is then rongeured off the inferior margin towards the middle fossa floor and anteriorly towards the temporal pole. A dural flap based superiorly is then elevated, exposing the temporal lobe. The authors then routinely perform EcoG, though not all surgeons subscribe to this.

A vertical cortical incision is made in the middle temporal gyrus at the posterior limit of the resection, staying anterior to the vein of Labbé and deepened down into the temporal horn of the lateral ventricle. In the next stage, the lateral neocortex (temporal operculum) is dissected sub-pially off the insula, maintaining the integrity of the arachnoid to protect the middle cerebral vessels. The dissection is then continued anteriorly down onto the floor of the middle fossa, following the curve of the sphenoid wing. Starting posteriorly, from the opening into the temporal horn, the white matter of the stem of the temporal lobe is progressively divided along the roof of the temporal horn, working anteriorly through the amygdala until the pia arachnoid of the pole of the temporal lobe is reached at the edge of the sphenoid wing. The previous incision in the middle temporal gyrus is then extended inferiorly towards the floor of the middle fossa, cutting through the remainder of the middle and inferior temporal gyri. The dissection is continued medially until the hippocampus is reached. This is the most difficult stage of the procedure, due to the proximity of the posterior cerebral vessels and third and fourth cranial nerves at the tentorial edge. The choroid plexus is retracted medially to expose the choroid fissure and fimbria. This can be divided either with a small sucker or the CUSA. The dissection then proceeds anteriorly along the tentorial edge, coagulating and dividing the hippocampal branches of the posterior cerebral artery. The specimen can then be removed and a post-resection ECoG performed.

It is also possible to carry out a restricted removal of the mesial temporal structures, described as selective amygdalo-hippocampectomy, using a number of techniques, including either the trans-sylvian technique described by Yasargil or the transcortical approach originally described by Niemeyer [14]. The trans-sylvian approach is a technically demanding procedure, with a potential risk of vascular and cranial nerve damage, and should be reserved for those individuals in whom the seizure focus is clearly limited to the mesial temporal lobe structures. It is possible, but not clearly proven in the literature, that there could be fewer cognitive changes, especially in the dominant hemisphere

Direct operative mortality following temporal lobe resection is rare and is 0.5% in the authors' series. In the latest review, it is less than 1%, with some centers reporting no deaths in over 500 consecutive operations. Late mortality is a different matter. In Falconer's material, 19% of patients suffered late deaths, half from seizures. In the authors' own material, there were 17 deaths in 305 patients (5.6%), of which six were sudden and unexpected (SUDEP) and the remainder were related to epilepsy. A summary of physical complications from temporal lobectomy in published series is shown in Table 34.4.

Early studies showed that recent memory was a material-specific function, mediated by the temporal lobes, and that bilateral medial temporal resections would produce global amnesia [15]. In general, the post-operative changes in intellectual function depend upon the preoperative state and the pathology. It was shown by Powell that those patients who were intellectually less able suffered less as a consequence of temporal lobe resection and, in general, these were patients with mesial temporal sclerosis who had undergone early brain reorganization [15]. It was hoped that selective amygdalo-hippocampectomy would produce better cognitive results but, with the exception of the study by the Oxford group, this has not been proven [16].

The overall seizure outcome for temporal lobe resections was quoted at the 2nd Palm Desert symposium as 68% seizure free, 24% improved and 9% not improved, using the Engel outcome scale [17]. The ILAE survey has similar figures – 57% seizure free, 27% improved and 10% not improved. The seizure outcome from temporal lobe surgery depends upon the type of resection and the pathology

Table 34.4. Complications from temporal lobe resections.

Complication	1975 (%)	1987 (%)	1993 (%)
Transient hemiparesis	4.2	0.7	4
Permanent hemiparesis	2.4	0.7	<2
Third nerve palsy	3.7	<1	
Complete hemianopia	5.6	0.6	3
Speech disturbance	5.2	0.37	2
Non-neurological	3		1.4
Mortality	0.8	0.47	<1

within the temporal lobe. MRI allows a better assessment of the pathology pre-operatively and the extent of removal post-operatively, both of which will influence seizure outcome and cognitive outcome. Cascino and his colleagues have demonstrated that there may be dual pathology in the temporal lobe, which could account for the failure of lesionectomy in this area. Pathology and outcome are clearly related, with the exception of cortical dysplasia. The resective procedure seems to make little difference to seizure outcome and overall results from anterior temporal lobectomy and selective amygdalo–hippocampectomy, summarized in two reviews, were almost identical (Table 34.5). The results in children tend to be better because these series contain a higher proportion of "positive" lesions.

Behavioral problems in patients with uncontrolled temporal lobe epilepsy (TLE) are well documented and they will often improve or disappear if seizure control is good.

Psychosis supervening upon chronic epilepsy is usually a late event. Temporal lobe surgery can produce a schizophreniform psychosis, often associated with left-sided resections, but this is rare – less than 1% in the authors' material. A depressive illness, more often associated with right-sided operations, occurs in 10–15% of our patients. It may be related to the size of the resection, being rare after amygdalo–hippocampectomy and in children.

Extra-temporal Resections

Lesionectomy is justified in extratemporal cases, since it produces good results, as described by the Mayo Clinic group in 1992. Studies have shown that if the extent of the resection is based upon the pathology rather than the neurophysiological abnormalities, then it is more likely to be successful. In the case of stereotactic lesionectomy, this is determined by the structural appearance of the lesion, whilst others use frozen sections.

Frontal-lobe resections are the most common extratemporal removals and a variety of pathological conditions are found with the overall complete seizure relief rate, reported in the literature to be around 20%. The Montreal Neurological Institute has the largest series of frontal-lobe resections and, in their last review of 257 patients with non-tumoral lesions, 26% had complete freedom from seizures and a further 30% had a marked reduction in seizures. Forty-seven percent of patients undergoing anterior frontal resections become seizure free compared with only 18% of those with parasagittal resections. This review is clearly well before the advent of direct brain imaging and it is now clear that the presence of a lesion on MRI alters the outcome favorably.

Resection from the central (parietal) region is rare. When there is a pre-existing deficit, then there is less likelihood of an increase as a result of operation and, therefore, it is more reasonable to attempt it. Surgical technique is important, especially care for the deep vessels, which may indeed have to be skeletonized to avoid deficits distant from the site of the resection. Modern methods of brain imaging, such as functional PET or functional MRI combined with surface rendering, including venous structures, can provide the surgeon with a precise map of the brain surface and pathology. The results of resections from the central and parietal areas are variable.

Occipital resections are also rare. There is a difficulty because seizure spread from the occipital lobe invariably involves the temporal lobe, often bilaterally, and temporal lobe seizures themselves can have visual components in their semiology. Modern brain imaging has made a considerable difference to the outcome of surgery in this area. It is now realized that most patients harbor either a low-grade tumor or a developmental abnormality. In 1998, Spencer reported 35 patients with either tumors or developmental abnormalities, reporting 85% good outcome in the tumors and 46% in the

Table 34.5. Outcome in large series of temporal lobe resections.

Outcome group	Operation	Palm Desert II (%)	ILAE Global Survey (%)
I (Seizure free)	ATL	67.9	57.3
	Selective AHE	68.8	60.1

Palm Desert II, refers to Pilcher et al., [35]. ILAE Global Survey, refers to Anonymous, [20].

developmental abnormalities. Location and surgical technique did not affect outcome. Williamson reported good results in 88%. Surprisingly, in many patients there was no increase in visual field defect and few patients acquired one.

Multi-lobar Resections, Hemispherectomy and Hemispherotomy

These procedures are performed in similar circumstances and for similar pathology. Multi-lobar resection is used to remove an epileptogenic area or pathology, which does not involve the whole hemisphere, and by means of which useful cortex may be spared. This technique is used for patients with widespread cortical neuronal migration disorder and gross destructive lesions consequent upon trauma or cerebral infarction. Multi-lobar resection is less common than hemispherectomy.

The indications for hemispherectomy are established unilateral hemisphere disease, causing intractable epileptic seizures, with an appropriate neurological deficit. The matter of the addition of a homonymous hemianopia is usually negotiable.

Surgical Technique

A number of techniques are employed for hemispherectomy, ranging from an anatomically complete operation in which the whole hemisphere is removed, preserving only the basal ganglia, to a hemispherotomy, in which the aim is to remove the smallest amount of brain tissue and still achieve complete hemispheric disconnection. The original operation, described by Krynauw in 1950, was, in effect, a hemi-decortication, usually described as an anatomically complete hemispherectomy.

There are three major steps involved in an anatomical hemispherectomy: ligation and division of the middle cerebral artery distal to the lenticulo-striate arteries; division of the remaining arterial supply and venous drainage of the hemisphere; and the removal of the hemisphere. This was abandoned in the 1970s because of the complication of late delayed bleeding (cerebral hemosiderosis) which occurred in up to a third of patients and was often fatal. The use of Adams' modification in which, amongst other features, the enormous cavity in contact with the sub-arachnoid space is converted into an extradural space led to a significant reduction of late hemosiderosis.

Rasmussen described a sub-total or functional hemispherectomy, in which blocks of cortex are left anteriorly and posteriorly but isolated functionally by callosal section. Hoffmann in Toronto has used a form of hemicorticectomy which only extends down to the white matter, in order to overcome the late risks, although these were less effective in the control of seizures.

In historical series of hemispherectomy, the overall results were good, with 70–80% of patients seizure free. The Palm desert experience, reported in 1993, gives 67.4% seizure free, with 21.1% improved and a failure rate of about 11.6%. The corresponding figures for multi-lobar resection are 45.2% seizure free, with a failure rate of 19.5% [17]. Other benefits include improved intellectual performance and behavior if the seizures are controlled.

Gradually, the extent of tissue resection in functional hemispherectomy has diminished so that the operation has become more and more of a disconnection. A new technique – hemispherotomy – has been reported, in which the major fiber tracts are divided with minimal removal of the pathological brain tissue [18]. The results are similar, at least in the short term, to those of hemispherectomy. The technique involves shorter operation times, much less operative trauma and less blood loss; these are all-important considerations when operating on infants.

A multi-center case study by Holthausen described 333 patients from 13 centers. The pathology and operative techniques were varied. Overall, 328 patients were available for follow-up and there were five pre-operative deaths (1.5%). Using a classification in which all the patients who fell within Engel group 1 were described as seizure free, there were 231 patients who fell into this group (70.4%). Detailed analysis suggested that surgical technique was important, with hemispherotomy and Adams techniques producing significantly better results than the others. Although pathology was not a significant factor, Holthausen notes that the various manifestations of cortical neuromigrational disorder did worse [19]. In a recent report, only 44% of children with hemimegalencephaly became seizure free compared with 77% of children with other pathologies.

Functional Procedures

Originally epilepsy surgery was based on physiological as well as structural principles. Increasing knowledge of the underlying pathology and improved direct brain imaging have resulted in less attention being paid to functional operations, especially stereotactic lesioning. Currently, the available procedures for epilepsy are stereotactic lesioning, cutting various fiber tracts or other connections, including the various methods of callosotomy and multiple sub-pial transection, and, finally, brain stimulation either with intracranial electrodes or VNS.

Stereotactic Lesions

In historical series, two targets for stereotactic lesions were involved: either areas within the deep gray matter, thought to be part of the circuit for centrencephalic epilepsy, popular in the 1950s, or targets within the medial temporal structures.

Callosal Section

This procedure was based upon observations in experimental models of epilepsy and a fortuitous observation that seizures improved in a patient whose glioma had invaded the anterior corpus callosum. Data from the Second Palm Desert meeting and the International League against Epilepsy (ILAE) survey show that no more than 3% of patients are seizure free but seizure control was improved, especially that of certain seizure types [17] [20]. Partial seizures and myoclonic jerks may not respond and may even be made worse by the procedure. In many patients subjected to callosotomy, there is no demonstrable structural lesion and, in these patients, the only absolute indication for callosal section seems to be bilateral synchronous EEG discharges. It is valuable to assess the degree of section post-operatively, using the MRI. Generally, complete callosotomy has been abandoned and an anterior two-thirds section substituted.

Callosotomy is performed under general anesthesia with the patient in the supine position, the head in the neutral position, neck slightly flexed and held in the 3-pin fixator. A right parasagittal craniotomy centered over the coronal suture is fashioned. A medially based dural flap is cut and held with stay sutures. The inter-hemispheric fissure needs to be opened up and fixed brain retractors are useful. The operating microscope is used to divide the adhesions and carefully preserve the pericallosal vessels. The corpus callosum is easily recognized by its glistening, pearly white appearance. Either a small sucker or the CUSA may be used to gently divide the anterior corpus callosum down to, but not through, the ependyma. The dissection is carried through the rest of the genu, rostrum and anterior body. On completion of the procedure, the anterior cerebral vessels are often visible around the divided genu. A fuller description of the operative techniques can be found in standard texts, e.g. Roberts (1995) [21]. In theory, carefully directed radiosurgery could be used but, at present, the location of the major midline vessels would make this potentially dangerous.

Complications from callosal section depend upon the extent of the section and the nature of the underlying disease process. In unilateral hemisphere disease, it is clearly sensible to approach the midline from the damaged side or otherwise from the known, or assumed, non-dominant side. Planning the approach will depend upon whether a total or partial section is intended and should avoid interruption of major tributaries to the superior sagittal sinus. The complications are acute and chronic and related to the extent of the resection, being minimal with a truncal section and greatest with a total section. Venous ischemia, or even thrombosis, when unilateral, may manifest itself as a hemiparesis, with the possible addition of focal seizures. There may be transient paresis due to retraction on the medial surface of the hemisphere. More serious, however, is akinetic mutism, probably the result of bilateral anterior cerebral artery spasm. However, even in recent series, there is a significant incidence of both general and neurological complications, although they tend to be transient. Overall, the risk of death at callosotomy seems to be between 0 and 6%, of permanent neurological deficit less than 5% and transient deficit up to 20%.

The outcome from callosal section cannot be assessed with the same criteria as those used for resective surgery. The patients usually have multiple seizure types. The response of some seizures may be dramatic, with an 80% or greater reduction or even complete abolition, leaving other seizure types unaffected or even increased. It is clear that atonic or drop attacks are well relieved, with permanent cure varying between 4 and 80%, and improvement in between 75 and 100% of patients. Other seizure types are less responsive; improvements of between 56 and 75% were seen for generalized tonic–clonic seizures and around 30–40% for partial complex seizures. In 17 series in the literature between 1990 and 2001, these figures remain broadly true. In a careful study of the long-term effects of callosal section in the authors' material, Pressler showed that there was some fall off in seizure control after 2 years.

Two cognitive complications may follow callosal section. Speech may be affected in patients of mixed cerebral dominance, where inter-hemispheric communication is essential for the proper comprehension and production of speech and related functions.

The second complication is the posterior disconnection syndrome, in which complex tasks requiring the utilization of information from both hemispheres become impossible. It is associated with division of the posterior fibers at a one-stage callosotomy and, when the operation is staged, it is said to be less severe.

Multiple Sub-pial Transsection (MST)

This technique, introduced by Morrell and Whisler, depends upon the observation that cortical organization is columnar. The functions of eloquent cortex are subserved by vertical columns, whereas the propagation of epileptic impulses occurs through horizontal fiber connections. Morrell reasoned that if multiple transsections of the cortex were made below the pia, preserving the cortical vessels, it would reduce epileptiform activity whilst preserving essential function [22].

The technique involves selective division, with specially constructed hooks under microscopic control, of the horizontal sub-pial fibres at 5-mm intervals along the gyri which exhibit epileptiform activity. It is important to maintain the integrity of the pia and avoid cortical blood vessels and also to be careful of vessels in the depths of the sulcus; the buried cortex of the insula is especially vulnerable.

Both Morrell and other authors describe using the technique both alone and in combination with resection. Published series show that the neurological consequences of MST are slight, the best results being achieved by the Chicago group. The effect on seizure control is variable; most series report reduction rather than abolition of seizures by MST alone. It is also very successful in Landau–Kleffner syndrome and has also been proposed to deal with patients with widespread multi-focal epilepsy.

Stimulation

This became practical with the miniaturization of electronic components and development of safe silicone polymers. Cooper applied stimulation to the surface of the cerebellum on the basis of work on cerebellar physiology, but a blinded trial showed this treatment to be ineffective and it fell into disuse. Theories relating to centrencephalic epilepsy and a thalamo–cortical relay had suggested that chronic thalamic stimulation might lead to better control of the epilepsy. Fisher has written a good review of these techniques [23].

Similar physiological considerations lead to intermittent retrograde stimulation of the left vagus nerve. Through a transverse or oblique cervical incision, the left vagus nerve is exposed in the neck. The stimulator consists of three elements – two stimulating electrodes and an anchoring wire – that have to be wrapped around the nerve. The lead is then tunnelled to the generator, which is placed in a subcutaneous pocket, just inferior to the clavicle.

The results of a number of trials have been published and the effects on seizure frequency have been mixed. There are inevitable minor side effects associated with this stimulation, including hoarseness and a sensation in the throat, and there is also the risk of electrode movement, cable fracture and receiver or generator failure. Deaths occur in patients with functioning VNSs in place, but the incidence of SUDEP is no greater than would occur in a group of severe epileptics. There have been reports of asystole during testing under general anesthesia and we now recommend that all patients have their VNS turned off during general anesthetic for other reasons. There is also evidence from our clinical experience, and from a study by Malow et al., that during VNS activation, there are decreases in airflow and respiratory effort, which are probably insignificant except in patients with pre-existing obstructive sleep apnoea.

A number of papers show that seizure frequency is reduced but seizures are seldom abolished by VNS. Binnie suggests that a better than 50% reduction in seizures occurs at 18 months in 50% of patients [24]. Similar figures (between 40 and 50%, with a greater than 50% reduction, showing an improvement with time) are given by other authors. Everyone is agreed that sustained freedom from seizures, equivalent to Engel I outcome in resective surgery, is rare, occurring in about 2% of patients. Results in children are also encouraging. In a group of 60 children, a greater than 50% reduction in 42% of them at 18 months has been reported and, in a group of 38 children, 26 had a greater than 50% reduction, 11 of whom had a greater than 75% reduction in seizure frequency. By contrast, the results have been unencouraging in a group of severely disabled children with epileptic encephalopathy. Boon and his colleagues in Ghent have reported a halving of direct epilepsy-related medical costs and reduction to one-third of hospital admissions for patients with VNS.

Re-operation

Re-operation is the use of a further surgical procedure intended to relieve a patient's drug-resistant epilepsy when a previous procedure for the same purpose has failed. The procedures do not necessarily have to be of the same kind.

There are two broad indications for re-operation, which, by their nature, define the candidates. The first is when a lesser procedure does not produce the expected result or is unsatisfactory to the patient or their relatives. The second is when seizures persist and there is reasonable evidence that further operation, usually a resection and often at the same site as the original surgery, will bring further benefit. The evaluation criteria must be the same as those used in assessing surgical candidates de novo. In passing from a functional operation such as callosotomy to a resective procedure, the same principles should apply. The goals of surgery should be similar to those expressed at a first operation but modified by a realistic reassessment of the situation. The most important element is a proper assessment of the underlying pathology. It is clear that, except in special circumstances, the complete removal of discrete pathology is most likely to produce complete freedom from seizures. The use of acute ECoG at re-operation is not clear.

The overall results of re-operation, as it affects seizure frequency, can be gleaned from the published papers. Three very crude groups were used: "seizure free", corresponding to Engel's group 1A; "significantly improved", corresponding to Engel groups 1B–1D, 2 and 3A; and "not improved", corresponding to Engel group 3B and worse. Overall, 44.3% were seizure free, 30.5% significantly improved and 25.2% were not improved. Temporal lobe resections tended to do better, with 55.7% seizure free and 16.5% not improved, whereas for other resections, only 24.5% were seizure free and 40% were not improved. When there is a structural lesion which has been missed or incompletely removed, then the seizure-free proportion rises to 80–90% [25]. A recent paper suggests that magnetic source imaging may aid selection for re-operation and showed epileptogenicity around the margin of a previous resection in ten patients. Five of these patients were selected for re-operation and three were rendered seizure free.

Radiosurgery

Stereotactic-guided radiotherapy for epilepsy has been described, using either a linear accelerator or the Leksell Gamma Knife. There is considerable experience using this method of treatment for obliteration of other lesions in the brain. It has come to the fore in the treatment of mesial temporal sclerosis and the largest experience has been reported by Regis and his colleagues. Their most recent report showed that, at 2 years, 81% of 16 patients were seizure free. Good results have also been reported with hypothalamic hamartoma [26]. Treatment of both AVMs and cavernomas with radiosurgery resulted in an improvement in seizure control.

Surgical Pathology

In many situations, the extent and nature of the cerebral pathology determine both the possible surgical intervention and the outcome of surgery. Certain kinds of pathology, including non-specific changes, have been seen regularly in resected specimens from a variety of centers around the world over a number of years. The occurrence of these various pathological entities in our series of 456 patients is shown in Table 34.6.

Atrophic and Destructive Lesions

These range very widely in site, extent and etiology. Cerebral infarction, the effects of infection both directly or as a consequence of secondary vascular changes, and the consequences of cranial trauma may all lead to such lesions. In general, to be amenable to resective surgery, such changes, whatever their origin, should be circumscribed and unilateral. If so, the solution is local resection.

Early pathological studies suggested that mesial temporal sclerosis was predominantly, rather than exclusively, unilateral [5]. The UCLA Group have shown that surgical outcome can be correlated with the completeness of the removal and others that it can be correlated with the severity of the neuronal loss and the existence of dual pathology.

Vascular Lesions

Cavernous malformations may present with either seizures (50% of cases), clinical hemorrhage (up to 10%) or a progressive neurological deficit (in about 25%). These lesions may be single or multiple. Another vascular pathology – Sturge–Weber syndrome – is susceptible to surgical treatment at several points in its natural history. Mostly unilateral in extent and generally based in the occipital or frontal regions, not only does its natural history include extension of the lesion itself, but the secondary neurophysiological consequences arising from processes such as kindling and secondary epileptogenesis may cause diversification of seizure type, increase in seizure severity and, with these, intellectual deterioration. Resections of various sizes can be used to treat epilepsy associated with these lesions but hemispherectomy may be the only effective solution if there is a gross hemiplegia. Some advise early hemispherectomy, accepting the resulting hemianopia and hemiplegia, which will probably develop anyway, as a reasonable trade-off for freedom from seizures and intellectual deterioration. Erba and Cavazutti suggested that although hemispherectomy was appropriate in some cases, in others between the ages of 2 and 5, where there is a localized lesion and only partial seizures, then partial resection may be more appropriate [27]. Brain plasticity and reorganization make the consequences of this major intervention at a very young age much less severe than if it is delayed. Occasionally, callosotomy is used to improve control of drop attacks and generalized seizures, where too great an increase in the neurological deficit would result from hemispherectomy or multilobar resection.

Malformation and Tumor-like Lesions, Including Cortical Neuronal Migration Disorder

This concept embraces a group of conditions previously described separately under a number

Table 34.6. Pathology in 456 resections, 1976–1995.

Pathology		All	Age > 16 years	Age < 16 years	Temporal resection	Other resection
MTS		169	149	20	169	0
Tumor-like	tumor	62	39	23	46	16
	malformation	33	17	16	29	4
Cortical dysplasia		42	20	22	9	33
Rasmussen's disease		24	9	15	2	22
Other pathology		78	56	22	22	56
Non-specific pathology		48	45	3	41	7
TOTAL		456	335	121	318	138

of headings, including hemi-megalencephaly, focal and diffuse cortical dysplasia, etc. The range of changes seen is wide and, when gross, they can be detected by structural and functional brain imaging. The detailed abnormalities found in these specimens not only demonstrate abnormal cells, but also a gross disruption of cortical lamination and organization. This probably accounts for two disappointing aspects of resective surgery in this group, which is, first, that the lesions may be impossible to remove completely and, secondly, even when seizures are controlled, these patients continue to show slow development and poor intellectual progress.

Malformations and similar lesions are a heterogeneous group and the surgeon must rely upon his neuropathological colleagues for a detailed classification of the lesions. More important are the location and size of the lesion, which determine outcome, rather than the precise nature. The DNET, if it can be completely removed outside of the temporal lobe or mostly removed as part of a temporal lobe resection, usually has a good outcome and long-term prognosis. Further treatment is seldom necessary, even when the removal is known to be incomplete surgically or pathologically [28]. Patients with tuberose sclerosis may develop large areas of focal change and some success in controlling epilepsy has been reported following their removal. Hypothalamic hamartomas are associated with precocious puberty and gelastic epilepsy. Recently, a number of treatments for these lesions have been reported, including radiosurgery, direct stereotactic ablation and open surgery. The group at the Austin Hospital in Melbourne has reported excellent results from a direct approach.

Rasmussen's Encephalitis or Chronic Encephalitis with Epilepsy

This rare but definite entity, first described from the Montreal Neurological Institute in 1958, was labelled "encephalitis" because this term most accurately described the pathological findings on light microscopy [29]. It is usually a progressive disease in childhood, affecting one cerebral hemisphere, but it is now known that it can occasionally burn out before the hemisphere and its functions are completely destroyed, that cases sometimes have a later onset and that there are a few well documented cases of bilateral occurrence. The pathophysiology is obscure. It has been linked, without definite proof, to a slow virus infection and with cytomegalic virus. It has also been proposed that it is linked to an autoimmune process related to the GluR receptor [30]. Medical treatment with anti-viral agents or steroids may be sporadically effective or coincide with the natural arrest of the disease. In some cases, temporary improvement has been seen with plasma exchange. Local resection early in the disease is ineffective, apart from as a biopsy, and later it is inappropriate. The only effective surgical therapy is hemispherectomy.

Miscellaneous Conditions

No account of the surgical pathology can include every condition found in this material. Two conditions deserve mention: arachnoid cysts and hydrocephalus. Neither of these will cause focal epilepsy, including partial complex seizures, so that if such epilepsy or focal elements such as an EEG focus exist, it must be attributed to some other condition.

In our series of 456 patients, there were no specific pathological changes in approximately 10.5% of the specimens.

Psychosocial Consequences of Epilepsy Surgery

There has been interest in the psychosocial results of epilepsy surgery since the 1950s, when the pre-operative assessment of such patients indicated that a high proportion of them suffered social, behavioral and personality disorders – over 70% in Taylor's material and 15–50% in Jensen's review of world literature in 1975. Recently, objective questionnaires to measure psychosocial outcome, known as quality-of-life measures, have been devised and applied to epilepsy [31]. Guldvog examined two groups of patients treated medically and surgically and followed them for 20 years. Significant improvement in the work situation was seen only in those who were in full-time education or work before surgery [32]. Similar findings were reported by McLachlan, in which patients treated both medically and surgically had improvement in quality of life if they were seizure free or had a 90% reduction at 2 years. The surgical group was more likely to attain this target [33]. Other authors report similar results but note that most patients probably have a sub-optimal post-operative performance because of the low profile given to post-operative rehabilitation.

The financial benefits to the state or community of epilepsy surgery are more difficult to assess because they are long-term, difficult to quantify and may well result in savings in one area of government spending which will not be appreciated by another [34].

Conclusions

Resective surgery for epilepsy, dependent upon the pathology, age of the patient and application of selection criteria, can result in cure of seizures in up to 80% of patients, with serious morbidity and mortality contained to within the 1–2% range.

Functional surgery suffers from two grave disadvantages when compared with resective surgery. First, the indications for the procedures are neither crisp nor rational and, secondly, the procedures only relieve epilepsy completely in less than 5% of cases, although they will produce significant and useful amelioration of the fits in between 30 and 80% of patients, depending upon the patient and the procedure.

The long-term psychosocial effects of epilepsy surgery are still unclear and the cost–benefit analysis of the results has yet to be carried out.

Key Points

- *Evaluation of patients being considered for epilepsy surgery requires a multidisciplinary team, with access to neuroimaging, neurophysiology, neuropsychology and functional imaging, in addition to careful clinical assessment.*
- *Successful epilepsy surgery consists of first identifying a seizure focus and then safely resecting it.*
- *Temporal resections represent the single largest group of patients and involve removal of both the neocortex as well as the medial structures.*
- *Functional operations modify the pathology of epilepsy and are less effective than resective procedures.*

References

1. Falconer MA. Genetic and related aetiological factors in temporal lobe epilepsy. Epilepsia 1971;12:13–31.
2. Chauvel P, Bartolomei F. Seizure symptoms and cerebral localization: frontal lobe and rolandic seizures. In: Oxbury J, Polkey CE, Duchowny M, editors. Intractable focal epilepsy. London: W.B. Saunders, 2000; 55–62.
3. Williamson PD. Parietal lobe epilepsy. In: Oxbury J, Polkey CE, Duchowny M, editors. Intractable focal epilepsy. London: W.B. Saunders, 2000; 69–76.
4. Guerrini R, Parmeggiani L, Berta E, Munari C. Occipital seizures. In: Oxbury J, Polkey CE, Duchowny M, editors. Intractable focal epilepsy. London: W.B. Saunders, 2000; 78–88.
5. Margerison JH, Corsellis JAN. Epilepsy and the temporal lobes: a clinical, electroencephalographic and neuropathological study of the brain in epilepsy, with particular reference to the temporal lobes. Brain 1966;89:499–534.
6. Prayson RA, Estes ML. Cortical dysplasia: a histopathologic study of 52 cases of partial lobectomy in patients with epilepsy. Human Pathology 1995;26:493–500.
7. Park SW, Chang KH, Kim HD, Song IC, Lee DS, Lee SK et al. Lateralizing ability of single-voxel proton mr spectroscopy in hippocampal sclerosis: comparison with mr imaging and positron emission tomography. AJNR Am J Neuroradiol 2001;22:625–31.
8. Ryvlin P, Bouvard S, Le Bars D, De Lamerie G, Gregoire MC, Kahane P et al. Clinical utility of flumazenil-PET versus [18F]fluorodeoxyglucose-PET and MRI in refractory partial epilepsy: a prospective study in 100 patients. Brain 1998;121(Pt 11):2067–81.
9. O'Brien TJ, So EL, Mullan BP, Cascino GD, Hauser MF, Brinkmann BH et al. Subtraction peri-ictal SPECT is predictive of extratemporal epilepsy surgery outcome. Neurology 2000;55:1668–77.
10. Jones Gotman M, Smith ML, Wieser HG. Intra-arterial amobarbital procedures. In: Engel JJ, Pedley TA, editors. Epilepsy: a comprehensive textbook. Philadelphia: Lippincott-Raven, 1998; 1767–75.
11. Spencer SS, Sperling MR, Shewmon DA. Intracranial electrodes. In: Engel J, Pedley TA, editors. Epilepsy: a comprehensive textbook. Philadelphia: Lippincott–Raven, 1997; 1719–47.
12. Wieser HG, Engel J, Williamson PD, Babb TL, Gloor P. Surgically remediable temporal lobe syndromes. In: Engel J, editor. Surgical treatment of the epilepsies. New York: Raven Press, 1993; 49–63.
13. Spencer DD, Spencer SS, Mattson RH, Williamson PD, Novelly RA. Access to the posterior medial temporal structures in the surgical treatment of temporal lobe epilepsy. Neurosurgery 1984;15:667–71.
14. Polkey CE. Amygdalo-hippocampectomy for drug-resistant temporal lobe epilepsy. In: Schmidek HH, Sweet WH, editors. Operative neurosurgical techniques:

indications, methods, results. Philadelphia: Saunders, 2000; 1295–304.
15. Oxbury S, Oxbury J, Renowden S, Squier W, Carpenter K. Severe amnesia: an usual late complication after temporal lobectomy. Neuropsychologia 1997;35: 975–88.
16. Powell GE, Polkey CE, McMillan TM. The new Maudsley series of temporal lobectomy. I: short term cognitive effects. Br J Clin Psychol 1985;24:109–24.
17. Engel J, Van Ness PC, Rasmussen T, Ojemann LM. Outcome with respect to epileptic seizures. In: Engel J, editor. Surgical treatment of the epilepsies. New York: Raven Press, 1993; 609–22.
18. Delalande O, Pinard JM, Basdevant C, Plouin P, Dulac O. Hemispherotomy: a new procedure for hemispheric disconnection [Abstract]. Epilepsia 1993;34 (Suppl. 2): 140.
19. Holthausen H, May TW, Adams CBT, Andermann F, Comair Y, Delalande O et al. Seizures post hemispherectomy. In: Tuxhorn I, Holthausen H, Boenigk H, editors. Paediatric epilpesy syndromes and their surgical treatment. London: John Libbey & Co. Ltd, 1997; 749–73.
20. Anonymous. A global survey on epilepsy surgery, 1980–1990: a report by the Commission on Neurosurgery of Epilepsy, the International League Against Epilepsy. Epilepsia 1997;38:249–55.
21. Roberts DW. Section of the corpus callosum for epilepsy. In: Schmidek HH, Sweet WH, editors. Operative neurosurgical techniques: indications, methods, results. Philadelphia: Saunders, 1995; 1351–8.
22. Morrell F, Whisler WW, Bleck TP. Multiple subpial transection: a new approach to the surgical treatment of focal epilepsy. J Neurosurg 1989;70:231–9.
23. Fisher RS, Mirski M, Krauss GL. Brain stimulation. In: Engel JJ, Pedley TA, editors. Epilepsy: a comprehensive textbook. Philadelphia: Lippincott–Raven, 1997; 1867–75.
24. Binnie CD. Vagus nerve stimulation for epilepsy: a review. Seizure 2000;9:161–9.
25. Germano IM, Poulin N, Olivier A. Reoperation for recurrent temporal lobe epilepsy. J Neurosurg 1994;81: 31–6.
26. Regis J, Bartolomei F, Hayashi M, Roberts D, Chauvel P, Peragut JC. The role of gamma knife surgery in the treatment of severe epilepsies. Epileptic Disord 2000;2: 113–22.
27. Erba G, Cavazutti V. Sturge Weber syndrome: natural history and indications for surgery. J Epilepsy 1990; 3:287–91.
28. Daumas-Duport C, Scheithauer BW, Chodkiewicz J-P, Laws ER, Vedrenne C. Dysembryoplastic neuroepithelial tumor. A surgically curable tumor of young patients with intractable partial seizures: report of thirty-nine cases. Neurosurgery 1988;23:545–56.
29. Rasmussen T, Obozewski J, Lloyd-Smith D. Focal seizures due to chronic localised encephalitis. Neurology 1958;8:435–45.
30. McNamara JO, Andrews PI. Autoimmune epilepsy: aspects of the pathogenesis of Rasmussen's encephalitis. Epilepsia 1995;36 (Suppl. 3):S172.
31. Vickrey BG, Hays RD, Engel J Jr, Spritzer K, Rogers WH, Rausch R et al. Outcome assessment for epilepsy surgery: the impact of measuring health-related quality of life [see comments]. Ann Neurol 1995;37:158–66.
32. Guldvog B, Loyning Y, Hauglie-Hanssen E, Flood S, Bjornaes H. Surgical versus medical treatment for epilepsy. II: outcome related to social areas. Epilepsia 1991;32:477–86.
33. McLachlan RS, Rose KJ, Derry PA, Bonnar C, Blume WT, Girvin JP. Health-related quality of life and seizure control in temporal lobe epilepsy. Ann Neurol 1997;41:482–9.
34. Silfvenius H. The health economics of epilepsy surgery. In: Oxbury J, Polkey CE, Duchowny M, editors. Intractable focal epilepsy. London: Saunders, 2000; 849–64.
35. Pilcher WH, Roberts DW, Flanigin HF, Crandall PH, Wieser HG, Ojemann GA et al. Complications of epilepsy surgery. In: Engel J, editor. Surgical treatment of the epilepsies. New York: Raven Press, 1993; 565–81.

35

Functional Neurosurgery for Movement Disorders

Ali Samii, Anna DePold Hohler and Robert Goodkin

Summary

In this chapter, the authors will provide an overview of movement disorders. It will begin with a review of nomenclature used to describe movement disorders, followed by a discussion of the basal ganglia circuitry. Neurosurgical treatment options for individual movement disorder syndromes will then be addressed.

Terminology Used in Describing Movement Disorders

The term "movement disorder" is used in two contexts: as a physical sign of involuntary movement or abnormal movement and to describe the syndrome that causes the involuntary movement [1].

In order to be able to discuss the different movement disorder syndromes, it is first imperative to define the types of movements that exist. This enables a common language among practitioners.

Tremor is defined as a rhythmic oscillation of a body part by alternating or synchronous contraction of agonist and antagonist muscles. It may be seen at rest or with action. It commonly affects the hands, but it may also involve the head, jaw, voice, tongue or lower limbs. Resting tremor occurs while the limb is not active. The typical resting tremor is the finger and wrist tremor in Parkinson's disease (PD). This is seen while the hand is resting on the patient's lap. Action tremor can be postural (seen during sustained posture, e.g. hands in the outstretched position), intention (during trajectory movement, e.g. finger–nose–finger), or task-specific (seen while performing a specific activity, e.g. only while writing).

Dystonia is an abnormal sustained muscle contraction, causing twisting or turning around one or multiple joints. It may be present in a variety of locations, including the neck (cervical dystonia/torticollis), eyelids (blepharospasm) or vocal cords (spasmodic dysphonia). Dystonia can be focal, segmental or generalized. An example of focal limb dystonia is writer's cramp. In segmental dystonia, an entire limb or trunk is involved. Generalized dystonia is multi-focal, involving several body parts.

Myoclonus is defined as a sudden, brief, shock-like involuntary muscle contraction or inhibition. Positive myoclonus occurs with active muscle contraction, while negative myoclonus causes inhibition of the activated muscle. An example of negative myoclonus is asterixis (brief interruption of muscle contraction in the extended arm and wrist). Myoclonus is classified by the body part involved (focal or multi-focal) and in relation to its etiology (e.g. post-anoxic) or site of origin (cortical or subcortical). Some types of myoclonus are stimulus sensitive or action induced.

Chorea is derived from the Greek word meaning "dance". Chorea consists of complex involuntary movements resembling exaggerated fidgetiness. The movements are usually generalized, purposeless and absent during sleep. Choreoathetosis is the term used when the movements are slow and writhing. In mild cases, the choreatic movements can be blended into natural movements and appear more purposeful.

Ballismus is characterized by large-amplitude, proximal chorea. At times, it can be quite violent. Onset is often sudden and typically related to an infarct in the contralateral subthalamic nucleus. It usually occurs on one side of body, hence the term hemiballismus. Hemiballismus usually evolves into the less violent hemichorea over time.

Tics are temporarily suppressible movements seen in Tourette's syndrome. The frequency and severity of tics are exacerbated after voluntary suppression. This is a rebound effect. Tics can be motor or vocal in nature. Simple motor tics are isolated, brief and sudden movements involving one body part. Complex motor tics may involve more than one body part and may have a component of dystonia or tremor. Complex motor tics may take the form of purposeful movements. A complex motor tic that is an obscene gesture is termed copropraxia. A simple vocal tic may be a grunt or a throat clearing. Complex vocal tics may be more elaborate vocalizations, words or phrases. When the words include profanities, the term coprolalia is used.

Bradykinesia literally means slowness of movement. It is a term used to describe slowness of voluntary movements, such as that seen in PD. The amplitude of fine movements is typically decreased. When there is a lack of movement, the term akinesia is used. Akinesia is frequently used interchangeably with bradykinesia.

Freezing is an arrest of gait and is usually associated with bradykinesia. It may occur during gait initiation, when approaching an obstacle or when attempting to turn. Freezing is a specific gait phenomenon that is often seen with PD.

Dyskinesia means abnormal involuntary movement. It is frequently seen in patients with PD receiving dopaminergic therapy. It is usually in the form of chorea or dystonia. Tardive dyskinesia refers to late-onset dyskinesia, secondary to long-term use of medications. Neuroleptic and anti-emetic medications are the usual culprits of tardive dyskinesia. Tardive dyskinesia and dyskinesia may be seen in PD and are usually in the form of chorea or dystonia.

Akathisia is defined as motor activity that is a result of a voluntary effort to relieve an uncomfortable sensation of inner restlessness. It is often manifested by an inability to remain seated, shifting weight or pacing. Akathisia usually occurs following the administration of neuroleptic medications. It may occur shortly after exposure (acute akathisia) or as a late complication of treatment (tardive akathisia).

Hyperekplexia is an exaggerated startle response to sudden unexpected stimulus. An individual may experience loss of postural control without loss of consciousness. It may be symptomatic or can be inherited as an autosomal-dominant condition.

Basal Ganglia Anatomy and Connections

There has been a significant amount of research involved in attempting to describe the mechanism by which movements, and hence movement disorders, occur. Here, we will briefly describe the most recent understanding of the function of the basal ganglia. It must be emphasized that the model of the basal ganglia circuitry presented here is simplistic (Fig. 35.1). Much work is needed to better elucidate the inconsistencies of this model [2].

The basal ganglia is composed of the striatum (caudate nucleus and putamen), the globus pallidus (internal and external), the substantia nigra (pars compacta and pars reticulata), and the sub-thalamic nucleus. The pedunculopontine nucleus is not traditionally included as a part of the basal ganglia, although it has significant connections with it.

The corpus striatum is composed of the caudate, the putamen and the globus pallidus.

The striatum is made up of the putamen and the caudate nucleus. The lentiform nucleus is made up of the putamen and both segments of the globus pallidus.

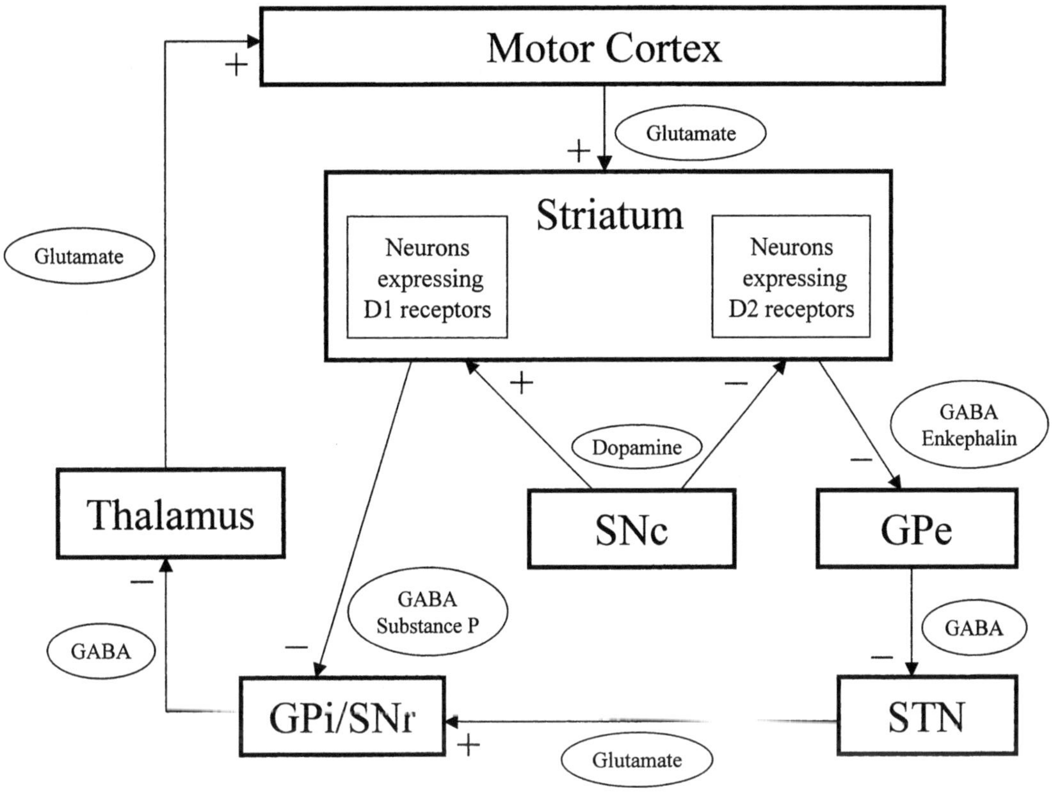

Fig. 35.1. Functional anatomy of the basal ganglia.

The striatum, particularly the putamen, receives excitatory glutamatergic input from the primary and secondary sensorimotor cortices. Medium spiny neurons (MSNs) make up 75% of the neurons in the striatum. Two major pathways, direct and indirect, arise from the MSNs. The population of MSNs rich in D1 dopamine receptors form the direct pathway and project to the globus pallidus internus (Gpi) and substantia nigra pars reticulata (SNr). These neurons co-express gamma-aminobutyric acid (GABA) and substance P. The population of MSNs rich in D2 dopamine receptors form the indirect pathway and project to the globus pallidus externus (Gpe). These neurons co-express GABA and enkephalin.

The GPi and SNr are the sensorimotor output nuclei of the basal ganglia. They have GABAergic projections to ventrolateral (VL), VA and centromedian (CM) nuclei of thalamus. GPi and SNr neurons have high spontaneous discharge rates (60–80 Hz).

The GPe is part of the indirect pathway. It receives input from the striatal MSNs that co-express GABA and enkephalin. The GPe has GABAergic projections mainly to the sub-thalamic nucleus (STN) and receives glutamatergic feedback from the STN. It also has GABAergic projections directly to GPi and SNr.

The STN is part of the indirect pathway. It receives inhibitory input from GPe and excitatory input from cortex. It has glutamatergic excitatory projections to the GPi and SNr.

The substantia nigra pars compacta (SNc) is the origin of the dopaminergic nigrostriatal pathway. Dopamine acts differently on the direct and indirect pathways. Activation of striatal MSNs that project to GPi and SNr (direct pathway) is achieved via activation of D1 receptors in the striatum. Suppression of striatal MSNs that project to GPe (indirect pathway) occurs via activation of D2 receptors in the striatum. The overall effect of dopamine release in the striatum is reduction of GPi and SNr's inhibition of thalamus, which leads to increased activity of excitatory thalamocortical projections. SNc also sends projections to the STN, GPi and SNr.

The pedunculopontine nucleus (PPN) receives mostly inhibitory collaterals from the GPi and SNr as they project to thalamus. It sends excitatory projections back to the GPi and SNr. The PPN also has connections to the STN, brainstem and spinal cord.

The basal ganglia and its connections are responsible for the orderly control of normal movements. As disease processes develop, different components of these circuits are affected. With an understanding of these abnormal circuits, the neurosurgeon can better conceptualize the mechanism behind the surgical interventions now available for the treatment of certain movement disorders.

Movement Disorder Syndromes

Essential Tremor

Essential tremor (ET) is the most common movement disorder. The tremor is present during action and absent at rest. (It may be postural, trajectory or occur while performing a task.) The pathophysiologic mechanism of tremor is not well understood. Mechanical, reflex oscillators and central neuronal pacemakers or circuits (e.g. olivo-cerebellar-thalamic circuit) have all been implicated in various types of tremor.

Essential tremor is more symmetric than the tremor of PD. Rigidity and bradykinesia are not seen with essential tremor. The tremor often involves the upper extremities, head and voice. Unlike PD, there is no significant response to anti-Parkinson medications. A family history is positive in half of patients. In patients with hereditary ET, there is autosomal-dominant inheritance. Men and woman are affected equally. Head tremor is usually mild and of a "no-no" type.

There are a number of surgical options for the treatment of tremor. The target for the treatment of isolated tremor with either ablative surgery or deep brain stimulation is the ventro-intermediate nucleus (VIM) of the thalamus. Unilateral thalamotomy improves contralateral tremor [3]. Bilateral thalamotomy is rarely performed, as it can cause cognitive and gait disturbances [4].

In contrast to ablative surgery, deep brain stimulation (DBS) is reversible and potentially adjustable. The goal of DBS is to render a target non-functional by stimulating it at high frequency. Unilateral thalamic DBS improves contralateral hand tremor. It is used mainly for essential tremor [5,6]. Bilateral thalamic DBS can improve tremor in both hands and in the head. Side effects may include serious cognitive and gait disturbances. The stimulation-related adverse effects of bilateral thalamic DBS may be more reversible than the adverse effects of bilateral thalamotomies.

DBS has several advantages over ablative surgery. It causes less brain trauma, is reversible and can be modified in terms of which of the four stimulation sites is active. Adjustments to the intensity, duration and frequency of the stimulation can also be made. The procedure can also be performed bilaterally. Side effects of the surgical procedure include brain hemorrhage, infarct, seizures and death. Adverse effects exclusive to DBS include the hours required to adjust the settings, lead damage or failure, the need to replace batteries after 3–5 years, the potential for infection and erosion of the device through the skin. Worsening dyskinesia (in the case of STN stimulation), paresthesias and subtle cognitive and mood changes have also been reported. Some of these side effects may be reversible by adjusting stimulation parameters, but hardware failure requires removal or replacement of parts or the entire device.

PD

The four cardinal features of PD are tremor, bradykinesia, rigidity and postural instability. Parkinsonism is a non-specific term, used to describe a constellation of signs on physical examination similar to those seen in PD. PD is defined as asymmetric Parkinsonism with no known cause, characterized by most of the four cardinal features and responsive to anti-Parkinson medications.

Tremor is typically the first symptom in PD patients. The tremor may result from dopamine loss unmasking pacemaker properties in the basal ganglia. The tremor is 3–5 Hz, with varying amplitude, described as pill rolling and seen at rest. Initially, it is distal more than proximal and may be intermittent. It is almost always asymmetric. It worsens with anxiety, contralateral motor tasks and during ambulation.

Bradykinesia and rigidity are believed to be due to the overactivity of the GPi and SNr. This leads to excessive inhibition of thalamus. The same symptoms may occur with overactivity of the STN. There is reduced activation of cortical areas by excitatory thalamocortical projections. In PD, there is a loss of dopaminergic input to the striatum. This leads to increased activation of the indirect pathway and decreased activation of the direct pathway. Rigidity is defined as an increased resistance to passive movement of joints. It may have a lead pipe or cogwheel quality and is also asymmetric.

Postural instability and gait abnormalities are the least specific cardinal features of PD. There is often loss of arm swing on one or both sides, neck and trunk flexion and shortened stride length. Gait is described as shuffling and there is an inability to turn quickly. Freezing may be seen in more advanced disease. Patients have an impaired ability to recover when pulled from behind.

Exclusion criteria for PD include exposure to drugs known to cause parkinsonism, such as neuroleptics and some anti-emetic medications. The presence of cerebellar deficits, corticospinal tract signs and oculomotor deficits, other than slight limitation of upward gaze, are also exclusion criteria. Finally, autonomic impairment independent of anti-Parkinson medications, early moderate to severe postural instability and early dementia also suggest an alternative diagnosis [7].

Surgical Options for Treatment of PD

There are several surgical options for treatment of PD. Ablative surgical procedures or DBS targeting the thalamus, globus pallidus or the sub-thalamic nucleus are currently available. Transplantation surgery for PD remains investigational. Thalamotomy is typically reserved for patients with isolated tremor, as this procedure has less impact on the rigidity and dyskinesias seen with PD [4].

Pallidotomy and sub-thalamotomy serve to decrease the tremor, rigidity and dyskinesias seen with PD. The target for pallidotomy is the postero–ventro–lateral portion of the globus pallidus. Unilateral pallidotomy mostly improves contralateral tremor and dyskinesia [8]. These results are sustained in 4-year follow-up studies [9]. These results are only seen in patients who are levodopa responders. As with all surgical interventions, there are risks. Surgical side effects include hemorrhage, infarct, aphonia, cognitive and gait disturbances. The side effects are increased for bilateral pallidotomies. Therefore, they are not typically recommended [10].

Sub-thalamotomy improves most of the contralateral motor symptoms of PD. Bilateral sub-thalamotomy also helps to reduce anti-PD medications. Rare but significant side effects of the surgery are irreversible ballism and chorea. This procedure is not done in the USA because of these potentially dangerous side effects.

DBS has several advantages over ablative surgery. It causes less brain trauma, is reversible and can be modified in terms of which of the four stimulation sites is active. Adjustments to the intensity, duration and frequency of the stimulation can also be made. The procedure can also be performed bilaterally. Side effects of the surgical procedure include brain hemorrhage, infarct, seizures and death. Adverse effects exclusive to DBS include the hours required to adjust the settings, lead damage or failure, the need to replace batteries after 3–5 years, the potential for infection and erosion of the device through the skin. Worsening dyskinesia (in case of STN stimulation), paresthesias and subtle cognitive and mood changes have also been reported. Some of these side effects may be reversible by adjusting stimulation parameters, but hardware failure requires removal or replacement of parts or the entire device.

Thalamic DBS, much like thalamotomy, is effective in reducing contralateral PD tremor [11]. As with thalamotomy, the dyskinesias seen with late-stage PD are not significantly improved. For this reason, PD patients are now typically recommended for globus pallidus or sub-thalamic surgical intervention. Unilateral thalamic DBS can also be performed on a patient who has already had a contralateral thalamotomy.

Similar to ablative surgery, the target for pallidal DBS is the GPi. However, the surgery is done bilaterally, which is an advantage over pallidotomy. With DBS there are fewer adverse effects than with bilateral pallidotomies. Bilateral GPi stimulation improves tremor, rigidity and dyskinesia. The benefit in tremor and bradykinesia is seen in the levodopa "off" state. There has been a trend toward improvement in the levodopa "on" state as well, mostly with reduction in dyskinesia [12]. Bilateral GPi stimulation usually does not allow a reduction in the overall dosages of anti-Parkinson medications. Unilateral pallidal DBS has been performed after contralateral pallidotomy in a few PD patients with positive results [13].

Sub-thalamic nucleus DBS is usually performed bilaterally and has shown improvement in levodopa "off" states [14]. Another advantage is that anti-PD medications are often reduced after the procedure. Some patients are even able to get off levodopa altogether [15]. The effects of the procedure appear to be present at 2-year follow-up assessment. Most of the motor symptoms of PD are improved by bilateral STN stimulation. Levodopa non-responders do not appear to respond to this procedure. Reported side effects include cognitive, speech and language deficits, eyelid-opening apraxia, confusion and hallucinations. Bilateral STN stimulation may be superior to bilateral GPi stimulation in PD patients [16], but the debate about the optimal stimulation target for PD continues. A large, randomized multicenter study comparing bilateral STN and bilateral GPi stimulation is currently under way.

Various combinations of different stereotactic neurosurgical procedures for advanced PD have been reported. Merello reported on the lack of efficacy of unilateral STN stimulation contralateral to a previous pallidotomy [17]. Moro et al. reported a patient who benefited from bilateral STN stimulation after unilateral pallidotomy and unilateral thalamotomy [18]. Houeto et al. reported on two patients in whom bilateral GPi stimulation failed to provide long-term improvement [19]. The GPi electrodes were then removed and bilateral STN electrodes were implanted, with improvement that was superior to that of bilateral GPi stimulation. Several patients have undergone bilateral STN stimulation after unilateral pallidotomy [20]. One patient has undergone bilateral STN stimulation after bilateral pallidotomies with no added benefit from DBS [21]. In summary, the efficacy of DBS after ablative surgery must be further studied.

Appropriate patient selection is extremely important for achieving a positive outcome from stereotactic surgery. Strict inclusion and exclusion criteria must be used. A recent large multicenter study by The Deep Brain Stimulation For PD Study Group [22] used specific criteria. These criteria included "a good response to levodopa". Table 35.1 summarizes basic guidelines for inclusion and exclusion criteria. Each patient must be considered individually.

Table 35.1. Basic guidelines for inclusion and exclusion criteria.

Patient inclusion criteria include:

1. Clinically definite PD.
2. Hoehn and Yahr stage 2–4 (patient should be ambulatory independently).
3. L-dopa responsive with clearly defined "on" periods (i.e. symptoms improve at least partially with L-dopa administration).
4. Persistent disabling symptoms (e.g. dyskinesias, motor fluctuations, disabling "off" periods of several hours per day), despite optimal medication therapy.
5. Age 20–80 years.

Patient exclusion criteria include:

1. "Parkinson's plus" syndromes, atypical parkinsonism or secondary parkinsonism (e.g. progressive supranuclear palsy, striato–nigral degeneration, multiple system atrophy, vascular parkinsonism and drug-induced parkinsonism).
2. Medical contraindications to surgery or stimulation (serious co-morbid medical conditions, chronic anticoagulation, pregnancy, etc.).
3. Contraindication to MRI (e.g. in-dwelling metal fragments or implants that might be affected by MRI).
4. Dementia or other active neuropsychiatric dysfunction (untreated depression, psychosis, etc.).
5. Intracranial abnormalities that would contraindicate surgery (e.g. stroke, tumor, vascular abnormality affecting the target area).

The goal of transplantation is to replace neuronal tissue lost to the neurodegenerative process of PD. Initial trials involved transplantation of the adrenal medulla. The initial positive results were short-lived and this procedure was abandoned. Dopaminergic transplant, in the form of fetal mesencephalic tissue, has been used. It is felt that neurotropic factors secreted by the implanted cells may contribute to the benefits seen with transplant [23]. Moderate or marked improvement was reported in these patients, although none had resolution of their PD symptoms. Graft survival is evident on PET scanning and on autopsy [24]. A side effect of the transplant seen in 15% of the patients is severe and disabling dyskinesias. In a randomized sham surgery-controlled study, there was some improvement in the medication-off state in younger patients, but disabling dyskinesia was again problematic [25]. Additional research is ongoing. Stem cell transplant is a current area of much interest. It is hoped that research will eventually enable cells from a patient to be de-differentiated into stem cells and then re-differentiated into dopamine-producing cells to be implanted in PD patients.

Wilson's Disease (WD)

WD is an autosomal-recessive disorder of copper metabolism. The term "hepatolenticular degeneration" is also used, as it affects the liver and causes movement disorders related to changes in the basal ganglia. The primary problem is a defect in copper metabolism, causing its build-up in the liver, brain and eye. Numerous cognitive, psychiatric and movement disorders may be seen with this disease. The neurologic manifestations include tremor (typically, a proximal or "wing beating tremor"), dystonia, dysmetria, dysrhythmia, ataxia and dysarthria. Testing for WD involves assessment of liver function, ceruloplasmin, serum and urine copper. Liver function abnormalities in the face of low ceruloplasmin and high urinary copper levels should prompt a diagnosis. Slit-lamp examination may reveal Kayser–Fleischer rings and MRI often shows abnormal T2 signal in the basal ganglia. It is important to be able to recognize this syndrome, as treatment is available. The typical patient presents in early or middle adulthood with hepatic, psychiatric and/or neurologic symptoms. The psychiatric or neurologic symptoms may rarely precede the diagnosis of hepatic dysfunction. Medical therapies include reducing copper in the diet, treatment with zinc, penicillamine or trientine. Liver transplantation also provides symptomatic benefit. Thalamotomy has been used in these patients, although, because of the progressive nature of the disease and the availability of medical options, it is rarely performed.

Huntington's Disease (HD)

HD is an autosomal-dominant inherited disorder, localized to the short arm of chromosome 4. It is characterized by a CAG trinucleotide repeat. Children of affected individuals that also express the gene show anticipation. Anticipation is an expansion of the trinucleotide repeat, resulting in earlier onset and more severe symptoms. Huntington's disease typically manifests in the third and fourth decades and is characterized by movement disorders and cognitive decline. Depression and high rates of suicide are also noted. The movement disorders can be varied, although most patients manifest with chorea.

Chorea, as seen in HD, is thought to result from loss of striatal projection neurons to the GPe. In early HD, there is reduced inhibition of GPe and increased inhibition of the STN. There is reduced inhibitory output from the GPi and SNr to the thalamus. In more advanced HD, striatal projections to the GPi also degenerate, causing reduced chorea and development of bradykinesia.

Pallidotomy has been attempted in HD with dystonia [26]. Although there was some symptomatic improvement, the background of dementia and the underlying progression of the disease make this a short-term solution. Surgical treatment with transplantation has been studied in a small number of patients [27]. Motor and cognitive functions were improved in three out of five patients who underwent bilateral fetal neuroblast transplantation in the striatum. Further work is needed in this area.

Dystonia

Dystonia is a symptom that may be seen as part of a variety of disorders. Dystonic contractions are often aggravated by purposeful actions and may be task specific. Dystonia is often worsened by stress. Dystonia may be classified according to age of onset, distribution or by etiology. Most recently, with the discovery of certain genes linked to types of dystonia, the classification is occasionally based on these genetics. Dystonia can be divided by this classification into primary, dystonia plus, secondary and heredodegenerative.

In primary dystonia, dystonia is the most pronounced symptom and no underlying injury or disease can be identified. The sporadic and many of the genetic dystonias fall into this category. In dystonia plus, patients have other symptoms such as tremor, myoclonus or parkinsonism associated with their dystonia. The disorders of dopamine synthesis are in this category, but not the neurodegenerative diseases. Secondary dystonia includes dystonia caused by a wide variety of insults to the CNS, including stroke and trauma to the brain, neck or limbs. In heredodegenerative dystonia, the dystonia occurs in conjunction with a progressive neurological disorder such as PD, MSA, WD or mitochondrial disorders.

Primary dystonia can be further divided into sporadic primary dystonia and genetic primary dystonia. Sporadic primary dystonia includes common forms of focal dystonia and is the most common type of dystonia encountered. Torticollis, blepharospasm, isolated hand and foot dystonias and task-specific dystonias would fall into this category. This is a diagnosis of exclusion. There are numerous genetically localized dystonia syndromes. These are subclassified into DYT categories.

Secondary dystonia can be related to a number of cerebral or peripheral insults. In evaluating a patient with dystonia, it is important to identify any possible underlying abnormalities, particularly ones that may be treatable. Secondary dystonias occur, related to perinatal cerebral injury, congenital malformations, central and peripheral nervous system insults or injuries, infections, inflammatory processes, paraneoplastic syndromes, drug or toxin exposure and metabolic disorders. Tardive dystonia results from exposure to neuroleptics. It may best be avoided by the use of low doses and slow increases of these medications.

There are a variety of treatments available for dystonia. Patients in whom a primary dystonia is identified or in whom there is a dystonia–parkinsonian syndrome should have a trial of levodopa. These dystonias are typically generalized and often present in childhood. Pharmacologic interventions for generalized dystonia include discontinuation of the offending agent (e.g. neuroleptic) and use of anti-cholinergic agents, benzodiazepines, muscle relaxants, anticonvulsants and clozapine. Other medical options for the treatment of severe generalized dystonia include intrathecal baclofen and tetrabenazine. Pallidotomy is superior to thalamotomy in relieving dystonia [28]. Now, bilateral pallidal DBS is being performed for severe cases of generalized dystonia, especially those associated with the DYT1 gene abnormality [29].

Myoclonus

Myoclonus can be classified according to its site of origin. It is also useful to sub-divide myoclonus according to its etiology. Physiologic myoclonus occurs in normal subjects and includes sleep jerks and anxiety- or exercise-induced myoclonus. Essential myoclonus is a category of myoclonus for which there is no known cause and no other gross neurologic deficit. There is a hereditary form and a sporadic form. In epileptic myoclonus, seizures dominate and, initially, there is no encephalopathy. Myoclonus can be related to fragments of epilepsy or it can manifest as childhood myoclonic epilepsy or benign familial myoclonic epilepsy. Finally, symptomatic myoclonus is a category that includes myoclonus, where a progressive or static encephalopathy dominates. Symptomatic forms of myoclonus include vascular, infectious, traumatic, autoimmune-related, metabolic, toxin-related, hereditary mitochondrial and storage diseases, and paraneoplastic etiologies.

Cortical, subcortical and spinal (including propriospinal) types of myoclonus are described. In cortical myoclonus, the abnormal activity originates in the sensorimotor cortex and is transmitted down the spinal cord via the pyramidal tract. Cortical myoclonus is thus a fragment of epilepsy.

Treatment of myoclonus is based on reversing the underlying pathology, as appropriate, and treating based on the localization of the myoclonus. If the myoclonus is related to an epileptic syndrome, anticonvulsant therapy is used. Valproic acid, clonazepam and primidone are often used in combination. The use of several anticonvulsants acting on different sites has also been advocated. Negative myoclonus (asterixis) does not appear to respond effectively to medical therapy. Stereotactic thalamotomy has been used in the past to treat myoclonus. Recently, thalamic stimulation has been successful in treating hereditary myoclonus [30]. Neurosurgical treatment of myoclonus has not been well studied.

Key Points

- *Neurosurgical options for essential tremor include thalamotomy and thalamic deep brain stimulation.*
- *Targets for lesioning or deep brain stimulation in PD include the thalamus, globus pallidus and sub-thalamic nucleus.*
- *Neurosurgical intervention is helpful for some types of dystonia and myoclonus.*
- *WD and HD have not shown a substantial response to surgical intervention.*

References

1. Kishore A, Calne DB. Approach to the patient with a movement disorder and overview of movement disorders. In: Watts RL, Koller W, editors. Movement disorders: neurologic principles and practice. New York: McGraw-Hill, 1997; 3–14.
2. Wichman T, DeLong M. Functional and pathophysio logical models of the basal ganglia. Curr Opin Neurobiol 1996;6:751–8.
3. Goldman MS, Kelly PJ. Stereotactic thalamotomy for medically intractable essential tremor. Stereotact Funct Neurosurg 1992;58:22–5.
4. Tasker RR. Thalamotomy for Parkinson's disease and other types of tremor. In: Tasker R, Gildenberg PL, editors. Textbook of stereotactic and functional neurosurgery. New York: McGraw-Hill, 1998; 1179–98.
5. Koller W, Pahwa R, Busenbark K, Hubble J, Wilkinson S, Lang A et al. High-frequency unilateral thalamic stimulation in the treatment of essential and parkinsonian tremor. Ann Neurol 1997;42:292–9.
6. Benabid AL, Pollak P, Seigneuret E, Hoffmann D, Gay E, Perret J. Chronic VIM thalamic stimulation in Parkinson's disease, essential tremor and extrapyramidal dyskinesias. Acta Neurochir Suppl 1993;53:39–44.
7. Gelb DJ, Oliver E, Gilman S. Diagnostic criteria for Parkinson Disease. Arch Neurol 1999;56:33–9.
8. Samii A, Turnbull IM, Kishore A, Schulzer M, Mak E, Yardley SE et al. Reassessment of unilateral pallidotomy in the treatment of Parkinson's disease: a two year follow-up study. Brain 1999;122:417–25.
9. Fine J, Duff J, Chen RM. Long-term follow-up of unilateral pallidotomy in advanced Parkinson's disease. N Engl J Med 2000;342:1708–14.
10. Hallett M, Litvan I. Scientific position paper of the Movement Disorder Society evaluation of surgery for Parkinson's disease. Task Force on Surgery for Parkinson's Disease of the American Academy of Neurology Therapeutic and Technology Assessment Committee. Mov Disord 2000;15:436–8.
11. Schuurman PR, Bosch DA, Bossuyt PM, Bonsel GJ, van Someren EJ, de Bie RM et al. A comparison of continuous thalamic stimulation and thalamotomy for suppression of severe tremor. N Engl J Med 2000;342:461–8.
12. Burchiel KJ, Anderson VC, Favre J, Hammerstad JP. Comparison of pallidal and subthalamic nucleus deep brain stimulation for advanced Parkinson's disease: results of a randomized, blinded pilot study. Neurosurgery 1999;45:1375–82.
13. Galvez-Jimenez N, Lozano A, Tasker R, Duff J, Hutchison W, Lang AE. Pallidal stimulation in Parkinson's disease patients with a prior unilateral pallidotomy. Can J Neurol Sci 1998;25:300–5.
14. Limousin P, Krack P, Pollak P, Benazzouz A, Ardouin C, Hoffmann D et al. Electrical stimulation of the subthalamic nucleus in advanced Parkinson's disease. N Engl J Med 1998;339:1105–11.
15. Moro E, Scerrati M, Romito LM, Roselli R, Tonali P, Albanese A. Chronic subthalamic nucleus stimulation reduces medication requirements in Parkinson's disease. Neurology 1999;53:85–90.
16. Krack P, Pollak P, Limousin P. Subthalamic nucleus or internal pallidal stimulation in young onset Parkinson's disease. Brain 1998;121:451–7.
17. Merello M. Subthalamic stimulation contralateral to a previous pallidotomy: an erroneous indication? Mov Disord 1999;14:890.
18. Moro E, Esselink RA, Van Blercom N, Caputo E, Pollak P, Limousin P et al. Bilateral subthalamic nucleus stimulation in a parkinsonian patient with previous unilateral pallidotomy and thalamotomy. Mov Disord 2000;15:753–5.
19. Houeto JL, Bejjani PB, Damier P, Staedler C, Bonnet AM, Pidoux B et al. Failure of long-term pallidal stimulation corrected by subthalamic stimulation in PD. Neurology 2000;55:728–30.
20. Mogilner AY, Sterio D, Rezai AR, Zonenshayn M, Kelly PJ, Beric A. Subthalamic nucleus stimulation in patients with a prior pallidotomy. J Neurosurg 2002;96:660–5.
21. Samii A, Giroux ML, Slimp JC, Goodkin R. Bilateral subthalamic nucleus stimulation after bilateral pallidotomies in a patient with advanced Parkinson's disease. Parkinsonism and Related Disorders 2003;9(3):159–62.
22. The Deep-Brain Stimulation for Parkinson's Disease Study Group. Deep-brain stimulation of the subthalamic nucleus or the pars interna of the globus pallidus in Parkinson's disease. N Engl J Med 2001;345:956–63.
23. Ahlskog JE. Cerebral transplantation for Pakinson's disease: current progress and future prospects. Mayo Clin Proc 1993;68:578–91.
24. Freed CR, Breeze RE, Rosenberg NL, Schneck SA, Kriek E, Qi JX et al. Survival of implanted fetal dopamine cells and neurologic improvement 12 to 46 months after transplantation for Parkinson's disease. N Engl J Med 1992;327:1549–55.
25. Freed CR, Greene PE, Breeze RE, Tsai WY, DuMouchel W, Kao R et al. Transplantation of embryonic dopamine neurons for severe Parkinson's disease. N Engl J Med 2001;344:710–19.

26. Cubo E, Shannon KM, Penn RD, Kroin JS. Internal globus pallidotomy in dystonia secondary to Huntington's disease. Mov Disord 2000;15:1248–51.
27. Bachoud-Levi AC, Remy P, Nguyen JP, Brugieres P, Lefaucheur JP, Bourdet C et al. Motor and cognitive improvements in patients with Huntington's disease after neural transplantation. Lancet 2000;356:1975–9.
28. Yoshor D, Hamilton WJ, Ondo W, Jankovic J, Grossman RG. Comparison of thalamotomy and pallidotomy for the treatment of dystonia. Neurosurgery 2001;48: 818–26.
29. Krack P, Vercueil L. Review of the functional surgical treatment of dystonia. Eur J Neurol 2001;8:389–99.
30. Kupsch A, Trottenberg T, Meissner W, Funk T. Neurostimulation of the ventral intermediate thalamic nucleus alleviates hereditary essential myoclonus. J Neurol Neurosurg Psychiatry 1999;67:415–6.

XII
Infection

36

Infections in the Central Nervous System

Joseph R. Zunt

Summary

This chapter will review the epidemiology, clinical presentation, recommended evaluation and treatment of Central Nervous System (CNS) infections associated with HIV infection and Neurocysticercosis (NCC). HIV infection is frequently complicated by opportunistic infection or neoplasm of the CNS. NCC, a parasitic infection of the CNS, is the most common cause of epilepsy in the developing world and may present clinically as obstructive hydrocephalus. Most opportunistic CNS infections and neoplasms are associated with headache, fever, meningismus, altered level of consciousness, or focal neurologic deficit. NCC is diagnosed by neuroimaging and serologic testing. Treatment of these CNS infections is mainly medical, but can include surgery for diagnostic purposes and surgical removal of lesions.

Introduction

HIV infection is frequently complicated by opportunistic infection or neoplasm of the CNS. Neurocysticercosis (NCC), a parasitic infection of the CNS, is the most common cause of epilepsy in the developing world and may present clinically as obstructive hydrocephalus. Stereotactic brain biopsy is at times necessary to determine or confirm the etiology of an HIV-associated CNS lesion or NCC. Ventricular shunting is occasionally required to relieve obstructive hydrocephalus associated with NCC. This chapter will review the epidemiology, clinical presentation, recommended evaluation and treatment of CNS infections associated with HIV infection and NCC.

HIV infection

Epidemiology

Neurologic illness affecting the peripheral or CNS occurs in 40–60% of HIV-infected people [1]. The most common opportunistic CNS infections and neoplasms associated with HIV infection are Toxoplasma encephalitis (TE), cryptococcal meningitis, primary CNS lymphoma (PCNSL), progressive multifocal leukoencephalopathy (PML), HIV-associated dementia and cytomegalovirus (CMV) encephalitis [2]. Focal brain lesions occur in up to 17% of people with AIDS and are most often due to TE, PML or PCNSL [3]. The incidence of CNS disorders appears to be declining since the introduction of potent antiretroviral therapy (previously called highly active antiretroviral therapy or HAART) [4].

A low absolute CD4 count is the most important risk factor for the development of an opportunistic CNS infection or neoplasm.

Cryptococcal meningitis, TE, PML, PCNSL, HIV-associated dementia and CMV encephalitis are uncommon if the CD4 count is greater than 200 cells/mm3. The incidence of each of these infections increases as the CD4 count drops from 200 to 100 cells/mm3 or less [2].

Clinical Presentation

Most opportunistic CNS infections and neoplasms are associated with headache, fever, meningismus, altered level of consciousness or focal neurologic deficit. The presence of one or more of these symptoms should alert the medical care provider to the possibility of CNS disease. Clinical and radiologic features of a CNS lesion may distinguish between the various opportunistic infections and neoplasms (Table 36.1).

Reactivation of previously acquired infection is responsible for the majority of opportunistic CNS infections and neoplasms. In the USA, 10–40% of people with AIDS are latently infected with *Toxoplasma gondii*, as determined by presence of serum anti-toxoplasma immunoglobulin G (IgG) antibodies. In France, the seroprevalence of anti-toxo IgG in people with AIDS is 80%. One-third of people with serum anti-toxo IgG antibodies will develop TE. The absence of serum anti-toxo IgG or IgM antibodies does not exclude the diagnosis of TE, as 22% of people with biopsy-confirmed TE do not have IgG antibodies and immunoglobulin M (IgM) antibodies are rarely present [5]. The incidence of TE is reduced in people who take TMP/SMX or dapsone/pyrimethamine as prophylaxis against pneumocystis carinii pneumonia (PCP).

Cryptococcus neoformans is a ubiquitous yeast that causes meningitis in 7% of people with AIDS living in the USA and 30% of those living in Africa. Cryptococcal polysaccharide capsular antigen (CrAg) is detectable in 99% of serum samples and 91% of CSF samples of people with cryptococcal meningitis [6]. Thus, a negative serum CrAg virtually excludes the diagnosis of cryptococcal meningitis.

Reactivation of latent Epstein-Barr virus (EBV) infection is associated with PCNSL and can be detected by polymerase chain reaction (PCR) assay in CSF of up to 100% of patients with PCNSL [7]. Reactivation of latent Jacob-Creutzfeldt (JC) virus infection is associated with PML and can be detected in the CSF of 92% of patients with PML [8]. The majority of people in the USA have serum antibodies against EBV and JC. Presence of antibodies against either EBV or JC in the serum is not associated with increased incidence of PCNSL or PML.

Recommended Evaluation

Evaluation of a focal CNS lesion in a person with AIDS should be guided by the following factors: CD4 count, serologic status to *T. gondii* and *C. neoformans*, findings on neurologic examination and presence or absence of headache or fever [9].

Opportunistic CNS infection or neoplasm is unlikely if the CD4 count is greater than 200 cells/ml. The differential diagnosis of CNS mass lesion in this setting should include bacterial or mycobacterial abcess, syphilitic gumma and stroke. People with an absolute CD4 count of less than 200 cells/ml are at risk for developing TE, cryptococcal meningitis or other opportunistic infection or neoplasm. If serum CrAg is negative, cryptococcal meningitis is unlikely. Fever is often present in patients with TE but serum anti-Toxo IgG may be negative in up to one-fifth of patients.

If a headache or focal neurologic deficit is present, evaluation should include neuroimaging with CT or MRI with and without administration of an intravenous contrast agent. Characteristic lesion location and contrast enhancement pattern can determine which infection or neoplasm is most likely (Table 36.2). If a solitary ring-enhancing mass lesion is present, lumbar puncture may help differentiate between TE and PCNSL (Fig. 36.1). Opportunistic infections most often associated with normal neurologic examination (a "non-focal" exam) include HIV-associated dementia, PML, cryptococcal meningitis and cytomegalovirus (CMV) ventriculitis. Bacterial or viral meningitis may occur at any stage of HIV infection and is typically accompanied by fever.

Invasive Diagnostic Tests

Lumbar puncture (LP) should be considered in any person presenting with new-onset headache or fever. If the patient is obtunded or comatose, or a focal deficit neurologic deficit is present, neuroimaging should be performed prior to LP. If a space-occupying CNS lesion is present in the posterior fossa or causes midline shift, LP

Table 36.1. Distinguishing features of neurologic disorders associated with HIV infection.

Etiology	CD_4 count (cells/mm^3)	Common clinical features	Neuroimaging findings by MRI or CT	Diagnosis
Fungal infections				
Cryptococcal meningitis	<200	Fever; bilateral headache; altered mental status; meningeal signs (photophobia, nuchal rigidity)	Normal; meningeal enhancement or enhancing lesion (cryptococcoma) may be present	Presence of cryptococcal polysaccharide capsular antigen (CrAg) in serum and CSF; positive CSF culture of *C. neoformans*; positive CSF india ink test
Parasitic infections				
Toxoplasma encephalitis	<200	Fever; unilateral or bilateral headache; altered mental status; seizures; focal neurologic deficit: hemiparesis, ataxia, facial weakness	Solitary or multiple ring-enhancing lesions located in the basal ganglia, deep white matter or hemispheric gray–white junction; MR more sensitive than CT and may detect more lesions	Serum anti-Toxoplasma IgG antibody usually present; definitive diagnosis by identification of trophozoiites on brain biopsy, but presumptive diagnosis by radiologic and clinical improvement after 10–14 days of anti-Toxoplasma therapy
Viral infections				
Progressive multi-focal leukoencephalopathy (JC virus)	<100	Unilateral or bilateral headache; visual field deficit; sub-acute onset of hemiparesis or other focal neurologic deficit; seizures	Solitary or multiple non-enhancing white matter lesions on CT or MRI; lesions most often in parieto–occipital region; on MRI, lesions hypointense on T1-weighted imaging and hyperintense on T2-weighted imaging	CSF–PCR for JC virus is sensitive and specific; brain biopsy
Primary CNS lymphoma (Epstein–Barr virus)	<100	Unilateral or bilateral headache; focal neurologic deficit; seizures	Solitary or multiple ring- or homogeneously enhancing lesions; may see nodular ventricular lesions or lesions that cross the midline	CSF–PCR for Epstein–Barr virus is sensitive and specific; brain biopsy
HIV-associated dementia	<200	Impaired memory and concentration; psychomotor slowing; apathy or withdrawal	Atrophy; on CT, diffuse white matter hypodensity; on MRI, white matter hyperintense on T2-weighted imaging; no contrast-enhancing lesions	Clinical diagnosis; CSF β_2 microglobulin > 3.8 mg/l specific, but not sensitive

Table 36.2. Characteristic findings of certain CNS infections and neoplasms with CT or MRI.

Finding on neuroimaging	Most common etiologies	Less common etiologies
Mass lesion with ring enhancement	Toxoplasma encephalitis Primary CNS lympoma Bacterial abscess	Cryptococcoma Mycobacterial or fungal abscess Kaposi's sarcoma Metastatic or primary malignancy
Non-enhancing lesion in white matter	Progressive multi-focal leukoencephalopathy	Multiple sclerosis Stroke
Meningeal enhancement	Herpes simplex virus Varicella zoster virus Bacteria	Atypical bacteria
Ventricular enhancement	Cytomegalovirus	Primary CNS lymphoma

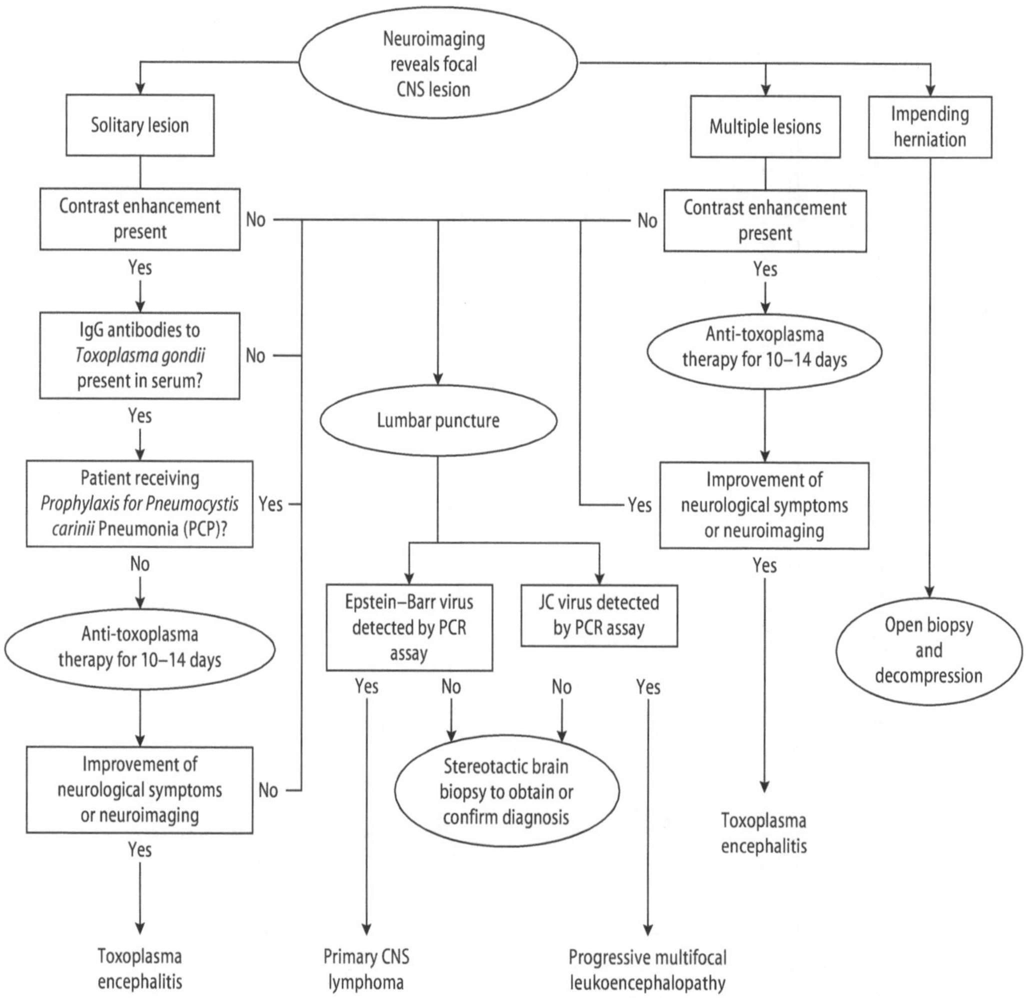

Fig. 36.1. Diagnostic algorithm for HIV-infected patient with neurologic deficit.

should not be performed as CNS herniation could result. Testing of CSF should include cell count with differential, glucose, protein, bacterial culture and VDRL. Other tests that should be considered include fungal cultures, CrAg (if serologic test results not available) and PCR assays. If PCNSL, PML, CMV ventriculitis or HSV encephalitis is suspected, PCR assay for the associated viral pathogen should be requested. The sensitivity and specificity of most PCR assays are high (Table 36.3).

Brain Biopsy

Toxoplasma encephalitis and PCNSL are the most common causes of CNS lesions in patients with AIDS. The differential diagnosis also includes fungal or atypical bacterial abscess, cryptococcoma, syphilitic gumma, tuberculoma, cerebrovascular disease and neoplasm other than PCNSL [10]. Stereotactic brain biopsy (SBB) of a CNS lesion may be necessary under certain clinical scenarios: if a solitary CNS lesion is accompanied by negative toxoplasmosis serology; if a contrast-enhancing lesion is atypical for TE or does not respond to anti-toxoplasma treatment; if a new lesion develops during anti-toxoplasma maintenance treatment; or if histopathologic diagnosis is required for entry into an experimental treatment protocol [9]. If CNS herniation is imminent, open biopsy and decompression should be considered, unless the patient is terminal or has previously requested no intervention. Stereotactic brain biopsy provides a diagnosis for 88–98% of contrast-enhancing lesions and 67% of non-enhancing lesions [10]. Studies that examined the effect of SBB upon treatment and outcome of CNS disease noted that biopsy results did influence treatment [11,12]. In addition, life expectancy was increased in patients who underwent SBB when compared to patients who did not undergo SBB.

Complications of SBB occur in 3–12% of patients with HIV infection and are most often associated with hemorrhage, but may also include neurologic deficit, seizures or infection. Mortality occurred in 2–8% of patients [10]. These rates are slightly higher than those associated with stereotactic biopsy in people without HIV infection.

Treatment

Most HIV-associated CNS infections are treatable. Toxoplasma encephalitis and cryptococcal meningitis require lifelong treatment. Treatment options and duration of therapy for the more common CNS infections are listed in Table 36.4.

NCC

NCC is a frequent cause of epilepsy in developing countries [13]. Ingestion of *Taenia solium* cysts, most often by fecal–oral transmission, results in NCC, while ingestion of *T. solium* tapeworms in undercooked pork results in taeniasis, but not infection of the CNS. Treatment of NCC with anthelmintics such as praziquantel and albendazole, with or without steroids, is controversial. If NCC occurs in the ventricular system or spinal cord, surgical extirpation may be necessary to relieve hydrocephalus or cord compression.

Epidemiology

T. solium infection is endemic throughout South and Central America. Seroprevalence rates range between 5 and 11% in Mexico, Perú and Ecuador [14]. In Brazil, the seroprevalence of antibodies to *T. solium* is 0.7–5.2%, with the highest rates in rural areas. In other parts of the world, seroprevalence rates vary from 13% in Bali to 4% in Korea and 18% in Madagascar.

Table 36.3. Sensitivity and specificity of PCR assays for selected opportunistic CNS infections.

Virus	Associated syndrome	Sensitivity (%)	Specificity (%)
Epstein–Barr virus	Primary CNS lymphoma	97	100
JC virus	Progressive multi-focal leukoencephalopathy	74–92	92–96
Cytomegalovirus	CMV ventriculitis and polyradiculopathy	80–100	75–100
Varicella zoster virus	VZV encephalitis and zoster	Unknown	100
Herpes simplex virus type 1	HSV encephalitis	<95	100

Table 36.4. Medical therapy of selected HIV-associated CNS infections.

Infection	Therapy	Dose and duration	Comment
Cryptococcal meningitis	Amphotericin B	0.6–0.8 mg/kg/day IV for 14 days, or until headache, fever, nausea and vomiting resolved	Initial therapy with fluconazole associated with delayed sterilization of CSF and more early deaths. For increased intracranial pressure, repeat lumbar punctures one to four times daily, with removal of 15–30 ml of CSF each time, until opening pressure consistently normal
	And		
	flucytosine (5-FC)	75–100 mg/kg/day PO	Flucytosine should be used concurrently with amphotericin B; may cause marrow suppression or leukopenia
	then		
	fluconazole	400 mg/day until CSF culture negative, then decrease to 200 mg/day and continue for life	Lumbar puncture should be repeated after amphotericin B, then every 2–4 weeks, or sooner if clinical deterioration occurs. Once CSF culture negative, fluconazole should be started. CSF CrAg can persist positive, even if culture negative, and should not guide therapy. If CSF CrAg titer rises above initial titer, repeat treatment with amphotericin B
Toxoplasma encephalitis	Pyrimethamine	100–200 mg load, then 75–100 mg/day PO	Alternatives to sulfadiazine: 1. Atovaquone: 750 mg PO qid 2. Clarithromycin: 1 g PO bid 3. Azithromycin: 1 g load, then 500 mg/day
	And	10–50 mg/day PO	
	folinic acid	4–8 g/day (100 mg/kg/day) PO divided into four doses	
	and		
	sulfadiazine	600–900 mg PO/IV qid	Consider sulfa desensitization for sulfa-allergic people
	or		
	clindamycin		Lifetime maintenance dose required: 1. Pyrimethamine: 25–50 mg/day 2. Folinic acid: 10–50 mg/day 3. Sulfadiazine: 1 g tid-qid, or clindamycin: 300–450 mg tid-qid

Table 36.4. continued

Infection	Therapy	Dose and duration	Comment
Primary CNS lymphoma	Radiotherapy	Whole-brain irradiation with 4,000 cGy with a "boost" of 1,000–2,000 cGy focused on the tumor bed	Radiation or combined modality treatments prolong life by several months (27 vs 119 days mean survival in persons receiving radiation therapy)
	Chemotherapy	Methotrexate (intravenous and intrathecal), thiotepa and procarbazine	Steroids (dexamethasone) may reduce edema associated with tumor, thereby improving symptoms
Progressive multi-focal leukoencephalo-pathy	Antiretroviral therapy Cidofovir/Ara-C	Potent antiretroviral therapy (previously called highly active antiretroviral therapy, or HAART)	Anecdotal reports of efficacy of cytosine arabinoside (Ara-C), and high-dose AZT (1,000 mg/day) Spontaneous remissions and prolonged survival in 5–10%, but average life expectancy is usually months
Cytomegalovirus ventriculitis or polyradiculitis	Gancyclovir Or Foscarnet	5 mg/kg BID or TID for 2–4 weeks (induction) then 5 mg/kg/day 5–7 times/week (maintenance) 60 mg/kg q8H for 2–3 weeks (induction), then 90–120 mg/kg/day IV 6–7 times/week (maintenance)	There may be synergy if gancyclovir and foscarnet used together. Resistance to gancyclovir has occurred in patients with polyradiculopathy. Poor prognosis associated with prior treatment for CMV retinitis, Karnofsky score less than 70, persistently positive CSF CMV PCR, persistent hypoglycorrhachia. Average life expectancy for CMVE or polyradiculopathy is weeks to months Recommended treatment for severely affected patients is induction with gancyclovir and foscarnet, then monotherapy after 2 weeks of therapy, if improvement in symptoms or lower quantitative CSF–CMV–PCR. Improvement of symptoms may take weeks or months

In the USA, government inspection usually identifies ten cases of cysticercosis in the 80 million hogs that are slaughtered each year [15]. During the first year of mandatory reporting of NCC in California, 134 cases were reported. The majority of infected people were immigrant Hispanics, but three people had never traveled outside the USA [16]. Neurocysticercosis has also been reported in Orthodox Jewish people with no travel outside the USA or exposure to pork products [17]. Presumptive infection through contact with infected immigrant food preparers illustrates that asymptomatic carriers of cysticercosis are an important factor in the development of NCC in developed countries.

Clinical Presentation

Symptoms and signs of NCC typically occur many years after initial infection and are associated with the release of *T. solium* antigens from the dying parasite (Table 36.5). A host-mediated inflammatory immune response causes the death of the parasite [14]. Neurologic symptoms of NCC may be acute, chronic or relapsing and are determined by the location of the cysts within the neuraxis (Table 36.6). Neurocysticercosis may also mimic stroke, tumor, carotid artery occlusion or intracerebral hemorrhage [18]. Extraneural cysticercosis may occur in skeletal musculature, conjunctiva or retina, but is rarely present in persons with NCC.

Table 36.5. Symptoms and signs of neurocysticercosis.

Presenting symptom or sign	%
Seizure	60
Increased intracranial pressure (headaches, vomiting, papilledema)	25
Meningitis	25
Altered mental status (including dementia, stupor or confusion)	15
Focal neurologic deficit (hemiparesis or paraparesis, visual loss or aphasia)	10
Asymptomatic	10

Diagnosis

Neurocysticercosis is diagnosed by neuroimaging and serologic testing. Del Brutto and colleagues proposed diagnostic criteria for NCC that combines histologic, radiographic, immunologic and clinical evidence [19]. Definitive diagnosis of NCC can be made if there is histopathologic diagnosis of NCC, a scolex within a cystic lesion visualized by CT or MRI or lesion(s) suggestive of NCC by neuroimaging, or clinical response to treatment of NCC, combined with serologic evidence of T. solium infection by serum enzyme-linked immunoelectrotransfer blot (EITB) or CSF enzyme-linked immunosorbent assay (ELISA) [19].

Laboratory Testing

The most common CSF abnormality in persons with NCC is pleocytosis (Table 36.7). Laboratory diagnosis of NCC can be made by EITB, ELISA, immunodot or immunoelectropheresis (IEF), but the test of choice is serum EITB. Serum ELISA may be more sensitive than CSF ELISA.

Table 36.6. Location of neurocysticercosis within the neuraxis and associated neurologic manifestations.

Location	Neurologic manifestations	Other
Parenchymal	Seizures or encephalitis; may be associated with dementia or behavioral abnormality	Most frequent site of NCC
Meningeal	Meningeal signs (photophobia, nuchal rigidity); cranial nerve palsy	If cysts proliferate at base of brain, basilar meningitis (racemose cysticercosis) occurs and can cause mental deterioration, coma, or death
Ventricular	With blockage of the Sylvian aqueduct, headache and vomiting (symptoms of intracranial hypertension) may occur	Most often occurs in fourth ventricle; obstructive hydrocephalus common
Spinal cord	May cause symptoms of transverse myelitis, spinal cord compression or radiculopathy	Rare occurrence; cysts most often in cervical cord

Table 36.7. Cerebrospinal fluid abnormalities in neurocysticercosis.

CSF findings	%
Normal	50
Elevated white count (>10 cells/mm^3)	45
Increased opening pressure	40
Elevated protein (>45 mg/dl)	40
Low glucose	25
Eosinophils in CSF	15

Radiologic Imaging

CT and MRI of persons with NCC typically reveal single or multiple cysts with variable calcification, cyst wall enhancement or surrounding edema [20]. Compared to CT imaging, MRI is superior for detection of the racemose form of NCC (basilar meningitis), the scolex of the parasite and additional cysts.

Escobar described four stages of NCC [21] (Table 36.8). Neurocysticercosis typically begins as one or more areas of non-contrast-enhancing areas of edema. This progresses to homogeneous contrast-enhancing lesions, then non-enhancing cystic lesions, then ring-enhancing cystic lesions with or without edema and, finally, to complete resolution or calcification. The majority of neurologic symptoms occur in people with cystic or calcified lesions.

Medical Treatment

Controversy exists regarding treatment of NCC. Most experts agree that the inflammatory response associated with the death of the cyst is usually responsible for the development of symptomatic NCC and that inactive infection does not require treatment. Some cases of NCC have lesions that are in different stages of infection. The most active stage of infection should determine if treatment is necessary. If a cyst is calcified or ring-enhancing on neuroimaging, treatment with anthelmintics is probably not necessary. The anthelmintics of choice for NCC are praziquantel and albendazole [19] (Table 36.9). Both medications are cysticidal. Some clinical trials favor the use of albendazole over praziquantel, especially if sub-arachnoid cysts are present [22]. Steroids can be given concomitantly with an anthelmintic to reduce edema that occurs with medical treatment, but may lower the plasma level of praziquantel or increase the plasma level of albendazole [23]. Treatment has been associated with long-term improvement of seizures and decrease in number and size of intraparenchymal lesions [24]. If treatment is not indicated, seizures should be treated with anticonvulsants. Close contacts of people with NCC should receive serologic testing for NCC. Treatment of intestinal *T. solium* infection is a single dose of niclosamide: 1 g for children weighing 25–75 lb, 1.5 g for children over 75 lb and 2 g for adults.

Surgical Treatment

Medical therapy alone may not be effective for ventricular or spinal cord cysts. Ventricular shunting or extirpation of cysts should be considered for patients with cysts in the ventricles, spinal cord or orbits, and for patients with encephalitic or racemose forms of NCC. Steroids and aggressive management of hydrocephalus, with ventricular shunting, if indicated, should be performed prior to administration of anthelmintics, as anthelmintics may exacerbate inflammation.

Fifteen percent of people with NCC have cysts in the ventricular system; the majority are located in the fourth ventricle. Cysts within the ventricles are often difficult to visualize with neuroimaging, but can usually be identified if imaging with intraventricular contrast is performed at the time of shunting [25]. Ventricular shunting for patients with NCC is frequently complicated by bacterial shunt infection and as many as 68% of patients may require shunt revision. Cysts in the spinal cord can cause symptoms of radiculopathy or myelopathy and are most often diagnosed at the time of extirpation. Surgical extirpation of cysts in the spinal cord or orbit is usually required, as medical treatment alone may not be effective and inflammation associated with medical treatment may cause worsening of symptoms or loss of vision. The encephalitic form of NCC is most often seen in young girls and is characterized by numerous intraparenchymal cysts and diffuse cerebral edema.

Table 36.8. Pathologic stages of Escobar correlated with radiographic findings and indications for treatment.

Escobar stage	Pathology	CT findings	MR findings	Treatment
Vesicular	Earliest stage. Larva alive, invaginated, cyst fluid translucent	No contrast enhancement or, rarely, homogeneous contrast enhancement	Increased signal on T2-weighted images; may see small nodule of gadolinium enhancement, or cyst with CSF-density fluid within	Patient asymptomatic; treatment with anthelmintic effective
Colloidal stage of the vesicular form	Parasite dying; degenerative changes present; cyst fluid jelly-like and white	Cystic lesions without contrast enhancement	Cystic lesion with thick capsule; on T1-weighted images, fluid signal higher than CSF	Patient usually asymptomatic; treatment with anthelmintic effective
Granular nodular	Cyst smaller; cyst fluid coarse granules	Cyst isodense or hyperdense to brain, ring-enhancement present; may have edema around cyst	Cystic lesion; fluid isodense to brain. Ring-enhancement with gadolinium	Patient symptomatic; treatment with anthelmintic probably not necessary; treat seizures with anticonvulsant
Nodular calcified	Complete mineralization of cyst fluid	Calcified lesions	Calcified lesions	Patient symptomatic; treatment with anthelmintic not indicated; treat seizures with anticonvulsant

Table 36.9. Dosages of medications for treatment of neurocysticercosis.

Medication	Recommended dosage	Notes
Albendazole	15 mg/kg/day for 8 days	Serum level may increase with use of steroids
Praziquantel	50 mg/kg/day divided TID for 8–15 days	Serum level may decrease with use of steroids
Steroids (dexamethasone)	12–24 mg/day in divided doses	May affect levels of anthelmintics

References

1. Levy RM, Bredesen DE, Rosenblum ML. Neurological manifestations of the acquired immunodeficiency syndrome (AIDS): experience at UCSF and review of the literature. J Neurosurg 1985;62:475–95.
2. Bacellar H, Munoz A, Miller EN et al. Temporal trends in the incidence of HIV-1-related neurologic diseases: Multicenter AIDS Cohort Study, 1985–1992. Neurology 1994;44:1892–900.
3. Anders KH, Guerra WF, Tomiyasu U, Verity MA, Vinters HV. The neuropathology of AIDS: UCLA experience and review. Am J Pathol. 1986;124: 537–58.
4. Maschke M, Kastrup O, Esser S, Ross B, Hengge U, Hufnagel A. Incidence and prevalence of neurological disorders associated with HIV since the introduction of highly active antiretroviral therapy (HAART). J Neurol Neurosurg Psychiatry 2000;69:376–80.
5. Luft BJ, Remington JS. AIDS commentary: toxoplasmic encephalitis. J Infect Dis 1988;157:1–6.
6. Powderly WG, Cloud GA, Dismukes WE, Saag MS. Measurement of cryptococcal antigen in serum and cerebrospinal fluid: value in the management of AIDS-associated cryptococcal meningitis. Clin Infect Dis 1994;18:789–92.
7. Cinque P, Brytting M, Vago L, et al. Epstein-Barr virus DNA in cerebrospinal fluid from patients with AIDS-related primary lymphoma of the central nervous system. Lancet 1993;342:398–401.
8. McGuire D, Barhite S, Hollander H, Miles M. JC virus DNA in cerebrospinal fluid of human immunodeficiency virus-infected patients: predictive value for progressive multifocal leukoencephalopathy [published erratum appears in Ann Neurol 1995;37:687]. Ann Neurol 1995;37:395–9.
9. Evaluation and management of intracranial mass lesions in AIDS: report of the Quality Standards Subcommittee of the American Academy of Neurology [see comments]. Neurology 1998;50:21–6.
10. Gildenberg PL, Gathe JC Jr, Kim JH. Stereotactic biopsy of cerebral lesions in AIDS. Clin Infect Dis 2000; 30:491–9.
11. Feiden W, Bise K, Steude U, Pfister HW, Moller AA. The stereotactic biopsy diagnosis of focal intracerebral lesions in AIDS patients. Acta Neurol Scand 1993;87: 228–33.
12. Hornef MW, Iten A, Maeder P, Villemure JG, Regli L. Brain biopsy in patients with acquired immunodeficiency syndrome: diagnostic value, clinical performance, and survival time. Arch Intern Med 1999;159:2590–6.
13. Senanayake N, Roman GC. Epidemiology of epilepsy in developing countries. Bull World Health Organ 1993;71: 247–58.
14. Pittella JE. Neurocysticercosis. Brain Pathol 1997;7: 681–93.
15. Schantz PM, McAuley J. Current status of food-borne parasitic zoonoses in the United States. Southeast Asian J Trop Med Public Health 1991;22 (Suppl.):65–71.
16. Ehnert KL, Roberto RR, Barrett L, Sorvillo FJ, Rutherford GWd. Cysticercosis: first 12 months of reporting in California. Bull Pan Am Health Organ 1992;26:165–72.
17. Moore AC, Lutwick LI, Schantz PM. Seroprevalence of cysticercosis in an Orthodox Jewish community. Am J Trop Med Hyg 1995;53:439–42.
18. Cantu C, Barinagarrementeria F. Cerebrovascular complications of neurocysticercosis: clinical and neuroimaging spectrum. Arch Neurol 1996;53:233–9.
19. Del Brutto OH, Wadia NH, Dumas M, Cruz M, Tsang VC, Schantz PM. Proposal of diagnostic criteria for human cysticercosis and neurocysticercosis [see comments]. J Neurol Sci 1996;142:1–6.
20. Rodriguez-Carbajal J, palacios E, Zee CS. Neuroradiology of cysticercosis of the central nervous system. In: Palacios E, Rodriguez-Carbajal J, Taveras JM et al., editors. Cysticercosis of the central nervous system. Springfield, IL: Charles C. Thomas, 1983; 101–43.
21. Escobar A. The pathology of neurocysticercosis. In: Palacios E, Rodriguez-Carbajal J, Taveras JM. Cysticercosis of the nervous system. Springfield, IL: Charles C. Thomas, 1983.
22. Takayanagui OM, Jardim E. Therapy for neurocysticercosis: comparison between albendazole and praziquantel. Arch Neurol 1992;49:290–4.
23. Jung H, Hurtado M, Medina MT, Sanchez M, Sotelo J. Dexamethasone increases plasma levels of albendazole. J Neurol 1990;237:279–80.
24. Vazquez V, Sotelo J. The course of seizures after treatment for cerebral cysticercosis [see comments]. N Engl J Med 1992;327:696–701.
25. Apuzzo ML, Dobkin WR, Zee CS, Chan JC, Giannotta SL, Weiss MH. Surgical considerations in treatment of intraventricular cysticercosis: an analysis of 45 cases. J Neurosurg 1984;60:400–7.

37

Infections in Neurological Surgery

Richard K. Osenbach and Stephen J. Haines

Summary

The incidence of brain abscess could be increasing due to the increased incidence of opportunistic infections in immunocompromised hosts. The bacteriological profile has changed over the past 50 years, with the most significant increase being in anaerobic infections. The infections presented here include cerebral, cranial epidural, subdural empyema, fungal, parasitic and postoperative, each of which depends on a timely diagnosis. The treatment options vary from surgery, i.e. stereotactic and non-surgical (i.e. antibiotic) therapy.

Pyogenic Brain Abscess

The incidence of brain abscess varies with geographic location and living standards within a given region. In underdeveloped countries, brain abscess constitutes a disproportionate percentage of space-occupying intracranial lesions compared with industrialized nations. It has been suggested that the incidence of brain abscess may be declining, although several authors have noted little change over two decades [1,2]. Indeed, the incidence of brain abscess may actually be increasing, owing to the increased incidence of opportunistic infections in immunocompromised hosts.

Microbiology and Pathogenesis

The bacteriological profile of brain abscess has changed significantly over the past 50 years. In the older literature, aerobic streptococci, pneumococci and *Staphylococcus aureus* predominated, with relatively few Gram-negative and anerobic infections reported [1,2]. More recent series have shown a significant increase in anerobic abscesses, the most common isolates being *Bacteroides spp.* and anerobic streptococci. The incidence of Gram-negative infections has also increased, sometimes comprising more than 20% of cases. Although most abscesses are caused by a single organism, mixed infections occur in up to 33% of cases, particularly otogenic abscesses. The incidence of negative cultures remains around 25%; however, the use of meticulous microbiological techniques can result in positive cultures in virtually 100% of brain abscesses, even in the face of antibiotic therapy [3].

The microbiological profile of a brain abscess is closely linked to the underlying etiology. Although the source of infection is usually apparent, a definitive underlying cause may be obscure in around 30% of patients. Anerobic organisms predominate in abscesses caused by underlying otogenic and dental infections, and are common in metastatic and cryptogenic abscesses. The most common organisms isolated from sinusitic abscesses include those that normally inhabit the para-nasal sinuses, including *S. aureus*, aerobic streptococci and *Hemophilus influenzae*, although anerobes may be identified in over 50% of sinusitic abscesses [3].

Suppurative processes of the air sinuses are the most common underlying cause of brain abscess, which develops by direct intracranial extension or through retrograde thrombophlebitis of diploic or emissary veins [1,2,4]. Sinusitic and otogenic abscesses are usually solitary and located superficially. Metastatic abscesses develop following hematogenous dissemination of micro-organisms from a systemic infection. Common primary foci include skin pustules, pulmonary infections, acute diverticulitis, osteomyelitis, periodontal abscess and sub-acute bacterial endocarditis (SBE). Interestingly, transient bacteremia alone is unlikely to result in abscess formation, owing to inherent resistance of the blood–brain barrier to infection. Metastatic abscesses are often multiple and are distributed in a manner proportionate to regional CBF, the middle cerebral artery territory being the most common location. They tend to occur at the corticomedullary junction but can also occur deep in the parenchyma.

Cerebral abscess is a leading cause of morbidity in patients with cyanotic congenital heart disease (CHD) [5]. Cardiac malformations that produce a right-to-left shunt allow bacteria to bypass the pulmonary capillary bed, where they are normally filtered. Additionally, long-standing hypoxemia results in polycythemia and increased blood viscosity that predispose to areas of microinfarction, thus providing favorable conditions for the growth of micro-organisms. Curiously, endocarditis is not thought to be an important factor in the pathogenesis of these lesions and, unlike many metastatic abscesses, those associated with CHD are generally solitary.

Finally, post-traumatic or post-operative abscesses may occur following direct inoculation of bacteria into the brain. Post-traumatic abscesses tend to develop relatively soon following trauma, although some cases have been described as presenting many years following injury. Post-traumatic abscess can be prevented in large measure by early, aggressive debridement of necrotic non-viable tissue at the time of the injury. Post-operative abscesses usually result from organisms introduced at the time of surgery or spread intracranially from an overlying wound or bone flap infection.

Brain abscess in neonates and infants deserves separate mention, since it differs from that in adults. In neonates, brain abscess frequently develops as a complication of meningitis – a feature atypical of brain abscess in older children and adults. Additionally, most abscesses in this population are caused by species of *Proteus* or *Citrobacter*, which is thought to be related to a deficiency of placentally transferred immunoglobulin and complement. Renier reviewed 30 neonatal abscesses and found that 90% were caused by *Proteus spp.* [6]. Graham et al. reviewed 53 cases of *Citrobacter* meningitis and found that 77% of cases resulted in brain abscess, compared with only 10% of 159 cases of non-*Citrobacter* meningitis [7].

Clinical Presentation

Contemporary clinical presentation of brain abscess differs negligibly from classical descriptions. Most cases occur in the first two decades, with an unexplained male predilection. Most patients present with generalized signs of elevated ICP and/or focal neurological findings that depend on the size, location and multiplicity of the lesions, virulence of the organism, host response and the severity of cerebral edema. Although the symptoms of brain abscess are largely indistinguishable from those of any other space-occupying lesion, the tempo of progression tends to be more rapid, with 75% of patients having symptoms for less than 2 weeks. However, immunocompromised patients may present more insidiously and a high index of suspicion is necessary to establish an early diagnosis [2].

Headache is prominent in 70–97% of patients, which is often constant, progressive and refractory to therapy. Nausea and vomiting due to elevated ICP occur in 25–50% of patients. Slightly over 50% of patients have a low-grade fever, but fever exceeding101.5°F is relatively unusual and may indicate a concomitant systemic infection or meningitis. Two-thirds of patients have varying degrees of altered sensorium and more than 60% of patients demonstrate focal neurological findings. Seizures occur in 30–50% of patients prior to any surgical intervention [2,8]. Infants present with a combination of enlarging head circumference, bulging fontanel, separation of the cranial sutures, vomiting, irritability, seizures and poor feeding [5].

Neuroimaging of Brain Abscess

The imaging characteristics of brain abscess using CT are time-dependent and roughly correlate with the histopathological findings [9] (Table 37.1). The evolution of a brain abscess progresses through four stages: early cerebritis, late cerebritis, early capsule formation and late capsule formation. During the cerebritis phases, there is progressive destruction of tissue, with formation of pus and cerebral edema. Capsule formation is exceedingly important, since it limits the destruction of brain parenchyma. Capsule formation is influenced by several factors, including the type of organism, the pathogenesis of infection and the use of steroids. Aerobic bacteria tend to promote the formation of a thick capsule, while anerobic organisms produce enzymes that may retard encapsulation and exacerbate cerebral edema. Post-traumatic abscesses are frequently better encapsulated than metastatic abscesses. The latter are often associated with vegetative emboli that produce micro-infarcts and secondary tissue hypoxia that impedes neovascularization and migration of fibroblasts. Corticosteroids also can impede capsule formation. However, the potential benefit of steroids on severe cerebral edema generally outweighs any disadvantage of their use in this setting.

Experience with MRI has shown it to be more sensitive than CT in detecting the very early changes of cerebritis and very early patterns of ring-enhancement. This advantage may be of limited benefit, since most patients present with an established lesion. Perhaps of more practical value is the suggestion that MRI is more specific than CT in differentiating cerebral edema from liquefactive necrosis, which would be valuable in planning timing of aspiration [10]. Diffusion weighted imaging (DWI) and magnetic resonance spectroscopy (MRS) have shown promise in differentiating abscess from a necrotic or cystic brain tumor. Abscess contents appear bright on DWI, while cystic tumors appear dark. Using MRS, tumor spectra are characterized by an elevated choline peak, while abscess spectra are not. Abscesses also demonstrate elevated acetate and amino acid resonances, which are not seen in tumor spectra. For maximum accuracy, spectra should be obtained so that the wall of the lesion is dominant in the acquisition voxel. Given that DWI and MRS may be performed simultaneously with routine MRI, a combination of MR techniques may provide the diagnostic study of choice in the evaluation of suspected abscesses [11].

Occasionally, CT and/or MRI may be inconclusive. In these cases, Indium^{111}-radiolabeled white blood cell (WBC) imaging may help clarify the diagnosis. Indium^{111} WBC imaging should theoretically be able to distinguish abscess from neoplasm. The technique is easy and non-invasive and can provide information that might influence management. The main disadvantage is that optimal images are obtained 24 hours following injection (although positive images are sometimes obtained at 6 hours) and, therefore, this test is best suited to patients who do not require emergent surgery. The diagnostic accuracy has been reported to be around 96%, with a sensitivity and specificity 100 and 94%, respectively [12]. In spite of the high sensitivity, false-negative scans may occur in tumors that have undergone extensive necrosis of such magnitude as to incite an inflammatory response sufficient to be detectable by labeled leukocytes. Other radionuclide scans such as thallium^{201} SPECT are useful for differentiating lymphoma from toxoplasmosis in AIDS patients. Thallium^{201} is taken up by lymphoma but not by toxoplasma abscesses. SPECT thallium may also help differentiate tumor from abscess in non-AIDS patients, although false-positive results have been reported [11].

Management of Cerebral Abscess

There are no randomized trials comparing treatment methods for brain abscess and optimal management continues to be a subject of controversy. However, in general, the treatment objectives in patients with brain abscess are:

- Identify the causative organism.
- Establish antibiotic sensitivities.
- Reduce intracranial pressure and mass effect.
- Prevent intraventricular rupture [13].

Table 37.1. Correlation of radiographic and histological findings in pyogenic brain abscess.

Abscess stage	Time course (days)	Histopathology	CT appearance	MRI appearance
Early cerebritis	0–3	Central zone of necrosis Local inflammatory response Marked peri-lesional edema Poor demarcation from adjacent brain	Poorly marginated area of hypodensity Minimal if any enhacnement with intravenous contrast	Edema may be more readily apparent
Late cerebritis	4–9	Enlargement of necrotic center Initial formation of pus Surrounding zone of inflammatory cells and macrophages Maximal cerebral edema Reticulin network as precursor to capsule	Hypodense area still may show poor margination Patchy enhancement during early part of phase Ring-enhancement begins later in phase Central hypodense areas fill in with contrast on delayed scans	Early patterns of ring-enhancement more easily detectable Surrounding edema hypointense compared to normal brain Rim of lesion may be mildly hyperintense to white matter on T1WI
Early capsule formation	10–14	Continued formation of pus Development of collagen capsule Cerebral edema surrounding capsule	Non-contrast CT-faint ring of increased density Early in phase, center may fill in with contrast on delayed scans Enhancement of well defined capsule Capsule usually thin, relatively uniform and smoothly contoured on inner surface	
Late capsule formation	>14	Five distinct histological zones: 1) necrotic center filled with pus 2) peripheral zone of inflammatory cells and fibroblasts 3) dense collagen capsule 4) neovascularity immediately external to capsule 5) peri-lesional edema and gliosis	Ring-enhancement of capsule, which becomes thicker Daughter abscesses may be seen budding from deep (medial) margin	Components on T2WI 1) hyperintense liquefied core 2) hypointense capsule 3) hypointense capsule with surrounding hyperintense area of vasogenic edema and gliosis

Principles of Antibiotic Therapy

The most important factor regarding antibiotic therapy for treatment of a cerebral abscess is to choose an agent(s) based on culture and sensitivity testing of the causative organism. Ideally, the culture should be obtained directly from the abscess. Given the ease and safety of stereotactic image-guided surgery, this should almost always be feasible, except in the presence of an uncontrolled bleeding diathesis. Other factors that influence antibiotic selection include spectrum of activity, bactericidal or bacteriostatic properties and the ability of a drug to penetrate into the abscess cavity to produce therapeutic concentrations at the site of action. Indeed, some abscesses may not be cured, in spite of antibiotic concentrations within the abscess cavity exceeding the minimum inhibitory concentration. Local factors within the abscess cavity such as pH or absolute number of microorganisms may produce a milieu in which drugs may be ineffective, despite seemingly adequate concentrations. In general, any abscess greater than 2.5–3.0 cm in diameter is unlikely to be cured by medical therapy alone and should be aspirated in conjunction with antibiotic therapy [13,14].

Non-surgical Management of Brain Abscess

Until the early 1970s, surgery was considered essential in the management of brain abscess. However, in 1971, it was suggested that brain abscess might be successfully treated non-operatively, using antibiotics alone. In 1986, a review was published of 67 cases of encapsulated brain abscess managed non-operatively [15]. The success rate of non-surgical therapy was 74% and the mortality 4%, although many of these lesions may have been treated during the cerebritis stage, which may have facilitated resolution. Antibiotics were chosen based on culture of organisms isolated from blood, CSF or other fluids in 49% of cases and by aspiration of one of multiple abscesses in 23% of patients, leaving 28% treated without a definitive diagnosis. This last figure is significant because a variety of intracranial processes (primary or metastatic tumors, resolving hematoma, infarction, etc.) can mimic both the clinical presentation and radiographic appearance of an abscess. Consequently, it is not inconceivable that a non-infectious process might be erroneously treated with antibiotics. It is especially critical to obtain cultures in immunocompromised patients who may harbor opportunistic infections not responsive to conventional antimicrobial therapy. Additionally, removal of purulent material provides a more favorable environment in which antibiotics can work and provides immediate reduction in mass effect and ICP. Therefore, with stereotactic techniques so readily available, it should be the rare case in which treatment is undertaken without obtaining a biopsy or culture material.

Operative Management

Contemporary surgical management of brain abscess consists of stereotactic aspiration or craniotomy and excision of the capsule. Each has its advantages, proponents and specific indications, and excellent outcomes have been achieved with both methods. Aside from personal bias, several factors may influence the choice of procedure, including age, neurological condition, location and stage of the abscess, type of abscess (fungal vs bacterial), the presence of multiple lesions and co-morbidity.

Aspiration using stereotactic image-guided techniques can be performed with precise localization, with minimal tissue damage. This is especially important for deep-seated abscesses, those located in eloquent areas and for drainage of multiple abscesses. Stereotactic aspiration can be performed under local anesthesia, even in very ill patients. Additionally, cultures can be obtained, even during the cerebritis stage, at a time when antibiotics are likely to be curative.

There are some circumstances where craniotomy and resection of the abscess may be more appropriate. Post-traumatic abscesses with a retained foreign body generally cannot be cured with aspiration. Abscesses that occur as a result of a CSF leak often require excision, along with repair of the CSF fistula. Air within the abscess may indicate the presence of a CSF leak and dictate the need for excision. Multiloculated abscesses may be appropriate for excision, due to difficulty in completely aspirating these lesions. Fungal abscesses often can only be cured by complete excision, since organisms may be present in the capsule of the abscess. Craniotomy and excision have been advocated for all cerebellar abscesses, since treatment failures in the posterior fossa can be rapidly fatal. Finally, it has been suggested that excision reduces the duration of antibiotic therapy, although this advantage would seem marginal.

Management of Multiple Brain Abscesses

Multiple abscesses occur in 10–50% of patients. However, few data exist regarding optimal management. Management strategies have included empirical use of antibiotics alone; aspiration of a single lesion followed by antibiotics; open excision combined with aspiration and antibiotics; and multiple repeated aspirations, when necessary. The following recommendations and conclusions can be made regarding the management of multiple brain abscesses [15]:

- Emergency surgery, preferably by stereotactic aspiration is indicated for all abscesses greater than 2.5 cm in diameter or for any lesion producing significant mass effect.
- If all lesions are less than 2.5 cm in diameter, then the largest abscess should be aspirated for culture material.
- Antibiotics should be withheld until samples are obtained for culture and/or biopsy.
- Once cultures are obtained, broad-spectrum antibiotics should be initiated; adjustments should be made once culture and sensitivity results become available.
- Duration of intravenous antibiotic therapy should be a minimum of 6–8 weeks, and often for at least a year in immunocompromised patients.
- CT or MRI should be obtained weekly during therapy, and then at monthly or bimonthly intervals, until the process has resolved radiographically.

Role of Corticosteroids

The use of corticosteroids as an adjunct in the management of brain abscess is controversial. While steroids clearly reduce the cerebral edema and mass effect that accompany an abscess, they may also have detrimental side effects. Experimentally, when administered during the early stages of cerebritis, steroids diminish the effectiveness of host defense mechanisms that help contain the infection. Overall, it would appear that steroids decrease both the rate and degree of capsule formation. Corticosteroids have also been shown to significantly reduce the degree of contrast enhancement on CT scans, particularly in the cerebritis stages. Therefore, in patients receiving steroids, reduction in contrast enhancement cannot be taken as a-priori evidence of abscess resolution. Corticosteroids should be reserved as a lifesaving measure for patients in whom significant mass effect and/or cerebral edema pose an imminent threat to survival or are significantly debilitating. They should be tapered rapidly, as the clinical condition permits.

Radiographic Follow-up of Brain Abscess

Frequent imaging is essential during treatment of patients with a brain abscess. MRI has no proven advantage over CT, but either is equally acceptable. Logically, for most accurate comparison, the same modality should be used consistently for each patient. Imaging should be performed weekly for the duration of treatment and for 1–2 weeks thereafter, followed by a study 1 month later. Bi-monthly examinations should then be performed until the process has radiographically resolved. The time course of abscess resolution is variable but, in general, radiographic evidence of resolution lags behind clinical improvement. In most cases, objective evidence of decrease in the size is first noticeable 2–3 weeks following initiation of therapy. However, complete resolution of the abscess cavity, mass effect and contrast enhancement may take 3–4 months and, occasionally, residual contrast enhancement may persist for up to 9 months. Indeed, prolonged enhancement should not, in and of itself, dictate the need for additional therapy. However, these patients bear close observation and follow-up. It should be noted that increase in contrast enhancement is commonly seen when patients are withdrawn from steroids, although, again, this does not necessarily indicate regrowth of the abscess.

Morbidity and Mortality

Advances in diagnosis and treatment have resulted in a drastic reduction in mortality related to brain abscess. Mortality rates of 50% were once commonplace but are now the exception rather than the rule. The reduction in mortality can be attributed to a number of factors. Advances in diagnostic imaging, most importantly the introduction of CT, have led to earlier diagnosis and treatment before neurological deterioration has occurred. Improved microbiological isolation techniques have dramatically reduced the incidence of negative cultures and significantly increased isolation rates of anerobic organisms. More effective antibiotics have become available, which have improved the treatment of Gram-negative and anerobic infections. Finally, the evolution of stereotactic image-guided techniques for aspiration of abscess contents has provided a simple and safe alternative to open surgery techniques.

Notwithstanding, brain abscess remains a serious illness that can result in death if misdiagnosed or managed improperly. The risk of death is directly related to the rapidity of progression and, *most importantly*, the neurological condition of the patient at the time of diagnosis. Patients who are alert at diagnosis have a mortality rate of around 20%. In sharp contrast, the mortality rate for patients who present with signs of herniation exceeds 60% and, for those in coma, it is around 90%. Other factors that might influence mortality include virulence of the organism, etiology of the abscess, size, the presence of multiple abscesses and intraventricular rupture. Abscesses of sinusitic or otogenic origin tend to have a better prognosis than do metastatic abscesses, which are more frequently deep-seated and multiple. The most important factor that appears to contribute to increased mortality is delay in diagnosis. Also, with recent trends towards non-surgical management, there may be an inappropriate delay in operative intervention that might otherwise prevent herniation or intraventricular rupture, which may prove fatal.

Even successfully treated brain abscesses can result in long-term neurological sequelae and disability, primarily related to seizures, cognitive dysfunction and focal neurological deficits [13,14]. Epilepsy is a common sequel of brain abscess, the incidence ranging from 30% to over 70%. The incidence may be influenced by several factors, including the presence of seizures prior to surgery, age at diagnosis, location of the abscess and choice of surgical procedure. Most patients who develop seizures pre-operatively go on to develop late epilepsy. Older patients generally have a shorter seizure-onset latency, with 50% suffering their initial seizure within 1 year of diagnosis. Although it has been suggested that seizure risk may be related to abscess location, this has not been substantiated. Finally, many series report a trend towards reduction in seizures in patients treated with aspiration as opposed to excision. Given the high incidence of seizures, it should probably be standard practice to place all patients with supratentorial brain abscesses on prophylactic anti-epileptic medications (AED). The AEDs should be continued for 1–2 years, following which they may be tapered, providing the EEG shows no epileptogenic activity.

Permanent neurological disability occurs in up to 50% of patients following treatment of brain abscess, most often the result of residual focal deficits or due to cognitive deficits, the latter particularly common in children [14]. The most important factors that influence long-term neurological outcome are age and abscess location. The incidence of focal deficits such as hemiparesis tends to be higher and more incapacitating in children. Morbidity is also higher in children, owing to the high incidence of abscesses caused by *Proteus* and *Citrobacter*, which are notorious for inducing a fulminant necrotizing reaction, with destruction of large amounts of brain parenchyma. Consequently, early aspiration is especially important in neonates and young children. The literature also suggests that permanent deficits may be more likely with excision than aspiration.

Recurrence occurs in 5–10% of cases, in spite of what is considered adequate therapy. Most recurrences become apparent within 6 weeks following therapy, although some have been reported many years following therapy. Reasons for recurrence include inadequate antibiotic therapy, incorrect choice of antibiotics, failure to aspirate large abscesses, presence of a retained foreign body or dural fistula and failure to eradicate underlying sources of infection.

Cranial Epidural Abscess (EDA)

Cranial EDA is a collection of pus that forms in the potential space between the dura and calvarium. Cranial EDA is relatively uncommon, accounting for only 5% of all localized intracranial infections [16,17]. Most cranial EDAs result from trauma with implantation of foreign material, following craniotomy or in association with infection of the para-nasal sinuses, although occasional cases are related to orbital cellulitis, sinus thrombophlebitis or congenital dermal sinuses. Rarely is cranial EDA related to invasive carcinoma of the head and neck that has eroded through the skull. Other conditions occasionally associated with cranial EDA include rhinocerebral mucormycosis, fetal monitoring and insertion of skull tongs for skeletal traction [16,17].

The bacteriology of cranial EDA correlates with the underlying cause of infection. Cases associated with para-nasal sinusitis, otitis and mastoiditis reflect the organisms of the underlying infection, most often hemolytic or microaerophilic streptococci and anerobes. Post-traumatic and or post-operative cases are most often caused by staphylococci.

As opposed to sub-dural empyema (SDE) (discussed later), the majority of patients with cranial EDA present with a relatively "benign" clinical course. A recent history of craniofacial trauma, sinusitis, ENT or neurosurgical procedure may provide an initial clue to the diagnosis. The typical patient reports a dull headache, which may be localized or diffuse. Periorbital swelling may occur, especially in cases related to frontal sinusitis. Signs of mild systemic illness such as fever are common and, while the patient may appear ill, signs of toxicity are usually conspicuously absent. Not infrequently, symptoms may be present for weeks to months, while the abscess slowly enlarges. Focal neurological signs are occasionally noted, usually due to mass effect from the epidural collection. Occasionally, an EDA located at the petrous apex can produce ipsilateral facial pain associated with sixth nerve palsy (Gradenigo's syndrome). However, the presence of progressive focal neurological deficit, seizures or a deteriorating sensorium should raise the suspicion of a concomitant SDE which is present in approximately 10% of patients.

Laboratory findings in EDA are non-specific and include elevation of the sedimentation rate (ESR), with or without an elevated blood leukocyte count. Lumbar puncture is potentially dangerous and adds little information. Plain skull radiographs may demonstrate bone destruction if there is an associated osteomyelitis, but the study of choice is either CT or MRI. EDA frequently involves a relatively large volume of fluid that usually appears as a lenticular-shaped extra-axial mass on both CT and MRI. The collection usually appears hypodense on CT with peripheral contrast enhancement. On MRI, EDA appears as a hyperintense signal abnormality on both T1WI and T2WI; the latter may be more sensitive than CT in detecting small collections early in the course of the disease.

The management of cranial EDA entails antibiotic therapy and surgical evacuation of the abscess. Not uncommonly, there will be a fluctuant sub-galeal component associated with the EDA that may be aspirated to obtain culture so that antibiotic therapy can be initiated. However, the notion that simple aspiration of the purulent material through the scalp, followed by antibiotics, might be adequate therapy should be condemned. Similarly, while burr-hole drainage may be attempted, it is usually inadequate. The optimum surgical management of EDA should consist of craniotomy or craniectomy, drainage of all purulent material, debridement of necrotic devitalized tissue and copious irrigation [18]. If there is an underlying frontal sinusitis, this can also be addressed with cranialization and exenteration of the sinus. Friable granulation tissue is usually encountered adherent to the dura and prudence must be exercised in attempting to remove this material. If it is not particularly adherent and can be easily removed, it should be done; however, this tissue is often quite vascular and adherent and the risk of creating a dural tear with contamination of the sub-dural space far outweighs the benefits of complete removal. Indeed, in the absence of compelling clinical and/or radiographic evidence to suggest the presence of an associated SDE, the sub-dural space should not be routinely explored [18]. Proper management of the bone flap following drainage of an EDA is debatable. If the bone appears "healthy" and radiographic signs of osteomyelitis are lacking, the bone flap can be soaked in an antiseptic solution and replaced [19]. It such instances, a suction–irrigation system can be employed for 48–72 hours. While this approach can undoubtedly be successful in some cases, the author generally advocates a craniectomy followed by cranioplasty, performed no sooner than 6 months and preferably 1 year following eradication of the EDA. This approach obviously commits the patient to a second operation but has been successful, without added morbidity. Intravenous antibiotics should be continued for a total of 6 weeks. With early aggressive treatment, the morbidity and mortality from isolated cranial EDA should be very low.

SDE

SDE is a purulent infection, occurring within the confines of the sub-dural space. SDE is less common than parenchymal brain abscess and accounts for roughly 12–25% of all intracranial infections, this figure being greater in underdeveloped countries. The disease is 2–3 times more frequent in males, the majority of cases occurring between 10 and 40 years of age [17,18].

SDE most commonly develops from direct spread from a para-nasal sinus or otogenic infection and is commonly associated with an intervening EDA [17]. Retrograde thrombophlebitis of mucosal sinus vessels, which communicate via emissary veins with the dural venous sinuses and hematogenous dissemination from a metastatic source of infection, can also result in an SDE. SDE may also occur following craniotomy, penetrating trauma or secondary to rupture of a brain abscess into the sub-dural space. SDE occurs as a complication in approximately 2% of children with meningitis, particularly *H. influenza*. The majority of cases of SDE occur as a complication of para-nasal sinus or otogenic infection [17]. The infection is located over the convexity in 70– 80% of cases; however, 10–20% of cases are parafalcine and may extend deep into the interhemispheric fissure. Posterior fossa collections also occur but are far less common than supratentorial collections.

SDE may be classified according to etiology and clinical features. Acute SDE most often occurs secondary to spread of a contiguous infection and, less often, through hematogenous dissemination [19]. A history of a recent or concurrent sinus or ear infection or a recent ENT procedure is not unusual. Patients with acute SDE frequently present with a rapidly progressive, fulminant clinical course that is fatal if not recognized and treated immediately. Patients with acute SDE typically complain of a severe intractable headache, along with nausea and vomiting in the early stages of the illness. Fever is often present and signs of meningeal irritation are noted in 70–90% of patients [17–20]. Sensorium is initially normal but, as the infection progresses, there is rapid declination in the level of consciousness. Focal neurological findings occur in up to 85% of patients and may be related to cortical dysfunction from thrombophlebitis and/or cerebral edema and mass effect, which can be considerable and is often out of proportion to the size of the purulent collection [18]. Indeed, cerebral infarction secondary to cortical venous thrombosis occurs in up to 90% of patients who succumbed to the illness. A concomitant brain abscess may be present in up to 25% of patients. Seizures occur in up to two-thirds of patients with SDE.

Sub-acute SDE is more common in cases that complicate craniotomy. The clinical course is somewhat more protracted and less fulminant. Patients often present with a history spanning several weeks and complain of chronic localized headache, along with a low-grade fever. The neurological examination is often unremarkable. In the post-craniotomy patient, inspection of the incision may reveal erythema and tenderness or a bulging burr hole. In these cases, the collection is usually contained by chronic membranes, in contrast to acute SDE, in which a thin layer of exudate spreads rapidly through the sub-dural space. Finally, SDE of infancy often occurs as a complication of bacterial meningitis. In infants, the clinical presentation is more non-specific and consists of high fever, irritability, poor feeding, vomiting, lethargy, bulging fontanel, nuchal rigidity and, finally, coma [19].

The microbiological spectrum of SDE mirrors that of the predisposing infection. Not surprisingly, then, most cases of SDE related to underlying para-nasal sinus or otogenic infections are caused by aerobic and anaerobic streptococci, especially *Streptococcus milleri*. Together, this group of organisms accounts for 45–75% of cases. Post-operative infections are most often due to staphylococci but are occasionally caused by Gram-negative bacilli. In infants and children, most cases are caused by the organisms responsible for meningitis in this age group, namely *H. influenza*, *E. coli* and *S. pneumoniae*.

Laboratory findings are non-specific and but include peripheral leukocytosis and/or positive blood cultures. Lumbar puncture is contraindicated, due to the risk of herniation, and adds little information, although there are considerable CSF data in the literature.

CT and MRI have become the cornerstones of diagnosis. The CT appearance of SDE is that of a hypodense, crescentic or lenticular, extra-axial fluid collection. If contrast is administered, a densely enhancing inner membrane, which displaces the gray–white junction, is often noted. There are frequently adjacent parenchymal edema and midline shift that may be dramatically out of proportion to the size of the collection – a feature that should raise the index of suspicion for an SDE. Early on, CT may miss a small collection, particularly a small parafalcine or interhemispheric collection or a posterior fossa empyema. In difficult cases, MRI is probably more sensitive in detecting small collections in difficult areas. An SDE typically appears hypointense on T1WI and hyperintense on T2WI. Administration of gadolinium may delineate a membrane similar to CT. The multiplanar imaging capabilities of MRI provide more precise anatomical localization than does CT without any bone-averaging artifact. It has been suggested that MRI is able to differentiate between SDE and a non-infected sub-dural effusion. Most often, MRI is capable of differentiating an EDA from an SDE and is more sensitive in detecting small, early empyemas [21].

Management of SDE involves emergent drainage of the purulent collection, along with antibiotics. There has been extensive debate regarding surgical management, with some authors advocating drainage through multiple burr holes, while others promote, de novo, a wide craniotomy [22]. Advocates of burr-hole drainage maintain that craniotomy has a higher risk and may necessitate performing a delayed cranioplasty. Furthermore, those favoring burr-hole drainage contend that extensive irrigation through multiple burr holes is sufficient, unless the collection is parafalcine. Advocates of craniotomy point out that incomplete drainage using burr holes often necessitates performing a craniotomy at a later time. Regardless of the type of surgery elected, timing of surgery is critical, with optimal results obtained when surgery is performed within 3–5 days of symptom onset. Following surgical evacuation, antibiotics should be administered for 4–6 weeks, based on culture and sensitivity testing.

Previously, the mortality from SDE has been as high as 40–50%, although more recent series report rates of between 10 and 20% [22]. Unfortunately, survivors often are left with significant neurological dysfunction and epilepsy may occur, either acutely or in a delayed fashion. The prognosis for patients with SDE is most closely associated with the degree of neurological dysfunction at the time of diagnosis, especially the level of consciousness. Mortality appears to be somewhat better in patients treated with craniotomy, although it is unclear whether this reflects an advantage of craniotomy or the better medical condition of these patients [22].

Fungal Infections of the CNS

Fungal infections are far less common than bacterial infections, yet their clinical presentations are often strikingly similar. Fungal involvement of the CNS most often takes the form of either meningitis or cerebral abscess. Host immune status is central in determining which organisms produce illness in a given patient. Coccidiomycosis, blastomycosis, histoplasmosis and most parasitic diseases generally occur in otherwise healthy individuals. Cryptococcosis occurs about equally in healthy and immunocompromised patients, while candidiasis, aspergillosis and mucormycosis are almost exclusively limited to immunocompromised or severely debilitated patients [23].

Cryptococcosis

Cryptococcosis is caused by *Cryptococcus neoformans*, an encapsulated yeast-like fungus. CNS disease occurs in 30–50% of patients with disseminated cryptococcosis and 90% of individuals who die of the disease show CNS involvement [24]. Typically, CNS involvement takes the form of chronic meningitis. The clinical presentation is variable, but usually is sub-acute. The typical patient presents with headache, nausea, vomiting and mental status changes, although the typical features of meningitis may be completely lacking. Occasionally, patients present with elevated ICP due to hydrocephalus caused by basal arachnoiditis. Cranial nerve deficits have been described in 20–30% of individuals, most commonly abducens or facial nerve palsy. The clinical course is usually steadily progressive over weeks to months, but may be remarkably indolent, punctuated by periods of clinical improvement interspersed among exacerbations. Cryptococcal meningitis may be complicated by basal arachnoiditis with communicating or obstructive hydrocephalus, meningovascular lesions that produce a stroke-like picture and, rarely, an expanding intraparenchymal granuloma.

The diagnosis hinges on identification of *Cryptococcus neoformans* in the CSF. Gram's stain sometimes reveals a Gram-positive spherical organism surrounded by a thick refractile capsule. India ink preparations are positive in 60% of cases. Although cryptococcus will usually grow in culture, both smears and cultures occasionally may be negative in which case latex cryptococcal agglutination is extremely beneficial. This test can rapidly identify the polysaccharide capsular antigen in 90–95% of cases. Antigen titers may have prognostic value, of which less than 1:256 is associated with a better prognosis.

Treatment of cryptococcal meningitis consists of administration of anti-fungal agents, including amphotericin B and/or flucytosine. Flucytosine may be a promising alternative to amphotericin B, since it has reduced toxicity and excellent CSF penetration. Indeed, when used as monotherapy, flucytosine has produced a cure in approximately two-thirds of patients. In uncomplicated cases, routine intrathecal administration of amphotericin displays little, if any, benefit over IV therapy and is generally reserved for patients with continued signs of active meningoencephalitis, despite adequate IV therapy. Weekly CSF surveillance should be performed during and for several months following discontinuation of therapy. With successful treatment, CSF studies normalize within 3 months; further CSF surveillance should be performed at 3-month intervals for an additional 2 years after therapy is stopped. Patients with solitary granulomas should undergo surgical excision followed by anti-fungal chemotherapy. Patients with symptomatic hydrocephalus require CSF shunting, despite the potential risk of cryptococcal peritonitis. Prior to the availability of amphotericin B, the mortality rate from CNS cryptococcal infection approached 80% but now, with aggressive medical and surgical therapy, 65–70% of patients are either improved or cured [23,24].

Candidiasis

Candida albicans is an opportunistic pathogen that rarely causes disease in healthy individuals, but becomes pathogenic when host defense systems become compromised or when the organism can accumulate in large numbers, such as during prolonged antibiotic therapy. CNS disease usually results from hematogenous dissemination and, less frequently, through direct invasion [24]. An extracranial focus of candidiasis is present in over 70% of patients with documented meningitis. Approximately 50% of patients with systemic candidiasis develop one of the following forms of CNS involvement:

- Meningitis.
- Cerebral abscess.
- Single or multiple granulomas.

The pathologic expression varies with age, meningitis being more common in children and neonates and micro-abscesses more prevalent in adults.

Candida produces a chronic, granulomatous meningitis, which, like cryptococcosis, can incite basal arachnoiditis with secondary cranial nerve dysfunction and/or hydrocephalus. Candida meningitis often occurs as a late complication of debilitating illness. Clinically, the typical clinical signs of meningitis may be present but, not infrequently, patients may be so ill and obtunded that they do not manifest the classic signs of meningitis. CNS involvement may also take the form of multiple miliary granulomas scattered throughout the brain, and presents clinically as a diffuse encephalopathy. Solitary or multiple cerebral abscesses can also occur. Because of the compromised host response, the capsule of a fungal abscess is often poorly developed and the abscess therefore less confined. The relative lack of capsule formation is often reflected on the CT image of a fungal abscess, which typically appears as a poorly circumscribed area of low density, with little contrast enhancement. Finally, *Candida* may occasionally invade large cerebral vessels and result in a mycotic aneurysm.

The treatment of CNS *Candida* infection is challenging. If patients are untreated or inadequately treated, the mortality rate approaches 80%. Intravenous amphotericin B has reduced the mortality rate by nearly 50%; the addition of IT therapy is even more effective [23,24]. Patients with frank cerebral abscess should undergo surgical drainage and/or excision, although the outcome is considerably poorer in these patients. Unfortunately, the extremely high mortality is more often the result of multi-system failure related to the underlying illness rather than the abscess per se.

Aspergillosis

Relatively few species of *Aspergillus* produce infection in man, *Aspergillus fumigatus* being the most common. Infection occurs through inhalation of spores that colonize the pulmonary system or para-nasal sinuses. Disseminated aspergillosis is almost uniformly encountered in debilitated or immunocompromised patients. Predisposing conditions include AIDS, organ transplant, leukemia, carcinomatosis, intravenous drug use, tuberculosis, hepatic cirrhosis and prolonged antibiotic therapy [23]. CNS involvement occurs in approximately 50% of patients with dissemintaed aspergillosis through hematogenous dissemination or direct invasion of a granulomatous lesion through the skull base.

Clinically, CNS aspergillosis may present as an acute necrotizing infection or a chronic granulomatous process. Intraparenchymal granulomas or cerebral abscesses produce findings typical of an intracranial mass. Granulomatous masses involving the meninges can produce cranial nerve deficits and/or brainstem dysfunction. Orbital infection may lead to proptosis, altered vision, external ophthalmoplegia and orbital apex syndrome. The organism has a propensity to invade cerebral vessels, causing occlusive vasculitis with cerebral infarction and/or hemorrhage. Vascular invasion of larger proximal vessels occasionally results in a mycotic aneurysm. *Aspergillus* meningitis is rare, except in intravenous drug users.

The diagnosis of CNS aspergillosis is difficult. Since meningitis is rare, CSF findings are non-specific; moreover, culture of the organism from CSF is almost impossible. Definitive diagnosis is based on identification of the fungus in tissue biopsies. The organism has septated hyphae with dichotomous branching, most readily seen using either periodic acid Schiff (PAS) or Gomori methenamine silver stains [24]. Management of CNS aspergillosis consists of surgical excision of fungal abscesses followed by treatment with amphotericin B. Unfortunately, in spite of aggressive therapy, prognosis is extremely poor and few patients survive.

Mucormycosis

Rhizopus is the genus responsible for most cases of mucormycosis in humans. It is part of the normal nasopharyngeal flora in less than 2% of normal individuals. Rhizopus is an opportunistic fungus that is non-pathogenic, except in patients with poorly controlled diabetes mellitus and especially diabetic ketoacidosis. The rhinocerebral form affects the para-nasal sinuses, orbit and brain and accounts for 80–90% of all cases. It usually begins in the sinuses and extends into the orbit, at which point the disease becomes clinically apparent. The characteristic clinical findings include headache, orbital pain, facial and/or peri-orbital swelling, proptosis and external ophthalmoplegia [25]. Visual loss secondary to occlusion of the central retinal artery may occur and represents an important feature which distinguishes mucormycosis from bacterial cavernous sinus thrombophlebitis, as vision is almost always preserved in the latter. Unchecked, continued invasion of the brain follows with rapid abscess formation. Mucormycosis, like *Aspergillus*, has a predilection for vascular invasion, leading to thrombosis, infarction and dissecting aneurysm. Rarely, dissemination from a pulmonary source may cause brain abscess, but this appears to be limited to immunocompromised patients.

Compared to other fungal diseases, which often follow a protracted clinical course, mucormycosis is a fulminant and rapidly fatal process, unless aggressive treatment is instituted. Treatment consists of aggressive drainage and debridement of involved tissue, along with control of the underlying illness. Amphotericin

B is administered, both intravenously and by local irrigation. Hyperbaric oxygen has been utilized, but its efficacy remains unproven. In spite of aggressive management, the mortality rate is about 15% but escalates to 50% in patients with carotid artery invasion.

Actinomycosis and Nocardiosis

Actinomycosis is most commonly caused by *Actinomyces israelii*, an atypical Gram-positive anaerobic bacterium that exists as part of the normal oral and intestinal flora in man. It is not an opportunistic pathogen, but needs devitalized tissue for the anaerobic milieu required to support its growth and, to this end, often coexists with a commensal bacterial infection [24]. Actinomycosis occurs following a break in the mucosal barrier and produces a chronic suppurative granulomatous infection, characterized by draining sinuses, intense fibrosis and purulent abscesses containing the characteristic multilobulated "sulphur granules".

CNS infection occurs in 2–5% cases. The organism reaches the brain through hematogenous dissemination or, less commonly, through direct extension from local cervicofacial disease, and most commonly results in a cerebral abscess [24]. Actinomycotic abscesses are usually solitary, multilobulated lesions, with a thick capsule. The clinical picture is that of a space-occupying lesion, causing focal neurological deficit and signs of increased ICP. Occasionally, an SDE or EDA may develop, following penetrating trauma or calvarial invasion from cervicofacial disease.

Actinomycosis is best diagnosed by microscopic examination of pus and infected tissue. The organism has long branching filaments that stain positively with Gram's stain, while hematoxylin and eosin (H&E) staining demonstrates basophilic filaments, terminating in eosinophilic "clubs". The characteristic "sulphur granules" consist of compact clumps of organisms. Culture of the organism is difficult and only possible under anaerobic conditions. There are no serologic or skin tests for *Actinomyces*.

Cranial imaging usually demonstrates a solitary, ring-enhancing lesion, with a thick capsule and surrounding edema. Management entails drainage and/or excision of the mass, followed by high-dose penicillin therapy (10–20 million units per day) for 3–4 months [23]. Luckily, with early diagnosis and optimum therapy, the prognosis is good.

Nocardia is another "fungus-like" atypical bacterium. However, *Nocardia* has little in common with *Actinomyces*, aside from their classification and tendency to produce brain abscess. Nocardiosis is most often due to *Nocardia asteroides*, a Gram-positive aerobe which is not part of the normal bacteriological flora, but is usually found in the soil and in decaying vegetable matter. Seventy-five percent of patients who develop Nocardiosis harbor an underlying disabling medical disorder (TB, COPD, carcinoma, diabetes, alcoholism, collagen vascular disease) and some form of immunocompromise is identified in 44% of patients [24]. Infection usually begins in the lung following inhalation of the airborne organisms. CNS disease in the form of single or multiple cerebral abscesses occurs from hematogenous dissemination in about 25% of cases. Nocardia abscesses tend to be multiloculated and poorly encapsulated due to the weak inflammatory response invoked by the organism.

The diagnosis of Nocardiosis may prove difficult. The organism is rarely recovered from CSF. Cranial CT is fairly sensitive but non-specific; it typically demonstrates a hypodense, enhancing lesion, with surrounding edema. The diagnosis is made by histological examination, which demonstrates beading, branching Gram-positive, acid-fast filaments; the organism is not seen using H&E or PAS techniques.

Mortality rates as high as 80% have been reported with CNS Nocardiosis [24]. However, in the absence of significant concomitant debilitating disease, prompt diagnosis and treatment are associated with an improved outlook. Treatment should consist of abscess drainage and/or excision along with intravenous sulfisoxazole. Relapse rates are high and prolonged antibiotic therapy (sometimes lasting 6–12 months) is required.

Parasitic Infections

NCC

NCC is the most common parasitic infection of the CNS. Cysticercosis is caused by infestation of the larva from *Taenia solium*, which, in humans, has a special affinity for the CNS. In some underdeveloped regions, NCC accounts for 33% of all intracranial mass lesions. There are several pathological forms of NCC, including racemose meningobasal disease, parenchymal lesions, intraventricular disease and mixed forms. Pathologically, NCC may result in meningoencephalitis, granulomatous meningitis, focal granulomas, space-occupying cysts, hydrocephalus and ependymitis [26,27].

The clinical presentation of NCC depends on multiple factors, including the size, number and location of cysts, as well as the toxicity of the parasite. Meningobasal disease occurs in 25% of patients with NCC and produces a syndrome typical of chronic granulomatous meningitis. Active growth of multiple small vesicles representing encysted larvae, which have a particular affinity for the basal cisterns, produces adherent or free-floating grape-like clusters that cause an intense basal arachnoiditis. This often results in secondary hydrocephalus and various cranial nerve palsies.

Parenchymal NCC occurs in 30–60% of patients. Viable parenchymal cysts produce little tissue reaction and are often asymptomatic. However, death of the parasite contained within the cyst produces an intense inflammatory response in adjacent brain and it is during this stage that patients frequently become symptomatic, with seizures and/or focal neurological findings. Large cysts may occasionally produce focal neurological findings, although the mass effect from even very large cysts is rarely life-threatening.

Intraventricular NCC affects 15–20% of patients. Larvae are believed to gain access to the ventricular system though the choroid plexus. Intraventricular cysts may be free-floating or pedunculated and, if sufficiently large or strategically positioned, can obstruct CSF flow, leading to obstructive hydrocephalus.

Diagnosis of NCC is based on serological testing and imaging. Peripheral eosinophilia may be seen, but is often inconsistent and unreliable. CSF may demonstrate findings of chronic meningitis, but can be entirely normal. However, the finding of more than 20% eosinophils is highly suggestive of parasitic infection. Antibody titers of greater than 1:64 in the serum or 1:8 in the CSF are significant. Serum titers of more than 1:64 are more sensitive for NCC, while elevated CSF titers have greater specificity. A new enzyme-linked immunoelectrotransfer blot is nearly 100% specific and highly sensitive in detecting NCC.

CT and MRI represent the most accurate imaging modalities available. CT is particularly beneficial in identifying parenchymal calcifications that occur in 65% of patients with NCC. Calcification is encountered more often in adults. In children, a diffuse, homogeneously enhancing lesion is more likely to be seen. Twenty-five percent of patients develop parenchymal or intraventricular cysts that are usually evident on CT and greater than 40% will have hydrocephalus. Intraventricular cysts are more readily seen in the presence of intraventricular contrast. Acute parenchymal NCC usually appears as a hypodense area that enhances following contrast administration. Large cystic lesions may show evidence of ring-enhancement. MRI, is also quite accurate in identifying lesions of NCC, and may be more sensitive for identifying intraventricular lesions than non-contrasted CT [26,27].

Treatment of NCC includes administration of anti-helminthic drugs and surgery in selected cases. Praziquantal is highly effective against cysticercosis [26]. The drug is well tolerated, the major side effect occurring from the intense inflammatory reaction produced by the dying parasite. Consequently, for patients with severe NCC, it has been recommended that praziquantal be given in conjunction with corticosteroids. The efficacy of praziquantal has undoubtedly altered the role of surgery in NCC. Indeed, 90% of patients with parenchymal lesions have a non-progressive course and can be successfully managed using praziquantal, corticosteroids and anti-epileptic agents to prevent or control seizures [27]. Nonetheless, there remain several indications for surgery. Occasionally, the diagnosis of NCC is unclear and diagnostic biopsy is necessary. Ventriculo-peritoneal shunting is necessary for patients with hydrocephalus, especially when related to racemose meningobasal disease, since CSF diversion is far safer than attempting to deal directly with the basal cysts. Surgical excision of large symptomatic space-occupying cysts is sometimes indicated. In fact, the best outcomes occur in this setting, with 75% of patients improved. In contrast, the poorest results are seen with basal meningeal disease, where improvement occurs in only 28% and the mortality rate is 67%. Finally, surgery is indicated for patients with intraventricular cysts that are minimally affected by drug therapy. Simple excision is usually sufficient for an unruptured intraventricular cyst. However, if there is a significant granular ependymal reaction, then CSF diversion may also be required as an adjunct to cyst removal.

Toxoplasmosis

Toxoplasmosis is caused by *Toxoplasma gondii*, an obligate intracellular protozoan. Up to 70% of adults have antibodies to *Toxoplasma*. The organism gains access to man through ingestion of contaminated food, although most infections are asymptomatic. However, immunocompromised patients, such as those with AIDS, organ transplants or malignancy, are predisposed to infection [28]. Pathologically, toxoplasmosis produces areas of tissue necrosis surrounded by an intense mononuclear reaction. Three patterns of CNS involvement have been described, including diffuse encephalopathy, meningoencephalitis and cerebral abscess. Many patients with abscess present with focal neurological signs and, in fact, toxoplasmosis is the single most common lesion, causing mass effect in AIDS patients. *Toxoplasma* abscesses are often multiple and bilateral. Intraparenchymal abscesses can be seen on CT and/or MRI. On CT, the lesions are characterized by a region of low density, variable adjacent edema and ring-enhancement. Most lesions are subcortical, often situated in the basal ganglia. Obstructive hydrocephalus sometimes occurs, especially with large lesions near the third ventricle.

The diagnosis of toxoplasmosis is made by a combination of serological testing and tissue biopsy. The organism is best seen in tissue sections stained by the Giemsa method.

Therapy for toxoplasmosis consists of a combination of pyrimethamine and sulfadiazine, along with folic acid. In AIDS patients with multiple intracranial lesions, toxoplasmosis is the most likely diagnosis and therefore it is reasonable to begin empiric therapy and observe the patient for clinical and radiographic response. If a response is not evident within 2 weeks, then biopsy should be considered, to confirm or refute the diagnosis. Even if a response does occur, cure is generally not possible and maintenance therapy is required indefinitely to achieve the goal of therapy, namely control of the disease. Prognosis depends on the extent and severity of brain involvement and, perhaps to a greater extent, on the underlying disease process.

Echinococcosis (Hydatid Disease)

Echinococcosis is caused by infestation of tissue with the encysted larval stage of *Echinococcus granulosa*, the dog tapeworm. Human infection occurs through ingestion of food contaminated by viable ova or by oral contamination from hands after handling infected dogs. The ingested larvae penetrate the intestinal tract, gain access to the bloodstream and are disseminated; they most commonly affect the lungs, liver, bone and brain. Following parasitic embolization, the larvae form a progressively enlarging uniloculated cyst and the cyst wall differentiates into an internal germinal layer from which daughter cysts form. This causes further growth of the cyst, which becomes filled with fluid and germinating parasitic particles known as "hydatid sand" [23].

CNS involvement occurs in 2–3% of patients with systemic echinococcosis. Children are most often affected and, in countries where echinococcosis is common, up to 50% of all childhood CNS "tumors" prove to be echinococcal cysts. Echinococcal cysts are customarily solitary and confined to the white matter of the cerebral hemispheres, although cerebellar, intraventricular and intrasellar cysts have been reported. Unlike NCC, there is negligible glial inflammatory reaction and, therefore, minimal peri-lesional edema. Clinically, children with echinococcal cysts most often present with signs of increased ICP and few focal findings. The clinical picture in adults mimics that of any other space-occupying lesion.

The diagnosis of echinococcosis is made in the presence of peripheral blood eosinophilia, a positive Casoni's intradermal skin test and Weinberg's complement fixation test. CT and/or MRI best demonstrate the parenchymal lesions. The appearance is that of a large, spherical cyst with sharply defined borders that rarely show fine enhancement – a paucity of surrounding edema. The cyst contents have imaging characteristics similar to those of CSF. Calcification of the cyst wall itself should raise the suspicion of a hydatid cyst [23].

Earlier reports have suggested surgical excision to be the treatment of choice [23,24]. Simple aspiration of the cyst was discouraged, unless removal was possible. The challenge of surgery is to remove the cyst intact, avoiding spillage of the contents, which can disseminate the disease process or, rarely, produce an anaphylactic reaction [24]. Removal is most easily accomplished by cortical incision and exposure of the cyst, followed by hydraulic dissection of the capsule, using gentle irrigation to separate the cyst wall from the surrounding brain to which the attachment is generally tenuous. The results of excision are variable, with poorer outcomes associated with inability to remove the cyst intact. More recently, it has been suggested that burr-hole aspiration, followed by systemic chemotherapy with mebendazole or albendazole, may be equally effective.

Post-operative Neurosurgical Infections

In spite of numerous improvements in aseptic technique and prophylaxis, post-operative infection following craniotomy continues to be a source of substantial morbidity. Post-craniotomy infection comprises a spectrum of infectious processes, including superficial wound infections, bone flap infection, bacterial meningitis, EDA, SDE and cerebral abscess. Assessment of the true incidence of post-operative infection is difficult and comparison of rates between studies is particularly problematic. Indeed, there is no consensus as to exactly what constitutes an infection. In some studies, infection is defined by a subjective impression, while in others, objective parameters such as positive bacterial cultures are required. Furthermore, notwithstanding the lack of a precise definition for infection, incidence rates are not calculated in a standard fashion. Various studies utilize different values for the denominator, including the number of procedures, incisions, discharges, admissions and patients undergoing a procedure. Similarly, the numerator differs; some studies include multiple infections in the same patient, patients with shunt infections and even patients with systemic infections.

The incidence of infection within 30 days of craniotomy ranges from 0 to 22%, with an average rate of around 5%. Lal et al. summarized post-craniotomy infection rates from a review of the neurosurgical literature reported between 1913 and 1992 [29]. If one series that did not provide data regarding total craniotomies and number of infections and a second series in which the results included all types of infection (urinary tract, pneumonia, etc.) are eliminated, 18 series that included 9,336 craniotomies are left. Among these patients, there were a total of 421 post-operative infections – an infection rate of 4.5%. Interestingly, the infection rates before and after 1940 are nearly indentical: 4.4% (91 infections in 2,054 procedures) and 4.5% (330 infections in 7,284 procedures), respectively.

Numerous studies have attempted to identify potential risk factors that might increase the rate of infection. Factors that have been felt to play a significant role include age, the presence of a concomitant systemic infection, duration of operation, re-operation, the use of externalized drains, surgeon experience, use of perioperative steroids and the use of perioperative antibiotics. Indeed, intuitively, all of these factors could conceivably contribute to a higher incidence of post-operative infection. However, the ability to measure some of these variables has caused a number of these studies to be questioned. Korinek et al. recently performed a prospective evaluation of 2,944 adult patients who underwent craniotomy [30]. Univariate analysis identified the following as predictive risk factors: emergency surgery, contaminated or dirty wound classification, duration of procedure being more than 4 hours, neurosurgical procedure within 30 days and post-operative CSF leak. This analysis assumes that the predictors act in isolation and are not influenced by other factors. However, following multivariate analysis, only post-operative CSF leak and re-operation proved to be independent risk factors.

Bacterial Meningitis in Neurosurgical Patients

Bacterial meningitis has been reported in up to 17% of neurosurgical patients. In contrast to most cases of pyogenic meningitis in the general population, the majority of cases of bacterial meningitis in the neurosurgical patient result from direct inoculation of micro-organisms into the CSF or, less commonly, through retrograde propagation from contiguous structures through emissary veins. Meningitis most commonly occurs in one of the following clinical settings:

- Post-operatively (mostly following craniotomy).
- Penetrating CNS trauma.
- Following basilar skull fracture associated with CSF leak.
- In association with CSF shunt devices.
- In association with spinal dysraphic states, such as ruptured myelomeningocele and persistent dermal sinus tracts [31–33].

Rarely, a lumbar puncture performed during an episode of bacteremia may precipitate bacterial meningitis. However, the overwhelming importance of obtaining CSF for rapid diagnosis and treatment should overshadow any concern for causing meningitis by performing a diagnostic lumbar puncture.

Post-operative Meningitis

It has been estimated that, in spite of the use of perioperative antibiotics, 0.5–0.7% of patients undergoing a clean neurosurgical procedure develop post-operative bacterial meningitis [32]. The incidence in clean-contaminated cases, such as transsphenoidal or surgical approaches that traverse air sinuses, ranges from around 0.4 to 2%. Although most cases probably occur as a result of direct inoculation of micro-organisms during the procedure, some cases occur from spread of infection from other nearby sites, such as a wound infection. It has been reported that the presence of a post-operative CSF leak results in a 13-fold increase in the risk of meningitis. Consequently, attempting a meticulous, water-tight dural closure should be a standard goal of any intradural procedure. It would appear that the other major independent risk factor would be early re-operation. Other potential risk factors for post-operative infection have been discussed previously. The microbiology of post-operative meningitis is consistent with the pathogenesis of infection, with staphylococcal organisms being the predominant pathogens. However, in procedures that traverse an air sinus, the most common organisms are, not surprisingly, those that customarily colonize these areas.

Meningitis Associated with CSF Leak

The incidence of bacterial meningitis following head trauma ranges from 0.2 to 18%. The incidence is greatly increased when there is an accompanying CSF leak, ranging anywhere from 3% to as high as 50% [32]. Direct implantation of organisms can occur with penetrating injuries, open depressed skull fractures or closed fractures that cross a chronically infected air sinus. Fractures of the cranial base are often associated with dural tears and often produce CSF rhinorrhea or otorrhea. Although meningitis can develop literally within hours after injury, the risk is highest within the initial few weeks following trauma. However, cases have been reported many years following injury.

Approximately 50–70% of cases of acute bacterial meningitis related to CSF leaks following basilar skull fracture are caused by pneumococcus; recurrent meningitis is highly correlated with head injury, with pneumococci accounting for 80% of these cases. The remaining cases are *Hemophilus influenza*, group A beta hemolytic streptococci and other genera. In cases of penetrating injury or open wounds of the brain, infection with Gram-negative organisms is more likely. In cases where there has been gross contamination, polymicrobial infections, especially involving anaerobes, are more common. Diagnosis and management of the bacterial infection are identical to those of other cases of acute bacterial meningitis. CSF leaks may spontaneously "seal" following treatment of meningitis, but those that persist require surgical repair.

An area of considerable controversy is the use of prophylactic antibiotics in patients with basilar skull fractures accompanied by CSF leaks. The premise supporting the use of prophylactic antibiotics is that CSF is exposed directly to pathogenic organisms and that infection is likely. However, interpretation of clinical studies is contaminated by multiple variables, including the definition of infection, patient selection and choice of antibiotics. Moreover, there exists no prospective randomized trial that examines this question. There are clearly those who advocate the routine use of prophylactic antibiotics, citing a reduction in the incidence of meningitis. On the other hand, there are many who have reported no apparent benefit from the use of prophylactic antibiotics. In fact, one study cited a 37% incidence of meningitis in patients who received prophylaxis [31]. On balance, based on the available evidence, it would appear that the routine use of prophylactic antibiotics in patients with post-traumatic CSF leaks cannot be supported and, in fact, may be responsible for the selection of more virulent and resistant organisms.

Key Points

- *The evolution of brain abscesses progresses through four stages: early cerebritis, late cerebritis, early capsule formation and late capsule formation.*
- *The microbiological profile of a brain abscess is closely linked to the underlying etiology.*
- *Surgical management of brain abscess consists of stereotactic aspiration or craniotomy and excision of the capsule.*
- *Frequent imaging is essential during treatment.*
- *Successful treatment of other infections of the nervous system requires prompt recognition, drainage in some cases and appropriate antibiotic therapy.*

References

1. Garfield J. Management of supratentorial intracranial abscess: a review of 200 cases. BMJ 1969;2:7–11.
2. Morgan H, Wood MW, Murphey F. Experience with 88 consecutive cases of brain abscess. J Neurosurg 1973;38:698–704.
3. deLouvois J. The bacteriology and chemotherapy of brain abscess. J Antimicrob Chemother 1978;4:395–413.
4. Beller AJ, Sahar A, Praiss I. Brain abscess: review of 89 cases over a period of 30 years. J Neurol Neurosurg Psychiatry 1973;36:757–68.
5. Fisher EG, McLennan JE, Suzuki Y. Cerebral abscess in children. Am J Dis Child 1981;135:746–9.
6. Renier D, Flandin C, Hirsch E, Hirsch JF. Brain abscesses in neonates: a study of 30 cases. J Neurosurg 1988;69:877–82.
7. Graham DR, Band JD. Citrobacter diversus brain abscess and meningitis in neonates. JAMA 1981;245: 1923–5.
8. Yang SY: Brain abscess: a review of 400 cases. J Neurosurg 1981;55:794–9.
9. Britt RH, Enzmann DR. Clinical stages of human brain abscesses on serial CT scans after contrast infusion: computerized tomographic, neuropathological, and clinical correlations. J Neurosurg 1983;59:972–89.
10. Brant-Zawadzki M, Enzmann DR, Placone RC, Sheldon P et al. NMR imaging of experimental brain abscess: comparison with CT. AJNR 1983;4:250–3.
11. Cure J. Imaging of intracranial infection. In: Batjer H, Loftus C, editors. Textbook of neurological surgery. Lippicott Williams and Wilkins (in press).
12. Bellotti C, Aragno MG, Medina M, Viglietti AL et al. Differential diagnosis of CT-hypodense cranial lesions with indium-111-oxine-labeled leukocytes. J Neurosurg 1986;64:750–3.
13. Gormley W, Rosenblum M. Cerebral abscess. In: Tindall G, Cooper P, Barrow D, editors. The practice of neurosurgery. Baltimore, USA: Williams and Wilkins, 1996; 3343–54.
14. Osenbach RK. Central nervous system infections. In: Grossman R, Loftus CML, editors. Principles of neurosurgery. 2nd Edition. Philadelphia, PA: Lippincott-Raven, 1999; 217–50.
15. Rosenblum ML, Mampalam TJ, Pons VG. Controversies in the manangement of brain abscesses. Clin Neurosurg 1986;33:603–32.
16. Harris LF, Haws FP, Triplett JN Jr. Subdural empyema and epidural abscess: recent experience in a community hospital. South Med J 1987;80:1254–8.
17. Krauss WE, McCormick PC. Infections of the dural spaces. Neurosurg Clin North Am 1992;3:421–33.
18. Hall WA. Cerebral infectious processes. In: Loftus CML, editor. Neurosurgical emergencies. Volume I. Neurosurgical Topics Series. AANS Publications, 1994; 165–82.
19. Haines SJ, Mampalam T, Rosenblum ML, Nagib MG. Cranial and intracranial bacterial infections. In: Youmans J, editor. Neurological surgery. Philadelphia, PA: W.B. Saunders, 1990; 3707–35.
20. Williams B. Subdural empyema. Adv Tech Stand Neurosurg 1982;9:133–170.
21. Weingarten K, Zimmerman RD, Becker RD et al. Subdural and epidural empyemas: MR imaging. AJR 1989;152:615–21.
22. Ackerman L, Traynelis V. Dural space infections. In: Osenbach RK, Zeidman SM, editors. Infections in neurological surgery: diagnosis and management. Philadelphia, PA: Lippincott–Raven, 1999; 85–99.
23. Martz RD, Hoff JT. Parasitic and fungal diseases of the central nervous system. In: Youman J, editor. Neurological surgery. 3rd Edition. Philadelphia, PA: W.B. Saunders, 1990; 3742–51. 24. Friedman AH, Bullitt E. Fungal and parasitic infections. In: Wilkins RH, Rengechary SS, editors. Neurosurgery. New York: McGraw-Hill, 1985; 2002–15.
25. Rangel-Cuerra R, Martinez HR, Saenz C. Mucomycosis: report of 11 cases. Arch Neurol 1985;2:578–81.
26. Sotelo J, Escobedo F, Rodriguez-Carbajal J, Torres B, Rubio-Donnadieu F. Therapy of parenchymal brain cycticercosis with praziquantel. N Engl J Med 1984;310:1001–7.
27. McCormick GF, Zee CS, Heiden J. Cysticercosis cerebri: review of 127 cases. Arch Neurol 1982;39:534–9.
28. Levy RM, Russel E, Yungbluth M et al. The efficacy of image-guided stereotactic brain biopsy in neurologi-

cally symptomatic acquired immune deficiency symdrome patients. Neurosurgery 1992;30:186–90.
29. Lal S, McCutcheon I. Infections after craniotomy. In: Hall W, McCutcheon I, editors. Infections in neurosurgery. Chicago, IL: American Association of Neurological Surgeons Publications Committee, 2000; 125–40.
30. Korinek AM, the French Study Group of Neurosurgical Infections, the SEHP et al. Risk factors for neurosurgical site infections after craniotomy: a prospective multicenter study of 2944 patients. Neurosurgery 1997;41: 1073–81.
31. Kaufman B, Tunkel A, Pryor J, Dacey R Jr. Meningitis in the neurosurgical patient. Infect Dis Clinics of North America 1990;4:677–701.
32. Abolnik I, Perfect J, Durack D. Acute bacterial meningitis. In: Wilkins R, Rengechary S, editors. Neurosurgery. 2nd Edition. New York: McGraw-Hill, 1996;3299–306.
33. Wilberger J Jr. Posttraumatic infectious complications. In: Hall W, McCutcheon I, editors. Infections in neurosurgery. Chicago, IL: American Association of Neurological Surgeons Publications Committee, 2000; 173–80.

38

Ischemic Stroke and Carotid Endarterectomy

Dennis A. Velez and David W. Newell

Summary

Ischemic stroke accounts for approximately 80% of all strokes, and most of the remainder are hemorrhagic subtypes. Most ischemic strokes are due to intracranial vessel occlusion, the majority resulting from embolism from the heart or extracranial vessels. Advances in medical treatment of ischemic stroke have included administration of thrombolytic substances, which have proven to be effective in improving outcome after ischemic stroke. Atheromatous disease of the cervical carotid artery is the most important source of embolic disease from extracranial cerebral vasculature. Prospective randomized trials of surgery versus medical therapy have established the role of carotid endarterectomy for stroke prevention in symptomatic and asymptomatic patients with high-grade carotid stenosis. Endovasular therapy, including angioplasty and stenting, is being investigated as an alternative to carotid endarterectomy for stroke prevention in these patients.

Introduction

Stroke continues to be the most common life-threatening neurologic disease and the third leading cause of death in the USA, after heart disease and cancer. It remains the most common neurological cause for hospital admission. Approximately 500,000 new or recurrent strokes occur every year in this country. It accounts for over 150,000 fatalities each year. Stroke is also the leading cause of intellectual and physical disability in adults and the most common cause of institutionalization for long-term care. It is estimated that there are over 3,000,000 stroke survivors, many of whom require chronic care. The economic costs of stroke due to healthcare expenses and lost productivity are estimated to be nearly $20 billion [1].

Ischemic stroke accounts for approximately 80% of all strokes, with the remainder being hemorrhagic strokes, with its different subtypes. This chapter will discuss the medical and surgical management of ischemic stroke, taking into consideration what is known about the pathophysiology of this condition. The focus will be on the knowledge acquired from basic science and clinical research, as well as the results of rigorous clinical trials which have helped to establish guidelines, which, in turn, have had an effect on the outcome of patients afflicted with this devastating condition.

Pathology and Pathophysiology of Ischemic Stroke and Extracranial Cerebrovascular Occlusive Disease

Ischemic Stroke: Pathophysiology

Although the human brain accounts for 2% of the total body weight, it utilizes 20% of the cardiac output to supply the required oxygen and glucose necessary for its incessant metabolic needs. Because the brain does not store or produce these substances, any interruption in their delivery results in some kind of dysfunction. Blood-flow alterations or limitations can, at times, be tolerated, because of compensatory mechanisms such as collateral circulation. Progressive ischemia can lead to brain infarction which, in turn, leads to local vasodilatation, edema, stasis of the blood column and segmentation of the red blood cells and, eventually, brain tissue necrosis. The local vasodilatation leads to an increase in cerebral blood volume and enhanced oxygen extraction from the capillaries.

Cellular edema occurs because of ischemic-induced changes in membrane permeability. This allows for a net ionic influx. There is an associated failure of the Na^+/K^+ pump, the release of excitatory neurotransmitters such as glutamate, and the opening of calcium channels. The opening of these calcium channels leads to further calcium influx, which results in cell injury, as a consequence of organelle dysfunction and disruption of neuronal metabolism. Calcium activates degradative enzymes, such as lipases, proteases and endonucleases. There is also an accumulation of free fatty acids from membrane phospholipid degradation, which are not oxidized by the cyclooxygenase or lipooxygenase pathways. As a result, prostaglandins, leukotrienes and free radicals are formed, which, in turn, lead to altered membrane permeability, vasoconstriction and the destruction of cellular membranes.

CBF regulation is an important mechanism, which plays a role in protecting the brain from ischemia. Blood-flow thresholds have been correlated to the degree of neuronal dysfunction and ischemic damage. Resting CBF is usually 50–55 ml/100 g/minute, with flow through gray matter higher than through white matter. Blood flow to the brain is coupled to neuronal activity and metabolism. There is an increase in cerebral blood flow during direct electrical excitation, seizure activity and the performance of certain intellectual tasks. Cerebral auto-regulation refers to the ability of the brain to maintain a constant CBF, despite changes in arterial perfusion pressure. During cerebral ischemia, auto-regulation is impaired [2]. At blood-flow levels of about 20 ml/100 g/minute, cortical electrical activity is not detectable. At levels of 10 ml/100 g/minute, there is an increase in extracellular potassium concentration – a finding consistent with membrane pump failure and cell death [3].

The ischemic penumbra is defined as that area of brain tissue surrounding the center of the infarct in which neuronal function is impaired but can be salvaged. Reduced perfusion or prolonged ischemia leads to incorporation of the penumbra region into the infarcted region, which, in turn, leads to more extensive tissue necrosis and death. Restoration of blood flow to this region allows for the delivery of vital substrates to the brain and eventual resolution of neuronal dysfunction. Most stroke therapy modalities now in use have as their goal the prompt restoration of blood flow to this region, so as to prevent the neurological dysfunction associated with massive tissue necrosis. Following infarction, the brain softens and liquifies and the necrotic tissue is removed by microglia. Astroglia from the surrounding brain tissue proliferate to occupy the remaining space.

The ischemic insult can be worsened by factors such as individual anatomical vascular variations and the presence and extent of collateral circulation. The vascular supply to the brain can vary from person to person, and arterial territories and their boundaries are even different within the same individual at different times. Changes in hemodynamic conditions can have an effect on these vascular territories and potentially worsen cerebral ischemia. Adequate supplementary blood flow through collateral vessels is also variable between individuals. In the presence of vessel occlusion or stenosis, pressure gradients help to supply, through anastomotic networks, blood to compromised territories.

Anastomotic networks exist in the adult circulation to help provide sources of collateral flow. The most prominent extracranial anastomotic channels are those between the external and the internal carotid artery. Occlusion of the proximal ICA results in retrograde blood flow in the ophthalmic artery, which serves to provide flow to the ICA region. The circle of Willis also serves as a collateral system. Its significance lies in its arrangement, which allows for flow to continue uninterrupted, despite complete occlusion of one of its constituent vessels. Variations in the anatomical arrangement are responsible for the limitations of the system to fully compensate and provide nourishment to the brain in cases of ischemic events. Leptomeningeal vessels constitute the primary anastomotic network on the surface of the cerebrum and cerebellum [4]. Although this system is usually quiescent, proximal vessel occlusion leads to a pressure differential, which allows blood to reach the areas with lowered cerebral perfusion pressure.

Extracranial Cerebrovascular Disease: Pathogenesis

Most ischemic strokes in the past were attributed to intracranial vessel occlusion. This was recognized by C. Miller Fisher, who found a clinicopathological association between atheromatous disease of the cervical carotid artery and an increase in the risk of stroke [5]; hence, the importance of the extracranial cerebral vasculature as a source of ischemic disease. The recent contributions from molecular biology, as well as improved vascular imaging, have increased our understanding of the diseases that affect this segment of the cerebral vasculature (Table 38.1).

Table 38.1. Conditions associated with extracranial cerebrovascular occlusive disease.

Atherosclerosis
Fibromuscular dysplasia
Radiation
Arterial dissection
Giant cell arteritis
Takayasu's arteritis
Mechanical compression of the subclavian and vertebral arteries

Atherosclerosis

Atherosclerosis is a diffuse disorder, which affects medium and large muscular and elastic arteries. The fatty streak, the initial lesion, is composed of discrete accumulations of intimal smooth muscle cells and lipids. These lead to the development of a fibrous plaque and, ultimately, a lesion associated with ulcerations, intramural hemorrhage and thrombosis. The great majority of ischemic strokes, in the setting of occlusive disease of the craniocerebral vasculature, are due to atherosclerotic disease. The most common extracranial sites for atherosclerosis are the carotid bifurcation, the sub-clavian arteries and the proximal vertebral arteries. Risk factors associated with the development of atherosclerosis include age, male gender, hypercholesterolemia, hypertension, family history, diabetes mellitus, chronic infection and smoking. Not only does atherosclerosis contribute to carotid artery stenosis, but also, more importantly, it can lead to thrombosis and subsequent embolization. These two processes depend on a series of factors, such as local blood flow, presence of turbulent flow and the state of the vessel lumen. Significant carotid stenosis at the site of a complex atherosclerotic lesion is thought to lead to thrombus formation. Endarterectomy is done to remove plaque and, hence, prevent stroke by removing the site of thrombosis rather than to increase blood flow through a stenotic segment in most instances.

Radiation-induced Atherosclerosis

Radiation-induced atherosclerosis can occur in patients treated with cervical supraclavicular and mediastinal radiation. Injury to the elastic membrane, intimal thickening and plaque formation and fibrosis have been described. Cholesterol deposition and plaque formation have also been documented after radiation exposure.

Dissection

Arterial dissection is a common cause of ischemic stroke in the young adult. These have been categorized as traumatic and spontaneous. Dissection along sub-intimal planes can cause luminal stenosis and hemodynamic and thromboembolic brain ischemia. Traumatic dissection usually involves the distal extracranial internal carotid artery, usually 2 cm from the carotid bifurcation. This portion of the carotid artery is thought to be tethered at the skull base and, hence, adjacent to the C2 transverse process. Hyperextension and rotation of the neck can then lead to carotid dissection. Spontaneous dissection can be associated with atherosclerosis or fibromuscular dysplasia (FMD). Other disorders of collagen and elastin, such as Marfan's syndrome, cystic medial necrosis and Type IV Ehler–Danlos syndrome, have also been associated with spontaneous arterial dissections. Clinically, these lesions typically present with headache, facial pain, oculosympathetic palsy (Horner's syndrome) and ipsilateral cerebral ischemia. The presumed mechanism is thought to be distal embolization. The characteristic angiographic pattern of these lesions includes a tapered stenosis or occlusion, beginning distal to the carotid bifurcation and ending at the skull base.

Fibromuscular Dysplasia

FMD is a vasculopathy characterized by arterial stenosis and is usually seen in young adult females. It affects the cervical carotid vessels in 25% of patients with symptomatic FMD. It is also the second most common cause of extracranial carotid stenosis. Pathologically, the lesions are characterized by fibroplasias of the media or, sometimes, the intima, with interspersed luminal constriction and segments of dilated, thinned media that produce a "string of beads" pattern on angiography. Regions of fibrosis may cause stenosis and dilated areas can cause low flow states, but ischemia is usually the result of dissection.

Inflammatory Conditions

Giant cell arteritis is the most common of the vasculitides. It usually affects vessels rich in elastic tissues, such as the superficial temporal and occipital arteries. Involvement of the subclavian and extracranial vertebral arteries, although rare, can cause infarction as a result of thrombotic vessel occlusion [6]. Takayasu's arteritis, an uncommon disease in the USA, can cause inflammation and occlusive disease of the aortic arch and great vessels. Dizziness, syncope and sub-clavian steal symptomatology is usually seen, but brain infarction is not.

Other Conditions

Tumors, infections, fibrous bands, osteophytes and fractures can also cause mechanical compression of the carotid, sub-clavian and vertebral arteries with the V2 segment commonly affected in the latter vessel.

Risk Factors for Ischemic Stroke

Ischemic stroke can occur in people of all ages, at any time and without predilection for sex or race. Age, however, is the most important determinant of stroke, with most strokes occurring in individuals older than 65. Atherosclerosis affecting the extracranial and intracranial circulation differs according to race and ethnic group. For example, extracranial atherosclerotic lesions are more common in whites, while intracranial lesions are more common in blacks, Hispanics and Asians.

Several disease processes and lifestyle habits can predispose or facilitate cerebral ischemia. For example, following age, hypertension is the most powerful stroke risk factor. People with cardiac disease, specifically with atrial fibrillation, valvular heart disease, coronary artery disease, myocardial infarction, congestive heart failure, as well as those with electrocardiographic evidence of left ventricular hypertrophy, are also at an increased risk for ischemic stroke. Other disorders, such as diabetes mellitus, hypercholesterolemia, sickle cell disease, coagulation deficiencies and non-atherosclerotic vasculopathies, have also been implicated as a cause of ischemic stroke. Physical inactivity, cigarette smoking and heavy alcohol use are also risk factors for ischemic stroke, which are amenable to lifestyle modifications.

Transient ischemic attacks (TIAs), defined as acute, non-convulsive, focal neurological deficit as a result of inadequate blood flow to a vascular distribution and which resolve in less than 24 hours, are strong predictors of subsequent stroke. Most TIAs typically last 2–15 minutes and their incidence increases with age [7]. The first year after a TIA portends the greatest risk of stroke, with an incidence of 1–15%.

Carotid artery disease resulting in a plaque or carotid stenosis has been found to confer an increased risk of stroke, especially in patients with greater than 75% stenosis. An annual stroke risk of 3.3% was found in this group of patients, which is higher than the 1.3% risk of stroke seen in patients with less than 75% stenosis. The combined risk of TIA and stroke was 10.5% per year in patients with greater than 75% stenosis. Also, the risk of ipsilateral stroke in this latter group was 2.5% [8].

Ischemic Stroke Subtypes

Hemodynamic factors, embolism and small vessel disease are the most common mechanisms by which ischemic strokes occur. The most frequent conditions leading to cerebral ischemia are atherosclerosis, embolism secondary to cardiac disease, small vessel disease and cryptogenic infarction.

Atherosclerosis

As previously noted, atherosclerotic plaques can lead to progressive vessel stenosis or occlusion. Ischemia leading to infarction is due to diminished blood flow distal to the site of stenosis or occlusion. The extent of infarction depends on collateral blood flow or re-establishment of blood flow through the affected region. Atherosclerosis can lead to infarct through dislodgement of an embolic fragment arising from an ulcerated vessel or from an unstable plaque.

Cardiac Embolism

Ischemic strokes caused by embolism usually have a cardiac source. It is estimated that cardioembolic events account for 15–20% of all ischemic strokes [9]. It is also estimated that 75% of cardiac emboli travel to the brain. Once in the brain, emboli can lodge themselves in arteries that are too small for them to pass, leading to vessel occlusion. Mural thrombi can form after a myocardial infarction (MI) and ischemic events follow an acute MI in 2–5% of cases [10]. Other common sources of cardiac embolism include atrial fibrillation, atrial myxoma, dilated cardiomyopathy, patent foramen ovale, atrial septal aneurysms, prosthetic heart valves, infective endocarditis, mitral valve prolapse and mitral annular calcification.

Small Vessel Lacunar Disease

Lacunes are small infarcts, which occur as a result of arterial disease of vessels supplying the deep aspects of the cerebrum and brain stem, such as the basal ganglia, the internal capsule, the thalamus, the corona radiata and paramedian regions of the brainstem. They account for 12–15% of ischemic strokes [11]. They can be silent or they can present with neurological deficits, such as pure motor hemiparesis, pure sensory syndrome, clumsy hand dysarthria, ataxic hemiparesis and sensorimotor stroke. The arterial damage is usually due to the effects of long-standing hypertension and diabetes. Many patients with radiographic evidence of lacunar infarcts do not present with the classic syndromes. Most patients are awake and their intellectual functions are not compromised. The mortality associated with this disease is low, but the morbidity can be significant.

Infarcts of Undetermined Cause

Despite complete diagnostic evaluation, the cause of cerebral ischemia cannot be identified in as many as 40% of ischemic strokes. Patients with these "cryptogenic strokes" usually have no prior TIAs, no bruits on physical examination and, usually, normal angiography. CT scanning or MRI may be normal or may show an infarct limited to a surface brain territory. Some of these infarcts have been attributed to conditions such as sickle cell disease, hypercoagulable states or protein C and protein S deficiencies, lupus anticoagulant or anticardiolipin antibodies.

Evaluation and Management of the Acute Ischemic Stroke Patient

The acute onset of a neurological deficit in a vascular distribution should prompt emergent clinical and radiographic evaluation to identify, treat and prevent recurrence of an ischemic stroke. Common neurological deficits include hemiparesis, aphasia, gaze palsies, hemianopia, dysarthria, confusion, hemineglect, hearing loss and ataxia.

The evaluation and management of the acute ischemic stroke patient begin in the ED, although efforts are underway to educate emergency medical technicians and paramedics so as to improve pre-hospital-phase care.

Once a patient arrives in the ED, a stroke team, already waiting for the patient, starts general therapeutic measures. These include obtaining vital signs such as temperature, blood pressure, pulse and oxygen saturation. Patients with severe deficits, including loss of consciousness, and those unable to protect their own airway should undergo emergent endotracheal intubation and mechanical ventilation. Adequate oxygen saturation is indispensable, as hypoxia can worsen cerebral ischemia. Appropriate laboratory studies (Table 38.2) and diagnostic studies (Table 38.3) should be obtained so as to determine the cause of the stroke. The most common and urgent condition to be differentiated in the setting of suspected ischemic stroke is intracerebral hemorrhage. A CT scan without contrast is the initial imaging modality of choice to help differentiate these two primary diagnostic considerations, since the clinical findings on these two groups of patients frequently overlap.

Patients suspected of having a stroke should have a thorough but concise history and a neurological examination of sufficient detail to assess the degree of dysfunction and to rule out other neurological conditions. Assessment of the level of consciousness, gaze, vision, dysarthria, aphasia, leg and arm strength, sensory loss or extinction, facial asymmetry and limb ataxia needs to be undertaken and clearly documented. Time of symptom onset is important to determine whether there is an opportunity for the patient to receive thrombolytic therapy, provided there are no contraindications (Table 38.4). Duration of symptoms beyond 3 hours excludes the patient from receiving thrombolysis using intravenous tissue plasminogen activator (t-PA) [12].

In order to optimize care and to prevent complications, patients with ischemic stroke probably should be admitted to an ICU or a specialized stroke unit. Neurological complications in the acute setting with the potential to worsen outcome include cerebral edema, hydrocephalus, elevated intracranial pressure, hemorrhagic transformation and seizures. Medical complications include aspiration, hypoxia, myocardial ischemia, cardiac arrhythmias, deep venous thrombosis (DVT), pulmonary embolism (PE) and urinary tract infections.

Blood pressure (BP) is usually elevated after a stroke and its optimal management is controversial. Since cerebral autoregulation is usually lost after an ischemic stroke, a fall in BP has the potential to exacerbate neurological symptoms, due to a decrease in CBF. The current American Heart Association (AHA) guidelines advise against using anti-hypertensive agents, unless the systolic blood pressure is greater than 220 mmHg or the mean arterial blood pressure (MABP) is greater than 130 [13]. It is also recommended that patients with signs of hypertensive emergency, such as hypertensive

Table 38.2. Routine laboratory studies to obtain in patients with ischemic stroke.

CBC with differential
Platelets
PT/PTT/INR
Serum electrolytes, glucose
BUN & Creatinine
Hepatic panel
Blood cultures
Urine toxicology, urine analysis, urine culture
Protein C, Protein S levels
Anti-thrombin III level
Antiphospholipid antibodies
Homocysteine levels
Arterial blood gases

Table 38.3. Immediate diagnostic studies in patients with acute ischemic stroke.

Head CT scan without contrast
Electrocardiogram
Chest X-ray

Table 38.4. Exclusion criteria for intravenous thrombolysis.

Current use of oral anticoagulants or prothrombin time > 15 seconds (INR > 1.7)
Use of heparin in the previous 48 hours and a prolonged PTT
Platelet count < 100,000/mm^3
Another stroke or serious head injury in the previous 3 months
Major surgery within the preceding 14 days
Pretreated systolic blood pressure > 185 or DBP > 110
Rapidly improving neurological signs
Isolated mild neurological deficits such as ataxia alone, sensory loss alone, dysarthria alone or minimal weakness
Prior intracerebral hemorrhage
Blood glucose < 50 mg/dl or > 400 mg/dl
Seizure at the onset of stroke
GI or GU bleeding within the preceding 21 days
Recent myocardial infarction

encephalopathy, retinal hemorrhage, cardiac ischemia, congestive heart failure or evidence of progressive renal dysfunction, should also be treated. Agents such as labetalol, esmolol and enalaprilat, which are short-acting, easily titratable and have a predictable response, are preferred [13]. Invasive arterial monitoring is necessary in patients treated with vasopressors or potent vasodilators.

Close monitoring of fluid status, electrolytes and blood sugar is necessary in the ischemic stroke patient. Normovolemia and euglycemia is the goal, since hyperglycemia is associated with increased morbidity and mortality after stroke [14]. Maintenance of normo- or hypothermia provides brain protection, since hyperthermia can worsen outcome in cerebral ischemia [15]. Fever after a stroke is a common occurrence. Acetaminophen and cooling blankets help in reducing acute increases in temperature. An infectious source for the fever should always be sought and treated with appropriate anti-microbial agents. Fever in the chronic phase of stroke is usually the result of aspiration pneumonia or urinary tract infection [16].

Cytotoxic and vasogenic edema can be seen after an ischemic stroke. Death during the first week after an ischemic stroke is usually the result of brain edema and elevated intracranial pressure. Cerebral edema usually peaks at between 3 and 5 days after a stroke and it warrants medical intervention in 10–20% of patients. Clinical signs of neurological deterioration secondary to brain edema and incipient herniation include a decrease in the level of consciousness, pupillary asymmetry, irregular breathing and a positive Babinski sign contralateral to the hemiparesis. Patients on mechanical ventilation may be hyperventilated to a PCO_2 of between 33 and 35 mmHg. Osmotic diuretics such as mannitol, which help to decrease the intracranial pressure, can be administered every 4–6 hours, with careful attention to volume status, serum electrolytes and serum osmolarity. In the case of refractory intracranial hypertension, CSF drainage via a ventriculostomy or surgical decompression via a hemicraniectomy with duraplasty might be indicated.

Seizures can occur during the acute stroke period in 4–43% of cases. They usually occur within 24 hours of a stroke and tend to be partial in nature. Recurrent seizures occur in approximately 73% of cases, usually within the first year. Seizure control can usually be achieved with antiepileptic monotherapy in the majority of cases.

Nutrition is important in both the acute and chronic phases of the ischemic stroke patient. Patients with ischemic stroke have increased caloric requirements. Nutritional support should be started as soon as possible after stroke and, preferentially, via the enteral route. This can be usually accomplished by placing either a nasogastric or feeding tube or, if long-term nutritional support is needed, either because of swallowing difficulties or increased aspiration risk, via a percutaneous gastrostomy tube.

The services of rehabilitation physicians, physical, occupational and speech therapists, as well as those from social workers and counseling professionals, should be implemented as soon as the patient is stabilized. Early mobilization of the stroke patient is desirable to prevent complications such as pneumonia, atelectasis, DVT, decubitus ulcers and PE, all of which are associated with increased morbidity and mortality.

Carotid Endarterectomy and Surgery for Cerebral Ischemia

Results of Clinical Trials

Carotid stenosis has been recognized to be a common cause of ischemic stroke. Carotid endarterectomy has been carried out in the past for a variety of clinical and radiographic findings, none of which were uniform up and until several prospective randomized trials were designed to determine the efficacy of this intervention as treatment modality in the prevention of ischemic stroke. Indications for carotid endarterectomy can be classified based on the presence or absence of symptoms. Classic asymptomatic findings include arterial narrowing found through a non-invasive study such as an ultrasound.

Symptomatic stenosis can present with transient monocular blindness, TIAs or a completed stroke in the distribution of the ipsilateral stenotic ICA. Trials for symptomatic and asymptomatic carotid stenosis are discussed.

Results of Trials for Symptomatic Carotid Stenosis

The European Carotid Surgery Trial (ECST) enrolled patients with mild (less than 30% stenosis), moderate (30–69% stenosis) and severe (70–99% stenosis) carotid stenosis and randomized them into a non-surgical group and a surgical group [17]. Among 374 randomized patients with mild stenosis, there was no difference in the risk of ipsilateral stroke between groups. Among those patients with severe stenosis, surgery proved beneficial in preventing stroke. A 7.5% risk of ipsilateral stroke or death within 30 days of surgery was found but, in follow-up at 3 years, the surgery group had an additional 2.8% risk of stroke compared with 16.8% risk for the non-surgical group. The risk of death or ipsilateral disabling stroke was reduced from 11% in the non-surgery group to 6% in the surgery group.

In the North American Symptomatic Carotid Endarterectomy Trial (NASCET), 659 patients with greater than 70% stenosis were randomized to surgical and non-surgical treatment [18]. At a mean follow-up of 24 months, ipsilateral stroke was noted in 26% of non-surgical patients compared to 9% of patients treated with endarterectomy. This trial was prematurely stopped as a result of the overwhelming risk reduction (17%) observed in the surgical group. The benefits of surgery were seen on a variety of outcomes, including major stroke, major stroke and death, and functional disability.

The Veterans Administration Symptomatic Stenosis Trial (VASST) [19] enrolled a total of 193 men aged 35–82 years. These were then randomized to a surgery group (n = 91) and a non-surgical group (n = 98). Although this study was also terminated prematurely as a result of the NASCET study findings, analysis demonstrated a significant reduction in ipsilateral stroke and crescendo TIAs for patients who had greater than 50% stenosis, two-thirds of whom demonstrated greater than 70% stenosis of their ICA by angiography. There was a risk reduction of 11.7% in the surgical group when compared to the non-surgical group. It was also observed that the greatest benefit was seen in patients who presented with hemispheric TIA rather than transient monocular blindness, although the difference was not statistically significant.

Results of Trials for Asymptomatic Carotid Stenosis

The CASANOVA Study [20] randomized patients who had 50–90% stenosis by non-invasive studies to either immediate surgery or no immediate surgery. In the no-immediate-surgery group, some underwent delayed surgery because of the development of ischemic symptoms or progressive stenosis. At a 3-year follow-up, no difference was found between the two groups, using death or new stroke as end-points.

The VASST randomized patients with greater than 50% stenosis to operative and non-operative therapy [19]. At a mean follow-up of 4 years, the combined incidence of TIA and stroke was reduced to 8% in the surgical group compared to 20.6% in the non-surgical group. The size of the sample for this study, however, was not large enough to give the study enough statistical power to show a difference in stroke as an end-point only.

The Asymptomatic Carotid Atherosclerosis Study (ACAS), the largest of the asymptomatic study trials, was capable of scientifically substantiating that carotid endarterectomy may prevent stroke in certain patients [21]. Patients with greater than 60% stenosis by were randomized to surgery versus medical management. At a mean follow-up of 2.7 years, the ipsilateral stroke risk was 5.1% in the surgical group and 11% in the medically treated group.

The Mayo Asymptomatic Carotid Endarterectomy Trial (MACE) randomized patients with greater than 50% carotid stenosis by non-invasive methods to operation versus medical management [22]. The study, however, was terminated because of the increased frequency of myocardial infarction in the surgical group.

Indications for CEA

Based on the data obtained from the different clinical trials, CEA has been found to offer protection against subsequent ipsilateral stroke or crescendo TIAs in patients with symptomatic high-grade stenosis. This risk reduction was accomplished with minimal morbidity, extended over time and was independent of other risk factors. Patients in the medically treated groups who did not receive an operation, even when taking aspirin, had stroke rates in the range of 15–20%, compared with 3–7% in the surgical group. The decision to institute surgical treatment in this group of patients was based not only on clinical findings, such as hemispheric TIAs or non-disabling stroke, but also on degree of stenosis as confirmed by cerebral angiography. This was seen in patients who underwent carotid duplex ultrasound and who had evidence of intermediate stenosis, which was then clarified by angiographic determination.

Finally, the efficacy of this procedure in symptomatic patients depends on an acceptable level of perioperative morbidity and mortality. Acceptable guidelines are 3% operative risk for asymptomatic patients, 5% for patients with TIAs, 7% for patients with ischemic stroke and 10% for patients with recurrent stenosis.

Treatment of carotid stenosis on asymptomatic patients is more controversial because the data are less conclusive. Based on the results of the above-mentioned trials, CEA in patients with asymptomatic stenosis needs to be determined taking into consideration multiple factors. The degree of ipsilateral and contralateral carotid stenosis, progression of stenosis, assessment of collateral flow, presence of silent infarcts on CT scanning, vessel ulceration and risk of stroke are some of the issues that need to be addressed prior to recommending a CEA as definitive therapy. Careful evaluation of the patient's risk factors, with attention to those factors that are modifiable and can, as a result, decrease the risk of surgery, need to be discussed as part of the pre-operative evaluation.

Pre-operative Evaluation and Risk Assessment

Patients who are being considered for undergoing CEA need a complete history and physical evaluation, with special attention paid to the history and timing of the neurological events. Risk factors, such as cardiac disease, diabetes mellitus, tobacco use, hyperlipidemia, family history and symptoms such as transient monocular blindness, TIAs or completed strokes, need to be elicited from the patient prior to any further evaluation. The prevalence of coronary artery disease is high in patients undergoing CEA; consultation with a cardiologist is recommended. Initial cardiac work-up should include electrocardiography and echocardiography. Medical therapy for concomitant medical conditions should be optimized before surgery. The efficacy of CEA depends on careful selection of patients who can benefit from the procedure with minimal associated morbidity and mortality.

Radiographic Assessment

Cerebral Angiography

The major clinical trials that identified which patients with cerebrovascular disease should undergo CEA relied on measurement of vessel stenosis based on angiography; hence, this invasive imaging modality is an essential component of the pre-operative evaluation.

Cerebral angiography should include visualization of both carotid bifurcations and the intracranial carotid circulation; this is because there can be tandem lesions situated in the same arterial tree as the carotid bifurcation stenosis. Because it can affect surgical therapy, visualization of the carotid siphon is also important. Angiography is not only useful in determining the percentage of cervical carotid stenosis, but also in assessing plaque ulceration and identifying areas of thrombosis. Assessment of anatomic variants and collateral flow patterns can also be accomplished with angiography.

Most carotid arteries harboring a high-grade stenotic area return to normal caliber distal to the stenotic segment. A high-grade ICA lesion with a tapering post-stenotic segment with a reduced caliber is usually referred to as the "string sign". This substantiated the concept that narrowing of the distal vessel past the stenotic segment occurs as a result of decreased perfusion pressure, because the diameter of the lumen always returns to normal after removal of the obstructing lesion. Conditions that can present with an angiographic "string sign" include radiation vasculopathy, moyamoya disease, FMD and congenital hypoplasia. The post-angiography stroke rate has been reported to be less than 1%. Cerebral angiography remains the "gold standard" for evaluating stenosis in patients with symptomatology suggestive of ischemic stroke. Recent data have shown that non-invasive evaluations may provide sufficient and accurate information regarding the degree of carotid stenosis [23].

It is important to consider that the degree of carotid stenosis was measured differently in the ECST versus the NASCET [17,18]. The degree of carotid stenosis is significantly higher if calculated by the NASCET rather than the ECST method [18] (see Fig. 38.1). The stroke rates in medically treated patients with carotid stenosis dramatically increase with stenosis by more than 80% as measured by the ECST method. This corresponds roughly to a 60% stenosis measured using the NASCET method.

MRA

MRA is a non-invasive imaging modality which can assess flow characteristics of the carotid circulation and define the degree of carotid stenosis. MRA resolution approaches a 90% sensitivity in detecting carotid stenosis when compared with angiography [24]. Two-dimensional MRA images are sensitive to low blood-flow states but are limited by their lower resolution. Three-dimensional images offer a better resolution and have a higher sensitivity to flow in any direction. Both of these images should be obtained in every evaluation, since it decreases problems associated with interpretation. MRA has the advantage of providing visualization of the entire carotid circulation, from the origin to the carotid siphon, along with the intracranial vasculature in one examination. The main disadvantage of MRA in this setting is its potential to overestimate the degree of stenosis. This is especially important in the mild to moderate group of patients who may have their degree of stenosis placed in a surgical category. Causes of this overestimation are due to loss of signal from disturbed flow or markedly decreased flow and distortion of the reconstructed images.

Ultrasound

Non-invasive evaluation of carotid stenosis usually begins with ultrasound studies. Doppler ultrasound, the most well established non-

Difference between NASCET and ECST in measurement of internal carotid artery stenosis

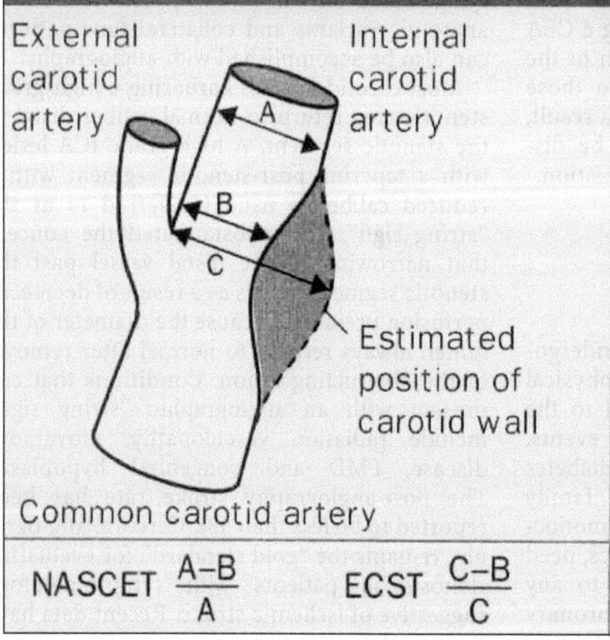

NASCET	ECST
30	65
40	70
50	75
60	80
70	85
80	91
90	97

Approximate equivalent degrees of internal carotid artery stenosis used in NASCET and ESCT according to recent direct comparisons

Fig. 38.1. The differences in measurement techniques used by the NASCET and ECST trials. Comparisons between the different severities of stenosis by the two methods are also illustrated (with permission).

invasive imaging study used to assess carotid stenosis, determines flow information on the basis of the change in frequency of the ultrasound signal reflected from moving red blood cells. B-mode ultrasound, another modality, examines blood vessel anatomy. It can help diagnose ulcerations in 50–95% of patients with carotid artery stenosis and has a higher sensitivity than angiography in the detection of ulceration and intraplaque hemorrhage [25]. Stenotic lesions, however, are difficult to visualize when the carotid bifurcation lies above the mandibular edge, with tortuous carotid arteries, and with a completely occluded carotid artery [25]. Duplex ultrasonography combines B-mode and Doppler ultrasound and helps to visualize vessel anatomy and blood flow velocity at various stages of the cardiac cycle. The study usually includes images of the common carotid artery (CCA), the ICAs and the ECA. High-grade stenosis or occlusion of the ICA is usually associated with a compensatory increase in blood-flow velocity in the ipsilateral ECA and contralateral carotid vessels. Duplex ultrasound, however, is highly technician-dependent and, although common with other non-invasive tests, cannot demonstrate the full extent of the carotid circulation. TCD ultrasonography allows for a non-invasive evaluation of blood velocity and can identify intracranial collateral flow patterns; it also has a high degree of sensitivity in identifying patients with severe ICA disease [26]. A reduction in ultrasound flow velocity in the middle cerebral artery (MCA) distribution can be typically observed distal to an ipsilateral stenotic carotid artery. Small, asymptomatic emboli can also be detected with TCD ultrasonography and can be of help not only in identifying the emboli locus, but also in assessing the response to anticoagulation.

CT

Spiral CT scanning is a non-invasive imaging modality that produces a three-dimensional reconstruction of the axial images and allows for evaluation of the cervical and intracranial vasculature after rapid contrast administration. One of its advantages is the ability to make a distinction between high-grade stenosis and total vessel occlusion, based on slight differences in contrast. Large ulcerations can be demonstrated, although calcification is still a source of error. Advantages of spiral CT angiography include its easy accessibility and tolerability by anxious patients and those with a large body habitus, who would have difficulty fitting in an MRI scanner. Disadvantages include exposure to ionizing radiation, allergic reactions to contrast material and potential nephrotoxicity.

Timing of Surgical Intervention

CEA has emerged as a validated surgical procedure, which has proven to be of benefit in preventing stroke in either asymptomatic patients or those with ischemic symptoms. Prospective studies have showed a high risk of stroke in close temporal proximity to presenting ischemic symptoms. Another retrospective study found that the risks of stroke for patients with untreated TIAs were greatly increased compared with those of an age-adjusted group in the first 30 days after symptom onset [7]. These studies suggest that patients with cerebral ischemic symptoms due to atherosclerotic carotid artery disease should be evaluated promptly after symptom onset for consideration of potential surgical intervention.

Controversy surrounding timing of surgical intervention for patients with recently completed stroke with neurological deficits is based on a study in which outcome was dismal after CEA [30]. In patients in which a previously auscultated bruit has disappeared with acute total carotid occlusion, those with stroke following angiography and those with stroke following CEA due to vessel thrombosis should undergo emergent surgical intervention [31,32].

Surgical Technique

Positioning and Anesthetic Considerations

With the patient in the supine position, with the neck slightly extended and the head turned away from the operative side, the surgical field is demarcated from the mastoid process superiorly to the sternal notch inferiorly. Towel rolls under the shoulder blades can also help keep the neck in slight extension (Fig. 38.2).

Carotid endarterectomy can be performed under general or local anesthesia. There are advantages for both approaches. The high-risk cardiac patient should have arterial lines and a

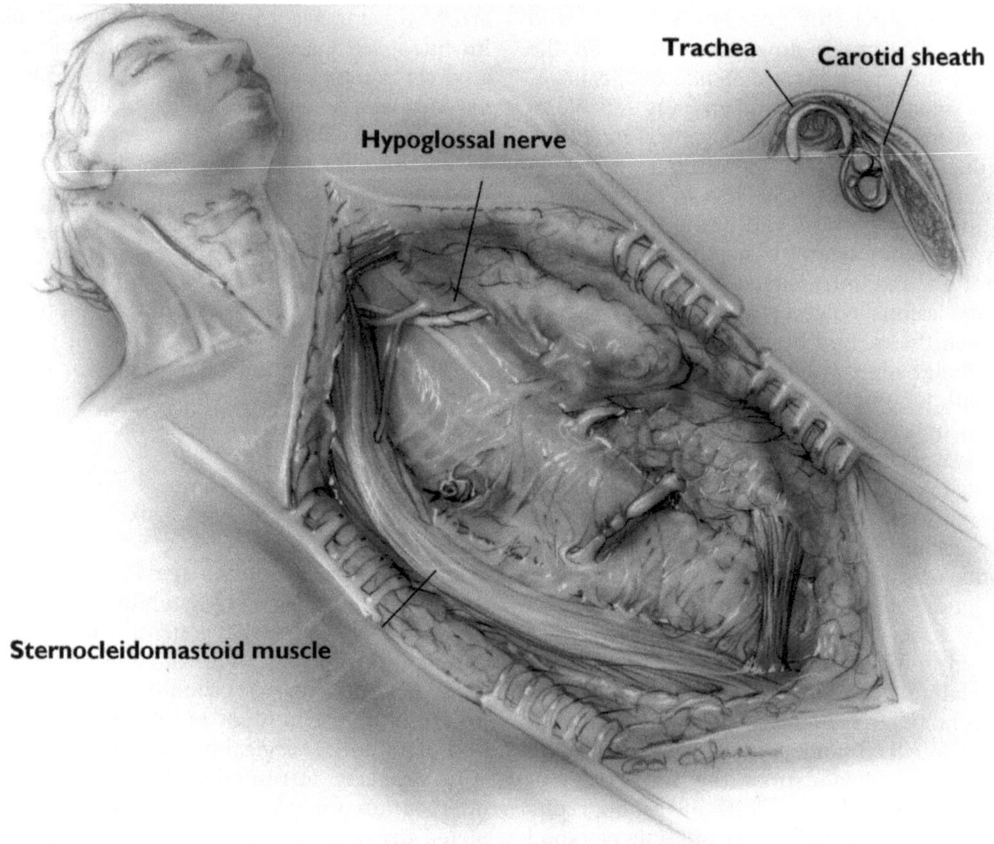

Fig. 38.2. Illustration of the positioning of the patient (upper left) and location of the surgical incision used for carotid CEA along the anterior border of the sternocleidomastoid muscle. The skin is divided sharply and the platysma muscle is also divided, exposing the sternocledomastoid and omohyoid muscle (middle). The dissection is then taken medial to the jugular vein and, often, one or two branches from the jugular vein need to be divided in order to expose the carotid artery. Most often, the common facial vein, which is a branch from the internal jugular vein, needs to be ligated in the upper third of the incision. The jugular vein is then retracted laterally with the sternocleidomastoid muscle. The relationship of the sternomastoid artery and the hypoglossal nerve is illustrated at the upper portion of the incision. The relationship of the carotid sheath to the trachea and overlying tissue planes are illustrated (upper right).

central venous pressure catheter placed. Anesthetic goals include preservation of adequate cerebral and myocardial perfusion, close attention to hemodynamic changes and maintenance of normocapnia with mechanical ventilation.

Operative Procedure

Under loupe magnification and headlight illumination, an incision is made along the anterior border of the sternocleidomastoid muscle; this may extend as high the retroaural region or as low as the suprasternal notch. With careful attention to hemostasis with the help of bipolar electrocautery, the skin and subcutaneous tissues are dissected sharply to the level of the platysma, which, once identified, is sharply divided as well. Self-retaining retractors are then placed and the underlying fat layer is dissected free from the anterior border of the sternocleidomastoid. Retractors are kept in the superficial wound layer, as deeper placement can cause injury to the recurrent laryngeal nerve or superior laryngeal nerve (Fig. 38.2).

Under the sternocleidomastoid, the internal jugular vein and the common facial vein, a branch of the internal jugular, are identified, double-ligated and divided. Care should be taken not to injure the spinal accessory nerve, which is at risk for transection and stretching. Gentle lateral retraction of the internal jugular exposes the carotid artery. Opening the carotid sheath then proceeds, starting inferiorly by the anterior surface of the artery to the level of the omohyoid muscle. Dissection of the CCA, ECA and ICA is gently carried out and vessel loops are placed around these vessels. Some surgeons, at this point, inject the carotid sinus with 2–3 cc of 2% plain lidocaine to minimize the potential bradycardia and hypotension that results from manipulating this structure. Proximal control of the CCA is obtained by dissecting the posterior wall to where the vagus is found. An 0-silk tie is passed through a wire loop, which is then pulled through a rubber sleeve (Rummel tourniquet). The superior thyroid artery, the ECA and the ICA are then dissected at the region of the bifurcation. Distal dissection along the ICA proceeds

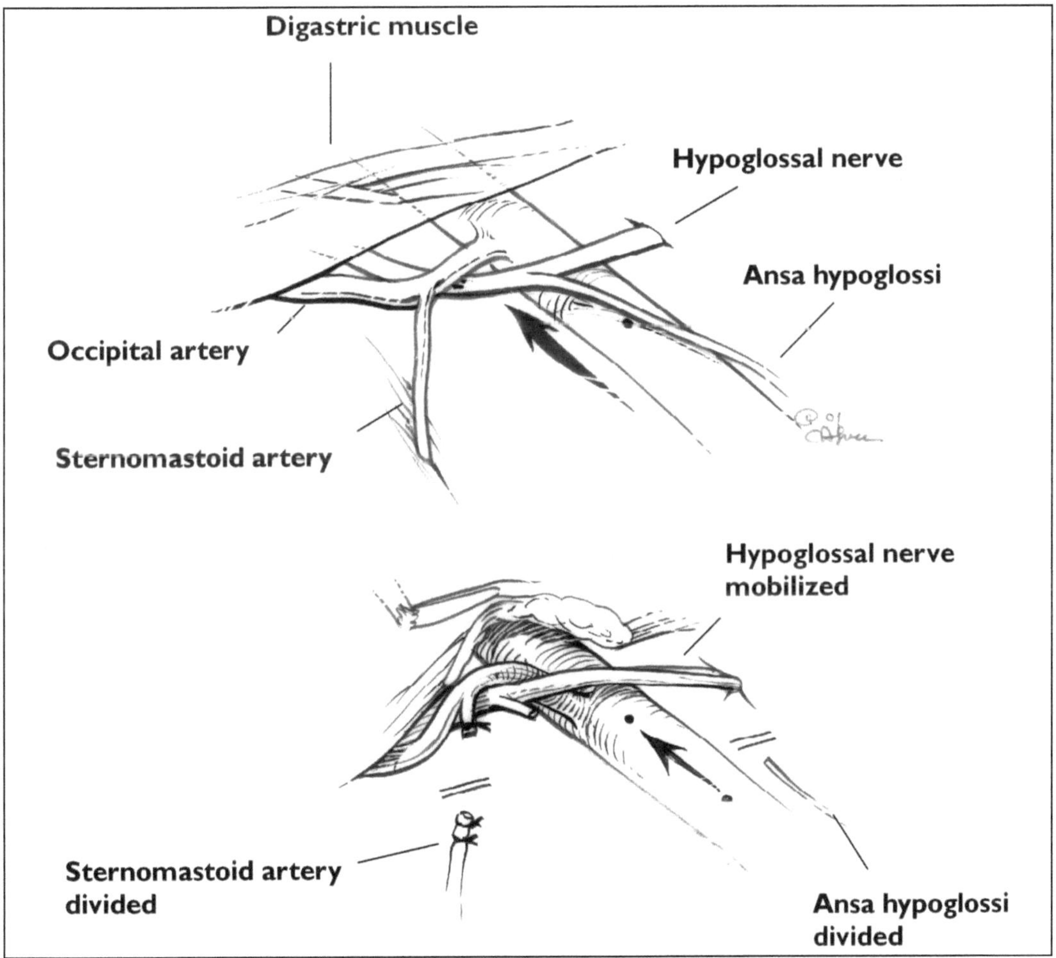

Fig. 38.3. Illustration of the maneuver used to expose the upper margin of the internal carotid artery by mobilizing the hypoglossal nerve. Normally, the hypoglossal nerve is tethered against the external and internal carotid artery by either the occipital artery or the first branch from the occipital artery after it emerges from the external carotid artery, the sternomastoid artery (upper). This small artery is usually associated with a small vein and enters the sternocleidomastoid muscle. Dividing the sternomastoid artery (lower) will allow mobilization of the occipital artery and the hypoglossal nerve. This allows dissection to proceed further distally along the internal carotid artery, allowing better exposure for more distal lesions or for shunt placement. If greater exposure is needed, then the digastric muscle can be divided.

with care not to injure the hypoglossal nerve as it crosses the distal ICA (Fig. 38.3). It is of vital importance to have adequate exposure of the ICA distal to the plaque before opening the vessel. The area of the plaque, on visual inspection, appears firm and yellow; distal to the plaque, the vessel becomes pinker. Dissection to at least 1cm distal to the end of the plaque is performed to allow for shunt placement if needed. The posterior belly of the digastric can be cut if higher exposure is needed. Circumferential dissection is completed so that the shunt clamp can be fitted, if needed. Similar dissection is then completed around the ECA and the superior thyroid artery. With the help of a sterile marking pen, a line is drawn along the vessel so as to delineate the arteriotomy site and prevent distortion (Fig. 38.4).

Prior to vessel clamping, intravenous heparin at a dose of 100 U/kg is given. The ICA is the first vessel clamped, because of the belief that it reduces the risk of embolization associated with cross-clamping. With a #11 blade, an arteriotomy is started 1 cm proximal to the bifurcation in the middle of the CCA. This incision can be extended, with the use of Pott's scissors, through the arterial wall until plaque is encountered. A smooth plane is then developed between plaque and arterial wall. Another technique, however, consists of incorporating the plaque into the incision (Fig. 38.5). A shunt may or may not be used but, with or without it, the

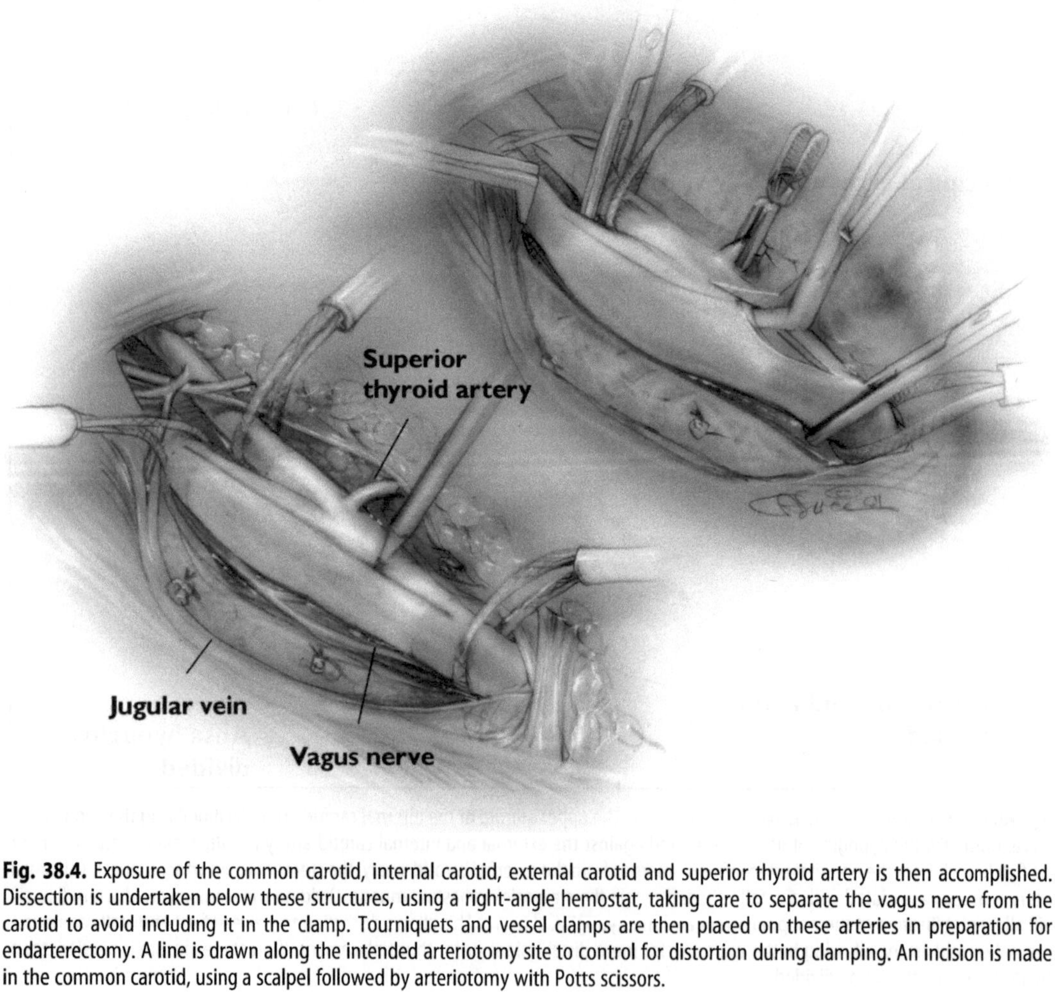

Fig. 38.4. Exposure of the common carotid, internal carotid, external carotid and superior thyroid artery is then accomplished. Dissection is undertaken below these structures, using a right-angle hemostat, taking care to separate the vagus nerve from the carotid to avoid including it in the clamp. Tourniquets and vessel clamps are then placed on these arteries in preparation for endarterectomy. A line is drawn along the intended arteriotomy site to control for distortion during clamping. An incision is made in the common carotid, using a scalpel followed by arteriotomy with Potts scissors.

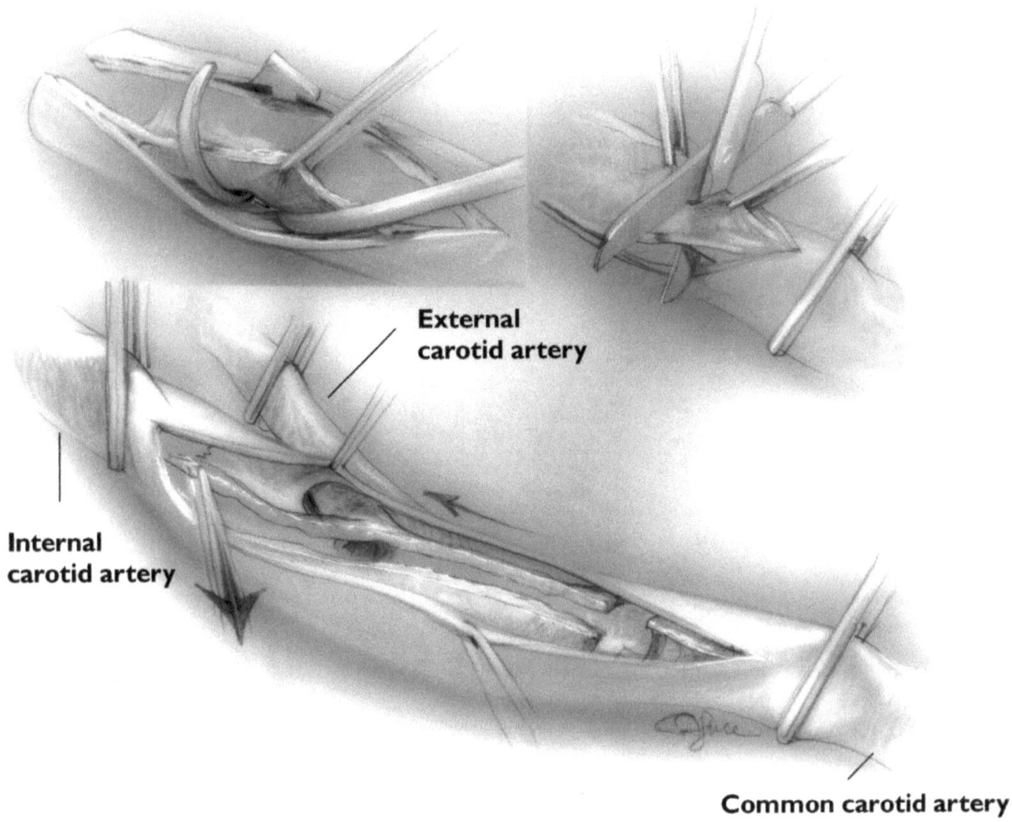

Fig. 38.5. Following completion of the arteriotomy, the plaque is identified using a #4 Penfield dissector or a Freier elevator. The plaque is divided sharply in the common carotid artery and dissected from the internal carotid artery. Most of the time, the plaque will thin and "feather" out, allowing it to be separated from the distal arterial wall with gentle traction. Occasionally, it will need to be sharply divided distally.

plaque is then removed from the arterial wall using a Freier elevator or a Penfield dissector. Plaque is removed from the lateral wall of the arteriotomy, then dissected medially on the CCA and then transected proximally. Attention is then turned to the ICA, where plaque is also dissected from lateral to medial and a concerted attempt is made to leave a smooth surface. Finally, attention is then focused on the orifice of the ECA and, with the use of vascular forceps, the entire plaque can be dissected off the vessel with gentle eversion in order to reach as distally as possible (Fig. 38.6). Inadequate ECA plaque removal can lead to thrombosis and complete occlusion of the carotid tree. The luminal surface is carefully inspected after plaque removal, while the site is being irrigated with heparinized saline. Visible debris should be meticulously removed so as to create a lumen that is as smooth as possible. Running 5-0 or 6-0 Prolene from distal to proximal end of the vessel is then used to close the site (Fig. 38.6). If a patch, such as a Hemashield, or a vein patch is used, it is placed over the arteriotomy site and cut to the exact length of the opening. The ends of the patch are anchored to the arteriotomy site and a running 6-0 Prolene suture used to close the patch. The internal carotid artery is briefly released just before the final sutures so as to assess the patency of the vessel and flush residual debris. The clamps are then removed in the following sequence: ECA, CCA and ICA. Once the clamps are removed, the suture lines are inspected for leaks. Surgicel, and sometimes a 6-0 Prolene, suture are needed to control a persistent arterial leak. The carotid sheath is then

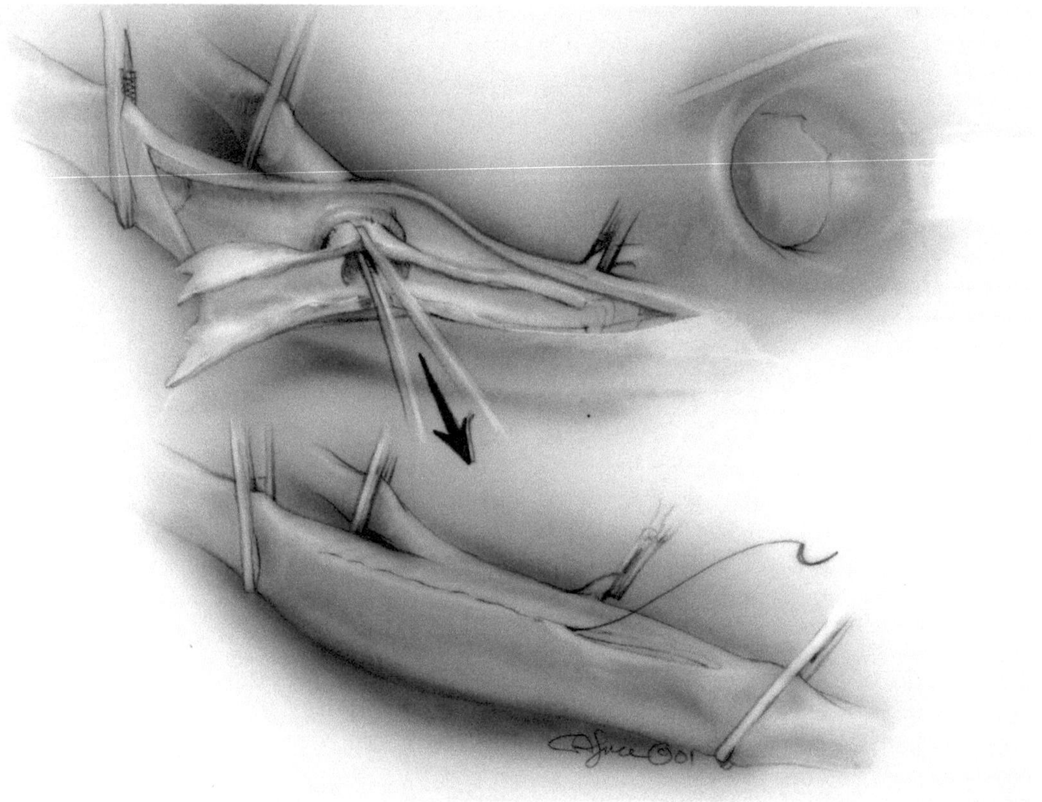

Fig. 38.6. The plaque can then be dissected from the external carotid artery by (upper) gentle traction and eversion of the artery, allowing the plaque to separate from the wall of the artery. The arteriotomy is then closed using a 6-0 or 5-0 proline suture. An alternative to primary closure is to use a vascular patch with a vein or artificial material.

approximated and the platysma is closed as a separate layer. Running sub-cuticular stitches approximate the skin and provide a good cosmetic result.

Patients are usually admitted to the ICU for overnight observation with serial neurological exams and for BP control. The aim is to keep the blood pressure as close to the pre-operative level as possible. Aspirin is resumed 1 day post-operatively and patients are usually discharged from the hospital in 1 or 2 days.

Intraoperative Monitoring: Transcranial Doppler Sonography and Electroencephalography

Stroke during CEA may result from embolization or thrombosis, as well as from a global reduction in CBF. Post-operative hyperperfusion can also result in stroke from intracranial hemorrhage. Intraoperative embolization can be reduced by minimizing the manipulation of the bifurcation during dissection, as well as by meticulous attention to the endarterectomy and arteriotomy part of the case. Intraoperative cerebral ischemia can be prevented with the use of an intraluminal shunt, although its use, in turn, can be associated with air and atheroma embolization.

Cerebral perfusion during carotid occlusion can be assessed by observing the patient while awake, as well as by a number of physiological parameters.

Electroencephalographic Monitoring

Since the EEG reflects the summated potentials of cortical neurons placed in the vicinity of the electrodes, it follows that the amplitude, frequency and power provide a measure of the amount and character of the activity present. Cortical ischemia results in smaller amplitudes and slower frequencies. Reductions in cerebral blood flow below 18 ml/100 g/minute usually produce EEG changes [33].

In cases in which there is a global reduction of EEG power after ICA clamping, an intraluminal shunt is placed. Marginally perfused regions and small areas of hypoperfusion cannot be detected by current EEG equipment. Brain mapping using multiple electrodes and computer integration may offer increased sensitivity.

Intraoperative TCD

TCD ultrasound is a valuable monitoring technique. It is non-invasive, relatively inexpensive, portable and provides more information than most other monitoring techniques. It provides continuous, real-time assessment of the blood flow velocity in the MCA during and after CEA. Changes in MCA blood-flow velocity during clamping of the carotid artery are proportional to blood-flow changes in this artery.

Intraoperative TCD use has proven to be beneficial by helping to differentiate thrombosis, embolism, hypoperfusion and hyperperfusion [34]. It has also proven beneficial in detecting cerebral ischemia during carotid cross clamping, hence, helping to avoid unnecessary shunting [35]. Occlusion of the ipsilateral carotid artery due to thrombosis or the development of an intimal flap can be detected by TCD ultrasound in the immediate post-operative period. This allows for early re-exploration and prevention of progression to an ischemic stroke.

Complications of CEA

Cerebral Infarction

Cerebral infarction is the most dreaded complication of CEA. Ischemic symptoms are seen in up to 5% of cases and can lead to major stroke in 1–3% of cases. Intraoperative monitoring and shunting can potentially minimize cerebral ischemia, due to hemodynamic factors. Thromboembolism with associated complete occlusion of the carotid artery is the most likely etiology of cerebral infarction following CEA. Prompt surgical exploration may be indicated. Diagnostic studies such as a CT scan to rule out an intracerebral hemorrhage and TCD to document hypoperfusion or emboli in the MCA territory are adjuncts when evaluating patients with new-onset neurological deficits in the post-operative period [34].

Cranial Nerve Injuries

Cranial nerve injury may be a complication of CEA. These injuries can be associated with significant morbidity. Injury is usually related to surgical technique and can be avoided. Use of magnifying instruments and careful attention to hemostasis with bipolar electrocautery, as well as gentle handling of the nerves that need to be mobilized, minimize this complication.

Injury to the hypoglossal nerve (CN XII) usually presents with unilateral tongue weakness, dysarthria and swallowing difficulties. Spinal accessory nerve injury needs to be considered in the patient who complains of ipsilateral shoulder drooping. Cutaneous anesthesia over the ear lobe and angle of the jaw may be due to injury to the greater auricular nerve and cutaneous branches. The vagus nerve can be injured in up to 6% of cases and presents with dysphagia or hoarseness caused by vocal cord dysfunction. Injury to the vagus by retraction on either the superior or recurrent laryngeal nerves can be prevented by identifying the vagus in the carotid sheath and by careful placement of the retractor blades. Most patients who develop dysphagia or hoarseness after CEA can be managed expectantly, since most recover spontaneously. It is important in the patient with bilateral carotid stenosis that, upon completion of one procedure, examination by an otolaryngologist, looking for occult vocal cord dysfunction, is performed prior to proceeding with the second procedure. Bilateral injury to the vocal cords can result in respiratory compromise and require a tracheostomy.

A transient or permanent injury to the mandibular branch of the facial nerve can produce a cosmetically disfiguring result. Curving the skin incision posteriorly towards the mastoid process so that it is 1–2 cm below the angle of the mandible can usually prevent this injury type. Injuries to the superficial cervical plexus and the greater auricular nerve produce a noticeable paresthesia as a result of transection but it is usually transient, since the nerve regenerates.

Myocardial Infarction

The incidence of cardiac morbidity and mortality ranges from 0.7 to 7.1%, although it represents 50% of all perioperative complications [36]. Careful patient selection and cardiac screening are important, especially in the high-risk patient. Coronary catheterization, angioplasty and even coronary artery bypass grafting (CABG) need to be considered pre-operatively, prior to CEA. Monitoring of cardiac enzymes might prove beneficial in patients at risk for silent ischemic episodes such as diabetics. Prompt identification of electrolyte abnormalities and aggressive treatment of dysrhythmias are carried out, as in all non-surgical patients.

Wound Complications

Wound hematomas and infections can occur after CEA. Post-operative hematomas may result from perioperative use of heparin and antiplatelet agents. Small neck hematomas usually have a benign course and resolve without complications. A rapidly enlarging hematoma, which compromises the airway, mandates surgical exploration to identify and control the sources of bleeding.

Wound infections are rare (less than 1%) and, when they occur, are usually superficial. Use of pre-operative antibiotics is instituted routinely. Patients with systemic conditions such as diabetes may be more at risk for post-operative infections.

Future Directions: Angioplasty and Stenting

Angioplasty and stent placement have gained some popularity for the treatment of atherosclerosis, dissection and other conditions leading to stenosis of the cerebral vasculature. It has become clear to most clinicians that angioplasty alone of cervical or cerebral arteries has a high complication and re-stenosis rate and, thus, has become much less frequently utilized. Advances in stent technology have resulted in more effective treatment methods for intracranial and extracranial lesions. Recently, angioplasty stenting of the carotid arteries has been advocated to treat internal carotid artery stenosis. There is a subgroup of patients with significant medical co-morbidities and high neurologic risk that might qualify for carotid angioplasty and stenting procedures. Several reports have indicated that high-risk patients and patients who meet strict criteria might benefit from stenting, with a minimum of morbidity and mortality [37,38].

Prospective randomized trials have begun to try to determine if angioplasty and stent placement in the internal carotid artery can be performed with equal or improved safety and efficacy as carotid endarterectomy in equivalent groups of patients; however, results have not been encouraging.

A trial in the UK was stopped due to the high stroke rate in the endovascular group.

Twenty-three patients with focal carotid territory symptoms and severe ICA stenosis (more than 70%) were randomized to either CEA or endovascular stenting [39]. CEA with patching or stenting were used as interventions. The main outcome measures were death or disabling or non-disabling stroke within 30 days. All ten CEA operations proceeded without complication, but five of the seven patients who underwent CA had a stroke (P = 0.0034). Results of the CAVATAS trial comparing endovascular treatment with conventional carotid surgery have also been reported. This trial assigned 504 patients with carotid stenosis to endovascular treatment (n = 251) or carotid endarterectomy (n = 253). The rates of major outcome events within 30 days of first treatment did not differ significantly between endovascular treatment and surgery (6.4 vs 5.9%, respectively, for disabling stroke or death; 10.0 vs 9.9% for any stroke lasting more than 7 days, or death). The stroke rate in both groups, however, was higher than previously reported results for endarterectomy and thus were associated with a diminished effect on stroke prevention in these groups of patients.

Newer endovascular devices are now being evaluated which prevent distal embolization associated endovascular treatment. It is believed that distal embolization is one of the major factors associated with stroke in patents undergoing stent procedures. Future trials will no doubt be conducted using these devices. Currently carotid endarterectomy remains the procedure of choice in otherwise uncomplicated patients with carotid stenosis who meet the criteria for treatment.

Key Points

- *Stroke continues to be the most common life-threatening neurologic disease and the third leading cause of death in the USA, after heart disease and cancer.*
- *The majority of ischemic strokes, in the setting of occlusive disease of the craniocerebral vasculature, are due to atherosclerotic disease. The most common extracranial sites for atherosclerosis are the carotid bifurcation, the sub-clavian arteries and the proximal vertebral arteries.*
- *Patients suspected of having a stroke should have a thorough but concise history and a neurological examination of sufficient detail to assess the degree of dysfunction and to rule out other neurological conditions. Assessment of the level of consciousness, gaze, vision, dysarthria, aphasia, leg and arm strength, sensory loss or extinction, facial asymmetry and limb ataxia needs to be undertaken and clearly documented. Time of symptom onset is important to determine whether there is an opportunity for the patient to receive thrombolytic therapy, provided there are no contraindications.*
- *Based on the data obtained from the different clinical trials, CEA has been found to offer protection against subsequent ipsilateral stroke or crescendo TIAs in patients with symptomatic high-grade stenosis.*

References

1. Heart and stroke facts: 1994 statistical supplement. Dallas, TX: American Heart Association, 1993.
2. Strandgaard S, Paulson OB. Cerebral autoregulation. Stroke 1984;15:413–16.
3. Branston NM, Hope DT, Symon L. Barbiturates in focal ischemia of primate cortex: effects of blood flow distribution, evoked potential and extracellular potassium. Stroke 1979;10:647–53.
4. Mishkin MM, Schreiber MN. Collateral circulation. In: Newton TH, Potts DG, editors. Radiology of the skull and brain: angiography. St Louis: CV Mosby, 1974; 2344–74.
5. Fisher CM. Transient monocular blindness associated with hemiplegia. Arch Ophthal 1952;47:167–203.
6. Busch H, Bohl J, Mattern R et al. Diseases of the vertebral arteries. Neurosurgery Review 1990;13:53–63.
7. Whisnant JP, Matsumoto N, Elvebach LR. Transient cerebral ischemic attacks in a community, Rochester, Minnesota, 1955 through 1969. Mayo Clinic Proceed 1973;48:194.
8. European Carotid Surgery Trialists Collaborative Group. Risk of stroke in the distribution on an asymptomatic carotid artery. Lancet 1995;345:209–12.
9. Hinckey J, Furlan A, Barnett H. Cardiogenic brain embolism: incidence, varieties and treatments. In: Bennet HJM, Mohr JP, Stein B et al., editors. Stroke: pathophysiology, diagnosis and management. 3rd Edition. Philadelphia, PA: Churchill-Livingstone, 1998; 1089.
10. Thompson PL, Robinson JS. Stroke after acute myocardial infarction: relation to infarct size. BMJ 1978;2:457.
11. Bayford J, Sandercoch P, Jones L et al. The natural history of lacunar infarction: The Oxfordshire Community Stroke Project. Stroke 1987;18:545.
12. Kiatkowski TG, Libman RB, Frankel M et al. Effects of tissue plasminogen activator for acute ischemic stroke at one year. NEJM 1999;340:1781–7.
13. Powers WJ. Acute hypertension after stroke: the scientific basis for treatment decisions. Neurology 1993; 43:461.
14. Baum A, Biller J, Adams HP Jr et al. Acute blood glucose level and outcome for ischemic stroke: Trial of ORG 10172 in acute stroke treatment (TOAST) investigators. Neurology 1999;52:280.
15. Dietrich WD, Busto R, Valdes I et al. Effects of normothermia versus mild hypothermia for brain ischemia in rats. Stroke 1990;26:1318.
16. Kalra L, Yu G, Wilson K et al. Medical complications during stroke rehabilitation. Stroke 1995;26:990.
17. European Carotid Surgery Trialists Collaborative Group. European Carotid Surgery Trial: interim results for symptomatic patients with severe (70–99%) or with mild (0–29%) carotid stenosis. Lancet 1991;337:1235–43.
18. North American Symptomatic Carotid Endarterectomy Trial Collaborators. Beneficial effects of carotid endarterectomy in symptomatic patients with high grade stenosis. NEJM 1991;325:445–53.
19. Mayberg MR, Wilson SE, Yatsu F et al. Carotid endarterectomy and prevention of cerebral ischemia from symptomatic carotid stenosis. JAMA 1991;266: 3289–94.
20. CASANOVA Study Group. Carotid artery surgery vs medical therapy in asymptomatic carotid stenosis. Stroke 1991;22:1229–35.
21. Executive Committee for the Asymptomatic Carotid Atherosclerosis Study (ACAS). Endarterectomy for asymptomatic carotid artery stenosis. JAMA 1995;273: 1421–8.
22. Mayo Asymptomatic Carotid Endarterectomy Study Group. Results of a randomized control trial of carotid endarterectomy for asymptomatic carotid stenosis. Mayo Clinic Proceed 1992;67:513–18.
23. Kuntz KM, Skillmann JJ, Whitemore AD et al. Carotid endarterectomy in asymptomatic patients: is contrast angiography necessary? J Vasc Surg 1995;22:706–16.
24. Mayberg MR. Extracranial occlusive disease of the carotid artery. In: Youman J, editor. Neurological surgery: a comprehensive reference guide to the diagnosis and management of neurosurgical problems. Philadelphia, PA: WB Saunders, 1996; 1159–80.
25. O'Donnel TF Jr, Erdoes L, Mackey WC et al. Correlation of B-mode ultrasound imaging and arteriography with pathologic findings at carotid endarterectomy. Arch Surg 1985;120:443–9.

26. Wilterdink JL, Feldman E, Furie KL et al. Transcranial Doppler ultrasound battery reliably identifies severe internal carotid artery stenosis [Comments]. Stroke 1997;28:133–6.
27. Pelz D, Rankin RN, Ferguson GG. Intravenous digital subtraction angiography and duplex ultrasonography in postoperative assessment of carotid endarterectomy. J Neurosurg 1987;66:88–92.
28. Dogan A, Dempsey RJ. Diagnostic modalities for carotid artery disease. Neurosurgery Clinics of North America 2000;11:205–20.
29. North American Symptomatic Carotid Endarterectomy Trial Collaborators. Beneficial effect of carotid endarterectomy in symptomatic patients with high grade stenosis. NEJM 1991;325:445–53.
30. Wylie E, Hein M, Adams J. Intracranial hemorrhage following surgical revascularization for treatment of acute strokes. J Neurosurg 1964;21:212–15.
31. Meyer FB, Sundt TM Jr, Piepgras DG et al. Acute carotid occlusion. In: Sundt TM Jr, editor. Occlusive cerebrovascular disease. Philadelphia, PA: W.B. Saunders, 1987; 269–79.
32. Loftus CM. Surgical management options to prevent ischemic stroke. In: Adams HP, editor. Handbook of cerebrovascular diseases. New York: Marcel Dekker Inc., 1993; 315–58.
33. Sundt TM, Sharbrough FW, Piepgras DG et al. Correlation of cerebral blood flow and electroencephalographic changes during carotid endarterectomy with results of surgery and hemodynamics of cerebral ischemia. Mayo Clinic Proceed 1981;56:533–41.
34. Naylor AR, Wildsmith JAW, McClure J et al. Transcranial Doppler monitoring during carotid endarterectomy. Br J Surg 1991;78:1264–8.
35. Lam AM, Newell DW. Intraoperative use of transcranial Doppler ultrasonography. Neurosurgery Clinics of North America 1996;7:709–22.
36. Gunel M, Awad IA. Carotid endarterectomy prevention strategies and complications management. Neurosurgery Clinics of North America 2000;11:351–64.
37. Diethrich EB, Ndiaye M, Reid DB. Stenting in the carotid artery: initial experience in 110 patients. J Endovasc Surg 1996;3:42–62.
38. Yadav JS, Roubin GS, Iver S et al. Elective stenting of the extracranial carotid arteries [Comments]. Circulation 1997;95:376–81.
39. Naylor AR, Bolia A, Abbott RJ, Pye IF, Smith J, Lennard N et al. Randomized study of carotid angioplasty and stenting versus carotid endarterectomy: a stopped trial. J Vasc Surg 1998;28:326–34.
40. Endovascular versus surgical treatment in patients with carotid stenosis in the Carotid and Vertebral Artery Transluminal Angioplasty Study (CAVATAS): a randomised trial. Lancet 2001;357:1729–37.

Index

B

J

K

L

M

O